S. MOTTO

CURRENT THERAPY IN SPORTS MEDICINE

CURRENT THERAPY SERIES

CURRENT THERAPY IN SPORTS MEDICINE

THIRD EDITION

JOSEPH S. TORG, M.D.
Professor of Orthopaedic Surgery
University of Pennsylvania School of Medicine
Director
University of Pennsylvania Sports Medicine Center
Philadelphia, Pennsylvania

ROY J. SHEPHARD, M.D., Ph.D., D.P.E., F.A.C.S.M.
Professor
School of Physical and Health Education
University of Toronto, Toronto
and
Health Studies Programme
Brock University, St. Catherine's
Ontario, Canada

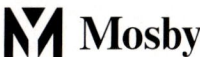 Mosby

St. Louis Baltimore Berlin Boston Carlsbad Chicago London Madrid
Naples New York Philadelphia Sydney Tokyo Toronto

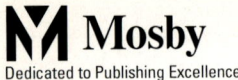
Mosby
Dedicated to Publishing Excellence

Executive Editor: *Susan M. Gay*
Senior Managing Editor: *Lynne Gery*
Production Supervisor: *Allan S. Kleinberg*
Manufacturing Supervisor: *Karen Lewis*

THIRD EDITION
Copyright © 1995 by Mosby–Year Book, Inc.

Composition by Graphic World, Inc.
Printed in the United States of America by Maple-Vail York

Mosby–Year Book, Inc.
11830 Westline Industrial Drive
St. Louis, Missouri 63146

NOTICE: The authors and publisher have made every effort to ensure that the patient care recommended
herein, including choice of drugs and drug dosages, is in accord with the accepted standards and practice at
the time of publication. However, since research and regulation constantly change clinical standards, the
reader is urged to check the product information sheet included in the package of each drug, which includes
recommended doses, warnings, and contraindications. This is particularly important with new or infrequently
used drugs.

ISBN 1-55664-384-5

95 96 97 98 99 / 9 8 7 6 5 4 3 2 1

JOHN ALBRIGHT, M.D.

Professor of Orthopaedic Surgery, University of Iowa College of Medicine; Director, Sports Medicine Service, Department of Orthopaedic Surgery, University of Iowa Hospitals and Clinics, Iowa City, Iowa

LOUIS C. ALMEKINDERS, M.D.

Assistant Professor of Orthopaedic Surgery, and Team Physician, University of North Carolina at Chapel Hill; Attending Surgeon, University of North Carolina Hospitals, Chapel Hill, North Carolina

MICHELE C. AMEY

School of Physical and Health Education, Queen's University, Kingston, Ontario, Canada

JAMES R. ANDREWS, M.D.

Clinical Professor of Orthopaedics and Sports Medicine, University of Virginia School of Medicine, Charlottesville, Virginia; Medical Director, American Sports Medicine Institute, and Orthopaedic Surgeon, Alabama Sports Medicine and Orthopaedic Center, Birmingham, Alabama

BERNARD R. BACH, Jr., M.D.

Associate Professor of Orthopaedic Surgery, Rush Medical College; Director, Sports Medicine Section, Rush-Presbyterian-St. Luke's Medical Center, Chicago, Illinois

CHAMP L. BAKER, M.D.

Clinical Assistant Professor of Orthopaedic Surgery, Tulane University School of Medicine, New Orleans, Louisiana; President, The Hughston Clinic, Columbus, Georgia

THOMAS J. BALSHI, D.D.S., F.A.C.P., F.A.O.

Director, Institute for Facial Esthetics, Fort Washington, Pennsylvania

RODNEY K. BEALS, M.D.

Professor, Division of Orthopaedics and Rehabilitation, Oregon Health Sciences University, Portland, Oregon

STEVEN N. BLAIR, P.E.D.

Director of Epidemiology and Clinical Applications, Cooper Institute for Aerobics Research, Dallas, Texas

MARK K. BOWEN, M.D.

Assistant Professor of Orthopaedic Surgery, Northwestern University Medical School; Team Physician, Chicago Bears, and Orthopaedic Consultant, Chicago Cubs; Active Attending, Northwestern Memorial Hospital, and Medical Director, Northwestern Memorial/Baxter, Inc. Physical Therapy Center, Chicago, Illinois

BRIAN T. BOYER, M.S.

Exercise Physiologist, Carolina Fitness and Sport Group, Greensboro, North Carolina

DAVID J. BOZENTKA, M.D.

Assistant Professor of Orthopaedic Surgery, Hand Surgery Section, University of Pennsylvania School of Medicine, Philadelphia, Pennsylvania

JAMES P. BRADLEY, M.D.

Clinical Assistant Professor, University of Pittsburgh Medical Center; Team Physician, Pittsburgh Steelers, Pittsburgh, Pennsylvania

ROBERT D. BRONSTEIN, M.D.

Assistant Professor, Section of Athletic Medicine, Department of Orthopaedics, University of Rochester School of Medicine and Dentistry; Attending Orthopaedist, Strong Memorial Hospital, Rochester, New York

ANDREW A. BROOKS, M.D.

Private Practice, Cedars-Sinai Medical Center, Los Angeles, California

DAVID E. BROWN, M.D.

Clinical Assistant Professor of Orthopaedic Surgery and Rehabilitation, University of Nebraska College of Medicine, Omaha, Nebraska

R. CHARLES BULL, M.D., B.Sc.(Med), F.R.C.S.(C)

Director, Eagleson Sports Clinic, York University; Chief Medical Officer, Team Canada (Hockey); Consultant, Humber Hospital and Orthopedic and Arthritic Hospital, Toronto, Ontario, Canada

R.S. BURNHAM, M.D., M.Sc., F.R.C.P.(C)

Assistant Professor, Division of Physical Medicine and Rehabilitation, Faculty of Medicine, Adjunct Professor, Faculty of Physical Education and Sport Studies, and Medical Consultant, Rick Hansen Center, University of Alberta, Edmonton, Alberta, Canada

GAIL BUTTERFIELD, Ph.D., R.D., F.A.C.S.M.

Visiting Assistant Professor of Human Biology, Stanford University, Stanford; Director of Nutrition Studies, Palo Alto VA Medical Center, Palo Alto, California

DAVID A. BUUCK, M.D.

Sports Medicine Fellow, University of Connecticut School of Medicine, Farmington, Connecticut

BERNARD R. CAHILL, M.D.

Clinical Professor of Orthopedics, University of Illinois College of Medicine at Peoria, and Ad Hoc Professor of Sports Medicine, Illinois State University; President and Medical Director, Orthopedic Institute of Illinois, and Director of Sports Medicine, Great Plains Sports Medicine and Rehabilitation Center, Peoria, Illinois

WILLIAM G. CARSON, Jr., M.D.

Assistant Clinical Professor of Orthopaedic Surgery, University of South Florida College of Medicine, Tampa, Florida

THOMAS R. CARTER, M.D.

Orthopaedic Consultant and Team Physician, Arizona State University, Tempe, Arizona

S.C. CHEN, M.D.†

Formerly Consultant Orthopaedic Surgeon, Chase Farm Hospitals, Enfield, Middlesex, England

---

†Deceased.

ANGELO J. COLOSIMO, M.D.

Assistant Professor of Orthopaedic Surgery, and Director, Division of Sports Medicine, University of Cincinnati College of Medicine, Cincinnati, Ohio

JOHN E. CONWAY, M.D.

Teaching Staff, Orthopedic Residency Program, Fort Worth Affiliated Hospitals, Fort Worth, Texas

DANIEL E. COOPER, M.D.

Associate Attending, Baylor University Medical Center; Staff, W.B. Carrell Memorial Clinic, Dallas, Texas

D.C. COVEY, M.D., M.S., Commander, U.S. Navy Medical Corps

Clinical Assistant Professor of Orthopaedic Surgery, University of Pennsylvania School of Medicine, Philadelphia, Pennsylvania; Chief of Orthopaedic Surgery, Naval Hospital, Bremerton, Washington

RICHARD S. CROW, M.D.

Associate Professor, Division of Epidemiology, University of Minnesota School of Public Health, Minneapolis, Minnesota

DONALD F. D'ALESSANDRO, M.D.

Chief, Sports Medicine and Shoulder Service, Carolinas Medical Center, and Associate, Miller Orthopaedic Clinic, Charlotte, North Carolina

CAROLINE DAVIS, Ph.D.

Associate Professor of Psychology, York University, North York; Associate Professor, Department of Psychiatry, The Toronto Hospital, Toronto, Ontario, Canada

KENNETH E. DeHAVEN, M.D.

Professor, Associate Chairman, and Director of Athletic Medicine, Department of Orthopaedics, University of Rochester School of Medicine and Dentistry; Attending Orthopaedist, Strong Memorial Hospital, Rochester, New York

STEVEN C. DENNIS, Ph.D.

Associate Professor of Physiology, University of Cape Town Medical School, Observatory, South Africa

LEITH G. DOUGLAS, M.D., F.R.C.S.(C), F.A.C.S.

Assistant Professor of Surgery, University of Toronto Faculty of Medicine; Plastic Surgeon, The Wellesley Hospital, Consultant in Plastic Surgery, Princess Margaret Hospital, and Team Plastic Surgeon, Toronto Maple Leafs Hockey Club, Toronto, Ontario, Canada

RICHARD V. DOWDEN, M.D., C.M., F.A.C.S.

Assistant Clinical Professor, Case Western Reserve University School of Medicine, Cleveland, Ohio

J. LARRY DURSTINE, Ph.D.

> Associate Professor of Exercise Science and Director of Clinical Exercise Program, University of South Carolina, Columbia, South Carolina

I.W.D. DYMOND, M.B.B.Ch., F.R.C.S.(Ed), F.C.S.(SA) Ortho, M. Med. Ortho

> Morningside Clinic, Morningside, Sandton, Republic of South Africa

MICHAEL EASTERBROOK, M.D., F.R.C.S.(C), F.A.C.S.

> Associate Professor of Ophthalmology, University of Toronto Faculty of Medicine; Consultant to Canadian Squash Racquets Association, United States Squash Racquets Association, Professional Squash Association, Canadian Badminton Association, Squash Ontario, and World Squash Federation; Eye Surgeon, Toronto Maple Leafs Hockey Team, Referees of National Hockey League, and National Team, Basketball Canada

JOHN C. EDWARDS, M.D.

> Interwest Sports and Orthopaedics, Bountiful, Utah

E. RANDY EICHNER, M.D., F.A.C.S.M.

> Professor of Medicine, University of Oklahoma College of Medicine; Attending Physician, University Hospital and VA Medical Center, Oklahoma City, Oklahoma

HARVARD ELLMAN, M.D.

> Associate Clinical Professor of Orthopaedics, University of California, Los Angeles, School of Medicine, Los Angeles, California

BO FERNHALL, Ph.D.

> Associate Professor of Exercise Science, The George Washington University School of Medicine and Health Sciences, Washington, DC

EDWARD P. FINK, M.D.

> Clinical Instructor of Orthopaedic Surgery, Harvard Medical School, Boston, Massachusetts

DAVID A. FISCHER, M.D.

> Clinical Assistant Professor of Orthopaedic Surgery, University of Minnesota Medical School—Minneapolis; Director, Minneapolis Sports Medicine Center Fellowship Program, Minneapolis, Minnesota

EVAN L. FLATOW, M.D.

> Herbert Irving Associate Professor of Orthopaedic Surgery; Columbia University College of Physicians and Surgeons; Associate Chief, The Shoulder Service, New York Orthopaedic Hospital, Columbia-Presbyterian Medical Center, New York, New York

LAWRENCE J. FOLINSBEE, Ph.D.

> Adjunct Associate Professor of Medicine, University of North Carolina at Chapel Hill School of Medicine; Research Physiologist, U.S. Environmental Protection Agency, Chapel Hill, North Carolina

AARON R. FOLSOM, M.D., M.P.H.

> Professor, Division of Epidemiology, University of Minnesota School of Public Health, Minneapolis, Minnesota

DAN FOSTER, M.A., A.T.C.

> Adjunct Assistant Professor and Director of Athletic Training in Exercise Science, and Associate Director of Athletic Training, University of Iowa College of Medicine, Iowa City, Iowa

BARRY A. FRANKLIN, Ph.D.

> Adjunct Professor of Physiology, Wayne State University School of Medicine, Detroit; Director, Cardiac Rehabilitation and Exercise Laboratories, William Beaumont Hospital, Royal Oak, Michigan

JONATHAN FRENCH, Ph.D.

> Research Physiologist, Armstrong Laboratory, Brooks Air Force Base, Texas

JOHN P. FULKERSON, M.D.

> Professor of Orthopaedic Surgery, University of Connecticut School of Medicine; Head Team Physician, NHL Hartford Whalers, Hartford, Connecticut

LeROY R. FULLERTON, Jr., M.D.

> Associate Clinical Professor, Department of Surgery, Section of Orthopaedics, Medical College of Georgia; Private Practice Orthopaedic Surgeon, Orthopaedic Associates of Augusta, Augusta, Georgia

GARY M. GARTSMAN, M.D.

> Clinical Associate Professor of Orthopedics, Baylor College of Medicine; Fondren Orthopedic Group, Houston, Texas

THOMAS A. GENNARELLI, M.D.

> Professor and Vice Chairman of Neurosurgery, and Director, Head Injury Center, University of Pennsylvania School of Medicine, Philadelphia, Pennsylvania

MICHELE GLASGOW, M.D.

> Assistant Professor of Orthopedic Surgery, School of Medicine, and Team Physician, University of Pennsylvania, Philadelphia, Pennsylvania

NORMAN GLEDHILL, Ph.D.

> Professor of Kinesiology, York University, North York, Ontario, Canada

ALLAN H. GOLDFARB, Ph.D.

Associate Professor, Department of Exercise and Sport Science, University of North Carolina, Greensboro, North Carolina

ROBERT C. GOODE, M.A., D.Phil.

Professor, Department of Physiology, Faculty of Medicine, and Graduate Programme in Exercise Sciences, School of Physical and Health Education, University of Toronto, Toronto, Ontario, Canada

JACK GOODMAN, Ph.D.

Associate Professor, School of Physical and Health Education, and Department of Community Health, Faculty of Medicine, University of Toronto; Consulting Exercise Physiologist, Department of Nuclear Cardiology, The Toronto Hospital, Toronto, Ontario, Canada

NAHUM HALPERIN, M.D.

Associate Professor of Orthopaedics, Sackler School of Medicine, Tel Aviv University, Tel Aviv; Head of Orthopaedic Department, Assaf Harofeh Medical Center, Zeriffin, Israel

WILLIAM G. HAMILTON, M.D.

Assistant Clinical Professor of Orthopedic Surgery, Columbia University College of Physicians and Surgeons; Senior Attending Orthopedic Surgeon, St. Luke's-Roosevelt Hospital, New York, New York

MARK L. HARTMAN, M.D.

Assistant Professor of Medicine, University of Virginia School of Medicine; Attending Physician, University of Virginia Hospital, Charlottesville, Virginia

SCOTT M. HASSON, Ed.D., P.T., F.A.C.S.M.

Associate Professor and Director of Advanced Studies, School of Physical Therapy, Texas Woman's University, Houston, Texas

JOHN A. HAWLEY, Ph.D., F.A.C.S.M.

Research Fellow and Senior Lecturer in Physiology, University of Cape Town Medical School, Observatory, South Africa

ELLIOTT B. HERSHMAN, M.D.

Assistant Director, Department of Orthopaedic Surgery, and Staff, Nicholas Institute of Sports Medicine and Athletic Trauma, Lenox Hill Hospital, New York, New York

CHERIE A. HOLMES, M.D.

Fellow, Sports Medicine Section, Rush-Presbyterian-St. Luke's Medical Center, Chicago, Illinois

CHRISTINE HUTTON, M.B., Ch.B.

Registrar, Auckland Hospital, Auckland, New Zealand

BRETT C. HYNNINEN, M.D.

Assistant Professor of Physical Medicine and Rehabilitation, University of Kentucky College of Medicine, Lexington, Kentucky

PETER A. INDELICATO, M.D.

Professor of Orthopaedics and Chief of Sports Medicine, University of Florida College of Medicine; Team Physician, University of Florida, and Associate Team Physician, Miami Dolphins, Gainesville, Florida

DAVID L. JACKSON, M.D., F.A.C.S.M.

Associate Professor, Departments of Physical Medicine and Rehabilitation and Sports Medicine, University of Kentucky College of Medicine, Lexington, Kentucky

DAVID R. JACOBS, Jr., Ph.D.

Professor, Division of Epidemiology, University of Minnesota School of Public Health, Minneapolis, Minnesota

ROLAND P. JAKOB, M.D

Professor and Vice Chairman, Department of Orthopaedic Surgery, Inselspital, Bern, Switzerland

CATHERINE M. JANKOWSKI, M.S.

Department of Kinesiology, Texas Woman's University, Denton, Texas

FRANK W. JOBE, M.D.

Clinical Professor of Orthopaedics, University of Southern California School of Medicine, Los Angeles; Orthopaedic Consultant, Los Angeles Dodgers and PGA Tour; Associate and President, Kerlan-Jobe Orthopaedic Clinic, and Medical Director, Biomechanics Laboratory, Centinela Hospital Medical Center, Inglewood, California

L.T. JOHNSON, M.D.

Clinical Assistant Professor of Orthopedic Surgery, University of Texas Southwestern Medical Center, Dallas, Texas

JILL A. KANALEY, Ph.D.

Research Associate, Department of Internal Medicine, University of Virginia Health Sciences Center, Charlottesville, Virginia

TERENCE KAVANAGH, M.D., F.R.C.P.(C), F.A.C.C., F.C.C.P.

Associate Professor of Medicine, University of Toronto Faculty of Medicine, Toronto, Ontario, Canada; Consultant Advisor, Cardiac Rehabilitation, Harefield Hospital, Middlesex, England

MARTIN J. KELLEY, M.S., P.T.

Adjunct Faculty, Department of Physical Therapy, Beaver College, Glenside; Director, University Sports Physical Therapy, University of Pennsylvania Sports Medicine Center, Philadelphia, Pennsylvania

JAMES P. KELLY, M.A., M.D.

Assistant Professor of Rehabilitation Medicine and Neurology, Northwestern University Medical School; Director, Brain Injury Program, Rehabilitation Institute of Chicago, and Consulting Neurologist, Northwestern Memorial Hospital, Chicago, Illinois

SIDNEY H. KENNEDY, M.D., M.R.C. Psych., F.R.C.P.(C)

Professor of Psychiatry, University of Toronto Faculty of Medicine, Toronto, Ontario, Canada

KIERAN J. KILLIAN, M.B., F.R.C.P.(I), F.R.C.P.(C)

Professor, Respiratory Division, Department of Medicine, McMaster University School of Medicine; Staff Physician, Respiratory Unit and Intensive Care, McMaster University Medical Centre, Hamilton, Ontario, Canada

THOMAS E. KLOOTWYK, M.D.

Clinical Instructor of Orthopaedics, Indiana University School of Medicine, Indianapolis; Team Physician, Department of Athletics, Indiana State University, Terre Haute, and Orthopaedic Consultant, Department of Athletics, Manchester College, North Manchester; Orthopaedic Surgeon, Methodist Sports Medicine Center, Indianapolis, Indiana

DANIEL E. KRAFT, M.D.

Clinical Instructor, Indiana University School of Medicine; Methodist Sports Medicine Fellowship Program, and Youth Sports Medicine Institute, Indianapolis, Indiana

JEFFREY R. KUHLMAN, M.D.

Orthopaedic Surgeon, Statesville Medical Group; Attending Surgeon, Iredell Memorial Hospital and Davis Community Hospital, Statesville, North Carolina

RONALD S. KVITNE, M.D.

Assistant Clinical Professor of Orthopaedics, University of Southern California School of Medicine, Los Angeles; Associate, Kerlan-Jobe Orthopaedic Clinic, Inglewood, California

LEWIS B. LANE, M.D.

Clinical Associate Professor of Surgery (Orthopaedics), Cornell University Medical College, New York; Chief of Hand Surgery and Associate Chief of Orthopaedic Surgery, North Shore University Hospital–Cornell University Medical College, Manhasset, and Assistant Attending, Hand Service, Hospital for Special Surgery, New York, New York

MICHAEL T. LEE, M.D.

Sports Medicine Fellow, University of Illinois College of Medicine, Peoria, Illinois

LARRY M. LEITH, Ph.D.

Associate Professor, School of Physical and Health Education, University of Toronto, Toronto, Ontario, Canada

BENJAMIN D. LEVINE, M.D.

Assistant Professor of Medicine, University of Texas Southwestern Medical School; Director, Institute for Exercise and Environmental Medicine, and Co-Medical Director, Finley Ewing Cardiovascular Center, Presbyterian Hospital, and Medical Director of Cardiac Rehabilitation, Parkland Memorial Hospital, Dallas, Texas

LAUREL TRAEGER MacKINNON, Ph.D., F.A.C.S.M.

Senior Lecturer in Exercise Physiology and Exercise Management, Department of Human Movement Studies, The University of Queensland, Brisbane, Australia

IAN MacNAB, M.B., Ch.B., F.R.C.S.†

Formerly Professor of Surgery, University of Toronto Faculty of Medicine, Toronto, Ontario, Canada

ROGER A. MANN, M.D.

Director, Foot Fellowship Program, Oakland, California

PETER MARSHALL, M.A., P.T.

Company Physical Therapist, American Ballet Theatre, New York, New York

MARC A. MARTENS, M.D.

Professor, University of Antwerp, Antwerp; Chairman, Orthopaedics Department, Hospital O.L.V. Middelares, Deurne, Belgium

SCOTT DAVID MARTIN, M.D.

Orthopaedic Sports Medicine Fellow, American Sports Medicine Institute, Birmingham, Alabama

JOHN R. McCARROLL, M.D.

Clinical Instructor of Orthopaedics, Indiana University School of Medicine, Indianapolis; Orthopaedic Consultant, Indiana University Athletics, Bloomington, and Orthopaedic Surgeon, Methodist Sports Medicine Center, Indianapolis, Indiana

---

†Deceased.

FRANK C. McCUE III, M.D.

Alfred R. Shands Professor of Orthopaedic Surgery and Plastic Surgery of the Hand, Director, Division of Sports Medicine and Hand Surgery, and Professor of Plastic Surgery, School of Medicine; Professor of Education, Curry School of Education; and Team Physician, Department of Athletics, University of Virginia, Charlottesville, Virginia

JOHN A. McCULLOCH, M.D., F.R.C.S.(C)

Professor of Orthopedics, Northeastern Ohio Universities College of Medicine, Rootstown, Ohio

J. SIMON McGRAIL, M.D., M.S., F.R.C.S.(C)

Professor of Otolaryngology, University of Toronto Faculty of Medicine; Consultant, Princess Margaret Hospital, and Active Staff, Wellesley Hospital and Central Hospital, Toronto, Ontario, Canada

MICHAEL J. McGRATH, M.D., F.R.C.S.(C)

Associate Professor and Chair, Division of Maternal-Fetal Medicine, Queen's University Faculty of Medicine, Kingston, Ontario, Canada

DOUGLAS B. McKEAG, M.D., M.S.

Professor of Family Practice, Associate Chair for Education, Coordinator of Sports Medicine, and Team Physician, Michigan State University, East Lansing, Michigan; President, American Medical Society of Sports Medicine, Middleton, Wisconsin

DONALD C. McKENZIE, M.D., Ph.D.

Professor, Division of Sports Medicine, University of British Columbia Faculty of Medicine, Vancouver, British Columbia, Canada

KEITH MEISTER, M.D.

Assistant Professor of Orthopaedics, Division of Sports Medicine, and Team Physician, University of Florida, Gainesville, Florida

JAN MELICHNA, Ph.D.

Associate Professor of Human and Exercise Physiology, Charles University, Prague, Czech Republic

LYLE J. MICHELI, M.D.

Associate Clinical Professor of Orthopaedic Surgery, Harvard Medical School; Director, Division of Sports Medicine, The Children's Hospital, Boston, Massachusetts

DAVID L. MONTGOMERY, Ph.D.

Professor of Physical Education, McGill University; Director, Seagram's Sports Science Centre, Montreal, Quebec, Canada

GEOFFREY E. MOORE, M.D.

Assistant Professor of Medicine, University of Pittsburgh School of Medicine, Pittsburgh, Pennsylvania

RODNEY E. MOUNTAIN, M.B., Ch.B., F.R.C.S.

Head and Neck Oncologic Surgery Fellow, Department of Otolaryngology, The Ohio State University, Columbus, Ohio

DAVID C. NIEMAN, Dr.P.H., F.A.C.S.M.

Professor of Health and Exercise Science, Appalachian State University, Boone, North Carolina

ROBERT P. NIRSCHL, M.D., M.S.

Assistant Clinical Professor of Orthopedic Surgery, Georgetown University School of Medicine, Washington, DC; Director, Orthopedic Sports Medicine Fellowship Program, Nirschl Orthopedic Clinic/Arlington Hospital, Arlington, Virginia

TIMOTHY D. NOAKES, M.B., Ch.B., M.D., F.A.C.S.M.

Liberty Life Chair of Exercise and Sports Science, University of Cape Town Medical School; Director, Medical Research Council/University of Cape Town Bioenergetics of Exercise Research Unit, Observatory, South Africa

FRANK NOFTALL, M.D., F.R.C.S.(C)

Assistant Clinical Professor of Surgery, Memorial University of Newfoundland Faculty of Medicine; Staff Orthopaedic Surgeon, Health Sciences Centre, General Hospital, and St. Clare's Mercy Hospital, St. John's, Newfoundland, Canada

GORDON W. NUBER, M.D.

Associate Professor and Vice Chairman of Orthopaedic Surgery, Northwestern University Medical School; Team Physician, Chicago Bears, and Orthopaedic Consultant, Chicago Cubs; Active Attending, Northwestern Memorial Hospital, and WOC Physician, VA Lakeside Medical Center, Chicago, Illinois

STEVEN J. O'BRIEN, M.D.

Associate Professor of Surgery (Orthopaedic), Cornell University Medical Center, New York, and Director of Continuing Education, Harvard University, Boston, Massachusetts; Assistant Team Physician, New York Football Giants; Assistant Scientist and Associate Attending in Orthopaedic Surgery, Hospital for Special Surgery, and Associate Attending in Orthopaedic Surgery, New York Hospital, New York, New York

DENIS E. O'DONNELL, M.D., F.R.C.P.(I), F.R.C.P.(C), F.C.C.P.

Associate Professor of Medicine, Division of Respirology and Critical Care Medicine, and Director, Respiratory Diseases Training Program, Queen's University; Attending Respirologist, Kingston General Hospital, Consulting Respirologist, Hotel Dieu Hospital and St. Mary's of the Lake Hospital, and Director, Pulmonary Rehabilitation Program, St. Mary's of the Lake Hospital, Kingston, Ontario, Canada

A. LEE OSTERMAN, M.D.

Professor of Orthopedics and Hand Surgery, Jefferson Medical College of Thomas Jefferson University, Philadelphia, Pennsylvania

JIRO OZAKI, M.D.

Assistant Professor of Orthopaedic Surgery, Nara Medical University, Kashihara City; Director and Chairman, Department of Orthopaedic Surgery, Nara Prefectural Hospital, Nara City, Nara, Japan

MICHAEL J. PAGNANI, M.D.

Clinical Assistant Professor of Orthopaedics and Rehabilitation, Vanderbilt University School of Medicine; Attending Orthopaedic Surgeon, The Lipscomb Clinic, Nashville, Tennessee

RANDAL A. PALMITIER, M.D.

Orthopaedic Associates of Grand Rapids, and Medical Director, Grand Rapids Sport and Spine Clinic, Grand Rapids, Michigan

KENT B. PANDOLF, Ph.D., M.P.H.

Adjunct Professor of Health Sciences, Sargent College of Allied Health Professions, Boston University, Boston, and Adjunct Clinical Professor of Sports Biology, Springfield College, Springfield; Director, Environmental Physiology and Medicine Directorate, U.S. Army Research Institute of Environmental Medicine, Natick, Massachusetts

J. SERGE PARISIEN, M.D.

Associate Professor of Clinical Orthopaedic Surgery, New York University School of Medicine; Chief of Arthroscopic Surgery Service and Attending Orthopaedic Surgeon, Sports Medicine Service, Hospital for Joint Disease, Orthopaedic Institute, New York, New York

ROBERT C. PASHBY, M.D., F.R.C.S.(C)

Assistant Professor of Ophthalmology, University of Toronto Faculty of Medicine; Active Staff, Department of Ophthalmology, Hospital for Sick Children and Mount Sinai Hospital, Toronto, Ontario, Canada

THOMAS J. PASHBY, C.M., M.D., C.R.C.S.(C)

Assistant Professor Emeritus of Ophthalmology, University of Toronto Faculty of Medicine; Honorary Consultant, Hospital for Sick Children, Centenary Hospital, and Toronto (Western) Hospital, Toronto, Ontario, Canada

HELENE PAVLOV, M.D.

Professor of Radiology, Cornell University Medical College; Attending Radiologist, Hospital for Special Surgery and New York Hospital, New York, New York

STEVEN J. PETRUZZELLO, Ph.D.

Assistant Professor of Kinesiology, University of Illinois at Urbana-Champaign, Urbana, Illinois

MICHAEL RAYMOND PIERRYNOWSKI, Ph.D.

Associate Professor, McMaster University, Hamilton, and Professor, University of Toronto, Toronto, Ontario, Canada

MICHAEL R. REDLER, M.D.

Visiting Consultant, Division of Sports Medicine and Hand Surgery, University of Virginia, Charlottesville, Virginia; Team Physician, Sacred Heart University, University of Bridgeport, and Connecticut Skyhawks; Staff, The Orthopaedic and Sports Center, Trumbull, Connecticut

DAVID COLLINSON REID, M.D., M.Ch.(Orth), F.R.C.S.(C)

Professor of Orthopaedic Surgery, University of Alberta Faculty of Medicine; Director, Glen Sather University of Alberta Sports Medicine Clinic, Edmonton, Alberta, Canada

PHILIP J. REILLY, M.D.

Gate Orthopedics, Warwick, Rhode Island

ARTHUR C. RETTIG, M.D.

Assistant Clinical Professor, Indiana University School of Medicine; Staff, Methodist Sports Medicine Clinic, Indianapolis, Indiana

DROR ROBINSON, M.D., Ph.D.

Assistant Professor of Orthopedics, Sackler School of Medicine, Tel Aviv University, Tel Aviv; Orthopedic Surgeon, Assaf Harofeh Medical Center, Zeriffin, Israel

SCOTT A. RODEO, M.D.

Fellow, Sports Medicine, The Hospital for Special Surgery, Cornell University Medical College, New York, New York

KENNETH J. ROGERS, A.T.C., M.S.

University of Pennsylvania Sports Medicine Center, Philadelphia, Pennsylvania

RICHARD ROST, M.D.

Director, Institute of Cardiology and Sports Medicine, German Sport University, Köln, Germany

GREGORY A. ROWDON, M.D.

Co-Director, Primary Care Sports Medicine Fellowship, Methodist Sports Medicine Center, Indianapolis, Indiana

CARTER R. ROWE, M.D.

Emeritus Associate Clinical Professor of Orthopaedic Surgery, Harvard Medical School; Senior Orthopaedic Surgeon (Retired), Massachusetts General Hospital, Boston, Massachusetts

G. JAMES SAMMARCO, M.D., F.A.C.S.

Volunteer Professor, Department of Orthopaedics, University of Cincinnati Medical Center, Cincinnati, Ohio

CHARLOTTE F. SANBORN, M.D.

Associate Professor of Exercise Physiology, Department of Kinesiology, and Director, Center for Research on Women's Health, Texas Woman's University, Denton, Texas

ALEXANDER A. SAPEGA, M.D.

Assistant Professor of Orthopaedic Surgery, University of Pennsylvania School of Medicine, Philadelphia, Pennsylvania

SCOTT P. SCHEMMEL, M.D.

Director of Sports Medicine, Medical Associates Clinic, Dubuque, Iowa

DAVID E. SCHULLER, M.D.

Professor and Chairman, Department of Otolaryngology, The Ohio State University, Columbus, Ohio

W. NORMAN SCOTT, M.D.

Director, Insall Scott Kelly Institute for Orthopaedics and Sports Medicine, New York, New York

GILES R. SCUDERI, M.D.

Attending Orthopedic Surgeon, Insall Scott Kelly Institute for Orthopaedics and Sports Medicine and Beth Israel Medical Center–North Division, New York, New York

BRIAN J. SENNETT, M.D.

Instructor in Sports Medicine and Hand Surgery, University of Pennsylvania School of Medicine, Philadelphia, Pennsylvania

BENJAMIN SHAFFER, M.D.

Assistant Professor of Orthopaedics, Georgetown University School of Medicine; Director, Division of Sports Medicine, Department of Orthopaedics, Georgetown University Medical Center, Washington, DC

K. DONALD SHELBOURNE, M.D.

Associate Professor, Indiana University School of Medicine, Indianapolis, Indiana

ROY J. SHEPHARD, M.D., Ph.D., D.P.E., F.A.C.S.M.

Professor, School of Physical and Health Education, University of Toronto, Toronto, and Canadian Tire Acceptance Limited Resident Scholar, Programme in Health Studies, Brock University, Saint Catherine's, Ontario, Canada

CLARENCE L. SHIELDS, Jr., M.D.

Associate Clinical Professor of Orthopaedics, University of Southern California School of Medicine, Los Angeles; Orthopaedic Consultant, Los Angeles Rams; Associate, Kerlan-Jobe Orthopaedic Clinic, Inglewood, California

CHRISTOPHER W. SIWEK, M.D.

Attending Physician, Susan B. Allen Memorial Hospital, El Dorado, Kansas

GEORGE A. SNOOK, M.D.

Senior Lecturer in Orthopedics, University of Connecticut Medical School, Farmington, Connecticut; Orthopedic Surgeon, Cooley Dickinson Hospital, Northampton, and Consultant in Orthopedics, University of Massachusetts, Amherst, Massachusetts

ROBERT J. SONSTROEM, Ph.D., F.A.C.S.M.

Professor of Physical Education, University of Rhode Island, Kingston, Rhode Island

KEVIN P. SPEER, M.D.

Assistant Professor of Orthopaedic Surgery, Duke University School of Medicine, Durham, North Carolina

PAUL WILLIAM STRATFORD, M.Sc., P.T.

Assistant Professor, School of Occupational Therapy and Physiotherapy, McMaster University, Hamilton, Ontario, Canada

JAMES STRAY-GUNDERSEN, M.D., F.A.C.S.M.

Assistant Professor of Orthopaedic Surgery, University of Texas Southwestern Medical School; Director, Baylor/UT Southwestern Sports Science Research Center, Dallas, Texas

LAWRENCE E. THIBAULT, Sc.D.

Professor of Bioengineering and of Bioengineering in Neurosurgery and Orthopaedic Surgery; Associate Director, Head Injury Center, Department of Neurosurgery, School of Medicine, and Executive Director, Laboratories for Injury Research and Prevention, Department of Bioengineering, University of Pennsylvania, Philadelphia, Pennsylvania

SCOTT G. THOMAS, Ph.D.

Assistant Professor of Physical Therapy, University of Toronto; Research Associate, Centre for Studies of Physical Function, Toronto, Ontario, Canada

JAMES E. TIBONE, M.D.

Associate Clinical Professor, University of Southern California School of Medicine, Los Angeles; Associate, Kerlan-Jobe Orthopaedic Clinic, Inglewood, California

PETER M. TIIDUS, Ph.D.

Assistant Professor and Chair, Department of Physical Education, Wilfrid Laurier University; Adjunct Assistant Professor, Department of Kinesiology, University of Waterloo, Waterloo, Ontario, Canada

NATHANIEL L. TINDEL, M.D.

Chief Resident in Orthopaedic Surgery, Lenox Hill Hospital, New York, New York

JOSEPH S. TORG, M.D.

Professor of Orthopaedic Surgery, University of Pennsylvania School of Medicine; Director, University of Pennsylvania Sports Medicine Center, Philadelphia, Pennsylvania

BEVERLY F. TREMAIN, M.Sc.

Professor of Health and Physical Education, and Wellness Coordinator, Collin County Community College, Plano, Texas

ELLY TREPMAN, M.D.

Associate Director, Boston Foot and Ankle Center, New England Baptist Hospital, Boston, Massachusetts

ROCCI V. TRUMPER, M.D.

Fellow, Rocky Mountain Associates in Orthopaedic Medicine, Fort Collins, Colorado

DAN TUNSTALL-PEDOE, M.D., D.Phil., F.R.C.P.

Consultant Cardiologist and Senior Lecturer, St. Bartholomew's Hospital; Medical Director, London Marathon, London, England

ANDRÉ L. VALLERAND, Ph.D.

Physiologist, Human Protective Systems Division, Defence and Civil Institute of Environmental Medicine, North York, Ontario, Canada

C. THOMAS VANGSNESS, Jr., M.D.

Associate Professor, University of Southern California, Los Angeles, California

WALTER P. van HELDER, M.D., Ph.D.

Professor, Departments of Preventive Medicine and Anaesthesia, University of Toronto Faculty of Medicine, Toronto, Ontario, Canada

JOSEPH J. VEGSO, M.S., A.T.C.

Area Manager, Health South Rehabilitation Corporation, Tucson, Arizona

ATKO VIRU, D.Sc.

Professor of Exercise Physiology, University of Tartu, Tartu, Estonia

JANET WALBERG-RANKIN, Ph.D.

Associate Professor, Human Nutrition and Foods, Virginia Polytechnic Institute and State University, Blacksburg, Virginia

MARY-BETH WALSH, P.T., Dip. M.P.T.

Physical Therapist and Clinical Education Coordinator, Department of Sports Medicine and Rehabilitation, Georgetown University Hospital, Washington, DC

RUSSELL F. WARREN, M.D.

Professor of Surgery (Orthopaedics), Cornell University Medical College; Attending Surgeon and Surgeon-in-Chief, The Hospital for Special Surgery, and Attending (Orthopaedic) Surgeon, The New York Hospital, New York, New York

KATHERINE A. WEBB, M.Sc.

Research Associate and Exercise Physiologist, Queen's University, Kingston, Ontario, Canada

GARRON G. WEIKER, M.D.

Associate Professor, Ohio State University College of Medicine, and Professor, Cleveland Clinic Education Foundation; Director of Graduate Medical Education and Staff Orthopaedic Surgeon, Cleveland Clinic, Cleveland, Ohio

R. PETER WELSH, M.B., Ch.B., F.R.C.S.(C), F.A.C.S.

Associate Professor of Surgery, University of Toronto Faculty of Medicine; Chief of Staff, Orthopaedic and Arthritic Hospital, Toronto, Ontario, Canada

ARTHUR WELTMAN, Ph.D.

Professor of Human Services and of Medicine, and Director, Exercise Physiology Laboratories, University of Virginia, Charlottesville, Virginia

EUGENE M. WOLF, M.D.

Director, Arthroscopy Laboratory, California Pacific Medical Research Institute, San Francisco, California

LARRY A. WOLFE, Ph.D., F.A.C.S.M.

Associate Professor, School of Physical and Health Education, Queen's University, Kingston, Ontario, Canada

SCOTT W. WOLFE, M.D.

Assistant Professor and Director, Hand and Upper Extremity Surgery, Department of Orthopaedics and Rehabilitation, Yale University School of Medicine, New Haven, Connecticut

ANDREW M. WONG, M.D.

Department of Orthopedics, University of Florida, Gainesville, Florida

LEE C. WOODS, M.D.

Attending Staff, Orthopaedic Hospital, Children's Rotational Abnormality and Clubfoot Clinics, Los Angeles, California

C. STEWART WRIGHT, M.D., F.R.C.S.(C)

Lecturer, University of Toronto, Toronto, Ontario, Canada

IRA ZALTZ, M.D.

Resident, Harvard Combined Orthopaedic Residency Program, Boston, Massachusetts

CHRISTIAN W. ZAUNER, Ph.D.

Professor of Exercise and Sport Science, Oregon State University, Corvallis, Oregon

An understanding of the discipline of sports medicine is becoming ever more important, not only for the certified specialist in this area of practice, but also for the general practitioner, the exercise physiologist, the trainer, the physical therapist, the coach: all of the team of health professionals who share in the delivery of medical care, not only to athletes, but also to that growing proportion of the general public who now regard regular physical activity as a part of a prudent lifestyle.

The present volume is designed to provide, in clear and readable form, a précis of the problems and disorders that are commonly encountered by the regular exerciser, offering effective methods of diagnosis, management, and treatment. Despite recent advances in preventive measures, participation in competitive sports inevitably remains associated with some risk of injury. A substantial part of this text thus addresses such problems. Maladies that were previously neglected or considered of little importance because no gross pathology was readily identifiable must now be considered and given appropriate treatment. As the population ages, the sports physician encounters a growing number of overuse injuries: lesions of the shoulder, the elbow, the knee, the foot, and the ankle. Some of these lesions are assuming growing socio-economic performance, not only on the sports field, but also in the workplace, as automation increases the replication of movements during the performance of daily tasks as diverse as word-processing and the gutting of chickens.

Like its predecessors, this Third Edition has drawn extensively upon the experience of current world leaders and experts in sports medicine. They cover recent advances in sports medicine itself and provide matching up-to-date information on exercise physiology and applied aspects of sports medicine. The latest details on arthroscopy of the shoulder, elbow, and wrist, and on arthroscopy-assisted knee ligament surgery are coupled with the presentation of important new concepts in the management of the many maladies encountered in daily practice. As in previous editions, a strong emphasis has been placed on prevention and training as well as on the current management of established disorders. The broad scope of the text continues to make it unique in its field. Individual chapters cover such important environmental topics as heat, cold, diurnal rhythms, and high altitude, as well as issues of sex, age, nutrition and concomitant medical problems ranging from diabetes to blood doping.

The scope of the text has expanded yet further with the production of this Third Edition. New illustrations and updated suggestions for further reading continue to enhance the value of what is becoming a standard resource for the well-informed practitioner in sports medicine. The contributors have been selected on a broad international basis; they have been chosen for their ability to provide authoritative information in their selected topic areas in a clear, concise, and practical manner. We are much appreciative of the succinct way in which they have succeeded in crystallizing their expertise and experience.

We have continued our original plan of directing the volume particularly to those who are involved in the day-to-day coaching, training, and treatment of athletes at all levels of competition. The text has been carefully reviewed to ensure that the material is appropriate to the needs of orthopaedists, physical medicine specialists, team physicians, trainers, physiotherapists, and physical educators. The broad scope of the text also makes it an important resource for the family physician who must provide sound advice and treatment to a population that is growing ever more interested in active and physically demanding leisure pursuits. Reference to this volume can be recommended as providing a rapid and concise update on the diverse issues that are encountered in managing the active patient, whether man, woman, or child.

Roy J. Shephard
Joseph S. Torg

CONTENTS

PSYCHOLOGICAL ASPECTS OF SPORTS MEDICINE

MEDICAL ASPECTS OF SPORTS MEDICINE

GENERAL

ATHLETIC INJURIES AND THE USE OF MEDICATION

LOUIS C. ALMEKINDERS, M.D.

Athletic injuries involving the musculoskeletal system are the most frequent cause of missed practice and competition in virtually every sport. Even though most of the injuries are mild and self-limited, there is a never-ending search for a form of treatment that will result in more rapid healing and an earlier return to full activities. Medication seems an ideal form of treatment, since it can generally be administered quickly and easily without the complications of surgical treatment. With this concept in mind, several types of medication are now used frequently, both during the rehabilitation of musculoskeletal injuries and in conjunction with surgical treatment for more severe athletic injuries. This chapter reviews these medications, their indications, side effects and efficacy.

NONSTEROIDAL ANTI-INFLAMMATORY DRUGS

Nonsteroidal anti-inflammatory drugs (NSAIDs) are probably the most commonly used medication in athletic injuries. They are presumed to act through inhibition of cyclo-oxygenase, with a resulting decreased production of prostaglandins. Prostaglandins are considered to be mediators of the "standard" inflammatory response to any traumatic disruption of tissue. The inflammatory response is classically associated with pain, swelling, erythema, and decreased function. NSAIDs are primarily aimed at decreasing the inflammatory response and thereby its symptoms. In this fashion they are used in both acute injuries (sprains, strains, and fractures) and chronic injuries (tendonitis, bursitis, and fasciitis).

Acute Injuries

The inflammatory response following acute injuries such as sprains, strains, and fractures is often clinically clearly evident through associated pain and swelling.

The most common examples of such injuries are muscle tears (strains) and ankle and knee ligament tears (sprains). Most of these strains and sprains are partial tears that will heal within 2 to 6 weeks without specific medical intervention. NSAIDs are often recommended in the immediate post-injury period. Double-blind, randomized studies have shown that NSAIDs give adequate control of discomfort during this period. It remains unclear whether this pain relief is associated with significant inhibition of the inflammatory reaction. Animal studies show only a mild delay in the inflammatory reaction. Human studies have not shown consistent anti-inflammatory effects such as an earlier decrease in swelling compared with placebo treatment. Drugs with little or no anti-inflammatory properties have been similarly effective in some studies. Fortunately, side effects such as gastrointestinal (GI) bleeding are relatively rare in this often young and otherwise healthy population. The analgesia that results from NSAID administration can be helpful during the rehabilitation of these injuries. Early, protected motion accelerates and improves the healing process of ligaments, muscles, tendons, and bones. The NSAID-induced analgesia may allow earlier institution of rehabilitation, thereby resulting in improved healing. Whether anti-inflammatory effects play a role in this healing process remains unclear.

Theoretically, NSAID therapy should begin as soon as the diagnosis is made. At that point, the inflammatory response may not have developed fully and it is more likely to be inhibited than later, when full-blown inflammation is present. Although a plausible hypothesis, this assumption has not yet been studied under controlled circumstances. Generally, it is recommended to prescribe the NSAID in an anti-inflammatory dose (Table 1). This is often based on animal studies, where anti-inflammatory effects were seen at doses two to three times higher than analgesic doses. Again, no human studies are available. The optimal duration of NSAID therapy also remains unclear. Most authors recommend a relatively short course of 5 to 10 days. Most of the inflammatory response usually subsides over that time. The use of NSAIDs following surgical treatment of athletic injuries is discussed in the section on analgesics.

Chronic Injuries

The use of NSAIDs in chronic injuries such as tendonitis or bursitis is also very common, but it is even

1

Table 1 Commonly Used Drugs in Athletic Injuries

Drugs	Usual Dose	Common Brand Name
Nonsteroidal Anti-inflammatory Drugs (NSAIDs):		
Aspirin	650 mg qid	
Ibuprofen	600-800 mg tid/qid	Motrin
Naproxen	250-500 mg bid	Naprosyn/Anaprox
Piroxicam	20 mg qd	Feldene
Diclofenac	50-75 mg bid/tid	Voltaren
Nabumetone	1000-1500 mg qd	Relafen
Corticosteroids (Local Injection):		
Methylprednisolone	10-40 mg per injection	Depomedrol
Betamethasone	3-6 mg per injection	Celestone
Triamcinolone	10-40 mg per injection	Kenalog
Analgesics:		
Aspirin	325 mg qid	
Ibuprofen	200-400 mg tid/qid	Motrin/Advil/Nuprin
Acetaminophen	325-650 mg qid	Tylenol
Ketorolac	60 mg IM loading dose 30 mg q6h	Toradol
Acetaminophen with codeine (30 mg)	1 or 2 tablets q4h	Tylenol #3
Acetaminophen with propoxyphene (50-100 mg)	1 or 2 tablets q4h	Darvon/Darvocet
Acetaminophen with oxycodone (5 mg)	1 or 2 tablets q4h	Percocet/Tylox
Acetaminophen with hydrocodone (5 mg)	1 or 2 tablets q4-6h	Vicodin

more unclear whether their anti-inflammatory properties truly play a role in the treatment of these injuries. These chronic injuries are often associated with prolonged repetitive motion and are common in endurance athletes. The repetitive motion is thought to result in cumulative microtrauma, to which the body responds with an inflammatory response. However, this concept of chronic athletic injuries remains unproven. Some studies suggest that such injuries are actually degenerative lesions, with a lack of healing response and no significant inflammatory response. Only occasionally is a clear inflammatory response seen in bursitis or involvement of the tendon sheath with visible swelling and pain. In spite of the lack of controlled studies, the use of NSAIDs in chronic injuries remains popular. If the anti-inflammatory effect is not part of their mechanism of action, NSAIDs can be as effective analgesics as they are in acute injuries. If actual swelling is present (as in bursitis or tendon sheath inflammation), they seem to be more effective, possibly due to their anti-inflammatory effect. In addition, some physicians have suggested that they are more effective early after the onset of tendonitis or bursitis than once the injury has been established for several weeks. However, such observations may be biased, since a number of these injuries are self-limiting without treatment. The dose of NSAID is generally similar to that used in acute injuries (see Table 1). Although there are no controlled studies, there seems a tendency to prescribe NSAID for a longer period of time (e.g., 2-4 weeks) than in acute injuries. This may be partly because NSAID-induced analgesia allows the athlete to continue sport participation, since the injury itself is often not disabling. However, continued sport participation may slow the recovery process, and often the injury only heals during the off season.

Contraindications to use of NSAIDs in these inju-ries are similar to those in acute injuries. Athletes with a history of peptic ulcer or previous GI problems with NSAID use should avoid repeated NSAID use. Athletes with suspected or proven stress fractures should also avoid NSAIDs, since NSAIDs can impede bone healing. Many stress fractures have a tendency to heal slowly, and it may thus be advisable to prescribe a non-NSAID analgesic for pain control in these athletes.

CORTICOSTEROIDS

Steroid hormones control many functions including sexual characteristics, glucose metabolism, mineral excretion, and stress reactions. Corticosteroids are normally produced by the adrenal gland and are of particular importance in the response of the body to many forms of physical stress. This response includes glucose metabolism, mobilization of fat stores, and regulation of inflammatory cells. Once corticosteroids had been isolated and produced on a large scale in the laboratory, these effects were studied extensively. Some of the chemical derivatives were especially effective in modifying the inflammatory response, both in inflammatory diseases and in the reaction to trauma. The synthetic corticosteroids are effective drugs to combat pathologic forms of inflammation. Drugs such as prednisone and hydrocortisone are commonly used in rheumatoid arthritis, many forms of vasculitis, and skin disorders such as psoriasis. The use of anti-inflammatory corticosteroids is more controversial following trauma such as athletic injuries. As explained in the section on NSAIDs, inflammation following athletic trauma is not necessarily pathologic. It may be an essential part of the initial healing response. It is clear that corticosteroids can modify this response significantly. One of their primary effects in this situation is the stabilization of the phospholipid cell membrane. This minimizes cell injury and results in decreased swelling, fewer inflammatory cells, and less erythema. Unfortunately, adverse effects have also been noted. A decrease in the fibroblastic response appears to result in a weaker scar formation, with less ultimate strength of the healed tissue. Healthy tissue can be affected by the presence of this stress hormone, leading to weakening of the surrounding tissues. Local atrophy of fatty tissue is also frequently noted. Clinically, this can present as problems in the healing of surgical or traumatic wounds. An increased risk of tendon ruptures has been reported after the use of corticosteroids. Permanent subcutaneous fat atrophy is often seen and can be a problem.

If corticosteroids are used systemically, they can cause adverse reactions elsewhere in the body. Alterations in fat metabolism are thought to contribute to the increased incidence of avascular necrosis of the femoral head, a potentially disastrous complication that can lead to severe hip arthritis. Prolonged systemic steroid use can also lead to chronic suppression of the adrenal gland, with a resulting Addisonian crisis.

Besides systemic use, corticosteroids can be used locally, through topical application or local injection. Both forms of application avoid the systemic side-effects, unless they are prescribed in massive doses. However, local side effects such as a weakening of surrounding tissue and a decrease in healing strength of the tissue may be more pronounced. In addition, repeated local application often causes a permanent local depigmentation of the skin, which may be cosmetically objectionable. Subcutaneous fat atrophy is a particular problem in regions where padding of the underlying bone by fatty tissue is needed, as in the heel pad.

In light of the above mentioned side effects, corticosteroids are rarely if ever indicated in acute athletic injuries during the early post-injury period. Soft tissue healing problems are common if corticosteroids are used in this setting, and inflammation and pain can usually be controlled by more conservative means such as physical modalities and NSAIDs. The only possible exception to this rule is an acute intramuscular hematoma following an acute muscle strain. Good results have been reported if corticosteroids are injected following local aspiration of the hematoma.

The main indication for corticosteroids is in the treatment of chronic injuries. Chronic soft tissue injuries such as tendonitis, bursitis, fasciitis, or synovitis may not respond to initial treatment with relative rest, NSAIDs, and physical therapy. Judicious use of corticosteroids may be of some help to affected athletes. Most of the structures concerned are superficial enough that they can be treated with local application, and there are few if any indications for the use of systemic steroid administration. In addition, the effects of systemically administered steroids are most likely blunted by factors relating to speed of absorption and excretion, and side effects can be disastrous. Local administration can be based on direct topical administration of steroid-containing cream. The absorption can be enhanced by modalities such as ultrasound (phonophoresis) or electrical stimulation (iontophoresis). The dose and depth of penetration that can be achieved in this manner is probably limited. In contrast, injection of the area with corticosteroid can yield very high local levels of the drug. Commonly used steroids and recommended doses are listed in Table 1. Systemic absorption from the site of injection is slow and is unlikely to result in systemic side effects. In order to prevent as many local side effects as possible, several things should be kept in mind. Repeated injections over a short period can result in clinically significant atrophy and complications in both surrounding and healing tissues. Although no scientific studies have investigated this issue, injections should probably be spaced 3 to 4 months apart. Intracutaneous and subcutaneous injection should be avoided if possible in order to decrease the risk of depigmentation, fat atrophy, and thinning of the dermis. If a tendon or ligament is to be treated, direct injection should be avoided to decrease the chance of mechanical weakening of the structure. Instead, the steroids should be infiltrated around the structure. Following injection, the athlete should be cautioned against excessive activity for 2 to 4 weeks. Inevitably, there will be some weakening of the involved structure. If competition is resumed too quickly, inadvertent rupture or further injury may occur.

The efficacy of local steroid injection in the treatment of chronic soft tissue injuries is unclear. It appears that the success rate is better in upper extremity injuries such as lateral epicondylitis (tennis elbow) or supraspinatus and biceps tendonitis of the shoulder than in lower extremity injuries. Injections into the foot for the treatment of plantar fasciitis or Morton's neuroma often lead to an initial flare-up of pain in the post-injection period before improvement is seen. Injection of major tendons in the lower extremity [for instance, the patellar tendon (jumper's knee) and Achilles tendon (Achilles tendonitis)] is often avoided, since in such locations a rupture following "steroid weakening" will likely be disastrous for the athlete. However, it remains to be proven that steroid associated ruptures are truly a result of steroid administration. Many of these forms of "tendonitis" are actually degenerative tendon lesions that can predispose to rupture even if they are left untreated.

ANALGESICS

The most prominent symptom of virtually all athletic injuries is pain. In many injuries pain is the main factor that keeps the athlete out of competition or practice. Generally this is a protective mechanism that prevents re-injury, and no attempt should be made to eliminate it completely. However, treatment with analgesic medication is indicated both to keep the athlete comfortable while he is at rest and to allow early supervised rehabilitative exercises. There are a few exceptions to this rule, including injuries that are medically of little significance but are associated with significant pain. In general, this includes localized bruises and contusions. If significant injuries such as a fracture have been ruled out, athletes can often return to their sport without significant risk of reinjury. Analgesia is usually obtained in such injuries by a local injection of anesthetic.

For most athletic soft tissue injuries, non-narcotic analgesics are adequate (see Table 1). Acetaminophen, aspirin, and NSAIDs are possible choices. Aspirin and NSAIDs carry the potential added advantage of an anti-inflammatory action, as discussed in the previous section. Fractures and dislocations may initially require narcotic analgesics such as codeine, propoxyphene, hydrocodone or oxycodone (see Table 1). During such medication, all exercises and practice should be strictly supervised, because these drugs have marked sedating effects. Constipation due to a combination of narcotics and rest is also a common side effect in athletes who are normally very active and are not used to taking this type of medication.

Athletes who undergo surgery for their athletic injuries often require narcotic medication initially. However, with the advent of arthroscopic surgery, they can often be switched to non-narcotic drugs within 24 to 48 h. Routine NSAIDs following arthroscopic surgery are no more effective than other analgesics. A new parenteral NSAID was marketed recently; this can be an effective analgesic in the immediate postoperative period, when oral intake is hampered by sedation and nausea.

ANTIBIOTICS

The use of antimicrobial agents should only be considered if an athletic injury results in an open wound or during and after surgery for athletic injuries. Among the few exceptions to this rule are a cellulitis or a septic bursitis such as olecranon bursitis. In such injuries, the entrance wound is often not visible. However, it is still likely that infection results from a direct inoculation of bacteria via a small breach in the skin surface.

Lacerations that occur during games or in practice generally do not require antibiotic treatment. A thorough irrigation and debridement of devitalized tissue under local anesthesia is generally sufficient to prevent infection. Most wounds can be sutured following such a procedure. However, deep and dirty wounds can potentially benefit from antibiotic treatment and delayed closure, particularly if the wound cannot be adequately debrided. Open wounds that communicate with fractures or joint cavities are routinely protected by the administration of antibiotic drugs following irrigation and debridement. Since such wound infections are most likely caused by gram-positive organisms, it is important to use a broad spectrum antibiotic with adequate gram-positive coverage. An oral cefalosporin derivative is often used for this purpose. Antibiotics to prevent wound infection are usually given for 3 to 5 days.

SUGGESTED READING

Almekinders LC. The efficacy of non-steroidal anti-inflammatory drugs in the treatment of ligament injuries. Sports Med 1990; 9:137–142.
Almekinders LC. Anti-inflammatory treatment of muscular injuries in sports. Sports Med 1993; 15:139–145.
Cox YS. Current concepts in the role steroids in the treatment of sprains and strains. Med Sci Sports Exercise 1984; 16:216–217.
Leadbetter WB, Buckwalter YA, Gordon S, eds. Sports induced inflammation. Park Ridge, IL: American Academy of Orthopaedic Surgeons, 1990.
Nelson WE, Henderson RC, Almekinders LC, et al. An evaluation of pre- and postoperative non-steroidal anti-inflammatory drugs in patients undergoing arthroscopy. Am J Sports Med 1993; 21: 510–516.
Woo SLY, Buckwalter JA, eds. Injury and repair of musculoskeletal soft tissues. Park Ridge, IL: American Academy of Orthopaedic Surgeons, 1988.

HUMAN IMMUNODEFICIENCY VIRUS IN SPORTS

KENNETH J. ROGERS, A.T.C., M.S.

The transmission of the human immunodeficiency virus (HIV) has been addressed with professional, student, and recreational athletes through various sources. This chapter focuses on the education that the athlete must receive both on and off the playing field. The current research on the pathophysiology of blood-borne pathogens is readily available in the literature and is not addressed here.

Most athletes participating in organized sports are covered by policies and procedures that safeguard against HIV transmission. Numerous sports organizations, including the National Collegiate Athletic Association (NCAA), United States Olympic Committee, National Federation of State High School Association, National Basketball Association, Major League Baseball, National Football League, and National Hockey League have adopted specific protocols to both educate athletes and help prevent the transmission of blood pathogens. Every individual associated with these organizations should be familiar with the policies regarding HIV. If your organization does not have a policy, make the effort to have a policy implemented.

The recreational athlete in the unorganized setting does not have any guidelines for handling blood during athletic competition. This area of the athletic population needs to be addressed in the future.

TRANSMISSION OF HIV IN ATHLETIC EVENTS

The risk of transmission of HIV during a game is thought to be extremely low (Table 1). The literature has shown only one reported case of possible transmission of HIV from athlete to athlete. This occurred when two soccer players collided and sustained scalp lacerations. After careful review from other researchers, the players' personal histories placed this theory of transmission in doubt. The rate of HIV transmission through cutaneous exposure is less than 0.04%, with no reported exposures occurring in athletics. The American Academy of Pediatrics, Canadian Academy of Sports Medicine, and the World Health Organization (WHO) have reported no cases of HIV infected athletes. The Centers for Disease Control (CDC) has reported no documented cases of HIV transmission during an athletic event as of June 1993.

A recent study by Brown and Drotman addressed the risk of HIV transmission during athletic competition. American professional football was studied to estimate the risk of HIV transmission during game conditions. An average of 3.75 blood injuries occurred during a game and 12% of the blood injuries were lacerations. It was assumed that lacerations exposed the athlete to possible blood contact with other athletes. The team physician was involved in 7.83 medical procedures that involved dressing wounds and injections. The rate of HIV infection among health care workers from exposure to an HIV infected person was 3 per 1000, comparable to the literature. Also comparable to the literature was the rate of 1 per 200 for HIV infection among the players. One interesting point is that blood injuries occurred significantly more often on artificial surfaces than on grass. The authors concluded that the risk of on-field HIV transmission is remote. The estimated risk found in this study of HIV transmission from one player to another was below one per one million games.

One area of concern is the sharing of needles among athletes who use steroids. Three cases have been reported in the literature. The three individuals did not engage in any other high-risk practice that might have led to HIV transmission. All athletes must be educated that the sharing of needles carries an inherent risk of transmission of HIV, as well as other blood-borne pathogens such as hepatitis B.

Even though the likelihood of HIV transmission is low, all athletes must be treated as being potentially HIV positive. An athlete may be HIV positive but not diagnosed or show any signs. The health care worker must take the necessary precautions with all athletes, in all settings, whenever the injury allows exposure to blood or body fluids.

EXERCISE AND HIV INFECTION

Exercise can be recommended as a healthy and safe activity for the HIV-infected athlete. As stated by Calabrese, psychological benefits may include reduced stress levels, decreased depression and anxiety, and increased self-esteem and body image, which all lead to a enhanced quality of life. The immunologic effects may include decreased corticosteroid levels and progression of HIV, plus enhanced immune response, which may increase the life span. The level of intensity of the exercise for different symptoms of HIV must be closely monitored, as this may improve or decrease the immune function levels. Emelyanov stated that many athletes tested at an anti-doping center had a decreased immune response resulting from physical overload.

POLICIES, PROCEDURES, AND THE EXPOSURE CONTROL PLAN

All institutions and organizations must have in place policies and procedures concerning HIV. NCAA institutions were surveyed by McGrew to measure their policies and universal precautions of HIV/AIDS. HIV testing was performed on a routine basis at 22 of the schools, with 2 schools performing mandatory testing and 20 schools having voluntary testing. Thirty three of the schools had a policy of restricting the participation of HIV-infected athletes. Athletes who were HIV-positive or AIDS diagnosed were reported at 12 schools. Six schools would not let a HIV-infected athlete participate in any sport. Three of eight institutions had HIV-diagnosed athletes participating in competition. At the time of the study, the NCAA had no data on HIV-infected athletes for any sports group. The college age group (18 to 24 years) shows a 0.08% prevalence of HIV infection. If the 0.08% is applied to the number of athletes participating in 1991 to 1992 (270,000), it can be estimated that 216 NCAA athletes are HIV infected. This survey made the valid point, also brought out in other studies, that the student athlete has a greater risk of contracting HIV through sexual contact than through sports. Student athletes use contraception less, have an increased number of sexual partners, and have a greater prevalence of sexually transmitted diseases than the non-student athlete population. The need for education is paramount among this population, because they perceive themselves as being immune to disease and think that contracting a "disease" will not happen to them.

The education of the athlete must include information on the prevention of HIV by explaining the modes of transmission of HIV, unsafe sexual practices and

---

Table 1 Risk Categories for Sports

Greatest risk: Boxing, Taekwondo, Wrestling, Rugby*
Moderate risk: Basketball, Field Hockey, Football,* Ice Hockey, Judo, Soccer, Team Handball
Lowest risk: Archery, Athletics, Badminton, Baseball, Bowling, Canoe/Kayak, Cycling, Diving, Equestrian, Fencing, Figure Skating, Gymnastics, Modern Pentathlon, Racquetball, Rhythmic Gymnastics, Roller Skating, Rowing, Shooting, Softball, Speed-skating, Skiing, Swimming, Synchronized Swimming, Table Tennis, Volleyball, Water Polo, Weight-lifting, Yachting

Data from U.S. Olympic Committee, 1991.
*Added by author.

intravenous drug use, especially steroid use and other high-risk behaviors. These issues must be handled in a nonthreatening, open, direct, and explicit manner with the athlete.

Many of the responding institutions did not have a HIV/blood-borne pathogen policy for infected student athletes. The survey noted that the athletic trainers and other health care providers demonstrated significant deficits in following the universal guidelines implemented by the Occupational Safety and Health Administration (OSHA). A large percentage of schools neither required student athletes to attend an educational session nor posted literature on the prevention of HIV transmission. The author notes that following the universal precautions in the health care setting would protect both the athlete and the health care provider.

The preceding study highlights an important component of preventing HIV transmission. The school, clinic, or other organization must institute and update annually policies for education on the prevention of transmission of HIV for all health care workers at the organization and affiliated agencies who may come into contact with an athlete. The education should include a discussion of universal precautions, transmission of HIV, and prevention of HIV infection. The supplies and equipment that pertain to universal precautions must be readily available and used properly when the need presents itself. This equipment, gloves, gowns and masks, must be provided at no cost to the employee and repaired and replaced when the need arises.

The exposure determination of each worker in that setting must be described in the exposure control plan. In the athletic setting, those at greatest risk for exposure to HIV are the physicians, athletic trainers, and other health care providers who have the possibility of direct blood contact on a frequent basis. Coaches and athletes would have infrequent contact with blood, while administrators would have no contact. This policy needs to be implemented to lay the groundwork of testing, counseling, education programs, handling of blood, and status of HIV among the athletes and health care workers.

An important fact of the federal OSHA guidelines is that they are intended to protect employees. The guidelines are not intended to protect athletes who are not employees. The federal OSHA guidelines for blood-borne pathogens are to be followed by all government and private employees in the states aligned with the federal OSHA. Not all states are federal OSHA states, but may have a separate state OSHA office that covers their state, municipal, and county employees. These workers are not required to follow the federal OSHA guidelines. This can promote confusion in the work setting where overlap may occur. It is your responsibility to determine what type of OSHA regulations, federal or state, apply in your work setting.

HIV TESTING

Student athletes from 11 Division I to III schools were asked in a Michigan State survey about their attitudes towards AIDS, alcohol, and drugs. The survey found that 64.4% of athletes in certain contact sports (football and men's and women's basketball) would ban HIV-positive athletes from competition. Only 54.7% of noncontact sport athletes would ban HIV-positive athletes. The author of the study noted that the results of the survey should not be generalized to all college student athletes. It is not known whether the athletes who would ban a HIV-positive athlete were involved in any educational programs regarding HIV in the athletic setting.

Garl mentions two important points when the question of testing for HIV/AIDS is approached. The first concern is to time the test to get a true positive result. If mandatory testing is done on a group of athletes, an infected athlete may not yet have seroconverted and would have a false negative result. Another point about testing that Garl makes is an athlete might be tested and that night or the following day participate in unsafe/risky behavior and become infected.

The second and more important point that Garl presents regards the American Disabilities Act of 1991. This act states that an HIV-infected person or a person with AIDS cannot be discriminated against and is considered disabled. Thus an athlete who is HIV positive cannot be prohibited from school activities. The mandatory HIV testing of athletes may not be allowed for legal reasons related to the act. Mandatory testing should not be an alternative; rather, education must be the top priority to prevent the transmission of HIV. The American Academy of Pediatrics, NCAA, CDC, and WHO do not recommend mandatory testing of athletes for HIV. Voluntary testing should be provided for those athletes who request it.

PARTICIPATION AND CONFIDENTIALITY

The athlete should not be denied participation in athletic competition because of HIV infection. The CDC recommends that the HIV-infected athlete's case be reviewed by the player, doctor, trainer, and coach. An athlete's participation in competition should be based only on a complete medical examination regarding the student-athlete's total health and fitness. If an athlete is able to fully participate in competition, without health compromises, he or she must be offered the opportunity to do so. The sport must be reviewed to ensure the safety of the athlete and other participants.

The athlete's confidentiality must be respected at all times. No harassment or discrimination must come about by any "accidental" announcement of an athletes serostatus. The athlete's primary health care provider must not allow information about the athlete's health to be released to the coaches, teammates, health care providers, administration, or public without written consent from the athlete. Many states have confidentiality laws to protect the rights of the HIV-infected person. It is the responsibility of the health care providers to know the federal, state, and local law as it applies to HIV and confidentiality.

GUIDELINES FOR PREVENTION OF HIV TRANSMISSION

HIV transmission can be prevented by following the universal precautions prepared by OSHA. These guidelines should be practiced by any individual coming into contact with blood or other body fluids.

1. Latex gloves, face masks/goggles, and nonabsorbent gowns must be available when there is exposure to blood, bloody fluids, mucous membranes, or broken skin (e.g., abrasions, dermatitis, puncture), also for handling items or surfaces soiled with blood or body fluids, or for performing venipuncture or other invasive procedures on the athlete.
2. Hands and all skin surfaces that come into contact with blood or other body fluids should be washed immediately with soap and/or antigermicidal agent.
3. Contaminated surfaces must be cleaned immediately with an EPA approved disinfectant or with a solution of one part bleach to 10 parts water (1:10). Linens or towels that become contaminated need to be isolated and then washed with hot water and detergent separate from the uncontaminated laundry. Gloves need to be worn during the bagging and cleaning of the contaminated linens or towels.
4. Needle stick injuries can be prevented by not bending, recapping, removing, or manipulating the needle after use. Needles should be placed in an appropriate puncture-resistant container after use and disposed of properly.
5. Emergency resuscitation must not be refused even if you suspect that an athlete is HIV positive. The risk of HIV transmission through saliva is very low. Oral airways or breathing bags can be used to minimize mouth-to-mouth contact.
6. The dressing of open wounds, abrasions, dermatitis, or other open skin conditions is mandatory and should be checked on a regular basis. The bleeding must be controlled.
7. Water bottles and towels that could be possibly contaminated are not to be shared among the athletes.
8. High contact sport athletes must be educated of the potential hazards of blood for the other athletes' protection. They must be taught to remove themselves from the game and receive proper medical attention.
9. The dressing should be checked periodically to determine if the bleeding is under control. The uniform should be replaced only when the blood saturates the underlying layer of skin. The health care professional should make this decision in consultation with a referee.
10. HIV testing should not be used as a screening tool to determine if an athlete may participate in sports.
11. If an employee is exposed to blood, confidential medical evaluation and counseling must be made available. The employee is not responsible for the cost of the laboratory tests and medical evaluation.

INFORMATION SOURCES

CDC National AIDS Hotline
English service 1-800-342-AIDS
Spanish service 1-800-344-7432
Deaf Service (TDD) 1-800-243-7889
CDC National AIDS Clearinghouse
1-800-458-5231, 9 AM – 7 PM Eastern time
National Collegiate Athletic Association
(913) 339-1906
National Federation of State High School Associations
1-800-366-6667
United States Olympic Committee
(719) 632-5551

SUGGESTED READING

American Academy of Orthopaedic Surgeons. Advisory statement. HIV-Infected Orthopaedic Surgeons.

American Academy of Pediatrics. Human immunodeficiency virus rome (AIDS) Virus in the athletic setting. Pediatrics 1991; 88:640-641.

Brown LS, Drotman P. What is the risk of HIV infection in athletic competition. International Conference on AIDS 1993. 1993; 9:PO-C21-3102.

Calabrese LH, LaPerriere A. Human immunodeficiency virus infection, exercise and athletics. Sports Med 1993; 15:6-13.

Centers for Disease Control and Prevention. HIV/AIDS and sports: A pathfinder to information. Atlanta, CDC, June 1993.

Emelyanov BA, Pokrovsky VV, Semenov VA, Socolov IA. Epidemiological danger of AIDS in sport. International Conference on AIDS 1992. 1992; 8:c378-Poc-4811.

Federal Register: Occupational exposure to bloodborne pathogens; final rule. Part II (Excerpts); Department of Labor, 29 CFR Part 1910.1030, p 64175.

Garl T. AIDS in athletics. Athletic Management 1993; May:18-22.

Garl T, Hrisomalos T, Rink L. Transmission of infectious agents during athletic competition. USOC Sports Medicine and Science Committee, 1991.

Gayle HD, Kelling RP, Garcia-Gunon M, et al. Prevalence of the human immunodeficiency virus among university students. N Engl J Med 1990; 323:1538-1541.

Goldsmith MF. When sports and HIV share the bill, smart money goes on common sense. JAMA 1992; 267:1311-1314.

Guidelines for prevention of transmission of human immunodeficiency virus and hepatitis B virus to health care workers and public safety workers. Morbid Mortal Weekly Report. 1989; 38(S-6):1-18.

Johnson RJ. HIV infection in athletes. Postgrad Med 1992; 92(7): 73-80.

McGrew CA, Dick RW, Schiedwind K, Gikas P. Survey of NCAA institutions concerning HIV/AIDS policies and universal precautions. Med Sci Sports Exerc 1993; 25: 917-921.

NCAA Policy No. 20: AIDS and intercollegiate athletics. Revised June 1991.

Nemechek PM. Anabolic steroid users-another potential risk group for HIV infection (letter). N Engl J Med 1991; 325:357.

Scott MJ, Scott MJ Jr. HIV infection associated with injections of anabolic steroids (letter). JAMA 1989; 262: 207.

Sklarek HM, Mantovani RP, Erens E, et al. AIDS in bodybuilder using anabolic steroids (letter). N Engl J Med 1984; 311:1701.

Torre D, Sampietro C, Ferraro G, et al. Transmission of HIV-1 infection via sports injury (letter) Lancet 1990; 335: 1105.

Woltiski RJ, Keeling RP. AIDS on the college campus: Athletics and HIV infection. A special report of the American College Health Association. 2nd ed. American Health Association, 1989: 113.

World Health Organization Consensus Statement. Consultation on AIDS and sports. JAMA 1992; 267: 1312.

SUDDEN CARDIAC DEATH IN THE ATHLETE

JOSEPH S. TORG, M.D.

The medical and lay communities have become increasingly aware of the instances of sudden cardiac death in athletes in the prime of their careers. On October 24, 1971, Chuck Hughes, wide receiver for the Detroit Lions, collapsed on the field after running a pass pattern. The cause of death was listed as premature atherosclerotic coronary artery disease. He had a history of type II hyperlipoproteinemia. In 1978, a professional tennis player died at the age of 28 of hypertrophic cardiomyopathy. During life, she had experienced episodes of chest pain and was thought to have "athletic heart syndrome." After her death, several family members were also found to have the disease but were asymptomatic. In 1980, a university star athlete, Tim Claxton, died after a pick-up basketball game. The cause of death was sarcoid heart disease. Len Bias, a top round draft pick of a pro basketball team in 1985, sustained a cardiac arrest secondary to cocaine abuse and died. Flo Hyman, an olympic volleyball player, died in 1986 of an aortic rupture secondary to Marfan's syndrome. A 7'2" center with Marfan's syndrome was recruited by Temple University. Although doctors prohibited him from playing college basketball, he died in his dormitory room in 1987, also from a ruptured aorta. Pete Maravich, a former NBA star, died suddenly in 1988 at the age of 40 following a pick-up game. He was found to have a congenitally absent left coronary artery. In 1986, a college basketball hopeful was restricted from intercollegiate athletics because of a history of heart disease. He left the country to play semi-pro ball in England and died on the court several years later. On March 4, 1990, NBA prospect Hank Gaithers died of an arrhythmia during a basketball game. More recently, Reggie Lewis, captain of the Boston Celtics, died while casually shooting baskets in the Brandeis University Gym 3 months after collapsing in the NBA playoffs.

Despite this long list of fallen athletes, sudden cardiac death in a competitive athlete is a rare event. Whenever such an event occurs, questions are raised as to whether the death was preventable and who is responsible. Unfortunately, in most instances, sudden cardiac death is not preventable because it is the first indication of underlying heart disease. In the case of athletes with known abnormalities, the question of responsibility is a clouded one. Not enough is known about the effects of exercise on different disorders to draw valid conclusions. The decision to compete becomes the responsibility of everyone involved with the athlete—the athlete himself, team physician, coach, and family.

This chapter identifies the causes of sudden cardiac death in athletes and what, if any, prodromal symptoms may exist. In addition, the work-up necessary to evaluate such symptoms and which abnormalities should preclude the athlete from competing will be discussed. The question of who makes the decision to return to sports will be raised. Finally, what, if any, preparticipation screening studies that may detect at-risk individuals will be presented.

CAUSES OF SUDDEN DEATH

The leading cause of sudden cardiac death among athletes is largely dependent on age. In those athletes aged 35 years or older, the number one cause is coronary artery disease (CAD), which in most cases was previously asymptomatic.

In younger athletes hypertrophic cardiomyopathy is the most common cause of sudden cardiac death. In the largest series on sudden cardiac death in young athletes, Maron et al reported that 14 of 29 athletes died from hypertrophic cardiomyopathy.

Hypertrophic cardiomyopathy is a disease characterized by an abnormal, nondilated hypertrophy of the left ventricle with the septum being asymmetrically hypertrophied. Histologically, one sees disorganization of the myocardial cells in both the septum and the left ventricular free wall. Typically, no evidence of disease predisposing to hypertrophy exist, e.g., systemic hypertension or aortic stenosis. The disease is thought to be genetically transmitted as an incompletely penetrant autosomal trait and can be detected in multiple family members. The diagnosis can be made by echocardiography and 90% to 95% of patients have abnormal electrocardiographic (ECG) findings.

Idiopathic concentric hypertrophy is another, less common, cause of sudden death. Unlike hypertrophic cardiomyopathy, this does not demonstrate the asymmetric hypertrophy of the septum nor the histologic findings; also it is not familial. Possibly, it represents a variant of hypertrophic cardiomyopathy.

Cystic medial necrosis of the ascending aorta with

eventual rupture can also lead to unexpected death. It is characterized by a decrease in the number of elastic fibers of the aortic media. Some patients with Marfan's syndrome are also known to have this abnormality. In Maron's study, 2 of 29 players, including one with Marfan's died from aortic rupture.

Congenital abnormalities of the coronary vasculature have also been implicated as a cause of sudden death. Presumably, because of the abnormality of the vessels, certain regions of the heart may be underperfused, leading to infarct or arrhythmia and death. Some of the abnormalities that have been reported include anomalous origin of the left coronary artery from the right sinus of Valsalva and vice versa, single coronary artery, hypoplasia of the coronary vessels, and anomalous origin of the coronary vessels from the pulmonary trunk. Some of these abnormalities may be detected by echocardiography.

Coronary atherosclerosis is another obvious cause of sudden death. Although it is most commonly seen in the older athlete, it has been reported in younger individuals, especially those with a family history of premature atherosclerosis or hypercholesterolemia. Typically, in these patients, sudden death is the first manifestation of CAD. Cardiac catheterization is the definitive test for this entity.

Disturbances of the normal conduction system have also been identified at autopsy in several individuals. Arrhythmias secondary to these abnormalities are the presumed cause of sudden death. Wiedermann in 1987 reported on sudden death in an athlete with Wolff-Parkinson-White syndrome.

Arrhythmias are also believed to be the etiologic factor in sudden death where no other evidence of cardiovascular disease is present. Detection of arrhythmias is difficult prior to death. Intracardiac electrophysiologic studies are usually needed.

Sudden death associated with more typical forms of congenital heart disease, e.g., aortic stenosis, ventricular septal defect, is not common in athletes, probably because such individuals are identified and treated early in life. Other diseases such as myocarditis, sarcoid or mitral valve prolapse are also rare causes of unexpected death in the young athlete.

One other "environmental" cause of death in athletes in all age groups is drugs, particularly cocaine. There have been many reports of acute myocardial infarction, arrhythmias and death secondary to drug abuse in the general population as well as in several highly competitive athletes. This possibility should not be overlooked in cases of unexplained death and, in fact, may be the most common cause in these instances.

PRODROMAL SYMPTOMS

Unfortunately sudden death is often the first manifestation of underlying cardiac disease. In Maron's study, 8 of the 29 athletes had antemortem symptoms—syncope, 3; presyncope, 1; chest pain, 2; fatigue, 1; and fatigue, palpitations, and presyncope, 1. Some of these complaints are relatively nonspecific, and only two of the eight athletes in this study were thought to have cardiac disease prior to death. In neither of these, however, was the correct diagnosis made prior to death. It is imperative to maintain a high index of suspicion when evaluating such symptoms and rule out potentially dangerous etiologies. A family history of sudden death or CAD is particularly important.

EVALUATION OF PREMONITORY SYMPTOMS

An athlete who presents with symptoms suggestive of cardiovascular disease should have a thorough investigation. This is most important if the athlete has experienced a true syncopal episode. Obviously the services of a cardiologist are required.

A careful history is the first step. Type and duration of symptoms as well as inciting factors all have prognostic significance. A family history of sudden death, premature atherosclerosis, or lipid disorders is also important. A history of drug abuse should be carefully sought.

Physical examination will concentrate on cardiac findings and some syndromes often have classic presentations. Clinical manifestations of Marfan's syndrome should be evaluated. Lab tests may reveal occult hypercholesterolemia.

Routine chest roentgenogram and ECG will help to detect some cases of hypertrophic cardiomyopathy, aortic dilation and arrhythmias. Echocardiography, to include 2-D and M-mode, is the most sensitive in detecting structural cardiac abnormalities and should be a routine part of the evaluation. Exercise stress testing and 24 hour ECG monitoring during competition are important to bring out abnormalities precipitated by activity. In rare instances, cardiac catheterization and electrophysiologic studies should be performed.

IMPLICATIONS FOR RETURN TO COMPETITION

Once a specific diagnosis has been established, a decision should be made about the individual's return to sports. In 1984, the Sixteenth Bethesda Conference was held by the American College of Cardiology and the National Institutes of Health. Its specific focus was to discuss the athlete with cardiovascular disease and to establish participation guidelines based on what definitive data are available and experience with the general population of cardiac patients. The authors emphasize that it has never been conclusively proven that exercise increases the likelihood of sudden death in an at-risk patient. These guidelines are essentially empiric recommendations; the ultimate decision to resume sports is the athlete's, after careful discussion with his or her physician about the possible risks including death.

Several task forces were established to deal with various subgroups of cardiac disease. These subgroups included hypertrophic cardiomyopathies and myopericardial disease, congenital heart disease, acquired valvular disease, hypertension, ischemic heart disease, and arrhythmias. Several conditions were considered to be absolute contraindications to competitive athletics. Many disorders, however, can be treated and the athlete allowed to resume sports after careful observation and evaluation of the treatment protocol. The reader is referred to the publications of this conference for implications regarding specific diagnoses.

PREPARTICIPATION SCREENING

The incidence of congenital heart disease in the population is estimated to be 0.5%. Of this group, approximately 1% are at risk for sudden death and only 1 in 10 in this group will actually die of congenital heart disease. Thus, to identify one individual in whom a sudden death will occur, 200,000 people would have to be screened.

The effectiveness of a preseason screening program is thus directly related to the financial resources of the particular team or athletic organization. Typically most preseason evaluations consist of a history and physical by the team physician who is often an orthopedist. Very few of the potentially fatal cardiac abnormalities will be picked up by such a screening process, although some classic cases of hypertrophic cardiomyopathy and Marfan's syndrome will be detected. Even if a routine chest x-ray, which is relatively inexpensive, is added, only a rare patient with hypertrophic cardiomyopathy or aortic dilatation will be found. Although ECG findings are often nonspecific, they do indicate which athletes may warrant further work-up. ECGs are abnormal in 90% of patients with hypertrophic cardiomyopathy and are probably positive in greater than 90% of those who will die suddenly.

Echocardiography is probably the most sensitive noninvasive test for detecting occult abnormalities. Unfortunately its cost prohibits its use as a routine screening procedure.

In 1987, Maron et al published a report on a large series of intercollegiate athletes who were screened preseason for cardiovascular disease. Initial screening in the 501 athletes consisted of history and physical by a cardiologist as well as 12 lead ECG. Ninety athletes had positive findings and were further evaluated. Of these, 84% had no definite evidence of cardiovascular disease, 15% had previously unsuspected mitral valve prolapse, and one athlete had systemic hypertension. The report concluded that a preparticipation screening program as described above was not an efficient means of detecting significant cardiovascular disease.

SUGGESTED READING

Cheitlin M, Bonow R, Parmley W, et al. Task force II: Acquired valvular heart disease. J Am Coll Cardiol 1985; 6:1209-1214.

Cheitlin M, DeCastro C, McAllister H. Sudden death as a complication of anomalous left coronary origin from the anterior sinus of valsalva. Circulation 1974; 50:780-787.

Coelho A, Palileo E, Ashley W, et al. Tachyarrhythmias in young athletes. J Am Coll Cardiol 1986; 7:237-243.

Cregler LL. Adverse health consequences of cocaine abuse. J Natl Med Assoc 1988; 81:27-38.

Epstein S, Blomquist C, Buja L, et al. Task force V: Ischemic heart disease. J Am Coll Cardiol 1985; 6:1222-1224.

Epstein S, Maron B. Sudden death and the competitive athlete: Perspectives on preparticipation screening studies. J Am Coll Cardiol 1986; 7:220-230.

Frohlich E, Lowenthal D, Miller H, et al. Task force IV: Systemic arterial hypertension. J Am Coll Cardiol 1985; 6:1218-1221.

Isner J, Estes N, Thompson P, et al. Acute cardiac events temporally related to cocaine abuse. N Engl J Med 1986; 315:1438-1443.

Maron B, Bodison S, Wesley Y, et al. Results of screening a large group of intercollegiate competitive athletes for cardiovascular disease. J Am Coll Cardiol 1987; 10:1214-1221.

Maron B, Epstein S, Roberts W: Causes of sudden death in competitive athletes. J Am Coll Cardiol 1986; 7:204-214.

Maron B, Gaffney A, Jeresaty R, et al. Task force III: Hypertrophic cardiomyopathy, other myopericardial diseases and mitral valve prolapse. J Am Coll Cardiol 1985; 6:1215-1217.

Maron B, Roberts W, McAllister H, et al. Sudden death in young athletes. Circulation 1980; 62:218-229.

McManus B, Waller B, Graboys T. Exercise and sudden death, Part I. Curr Probl Cardiol 1981; 6:17-78.

McNamara D, Bricker T, Galioto F, et al. Task force I: Congenital heart disease. J Am Coll Cardiol 1985; 6:1200-1208.

Menke D, Waller B, Pless J. Hypoplastic coronary arteries and high takeoff position of the right coronary ostium. A fatal combination of congenital coronary artery anomalies in an amateur athlete. Chest 1985; 88:299-301.

Mitchell J, Maron B, Epstein S. Sixteenth Bethesda Conference: Cardiovascular abnormalities in the athlete: Recommendations regarding eligibility for competition.

Roberts W, Maron B. Sudden death while playing professional football. Am Heart J 1981; 102:1061-1063.

Roberts W, Siegel R, Zipes D. Origin of the right coronary artery from the left sinus of valsalva and its functional consequences: Analysis of ten necropsy patients. Am J Cardiol 1982; 49:863-868.

Thiene G, Pennell N, Rossi L. Cardiac conduction system abnormalities as a possible cause of sudden death in young athletes. Hum Pathol 1983; 14:706-709.

Warren S, Boice J, Bloor C, Vieweg W. The athletic heart revisited: Sudden death of a twenty-eight year old athlete. West J Med 1979; 131:441-447.

Wiederman C, Becker A, Hopferwieser T, et al. Sudden death in a young competitive athlete with Wolff-Parkinson-White syndrome. Eur Heart J 1987; 8:651-655.

Zipes D, Cobb L, Garson A, et al. Task force VI: Arrhythmias. J Am Coll Cardiol 1985; 6:1225-1232.

HEAD AND FACIAL INJURIES

EMERGENCY MANAGEMENT OF HEAD AND CERVICAL SPINE INJURIES

JOSEPH S. TORG, M.D.

Although all athletic injuries require careful attention, the evaluation and management of injuries to the head and neck should proceed with particular consideration. The actual or potential involvement of the nervous system creates a high-risk situation in which the margin for error is low. An accurate diagnosis is imperative, but the clinical picture is not always representative of the seriousness of the injury. An intracranial hemorrhage may initially present with minimal symptoms, yet follow a precipitous downhill course, whereas a less severe injury, such as neurapraxia of the brachial plexus that is associated with alarming paresthesias and paralysis may resolve swiftly and allow for quick return to activity. Although the more severe injuries are rather infrequent, this low incidence results in little, if any, management experience for the on-site medical staff.

Several principles should be considered by individuals responsible for athletes who may sustain injuries to the head and neck:

1. The team physician or trainer should be designated as the person responsible for supervising on-the-field management of the potentially serious injury. This person is the "captain" of the medical team.
2. Prior planning must ensure the availability of all necessary emergency equipment at the site of potential injury. At a minimum, this should include a spineboard, stretcher, and equipment necessary for the initiation and maintenance of cardiopulmonary resuscitation (CPR).
3. Prior planning must ensure the availability of a properly equipped ambulance, as well as a hospital equipped and staffed to handle emergency neurologic problems.
4. Prior planning must ensure immediate availability of a telephone for communicating with the hospital emergency room, ambulance, and other responsible individuals in case of an emergency.

Managing the unconscious or spine-injured athlete should not be done hastily or haphazardly. Being prepared to handle this situation is the best way to prevent actions that could convert a repairable injury into a catastrophe. Be sure that all the necessary equipment is readily accessible, in good operating condition, and that all assisting personnel have been trained to use it properly. On-the-job training in an emergency situation is inefficient at the least. Everyone should know what must be done beforehand, so that on a signal the game plan can be put into effect.

A means of transporting the athlete must be immediately available in a high-risk sport such as

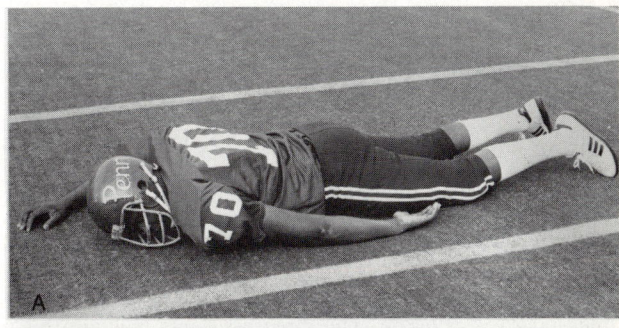

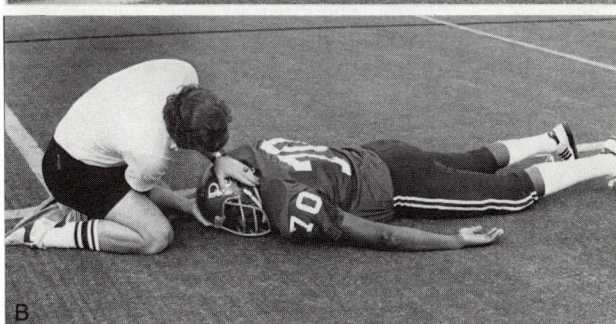

Figure 1 *A*, Athlete with suspected cervical injury may or may not be unconscious. However, all who are unconscious should be managed as though they have significant neck injury. *B*, Immediate manual immobilization of the head and neck unit. First check for breathing. (From Torg JS, ed. Athletic injuries to the head, neck and face. St. Louis: Mosby–Year Book, 1991; with permission.)

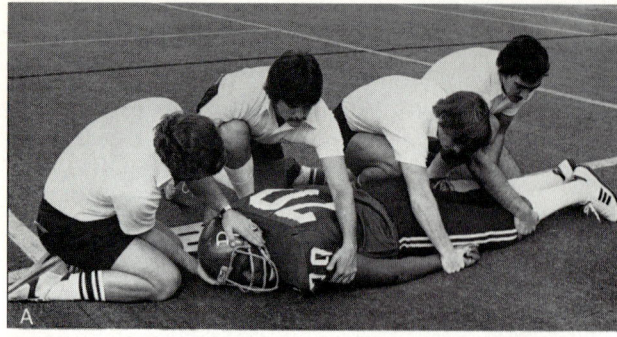

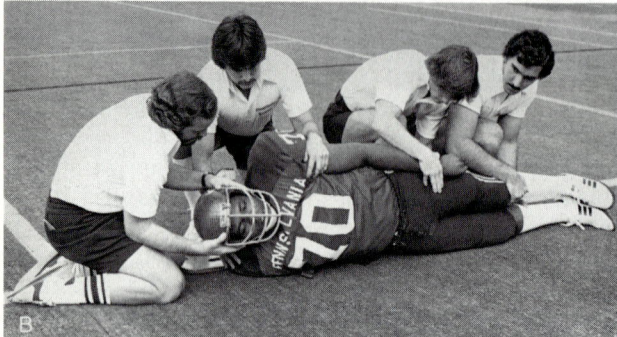

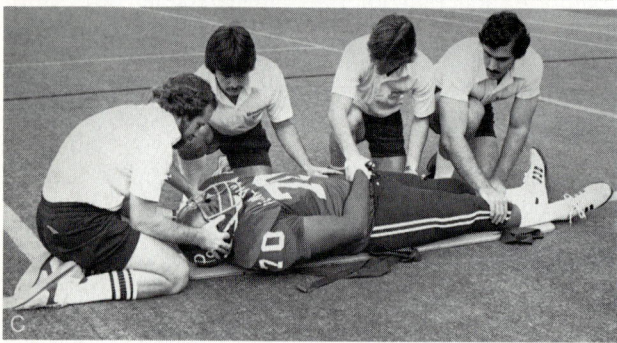

Figure 2 *A,* Logroll to a spine board. This maneuver requires four individuals; the leader to immobilize the head and neck and command the medical-support team, and the remaining three individuals positioned at the shoulders, hips, and lower legs. *B,* Logroll. The leader uses the crossed-arm technique to immobilize the head. This technique allows the leader's arms to "unwind" as the three assistants roll the athlete onto the spine board. *C,* Logroll. The three assistants maintain body alignment during the roll. (From Torg JS, ed. Athletic injuries to the head, neck and face. St. Louis: Mosby–Year Book, 1991; with permission.)

football and "on-call" in other sports. The medical facility must be alerted to the athlete's condition and estimated time of arrival so that adequate preparation can be made.

Having the proper equipment is essential! A spine-board is necessary and is the best means of supporting the body in a rigid position. It is essentially a full body splint. By splinting the body, the risk of aggravating a spinal cord injury, which must always be suspected in the unconscious athlete, is reduced. In football, bolt cutters and a sharp knife or scalpel are also essential if it becomes necessary to remove the face mask. A telephone must be available to call for assistance and to notify the medical facility. Oxygen should be available and is usually carried by ambulance and rescue squads, although it is rarely required in an athletic setting. Rigid cervical collars and other external immobilization devices can be helpful if properly used.

ON-SITE MANAGEMENT

Properly trained personnel must know, first of all, who is in charge. All personnel should know how to perform CPR and how to move and transport the athlete. They should know where emergency equipment is located, how to use it, and the procedure for activating the emergency support system. Individuals should be assigned specific tasks beforehand, if possible, so that duplication of effort is eliminated. Being well prepared helps to alleviate indecisiveness and second-guessing.

Prevention of further injury is the single most important objective. Do not take any action that could possibly cause further injury. The first step should be to immobilize the head and neck by supporting them in a stable position (Fig. 1). Then, in the following order, check for breathing, pulse, and level of consciousness.

If the victim is breathing, simply remove the mouth guard, if present, and maintain the airway. It is necessary to remove the face mask only if the respiratory situation is threatened or unstable, or if the athlete remains unconscious for a prolonged period. Leave the chin strap on.

Once it is established that the athlete is breathing and has a pulse, evaluate the neurologic status. The level of consciousness, response to pain, pupillary response, and unusual posturing, flaccidity, rigidity, or weakness should be noted.

At this point, simply maintain the situation until transportation is available, or until the athlete regains consciousness. If the athlete is face down when the ambulance arrives, change his position to face up by logrolling him onto a spineboard (Fig. 2). Gentle longitudinal traction should be exerted to support the head without attempting to correct alignment. Make no attempt to move him except to transport him or to perform CPR if it becomes necessary.

If the athlete is not breathing or stops breathing, the airway must be established. If he is face down, he must be brought to a face-up position. The safest and easiest way to accomplish this is to logroll the athlete into a face-up position. In an ideal situation the medical-support team is made up of five members: the leader, who controls the head and gives the commands only; three members to roll; and another to help lift and carry when it becomes necessary. If time permits and the spineboard is on the scene, the athlete should be rolled directly onto it. However, breathing and circulation are much more important at this point.

With all medical-support team members in position, the athlete is rolled toward the assistants—one each at the shoulders, hips, knees. They must maintain the body in line with the head and spine during the roll. The leader maintains immobilization of the head by applying

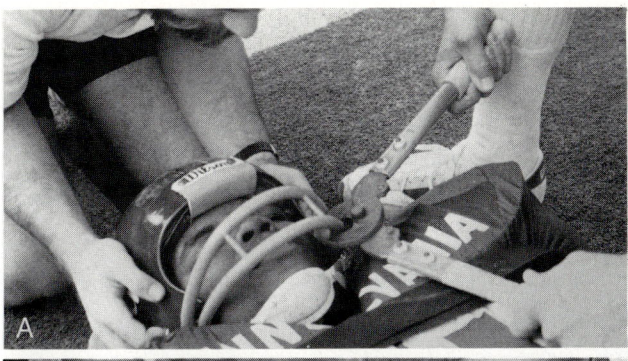

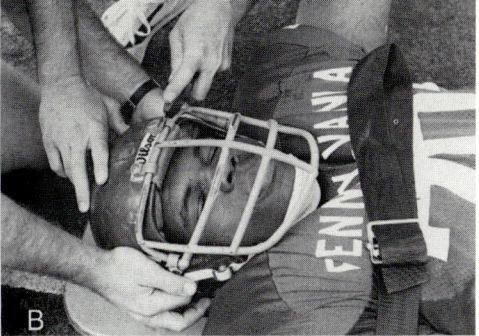

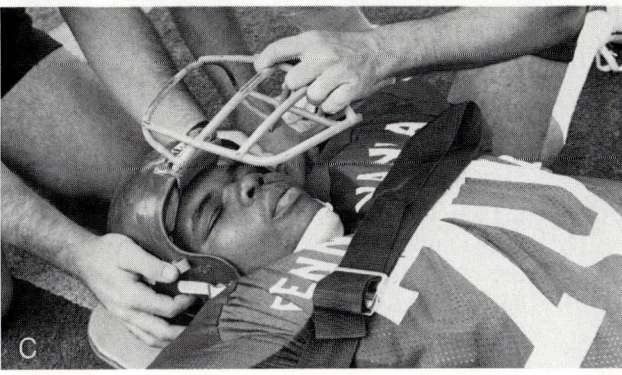

Figure 3 *A,* Remove double and single masks with bolt cutters. Head and helmet must be securely immobilized. *B,* Remove "cage"-type masks by cutting the plastic loops with a utility knife. Make the cut on the side of the loop away from the face. *C,* Remove the entire mask from the helmet so that it does not interfere with further resuscitation efforts. (From Torg JS, ed. Athletic injuries to the head, neck and face. St. Louis: Mosby–Year Book, 1991; with permission.)

slight traction and by using the crossed-arm technique. This technique allows the arms to unwind during the roll (Fig. 2).

The face mask must be removed from the helmet before rescue breathing can be initiated. The type of mask that is attached to the helmet determines the method of removal. Bolt cutters are used with the older single- and double-bar masks. The newer masks that are attached with plastic loops should be removed by cutting the loops with a sharp knife or scalpel. Remove the entire mask so that it does not interfere with further rescue efforts (Fig. 3).

Once the mask has been removed, initiate rescue breathing following the current standards of the American Heart Association.

Once the athlete has been moved to a face-up position, quickly evaluate breathing and pulse. If there is still no breathing or if breathing has stopped, the airway must be established. The jawthrust technique is the safest first approach to opening the airway of a victim who has a suspected neck injury, because in most cases it can be accomplished by the rescuer grasping the angles of the victim's lower jaw and lifting with both hands, one on each side, displacing the mandible forward while tilting the head backward. The rescuer's elbows should rest on the surface on which the victim is lying.

If the jaw thrust is not adequate, the head tilt-jaw lift should be substituted. Care must be exercised not to overextend the neck. The fingers of one hand are placed under the lower jaw on the bony part near the chin and lifted to bring the chin forward, supporting the jaw and helping to tilt the head back. The fingers must not compress the soft tissue under the chin, which might

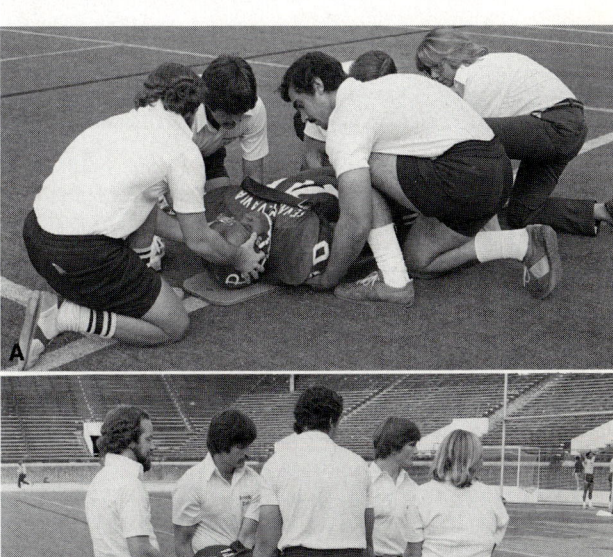

Figure 4 *A,* Four members of the medical support team lift the athlete on the command of the leader. *B,* The leader maintains manual immobilization of the head. The spine board is not recommended as a stretcher. An additional stretcher should be used for transporting the patient over long distances. (From Torg JS, ed. Athletic injuries to the head, neck and face. St. Louis: Mosby–Year Book, 1991; with permission.)

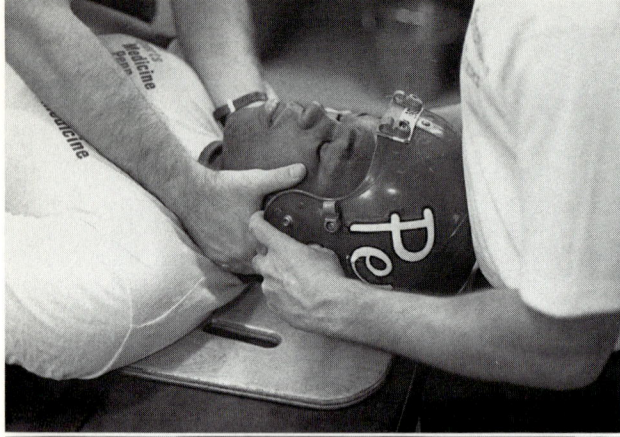

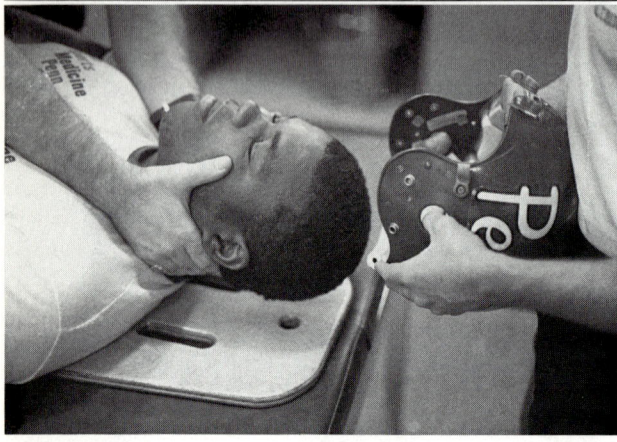

Figure 5 *A,* The helmet should be removed only when permanent immobilization can be instituted. The helmet may be removed by detaching the chin strap, spreading the earflaps, and gentle pulling the helmet off in a straight line with the cervical spine. *B,* The head must be supported under the occiput during and after removal of the helmet. (From Torg JS, ed. Athletic injuries to the head, neck and face. St. Louis: Mosby–Year Book, 1991; with permission.)

obstruct the airway. The other hand presses on the victim's forehead to tilt the head back.

The transportation team should be familiar with handling a victim with a cervical spine injury and they should be receptive to taking orders from the team physician or trainer. It is extremely important not to lose control of the care of the athlete; therefore, be familiar with the transportation crew that is used. In an athletic situation, prior arrangements with an ambulance service should be made.

Lifting and carrying the athlete requires five individuals; four to lift, and the leader to maintain immobilization of the head. The leader initiates all actions with clear, loud verbal commands (Fig. 4).

MANAGEMENT IN THE MEDICAL FACILITY

The same guidelines apply to the choice of a medical facility as to the choice of an ambulance: Be sure it is equipped and staffed to handle an emergency head or neck injury. There should be a neurosurgeon and an orthopedic surgeon to meet the athlete upon arrival. Roentgenographic facilities should be standing by.

Once the athlete is in a medical facility and permanent immobilization measures are instituted, the helmet is removed. The chin strap may now be unfastened and discarded. The athlete's head is supported at the occiput by one person while the leader spreads the earflaps and pulls the helmet off in a straight line with the spine (Fig. 5).

Despite the advent of such high-tech imaging modalities as computed tomography (CT) and magnetic resonance imaging (MRI), the initial radiographic examination of a patient with suspected or actual cervical spine trauma remains a routine, roentgenographic examination.

The preliminary study, while immobilization of the head, neck, and trunk are maintained, includes an anteroposterior and lateral examination of C1-C7. If a major fracture, subluxation, dislocation, or evidence of instability are not evident, the remainder of routine examination including open mouth and oblique views should be obtained. Depending on the neurologic and comfort status of the patient, lateral flexion and extension views should at some point be obtained. CT and MRI may provide more detailed information, however, horizontally oriented fractures and subtle subluxations are best identified on the routine radiographs. The choice of imaging technique will depend on the results of routine examination, neurologic status of the patient, preference of the responsible physician, and availability of the imaging modalities.

CLOSED HEAD INJURIES

THOMAS A. GENNARELLI, M.D.
JOSEPH S. TORG, M.D.

The athlete who receives a blow to the head, or a sudden jolt to the body that results in a sudden acceleration-deceleration force to the head, should be carefully evaluated. If the individual is ambulatory and conscious, the entire spectrum of intracranial damage, ranging from concussion to a more severe intracranial condition, must be considered. Initial on-field examination should include an evaluation of: (1) facial expression; (2) orientation to time, place, and person; (3) presence of post-traumatic amnesia; (4) presence of retrograde amnesia; and (5) abnormal gait.

Traumatic injuries to the brain can be classified as diffuse or focal.

The immediate and definitive management of athletically induced trauma to the brain depends on the nature and severity of the injury. Those responsible for managing such injuries must understand the problems from the standpoint of basic pathomechanics.

DIFFUSE BRAIN INJURIES

Diffuse brain injuries are associated with widespread or global disruption of neurologic function and are not usually associated with macroscopically visible brain lesions. Diffuse brain injuries result from shaking of the brain within the skull, and thus are lesions caused by the inertial or acceleration effects of a mechanical input to the head. Both theoretic and experimental evidence points to rotational acceleration as the primary injury mechanism for diffuse brain injuries.

Since diffuse brain injuries, for the most part, are not associated with visible macroscopic lesions, they have historically been lumped together to include all injuries not associated with focal lesions. More recently, however, diagnostic information has been gained from computed tomography (CT) and magnetic resonance imaging (MRI), as well as from neurophysiologic studies, that make it possible to define more clearly several categories within this broad group of diffuse brain injuries.

Three categories of diffuse brain injury are recognized:

1. *Mild Concussion*—Several specific concussion syndromes involve temporary disturbances of neurologic function without loss of consciousness.
2. *Classic Cerebral Concussion*—This is a temporary, reversible neurologic deficiency caused by trauma that results in temporary loss of consciousness.
3. *Diffuse Axonal Injury* (DAI)—This takes the form of prolonged traumatic brain coma with loss of consciousness lasting more than 6 hours. Residual neurologic, psychological, or personality deficits often result because of structural disruption of numerous axons in the white matter of the cerebral hemispheres and brain stem.

Mild Cerebral Concussion

The syndromes of mild cerebral concussion are included in the continuum of diffuse brain injuries; they represent the mildest form of injury in this spectrum. Mild concussion syndromes are those in which consciousness is preserved but with some degree of noticeable temporary neurologic dysfunction. These injuries are exceedingly common and, because of their mild degree, often are not brought to medical attention; however, they are the most common brain injuries encountered in sports medicine.

A grade I mild concussion, the mildest form of head injury, results in confusion and disorientation unaccompanied by amnesia. This temporary confusion, without loss of consciousness, lasts only momentarily after the injury. This concussion syndrome is completely reversible and there are no associated sequelae. An individual with a grade I mild concussion is confused, has a dazed look, and may exhibit mild unsteadiness of gait. However, post-traumatic and retrograde amnesia are not prominent features. This clinical picture is best described by the athletes themselves who say, "I had my bell rung." Usually the state of confusion is short lived and the athlete is completely lucid in 5 to 15 minutes. When the athlete's mind is clear, he may return to the activity under the watchful supervision of the team physician or trainer. However, associated symptoms such as vertigo, headaches, photophobia, and labile emotions should preclude returning to the game.

A grade II mild concussion is characterized by confusion associated with retrograde amnesia that develops after 5 to 10 minutes. Again, this is an extremely frequent event. Athletes may experience a "ding", and although confused, continue coordinated sensorimotor activities after the injury. If examined immediately, these players have total recall of the events immediately before impact. However, retrograde amnesia develops 5 to 10 minutes later, and thereafter they do not remember the impact or events immediately before impact. The amnesia usually covers only several minutes before the injury; it may diminish somewhat, but players always have some degree of permanent, though short, retrograde amnesia despite resumption of completely normal consciousness. The confusion and disorientation completely resolve.

Individuals manifesting amnesia should not be permitted to return to play that day. These athletes require careful postinjury evaluation. They may develop the "postconcussion syndrome," characterized by persistent headaches, inability to concentrate, and irritability. In some instances, these symptoms may last for several weeks after the injury, and participation in the sport is precluded as long as symptoms are present.

As the mechanical stresses to the brain increase in the grade III mild concussion, confusion and amnesia are present from the time of impact. Athletes can usually continue to play while having no recollection of previous events. By this stage, some degree of post-traumatic amnesia (forgetting events after the injury) also occurs in addition to retrograde amnesia (forgetting events before the injury). The patient's confusion may last many minutes, but then the level of consciousness returns to normal, usually with some permanent degree of retrograde and post-traumatic amnesia.

These three syndromes of mild cerebral concussion have been frequently witnessed and described in detail. Although consciousness is preserved, it is clear that some degree of cerebral dysfunction has occurred. The fact that memory mechanisms appear to be the most sensitive to trauma suggests that the cerebral hemispheres, rather than the brain stem, are the location of the mild injury forces. The degree of cerebral cortical dysfunction, however, is not sufficient to disconnect the influence of the cerebral hemispheres from the brain stem activating system, and therefore consciousness is preserved. No other cortical functions except memory seem in jeopardy, and the only residual deficits that patients with mild concussion syndromes have is the brief retrograde or post-traumatic amnesia. However, since definite alteration of brain function has occurred, athletes who sustain grades II and III mild cerebral concussions should not be permitted to participate in the remainder of the contest.

Classic Cerebral Concussion

Classic cerebral concussion is seen in the "knocked-out" player. This individual is in a paralytic coma, usually recovering after a few seconds or minutes, and then passing through stages of stupor, confusion with or without delirium, and finally an almost lucid state with automatism before becoming fully alert. This individual will most certainly have retrograde and post-traumatic amnesia. If the loss of consciousness lasts for more than several minutes or if there are other signs of a deteriorating neurologic state, the patient should be immediately transported to a hospital.

Initial evaluation of the athlete who has been rendered unconscious should involve determining whether he is breathing, whether there is a pulse, and the level of consciousness. If unobstructed respirations and an adequate pulse are present, there is no immediate need to do anything except keep in mind that head and neck injuries are frequently associated. Therefore, the player should be protected from injudicious manipulation or movement.

Such patients frequently remain semistuporous for more than several minutes. They should be removed from the field on a spine board or stretcher rather than be permitted to stagger off. An athlete who has been rendered unconscious for any length of time should not be allowed to return to contact activity that day, even if mentally clear. Overnight observation in a hospital should be considered for those who experience more than a transient loss of consciousness.

Insufficient attention has been given to the precise stages of recovery form classic cerebral concussion. Although, by definition, loss of consciousness is transient and reversible, the sequelae of concussion are commonplace. Some sequelae such as headache or tinnitus may reflect injuries to the head, the inner ear, or other noncerebral structures. However, subtle changes in personality and in psychologic or memory functioning have been documented and must have a cerebrocortical origin. Thus, although most patients with classic cerebral concussion experience no sequelae other than amnesia for the events of impact, some individuals may have other long lasting, although subtle, neurologic deficiencies that must be investigated further.

FOCAL BRAIN SYNDROMES

In discussing the occurrence of intracranial hematoma resulting from athletic injury, two major points must be emphasized. First, owing to recent developments in the clinical evaluation of patients and correlated animal research, there is a satisfactory understanding of the mechanism of occurrence of focal intracranial hematoma, which is somewhat different from older concepts of patients with head injuries. Second, management of such patients has advanced rapidly and changed dramatically over the last decade from what was accepted medical practice in the past.

The entire spectrum of traumatic intracranial hematomas occurs in sports injuries. These include cerebral contusions, intracerebral hematomas, epidural hematomas, and acute subdural hematomas. The presentation of athletes with head injuries who have had serious trauma is similar in most instances. Management depends on definitive diagnosis, and varies according to the underlying pathologic process.

Intracerebral Hematoma and Contusion

These injuries occur in patients with a significant intracerebral pathologic condition who have not suffered loss of consciousness or focal neurologic deficit, but who do have persistent headache or periods of confusion after head injury and post-traumatic amnesia. As with any patients who have suffered head injuries, athletes with such symptoms should undergo a CT scan to permit early differentiation between solid intracerebral hematoma and hemorrhagic contusion with surrounding edema.

Epidural Hematoma

Epidural hematoma results when the middle meningeal artery, which is imbedded in a bony groove in the skull, tears as a result of a skull fracture, crossing this groove. Because the bleeding in this instance is arterial, accumulation of clot continues under high pressure and, as a result, serious brain injury can occur.

The classic description of an epidural hematoma is

that of loss of consciousness at the time of injury, followed by recovery of consciousness in a variable period, after which the patient is lucid. This is followed by the onset of increasingly severe headache, decreased level of consciousness, dilation of one pupil, usually on the same side as the clot, and decerebrate posturing and weakness, usually on the side opposite the hematoma. In our experience, however, only one-third of the patients with epidural hematoma present with this classic history. Another one-third of patients do not become unconscious until late in their course, and the remaining one-third are unconscious from the time of injury and remain unconscious throughout their course.

The absence of a classic clinical picture of epidural hematoma cannot be relied on to rule out this diagnosis, and the best diagnostic test for evaluating these patients is a CT scan.

Acute Subdural Hematoma

Athletic head injuries result from inertial loading, which is lower than that of serious head injuries caused by vehicular accidents or falling from heights. Also, acute subdural hematomas occur much more frequently than epidural hematomas in athletes. In patients with head injuries in general, approximately three times as many acute subdural hematomas occur as do epidural hematomas.

Two main types of acute subdural hematomas have been clearly identified: (1) those with a collection of blood in the subdural space, apparently not associated with underlying cerebral contusion or edema; and (2) those with collections of blood in the subdural space, but associated with an obvious contusion on the surface of the brain and hemispheric brain injury with swelling. The mortality rate for simple subdural hematomas is approximately 20%, but this increases to more than 50% for subdural hematomas with an underlying brain injury.

Patients with an acute subdural hematoma typically are unconscious, may or may not have a history of deterioration, and frequently display focal neurologic findings. Patients with simple subdural hematomas are more likely to have a lucid interval following their injury and are less likely to be unconscious at admission than patients with hemispheric injury and brain swelling. It is necessary to obtain a CT or MRI scan to diagnose an acute subdural hematoma. The size of the subdural clot relative to the size of the midline shift of the brain structures can be evaluated best by CT scan. Of patients with acute subdural hematoma, 84% also have an associated hemorrhagic contusion or intracerebral hematoma with associated brain swelling.

The term *acute subdural hematoma* raises the image of a large collection of clotted blood in the intracranial cavity, compressing the brain substance and causing compromise due to the space occupied by the hematoma. This is not an infrequent consequence of closed head trauma, but this type of subdural hematoma is more common in adults who have a degree of cortical atrophy.

Young athletes, and especially children, frequently develop only minimal subdural hematomas with under-lying cerebral hemispheric swelling. This type of brain injury is not the result of a space-occupying mass from clotted blood causing brain compression, but rather swollen brain tissue causing consequent rises in intracranial pressure. The advent of CT and MRI permit accurate differential diagnosis between these two conditions, which frequently cause similar clinical pictures. The modalities of treatment for these two distinct types of acute subdural hematomas are quite different.

Brain Swelling

Brain swelling is a poorly understood phenomenon that can accompany any type of head injury. Swelling is not synonymous with cerebral edema, which refers to a specific increase in brain water. Such an increase in water content may not occur in brain swelling, and current evidence favors the concept that brain swelling is due in part to increased intravascular blood within the brain. This is caused by a vascular reaction to head injury that leads to vasodilation and increased cerebral blood volume. If this increased cerebral blood volume continues long enough, vascular permeability may increase and true edema may result.

Although brain swelling may occur in any type of head injury, the magnitude of the swelling does not correlate well with the severity of the injury. Thus, both severe and minor head injuries may be complicated by brain swelling. The effects of brain swelling are thus additive to those of primary brain injury, and may in certain instances be more severe than the primary injury itself.

Despite the lack of knowledge of the precise mechanism that causes brain swelling, it can be conceptualized in two general forms. It should be remembered that many different types of brain swelling exist and that acute and delayed brain swelling represent phenomenologic, rather than mechanistic entities.

Acute brain swelling occurs in several circumstances. Swelling that accompanies focal brain lesions tends to be localized, whereas diffuse brain injuries are associated with generalized swelling. Focal swelling is usually present beneath contusions but does not often contribute additional deleterious effects. On the other hand, the swelling that occurs with acute subdural hematomas, although principally hemispheric in distribution, may cause more mass effect than the hematoma itself. In such circumstances, the small amount of blood in the subdural space may not be the entire reason for the patient's neurologic state. If the hematoma is removed, the acute brain swelling may progress so rapidly that the brain protrudes through the craniotomy opening. Every neurosurgeon is all too familiar with external herniation of the brain, which, when it occurs, is difficult to treat.

The more serious types of diffuse brain injuries are associated with generalized, rather than focal, acute brain swelling. Although not all patients with DAI have brain swelling, the incidence of swelling is higher than in patients with either classic cerebral concussion or one of the mild concussion syndromes. Because of the serious nature of the underlying injury, it is difficult to determine the extent of swelling in these patients. The swelling, although widespread throughout the brain, may not cause a rise in intracranial pressure (ICP) for several days. This late rise in pressure probably reflects the formation of true cerebral edema, and it may be that diffuse swelling associated with severe diffuse brain injuries is harmful because it produces edema. In any event, this type of swelling is different from the type of swelling associated with acute subdural hematomas.

Delayed brain swelling may occur minutes to hours after head injury. It is usually diffuse and is often associated with the milder forms of diffuse brain injuries. Whether delayed swelling is the same as or a phenomenon different from the acute swelling of the more serious diffuse injuries is unknown. However, in less severe diffuse injuries there is a distinct time interval before delayed swelling becomes manifest, thus confirming that the primary insult to the brain was not serious. Considering the high frequency of the mild concussion, the incidence of delayed swelling must be low. However, when it occurs, delayed swelling can cause profound neurologic changes or even death.

In its most severe form, severe delayed swelling can cause deep coma. The usual history is that of an injury associated with a mild concussion or a classic cerebral concussion from which the patient recovers. Minutes to hours later the patient becomes lethargic, then stuporous, and finally lapses into a coma. The coma may be either a light coma with appropriate motor responses to painful stimuli, or a deep coma associated with decorticate or decerebrate posturing.

The key differences between these patients and those with DAI is that in the latter the coma and abnormal motor signs are present from the moment of injury, whereas with delayed cerebral swelling there is a time interval without these signs. This distinction is significant, however, since with DAI a certain amount of primary structural damage has occurred at the moment of impact, but this is not present in cases of pure delayed swelling. Therefore, the deleterious effects of delayed swelling should be potentially reversible, and if these effects are controlled the outcome should be good. However, such control may be difficult. Vigorous monitoring of and attention to ICP is necessary, and prompt and vigorous treatment of raised ICP is required in order to control brain swelling. If this is successfully accomplished, the mortality rate from increased ICP associated with diffuse brain swelling should be low.

MANAGEMENT OF FOCAL BRAIN SYNDROMES

As knowledge of physiology and pathophysiology has increased, so has the ability to resuscitate seriously ill or severely injured people successfully. The 1950s saw the start of successful treatment of acute respiratory and postoperative problems, followed by satisfactory cardiac resuscitation and emergency cardiac care in the 1960s. Innovations in critical care medicine were extended in the form of brain resuscitation in the 1970s. Such care is based on the concept that the degree of permanent neurologic, intellectual, and psychological deficit after brain trauma with coma is only partly the result of the initial injury, and is certainly in part due to secondary changes, which can be worsened or improved by the quality of the supportive care received. Head injuries, by their very nature, require resuscitation, i.e., therapy initiated after the insult. The proper care of patients with head injuries, athletic or otherwise, depends on the full appreciation and use of brain resuscitation measures in an intensive care setting.

Present management of focal intracranial hematoma resulting from athletic injury includes not only treatment for, and removal of, hematoma, but also recognition of, and treatment for, the underlying brain injury, which is resuscitation of the brain. This is therapy designed to have specific neuro-saving potential once general resuscitation methods and supportive care have begun. Our concerns in management of the athletic-injured patient are the same as those for any patient who has received severe head injuries.

First Aid and Emergency Care

First aid should consist of getting the patient safely into a supine position and determining vital signs and the significance of any associated injuries. Initial treatment should be to establish an adequate and useful airway and begin oxygenation maneuvers. This can be accomplished by using a manual resuscitation bag with supplemental oxygen, if available. The patient should then be transferred as quickly as possible to medical facility where diagnosis and treatment of brain injury can begin. Although these measures are important for all patients who have suffered concussion, they are vital for patients who remain comatose after trauma. Also, consideration must be given for a concomitant cervical spine injury and appropriate measures taken. Once patients arrive in the emergency room and it is determined that their cardiorespiratory status is stable, endotracheal intubation is immediately performed on comatose patients. A CT or MRI is obtained as soon as possible to provide an immediate diagnosis of the intracranial condition. Patients are then categorized as either surgical or nonsurgical cases, depending on the size of the intracranial hematoma.

Initial evaluation of all head trauma patients includes determination of their coma state by numerical ranking on the Glasgow Coma Scale (Table 1). This coma scale is based on the patient's response to stimulation by eye opening, best motor response, and best verbal response. Scores of 15 to 3, from normal neurologic status to deeply comatose, are possible.

Intracranial Pressure Monitoring and Control

Patients with a Glasgow Coma Scale of 7 or lower should have immediate ICP monitoring as part of their treatment. Intracranial hypertension, defined as a pressure of more than 15 mm Hg, is seen in 50% or more of patients with severe head injuries. The correlation between alterations in ICP and the patient's neurologic

Table 1 Glasgow Coma Scale

Eyes	Open	Spontaneously	4
		To verbal command	3
		To pain	2
		No response	1
Best motor response	To verbal command	Obeys	6
	To painful stimulus*	Localizes pain	5
		Flexion-withdrawal	4
		Flexion-abnormal (decorticate rigidity)	3
		Extension (decerebrate rigidity)	2
		No response	1
Best verbal response†		Oriented and converses	5
		Disoriented and converses	4
		Inappropriate words	3
		Incomprehensible sounds	2
		No response	1
Total			3-15

The Glasgow Coma Scale, based upon eye opening, verbal, and motor responses, is a practical means of monitoring changes in level of consciousness. If response on the scale is given a number, the responsiveness of the patient can be expressed by summation of the figures. Lowest score is 3; highest is 15.
*Apply knuckles to sternum; observe arms.
†Arouse patient with painful stimulus if necessary.

status has been well described in the past. Therapy for intracranial hypertension can be given correctly only when the pressure is known. We are firmly convinced of the usefulness of continuous ICP monitoring in the intensive care of the patient with severe head injuries. Because intermittent waves of increased pressures, which commonly occur without other signs or symptoms, can be diagnosed and treated before significant neurologic deterioration occurs, ICP monitoring facilitates titration of therapy.

When muscle paralysis or barbiturates are used to control elevated ICP, it is impossible to follow the patient's neurologic state and ICP is a more useful parameter to be followed. It would be inappropriate to use muscle paralysis or barbiturates without continuously recording ICP. Ideally, the ICP should be monitored from the earliest possible time after the patient's arrival in the hospital. In our unit it is usually possible to obtain a CT scan within 1 hour of admission in all severe head injuries. The ICP monitor is usually inserted after the CT scan and within 2 hours of admission.

However, if any delay in diagnosis is foreseen, or if the patient is rapidly deteriorating, an ICP monitor is inserted immediately after emergency resuscitation. This early insertion is especially important in patients with signs of shock from other injuries who require rapid fluid replacement. In these cases, we begin to monitor pressure in the emergency room with a portable recording system.

We monitor ICP in comatose patients with head injuries whether they are operated on initially for decompression or not. We rarely intervene surgically to remove contused brain, believing that if ICP can be controlled, the removal of potentially functional brain tissue is unacceptable because it may limit the patient's recovery. After surgical intervention in patients with hematoma, we routinely monitor ICP for possible further therapy. The following principles of management of patients with head injuries apply to those who do not have indications for surgical intervention and to postoperative patients. This management is guided by the monitored variables, and its goals are to prevent three major complications that cause more deaths if the patient is alive on arrival at the hospital: (1) intracranial hypertension, (2) inadequate cerebral oxygenation, and (3) systemic medical complications. These must be attacked vigorously for optimum results. Treatment for intracranial hypertension is also designed to maximize cerebral oxygenation, and the modalities are those previously listed.

Of all therapies for high ICP, hyperventilation is the first that we use, and it is extremely effective. A rapid and persistent fall of the ICP is anticipated in most circumstances and occurs without changes in the mean arterial blood pressure (MAP). This is important because it is the cerebral perfusion pressure (MAP-ICP) that is the true driving force for cerebral oxygenation and perfusion and it is really the cerebral perfusion pressure that must be kept normal (i.e., > 70-80 mm Hg). Hyperventilation must be carefully monitored, however, because too much hyperventilation can worsen or even cause cerebral ischemia. The best way to monitor hyperventilation is to place a jugular venous catheter and keep jugular venous saturation within normal limits. This will assure that adequate cerebral oxygenation is present during hyperventilation treatment and allows safer and more individualized treatment than if an arbitrary pCO_2 level is targeted.

Hyperosmotic agents decrease ICP by removing brain water resulting from an induced osmotic gradient from the brain to the intravascular component. Although slightly less rapid in its action, 20% to 25% mannitol has largely replaced 30% urea in the United States because of less rebound after administration. Two forms of hyperosmotic therapy are available; intermittent bolus use and continuous infusion therapy. High-dose bolus therapy, 1 to 2 g/kg of mannitol, is reserved for initial emergency control of ICP, usually in patients who have rapid decrease in level of consciousness, dilating pupils, or decerebration. Maintenance therapy can then be carried out with smaller boluses of 0.15 to 0.3 g/kg of mannitol every 1 to 2 hours, or whenever the ICP exceeds 15 mm Hg. Close attention must be given to the serum osmolality so that it does not rise above 320 mOsm/L. Significant cardiopulmonary and renal complications are frequent and often irreversible with serum osmolality above levels. Clincians utilizing this therapy should have a thorough understanding of the hyperosmolar state.

A late step for ICP control is the use of barbiturates. When initially used to protect the brain by lowering metabolism, it became apparent that reductions of ICP occurred regularly. Although the mechanism of barbiturate action on elevated ICP is not known, its successful use when other forms of therapy have failed to lower ICP is encouraging. The doses of barbiturates required have varied. Pentobarbital has been the most widely used agent, usually with loading doses of 10 to 30 mg/kg. Thereafter, infusions of 0.5 to 3 mg/kg/hr are maintained. Because of the wide variation of serum levels obtained by similar doses in different patients we no longer rely solely on serum levels as criteria. We prefer to titrate the dose until a burst-suppression pattern is present on the electroencephalogram monitor. Therapy is then closely regulated to keep the burst-suppressions of equal length. At this physiologic end-point, the serum pentobarbital level may vary from 2.5 to 5.0 mg/dl. Care must be taken to prevent barbiturate cardiac toxicity and subsequent hypotension. This has not been a problem except in older patients, and the cerebral perfusion pressure can be adequately maintained without the use of pressor agents.

For the duration of barbiturate therapy, monitoring must be intensive because neurologic signs are abolished. Spontaneous respiratory activity is not present and all other neurologic signs are generally absent. Although we have continued barbiturate therapy for as long as 21 days, the usual course is less than 5 days. By this time the ICP rarely rises when an attempt is made to discontinue the barbiturate infusion. Once a patient's ICP is less than 15 mm Hg for longer than 48 hours, we discontinue therapy in a sequential manner, stopping barbiturates first, then decreasing hyperosmolar therapy, and, finally, ceasing hyperventilation.

Treatment of Subdural Hematoma

The treatment of a patient with acute subdural hematoma remains controversial. Some neurosurgeons believe that most patients with acute subdural hematomas are not helped by an operation, and that the major problems are the control of brain swelling and elevated ICP. Others believe that evacuation of the hematoma, no matter how small, improves intracranial compliance and the neurologic state.

In those patients whose CT scans show a large, localized subdural clot with an equal or larger shift of the midline structures, we surgically evacuate the hematoma. In patients with a "smear subdural hematoma", a few millimeters thick over the entire lateral aspect of one hemisphere, with the midline shift greater than the thickness of the subdural hematoma, we probably would not operate but would aggressively control ICP. Disagreements arise when a state between these two is seen. The argument against surgical intervention is that the major cerebral problem is brain injury, which cannot be helped by an operation. If there is a disruption of the blood-brain barrier with vasogenic edema, craniotomy decreases tissue pressure, increases hydrostatic pressure gradients between capillaries and tissue, and may therefore cause a marked increase in edema in the decompressed hemisphere. Thus, even if the clot is removed, the increased edema may cause swelling of the hemisphere, which rapidly returns the intracranial volume-pressure relationship to where they were before the operation.

If an operation is performed, we recommend a large temporofrontoparietal craniotomy flap with evacuation of the clot and control of the hemorrhage from bridging veins and cortical laceration. The patient with a sizable subdural hematoma should have an operation for evacuation of the clot followed by management of ICP. A patient with a subdural hematoma along the outside of the hemisphere is best managed by aggressive treatment of brain swelling and therapy for increased ICP.

The mortality rates for the surgical treatment of acute subdural hematoma reported in the last 10 years vary from 42% to 63%. One important variable seems to be the level of consciousness of the patient at the time of the operation. We do not believe that an operation is necessary in all patients with acute subdural hematoma, but we do believe it is vital that all patients, including those who have had surgical intervention, have postoperative ICP monitoring and control. Of patients who died after surgical intervention, 25% died from uncontrollable elevated ICP. Thus, postoperative ICP monitoring plays a major role in the care of patients with acute subdural hematomas. We believe strongly that this will improve mortality rates but also quality of life.

RECOMMENDATIONS

We have come to recognize that in all patients with serious head injuries, including athletic head injuries, pathologic damage is usually diffusely distributed throughout the cerebral hemispheres and brain stem. Ideally, therapy should prevent secondary damage rather than modify any secondary injury once it occurs. With this approach it should be possible to limit patient disability to the results of the primary biomechanical injury alone. Theoretically, no patient who is conscious after injury should die or suffer major disability.

Comatose patients require immediate and intensive therapy after injury. The triage must include transport to a medical facility where rapid diagnosis and intensive care are available and routine.

Early effective diagnosis of surgically correctable lesions by CT scanning has reduced mortality from epidural and surgically treatable subdural hematomas. With no mass lesion, aggressive management can be started without undue concern that a mass lesion has been missed, and negative exploratory surgery can be avoided. The use of ICP monitoring and monitoring of the systemic arterial pressure and blood gases, serum osmolality, and electrolytes allow any trend away from normal to be detected and corrected at the earliest possible time. The use of barbiturates is another way to control intracranial hypertension when other more common modes of treatment have failed.

Any athlete who has suffered loss of consciousness from head injury for more than 1 minute, or who has persistent headache with confusion or any disorientation that persists longer than 1 hour after trauma, or an athlete who has more than one episode of unconsciousness, however momentary, during any one playing season should be referred for neurologic examination and CT evaluation. With the proper diagnosis and management of patients with head injuries, we are convinced that the present distressingly high mortality and morbidity from severe head injury can be lowered without a decrease in the quality of life.

CONCUSSION

JAMES P. KELLY, M.A., M.D.

Concussion is a common experience in athletic and recreational activities, especially in contact sports. Surveys have found that 10% of college football players and 20% of high school football players experience concussions in a given football season. That translates to more than 250,000 concussions per year in football alone. While football serves as a good model of the incidence and characteristics of concussion, other sports are also vulnerable to this problem including martial arts, ice hockey, gymnastics, rugby, soccer, cycling, horseback riding, swimming, and other recreational and competitive activities. Boxing serves as a model of traumatic brain injury in that the objective of this "sport", at least at the professional level, is to produce concussion in one's opponent.

The most important step in the management of concussion in athletes is its recognition. Some typical features that might be observed in the athlete who has suffered concussion are listed in Table 1. Concussion should be defined as an alteration in mental status induced by mechanical forces affecting the brain. These forces may be applied directly to the head, or they may be induced by sudden acceleration-deceleration changes without a direct blow to the head. The hallmarks of concussion are confusion and amnesia. Even though most athletes will recover spontaneously and completely from concussion, there are serious considerations in the identification and management of this type of mild traumatic brain injury (TBI).

First, concussion itself can be associated with the development of intracranial pathology that requires neurosurgical intervention. Intracranial bleeding can occur even with relatively mild TBI, the most common pathology being subdural hematoma. Epidural hematomas, intracerebral hematomas, and cerebral contusions can also occur. These should be viewed as potential

Table 1 Frequently Observed Features of Concussion

Vacant stare (befuddled facial expression)
Delayed verbal and motor responses (slow to answer questions or follow instructions)
Inability to focus attention (easily distracted and unable to follow through with normal activities)
Disorientation (walking in the wrong direction, unaware of time, date, place)
Slurred or incoherent speech (making disjoint or incomprehensible statements)
Gross observable incoordination (stumbling, inability to walk tandem/straight line)
Emotionality out of proportion to circumstances (appearing distraught, crying for no apparent reason)
Memory deficits (exhibited by repeatedly asking the same question that has already been answered or inability to memorize and return 3/3 words and 3/3 objects for 5 minutes)
Any period of loss of consciousness (paralytic coma, unresponsiveness to arousal)

neurosurgical emergencies, and must be detected early in order to minimize morbidity and even the risk of mortality.

Secondly, repeated concussions that are spaced near in time to each other can lead to catastrophic neurologic injury. This has been reported in the literature as the "second impact syndrome," which is the development of brain swelling after a second concussion while an individual is still symptomatic from an earlier concussion. This form of brain swelling is due to cerebrovascular congestion and dilation of the blood vessels of the brain due to diminished vasomotor control. This loss of autonomic regulation of blood vessel diameter causes increased blood volume within the cerebrovascular system leading to increased intracranial pressure (ICP). Diminished cerebral perfusion pressure can result, along with herniation syndromes. This phenomenon is reported primarily in children and young adults. Death or severe disability from the consequences of massively elevated ICP are the rare but devastating sequelae of repeated concussions in these cases.

And third, even repeated concussions spaced distant in time from each other can impart cumulative neurological damage reflected in documented neuropsychological decline in mental performance, atrophy on repeated neuroimaging studies, and the development of dementia (global intellectual decline) with Parkinsonian features first noted in boxers and termed *dementia pugilistica*.

There is a common misconception that an individual must be rendered unconscious to have suffered a concussion. In fact, the Congress of Neurological Surgeons stated in 1964 that concussion is an alteration in mental status produced by mechanical forces, with no mention of loss of consciousness in the criteria for diagnosis. Thoughtful articles appeared in the literature around the same time identifying confusion and amnesia as the most consistent clinical features of concussion. Loss of consciousness is a clear sign that TBI has occurred with sufficient force to affect bilateral hemispheric or brain stem functions. Common symptoms experienced by the athlete after concussion are listed in Table 2.

Mild TBI in sports can result from rotational (angular) or translational (linear) force that affects the brain. Frequently, both forces act in combination. Rotational forces are more commonly associated with deep shearing injuries affecting the vulnerable axons in a pattern known as *diffuse axonal injury*. Translational forces may also cause deep injuries, but are more commonly associated with skull fractures and intracranial bleeding on the surface of the brain in the form of cerebral contusions.

The modern neuroimaging technique of magnetic resonance imaging (MRI) is superior to computed tomography (CT) in the detection of pathologic changes related to TBI. However, the CT scan is still the most widely available study, and it is usually able to detect worrisome neurosurgical concerns.

Recent research shows that even mild forms of TBI are associated with axonal injury on electron microscopic evaluation. The swelling and anatomical disruption of the axon appears to evolve within minutes or hours after the traumatic injury itself, suggesting that the clinical observation of gradual worsening of certain mental functions in the concussion victim may be the manifestation of this delayed axonal swelling seen in animal research models of TBI.

The threshold of force necessary to produce concussion has not been clearly defined, even though elaborate experiments have been conducted using animals and physical model gels to simulate mild TBI. Most authors seem to agree that the observation of transient confusion is the clinical manifestation of the threshold of injury producing enough disruption of brain function to cause concussion effect. The appearance of posttraumatic amnesia is even more convincing when combined with transient confusion or disorientation. Any period of loss of consciousness, no matter how brief, is clear evidence for biomechanical injury to the brain, and there seems to be uniform agreement that this constitutes what had traditionally been called *classical concussion*.

The point at which concussion becomes some other more severe form of brain injury is equally unclear. As

Table 2 Symptoms of Concussion*

Early
  Headache
  Dizziness or vertigo
  Lack of awareness of surroundings
  Nausea and vomiting
Late
  Persistent low grade headache
  Lightheadedness
  Poor attention and concentration
  Memory dysfunction
  Excessive sleepiness or easy fatigue
  Irritability and low frustration tolerance
  Intolerance of bright night lights or difficulty focusing vision
  Intolerance of loud noises, sometimes ringing in the ears
  Anxiety and depressed mood

---

*Symptoms that the athlete may experience are divided into "early" and "late" categories, although they may not confine themselves in all cases to a typical time course.

mentioned above, even a mild form of concussion without loss of consciousness can lead to massive brain swelling and severe neurological dysfunction or death. We must learn from these unfortunate cases and regard every concussion as carrying the potential risk of such catastrophic outcome. If an athlete is rendered unconscious and remains unconscious at the time of emergency department evaluation, the "concussion" might very well be evaluated in the category of severe TBI with a Glasgow Coma Scale score of 8 or less. For the purposes of this discussion, a concussion must include at least transient confusion as a threshold at the mild end, and cannot be associated with loss of consciousness lasting longer than 1 hour or with post-traumatic amnesia of more than 24 hours' duration.

MANAGEMENT GUIDELINES

In the late 1980s, members of the Colorado Medical Society reviewed existing sports concussion grading scales and management guidelines, concluding that a mixture of old and new medical literature supported the notion that a different grading scale should be created (Table 3). The Sports Medicine Committee of this organization drafted "Guidelines for the Management of Concussion in Sports," which have subsequently been endorsed by several national physician organizations and widely distributed for the use of coaches, trainers, and allied health personnel as well as physicians.* These guidelines are offered to the reader as most consistent with available evidence in clinical and research literature as well as consensus formed by medical experts.

The history of recent head trauma outside the sports setting, e.g., motor vehicle accident, should be considered in the "Return to Play" section for each grade of concussion (Table 4).

---

*An educational videotape offering instruction on the use of these guidelines is available through the Rehabilitation Institute of Chicago (312/908-6179).

Table 3 Grading Scale for Concussion in Sports

Grade 1	Confusion without amnesia No loss of consciousness
Grade 2	Confusion with amnesia No loss of consciousness
Grade 3	Loss of consciousness

Table 4 Guidelines for Return to Competition

Grade 1 – Remove from contest. Examine immediately and every 5 minutes for the development of amnesia or post-concussive symptoms at rest and with exertion (see Table 1). May return to contest if amnesia does not appear and no symptoms develop for at least 20 minutes.

Grade 2 – Remove from contest and disallow return. Examine frequently for signs of evolving intracranial pathology. Re-examine the next day. May return to practice only after 1 full week without symptoms at rest and with exertion.

Grade 3 – Transport from field by ambulance (with cervical spine immobilization if athlete remains unconscious) to nearest hospital. Thorough neurological evaluation immediately. Hospital confinement if signs of pathology are detected. If findings are normal, give instructions to family for overnight observation. May return to practice only after 2 full weeks without symptoms at rest and with exertion.

Prolonged unconsciousness, persistent mental status alterations, worsening postconcussion symptoms, or abnormalities on neurological examination require urgent neurological consultation or transfer to a trauma center.

Table 5 Sideline Evaluation

Mental Status Testing

Orientation:	Time, place, person, and situation (circumstances of injury)
Concentration:	Digits backward 3-1-7 4-6-8-2 5-9-3-7-4 Months of year in reverse order
Memory:	Names of teams in prior contest, President, Governor, Mayor; recent newsworthy events; 3 words and 3 objects at 0 and 5 minutes; details of contest (plays, moves, strategies, etc., as applicable)

Neurologic Tests

Pupils:	Symmetry and reaction
Coordination:	Finger-nose-finger and tandem
Sensation:	Finger-nose (eyes closed) and Romberg

Exertional Provocative Tests

40 yard sprint
5 push-ups
5 sit-ups
5 knee bends

(Any appearance of associated symptoms is abnormal, e.g., headache, dizziness, nausea, unsteadiness, photophobia, blurred or double vision, emotional lability, or mental status changes.)

Grade 1

This is the most common yet the most difficult form of concussion to recognize. The athlete is not rendered unconscious and suffers only momentary confusion. Most concussions in sports are of this type, and players commonly refer to it as having been "dinged" or having their "bell rung". All athletes with Grade 1 concussions should be removed from the game and evaluated (Table 5) before re-entering the contest.

Return to Play After Grade 1 Concussion

After a first Grade 1 concussion, if the athlete has no symptoms at rest or with exertion, return to the game may be permissible after at least 20 minutes observation. In every instance when the athlete is symptomatic, removal from the game is mandatory. All symptoms (headache, dizziness, impaired orientation, impaired concentration, memory dysfunction) must have disappeared, first at rest and then with exertional provocative testing before return to competition (see Table 5). Return is allowed only if the athlete is asymptomatic during rest and exertion for at least 20 minutes. A second Grade 1 concussion in the same contest eliminates the player from competition that day. CT or MRI scanning is recommended in all instances in which headache or other associated symptoms either worsen or persist longer than 1 week. It is recommended that three Grade 1 concussions terminate a player's season. No further

contact sports are permitted for at least 3 months, and then only if the athlete is asymptomatic at rest and with exertion.

Grade 2

With a Grade 2 concussion, the athlete is not rendered unconscious but exhibits confusion and has amnesia for the events following the impact (post-traumatic amnesia). Amnesia for events preceding the injury (retrograde amnesia) may be seen along with post-traumatic amnesia in more severe cases. After a Grade 2 concussion the athlete should be removed from the game and given a thorough neurological evaluation. The athlete should be evaluated frequently over the next 24 hours for signs of evolving intracranial pathology by direct medical observation or with explicit, written instructions given to the family for monitoring the athlete at home.

Return to Play After Grade 2 Concussion

Return to competition after a first concussion may be as soon as 1 week after the athlete is asymptomatic at rest and with exertion. A neurological examination should be performed by a physician before return to practice. CT or MRI scanning is recommended in all instances in which headache or other associated symptoms either worsen or persist longer than 1 week. Return to contact play should be deferred for at least 1 month after a second Grade 2 concussion, and termination of the season should be considered. Terminating the season for that player is mandated by three Grade 2 concussions, as would any abnormality on CT or MRI scan consistent with brain swelling, contusion, or other intracranial pathology.

Grade 3

It is usually quite easy to recognize a Grade 3 concussion. This level of head injury applies to any athlete who is rendered unconscious for any period of time. Initial treatment includes transport to the nearest hospital by ambulance, with the cervical spine immobilized if the athlete remains unconscious and cannot be fully evaluated. A thorough neurologic evaluation should be performed immediately. A neuroimaging study (CT or MRI scan) of the head should be performed in all athletes rendered unconscious even for brief periods of time. Hospital confinement is indicated if any signs of pathology are detected or if the mental status of the athlete remains abnormal. If findings are normal, explicit written instructions may be given to the family for overnight observation. Neurologic status should be assessed daily thereafter until all symptoms have resolved.

Return to Play After Grade 3 Concussion

The athlete is typically held from contact sports for 1 month after a Grade 3 concussion. Return to play before 1 month is allowed only if the athlete has been asymptomatic at rest and with exertion for at least 2 weeks. CT or MRI scanning is recommended in all instances in which headache or other associated symptoms either worsen or persist longer than 1 week. A season is terminated by two Grade 3 concussions or by any abnormality on CT or MRI consistent with brain swelling, contusion, or other intracranial pathology. Return to any contact sport should be seriously discouraged in discussions with the athlete.

In most instances when an athlete has suffered a head injury that requires intracranial surgery, return to contact sports is contraindicated. However, the final determination as to whether an athlete may return to competition is the team physician's clinical decision.

TREATMENT

It is not my intention to review those neurosurgical interventions performed in athletes suffering severe intracranial trauma. These considerations are discussed in the chapter on Closed Head Injuries in this text, and other authoritative texts on the subject. However, the treatment of postconcussion symptoms may be of interest to the reader and allow the athlete to recover more quickly and return to the sport or recreational activity. The most common symptoms of postconcussion syndrome are listed in Table 2.

The physician must avoid the use of antiplatelet aggregation agents such as aspirin and ibuprofen in the acute setting in order to avoid exacerbating intracranial bleeding that may have gone undetected. Acetaminophen products are a better choice for the management of headache or other pain syndromes. The athlete sometimes reports difficulty with sleep, not uncommonly finding sleepless nights quite disruptive and exhausting. It might be useful to try a very low dose of tricyclic antidepressant at bedtime, which often relieves this symptom by offering better sleep and improving daytime mood as well as fortuitously treating neurologic pain syndromes such as post-traumatic migraine. Insomnia refractory to this approach is best treated with a short course of chloral hydrate as a sedative hypnotic at bedtime until more normal sleep patterns have developed. Exertional headaches in the absence of intracranial pathology are best treated in many cases with cyproheptadine, which may be necessary for 2 to 4 weeks and then tapered off.

Again, it is essential that any athlete who has ongoing symptoms from concussion be restricted from any activities that run the risk of additional concussion. It is advisable to avoid alcoholic beverages during this phase of recovery because it can exacerbate symptoms, delay recovery, and put the athlete at greater risk of additional injury.

SUGGESTED READING

Barth JT, Alves WM, Thomas VR, et al. Mild head injury in sports: Neuropsychological sequelae and recovery of function. In: Levin HS, Eisenberg HM, Benton AL, eds. Mild head injury. New York: Oxford University Press, 1989.

Jordan BD. Head injury in sports. In: Jordan BD, Tsairis P, Warren RF, eds. Sports neurology. Rockville, Md: Aspen Publishers, 1989.

Kelly JP, Nichols JS, Filley CM, et al. Concussion in sports: Guidelines for the prevention of catastrophic outcome. JAMA 1991; 266(20): 2867-2869, 1991.

Mueller FO, Schindler RD. Annual survey of football injury research. National center for catastrophic sports injury research, Chapel Hill, NC. Submitted February, 1994.

Report of the Ad Hoc Committee to Study Head Injury Nomenclature. Proceedings of the Congress of Neurological Surgeons in 1964. Clin Neurosurg 1966; 12:386-394.

The Sports Medicine Committee, Colorado Medical Society. Guidelines for the management of concussion in sports. Revised May, 1991.

OCULAR INJURIES

ROBERT C. PASHBY, M.D., F.R.C.S.(C)
THOMAS J. PASHBY, C.M., M.D., C.R.C.S.(C)

Eye injuries account for 1% of total sports-related injuries. They can end the career of a professional athlete and change the life-style and earning power of others. Prevention of eye injuries is possible, as proved first in hockey and now in racquet sports. When they do occur, they must be recognized, their severity assessed, and treatment instituted. The team physician, trainer, or first aid attendant should have a basic knowledge of eye anatomy and physiology (Fig. 1) and the necessary equipment to carry out on-the-spot examination. He or she must decide whether the injury can be treated, and the patient released or whether ophthalmologic consultation is necessary.

EXAMINATION

A minimal list of equipment required for ophthalmologic examination includes the following:

1. Vision card
2. Pen light
3. Sterile flourescein strips
4. Sterile eye pads
5. Eye shield
6. Tape
7. Sterile cotton-tipped swabs
8. Sterile irrigating solution

To determine the severity of an eye injury, a routine eye examination is carried out. By oblique illumination of the eye with a pen light, damage to the conjunctiva, cornea, anterior chamber, iris, pupil, and lens can be determined. Intraocular examination behind the lens requires the use of an ophthalmoscope and the ability to interpret findings.

The steps in the examination are as follows:

1. Inspection of the soft tissues for laceration, bruising, or hematoma.
2. Inspection of the conjunctival sac for hemorrhage, laceration, and foreign bodies. In many cases eversion of the upper eyelid reveals a foreign body, which is easily brushed away. Displaced contact lenses often are found.
3. Examination of the cornea by oblique illumination for foreign bodies, abrasions, and lacerations. Abrasions are readily outlined by a flourescein strip dipped into the tears exposed as the lower lid is pulled downward.
4. The clarity and depth of the anterior chamber with that of the fellow eye.
5. Pupillary size, shape, and reaction to light are compared with those of the other eye.
6. The iris colors of each eye are compared.
7. Intraocular examination with an ophthalmoscope (if available) may reveal lens, vitreous, and retinal damage.
8. Visual acuity is tested in each eye separately, using a reading card or book; corrected vision less than 20/40 is referred.
9. Peripheral vision is tested by having the patient fix on the examiner's nose and, after occluding the other eye, asking for identification of the number of fingers held up in all fields of gaze. A normal visual field extends to 90 degrees temporally, 65 degrees downward, 60 degrees nasally, and 45 degrees upward. Any loss of field demands referral.
10. Ocular movements are tested by having the patient follow a light to his right, then upward, then downward, then similarly to his left. Both eyes should move together. Any diplopia must be referred.
11. Facing the patient, determine whether one eye is sunken (narrowing the palpebral aperture) or proptosed (enlarging it). The former suggests an orbital floor fracture while the latter suggests an orbital hemorrhage. Should there be any doubt about the function of the eye or seriousness of the injury, referral is indicated.

In our series of almost 4100 eye injuries caused by sports, gathered over the past 16 years, all of which required ophthalmologic care, 11% resulted in a legally blind eye (20/200 or less) and most suffered severe intraocular damage.

The sport causing most eye injuries varies from country to country (Table 1). In Canada, hockey has been responsible for most eye injuries, although since the hockey mask was introduced, racquet sports are rapidly catching up (Table 2).

Examining the hockey injuries in more detail proves the benefit of wearing certified protective equipment. Before hockey face masks were introduced, an average

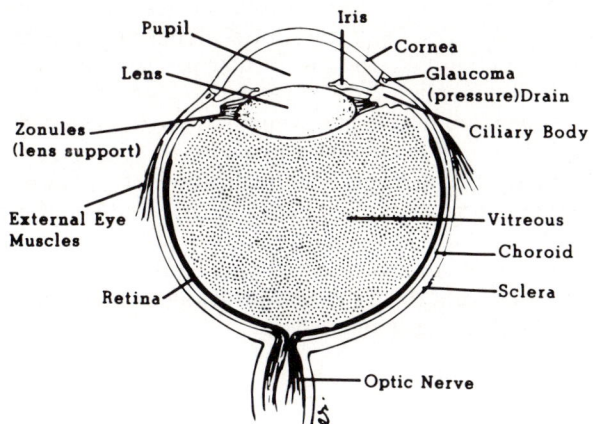

Figure 1 Cross section of the eye.

Table 1 Causes of Sports-Related Eye Injuries in United States and Canada

Canada (COS Study)*	Sport	United States (CPSC)†
39%	Hockey (post, mask)	4%
30%	Racquet sports	20%
11%	Baseball	27%
8%	Ball hockey	1%
4%	Football and soccer	7%
1%	Basketball	20%

*Canadian Ophthalmological Society
†Consumer Product Safety Commission

Table 2 Number of Eye Injuries According to Sport

Sport	Injuries	Blind Eyes
Hockey (18 years)	1754	271
Racquet sports (16 years)	997	44
Baseball (16 years)	409	23
Ball hockey (16 years)	320	27
Football (16 years)	167	7
Golf (16 years)	52	15
Skiing (16 years)	31	9
War games (8 years)	60	23
Other sports (16 years)	232	30

Table 3 Types of Sports-Related Eye Injuries

Injury	Percent
Soft tissue	34%
Orbital fractures	4%
Corneal injuries	9%
Hyphemas	27%
Other intraocular injuries	23%
Ruptured globes	3%

272 hockey eye injuries, including 32 blinding injuries, were reported annually. Since masks have been required in minor hockey, the annual average number of eye injuries has dropped to 94 and the number of blinding injuries to 14. No eye injury has been reported to a player wearing a Canadian Standards Association certified mask.

An analysis of 4027 sports-related eye injuries reveals that over 50 percent are intraocular in type (Table 3).

TREATMENT AND MANAGEMENT

Orbital Hemorrhage

Orbital hemorrhage usually results from blunt trauma. Bleeding into the orbit causes swelling and proptosis. It is wise to check for intraocular damage before the swelling becomes extensive. Central and peripheral vision, pupils, iris color, and the presence of diplopia must be recorded. Most injuries resorb without treatment, but severe hemorrhage may embarrass the blood supply to the optic nerve and cause visual loss. Such injuries must be referred to an ophthalmologist. Application of an ice pack is suggested.

Corneal lacerations present, again, with similar symptoms. If the eye can be gently opened without undue squeezing and without pressure on the globe, the pupil appears irregular, the anterior chamber shallow, and the iris probably attached to or prolapsed outside the corneal wound. A sterile eye pad is gently applied, and the patient is referred to the hospital for immediate ophthalmologic repair.

Injuries to the Lens

The lens can be injured by blunt trauma interfering with lens metabolism or causing a split in the lens capsule, allowing aqueous to enter the lens, rending it opaque. The lens may also be involved in penetrating injuries. Cataract changes may occur immediately or develop over weeks or months. The lens is suspended within the eye by radiating zonular fibers attached to the ciliary body. Zonular rupture is not unusual following injury, and this allows vitreous to herniate into the anterior chamber. If the zonular rupture is extensive, the lens may subluxate. The iris will jiggle (iridodonesis).

Removal of the cataractous or dislocated lens and replacement with an implant or the fitting of a contact lens usually restores vision to normal. Lens injuries, of course, demand specialized care.

Traumatic Glaucoma

Intraocular tension often fluctuates above and below normal for days after ocular trauma. If there is not structural damage inside the eye, intraocular tension then settles back to normal. More severe trauma may produce a recession in the anterior chamber angle. The ciliary body is damaged, the anterior chamber is deepened, and the aqueous outflow channels are embarrassed. Should the remaining undamaged aqueous outflow channels be unable to adequately handle aqueous production, ocular hypertension ensues. Glaucoma will develop in 10 percent of split angles early or even after many years. Once anterior chamber angle damage has been identified, the intraocular pressure should be followed annually.

Secondary glaucoma commonly complicates lens dislocation and occurs with hyphemas, especially after secondary hemorrhages. Normalization of pressure is necessary to prevent optic nerve damage and peripheral field loss. Secondary glaucoma complicating hyphema requires early attention to prevent blood staining of the cornea. Evacuation of the blood and blood clots from the anterior chamber is indicated.

Hyphema

Hyphema is a collection of free blood in the anterior chamber. It is a very common ocular sports injury. Over 900 hyphemas are listed in our series. It is important that

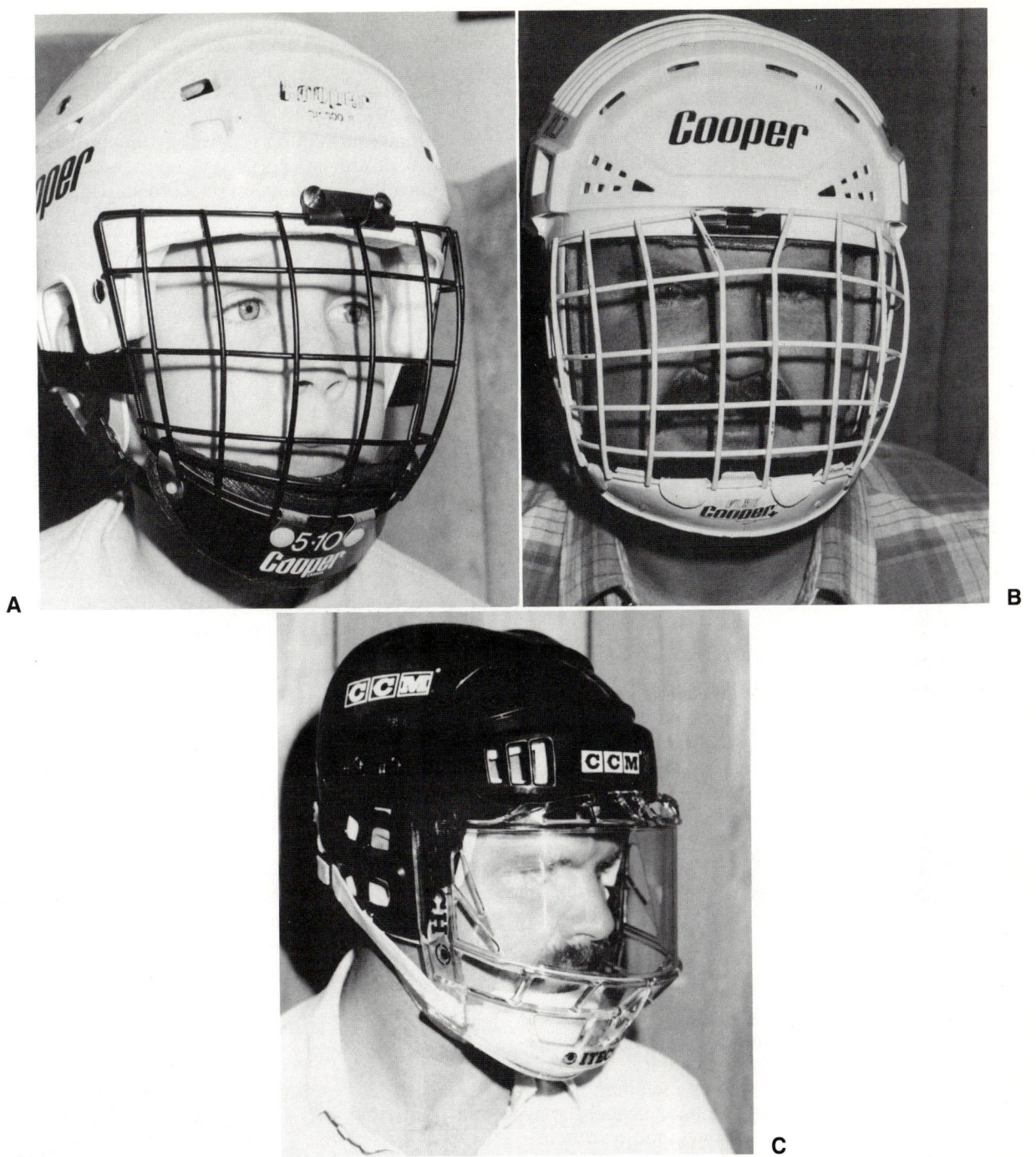

Figure 2 *A*, Certified mask-helmet for 5- to 10-year-old hockey players. *B* and *C*, Certified mask-helmets for older players.

the person rendering first aid recognized this type of injury, because immediate referral and hospitalization is required. Aspirin should be avoided.

When the injured eye is first examined, the blood appears as a haze in the anterior chamber. The pupil is usually irregular in shape and sluggish in reaction to light. The anterior chamber may be deepened. These diagnostic points are readily appreciated by comparing the injured with the fellow eye. Vision is blurred. On bed rest the blood settles down by gravity and appears the next day as a level in the anterior chamber. Continued bleeding may occur, however, and if it is severe the anterior chamber appears black, the so-called "8-ball eye." Most hyphemas clear in 5 days, but 15% suffer secondary bleeds, usually within 2 to 5 days. Prompt recognition and referral is necessary. Conservative treatment may include hospitalization and patching the injured eye for children or simply bed rest at home with daily reexamination by the ophthalmologist. Secondary glaucoma occurs in 50% of secondary hemorrhages.

Irrigation of the anterior chamber and clot evacuation may be indicated to relieve the increased intraocular pressure and prevent blood staining of the cornea.

Lid Lacerations

With any lid laceration, damage to the globe, ocular muscles, and orbit must be ruled out. Bleeding can be controlled by direct pressure. Close inspection is necessary to reveal lacerations of the lid margin, of the puncta, or into the lacrimal apparatus. Such lacerations demand meticulous closure to prevent epiphora. Primary repair using the microscope is indicated. Examination of the globe and a record of visual function is necessary.

Conjunctival Injuries

Minor lacerations of the conjunctiva do not require suturing. Foreign bodies may be removed with a moist, sterile cotton-tipped swab. A sterile eye pad is applied for 24 hours when follow-up examination is made.

Foreign bodies commonly lodge under the upper lid margin. Eversion of the upper eyelid will expose them. They too can be wiped away with a moist cotton-tipped swab.

Subconjunctival Hemorrhage

Although the bright red blood covering the white sclera is an alarming sight, such uncomplicated injuries are not serious. Eye function is recorded, and if it is normal, no treatment is needed. The redness gradually disappears over 10 days.

Orbital Fractures

Orbital fractures usually result from blunt trauma. The most common fracture occurs to the orbital floor where the bone is thinnest. Blunt trauma forces the eye back into the orbit, increasing the orbital pressure and causing a "blow-out" fracture of the orbital floor. The inferior ocular muscles may be caught in the fracture, causing limitation of upward and downward gaze with resulting diplopia. Enophthalmos is usual. Eye function is recorded, and radiographic studies including computed tomography or magnetic resonance imagery are arranged. Some patients recover spontaneously; others require freeing of the inferior ocular muscles if trapped in the fracture and insertion of a Teflon plate or bone graft along the orbital floor to cover the fracture. Fractures into the sinuses cause leakage of air into the orbit, producing crepitus, a crackling sound, with finger pressure over the swelling. Radiographic examination reveals air in the tissue. Spontaneous resolution is usual. Roof fractures require immediate neurosurgical assessment because they involve the anterior cranial fossa.

Corneal Injuries

Corneal injuries cause sudden, severe pain accompanied by tearing, photophobia, and blepharospasm.

Superficial corneal foreign bodies can be irrigated off with sterile solution or brushed off with a moist cotton-tipped swab. Eye function is recorded, a sterile eye pad applied, and the eye re-examined in 24 hours. Embedded foreign bodies will not irrigate or brush off the cornea and require removal by an ophthalmologist using a sterile needle or eye spud under slit lamp magnification. Eye function is recorded, a sterile eye pad applied, and recheck in 24 hours arranged.

Corneal abrasions produce similar symptoms. fluorescein outlines the denuded area. Should no foreign body be present, visual function is recorded, a sterile eye pad applied, and follow-up examination in 24 hours carried out.

Injuries to the Posterior Pole

Injuries to the posterior pole commonly result from a blunt blow to the front of the eye, producing a pressure wave that travels to the posterior pole and crushes the choroid and retina against the tough sclera. This contra-coup force commonly causes a choroidal split or tear. Should the split occur across the macular area, visual acuity is markedly reduced. Less severe contra-coup forces may cause macular edema with reduced visual acuity. Depending on the severity of the blow, resolution may occur, but usually the edema creates a macular cyst, which then may rupture and leave a macular hole. Central vision is then markedly reduced.

Retinal injuries may result in hemorrhages or detachments. One-third of traumatic retinal detachments are sports related. Recovery of visual function depends on early recognition and treatment. Once the detachment involves the macula, normal vision will not be restored, although the retina is successfully reattached.

No outward sign of retinal detachment is evident. Some blurring of vision, when tested, with some loss of peripheral field is diagnostic. For this reason, eye injuries of even moderate degree deserve ophthalmoscopic

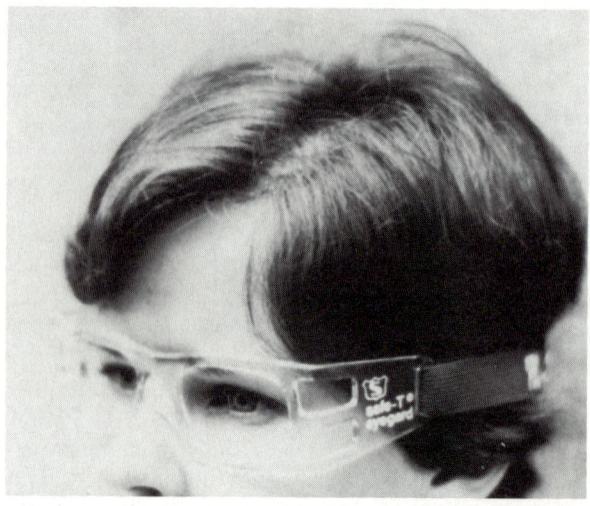

Figure 3 Eye protector for racquet sports participants.

examination at the time of injury, and certainly recheck the following day. The patient is warned to report any loss of visual function, namely acuity or visual field loss.

Ruptured Globe

Ruptured globe injuries destroy vision and usually result in removal of the eye. Over 100 such injuries have been recorded in our series. The offending weapon is usually a hockey stick or puck, a golf ball or club, a ski tip, a squash ball or racquet, or a tennis ball or baseball. At the time of injury, pain causes orbicularis spasm. If the lids can be gently opened, the eye will appear soft and sunken in the orbit. Vision will usually be reduced to perception of hand movement or light. Treatment requires gentle application of a sterile eye pad and transport to a hospital for immediate ophthalmologic care.

Prevention

Prevention is the key. Modifying rules and the wearing of certified protective equipment have done much to reduce the number of eye injuries in Canadian hockey. (Racquet sports eye protectors with polycarbonate lenses are saving eyes in squash and racquetball as well) (Figs. 2 and 3).

EYE PROTECTORS IN RACQUET SPORTS

MICHAEL EASTERBROOK, M.D., F.R.C.S.(C), F.A.C.S.

This chapter summarizes our experience over the last 15 years with eye protectors, specifically in racquet sports.

BADMINTON

It has been apparent for some time that the badminton shuttlecock is ideally suited to produce an eye injury. Indeed, speeds of 130 to 135 miles per hour have been recorded, using high-speed film (Table 1).

Table 2 demonstrates the increasing percentage of badminton injuries in racquet sports in Canada over a 5 year period, as more and more racquetball and squash players are wearing eye protection.

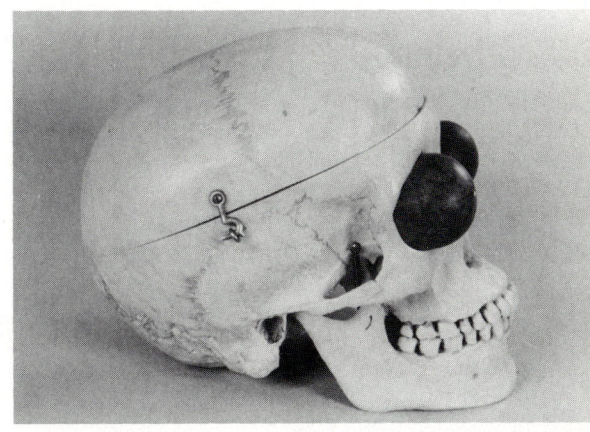

Figure 1 Skull containing an international yellow dot soft ball in the right orbit, and a 70+ American ball in the left orbit.

Table 1 Ball and Racquet Velocities

	Speeds (mph)
Racquetball	
Ball	85-110
Racquet	85-90
Squash	
Ball	130-140
Racquet	95-110
Tennis ball	90-110
Handball	60-70
Badminton shuttlecock	130-135

Table 2 533 Eye Injuries in Racquet Sports in Canada

Year	Number of Injuries	Raquetball and Squash (%)	Badminton (%)	Tennis (%)
1982	90	73	13	14
1983	87	59	22	19
1984	115	58	16	26
1985	82	50	33	17
1986	83	36	35	29
1987	66	38	38	24

Table 3 Canadian Racquets Survey 1978-1987

Injury	Squash	Racquetball
Lid hemorrhage	57	42
Lid laceration	36	19
Subconjunctival hemorrhage	31	14
Corneal abrasion	44	32
Corneal lacerations requiring surgery	6	2
Iritis	26	26
Iris tear or dialysis	10	8
Angle recession	18	4
Hyphema	114	106
Secondary hemorrhage	5	4
Cataract	8	6
Vitreous/retinal hemorrhage	17	21
Macular scar	8	5
Retinal detachment	10	3
Orbital fracture	3	1
Number of patients	393	293

Table 4 Energy Levels in Racquet Sports

ANSI Z87 STANDARD (Industrial safety lenses)	0.6 ft/lb
RACQUETBALL	
1.4 oz at 128 mph	29.0 ft/lb
1.4 oz at 78 mph	17.8 ft/lb
SQUASH	
70+: 1.25 oz at 100 mph	23.63 ft/lb
Yellow dot: 0.846 oz at 100 mph	17.76 ft/lb

Table 5 Injuries Sustained by 80 Athletes Wearing Open Eyeguards

Injury		
Lid hemorrhage		11
Lid lacerations		3
Corneal abrasions		10
Iritis		8
Hyphemas		56
Mechanism of injury		
Ball		77
Racquet		3
Ball penetrated eyeguard		69
Eyeguard displaced		11
Eyeguard	Squash	Racquetball
Protec	14	22
Ektelon	1	15
Rainbow	5	2
Voit	2	13
Solari	1	2
Champion	1	—
Duraguard	0	2
	24	56

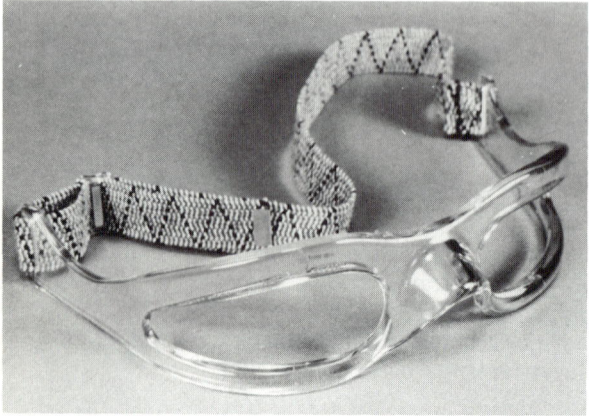

Figure 2 Protec, one of the initial open eyeguards widely distributed for squash and racquetball.

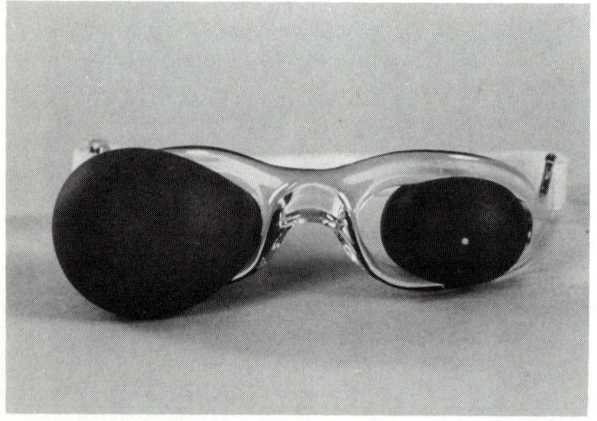

Figure 3 Penetration of an open eyeguard by a racquetball ball and squash ball.

Although no surveys have been performed in recent years, it appears that the incidence of injuries in badminton is relatively high in doubles. The badminton community is becoming concerned that national and provincial organizations and local clubs may be liable if a strong educational program is not designed to promote the use of eyeguards.

Although testing by the Canadian Standards Association (CSA) has not yet been carried out for eye protectors in badminton, it appears that the polycarbonate eye protectors used in squash and racquetball may

well suffice to prevent eye injuries in this very active sport.

RACQUETBALL AND SQUASH

Racquetball and squash are ideally suited to produce an eye injury: the balls and racquets either fit exactly or can be compressed to fit into the human orbit (Fig. 1). Table 3 lists some of the injuries seen over a 10 year period in Canada. Table 1 lists the speeds of squash, racquetball, and tennis balls; it is not surprising that eye injuries are occurring on a regular basis.

It is apparent that energy levels in racquet sports are significant (Table 4). To pass the industrial lens safety standard in the United States, a lens must not break after a 1-lb ball is dropped on it from a distance of only 0.6 foot. This is grossly inadequate to resist the enormous energy levels in squash and racquetball. A novice racquetball player hits the ball at 78 miles per hour; an "A" player hits the ball at speeds of 125 to 140 miles per hour.

OPEN EYEGUARDS

A variety of open eyeguards that were unbreakable and did not restrict peripheral vision, but allowed eye penetration, entered the market in the late 1970s (Fig. 2). It was apparent, without formal testing, that squash and racquetball balls readily penetrated these open eyeguards (Fig. 3). Table 5 gives details of the first 80 patients who sustained an injury while wearing open eyeguards.

These eyeguards were of no use in racquetball, in which 95% of the injuries were caused by the ball. Indeed, players have indicated that they had a false sense of security, since players who feel protected watch the ball more closely. It might be argued that these open

Table 6 Canadian Standards Association Approved Eyeguards

Model	Manufacturer/Distributor	Address (Canada)	Address (United States)
1. Defender 600	Peepers	Peepers, Inc. P.O. Box 951, Station A 150 Chatham Steel Hamilton, Ontario L8N 3P9 416-525-3363	Peepers International 417 Fifth Ave. New York, NY 10016 212-696-9797
2. CRS 300	CRS Sports	CRS Sports International, Inc. 10021 169th Street Edmonton, Alberta T5P 4M9 403-483-5149	Same address as Canada
3. Sports Scanners	American Optical	AOCO Ltd. 80 Centurian Dr. Markham, Ontario L3R 5Y5 416-479-4545	American Optical Mechanic Optical Southbridge, MA 01550 617-765-9711
4. Safe-T Eyegard	Imperial Optical	Imperial Optical Canada 21 Dundas Square Toronto, Ontario M5B 1B7 416-595-1010	Embassy Creations P.O. Box 143 234 Holmes Rd. Holmes, PA 19043 215-586-9640
5. Albany	Leader	International Forums, Inc. (Leader Sports) 1150 Marie Victoria Longuevil, Quebec J4G 1A1 514-651-2300	LST Leader Sports Products Inc. P.O. Box 271 Main Street, Route 22 Essex, NY 12936 518-963-4268
6. New Yorker	Leader	Same address as no. 5	Same address as no. 5

Table 7 Eyeguards That Meet United States ASTM Standard

Model	Manufacturer/Distributor	Address (Canada)	Address (United States)
1. Action Eyes	Viking Sports	Black Knight Enterprises 3792 Commercial Street Vancouver, British Columbia V5N 4G2 604-872-3123	Viking Sports 5355 Sierra Road San Jose, CA 95132 408-923-7777
2. Albany	Leader	International Forums, Inc. (Leader Sports) 1150 Marie Victoria Longuevil, Quebec J4G 1A1 514-651-2300	LST Leader Sports Products Inc. P.O. Box 271 Main Street, Route 22 Essex, NY 12936 518-963-4268
3. New Yorker	Leader	Same address as no. 2	Same address as no. 2
4. Sierra	Ektelon	Paris Glove of Canada Ltd. 9200 Rue Meilleur St. #101 Montreal, Quebec B2N 2A8 514-381-8611	Ektelon 8929 Aero Dr. San Diego, CA 92123 619-560-0066
5. Court Goggles	Ektelon	Same address at no. 4	Same address as no. 4
6. Safety Lites (tested and approved for racquetball, not squash)	Penn	Same address as US	306 South 45th Avenue Phoenix, AZ 85043 602-269-1492

eyeguards, being unbreakable, only funnel a compressible squash or racquetball ball directly into the eye, increasing the risk of ocular injury. On the basis of these reports of inadequate eye protection, standards were set in Canada and the United States. Table 6 lists the eyeguards that have passed CSA standard. Table 7 lists the eyeguards that have met the ASTM standard in the United States.

CLOSED EYEGUARDS

The present Canadian and American standards relate to performance, not design. An eyeguard is positioned on a head form (Fig. 4), which is placed in a testing device (Fig. 5) whereby balls are projected at speeds of 90 miles per hour at the lens and at the hinge.

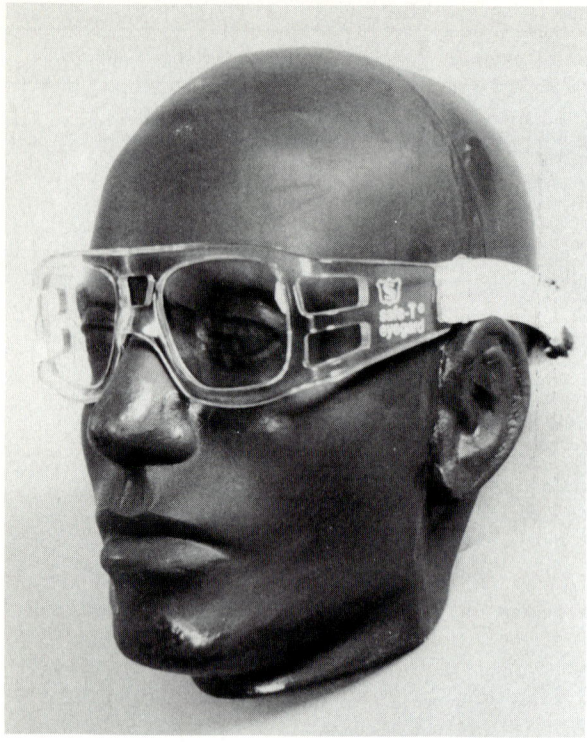

Figure 4 Eyeguard on Alderson head form.

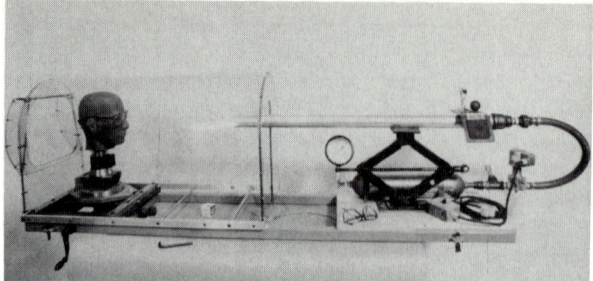

Figure 5 Testing device at Canadian Standards Association.

SUGGESTED READING

Barrell GV, Cooper PJ, Elkington AR, et al. Squash ball to eye ball: the likelihood of squash players incurring an eye injury. Br Med J 1981; 283:893-895.

Bishop PJ, Kozey J, Caldwell G. Performance of eye protectors for squash and racquetball. Phys Sports Med 1982; 10:63-69.

Diamond GR, Quinn GE, Pashby TJ, Easterbrook M. Ophthalmologic injuries. Clin Sports Med 1982; 1:469-482.

Diamond GR, Quinn GE, Pashby TJ, Easterbrook M. Ophthalmological injuries. Primary Care 1984; 11:161-174.

Doxanas MT, Soderstrom C. Racquetball as an ocular hazard. Arch Ophthalmol 1980; 98:1965-1966.

Easterbrook M. Eye injuries in racquet sports; a continuing problem. Phys Sports Med 1981:91-101.

Easterbrook M. Eye injuries in racquet sports. Int Ophthalmol Clin 1981; 21:87-119.

Easterbrook M. Eye injuries in squash and racquetball players: an update. Phys Sports Med 1982; 10:47-56.

Easterbrook WM. Eye protection in racquet sports: an update. Phys Sports Med 1987; 15:180-186.

Easterbrook M. Eye protection in racquet sports. Int Ophthalmol Clin 1988; 28:232-237.

Feigelman M, Sugar J, Rednock N, Read J, Johnson PL. Assessment of ocular protection for racquetball. JAMA 1984; 250:3305-3309.

Fowler BJ, Seelenfreund M, Newton JC. Ocular injuries sustained playing squash. Am J Sports Med 1980; 8:126-128.

Kennerley-Bankes JL. Squash rackets: a survey of eye injuries in England. Br Med J 1985; 291:1539-1540.

Maberley AL. Retinal detachments and athletic eye injuries. BC Med J 1981; 23:70-73.

Seelenfreund MH, Freilich DS. Rushing the net and retinal detachment. JAMA 1976; 235:2723-2726.

Vinger PF. Sports eye injuries—a preventable disease. Ophthalmology 1981; 108-113.

Vinger PF. The incidence of eye injuries in sports. Int Ophthalmol Clin 1981; 21:21-46.

If contact is made between the lens and the head form, the eyeguard fails.

There are eye protectors currently on the market that protect players at speeds in excess of 90 miles per hour. No significant ocular injury has been reported in North America to players wearing polycarbonate eyeguards that meet CSA and/or ASTM standards.

Any player can wear sunglasses; any player can wear a closed eyeguard. Newer eyeguards are meeting standards designed as performance standards. Antifog coating is available on many of the new eyeguards.

Excellent eye protection is now available. It behooves all physicians and those interested in the prevention of vision loss to encourage all recreational racquet players to wear eyeguards certified for competitive racquet sports.

FACIAL INJURIES

LEITH G. DOUGLAS, M.D., F.R.C.S.(C), F.A.C.S.

Injuries to the face are common in many sports, particularly those involving body contact. In my experience as team plastic surgeon with the Toronto Maple Leafs of the National Hockey League (NHL) for some 25 years, I have seen approximately 100 per season. The main instrument of injury has been the hockey stick, accounting for about 80% of cases. The puck, the ice, skates, goalposts, the glass surrounding the rink, and fists accounted for the remainder. The incidence has remained approximately the same, but the seriousness of the injuries has decreased now that almost everyone in the NHL wears a helmet.

PREVENTION

Body contact sports will always be responsible for some facial trauma. This probably can still be reduced to some degree. The use of properly fitting helmets in hockey and football is mandatory, and their value is self-evident. Face guards may become popular in hockey in the future if they can be made lighter and easier to wear. Penalties for improper use of hockey sticks and deliberate attempts to injure in any way should be increased and will act as a deterrent to violence-minded players. Football goalposts have been made much safer, so consideration might be given to altering the construction of the goalposts in hockey. The removal of the deep central tongue of the hockey net and the introduction of the new magnetically seated net are steps in the right direction.

Facial injuries can be broadly classified into those involving soft tissue only and those involving the facial bones.

SOFT TISSUE INJURIES

The types of soft tissue injury are (1) contusions, (2) abrasions, (3) puncture wounds, and (4) lacerations (simple and complicated). Each type is discussed in the sections below.

Contusions

Most contusions are simple and require no treatment other than the application of an ice bag. However, some may result in hematoma formation. A small hematoma is completely absorbed in a few weeks, but larger ones that become encapsulated require incision and drainage. Incisions for these should be placed so that the resulting scar is minimized and no vital structures are damaged. Sometimes it is necessary to insert a small Penrose drain in the incision for 24 to 48 hours. It is best to evacuate hematomas at the "currant jelly" stage rather than go on for many weeks waiting for full liquefaction.

Hematomas of the external ear must be promptly and properly drained and prevented from reaccumulating or developing a seroma. Failure to do so results in the formation of a cauliflower ear.

Abrasions

Abrasions vary from simple brush burns of the epidermis to those that go through the epidermis and into the dermis. The former require nothing other than cleansing with a good detergent and the application of an antibiotic cream for a few days. With deeper abrasions the area should be fully cleansed and any foreign material removed. The time to do this is at the initial treatment. Foreign material left in a wound not only contributes to the incidence of infection, but may result in traumatic tattooing. It becomes fixed to tissues in about 12 hours and becomes extremely difficult to remove without a formal surgical abrasion procedure. The use of local, and even general, anesthesia may be necessary to permit proper cleansing. A soft brush may be required to remove deeply embedded material. The area should then be covered with an antibiotic ointment

and suitably dressed. Most abrasions heal in about a week unless they become infected.

Puncture Wounds

The principles of treatment are the same as for puncture wounds anywhere on the body. The track of the puncture should be followed and the possibility of deep injury to nerves, vessels, or other vital structures ruled out. It is particularly important to determine whether foreign bodies are retained in the wound. X-ray examination should be done as indicated. Narrow puncture wounds are best not sutured, particularly if they are deep and if there is a possibility of the development of infection. The track should be irrigated with saline or hydrogen peroxide and covered with a dry dressing.

Bite wounds are a special type of puncture wound. They may occur when a player strikes his face on an opponent's teeth or, fortunately infrequently, as a result of malicious intent. These are very serious wounds and have a very high potential for infection. They should be copiously irrigated with hydrogen peroxide and saline, getting to the depths of the wound with the liquid. They should be left open in all except the rare case in which a vital function is compromised as, for example, in a complete tear of a lower lip. In these cases, loose closure is done, with definitive repair carried out secondarily or as a delayed primary procedure.

Penicillin and cloxacillin are started immediately in moderately high dosage; cephalosporins are used in patients with penicillin allergy. The wound is re-examined in 24 hours, and may be secondarily closed in a few days if it remains clean. Evidence of developing infection warrants admission to the hospital, where high-dose intravenous antibiotic therapy is administered.

Lacerations
Simple Lacerations

These may be linear lacerations due to hockey sticks and other sharp objects, but are frequently of the bursting type caused by a bony prominence of the face coming in contact with a blunt object. With these there is also an element of contusion.

They should be cleansed with a good antiseptic solution, such as aqueous Hibitane, then irrigated with saline. Needless to say, no material should be used on the face that is poisonous, stains the skin, or is dangerous to the eyes.

Examination of the wound for foreign material and damage to blood vessels and nerves is then carried out. A judicious debridement may be necessary if there are small tags of nonviable tissue or ragged edges in bursting wounds, but this should be very judicious.

The vast majority of simple facial lacerations may be repaired under local anesthesia. I usually use 1% lidocaine without epinephrine. Infiltration with a No. 25 or 27 needle through the wound is adequate.

If an adequate clinic room is available at the arena or stadium, most simple facial lacerations can be repaired there without compromising good medical practice. There should be adequate space with a good light and a quiet environment. One must have an assistant to help with the supplying of materials and possibly to cut sutures and sponge as indicated. Antiseptic solutions, saline, gauze dressings, drapes, and sterile instruments are required. I have been using disposable paper drapes with a small window cut out for some time, and they are excellent for this purpose. Instruments needed are a suitable needle holder, Adson forceps, about six hemostats, curved and straight iris scissors, the necessary syringes and needles, and suture material.

My choice of suture material for facial lacerations is 5-0 or 6-0 nylon on the surface, sometimes supplemented by deep sutures of 4-0 or 5-0 polyglycolic acid material.

Any small bleeders should be caught and ligated as necessary. Wound closure should be done somewhat more loosely than in a clean surgical wound, because the element of contusion leads to more swelling, causing the sutures to tighten and cut in. Interrupted suture technique is usually employed, although subcuticular closure with a continuous suture may be possible in some clean, incised linear wounds.

Simple lacerations are usually dressed with a small adhesive dressing strip. Sometimes an antibiotic ointment may be applied over the suture line. When there is contusion, the application of ice over the dressing is indicated.

I recommend removal of dressings in 24 hours and gentle daily washing after that. My infection rate in such wounds has been practically zero.

Complicated Lacerations

These include more extensive lacerations requiring more than 10 or 12 sutures as well as those involving specialized structures.

Lacerations of the eyelids and of the alar margin and complex lacerations of the ears are probably best dealt with in the Emergency Department of a hospital rather than in a clinic room. The technique remains the same, i.e., cleansing, anesthetizing properly, very judicious debridement, and accurate closure. Closure of lacerations crossing anatomic boundaries, such as the vermilion border of the lip and the eyebrow, should be done very carefully, in order to restore the anatomy as perfectly as possible. This is not always as easy as it sounds and frequently requires considerable effort. Incidentally, one *never* shaves an eyebrow!

Also included in this group are lacerations with actual soft tissue loss. If this is minimal the wound may be closed by simply advancing the edges. Other more complicated situations with avulsion of flaps should be treated in the hospital and, in rare instances, may require skin grafting to restore the deficit.

The trap door flap or U-shaped laceration is always a problem. The dimensions of the flap may be such that the length-to-width ratio leads to compromising of its circulation. It may therefore be necessary to excise the questionable part and close it by advancing the edges. In curved lacerations, direct closure frequently leads to a pincushion effect with the central part becoming heaped up in relation to the surrounding tissues. This is due to contracture along the line of the scar and sometimes to a degree of edema, which makes it stand out even more prominently. This is particularly true if the flap is in a true U shape based superiorly rather than an inverted U shape, as this tends to act as a barrier to normal lymphatic drainage. Despite this problem, there is no place for Z-plasties and excisions of tissue at the initial procedure. The best plan is simply to close the wound as carefully as possible, revising it later only if necessary. Since it is not possible to predict just how good or how bad a given flap is going to be, it is always the wisest course to wait.

With simple lacerations the player is usually able to return to the game, but with the more complicated ones it is prudent to give them a chance to heal without danger of further trauma. A simple laceration heals in a few days, sutures being removed at 4 or 5 days. In more complicated ones a few sutures may be left in place for 2 or 3 days more. Lacerations that have transgressed the facial nerve or parotid duct and other such serious injuries are beyond the scope of this discussion. They should be dealt with in the same manner as they would be in nonsports practice.

Antibiotics are employed only when dictated by common sense. In simple lacerations they are not indicated unless there is gross contamination. They should be employed in the more complicated ones, those involving eyelids and ears, and those in which there has been considerable contamination or in which there is a doubt whether the wound has been cleansed adequately.

The patient's tetanus immunization status should be determined and supplemented as indicated.

It is necessary to carry out a proper examination of vital structures, such as the eyes if the eyelids are injured, the internal structure of the nose if the nose is injured, or the teeth and underlying bone if the mouth area is involved. Facial nerve injuries do not occur frequently, but function should be tested if there is any possibility of damage.

The cardinal principles are (1) a full assessment of the injury, (2) thorough cleansing, (3) hemostasis, (4) judicious debridement, and (5) anatomic closure with fine sutures.

FRACTURES OF THE FACIAL BONES

These may be classified as closed (simple) and open (compound) fractures. By far the greater majority are compound. This compounding is from within rather than from without in most cases. For example, nasal bone fractures and fractures of the zygoma and maxilla almost invariably involve tears of the mucoperiosteum of the nasal cavity or the maxillary antrum. Most fractures of the mandible, being through tooth-bearing areas, are also compound. Fractures may be further classified as linear or comminuted, displaced or undisplaced, and stable or unstable.

The Nose

The nose is the most commonly injured bone structure on the face. Fractures may be due to blows from the side or directly end-on. The former type of injury usually produces simple fracturing with deviation to one side, whereas end-on blows may result in comminution of both bone and cartilage.

Diagnosis usually is not difficult. The patient may have heard or felt a crack in the nose at the time of the injury. There is usually epistaxis, which may be profuse, and a clinical deformity of the nose may be obvious to both the patient and the attending physician. Roentgenograms are helpful, but the decision to treat and the assessment of the results of treatment are a matter of clinical judgment.

It may be possible to manipulate a fractured nose quickly back into position in a relatively painless manner if the physician sees the patient immediately after the injury. This has the effect of reducing the bleeding, reducing bruising and edema, and affording considerable comfort to the patient.

A good clinical examination of the internal as well as the external nose is mandatory. If the nasal septum is fractured, it is possible to develop a septal hematoma. The characteristic bluish bulge on the septum should alert the physician, and appropriate drainage with packing should be carried out without delay. The mucoperichondrium may be dissected off the underlying cartilaginous septum by the hematoma. This can lead to resorption of the cartilage and loss of tip support. In some cases, cartilage is laid down as it is in a cauliflower ear, producing a mass that obstructs the airway. Septal abscess formation is also possible. Septal hematomas are of vital importance in children, because loss of cartilaginous tip support in a growing nose may lead to severe "snub-nose" deformity.

Reduction of the fracture, if necessary, may be done under local or general anesthesia after the swelling has subsided—usually within 4 or 5 days. Intranasal packing and plaster splinting are usually necessary in complex injuries involving comminution or septal hematomas, but the simpler fractures may be treated without them.

It is usually inadvisable for players to resume playing for at least a week after a nasal fracture of any consequence. Before they return it is necessary to be sure that there is no significant swelling and no possibility that bleeding will recur, and that the fracture is stable and does not require external support.

An external protective device is usually required for at least 4 weeks after such an injury. The wearing of helmets in hockey facilitates the attachment of a face guard, and in football, of course, it is already worn.

Antibiotics usually are not necessary in the treatment of nasal fractures unless there has been gross comminution or operative intervention such as the drainage of a septal hematoma.

The Zygoma and Orbit

Blows to the prominence of the cheek may result in zygomatic fractures. These may involve only the arch laterally or, more commonly, may cause the classic fracture through the frontozygomatic, zygomaticomaxillary, and zygomaticotemporal suture lines, the zygoma being displaced medially and inferiorly.

Diagnosis may be made by inspection alone when there is obvious flattening of the cheek on the affected side. Patients complain of pain and, frequently, of trismus due to the impingement of the displaced zygomatic arch on the coronoid process of the mandible. They may also complain of diplopia due to displacement of the lateral canthal ligament of the eye, which is attached to the zygoma. There may be loss of sensation on the tip of the nose and the upper lip on the affected side due to impingement of the fracture site on the infraorbital nerve. Unilateral epistaxis is also seen due to the fracture crossing the antrum and thus tearing its mucoperiosteum and causing bleeding, which spills over through the ostium into the nose. In addition to these symptoms and signs, palpation over the fracture sites will reveal the characteristic steps in the bone.

X-ray examination shows the fractures at these three sites, opacification of the antrum due to blood, and an alteration of the contour of the lateral wall of the maxilla.

The majority of these are sufficiently displaced to warrant surgical intervention. Most can be managed by simple elevation, an elevator being passed down behind the zygomatic arch in the temporal area and the bone levered up into normal position. Although this measure is usually sufficient, some of these fractures may be unstable, and interosseous fixation may be required.

Blow-out fractures of the orbital floor also occur. The surrounding bony framework of the orbit itself need not be fractured, and the damage may be confined to the orbital floor. This occurs when a blow to the eyeball forces it backward, compressing the orbital fat so that it finally bursts out through the inferomedial part of the floor, which is its weakest part. Herniation of the orbital contents into the antrum may occur, producing enophthalmos. This constitutes a significant cosmetic deformity and may also produce diplopia. It is also possible for the extraocular muscles to become caught up on the bony margin of the blown-out segment, thereby becoming tethered and limiting upward gaze. The presence of these signs and symptoms should be sought in any player after a blow to the eye. Facial roentgenograms show antral opacity and air in the orbit suggesting the injury, but tomograms are necessary to delineate fully the damage. Surgical exploration is usually required. The defect in the floor may be repaired by replacing the fracture fragments with bone from the anterior wall of the antrum or with a sheet of silicone rubber. Obviously, a full ophthalmologic examination is mandatory in such cases. Sometimes the blow may cause only a small crack between the ethmoid sinus and the orbit. When the patient blows the nose, air is forced back up through this into the orbit, and the eyelids rapidly inflate with surgical emphysema, causing the patient considerable alarm. There is no specific treatment other than to refrain from blowing the nose for 2 weeks or so while the opening closes spontaneously. Antibiotic cover is prescribed. This phenomenon may sometimes be seen in fractures of the zygoma, particularly if the patient has engaged in vigorous nose blowing.

Players with a fractured zygoma or orbit should not engage in contact sports for at least 3 weeks, and then should wear a protective face mask to avoid further injury for at least another 3 weeks.

The Maxilla

Fractures of the maxilla are classically divided into three types:

1. *LeFort Type I* — This extends horizontally across the maxilla at the level of the floor of the nose, thereby shearing off the hard palate and upper dental alveolus.

2. *LeFort Type II* — Also called a pyramidal fracture, this extends obliquely upward and medially through the body of the maxilla toward the apex of the nose on both sides, thereby fracturing out a pyramid-shaped section of bone.

3. *LeFort Type III* — Also called a craniofacial separation, this describes the injury in that the fracture extends from one frontozygomatic suture line across the craniofacial junction to the other side. This shears the facial bones completely away from the cranium. It is usually due to a blow from straight ahead, and the wedge-shaped face is driven posteriorly and downward along the inclined plane of the base of the skull, producing a dish-face deformity or an "equine facies."

Combinations of these types may occur, e.g., LeFort II on one side and III on the other or bilateral II and III. The deformities may be evident on inspection, and palpation of the bones reveals the fracture sites. In most cases mobility may be demonstrated in the fractured segment. X-ray examination confirms the clinical findings.

These are very serious injuries, particularly the craniofacial separation, and require reduction and appropriate interosseous fixation and suspension of the fracture fragments. A tracheotomy is frequently necessary at surgery. It may be many months before any consideration can be given to a return to sports following such an injury. Residual deformity is frequent despite adequate surgery. Loss of sense of smell is also common owing to tearing of the olfactory bulbs.

It is obviously possible to suffer an associated craniocerebral injury with fractures of the maxilla or, indeed, with any facial injury. One extremely important finding, which should be sought at the time of the original examination, is the presence of cerebrospinal fluid rhinorrhea, indicating a fracture in the area of the cribriform plate of the ethmoid and tearing of the dura mater. Neurosurgical consultation should be sought in all patients with significant facial trauma whether or not they show signs of head injury.

The Mandible

Fractures of the mandible may be simple or compound. The latter is the rule, since most of them occur through the tooth-bearing area, thus opening a free passage from the mouth down to the root level. They may be unilateral or bilateral, or may have multiple sites. They may also be classified anatomically, i.e., condylar neck, ascending ramus, angle, body, coronoid process, or parasymphyseal.

The diagnosis is usually straightforward. The patient may have actually heard or felt the bone fracturing at the time of the injury. There is usually significant pain. In the case of a compound fracture, bleeding may be noted in the mouth. The patient may complain of malocclusion, and crepitus and mobility may be noted at the fracture site. X-ray examination usually confirms the diagnosis. It is sometimes necessary to employ special x-ray techniques, such as the Panorex view.

Single undisplaced fractures of the condylar neck and the ascending ramus, or of the body in an edentulous patient, may warrant a trial period of conservative management employing only soft diet and avoidance of trauma without wiring of the teeth. This is sufficient if the patient is comfortable. The majority, and certainly all compound fractures, should be immobilized in some way. The simplest form of immobilization for single undisplaced fractures is the application of islet loops with cross-wiring to hold the teeth in occlusion. With instability or displacement, some form of arch is necessary to hold the fragments in place before the teeth are wired into occlusion. A cable arch made up of twisted 24 gauge wire (Risdon's method) or patent arches of the Erich or Winter type may be used. These latter have an added advantage in that elastic band traction may be employed with them and the cross-elastics or wires may be more readily removed for access to the mouth in an emergency. In fractures that are unstable or unfavorable in their angulation, an open reduction with interosseous fixation as well as interdental wiring is done. Patients with partial or full dentures should have them in place to maintain spacing and for stability during the period of immobilization.

The presence of fractures of the roots of teeth is significant, and a dental consultation may be sought to determine whether certain teeth are salvageable and to extract fractured roots. Fragments of teeth, fillings, and dentures should always be sought in the patient's mouth at the time of injury to prevent his swallowing or aspirating them. It is necessary to obtain a chest roentgenogram of a patient with a missing tooth, denture, or tooth fragment to rule out the possibility of its having been aspirated, particularly if he has been unconscious.

Fractures of the mandible may constitute a life-threatening injury under some circumstances, particularly in patients with bilateral, displaced, unstable fractures of the body. The patient, in effect, loses control of the tongue and may be unable to swallow properly. This, plus the presence of blood and saliva, and possibly vomitus in the mouth, may constitute a threat to the airway. Such patients should be cared for initially in the sitting position or, failing this, while prone with their face turned to one side to allow free drainage from the mouth. A tensor bandage around the face under the chin may temporarily hold the mandible immobilized in occlusion, thus affording considerable comfort to the patient and helping him to retain some control over the airway.

Compound fractures of the mandible rarely become infected nowadays, but this is indeed possible. All patients require appropriate antibiotic coverage.

Immobilization of most fractures is required for approximately 6 weeks. In simpler fractures in which an arch bar has been applied to the lower dentition, it may be possible to open the interdental fixation earlier and rely on the arch alone for stability.

Contact sports are out of the question during this 6 week period, and the patient should wear an appropriate face protector for at least a further 6 weeks to prevent another injury.

Maintenance of proper nutrition may be a problem with patients who have their teeth wired into occlusion, particularly those who do not have any gaps due to missing teeth through which solid food can be passed. Food reduced to the fine consistency of baby food by a food processor is required.

Dislocations of the Mandible

These may occur if the patient is struck while the mouth is open wide. They may also result from simply opening the mouth very widely in a shout or a yawn, as in nonsports practice.

To reduce a dislocated mandible, first be seated behind the patient, cradling his head against the chest. Place both *well-padded* thumbs just posterior to the last lower molars. Then, exert downward and posterior traction with the thumbs, at the same time rolling the mandible upward and anteriorly so that the condyles slip back into position.

Some persons have very lax temporomandibular joints and suffer periodic dislocations. Reduction is usually easy in them.

It may be necessary to employ sedation for sufficient relaxation to carry out the reduction in some patients, particularly if they are having a considerable amount of pain or are very apprehensive.

After-care includes resting the mandible and avoidance of maneuvers that might lead to another dislocation.

SUGGESTED READING

McCarthy JG. Plastic surgery. Philadelphia: WB Saunders, 1990.
Schultz RC. Facial injuries. 3rd Ed. St. Louis: Mosby–Year Book, 1988.
Torg JS. Athletic injuries to the head, neck and face. 2nd Ed. St. Louis: Mosby–Year Book, 1991.

EAR, NOSE, AND THROAT INJURIES

J. SIMON McGRAIL, M.D., M.S., F.R.C.S.(C)

The head and neck areas of the body are vulnerable to injury in sports that involve bodily contact. This contact can be with an opponent's head, fist, or other parts of his anatomy, or with a foreign object held by the opponent, such as a hockey stick.

Like injuries from any cause, these can be classified into soft tissue injuries with or without involvement of the underlying bone or cartilage. Soft tissue injuries include injuries to skin, subcutaneous tissue, muscles, nerves, and blood vessels. Each of these must be considered when an injury is being evaluated.

THE NECK

Injuries to the neck are usually blunt injuries and do not involve laceration of the skin and underlying soft tissues. By far the most important structure in the neck to consider is the airway. The larynx can be injured by blunt trauma, e.g., a cross-check from a hockey stick or a karate chop.

In this type of injury the head is usually extended, bringing the larynx closer to the surface where it is much more vulnerable to the assault. Immediately the player complains of discomfort in the neck, but more important, there can be different degrees of airway obstruction. If there is immediate hemoptysis a mucosal tear is present, and with this combination of events the player must be immediately removed from the scene of activity and carefully and thoroughly assessed.

The first consideration is the adequacy of the airway. If his breathing is noisy but he can inflate his chest well, there is time to get this player to a hospital where he can be properly examined. If his breathing is such that he has gross airway obstruction, indicating a badly smashed larynx, an airway has to be secured. Fortunately, most laryngeal fractures involve the thyroid cartilage, and placing an airway into the cricothyroid membrane alleviates most of the obstruction. A hypodermic needle placed in the cricothyroid membrane can act as a very adequate first aid measure until the player can be moved to a hospital. Alternatively, in the past I have employed a stab incision over the cricothyroid membrane and inserted the outer casing of a ballpoint pen, which gives a very adequate airway. Any time a cricothyrotomy is carried out, a tracheostomy must be done later in an orderly manner, but there is no urgency in this, provided that the revision is done within 24 hours. However, in the case of a badly smashed larynx, a tracheostomy almost certainly would be necessary anyway to assist in the rebuilding process.

An alternative cricothyrotomy instrument is the Fisher tube, which is part of a standard intravenous set.

Most sports injuries to the neck fall short of this dire emergency, but certainly can be worrisome to the attending physician or trainer. Any player who has received a neck injury and has any degree of airway problem should be sent as soon as possible to the nearest hospital where indirect laryngoscopy can be carried out. The usual finding in such a case is some degree of laryngeal edema, with or without submucosal hemorrhage, the degree of edema being reflected in the amount of airway obstruction present. As the edema is likely to progress for up to 12 to 24 hours, these players should be kept under close observation in a hospital setting until the airway has returned to normal.

Most such injuries do not require surgical intervention. They subside with rest, steam, and reassurance. I do not advocate sedatives in these cases because of their respiratory depressant action, and I find that most players respond well to a full explanation of this, together with the reassurance already mentioned. Most patients need a 3 to 4 day stay in the hospital. As soon as the larynx has returned to normal, the player can resume full normal activities.

If a mucosal tear is suspected because of hemoptysis, nothing further need be done unless the tear can be seen. If it can be visualized on indirect laryngoscopy, the larynx should be carefully assessed under general anesthesia, because a compound fracture of this nature may require an open reduction.

Finally, I would not recommend intubation of a suspected laryngeal fracture until the extent of the injuries can be assessed fully. It is better to establish an airway below the area of fracture, and then assess the degree of damage. Intubation may be difficult because of edema, and also may cause further damage and displacement of laryngeal fragments. If available, Heliox is always useful in the treatment of airway obstruction, but the vast majority of such injuries subside without heroic measures, particularly if a calm reassuring attitude can be maintained.

Sharp injuries (e.g., from a skate blade) can cause significant lacerations to the neck and, if deep enough, can cut the sternocleidomastoid muscle and the underlying jugular vein. Fortunately, this type of injury is relatively uncommon, but it is a very dramatic one when it does occur. In one case a jugular vein was cut during a hockey game, and the player's life was saved by the quick action of the trainer, who was able to exert pressure on both sides of the laceration and occlude the jugular vein until this could be surgically repaired.

A more common injury is the superficial laceration, which usually can be primarily sutured. As with all lacerations, care should be taken to clean the wound to ensure that no foreign particles have been left behind.

Lacerations around the upper neck, the ear, and the face may damage the facial nerve. In the immediate evaluation of the injury, it is sufficient to document whether facial nerve function has been affected. If the player is asked to close the eyes tight, wrinkle the forehead, screw up the nose, smile, and whistle, any facial asymmetry should be recognized during these maneuvers. If there is injury to the facial nerve, this should be mentioned so that appropriate exploration and nerve repair can be carried out within a few hours of the injury.

THE MOUTH

Injuries to the mouth include those of the lips, teeth, and tongue.

Injuries to the lip follow the principles outlined in the chapter on *Facial Injuries,* and it is worth noting that most mucosal injuries heal spontaneously, often with minimal morbidity. If a laceration includes skin and mucosa, this must be carefully sutured, preferably in a hospital setting.

Trainers of sports teams are usually taught good first aid procedures, and for a lip laceration the most important measure is to squeeze it tightly on either side of the laceration to cut down on what is often very free bleeding. Having the patient suck an ice cube and placing this next to the laceration also helps. Similar principles apply to lacerations of the tongue, which are not uncommon hockey injuries. They usually occur in a player who, while skating hard with mouth open and tongue out, receives a blow under the jaw to cause a self-inflicted bit injury to the tongue.

These bleed freely, but firm pressure on either side of the cut controls the bleeding until hemostasis can be secured and the tongue sutured. Because of the possible edema that can result from this type of injury, it should be treated in a hospital setting and the player kept under observation for 24 hours to ensure that there is no airway problem.

THE EAR

Injuries to the ear are relatively uncommon, occurring most often in wrestlers. We are all familiar with the classic cauliflower ear of the wrestler and boxer, and this should be an entirely preventable result of injury. It follows from a subperichondrial hematoma that is not treated and finally absorbs the underlying cartilage, resulting in a grotesque abnormality. If a hematoma is recognized in the auricle, the correct treatment is immediate incision. The hematoma is drained, and to prevent its recurrence careful localized packing is placed in the different nooks and crannies of the auricle, and a firm pressure bandage applied over the ear and head. This should be inspected daily until it is clear that the hematoma is not forming again. If this treatment is carried out expeditiously, the ear will suffer no anatomic damage. The patient should be given antibiotics because the danger of perichondritis is high, and this in itself can cause severe deformities.

THE NOSE

Lacerations to the nose are discussed in the chapter on *Facial Injuries.* I mention them here only to reinforce the view that a laceration to the nose that involves a through-and-through injury with underlying mucosal damage must be treated in a hospital setting. Treatment consists of careful intranasal mucosal approximation by suturing, followed by suturing of the skin laceration. If this type of injury is neglected, adhesions within the nose can cause significant nasal obstruction in the future.

Perhaps the most important injury of the nose is that affecting the nasal septum. Careful evaluation is necessary to see whether a septal hematoma is forming. If a bulge in the septum is noticed, particularly bilaterally, this must be drained immediately. This is done by a sharp incision through the nasal septal mucosa and suctioning out the blood that is present. Through this incision a small wick is inserted, and the nose is packed fairly firmly to hold the septal mucosa together and prevent recurrence of the hematoma. If a hematoma is overlooked or neglected, a septal abscess is likely to develop, causing loss of bone and cartilage in the nose and leaving a nose that is difficult to correct from both a cosmetic and a functional point of view. Antibiotics should be given when a septal hematoma is diagnosed, in an effort to prevent infection.

After any injury to the nose with epistaxis, the player is instructed to sit forward with head down and to gently blow one nostril at a time. This measure is expected to remove clots, allow the vessels to contract and retract, and stop the nosebleed. The nose is then gently pinched, if this is possible (i.e., if there is no associated fracture), and the nosebleed stops quickly, in which case the player can probably resume activity. If there is an associated fracture that prevents pressure from being applied, ice is applied to the back of the neck in the hope of causing a reflex vasoconstriction, and a small amount of packing into both sides of the nose usually helps. When there is an associated fracture, the player is sent to the hospital where the fracture can be reduced, either within 24 hours or within the next 7 to 10 days, depending on the degree of edema and bruising.

Although most nosebleeds are caused from septal blood vessels, a significant nosebleed can be caused by injury to the anterior ethmoidal artery. This is seen with a blunt injury to the root of the nose and the medial canthal area of the eye, as from a fist or hockey puck. This can result in a brisk hemorrhage, which needs careful and thorough packing in the roof of the nose to control it. This type of bleeding tends to persist even after adequate packing, and it is not unusual to explore the ethmoid sinuses through an external incision and clip the anterior ethmoidal vessel.

AURICULAR INJURY

DAVID E. SCHULLER, M.D.
RODNEY E. MOUNTAIN, M.B., Ch.B.

Although auricular injury can occur in a variety of sports, the greatest incidence of such injuries occurs in wrestling. Auricular hematoma resulting from blunt compression or shearing injury is by far the most common injury in this sport. By contrast, auricular lacerations are surprisingly infrequent. As with many sports injuries, the challenge is in both prevention and treatment. When auricular injury occurs, the goal of treatment is to resolve the injury with minimal negative impact on the athlete's training and competition schedule. Attempts to prevent auricular injuries are also critically important.

PREVENTION

As we have gained experience treating athletes with auricular injuries, it has become apparent that most injuries occur in athletes who are not wearing headgear. It seems that a simple preventative measure would be for the athlete to wear protective headgear. However, after further investigation, we identified several deterrents to the routine use of protective headgear by wrestlers. Various types of headgear have been developed and are readily available. The National Collegiate Athletic Association (NCAA) and most state high school athletic associations require that headgear be worn during competitive events. But there are no requirements for headgear to be worn during practice. We undertook an evaluation to ascertain patterns of utilization and athletes' attitudes toward headgear. The investigation also measured whether use of the headgear resulted in decreased frequency of auricular injuries. The following information is based on a survey that was completed by 537 NCAA Division I wrestlers.

The responses to this questionnaire verified that the headgear provides some protection. There was a greater frequency of auricular injury in wrestlers who were not wearing headgear than in those who had headgear in place. This increased frequency of injury was statistically significant. However, headgear does not provide 100% protection. About one fourth of wrestlers using headgear develop an auricular injury.

In addition, relatively few of the wrestlers (about

35%) used the headgear during both competition and practice. When wrestlers competed in events other than school team competitions, the percentage wearing headgear decreased to 22%. Thus, it appears that wrestlers use the headgear in response to written mandates rather than personal preference.

The most common reason cited for not using headgear is that the apparatus is uncomfortable. The heat generated by the headgear as well as the decrease in hearing were also frequent explanations specified for nonuse. Finally, we were alarmed to note that almost 40% of Division I collegiate wrestlers report that one or both of their auricles are permanently deformed because of wrestling injuries.

One potential positive influence on prevention could be the coaches. Accordingly, NCAA Division I coaches were polled to learn more about the influence of coaches' attitudes on athletes' use of this equipment. Almost 80% of these coaches believe that auricular injuries occur more often when the headgear is not worn. These same coaches also responded that only about 20% of the wrestlers wear the headgear during practice. More than 80% of the coaches responded that they have no policy of mandatory headgear use during contact phases of practices.

Prevention can be improved by legislating use of the headgear during all wrestling activities, in practice and in actual competition, or by developing more comfortable head gear. Until either or both of these goals are realized, auricular injury among wrestlers will continue to be commonplace.

PATHOPHYSIOLOGY

Auricular injury is most frequently associated with some type of blunt trauma that is a compressive and/or shearing force. There are actually some legal wrestling maneuvers (Fig. 1) that create these types of forces, predisposing wrestlers to auricular injury. This compression or shearing effect creates subcutaneous bleeding. There has been some disagreement in the past about the plane of the bleeding. But, it is now established that the predominant blood collection is deep to the perichondrium of the auricular cartilage. This perichondrium provides the sole blood supply to the auricular cartilage. The separation of the tissue that provides the blood supply from the cartilage can predispose to a variety of negative events. If there is a collection of blood in the form of a hematoma or a seroma, this could potentially become infected. Such an infection could subsequently involve the devascularized auricular cartilage, eventually requiring the removal of the infected cartilage, with permanent auricular deformity as the result. Another possible series of events is the development of excessive fibrosis of the blood clot with the creation of the "cauliflower" deformity, where the auricle becomes distorted by the accumulation of scar tissue.

Auricular hematoma has a propensity for reaccumulation after the hematoma/seroma has been removed. This high frequency of recurrence can happen until the

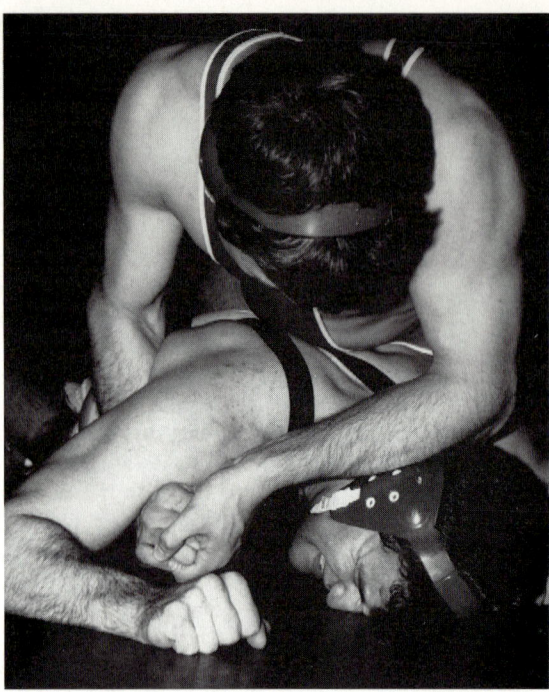

Figure 1 Headgear can move during certain wrestling maneuvers, causing trauma to auricle. (From Schuller DE, Dankle SD, Strauss RH. A technique to treat wrestlers' auricular hematoma without interrupting training or competition. Arch Otolaryngol Head Neck Surg 1989; 115:202-206. Copyright 1989, American Medical Association; with permission.)

detached perichondrium has reattached to the underlying auricular cartilage. Any of these pathophysiologic events of blood/seroma accumulation, infection, reaccumulation, or fibrosis, can have a negative impact on the athlete's ability to train and compete. This injury has the potential to create a life-long deformity, which is not easily surgically reconstructed after the athlete's competitive days have been completed. Knowledge of the potential course of events makes it easy to recognize the importance of prompt and vigorous treatment.

DIAGNOSIS

The diagnosis of auricular hematoma is made with primary reliance on the principles of physical diagnosis. No radiographs are necessary. History taking, inspection, and palpation are the cornerstones of an accurate diagnosis. As stated earlier, this injury is temporally related to blunt trauma that contains a compressive and/or shearing force to one or both auricles, and it usually, although not always, occurs when the wrestler is not wearing protective headgear. A portion of the lateral surface of the auricle will have a fullness (Fig. 2) that obliterates the usual normal auricular contour. There is usually no overlying skin erythema or edema unless infection has already occurred. Palpation of the full area reveals it to be somewhat compressible, with mild to moderate tenderness. It is important to determine if

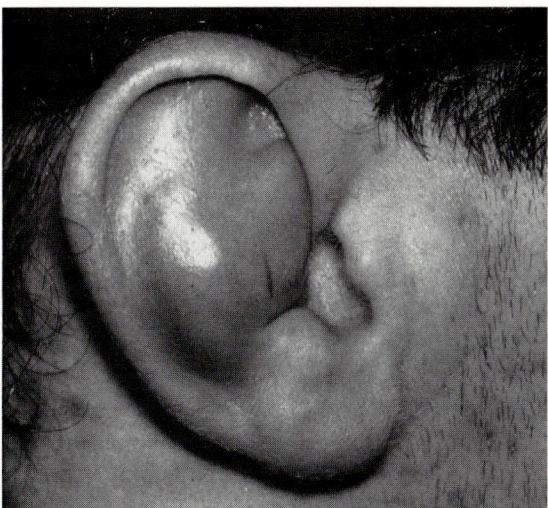

Figure 2 An auricular hematoma separates cartilage from overlying perichondrium. (From Schuller DE, Dankle SD, Strauss RH. A technique to treat wrestlers' auricular hematoma without interrupting training or competition. Arch Otolaryngol Head Neck Surg 1989; 115:202-206. Copyright 1989, American Medical Association; with permission.)

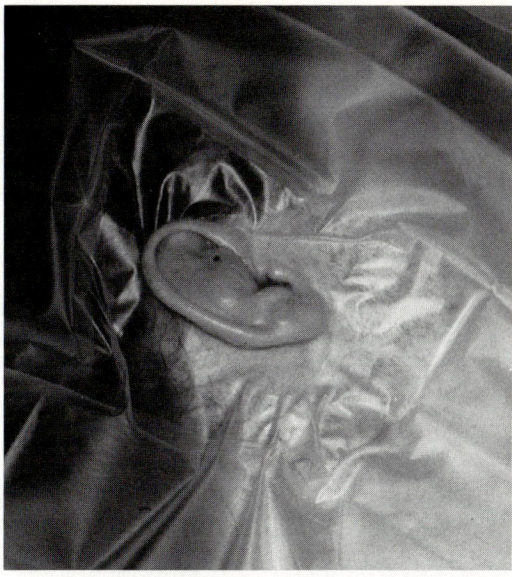

Figure 3 An ear drape is an effective means of isolating the auricle from surrounding hair. (From Schuller DE, Dankle SD, Strauss RH. A technique to treat wrestlers' auricular hematoma without interrupting training or competition. Arch Otolaryngol Head Neck Surg 1989; 115:202-206. Copyright 1989, American Medical Association; with permission.)

there are any portions of the full area that are firm and nontender. It is not unusual for a wrestler to have an older auricular hematoma that has undergone fibrosis in the same area as a new hematoma. That component of the fullness will not respond to the treatment of the acutely injured region. Although not as common, hematomas can develop on the medial surface of the auricle. However, we have not personally encountered a hematoma isolated to the medial surface in the absence of hematoma involving the lateral surface. It is rare for auricular hematoma to alter hearing unless the hematoma has occluded the external auditory meatus.

TREATMENT

The goals of treatment are to completely remove the blood or seroma, reapproximate the perichondrium to the underlying auricular cartilage, and prevent reaccumulation of fluid. The small (less than 1 cc) hematoma can be treated solely by aseptic aspiration of the fluid without the need for application of any sustained pressure. For any hematoma that is larger or for the recurrent small hematoma, an aggressive treatment approach is recommended. Another primary goal of treatment should be to minimize missed practice and/or competition time for the athlete. It is this latter consideration that makes some of the standard approaches to treatment unrealistic. Any treatment that has the likelihood of significantly interfering with practice or competition schedules will increase the probability of noncompliance. We have developed a treatment program that resolves the problem without impacting practice and competition schedules.

The treatment does not require an operating room

setting. It can be performed in a physician's office or in a trainer's room. The only instruments required are a needle holder and forceps. It is necessary to have a 3-0 silk suture, cotton dental roll, 10 cc syringe with an 18 gauge needle as well as a 27 gauge needle, adhesive, plastic ear drape, antibacterial ointment, aseptic preparation solution, sterile gloves, and gauze dressings. The patient is placed in a supine position with the involved ear exposed. The initial step is to infiltrate the overlying skin with a local anesthetic containing 1/100,000 epinephrine. In addition to the skin overlying the hematoma, the skin in the corresponding medial surface of the auricle is also infiltrated and a small amount of the anesthetic is instilled into the cavity of the hematoma. After infiltration, the auricle and the surrounding area are prepped and draped using the clear plastic ear dressing (Fig. 3), which effectively keeps hair away from the sterilized region. By the time the ear has been prepped and draped, the epinephrine in the local anesthetic has caused maximal vasoconstriction.

The syringe with the local anesthetic is emptied, and the 27 gauge needle is replaced with the 18 gauge needle. The hematoma is aspirated until it has been completely evacuated (Fig. 4). It is not unusual to aspirate in more than one region on the lateral surface and even to aspirate on the medial surface to ensure that complete evacuation has been achieved. Formerly, we incised the overlying skin and perichondrium to ensure complete evacuation. However, in the past few years, we have determined that needle aspiration can achieve the same without the creation of the scar secondary to an incision. Local anesthetic enables the aspirator to provide vigor-

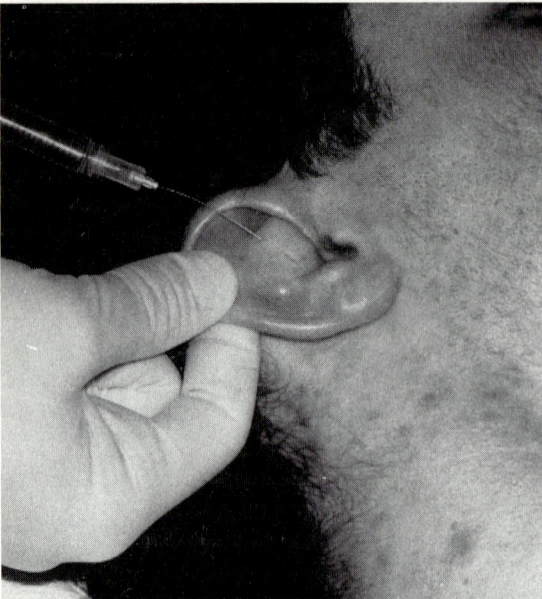

Figure 4 The hematoma is aspirated until it has been completely evacuated. (From Schuller DE, Dankle SD, Strauss RH. A technique to treat wrestlers' auricular hematoma without interrupting training or competition. Arch Otolaryngol Head Neck Surg 1989; 115:202-206. Copyright 1989, American Medical Association; with permission.)

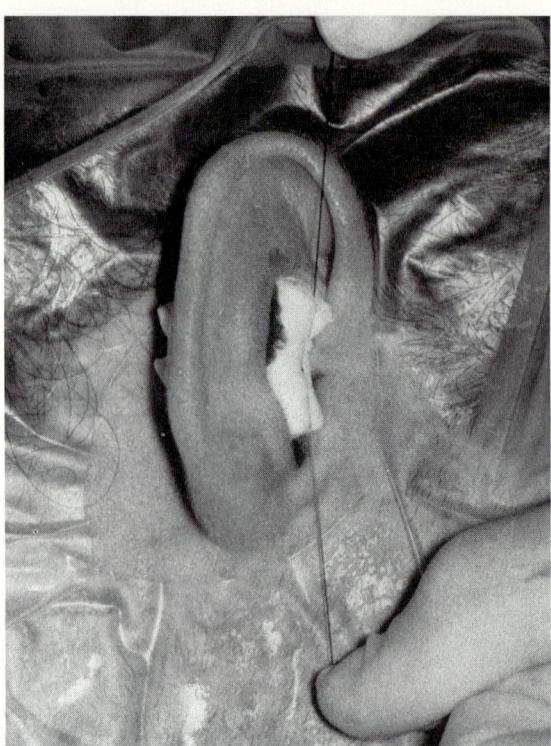

Figure 6 Suture is tightened securely using dental rolls to oppose skin to underlying cartilage with minimal chance of underlying skin necrosis. (From Schuller DE, Dankle SD, Strauss RH. A technique to treat wrestlers' auricular hematoma without interrupting training or competition. Arch Otolaryngol Head Neck Surg 1989; 115:202-206. Copyright 1989, American Medical Association; with permission.)

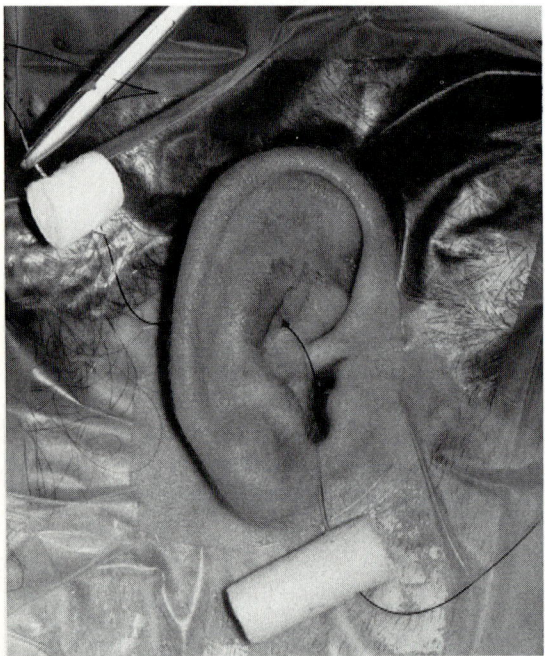

Figure 5 Suture is passed back and forth through smaller dental roll to be placed on medial surface of auricle. (From Schuller DE, Dankle SD, Strauss RH. A technique to treat wrestlers' auricular hematoma without interrupting training or competition. Arch Otolaryngol Head Neck Surg 1989; 115:202-206. Copyright 1989, American Medical Association; with permission.)

ous compression with the other hand to assure complete evacuation.

The next phase of treatment consists of a maneuver that will apply pressure over the involved area to decrease the chances of fluid reaccumulation. This is achieved with the application of dental rolls that are sutured into position to ensure that uniform pressure is achieved. To facilitate the passage of the needle through the dental roll and the auricle, the arc of the needle of a 3-0 silk suture is widened with digital pressure. The dental roll is cut so that its length corresponds to the amount of skin and perichondrium that has been undermined by the hematoma. The remaining shorter piece of the cut dental roll can be used as the counterpart to provide pressure to the medial surface of the auricle. The "stitch dressing" is applied by passing this 3-0 silk suture through the longer length of the dental roll and subsequently through the full thickness of the auricle in a lateral to medial direction at a level that corresponds to the superior extent of the undermined skin and perichondrium. This suture is passed back and forth through the smaller length of dental roll and then advanced in the opposite direction from the medial to lateral surface through the full thickness of the auricle near the inferior extent of the undermined skin and perichondrium (Fig. 5). This suture is advanced through the lower portion of the larger longer length dental roll and creates a mattress suture that, when tightened, compresses the auricular skin, perichondrium, and cartilage between these two rolls (Fig. 6). Before the mattress suture is tightened, a generous amount of antibacterial ointment is placed over the dental rolls and over the aspiration site(s). The dental rolls are subsequently covered with a generous amount of antibacterial ointment. Finally, the auricle is protected with the application of a mastoid dressing.

Oral systemic antibiotics are prescribed for the duration of the application of the "stitch" dressing (14 days). The athlete is permitted to run and lift weights on the day of treatment. The mastoid dressing is removed on the following day and regular practice and competition schedules can immediately resume.

The patient is instructed to keep the dental rolls covered with antibacterial ointment at all times, to wear protective head gear at all times in practice and in competition, and to use an extra amount of antibacterial ointment over the dental rolls prior to showering. Nonprescription mild analgesics are recommended. The athlete is directed to notify the physician if the auricle becomes increasingly tender, red, or edematous, or if there are other questions during the time of wearing the "stitch" dressing. The "stitch" dressing is removed at the end of 2 weeks. No anesthetic is required during removal of the dressing. The auricle will have some transient mild edema surrounding the area of the "stitch" dressing.

There are times when the fluid collection is so large that it encompasses more than one region of the auricle. In this situation, more than one pair of dental rolls is used to provide sufficient pressure over all the involved regions of the auricle. On a few occasions we have used three pairs of dental rolls to provide sufficient pressure over all areas involved with hematoma.

The approach described has been utilized for several years and provides uniformly positive results in most patients. Infection is the primary threat to this and other treatment programs. If infection arises, its severity determines whether it can be treated with antibiotics alone or with antibiotics and removal of the "stitch" dressing.

SUGGESTED READING

Bull PD, Lancer JM. Treatment of auricular haematoma by suction drainage. Clin Otolaryngol 1984; 9:355–360.

Giffin CS. The wrestler's ear (acute auricular hematoma). Arch Otolaryngol Head Neck Surg 1985; 111:161–164.

Savage R, Bevivino J, Mustafa E. Treatment of acute otohematoma with compression sutures. Ann Emerg Med 1981; 10:641–642.

Schuller DE, Dankle SK, Martin M, Strauss RH. Auricular injury and the use of headgear in wrestlers. Arch Otolaryngol Head Neck Surg 1989; 115:714–717.

Schuller DE, Dankle SD, Strauss RH. A technique to treat wrestlers' auricular hematoma without interrupting training or competition. Arch Otolaryngol Head Neck Surg 1989; 115:202–206.

Talaat M, Azab S, Kamel T. Treatment of auricular hematoma using button technique. ORL J Otorhinolaryngol Relat Spec 1985; 47:186–188.

ORAL PROSTHODONTIC REHABILITATION

THOMAS J. BALSHI, D.D.S., F.A.C.P.

Implant prosthodontic treatment has been available for the replacement of missing teeth for several decades. The benchmark of scientifically studied implants is the Branemark titanium screw, which has proven that osseointegrated fixtures (implants) provide excellent long-term favorable prognosis for fixed bone-anchored replacement teeth. The use of osseointegrated Branemark implants for patients who have sustained traumatic tooth loss takes on some very special considerations.

The entire procedure of osseointegration is based on a biocompatable coexistence between living tissues and titanium components that these tissues were never genetically coded to accept. Osseointegration relies on a situation where we create a predictable tissue to titanium interface through a very carefully controlled surgical procedure.

ETIOLOGY OF TOOTH LOSS

Contact sports such as football, basketball, hockey, and boxing have produced a myriad of dental problems, the most serious of which is the loss of natural dentition. Other more genteel sports such as tennis, golf, horse back riding, and swimming have also led to inadvertent tooth loss. A recent review of our clinical data on sports related injuries indicate that 90% of tooth loss occurs in the anterior part of the mouth. In most of these situations the injury occurs on impact when the player is moving toward an inanimate object or receives a blow from an oncharging competitor.

CHARACTER OF THE INJURY

A traumatic blow to the anterior part of the mouth creates a variety of hard and soft tissue lesions. Facial lacerations frequently cover deep seated fractures of the teeth and/or alveolar bone. If the impact is of sufficient magnitude, avulsion of anterior teeth is the most frequent form of permanent trauma. With severe impact, fractured roots and compound fractures of the alveolar bone are more complicated and create biologic devastation and post-trauma prosthodontic challenges. Social implications are worthy of note in as much as unreplaced tooth loss is viewed as a social stigma.

PROSTHETIC TREATMENT FOR LOST TEETH

There are five types of prosthetic approaches to replacing missing teeth (Table 1).

Temporary Removable Partial Dentures (Provisional Restoration)

Traditionally the simplest form of tooth replacement has been the use of removable dental appliances (Fig. 1). Easily fabricated, light weight, temporary removable appliances provide the partially edentulous patient with immediate esthetic replacement. This form of treatment gives the athlete psychological and often physical comfort, but limited functional ability.

Long-Term Removable Partial Dentures

When the hard and soft tissues have healed after traumatic tooth loss, a stronger removable prosthesis can be constructed using chrome cobalt castings to fasten the prosthesis to the remaining dentition. This is an inferior alternative form of treatment to "permanent" tooth replacement.

Another indication for the use of removable partial dentures is replacement of multiple missing teeth. When

five or six consecutive teeth are avulsed, the adjacent abutment teeth are widely spaced. In this condition, the use of a traditional fixed partial denture may be contraindicated. For example, the loss of all of the maxillary anterior teeth (six teeth) would require the use of multiple posterior teeth for the construction of a fixed prosthesis. This prosthetic design would place the remaining abutment teeth under severe strain because of the forces applied to the anterior cantilevered pontic (tooth replacement) section. A removable partial denture may put less stress on these abutment teeth. Likewise it is not uncommon when large numbers of teeth are traumatically lost that portions of the alveolar ridge are also lost. When this occurs the removable partial denture also provides an esthetic replacement for the missing residual ridge tissue.

Fixed Partial Dentures (Traditional Crown and Bridge)

With technologic advances, nonremovable prosthodontics for the replacement of missing teeth is preferred over removable appliances. Using crowns and fixed bridges (Fig. 2) to replace avulsed maxillary anterior teeth can generally be considered after a preparatory treatment program.

A thorough diagnosis is required when considering a fixed prosthesis of this nature. A traumatic impact to the mouth, creating the loss of some teeth, may also have an impact on the remaining teeth. Teeth and bone adjacent to a trauma site may sustain fractures. Complete radiographic examination is necessary to determine the condition of the potential abutment teeth, their nerves, and surrounding bone. Testing these teeth for mobility will effect the number required as support for a nonremovable prosthesis.

Diagnostic pulp testing for nerve vitality in the proposed abutment teeth is also important after traumatic injury. If the supporting abutment teeth for a fixed prosthesis are traumatically injured or sustain partial fractures, root canal therapy for the abutment teeth and the use of a post and core restoration will be a necessary part of the prosthetic treatment.

Table 1 Prosthetic Treatment for Lost Teeth

Temporary removable partial dentures (provisional restoration)
Long-term removable partial dentures
Fixed partial dentures (traditional crown and bridge)
Resin bonded fixed partial denture (Maryland bridge)
Osseointegrated implants (tissue integrated prosthesis)

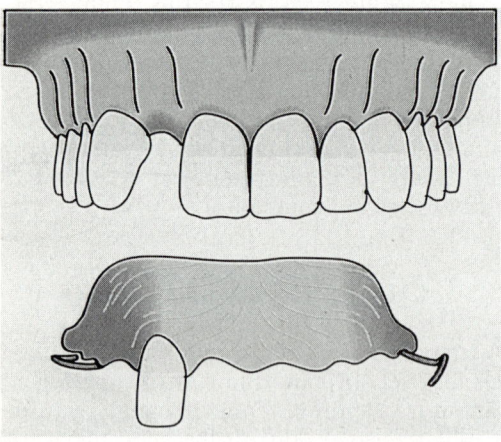

Figure 1 Temporary removable partial denture, constructed of acrylic, provides interim esthetics but limited function. (Courtesy of Nobelpharma U.S.A., Inc., Westmont, Il.)

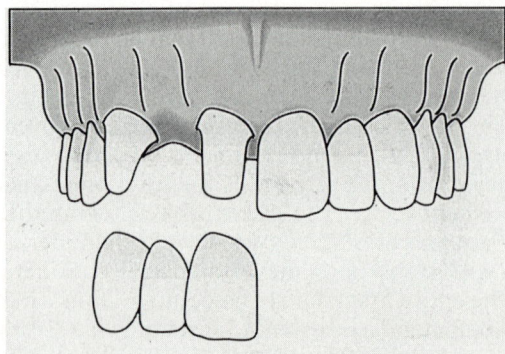

Figure 2 Traditional fixed partial denture firmly replaces a missing tooth but requires the removal of enamel from adjacent healthy teeth. (Courtesy of Nobelpharma U.S.A., Inc., Westmont, Il.)

Following trauma, the soft tissue morphology changes as the edema diminishes. Therefore, an interim restoration is recommended before the construction of a final fixed prosthesis. This healing time serves well to permit the patient time to accommodate to both the concept of a fixed prosthesis, as well as the physical change in the mouth. The complete reduction of edema in the healing edentulous ridge is necessary to establish a physiologic relationship between fixed replacement teeth and the remaining vital tissues. This period also provides the patient an opportunity to learn new oral hygiene methods required to maintain a healthy mucosal response to the prosthesis.

The *advantage* of a traditional fixed partial denture is the stability of the restoration and its esthetic value. The greatest *disadvantage* of this prosthesis is the biologic insult to the abutment teeth. Removal of enamel and dentin frequently lead to insult of the pulp requiring subsequent endodontic (root canal) treatment. In addition, the margins of the crowns, when placed subgingivally (below the gum lines), can lead to periodontal insult and subsequent gingival irritation and alveolar bone loss.

Resin-Bonded Fixed Partial Denture (Maryland Bridge)

Advancement in enamel bonding during the past 3 decades permits the replacement of small numbers of teeth with resin bonded retainers. These fixed bridges can be used as an interim form of tooth replacement, and, in some rare cases, as a long-term form of prosthetic treatment.

Resin bonded retainers rely on the ability to isolate healthy, clean enamel on the adjacent abutment teeth and produce a mechano-chemical bond between the metallic wings of the prosthesis and the abutment tooth enamel (Fig. 3).

Bonded Strength

Careful patient selection is essential for the effective use of a resin bonded fixed partial denture. Adequate occlusal (bite) clearance for the lingual retentive wings

must be determined in advance. The strength and longevity of this prosthesis is only as strong as the resin bond between the enamel and the base metal alloy of the restoration. When the design relies totally on the bond strength, these bridges become loose and often fall out within 5 years.

Alloy Allergies

Resin bonded bridges are generally constructed with base metal alloys usually containing nickel. Patients with known allergies to the contents of the base metal alloys

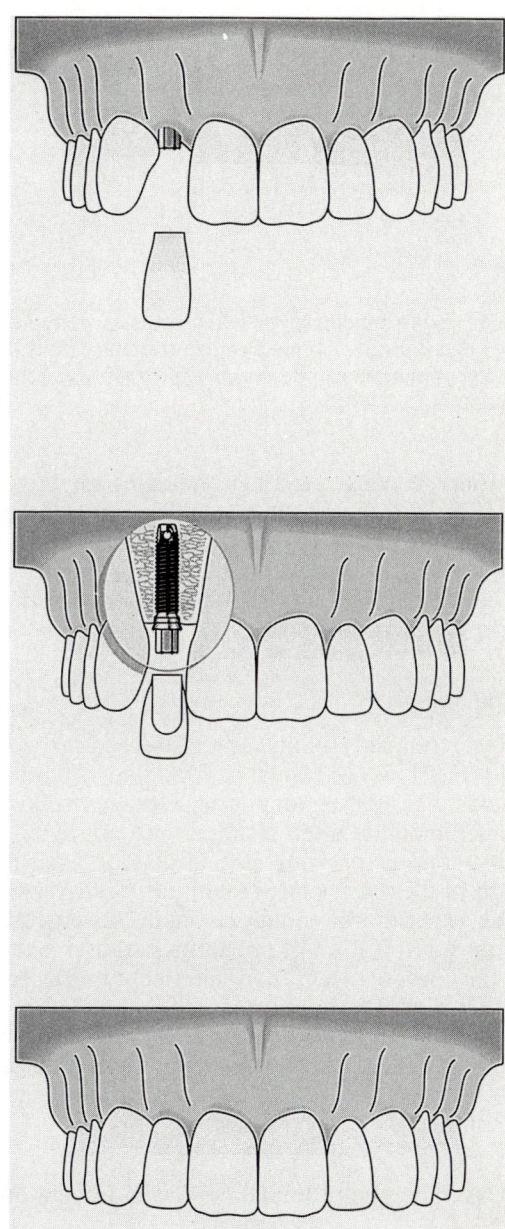

Figure 4 State-of-the-art replacement of a traumatically lost tooth relies on osseointegration of a Branemark implant in the alveolus followed by the placement of a ceramic crown. (Courtesy of Nobelpharma U.S.A., Inc., Westmont, Il.)

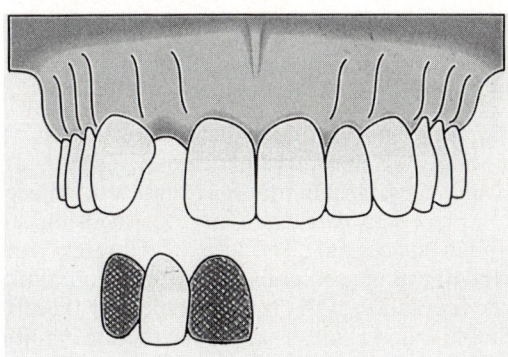

Figure 3 A resin bonded fixed partial denture relies on the bond strength of resin between enamel and the base metal alloy. (Courtesy of Nobelpharma U.S.A., Inc., Westmont, Il.)

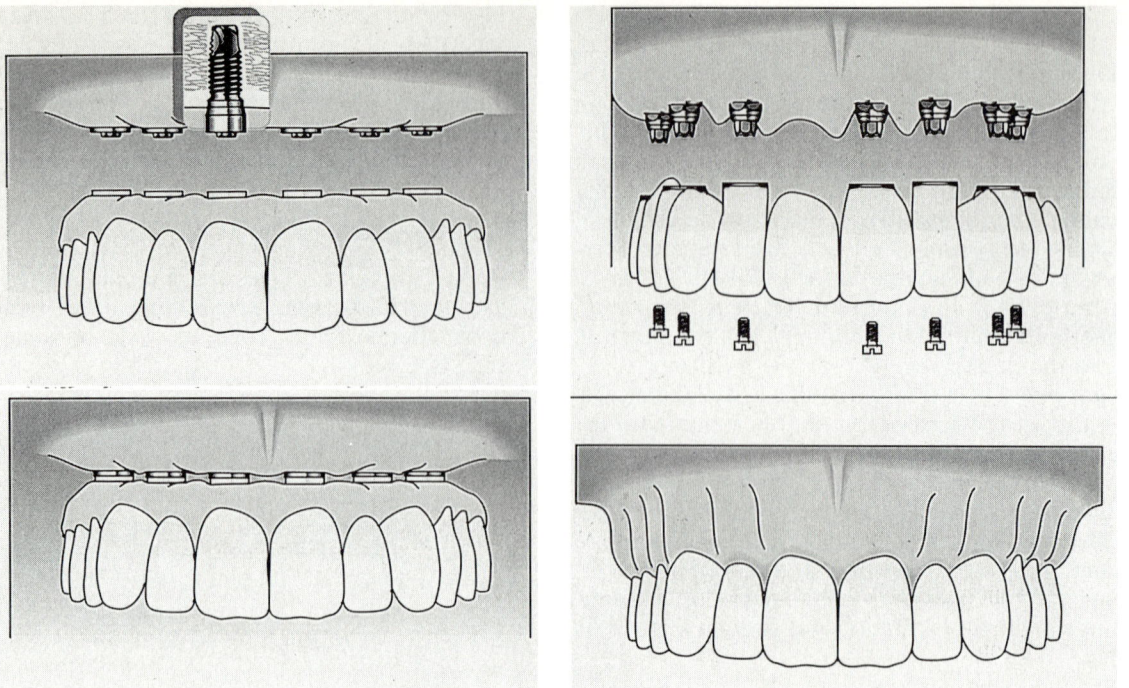

A   B

Figure 5 *A,* An implant supported prosthesis can replace not only missing teeth but missing alveolar bone and mucosal tissue (gum tissue) when these structures have been traumatically lost. *B,* When only tooth is lost and overlying mucosa retained, an implant supported prosthesis can be constructed simply to replace the missing tooth structure. (Courtesy of Nobelpharma U.S.A., Inc., Westmont, Il.)

should not be considered as candidates for this treatment. Increased allergies to metals containing nickel and beryllium have been reported particularly in females. Patients who brux or clench are not good candidates for resin bonded bridges and should be treated with more strongly retained prostheses.

Bonded Splints

Resin bonded splints are also used to stabilize mobile teeth as a result of traumatic injuries. In situations like these, long-term root resorption and continued mobility often result.

The concept of using a resin bonded fixed partial denture, or the resin bonded retaining splints, have many positive aspects and equally as many drawbacks. The advantage of this form of prosthesis is that it is thought to be the conservative form of abutment tooth preparation. Historically, however, it is well noted that frequent maintenance problems are often found with inadequately designed resin bonded fixed partial dentures or splints unless extensive abutment preparation has been accomplished.

Osseointegrated Implants (Tissue Integrated Prosthesis)

Osseointegration is the long-term intimate relationship of ordered living bone fusing to the surface of a load bearing titanium implant. The use of osseointegrated implants today may be considered the most biologically

conservative form of replacement for patients who have sustained traumatic tooth loss (Fig. 4).

Implant Placement Secondary To Alveolar Ridge Healing

Following severe traumatic loss of numerous teeth and the alveolar ridge, as often seen in high speed impact accidents, the edentulous ridge should usually be allowed to heal initially before fixture (implant) placement. This permits complete mucosal closure over the remaining alveolar bone. Careful treatment planning is necessary to determine precise fixture position, long axis angulation, and implant distribution relative to the potential loading forces created by the implant supported prosthesis.

Guided Bone Regeneration Around Implants

Recently some studies have shown that various barrier materials used to enhance osseous generation in areas of voids, frequently encountered adjacent to fixtures placed in extraction or root avulsion sockets, have been successful. The use of Goretex has been reported to produce osseous generation around titanium fixtures (implants). Others have reported the effect of resorbable Vicryl mesh as a barrier to inhibit the ingrowth of epithelium around Branemark fixtures where osseous voids are encountered at the time of initial fixture placement.

Generally sports injuries to the teeth are nonrepeti-

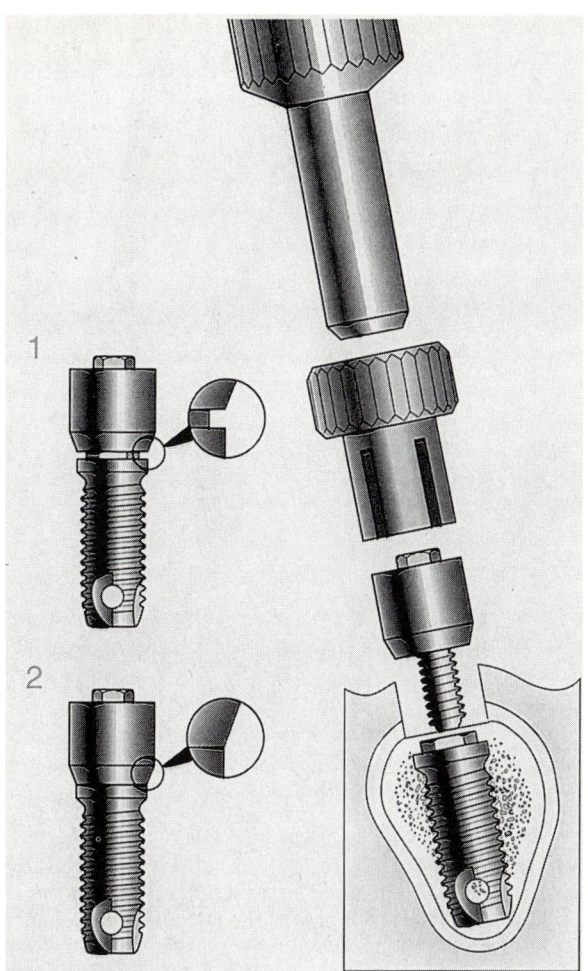

Figure 6 After the appropriate healing time the fixture is reexposed and the titanium abutment securely fastened after aligning the interlocking hex between the cylinder and the top of the implant. (Courtesy of Nobelpharma U.S.A., Inc., Westmont, Il.)

tive and permit the patient to proceed with complete prosthodontic rehabilitation after a normal course of healing. In light of this biologic conservatism, however, one must also consider the professional athlete where the potential for repeated injury does exist.

Removable Prostheses Versus Fixed Implant Supported Prostheses

In some circumstances professional athletes who have lost some of their anterior teeth can benefit greatly from permanent tooth replacement with osseointegrated implants. Such examples might be professional boxers and hockey players who sustain high-impact trauma to the anterior dentition. When such athletes continue in their professional careers, careful consideration should be given to whether or not the use of a fixed implant supported prosthesis is advisable. Because osseointegration by definition is the intimate contact of ordered living bone on the surface of a load carrying implant, without a soft tissue interface, there is absolutely no mobility to

the implant fixture. Without a ligament, any impact to the implant supported bridge will convey the same impact to the underlying bone. A sudden blow to the prosthesis can create microfractures to the bone, thereby destroying osseointegration, leading ultimately to the failure of the bone anchored unit through the development of fibrous encapsulation.

When professional athletes continue to compete, the clinician may consider the use of osseointegrated implants to support a removable appliance with a resilient interface between the prosthetic teeth and the osseointegrated fixtures. Such appliances can be constructed in the form of overdentures with soft tissue liners. Gold clip bars frequently serve as one of the best mechanisms for overdenture retention.

Athletes should be warned that severe impact to the implants can destroy the bone implant interface. Under these circumstances, a secondary appliance should be constructed to prevent implant impact. Mouth guard appliances serve well to protect these implants. During competition, the professional hockey player, the boxer, and other contact sport athletes might do well to remove the implant supported overdenture and replace it with a specially designed mouth guard to avoid implant fractures caused by impact. For these same athletes a nonremovable prosthesis may be constructed to be used during the off season.

Because the Branemark implant system uses gold set screws to retain the prosthetic components, the bar retainer for the overdenture may be very easily unscrewed and removed at the end of the season and a fixed prosthesis secured with the same fastening screws. At the end of the off season, the athlete may again change from a nonremovable prosthesis to the removable overdenture.

A variety of implant prostheses can be constructed to provide prosthetic replacement for missing dentition as well as supporting alveolar and mucosal tissues. Figure 5 shows two types of prostheses supported by Branemark osseointegrated implants; one requires prosthetic replacement of lost alveolar tissue (Fig. 5, *A*), the other takes advantage of adequate alveolar and mucosal support (Fig. 5, *B*).

BRANEMARK IMPLANT TREATMENT PROCESS

In order to attain osseointegration, implants must be placed in the alveolar or basal bone and allowed to remain undisturbed for 5 to 6 months in the maxillary (upper) jaw and 3 to 4 months in the mandibular (lower) jaw. During this initial healing stage the patient can be temporarily restored with a provisional light weight acrylic removable denture. Alternative forms of temporary prosthesis also include resin bonded teeth or fixed provisional crown and bridge restorations. After the prescribed healing period, a second stage surgery is performed to re-expose the implant and add an extension called the abutment, to which the permanent teeth are ultimately fastened (Fig. 6).

The hardware consists of very special sharp instru-

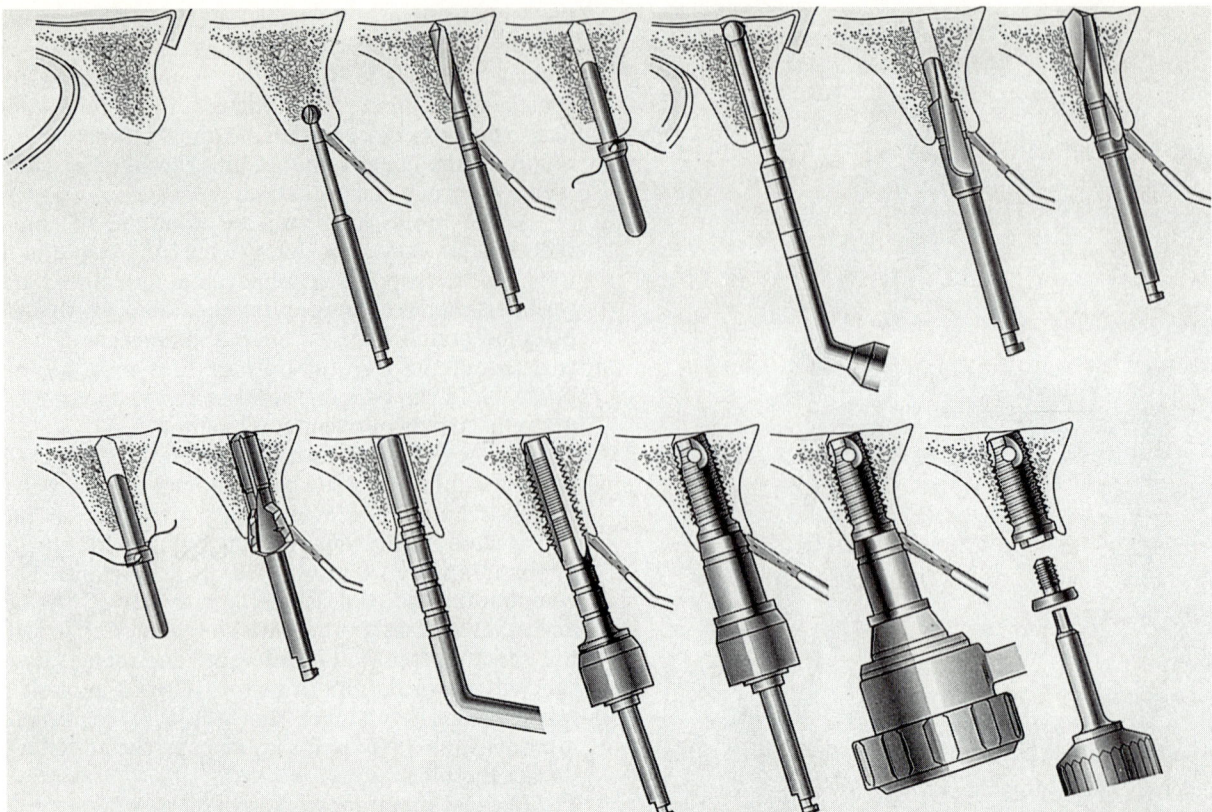

Figure 7 Fixture installation. Sequential drilling to prepare the osteotomy site is performed with single use disposable carbon steel drills and taps. *Top row:* Mucoperiosteal flap, round pilot drill perforates cortical plate, 2 mm diameter twist drill establishes implant depth, guidepin confirms long axis angulation, measuring instrument used to determine exact length of the implant, 3 mm diameter pilot drill starts the final preparation, 3 mm twist drill completes the depth of preparation. *Bottom row:* 3 mm diameter guidepin confirms angulation, counter sink prepares the crestal bone, the final measurement determined, titanium tap establishes threads in areas of dense bone, implant placed at 15 to 20 RPM, final hand tightening of implant in bone, removal of carrying device and placement of cover screw prior to mucosal closure. (Courtesy of Nobelpharma U.S.A., Inc., Westmont, Il.)

ments (Fig. 7) and noncontaminated, commercially pure titanium implants (Fig. 8) and abutments (Fig. 9) with a particular surface microarchitecture. These components must be manufactured from a correct bulk metal (CP titanium) and must have an oxide cover with the right characteristics down to the molecular level. Even minor deviations in the titanium oxide can result in the incorrect attachment or arrangement of the early proteins in the wound as it heals.

The software consists of procedures that assure a very gentle tissue handling and careful preparation, recognizing the fact that we are dealing with a wound and that we are creating a defect in the bone that is similar to a fracture. We have to respect that the tissue needs undisturbed healing until the young bone tissue can be made to remodel under functional load (see Fig. 7).

SURGICAL PROCEDURE

Stage I: Implant Installation

A mucoperiosteal flap generally in the labial fold permits access to the area of the jaw bone where the

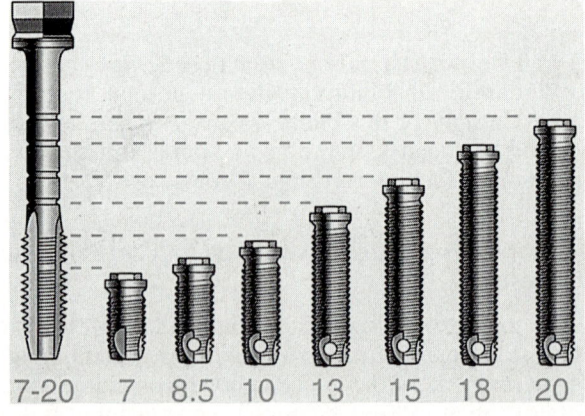

Figure 8 Proper depth for different fixtures is indicated on the screw taps as well as various measuring instruments used during stage I surgery. (Courtesy of Nobelpharma U.S.A., Inc., Westmont, Il.)

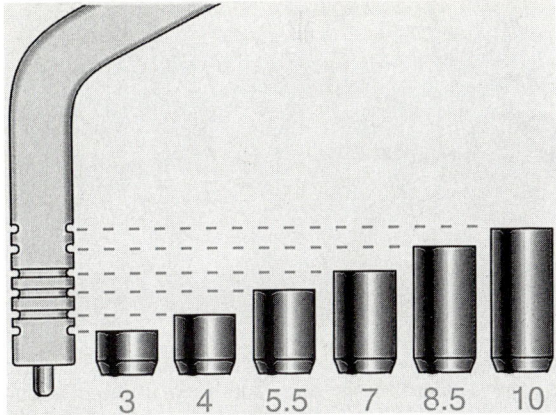

Figure 9 Standard abutments. At stage II surgery, a variety of both standard and special abutments are available. The depth gauge has six markings to indicate the different heights for standard abutments. (Courtesy of Nobelpharma U.S.A., Inc., Westmont, Il.)

implants will be installed (see Fig. 1). Anterior borders of the maxillary sinuses and the lower border of the piriform aperture should be identified. Evaluate any concavities on the buccal aspect of the alveolar crest, especially in the region of the lateral incisors.

All of the "drills" are single use carbine steel with maximum sharpness to minimize heat of friction. The entire procedure is accompanied by copious saline irrigation for cooling. The cortical layer and a small amount of trabecular bone are penetrated with a round guide drill. Then a 2 mm diameter twist drill is used to prepare the initial long axis angulation for implant placement. The implant site is then widened with a pilot drill and finally a 3 mm twist drill prepares the receptor site (see Fig. 7, *top row*). Assuming there is sufficient cortical bone, countersinking the fixture site should be performed. If the maxillary bone is dense, pretapping threads into the bone may be necessary (Fig. 7, *bottom center*). The implant with attached fixture mount is picked up with the drill machine and rotated into the alveolar bone at 15 to 20 RPMs. When the fixture is fully seated, the fixture mount is disconnected and removed. A cover screw is then manually tightened onto the top of the fixture to prevent bone from growing into the internal threads (see Fig. 7, *bottom right*). The area is then thoroughly cleansed and the mucoperiosteal flap sutured closed.

Stage II: Abutment Connection

After the prescribed healing period for osseointegration, generally 5 to 6 months in the maxilla and 3 to 4 months in the mandible, the second stage surgery is performed to expose the implant. The cover screw is removed and the appropriate titanium abutment placed.

A variety of abutments are available for various prosthetic purposes. Standard abutments, however, are most commonly used (see Fig. 9) and are available in sizes ranging from 3 to 10 mm in height depending on

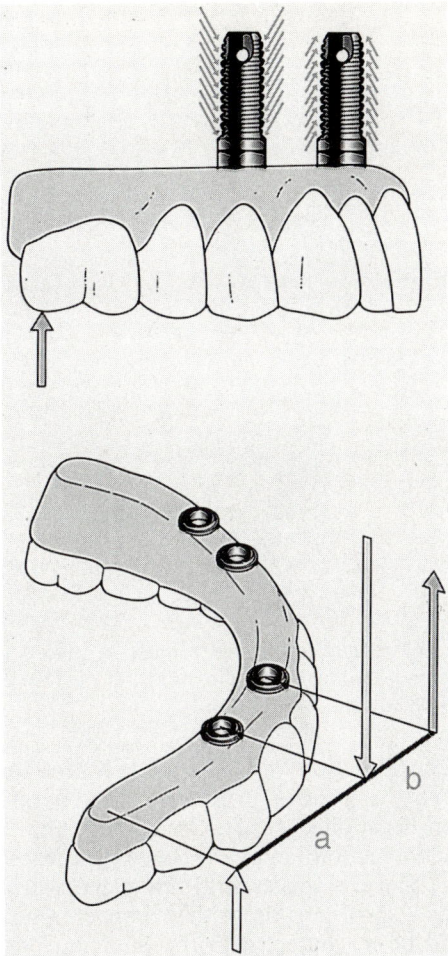

Figure 10 Spreading the implants across the edentulous area is important for load distribution to the underlying alveolar bone. (Courtesy of Nobelpharma U.S.A., Inc., Westmont, Il.)

mucosal thickness. The titanium abutment is retained to the fixture with a titanium abutment screw. Interlocking male and female hexagonal components must be aligned to fit on top of the fixture properly (see Fig. 6). Before final tightening an abutment clamp should be used to rotate the abutment cylinder to ensure the appropriate interlocking of the hexagonal faces. After the abutments are installed the mucosal tissue is sutured, if necessary, to achieve a close adaptation between the soft tissue and the titanium abutments. The precision fit of the implants to the abutments must be verified radiographically. The prosthetic reconstruction can then be carried out. The final prosthesis is retained using small gold set screws as illustrated (see Fig. 5, *B*).

BIOMECHANICAL CONSIDERATIONS

Biomechanical considerations for construction of a tissue integrated prosthesis are important for patients who have sustained traumatic injuries to the alveolar bone. When alveolar bone is weakened through trauma, fracture, or because of the nature of the bone itself,

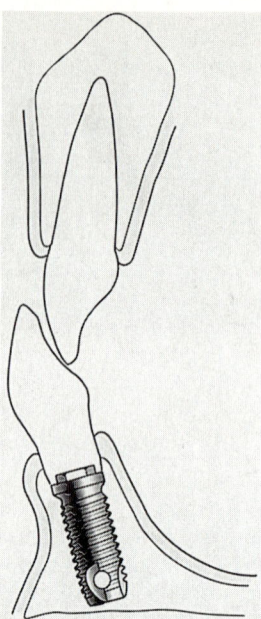

Figure 11 A single tooth fixture must be placed to permit optimal bone loading in all directions. (Courtesy of Nobelpharma U.S.A., Inc., Westmont, Il.)

special consideration should be made for loading forces applied to the implant prosthesis. In general, several rules can be applied easily. Osseointegration is direct bone anchorage to titanium. If the implant receptor site has large marrow spaces with few osseous trabeculae, then only a small portion of the compact bone (trabeculae) will be in contact with the implant. Under such circumstances multiple fixtures should be used to attempt to increase the bone volume in contact with the titanium fixtures. The more fixtures, the more bone surface will be osseointegrated in that arch.

BONE REMODELING

The concept of gradual loading is combined surgical/prosthodontic methodology. Knowledge of the bone quality and quantity is integrated in an empirical formula with the number of fixtures used to support any given prosthesis.

Should a patient present with evidence of parafunctional habits, such as bruxing and clenching, soft loading of the newly uncovered implants with a soft denture liner will limit the amount of force applied to the fixtures. Gentle loading creates a remodeling stimulus to the bone surrounding the implants. As the remodeling increases the density and amount of cortical bone around the fixtures over the loading time, other more rigid prosthesis attachment methods may be employed.

In the large prosthesis used to replace multiple missing teeth, the implants constitute bridge posts that share the applied functional loads as axial forces between them. Spreading implants evenly along the arch enables this axial load distribution (Fig. 10). In smaller restorations with shorter spans, this geometric implant

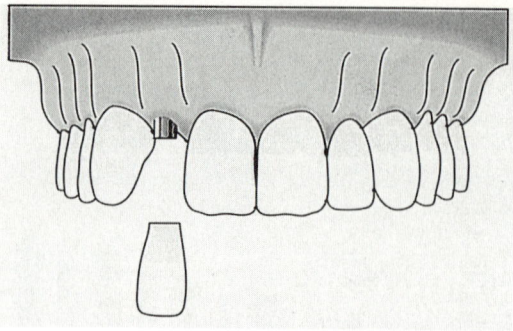

Figure 12 A crown consisting of an aluminum oxide ceramic core is constructed for the single tooth replacement. (Courtesy of Nobelpharma U.S.A., Inc., Westmont, Il.)

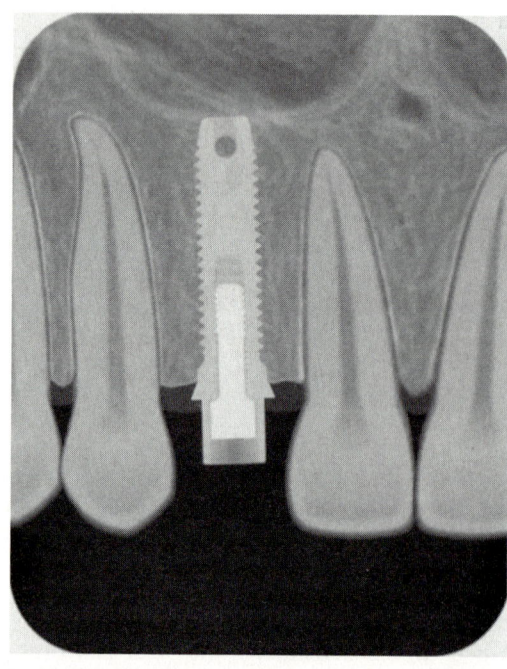

Figure 13 Radiographic illustration of the ideal implant position with the titanium abutment in place. (Courtesy of Nobelpharma U.S.A., Inc., Westmont, Il.)

spread is not always possible. In such cases, it is appropriate to look at the implant as being an artificial tooth root rather than a bridge post, because it may have to withstand load in all directions from the connected prosthesis. A small implant supported partial prosthesis, or a single tooth implant (Fig. 11), is more sensitive to the precise and detailed placement and anchorage of the fixtures than are full arch, or large multiple fixture supported prostheses.

SINGLE TOOTH REPLACEMENT WITH TITANIUM IMPLANTS

A single tooth replacement in the maxillary anterior part of the jaw means the replacement of a missing natural tooth with a fixture approximately the same dimension as the missing tooth root. If the fixture in such a case is as long as the missing natural root and has the same amount of bone support as the natural root once did, sufficient bone strength can be expected. Generally, ample bone is available for the placement of an implant, which can be considerably longer than the natural root, providing exceptionally good anchorage.

Single tooth replacement is used most frequently for traumatic injuries where tooth avulsion occurs and the alveolar bone remains relatively intact. The placement of a Branemark fixture into the alveolar ridge beyond the apex of the missing tooth provides ideal anchorage for a single tooth replacement (Figs. 12 and 13). The prosthesis itself can be constructed of porcelain fused to a high gold content substructure or to high strength ceramic core.

In the posterior part of the jaw, a single fixture does not correspond to the lost root support of a molar, which ordinarily has multiple roots of approximately the same dimension as the implants. In this situation, if space is available, multiple implants should be used to replace a single molar. Considering these factors, in combination with the fact that loading forces are at their greatest in the posterior region of the mouth, it is easy to understand that a single fixture used in the molar region may be subjected to excessive forces that may fracture the bone/implant interface.

SUGGESTED READING

Adel R, Lekholm U, Rockler B, et al. A 15 year study of osseointegrated implants in the treatment of the edentulous jaw. Int J Oral Surg 1981; 10:327-416.

Albrektsson T, Zarb G, Worthington P, et al. The long-term efficacy of currently used dental implants: A review and proposed criteria of success. Int J Oral Maxillofac Implant 1986; 1:11-25.

Balshi T. Preventing and resolving complications with osseointegrated implants. Dent Clin North Am 1989; 33:821-868.

Balshi T: First molar replacement with an osseointegrated implant. Quintessence Int 1990; 21:61-65.

Becker B. The use of guided tissue regeneration for implants placed in immediate extraction sockets. Presented at the 2nd International Congress on Tissue Integration in Oral, Orthopedic, and Maxillofacial Reconstruction. Mayo Medical Center, Rochester, MN, Sept, 1990.

Branemark P-I. Surgical procedure manual. The Branemark system. Gothenburg, 1992.

Branemark P-I, Zarb G, Albrektsson T. Tissue integrated prosthesis — Osseointegration in clinical dentistry. Chicago: Quintessence, 1985.

van Steenberghe D. A retrospective multicenter evaluation of the survival rate of osseointegrated fixtures supporting fixed partial prostheses in the treatment of partial edentulism. J Prosthet Dent 1989; 61:217-223.

SPINAL INJURIES

CERVICAL SPINE INJURIES

JOSEPH S. TORG, M.D.

Athletic injuries to the cervical spine may involve the bony vertebrae, intervertebral discs, ligamentous supporting structures, the spinal cord, roots, and peripheral nerves, or any combination of these structures. The panorama of injuries observed runs the spectrum from the "cervical sprain syndrome" to fracture-dislocations with permanent quadriplegia. Fortunately, severe injuries with neural involvement occur infrequently. However, those responsible for the emergency and subsequent care of the athlete with a cervical spine injury should possess a basic understanding of the variety of problems that can occur.

The various athletic injuries to the cervical spine and related structures are (1) nerve root-brachial plexus neurapraxia, (2) stable cervical sprain, (3) muscular strain, (4) nerve root-brachial plexus axonotmesis, (5) intervertebral disc injury (narrowing-herniation) without neurologic deficit, (6) stable cervical fractures without neurologic deficit, (7) subluxations without neurologic deficit, (8) unstable fractures without neurologic deficit, (9) dislocations without neurologic deficit, (10) intervertebral disc herniation with neurologic deficit, (11) unstable fracture with neurologic deficit, (12) dislocation with neurologic deficit, (13) quadriplegia, and (14) death.

Criteria for return to contact activities following congenital and traumatic problems of the cervical spine are included in a subsequent chapter.

NERVE ROOT-BRACHIAL PLEXUS NEURAPRAXIA

The most common and poorly understood cervical injuries are the pinch-stretch neurapraxias of the nerve roots and brachial plexus. Typically, after contact with head, neck, or shoulder, a sharp burning pain is experienced in the neck on the involved side that may radiate into the shoulder and down the arm to the hand. There may be associated weakness and paresthesia in the involved extremity lasting from several seconds to several minutes. Characteristically, there is weakness of shoulder abduction (deltoid), elbow flexion (biceps), and external humeral rotation (spinati). The key to the nature of this lesion is its short duration and the presence of a full, pain-free range of neck motion. Although most of these injuries are short-lived, they are worrisome because of the occasional plexus axonotmesis that occurs. However, the youngster whose paresthesia completely abates, who demonstrates full muscle strength in the intrinsic muscles of the shoulder and upper extremities, and who, most importantly, has a full, pain-free range of cervical motion, may return to activity.

Persistence of paresthesia, weakness, or limitation of cervical motion requires that the individual be protected from further exposure and that neurologic, electromyographic, and roentgenographic evaluations are performed.

ACUTE CERVICAL SPRAIN SYNDROME

An acute cervical sprain is a collision injury frequently seen in contact sports. The patient complains of having "jammed" the neck, with subsequent pain localized to the cervical area. Characteristically, the patient presents with limitation of cervical spine motion, but without radiation of pain or paresthesia. Neurologic examination is negative and roentgenograms are normal.

Stable cervical sprains and strains eventually resolve with or without treatment. Initially, the presence of a serious injury should be ruled out by a thorough neurologic examination and determination of the range of cervical motion. Range of motion is evaluated by having the athlete actively nod his head; touch his chin to his chest; extend his neck maximally; touch his chin to his left shoulder; touch his chin to his right shoulder; touch his left ear to his left shoulder; and touch his right ear to his right shoulder. If the patient is unwilling or unable to perform these maneuvers actively while standing erect, proceed no further. The athlete with less than a full, pain-free range of cervical motion, persistent paresthesia, or weakness should be protected and excluded from activity. Subsequent evaluation should include appropriate roentgenographic studies, including flexion and extension views, to demonstrate fractures or instability.

In general, treatment of athletes with "cervical sprains" should be tailored to the degree of severity. Immobilizing the neck in a soft collar and using analgesics and anti-inflammatory agents until there is a full, spasm-free range of neck motion is appropriate. It should be emphasized that individuals with a history of collision injury, pain, and limited cervical motion should have routine cervical spine roentgenograms. Also, lateral flexion and extension roentgenograms are indicated after the acute symptoms subside. Marked limitation of cervical motion, persistent pain, and/or radicular symptoms or findings may require a MR scan to rule out intervertebral disc injury.

INTERVERTEBRAL DISC INJURIES

Acute herniation of a cervical intervertebral disc associated with neurologic findings occurring as an isolated entity is rare in the athlete. However, with an acute onset of quadriplegia occurring in an athlete who has sustained head impact with negative cervical spine roentgenograms, an acute rupture of a cervical intervertebral disc should be considered. The syndrome of acute anterior spinal cord injury, as described by Schneider, may be observed: "an immediate acute paralysis of all four extremities with a loss of pain and temperature to the level of the lesion, but with preservation of posterior column sensation of motion, position, vibration and part of touch." The pressure of the disc is on the anterior and lateral columns, while the posterior columns are protected by the denticulate ligaments. MRI should be performed to substantiate the diagnosis. Anterior discectomy and interbody fusion for a patient with neurologic involvement or persistent disability because of pain should be considered.

Albright et al studied 75 University of Iowa freshmen football recruits who had roentgenograms of their cervical spines after having played in high school, but before playing in college. Of the group, 32% had one or more of the following: "occult" fracture, vertebral body compression fractures, intervertebral disc-space narrowing, or other degenerative changes. Of this group, only 13% admitted to a positive history of neck symptoms. The development of early degenerative changes or intervertebral disc-space narrowing in this group was attributed to the effect of repetitive loading on the cervical spine as a result of head impact from blocking and tackling.

Acute and chronic cervical intervertebral disc injury without frank herniation or neurologic findings occur with considerable frequency in the athlete. Associated with a history of injury are neck pain and limited cervical spine motion. Roentgenograms may demonstrate disc space narrowing and marginal osteophytes. MR scans frequently demonstrate disc bulge without herniation. In general, management is conservative with the youngster being precluded from activity until he or she is asymptomatic and has achieved a full range of cervical spine motion.

CERVICAL VERTEBRAL SUBLUXATION WITHOUT FRACTURE

Axial compression-flexion injuries incurred by striking an object with the top of the helmet can result in disruption of the posterior soft-tissue supporting elements with angulation and anterior translation of the superior cervical vertebrae. Fractures of the bony elements are not demonstrated on roentgenograms, and the patient has no neurologic deficit. Flexion-extension roentgenograms demonstrate instability of the cervical spine at the involved level manifested by motion, anterior intervertebral disc-space narrowing, anterior angulation and displacement of the vertebral body, and fanning of the spinous processes. I believe that demonstrable instability on lateral flexion-extension roentgenograms in a young, vigorous individual requires aggressive treatment. When soft-tissue disruption occurs without an associated fracture, it is likely that instability will result despite conservative treatment. When anterior subluxation greater than 20% of the vertebral body is due to disruption of the posterior supporting structures, a posterior cervical fusion is recommended.

UPPER CERVICAL SPINE FRACTURES AND DISLOCATIONS

Upper cervical spine lesions involve C1 through C3. Although rarely occurring in sports, several specific injuries to the upper cervical vertebrae deserve mention. The transverse and alar ligaments are responsible for atlantoaxial stability. With rupture of these structures resulting from a flexion injury, with translation of C1 anteriorly, the spinal cord can become impinged between a posterior aspect of the odontoid process and the posterior rim of C1. The patient gives a history of head trauma and complains of neck pain, particularly with nodding, and may or may not present with cord signs. Roentgenographically, lateral views of the C1-C2 articulation demonstrate increase of the atlantodens interval (ADI). This interval is normally 3 mm in the adult. With transverse ligament rupture it may increase up to 10 to 12 mm, depending on the status of the alar and accessory ligaments. Note that increase in the ADI may only be seen with the neck flexed. Fielding states that atlantoaxial fusion may be the "conservative" treatment for this lesion. He recommended posterior C1-C2 fusion using wire fixation and iliac bone graft.

Fractures of the atlas were described by Jefferson in 1920. These may be of two types: posterior arch fractures and burst fractures. Posterior arch fractures are the more common of the two, and with a brace support go onto satisfactory fibrous or bony union. Burst fractures result from an axial load transmitted to the occipital condyles, which then disrupt the integrity of both the anterior and posterior arches of the atlas. Roentgenograms demonstrate bilateral symmetric overhang of the lateral masses of the atlas, in relationship to the axis, with increase in the paraodontoid space on the open-mouth view. Clinically, the patient characteristically demonstrates pain and imitation of the nodding motion. These fractures are considered stable when the combined lateral overhang of the atlas measures less than 7 mm. When the transverse diameter of the atlas is 7 mm greater than that of the axis, a transverse ligament rupture should be suspected.

Treatment, as recommended by Fielding, includes head-halter traction until muscle spasm resolves, followed by a brace support. If flexion-extension roentgenograms subsequently demonstrate significant instability, fusion may be indicated.

Fractures of the odontoid have been classified into three types by Anderson and D'Alonzo. Type I is an avulsion of the tip of the odontoid at the site of the attachment of the alar ligament and is a rare and stable lesion. Type II is a fracture through the base, at or just below the level of the superior articular processes. Type III involves a fracture of the body of the axis. When not displaced, planograms may be required to identify the lesion.

The mechanism of odontoid fractures has not been clearly delineated. However, they appear to be due to head impact. All routine cervical spine roentgenographic studies should include the open-mouth view to identify lesions involving the odontoid as well as the atlas. If these are negative, and if a lesion in this area is suspected, planograms or bending films may further delineate pathologic changes in this area.

Managing Type II fractures is a problem. It has been reported that 36% to 50% of these lesions treated initially with plaster casts or reinforced cervical braces fail to unite. Cloward has reported that 85% of his patients heal within 3 months when treated with the halo brace.

It is necessary to surgically stabilize fibrous unions or nonunited fractures of the odontoid if they are demonstrated to be unstable on flexion and extension views. Stabilization may be effected either through posterior C1-C2 wire fixation and fusion or anterior fusion of C1-C2 by a dowel graft through the articular facets, as described by Cloward.

Fractures through the arch of the axis are also known as traumatic spondylolisthesis of C2 or hangman's fracture. These are relatively rare lesions. The mechanism of injury is generally recognized to be hyperextension. This injury is inherently unstable. However, it has been shown to heal with predictable regularity without surgical intervention.

MIDCERVICAL SPINE FRACTURES AND DISLOCATIONS

Acute traumatic lesions of the cervical spine at the C3-C4 level are rare and are generally not associated with fractures. These lesions are classified as follows: (1) acute rupture of the C3-C4 intervertebral disc; (2) anterior subluxation of C3 on C4; (3) unilateral dislocation of the joint between the articular processes; and (4) bilateral dislocation of the joint between the articular processes.

An episode of transient quadriplegia in an athlete who has sustained head impact with a negative cervical spine roentgenogram suggests acute rupture of the C3-C4 intervertebral disc. The syndrome of acute anterior spinal cord injury may be observed. A cervical myelogram or MRI will substantiate the diagnosis. Anterior discectomy and interbody fusion may be the most effective treatment of this lesion.

Anterior subluxation of C3 on C4 is a result of a shearing force through the intervertebral disc space, disrupting the interspinous ligament, as well as the posterior supporting structure. Roentgenograms demonstrate narrowing of the intervertebral disc space, anterior angulation and translation of C3 and C4, an increase in the distance between the spinous processes of the two vertebrae, and instability without fracture of the bony elements. Spine fusion may be necessary for adequate stabilization in such cases, in contrast with instances of cervical spine instability caused by fracture in which adequate reduction and subsequent bony healing results in stability. When the patient has posterior instability, posterior fusion is preferable to an anterior interbody fusion.

Unilateral facet dislocation at C3-C4 may result in immediate quadriparesis. This injury involves the intervertebral disc space, the interspinous ligament, the posterior ligamentous supporting structures, and the one facet with resulting rotatory dislocation of C3 on C4 without fracture. At this level, strong skeletal traction does not yield a successful reduction, and closed manipulation under general anesthesia is necessary to disengage the locked joint between the articular processes.

Bilateral facet dislocation at the C3-C4 level is a grave lesion. Skeletal traction may not reduce the lesion, and the prognosis for this injury is grave.

LOWER CERVICAL SPINE FRACTURES AND DISLOCATIONS

Lower cervical spine fractures or dislocation are those involving C4 through C7. In those injuries that result from various athletic endeavors, the majority of fractures and/or dislocation of the cervical spine, with or without neurologic involvement, involve this segment. Although unilateral and bilateral facet dislocations occur, they are relatively rare. The vast majority of severe athletically incurred cervical spine injuries are fractures of the vertebral body with varying degrees of compression or comminution.

UNILATERAL FACET DISLOCATIONS

Unilateral facet dislocations are the result of axial loading, flexion-rotation type of mechanisms. The lesion may be truly ligamentous without associated vertebral fracture. In such instances, the facet dislocation is stable and is usually associated with neurologic involvement. Roentgenograms demonstrate less than 50% anterior shift of the superior vertebra on the inferior vertebra. Attempts should be made to reduce the facet dislocation by skeletal traction. However, as with similar lesions described at the C3-C4 level, it may not be possible to effect a closed reduction. In this instance, open reduction under direct vision through a posterior approach with supplemental posterior element bone grafting should be performed.

BILATERAL FACET DISLOCATIONS

Bilateral facet dislocations are almost always associated with neurologic involvement. These injuries are associated with a high incidence of quadriplegia. Lateral roentgenograms demonstrate greater than 50% anterior displacement of the superior vertebral body on the inferior vertebral body. Immediate treatment, as previously delineated, is closed reduction with skeletal traction. Such lesions are generally reducible by skeletal traction and then treated by halo-cast stabilization and posterior fusion. It should be noted that instability is directly related to the ease with which the lesion is reduced, since the easier it is to reduce, the easier it is to redislocate. If skeletal traction is unsuccessful, either manipulative reduction under sedation or general anesthesia, or open reduction under direct vision is recommended. When the dislocation is reduced closed, and the reduction maintained, immobilization should be effected by use of the halo cast for 8 to 12 weeks. Corrective bracing should continue for an additional 4 weeks.

VERTEBRAL BODY COMPRESSION FRACTURES

Compression fractures of the vertebral body are a result of axial loading. Vertebral body fractures of the cervical spine can be classified into the following five types:

Type I — Simple wedge or vertebral end plate compression fractures of the cervical vertebrae are common injuries that respond to conservative management and rarely, if ever, are associated with neurologic involvement. It is important that these lesions be differentiated from compression fractures that are associated with disruption of the posterior element soft-tissue supporting structures. The latter lesions are unstable and frequently associated with neurologic involvement, including quadriplegia.

Type II — An isolated anterior-inferior vertebral body or "tear drop" fracture is without displacement, has intact posterior elements, and is not associated with neurologic involvement. This is a relatively stable fracture and may be treated conservatively.

Type III — Comminuted burst vertebral body fractures with intact posterior elements, but displacement of bony fragments into the vertebral canal, may place the cord in jeopardy. Late settling of the fracture with deformity can occur. Surgical stabilization is recommended.

Type IV — The axial load three part-two plane vertebral body fracture consists of three fracture parts: (1) an anteroinferior "teardrop"; (2) sagittal vertebral body fracture; and (3) disruption of the posterior neural arch. This lesion is unstable and almost always associated with quadriplegia. Careful evaluation of the routine anteroposterior roentgenogram or a CT scan is necessary to appreciate the sagittal vertebral body fracture, a finding that portends a grave prognosis.

Type V — Vertebral body three part-two plane compression fracture associated with disruption of posterior elements of an adjacent vertebra. This is an extremely unstable fracture.

CERVICAL FRACTURES AND/OR DISLOCATIONS: MANAGEMENT PRINCIPLES

Fractures and/or dislocations of the cervical spine may be stable or unstable, and may or may not be associated with neurologic deficit. When fracture or disruption of the soft-tissue supporting structure immediately violates or threatens to violate the integrity of the spinal cord, implementation of certain management and treatment principles is imperative. These include (1) protecting the cord from further injury; (2) expeditious reduction; (3) effect rapid and secure stability; and (4) implement an early rehabilitation program (discussed in the chapter *Rehabilitation of the Postinjured/Postoperative Cervical Spine*).

Protection

It has been estimated that many neurologic deficits occur after the initial injury. That is, if a patient with an unstable lesion is carelessly manipulated when being transported to a medical facility or subsequently inappropriately managed, further encroachment on the spinal cord can occur.

Reduction

Once appropriate roentgenograms are obtained and qualified orthopedic and neurosurgical personnel are available, the malaligned cervical spine should be reduced as quickly and gently as possible. This will effectively decompress the spinal cord. When dislocation or anterior angulation and translation are demonstrated roentgenographically, immediate reduction is attempted with skull traction utilizing Gardner-Wells tongs. These tongs can be easily and rapidly applied under local anesthesia, without shaving the head, in the emergency room or in the patient's bed. Since these tongs are spring-loaded, it is unnecessary to drill the outer table of the skull for their application. The tongs are attached to a cervical-traction pulley and weight is added at a rate of 5 lbs/disc space or 25 to 40 lbs for lower cervical injury. Reduction is attempted by adding 5 lbs every 15 to 20 minutes and is monitored by lateral roentgenograms.

Unilateral facet dislocations, particularly at the C3-C4 level, are not always reducible using skeletal traction. In such instances, closed skeletal or manipulative reduction under nasotracheal anesthesia may be necessary. The expediency of early reduction of cervical dislocations must be emphasized.

It has been proposed that the presence of a bulbocavernous reflex indicates that spinal shock has worn off and that, except for the recovery of an occasional root at the injury, neither motor nor sensory paralysis will resolve regardless of treatment. The bulbocavernous reflex is produced by a pulling on the urethral catheter. This stimulates the trigone of the bladder, producing a reflex contraction of the anal sphincter around the examiners gloved finger. Although the presence of a bulbocavernous reflex is generally a sign that there will be no further neurologic recovery below the level of injury, this is not always true. The presence of this reflex does not give the clinician license to handle the situation in an elective fashion. The cervical spine malalignments and dislocations associated with quadriparesis should be reduced as quickly as possible, by whatever means necessary, if maximum recovery is to be expected.

In most instances in which a vertebral body burst fracture is associated with anterior compression of the cord, decompression is logically effected through an anterior approach with an interbody fusion. Likewise, intervertebral disc herniation with cord involvement is best managed through an anterior discectomy and interbody fusion. In cervical fractures and dislocations, posterior cervical laminectomy is indicated only rarely when excision of foreign bodies or bony alignment of the spine is the most effective method for decompression of the cervical cord.

Indications for surgical decompression of the spinal cord have been delineated. A documented increase in neurologic signs is the clearest mandate for surgical decompression. Further observation, expectancy, and procrastination in this situation is contraindicated. Persistent partial cord or root signs, with objective evidence of mechanical compression, is also an indication for surgical intervention.

The use of parenteral corticosteroids to decrease the inflammatory reactions of the injured cord and surrounding soft-tissue structures is indicated in the management of acute cervical spinal cord injury. The efficacy of methyl prednisolone in improving neurologic recovery when given in the first 8 hours has been recently demonstrated. The recommended regiment is a bolus of 30 mg/solidus kg of body weight of methyl prednisolone administered intravenously followed by an infusion of 5.4 mg/kg/hour for 23 hours.

Stabilization

White recognized that the literature is not always clear or consistent in describing what constitutes an unstable cervical spine. Using fresh cadaver specimens, he performed load displacement studies on sectioned and unsectioned two-level cervical spine segments to determine the horizontal translation and rotation in the sagittal plane after each ligament was transected. The experiments constituted a quantitative biomechanical analysis of the effects of destroying ligaments and facets on the stability of the cervical spine below C2 in an attempt to determine cervical stability. The express purpose of the study was to establish indications for treatment methods to stabilize the spine. Although the intent of the study was to define clinical instability to formulate treatment standards and was not intended to establish criteria for a return to contact athletics, it does appear that their findings are relevant to this latter issue.

White described clinical stability as the ability of the spine to limit its patterns of displacement of physiologic loads so as not to damage or irritate the spinal cord or the nerve roots.

White delineated four important findings. First, in sectioning the ligaments, there were small increments of change in stability followed without warning by sudden, complete disruption of the spine under stress. Second, removal of the facets alters the motion segment such that in flexion there is less angular displacement and more horizontal displacement. Third, the anterior ligaments contribute more to stability in extension than the posterior ligaments and in flexion the posterior ligaments contribute more than the anterior ligaments. The fourth and most relevant finding from the standpoint of parameters for return to contact sports is as follows: The adult cervical spine is unstable, on the brink of instability, when any of the following conditions are present: (1) all of the anterior or all of the posterior elements are destroyed or unable to function; (2) more than 3.5 mm horizontal displacement of one vertebra in relationship to an adjacent vertebra measured on lateral roentgenograms (resting or flexion-extension), and/or (3) more than 11 degrees of rotation difference to that of either adjacent vertebra measured on a resting lateral or flexion-extension roentgenogram.

The method of immobilization depends on the postreduction status of the injury. Thompson et al have concisely delineated indications for nonsurgical and surgical methods for achieving stability. These concepts for managing cervical spine fractures and dislocations may be summarized as follows:

1. Patients with stable compression fractures of the vertebral body, undisplaced fractures of the lamina or lateral masses, or soft-tissue injuries without detectable neurologic deficit can be adequately treated with traction and subsequent protection with a cervical brace until healing occurs.
2. Stable, reduced facet dislocation without neurologic deficit can also be treated conservatively in a Halo jacket brace until healing has been demonstrated by negative lateral flexion-extension roentgenograms.
3. Unstable cervical spine fractures or fracture-dislocations without neurologic deficit may require either surgical or nonsurgical methods to insure stability.
4. Absolute indications for surgical stabilization of an unstable injury without neurologic deficit are late instability following closed treatment, and

flexion-rotation injuries with unreduced locked facets.

5. Relative indications for surgical stabilization in unstable injuries without neurologic deficit are anterior subluxation greater than 20%, certain atlantoaxial fractures or dislocations, and unreduced vertical compression injuries.

6. Cervical spine fractures with complete cord lesions require reduction followed by stabilization by closed or open means, as indicated.

7. Cervical spine fractures with incomplete cord lesions require reduction followed by careful evaluation for surgical intervention.

CERVICAL SPINAL STENOSIS WITH CORD NEURAPRAXIA AND TRANSIENT QUADRIPLEGIA

JOSEPH S. TORG, M.D.

In the syndrome of neurapraxia of the cervical spinal cord with transient quadriplegia, the sensory changes include burning pain, numbness, tingling, and loss of sensation, and motor changes range from weakness to complete paralysis in both upper and/or lower extremities. The episodes of transient and complete sensory and motor recovery usually occur in 10 to 15 minutes, although in some patients gradual resolution may occur over 24 to 36 hours. Except for burning paresthesias, pain in the cervical area is not present at the time of injury and there is complete return of motor function and full, pain-free motion of the cervical spine.

Routine roentgenograms of the cervical spine are negative for fracture, subluxation, and dislocation. However, in every instance, roentgenographic findings include developmental cervical spinal narrowing, either as an isolated finding or associated with congenital fusions, ligamentous instability, or intervertebral disc disease (Fig. 1, *A* and *B*).

A review of the literature has revealed few reported cases of transient quadriplegia occurring in athletes. Attempts to establish the occurrence rates indicate that the problem is more prevalent than expected. Specifically, in the population of 39,377 exposed football participants the reported incidence rate for transient paresthesia in all four extremities was six per 10,000 while the incidence rate reported for paresthesia associated with transient quadriplegia was 1.3 per 10,000 in one season surveyed. From these data it appears that the problem is relatively common and an awareness of the etiology, manifestations, and appropriate management principles are warranted.

There has been sparse documentation in the literature of the syndrome that we call cervical spinal cord neurapraxia. Grant and Puffer reported a case of quadriplegia that occurred in an 18-year-old football player with developmental cervical stenosis. Stratford published an account of a professional football player who had a minimal transient neurologic deficit following a hyperextension injury to his cervical spine. Funk presented two cases of temporary quadriplegia occurring in football players. One, who had suffered two episodes of generalized numbness and paralysis that lasted only a few seconds following hyperextension of his neck, had reportedly normal roentgenogram, myelogram, and neurologic examination. The second, a professional player, was temporarily rendered quadriplegic following neck hyperflexion.

Multiple investigators have reported the measurement of the sagittal diameter of the cervical spinal canal as a means to diagnose spinal stenosis. These reports have resulted in inconsistencies in "normal" and "abnormal" values for the sagittal diameter of the cervical spine. Of the various techniques and measurements reported, the most commonly employed method for determining the sagittal spinal canal diameter utilizing the lateral roentgenographic view of the cervical spine measures the distance from the middle of the posterior surface of the vertebral body to the nearest point of the corresponding spinal laminar line, which Wilkinson called the pre-existing sagittal diameter. The actual millimeter measurement of the sagittal diameter as determined by the conventional method is misleading both as reported in the literature and in actual practice due to variations in the target distance used in obtaining the roentgenogram and the landmarks used for obtaining the measurement.

Boijsen investigated the cause of variation in the reported radiographic measurements of the sagittal diameter of the cervical spinal canal and evaluated the effects of the following two factors: (1) the focus to film (F/F), distance, i.e., the target distance, and (2) the object to film (O/F) distance, i.e., the cervical spine to cassette, the object distance. He reported that the effect of a difference between a 1 m and 1.5 m F/F distance on the resultant sagittal canal measurement is 0.5 mm. To evaluate the effects of the O/F distance, he calculated that the average difference in shoulder breadth between men and women is 10 cm or approximately a 5 cm difference in the O/F distance. The effect of a 5 cm difference in the O/F distance on the resultant sagittal canal measurement is 1.2 mm at a F/F distance of 1.0 m and 0.7 mm at a F/F distance of 1.5 m.

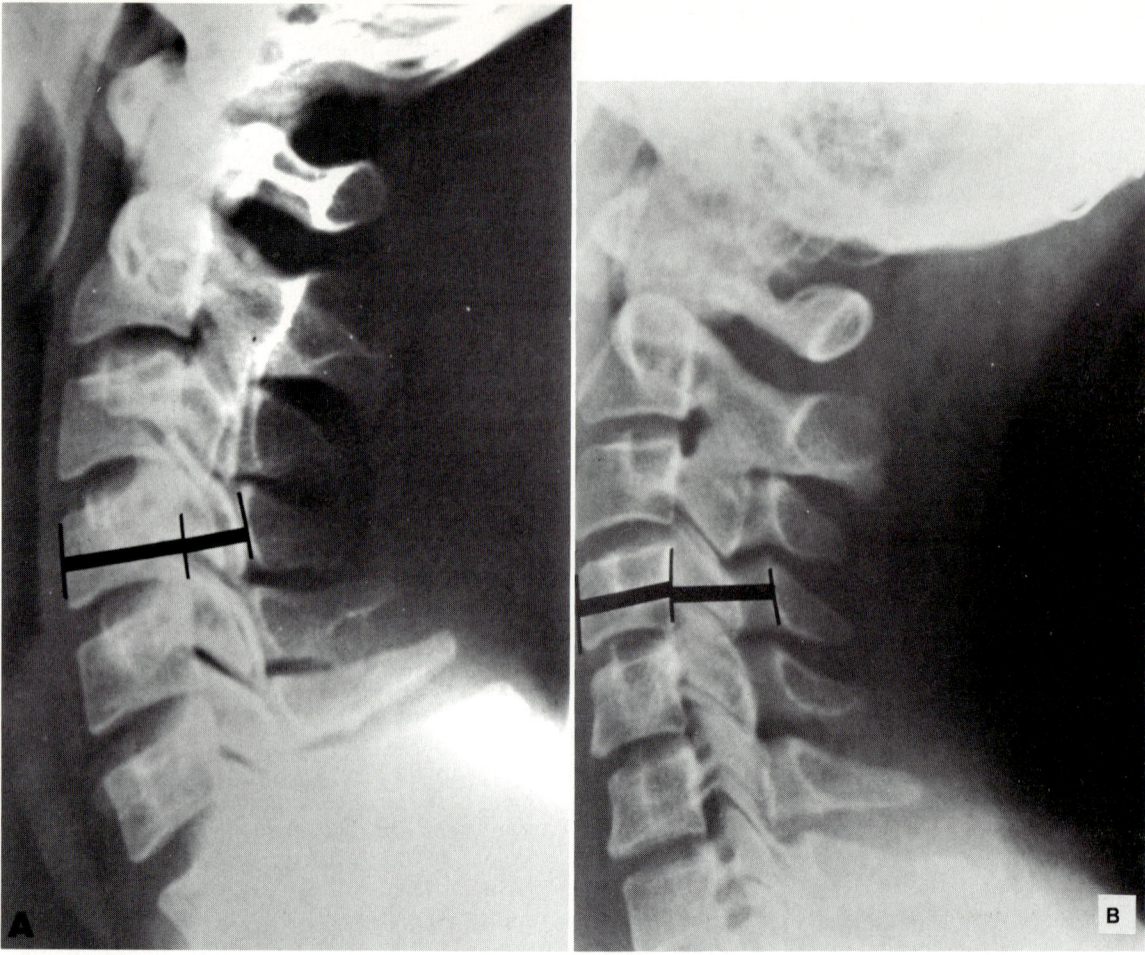

Figure 1 Comparison between the ratio of the spinal canal to the vertebral body of a "normal" control subject with that of a stenotic patient demonstrated on lateral-view roentgenograms of the cervical spine. Pavlov's ratio is 1:1 (1.00) in the control subject *(A)* compared with 1.2 (0.50) in the stenotic patient *(B)*. (From Torg JS, Pavlov H, Genuario S, et al. Neurapraxia of the cervical spine cord with transient quadriplegia. J Bone Joint Surg 1987; 68(A):1370; with permission.)

The ratio method for determining the sagittal spinal canal diameter was devised by Pavlov and compares the standard measurement of the canal with the anteroposterior (AP) width of the vertebral body at the midpoint of the corresponding vertebral body (Fig. 2). This method is independent of magnification factors caused by differences in target distance, O/F distance, or body type because the sagittal diameter of the spinal canal and that of the vertebral body are in the same anatomic plane and are similarly affected by magnification. There is normally a one to one relationship between the sagittal diameter of the spinal canal and that of the vertebral body, regardless of sex. A spinal canal–vertebral body ratio of less than 0.82 was recorded at one or more levels in all patients who experienced cervical cord neurapraxia.

Our experience has clearly indicated that those individuals who experienced an episode of cervical cord neurapraxia manifested by sensory and/or motor symptoms have, with very few exceptions, a spinal canal–vertebral body ratio of 0.80 or less at one or more levels. The sensitivity of the ratio, i.e. the probability

of getting a positive result in a symptomatic individual, was 100% in our reported series. To be noted, our initial report was based solely on roentgenographic findings, all the patients having been evaluated before magnetic resonance imaging (MRI) became widely available. The importance of roentgenographic ratio determination, in addition to standardizing the films that had been taken by varying techniques, has been to explain the pathophysiologic basis for the occurrence of cord neurapraxia. That is, developmental narrowing of the spinal canal in the AP plane associated with extreme flexion or extension of the spine can result in a transient compression of the cord. This has been described by Penning as the "pincer mechanism" (Fig. 3). Specifically, with hyperextension of the cervical spine, the posterior inferior aspect of the superior vertebral body and the anterior superior aspect of the spinolaminar line of the subjacent vertebra (and conversely, in flexion, the spinolaminar line of the superior vertebra and the posterior superior aspect of the subjacent vertebral body) approximate with a sudden decrease in the AP diameter of the canal at that point,

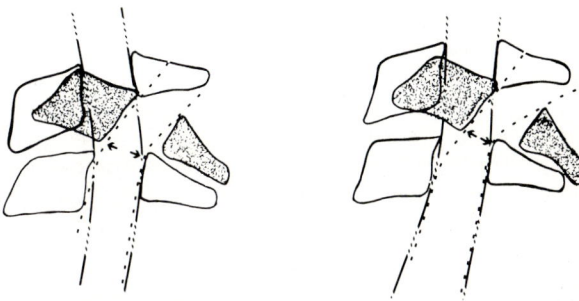

Figure 3 The pincers mechanism, as described by Penning, occurs when the distance between the posteroinferior margin of the superior vertebral body and the anterosuperior aspect of the spinolaminar line of the subjacent vertebra decreases with hyperextension, with compression of the cord occurring. With hyperflexion, the anterosuperior aspect of the spinolaminar line of the superior vertebra and the posterosuperior margin of the inferior vertebra would be the "pincers."

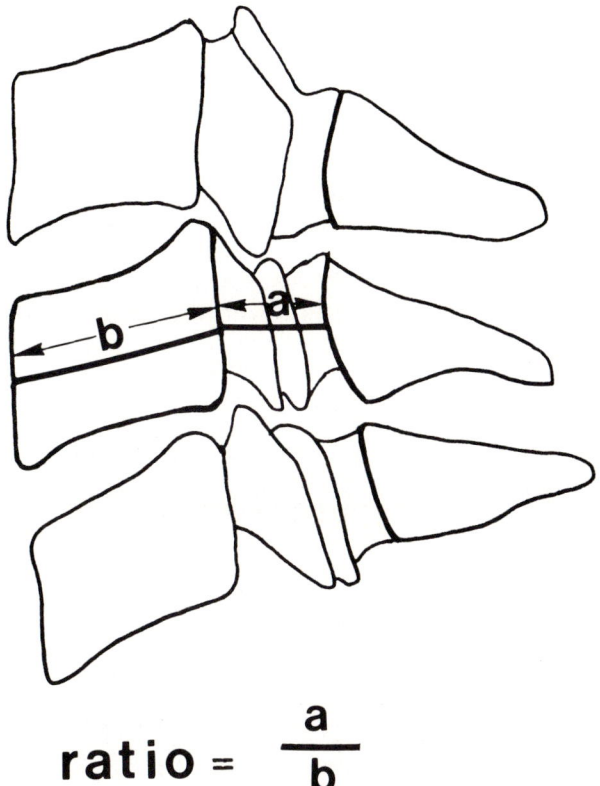

$$ratio = \frac{a}{b}$$

Figure 2 The spinal canal–vertebral body ratio is the distance from the midpoint of the posterior aspect of the vertebral body to the nearest point on the corresponding spinolaminar line (*a*) divided by the anteroposterior (AP) width of the vertebral body (*b*). Pavlov's ratio is *a/b*. (From Torg JS, Pavlov H, Genuario S, et al. Neurapraxia of the cervical spine cord with transient quadriplegia. J Bone Joint Surg 1986; 68(A): 1354–1370, with permission.)

resulting in compression of the spinal cord. In every instance of symptomatic developmental narrowing uncomplicated by instability or disc herniation, the neurologic manifestations are transient and completely reversible.

The low specificity of the ratio method in the elite college and professional cohorts are due to anthropomorphic differences. Specifically, the physical characteristics of the cervical spine in individuals in two groups is characterized by relatively larger vertebral bodies with subsequent lower ratios.

Permanent neurologic loss resulting from cervical spine injuries sustained in tackle football is a function of playing technique in which the cervical spine is axial loaded, resulting in unstable fractures and/or dislocations and irreversible neurologic compromise. The question of whether individuals who have experienced an episode of cord neurapraxia are predisposed to injury with permanent neurologic residual has been answered. None of the 117 known quadriplegics in The National Football Head and Neck Injuries Registry had experienced prior episodes of cord neurapraxia and none of the 45 patients in the transient cohort have gone on to become quadriplegic. On the basis of the random

distribution of ratio determinations as well as the lack of correlation between the occurrence of permanent quadriplegia and prodromal episodes of cord neurapraxia, it is clear that the occurrence of cord neurapraxia does not predispose an individual to an injury associated with permanent catastrophic neurologic sequelae. There is no correlation between occurrence of permanent quadriplegia and prodromal episodes of cord neurapraxia in a tackle football population. Therefore, we believe that the presence of uncomplicated developmental narrowing of the stable cervical spine is neither a harbinger of nor predisposes to permanent neurologic injury.

Our finding of no correlation between developmental narrowing (stenosis) of the spinal canal and irreversible neurologic loss is in direct conflict with a previously published report. Eismont et al have reported a series of cervical spinal fracture/dislocations in which the severity of the neurologic injury was inversely proportional to the AP diameter of the cervical canal. To be noted, 49 of the 98 reported injuries were a result of vehicle accidents and only 15 were secondary to sports participation; football was not specifically mentioned. An excellent case is made for the protective effect of a large cervical canal. The pooled mean AP canal diameters C3-C7 for all 98 patients was 17.9 mm. The pooled mean AP canal diameters C3-C7 for Eismont's "no neurologic deficit" group and "complete deficit" group were 18.9 mm and 16.3 mm respectively ($p < 0.001$). In his patient population there were only 14 patients in the "complete deficit" group. They had a mean AP canal diameter 1.6 mm less than the group overall and none had what they described as a large spinal canal, i.e., mean diameter of 18.9 mm or greater.

In comparison, in the 77 quadriplegic patients from our Registry who were injured while playing tackle football, the pooled mean AP diameter was 18.9 mm. This is virtually identical to the AP canal diameters of the 212 intercollegiate, 97 professional, and 100 control subjects that we have studied. If Eismont's conclusions are to be applied to cervical spine injury resulting from tackle football, the mean canal measurement of the quadriplegic cohort should be much less than those of the collegiate, professional, and control groups. The conclusion of Eismont that a narrow canal predisposes to "complete neurologic deficit," is not reflected in our data. Specifically, the mean AP canal diameter of C3-C6 of the quadriplegic cohort of 18.9 mm is the same as other groups and more consistent with the mean AP canal diameter C3-C6 of Eismont's "no neurologic deficit" group, i.e., 18.9 mm. Clearly, Eismont's conclusions cannot be applied to tackle football-induced quadriplegia.

We know of one intercollegiate defensive back with a history of one episode of cord neurapraxia with both sensory and motor symptoms and developmental narrowing who was subsequently rendered quadriplegic as a result of a clearly documented spear tackle. Rather than implicate his premorbid status of a cervical spine with the occurrence of quadriplegia, we believe that this case emphasizes the role of technique in the occurrence of football-induced cervical quadriplegia. This position is further supported by the chance distribution of the ratio of those individuals in the quadriplegic cohort, the lack of correlation between premorbid manifestations of cord neurapraxia and permanent lesions, and, with the exception cited, the failure to demonstrate the subsequent occurrence of a permanent lesion in those who have experienced a transient episode.

DISCUSSION

1. The extremely high sensitivity of the spinal canal–vertebral body ratio of less than 0.8 at one or more levels supports the concept of the manifestations of cord neurapraxia resulting from transient, reversible, compression deformation of the spinal cord.
2. The extremely low predictive value of the ratio precludes its use as a screening mechanism for determining suitability for participation in contact activities.
3. Uncomplicated developmental narrowing of the cervical canal in a stable spine does not predispose to permanent neurologic injury. Our data do not indicate that there is a correlation between developmental narrowing and permanent neurologic sequelae in a spine rendered unstable by football-induced trauma.
4. Absolute contraindications of continued participation in contact activities apply to those individuals who have had a documented episode of cervical cord neurapraxia associated with: ligamentous instability; intervertebral disc disease with cord compression; significant degenerative changes; MRI evidence of cord defects or swelling; symptoms of positive neurologic findings lasting more than 36 hours; and more than one recurrence.

SUGGESTED READING

Boijsen E. Cervical spinal canal in intraspinal expansive processes. Acta Radiol 1954; 42:101–115.

Eismont FJ, Clifford S, Goldberg M, Green B. Cervical sagittal spinal size in spine injury. Spine 1983; 9:663–666.

Funk PJ, Wells RE. Injuries of the cervical spine in football. Clin Orthop 1975; 109:50–58.

Grant T, Puffer J. Cervical stenosis: A developmental anomaly with quadriparesis during football. Am J Sports Med 1976; 4:219–221.

Herzog RJ, Wiens JJ, Dillingham MF, Sontag MJ. Normal cervical spine morphometry and cervical spinal stenosis in asymptomatic professional football players: Plain film radiography, multiplanar computed tomography, and magnetic resonance imaging. Spine 1990; 16:178–186.

Pavlov H, Torg JS, Robie B, Jahre C. Cervical spinal stenosis: Determination with vertebral body ratio method. Radiology 1987; 164:771–775.

Penning L. Some aspects of plain radiography of the cervical spine in chronic myelopathy. Neurology 1962; 12:513–519.

Stratford J. Congenital cervical stenosis: A factor in myelopathy. Acta Neurochir (Wien) 1978; 41:101–106.

Torg JS, Pavlov H, Genuario S, et al. Neurapraxia of the cervical spinal cord with transient quadriplegia. J Bone Joint Surg 1986; 68(A): 1354–1370.

Wilkinson HA, LeMay ML, Ferris EJ. Roentgenographic correlation in cervical spondylolysis. Am J Roentgenol 1969; 105:370–374.

ATHLETIC INJURY TO CERVICAL NERVE ROOTS AND BRACHIAL PLEXUS

JOSEPH S. TORG, M.D.
PHILIP J. REILLY, M.D.

Injury to the cervical spine, cervical discs, brachial plexus, and peripheral nerves can all result in neurologic signs and symptoms involving the upper extremity. The most common and difficult injuries to differentiate are the cervical pinch–stretch neurapraxias of the nerve roots and brachial plexus. Commonly called "burners" or "stingers" by players and trainers, these injuries often go unreported and untreated.

Injury to the cervical nerve roots and brachial plexus most frequently occur in contact sports, particularly football, as well as rugby, wrestling, and soccer. In football, burners are usually diagnosed in defensive players and offensive lineman. Clancy reported that 49% of University of Wisconsin football players had experienced at least one burner at some time during their playing career. Sallis, in a survey of six division III football teams, reported an incidence of 52% in 1 calendar year. In this survey, only 10% of players were evaluated by the team physician, 65% reported at least

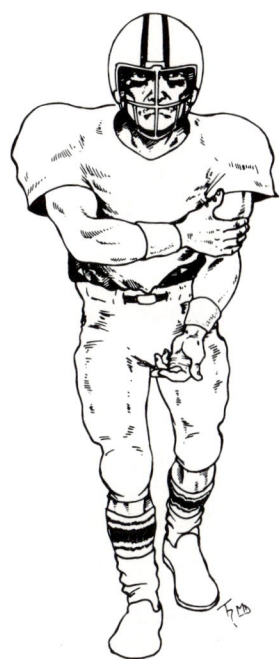

Figure 1 The "burner" syndrome is characterized by lancinating pain in the involved extremity, often with accompanying paraesthesias. There may be concomitant weakness of the deltoid, biceps, and spinati. The player will often be seen leaving the field holding the involved upper extremity to his side.

one burner during their career, and of those players experiencing burners, 87% reported recurrences.

Burners typically occur following head and shoulder contact. The player often leaves the playing field complaining of pain and numbness and inability to move the involved upper extremity (Fig. 1). Pain is usually experienced radiating from the base of the neck into the shoulder and down the arm, including the hand. Burning paraesthesias and numbness may accompany the pain and also radiate into the arm and hand. Most often these symptoms are not dermational in distribution. Weakness may occur, characteristically affecting the deltoid, spinati, and biceps. Motor weakness is often not initially apparent, and may not manifest until a few days after injury. Hence repeat neurologic evaluation is mandatory.

ETIOLOGY

The burner syndrome has been attributed to different mechanisms. Bateman believed that in athletic injuries root lesions were rare, whereas peripheral nerve lesions were common. He recognized that direct blows as well as other mechanisms could result in varying peripheral nerve injuries about the shoulder.

Chrisman described lateral neck flexion away from the involved side, resulting in cervical sprain and traction injury to the cervical nerve roots. Rockett reported operative findings in patients with persistent burners. He

noted scarring of the C5 and C6 nerve roots at their point of emergence from the vertebra between the anterior and middle scalene. He suggested that repetitive tightening of the scalenes causes trauma to the nerve roots, with resultant scarring.

Clancy et al suggested a more distal injury. They believe that burners are brachial plexus injuries. Electrodiagnostic evidence indicated that a plexus axonotmesis involved only the upper trunk. They noted different mechanisms of injury and suggested that the point of plexus injury may vary depending on neck, arm, and shoulder position. Neck hyperextension, shoulder depression, neck hyperextension with lateral bend to the side of injury, and contralateral lateral neck flexion with ipsilateral shoulder depression were all reported mechanisms.

Clancy et al also recommended classifying these injuries based on the staging system of Seddon. Neurapraxia, the mildest form of injury, represents a reversible aberration in axonal function. Focal demyelinization can occur, producing an electrophysiologic conduction block or conduction slowing. Complete recovery usually occurs immediately and at most within 2 weeks. Axonotmesis describes an injury where the axon and myelin sheath are disrupted, but the epineurium remains intact. Wallerian degeneration occurs distal to the point of injury; functional recovery may occur, but it can be incomplete and unpredictable. The most severe injury, neurotmesis, is rarely seen in athletics and results in complete disruption of the nerve. Prognosis is poor, and recovery generally does not occur.

Clancy et al define cervical nerve pinch syndrome as those injuries that recover within 2 weeks and recognize that they most likely represent neurapraxia. The term *brachial plexus injury* is reserved for injuries with weakness or sensory changes lasting longer than 2 weeks. In our opinion, the term *brachial plexus injury* should be reserved for anatomic localization. Practically, many of these injuries are mixed lesions, and classification by Seddon's system serves mainly to aid in describing potential recovery course and prognosis.

Robertson et al indicated the point of brachial plexus injury most likely to be a stretch injury occurring at Erb's point (Fig. 2). They reported all patients became symptomatic after contact causing ipsilateral shoulder depression and lateral neck flexion to the opposite side. Sallis has described how brachial plexus injury may occur by traction or compression.

Poindexter and Johnson believe the lesion is at the root level. In their series of 12 patients undergoing electromyography (EMG), 7 had evidence of C6 radiculopathy. They reported hyperextension as a common mechanism of injury.

Kelly et al investigated the relationship between burners and cervical stenosis in younger patients, age 15 to 18 years. Review of 69 cervical spine radiographs demonstrated a significant decrease in the Torg ratio when compared to controls. They hypothesized that developmental cervical stenosis predisposes to burners due to concomitant foraminal narrowing, with nerve root compression.

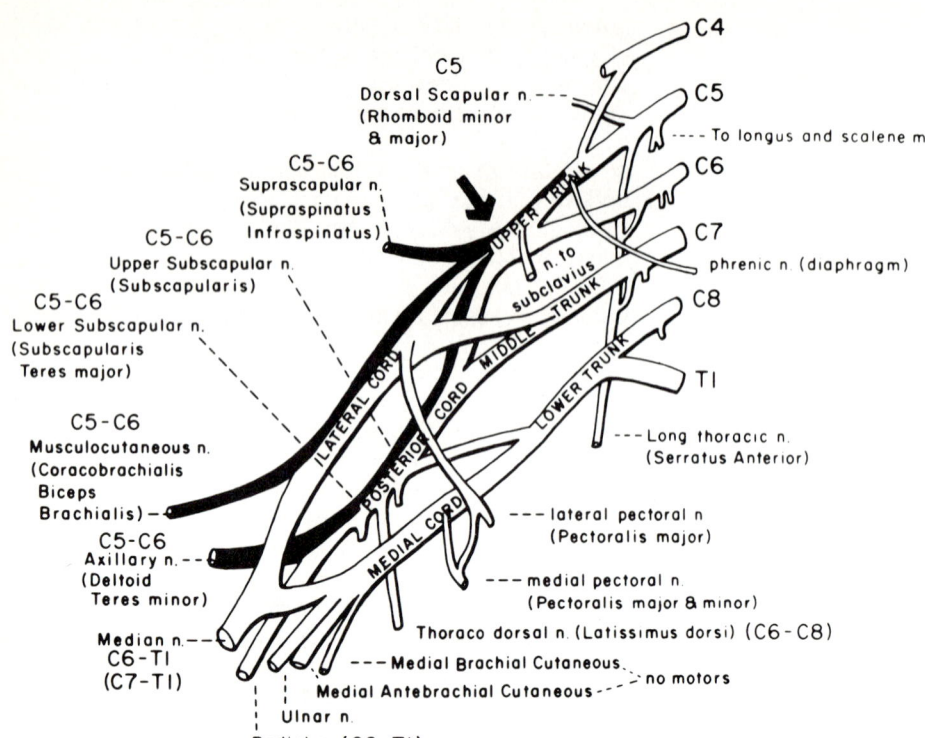

Figure 2 Diagram of the brachial plexus demonstrating the location of Erb's point *(arrow)*. Presumably, brachial plexus stretch injuries are due to traction of the plexus at this point.

Meyer et al studied 40 patients with stingers at the University of Iowa from 1987 to 1991. The mechanism was reported as extension-compression in 34 and brachial plexus stretch in six subjects. Analysis of cervical spine radiographs were performed and compared to a control group of asymptomatic football players. Players with stingers demonstrated a statistically significant incidence of spinal stenosis of at least one cervical segment as defined by a Torg ratio of less than 0.8. For the stinger group, 47.5% had a ratio less than 0.8 for at least one level versus 25.1% in the asymptomatic group. No patient in the brachial plexus stretch injury group had a Torg ratio less than 0.8. They concluded there is a relationship between cervical stenosis and the occurrence of nonparalyzing extension-compression injuries.

BRACHIAL PLEXUS VERSUS CERVICAL ROOT INJURY

It is clear that the typical burner can result from different injury mechanisms. History, physical examination, and appropriate diagnostic studies help to differentiate between brachial plexus and cervical nerve root lesions.

Brachial plexus injuries are more likely to occur in younger patients with less well developed neck musclature. Usually these are traction injuries resulting from lateral neck flexion away from and/or shoulder depression to the side of involvement. Neck pain can be present but is usually not a prominent feature. When present, cervical spine radiographs are necessary. Typically, pain and paresthesias involving the arm and shoulder are

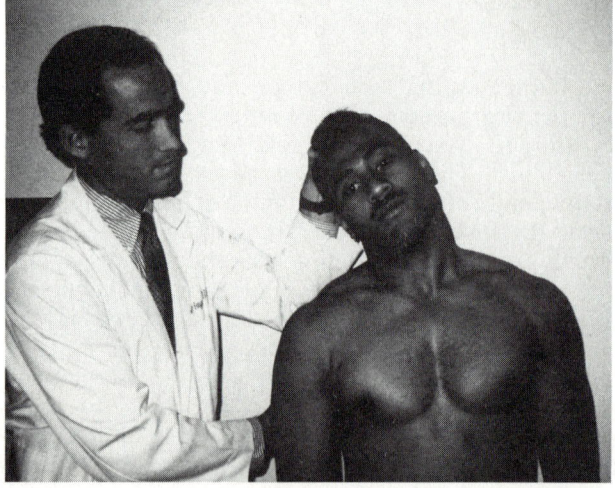

Figure 3 Spurling's maneuver: The examiner applies pressure to the head forcing the cervical spine into extension and lateral flexion towards the symptomatic side. This reproduces the pathomechanics of those injuries due to compression of the cervical nerve root and/or dorsal root ganglion in the involved intervertebral foramen.

transient. On examination Spurling's test is negative (Fig. 3). Weakness is in the characteristic distribution, typically involving the deltoid, spinati, and biceps. Weakness may not be initially evident on clinical exam and follow-up exam is necessary.

Root lesions result from compression of the nerve root and/or dorsal root ganglion in the intervertebral foramen and are generally associated with radiologic

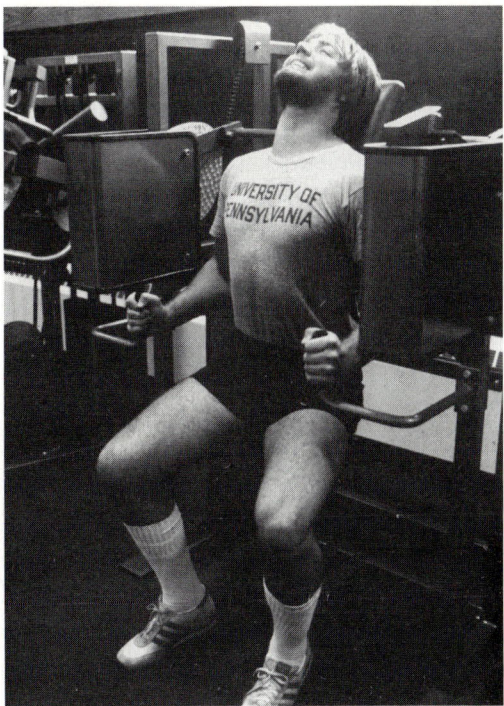

Figure 4 Crucial in the effective management of the athlete with recurrent burners is the implementation of an aggressive, year round neck and shoulder muscle strengthening program. Effective are variable resistant isotonic "neck machines."

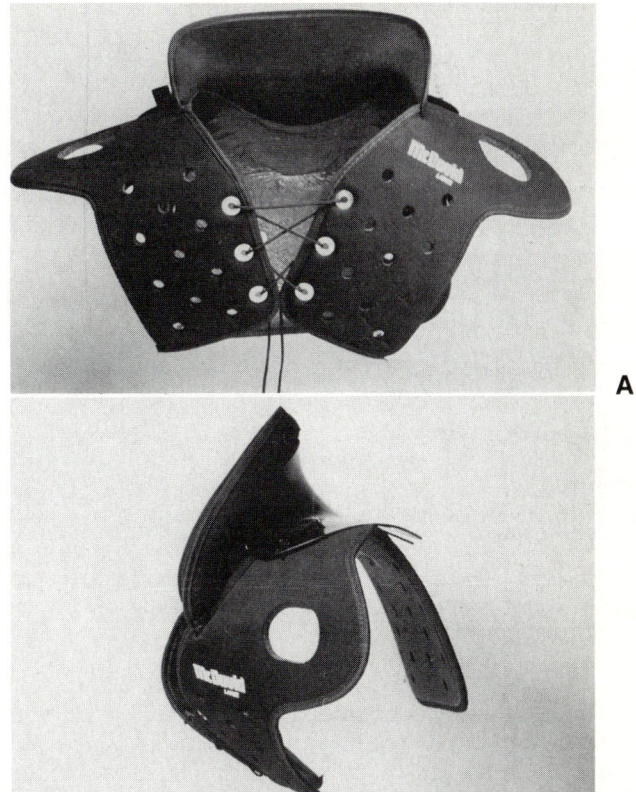

Figure 5 Frontal *(A)* and lateral *(B)* views of the cowboy collar. This device, which is worn under the shoulder pads, effectively limits the extremes of extension and lateral bending of the cervical spine.

evidence of cervical disc disease and/or developmental stenosis. In football players these injuries usually occur at the college and professional levels. Hyperextension or hyperextension with lateral neck flexion are the common mechanisms of injury. Neck pain and a decreased cervical range of motion may be present. Spurling's test is positive. Plain radiographs may be normal or demonstrate loss of normal cervical lordosis and changes of degenerative disc disease. Magnetic resonance imaging (MRI) is indicated in patients with a persistent neurologic deficit and/or prolonged or recurrent symptoms. MRI will demonstrate either acute disc herniation or degenerative disc disease with asymmetric disc bulging. In our experience, patients often have developmental spinal stenosis, degenerative disc disease, and asymmetric disc bulging, which results in root irritation with cervical hyperextension.

MANAGEMENT

Initial management must be directed towards thorough evaluation of the cervical spine, shoulder girdle, affected upper extremity, and peripheral nervous system. The first obligation of the physician is to rule out a serious cervical spine injury. A history of bilateral symptoms or symptoms including the lower extremities should alert the physician to the possibility of cord neurapraxia, cervical spine fracture, or ligamentous injury. In this instance the spine should be immobilized

until injury is ruled out. If a player complains of neck pain, a complete cervical spine evaluation is mandatory, including radiographic examination.

Characteristically the signs and symptoms are transient and resolve within minutes. The athlete whose pain and paresthesias abate, demonstrates a normal neurologic examination, and, most importantly, has a full, pain-free range of cervical motion may return to activity. Also, players must demonstrate normal strength on clinical exam before return to participation. Recurrent symptoms without weakness does not preclude participation, however, these individuals require careful follow-up. Continued symptoms associated with weakness precludes further athletic participation.

In brachial plexus injuries prevention is based on an aggressive neck and shoulder strengthening program (Fig. 4). Chrisman observed that lateral neck flexion injuries were less frequent in individuals with thick, short necks. Neck rolls, or devices such as the Cowboy collar, and high profile shoulder pads also help prevent injury by limiting lateral flexion and extension (Fig. 5).

Electrodiagnostic studies may be helpful but are not mandatory in the management of burners secondary to brachial plexus injury. Speer et al demonstrated that although there was no correlation between initial physical findings and the results of electrodiagnostic

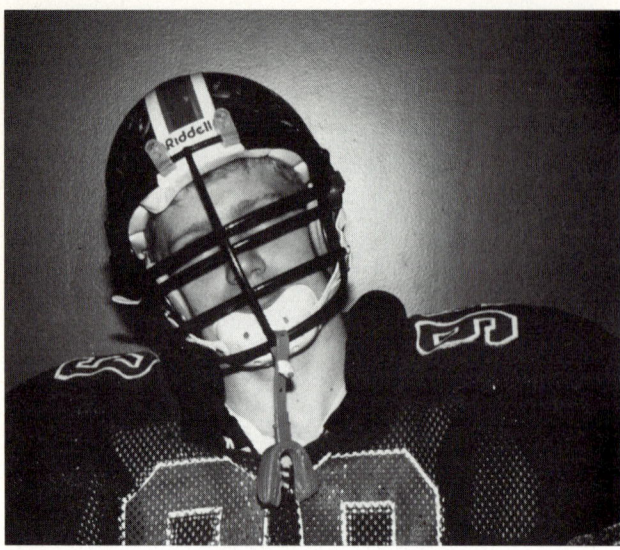

Figure 6 The combined action of the football helmet, "cowboy collar", and shoulder pads effectively limits the extremes of lateral bend of the neck.

testing, evidence of muscular weakness at 72 hours postinjury did correlate with a positive EMG. Bergfeld reported that EMG findings persist long after weakness has resolved by clinical exam and therefore abnormal EMG findings should *not* be used as a criteria for exclusion from athletic participation.

EMG examination should be reserved for severe injuries and to aid in diagnosis in difficult cases, and can be helpful in the prognosis of injuries associated with significant weakness, i.e., axonotmesis or neurotmesis. In selected cases, such data may help delineate the extent of injury and aid in differentiation of brachial plexus versus cervical root injury. Wilbourn cautions that the absence of paraspinal fibrillation potentials does not necessarily allow one to exclude root pathology. He further cautions that one be familiar with the EMG examination when interpreting data. MRI of the cervical spine is the preferred modality for the diagnosis of cervical disc disease.

In these individuals with cervical disc disease, the criteria for return to sports is identical as for brachial plexus injuries. Again, neck and shoulder strengthening is the key to prevention. A neck roll or "cowboy collar" by limiting extension, help control recurrences (Fig. 6).

Athletes with large, acute herniations or with large central disc components should be withheld from participation. Players with chronic symptoms and degenerative disc disease should be counseled as to the likelihood of continued symptoms with athletic participation. In those patients with subjective symptoms but normal strength, participation is not contraindicated as long as the player understands the possible implications of repetitive root trauma. In rare instances discectomy and fusion may be considered if symptoms persist. A one level fusion is not an absolute contraindication to athletic participation.

SUGGESTED READING

Bateman JE. Nerve injuries about the shoulder in sports. ICLS 1967; 49(4).

Bergfeld JA. Brachial plexus injury in sports: A five year follow-up. Orthop Trans 1988; 12:743–744.

Chrisman OD. Lateral-flexion neck injuries in athletic competition. JAMA 1965; 192:613–615.

Clancy WG, Brand RL, Bergfeld J. Upper trunk brachial plexus injuries in contact sports. Am J Sports Med 1977; 5:209–214.

Hershman EB. Brachial plexus injuries. Clin Sports Med 1990; 9:311–329.

Kelly JD. The relationship of transient upper extremity paresthesias and cervical stenosis. Orthop Trans 1988; 12:732.

Maroon JC. 'Burning hands' in football spinal cord injuries. JAMA 1977; 238:2049–2051.

Meyer SA. The incidence of cervical spinal stenosis in college football players with stingers. Abstract. Am Soc Orthop Sports Medicine Fellowship Directors, July 1992.

Poindexter DP, Johnson EW. Football shoulder and neck injury: A study of the "stinger." Arch Phys Med Rehab 1984; 65:601–602.

Robertson WC. Upper trunk brachial plexopathy in football players. JAMA 1979; 241:1480–1482.

Rockett FX. Observations on the "burner." Traumatic cervical radiculopathy. CORR 1982; 164:18–19.

Sallis RE. Burners. Offensive strategy for an underreported injury. Physician Sports Med 1992; 20(11):47–55.

Seddon H. Surgical disorders of the peripheral nerves. Edinburgh: Churchill-Livingstone, 1972.

Speer KP. The prolonged burner syndrome. Am J Sports Med 18:591–594.

Torg JS. Criteria for return to contact activities following cervical spine injury. Clin J Sports Med 1991; 1(1):12–26.

Warren RF. Neurologic injuries in football. In: Jordan BD, ed. Sports neurology. Rockville, Md: Aspen, 1989:235.

Watkins RG. Neck injuries in football players. Clin Sports Med 1986; 5:215–245.

Wilbourn AJ. Electrodiagnostic testing of neurologic injuries in athletes. Clin Sports Med 1990; 9:229–245.

ACUTE BRACHIAL NEUROPATHY

NATHANIEL L. TINDEL, M.D.
ELLIOTT B. HERSHMAN, M.D.

Shoulder pain is a common complaint among athletes. The commonly considered differential diagnoses include impingement syndrome, rotator cuff tear, glenohumeral instability, tendinitis, nerve entrapment, "burner" syndrome, and fracture. Acute brachial neuropathy (ABN) is an uncommon cause of symptoms related to the shoulder. Nevertheless, ABN should be included in the differential diagnosis of shoulder pain because both the treatment and prognosis are unlike other more common causes of shoulder disability in the athlete. Correct identification of this disorder will prevent interventions based on an incorrect diagnosis.

ABN is characterized by the acute or subacute onset of shoulder pain, weakness, and atrophy of various shoulder girdle muscles. ABN is not limited to athletes, as they clearly represent the minority of cases. In fact, a variety of names have been used to describe the same syndrome, including multiple neuritis, neuralgic amyotrophy, shoulder girdle syndrome, serum brachial neuritis, and Parsonage-Turner syndrome.

The cause of ABN is unknown. Although hereditary types have been described, most cases are sporadic. Proposed etiologies include an immune response to preceding infection, allergic reaction to immunization, radiation therapy, chemotherapy reaction, vasculitis, and pregnancy/postpartum reaction. Although the onset may be associated with athletic activity, it is not believed that ABN is truly an athletic injury. The most common age of onset is during the third through sixth decades. Males are more commonly afflicted than females. Roughly 25% of patients have bilateral involvement without any right/left sided predominance. Interestingly, however, in almost 50% of the unilaterally affected patients, electromyographic studies have shown evidence of subclinical involvement in the contralateral side. In bilateral cases, there is often a symptom-free interval between the involvement of the two sides.

DIAGNOSIS

The predominant feature of ABN is pain localized to the shoulder. The pain has been described as throbbing, aching, and even burning. The symptoms are unrelenting and can last from several hours to several weeks. The pain is often so intense as to require narcotic analgesia. Occasionally, symptoms may extend up to the neck and down to the elbow and forearm. In the athlete, weakness often only becomes apparent during athletic activity. Attempted movement of the shoulder girdle on examination generally exacerbates the pain. In fact, the patient is most comfortable with the shoulder adducted and the elbow flexed, a position described by Waxman as the flexion-adduction sign.

Weakness of the shoulder usually follows the onset of pain. On average, weakness can be documented 4 to 5 days after the onset of pain. Due to the severity of the pain, the degree of weakness on initial examination may be underestimated. In addition, the distribution of weakness can be quite variable. The paralysis is characterized by muscle flaccidity and wasting without a true motor, radicular, or nerve trunk pattern. In order of decreasing frequency the most often affected muscles include the deltoid, supraspinatus, infraspinatus, serratus anterior, biceps, triceps, and wrist extensors. When there is whole nerve root involvement, C5 and C6 are most commonly affected.

Frequently, cutaneous sensation is lost but this rarely matches the neurologic distribution of the motor loss. Most commonly, a small area of hypesthesia can be detected on the outer surface of the arm in the distribution of the axillary nerve. Likewise, sensation served by the C5 and C6 nerve roots are most likely to have sensory loss.

Deep tendon reflex changes are related to the severity of the muscle paralysis. Most commonly, hypoactive biceps and triceps reflexes are noted. Hyperreflexia and upper motor neuron findings are not seen.

There are generally no constitutional symptoms or fever at the time of onset of pain. In addition, laboratory studies including blood count, sedimentation rate, rheumatoid factor, antinuclear antibody, serum electrophoresis, and examination of the cerebrospinal fluid generally yield normal results. Radiographs of the neck and shoulder and myelogram likewise only rule out other common injuries.

Electrophysiologic studies are of major benefit in the athlete suspected of ABN. Characteristically, involved muscles demonstrate fibrillation potentials with axon degeneration in the associated peripheral nerves. As a result, diminished amplitudes of the motor and sensory nerves involved are the most commonly detected nerve conduction study parameter. Of most importance, electromyography can be used to differentiate ABN from traumatic upper trunk or other plexus lesions. These findings include: (1) involvement of muscles not innervated by the brachial plexus (e.g., serratus anterior, diaphragm, trapezius); (2) severe denervation of muscles innervated by only one or two peripheral nerves (e.g., suprascapular nerve or axillary nerve); (3) severe denervation restricted to a single muscle, with sparing of muscles innervated by the same portion of the plexus (e.g., supraspinatus involvement with normal infraspinatus function); and (4) severe motor involvement of a particular mixed motor–sensory peripheral nerve with sparing the of the sensory action potentials in the same nerve (e.g., denervation of biceps and deltoid with intact lateral antebrachial cutaneous sensory nerve action potentials).

TREATMENT

Treatment is generally divided into two phases. During the first phase, the extremity is rested, as activity may be associated with increased symptoms. A sling for immobilization is often all that is needed with analgesics to control the pain. Once the pain is resolved, the second phase of rehabilitation can begin. Passive range of motion exercises followed by active strengthening programs are instituted to regain strength in the involved muscles. Rehabilitation should emphasize all muscles of both upper extremities, as subclinical involvement is common. Corticosteroids have not been found to be effective in the treatment of this disorder.

OUTCOME

The prognosis for functional recovery is fairly good. Most patients show evidence of recovery within 3 years. Nevertheless, residual motor weakness is a frequent finding. This corresponds to those muscles most severely affected early in the course of the disease. Scapula winging and deltoid weakness in particular often persist. Nevertheless, most athletes return to participating in sports, probably because of the limited disability associated with a winging scapula or mild proximal shoulder weakness. It is important to warn athletes who present with scapula winging on examination of the probability of its persistence. Athletes may be allowed to return to sports once a plateau in their strength recovery has been reached. Certainly, athletes who do not regain sufficient strength to control the extremity should modify their athletic endeavors. Permission for an athlete to return to sports is based on individual ability and the requirements of the sport and likewise should be a decision made on a case by case basis.

SUGGESTED READING

Dillin L, Hoaglund FT, Scheck M: Brachial neuritis. J Bone Joint Surg 1985; 67A:878–880.
Flaggman PD, Kelly JJ. Brachial plexus neuropathy: an electrophysiologic evaluation. Arch Neurol 1980; 37:160–164.
Hershman EB. Brachial plexus injuries. Clin Sports Med 1990; 9:311–329.
Hershman EB, Wilbourn AJ, Bergfeld JA. Acute brachial neuropathy in athletes. Am J Sports Med 1989; 17:655–659.
Tsairis P, Dyck PJ, Mulder DW. Natural history of brachial plexus neuropathy: report of 99 patients. Arch Neurol 1972; 27:109–117.
Wilbourn AJ. Electrodiagnosis of plexopathies. Neurol Clin 1985; 3:511–529.
Yang SS, Hershman EB. Idiopathic brachial plexus neuropathy: a review. Crit Rev Phys Rehab Med 1993; 5:193–201.

SPINAL CORD RESUSCITATION

JOSEPH S. TORG, M.D.
LAWRENCE E. THIBAULT, Sc.D.

Twenty years ago head injured patients who were deeply comatose or showed signs of neurologic deterioration routinely underwent burr hole surgery. Often bilateral burr holes were performed as an emergency procedure to assess and treat possible significant intracranial hematoma. Patients were assumed, for all intents and purposes, to have subdural or epidural hematoma until proven otherwise. Essentially, intracranial injury was thought to result from mechanical damage to the brain with subsequent neural insult. With improved diagnostic modalities and research findings, it became apparent that permanent brain injury was the result of both primary and secondary mechanisms.

Primary brain injury mechanisms produced mechanical damage to the brain either by the mechanical energy input or the effects of increased intracranial pressure. Fortunately, in most instances, the mechanical injury to the brain substance is not overwhelming. Secondary brain injury is caused by cerebral ischemia or hypoxia resulting from increased intracranial pressure, hemorrhage, brain swelling, or the indirect consequence of hypotension or respiratory compromise. Secondary brain injury has come to be recognized as the most important problem in the care and treatment of patients with closed head injuries. Thus, the major focus in the management of closed head injury now deals with implementation of the evolving principles of brain resuscitation.

On the basis of recent published reports, as well as our own anecdotal clinical experience and laboratory observations, it is apparent that the time has arrived for consideration of the concept of spinal cord resuscitation.

REDUCTION OF SPINAL CORD DISLOCATION

Case Histories

The value of prompt reduction of traumatic cervical vertebral malalignment was made evident while managing two youngsters rendered quadriplegic in 1975 as a result of football injuries.

Case 1

A 19-year-old defensive back was injured while participating in an intercollegiate game. He tackled an opposing ball carrier by striking him with the top or crown of his helmet and was immediately rendered quadriplegic for both motor and sensory function distal to C4. There were no reflexes, either physiologic or pathologic, and there was no evidence of sacral sparing. These findings were consistent with spinal shock. Initial cervical spine roentgenograms on admission to the hospital demonstrated a unilateral facet dislocation of C3 on C4 without evidence of fracture.

Gardner skull tongs were applied and a reduction of the dislocation attempted by applying a total of 18 kg in progressive increments over 30 minutes. Reduction by this method was unsuccessful. The patient was then taken to the operating room and under nasotracheal anesthesia a satisfactory reduction by closed manipulation was obtained within 3 hours of his injury. Also, corticosteroids were administered intravenously. The following morning, neurologic examination revealed persistence of complete motor paralysis. There was evidence of return of some posterior column function, specifically position and vibratory sensation. Four days after injury, a cervical myelogram was performed by way of lateral C1–C2 puncture. The myelogram demonstrated a complete block at the C3–C4 level. The following day the patient was taken to the operating room where, under general nasotracheal anesthesia, a C3–C4 diskectomy and anterior interbody fusion was performed.

The patient's subsequent course was gratifying, with progressive improvement in both motor and sensory function. Approximately 1 month after injury motor return first became evident in the long toe extensors in the right foot. One year after injury the patient had significant return of motor function to all of the major muscle groups of the lower extremities. There was also return of motor function to the muscle groups of both upper extremities to a lesser degree. He had bilateral intrinsic minus hands. In general, motor return on the left side of the body was greater than on the right side of the body. He was able to ambulate with bilateral Loptstrand crutches and could manage stairs with one rail and one crutch. Return of sensory function was complete with the exception of decreased pain–temperature sensation. Although he has a neurogenic bladder, he has been successfully employed and recently married.

Case 2

A 15-year-old high school student sustained a C3–C4 dislocation while participating in a sandlot tackle football game. Circumstances surrounding the injury were unclear, but it appeared that he was running with the ball and head-butted a tackler and was immediately rendered quadriplegic. He was taken to a local hospital, and was subsequently transferred to the University hospital. Initial examination demonstrated complete motor and sensory quadriplegia below C4. He was conscious, alert, and oriented to time, place, and person. Roentgenographic examination demonstrated unilateral facet dislocation with anterior translation of C3 and C4 without evidence of fracture.

Gardner skull tongs were inserted and attempts to reduce the dislocation with 18 kg of skeletal traction under radiographic guidance over 30 minutes were unsuccessful. General nasotracheal anesthesia was then administered, and reduction of the C3–C4 dislocation was accomplished by closed manipulation within 4 hours of the injury.

Subsequent roentgenograms demonstrated instability of the reduction. The patient was placed on a circle electric bed and intravenous steroids were administered. Over the subsequent 48 hours there was return of touch, position sense, and vibrating sensations in an inconsistent fashion. Motor function, light touch, and temperature sensation remained absent. A cervical myelogram was negative. Subsequently, the patient's course was complicated by development of gastric stress ulcers and protracted delayed gastric emptying, with ensuing debilitating malnutrition requiring hyperalimentation. Subsequent roentgenograms at 4 and 6 weeks after injury demonstrated persistent instability at C3–C4.

Two months after the injury, under general nasotracheal anesthesia, a C3–C4 anterior cervical interbody fusion was performed. Following stabilization of the spine there was progressive increase in motor and sensory function. The patient was able to ambulate on parallel bars 6 months after injury and independently 8 months after injury.

Examination 1 year after injury revealed excellent strength of all muscle groups of lower extremities. The strength of muscle groups in the left shoulder girdle and the left upper extremity was good, whereas the strength of those on the right was graded as fair plus. The patient had bilateral intrinsic deficient hands. However, he stated that he can perform all tasks but is "somewhat clumsy." All sensation had returned with the exception of spotty decrease in temperature. He regained bowel and bladder function. The true measure of his recovery is evidenced by the fact that he is currently a practicing physical therapist.

Other Experience

Our experience in managing these two cases has emphasized the difficulty in reducing unilateral facet dislocation at the C3–C4 level by skeletal traction as well as the urgency in effecting immediate reduction in order to obtain maximum neurologic return. The protracted period for maximum neurologic recovery is noteworthy.

Bohlman and Anderson have documented the degree of neurologic improvement patients can have after sustaining an incomplete spinal-cord injury. The medical records of 68 patients having an incomplete spinal cord injury were reviewed, with 58 selected for the study. Of these 58, three patients died within 2 to 18 months after surgery. Cervical myelography with or without computed tomography documented the presence of compression of the anterior portion of the cord. At the time of surgery, the patient population had an average age of 40 years. The time from injury to decompression was 13 months. Forty-four of the 58 patients could not walk before the operation and 14 had lower-extremity problems before surgery.

The long-term results compared with the neurologic

examination and ambulatory status before the operation and at follow-up demonstrated that 29 patients experienced an excellent outcome, 13 a good, 6 a fair, and 10 a poor result. Motor function improved distally for 24 patients, while 18 had not improved after the operation. Of the 42 patients who had a decompression within 12 months of the injury, 34 had a good or excellent outcome, which was significantly better than for those patients who had their decompression more than 12 months postinjury. No relationship was observed between the amount of anterior decompression and the neurologic improvement.

These results indicate that even late anterior decompression and arthrodesis can improve a patient's neurologic function in both the upper and lower extremities. As a result of these findings the authors presently initiate immediate skeletal traction and spinal realignment without waiting for the patient's neurologic status to stabilize in an effort to prevent irreversible neurologic changes from occurring.

Anderson and Bohlman have also documented the extent of neurologic and functional improvement with anterior decompression and arthrodesis in 51 patients with complete motor quadriplegia resulting from a fracture or dislocation of the cervical spine, most from a motor vehicle or diving accident. All underwent anterior cervical decompression and arthrodesis using iliac bone grafting. All had myelographically confirmed compression of the anterior aspect of the spinal cord by displaced fragments of bone and disk. This operation was done an average of 15 months after injury. Improvement in ability to carry out activities of daily living was assessed by the modified Barthel index.

Five patients died, leaving 46 patients who were followed for an average of 5 years. Eighteen patients had documented neurologic improvement of at least one new functional level and seven had improvement of at least two levels. The others had no remarkable improvement in motor function. Mean score on the modified Barthel index improved from 17 to 33 points out of a possible 100. One patient had functionally significant improvement of the caudad part of the cord; another patient had neural injury with loss of one motor root level and only partial improvement. The result was poor in nine of eleven patients who had decompression 1.5 years or more after injury, with only modest functional improvement in the other two patients. Results were poor in all five patients over 53 years old.

These authors concluded that anterior decompression and arthrodesis of the cervical spine can result in neurologic and functional improvements for some patients with complete traumatic quadriplegia. Currently, the authors perform anterior decompression of the cord and arthrodesis if myelography reveals anterior compression of the cord or motor roots. They believe this procedure is contraindicated for older patients and those with significant loss of pulmonary function.

The pathomechanics of reversible, incompletely reversible, and irreversible cervical spinal cord injury are currently being investigated in the Bioengineering Laboratory at the University of Pennsylvania. Specifically, clinical observation of 1,200 cervical spine injuries have been correlated with the response of an in vitro model of isolated neural elements subjected to control mechanical deformation. The pathophysiology of cervical cord injury includes a spectrum from transient neurapraxia to permanent quadriplegia. The laboratory application of microdeformation of an in vitro axon model has resulted in the histomechanical explanation of this phenomenon as it occurs at the cellular level. Correlation of data obtained from the axon injury model with analysis of selected cervical cord injuries has resulted in a schematic that explains one of the major components of reversible, incompletely reversible, and irreversible spinal cord injury. In addition, both clinical and laboratory data clearly delineate the relationship of injury mechanisms, spinal instability, cord deformation, rate of loading, duration of deformation, and local anoxia to ultimate cord function. In most instances of acute spinal cord injury, interruption of neural function is not due to instantaneous axonal disruption, but rather a functional response that without therapeutic intervention will ultimately become structural, i.e. axotomy, secondary to the result of aberrations in histomechanical function (Fig. 1). It is proposed that measures initiated to obviate the effects of local anoxia and increased concentrations of intra-axonal calcium will result in significant recovery of neural function.

In both clinical and laboratory situations return of neurologic function is related to factors affecting neural element deformation. Clinical-laboratory correlation clearly supports the concept of cord resuscitation (i.e., immediate reduction, administration of intravenous steroids, and initiation of pharmacologic measures that will increase spinal cord perfusion).

A recent study by Bracken and colleagues, performed under the auspices of the National Institute of Neurological Disorders and Stroke, has demonstrated that patients sustaining spinal cord injury showed significant improvement in muscle function and sensation if administered methylprednisolone intravenously within 8 hours of injury. Specifically, the initial dose of methylprednisolone is administered in a bolus of 30 mg/kg of body weight intravenously with an infusion pump for 15 minutes. Forty-five minutes after this, a maintenance dose of 5.4 mg/kg/hr is administered intravenously with an infusion pump for 23 hours.

RECOMMENDATIONS

We believe that with particular regard to resulting morbidity, the same phenomenon occurs in acute spinal cord injury as that observed in closed head injury. Specifically, the primary injury is the product of mechanical damage that occurs as a result of traumatic spinal instability. Whether the resulting pathology is due to plastic deformation and/or anatomic disruption of neural structures, irreversible neurologic injury results. Fortunately, in most instances of acute spinal cord injury, interruption of neural function is not due to axonal disruption. Rather, as in closed head injury it is

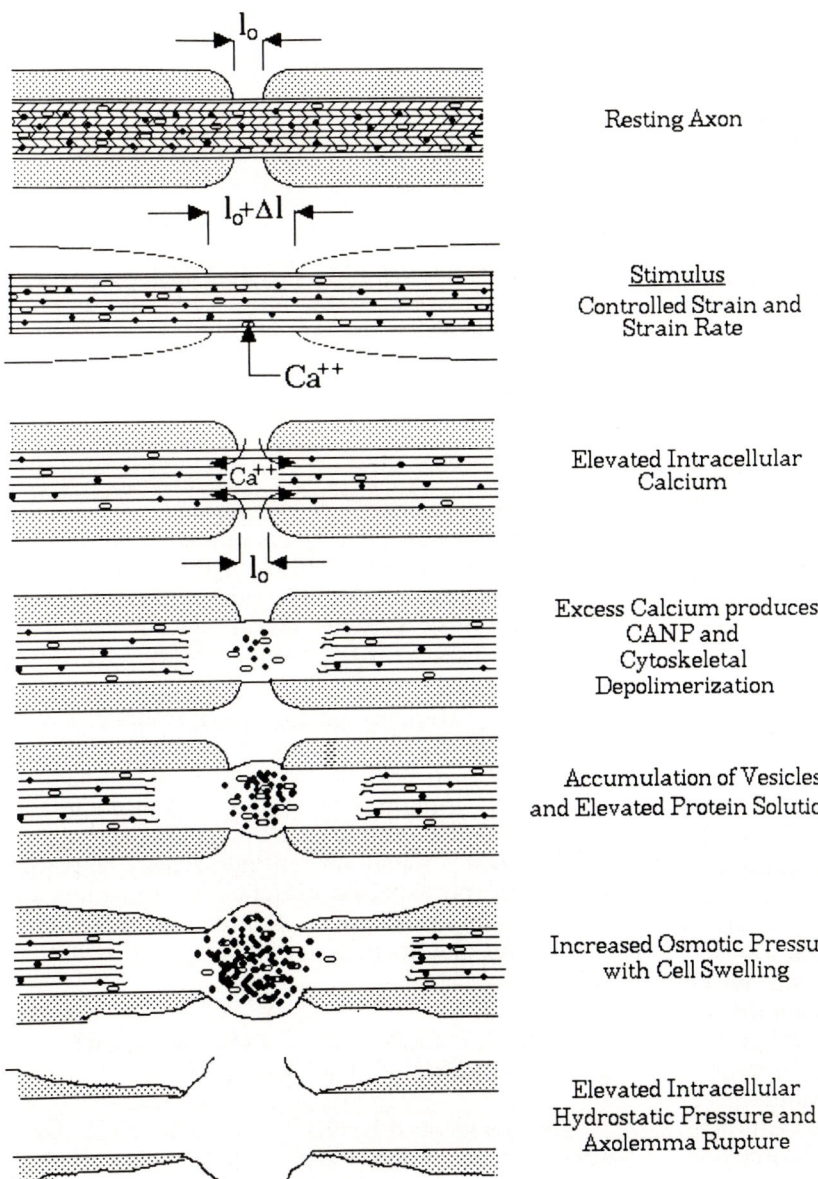

Resting Axon

Stimulus
Controlled Strain and
Strain Rate

Elevated Intracellular
Calcium

Excess Calcium produces
CANP and
Cytoskeletal
Depolimerization

Accumulation of Vesicles
and Elevated Protein Solution

Increased Osmotic Pressure
with Cell Swelling

Elevated Intracellular
Hydrostatic Pressure and
Axolemma Rupture

Figure 1 Deformation of the in vitro axonal injury model intension results in depolarization of cell membrane potential with a dramatic rise in intracellular calcium concentration. Intracellular free calcium concentration exceeding 50 micromolar results in calcium activated neutral protease production and cytoskeletal depolimerization. Subsequent increased osmotic pressure leads to elevated intracellular hydrostatic pressure and axolemma. This process is potentiated by the effects of local anoxia. The goals of cord resuscitation are to reverse: (1) cord deformation, (2) cell membrane depolimerization, (3) calcium pump failure, and (4) local tissue anoxia.

secondary cord injury caused by hypoxia, edema, and aberrations in cell membrane potential that is largely responsible for the resulting neurologic deficit. In view of this, spinal cord resuscitation is proposed as an attempt to reverse the secondary changes that occur in order to obtain maximal neurologic recovery. Measures in keeping with this concept include:

1. Treatment of any aberrations in cardiovascular function with particular regard to maintaining blood pressure and respiratory function.
2. Prompt initiation of measures to affect reduction of spinal deformity so as to relieve cord deformation.
3. Prompt decompression and stabilization of the injured cervical segment.
4. Administration of cordicosteroids intravenously in doses recommended by Bracken et al.

To be defined on the basis of future clinical and laboratory investigational efforts are a determination of pharmacologic measures that will increase spinal cord perfusion.

SUGGESTED READING

Anderson PA, Bohlman HH. Anterior decompression and arthrodesis of the cervical spine: Long-term motor improvement: Part II—Improvement in complete traumatic quadriplegics. J Bone Joint Surg 1992; 74A:683–692.

Bohlman HH, Anderson PA. Anterior decompression and arthrodesis of the cervical spine: Long-term motor improvement: Part I—Improvement in incomplete traumatic quadriparesis. J Bone Joint Surg 1992; 74A:671–682.

Bohlman HH, Bahniuk E, Raskulinecz G, Field G. Mechanical factors affecting recovery from incomplete cervical spinal cord injury: A preliminary report. Johns Hopkins Med J 1979; 145:115–125.

Bracken MB, Shepard MJ, Collins WF, et al. A randomized, controlled trial of methylpredinisolone or naloxone in the treatment of acute spinal-cord injury. N Engl J Med 1990; 322:1405–1411.

Dolan EJ, Tator CH, Endrenyi L. The value of decompression for acute experimental spinal cord compression injury. J Neurosurg 1980; 53:749–755.

Ducker TB, Salcman M, Daniell HB. Experimental spinal cord trauma: III—Therapeutic effect of immobilization and pharmacologic agents. Surg Neurol 1978; 10:71–76.

Rivlin AS, Tator CH. Effect of duration of acute spinal cord compression in a new acute cord injury model in the rat. Surg Neurol 1978; 10:39–43.

Tarlov IM. Acute spinal cord compression paralysis. J Neurosurg 1972; 36:10–20.

Thibault L, Torg JS. The biomechanics of injury to the neural and neurovascular elements of the cervical spine as it relates to spinal cord resuscitation. Book of Abstracts, Cervical Spine Research Society Annual Meeting, Philadelphia, Pa, 1991.

Torg JS, Sennett B, Vegso JJ, et al. Axial loading injuries to the middle cervical spine segment: A analysis and classification of twenty-five cases. Am J Spine Med 1991; 19:6–20.

Torg JS, Thibault L. The epidemiology, pathomechanics and pathophysiology of reversible, incompletely reversible and irreversible cervical spinal cord injury: The case for cord resuscitation. Cervical Spine Research Society Annual Meeting Book of Abstracts, Philadelphia, Pa, 1991.

Torg JS, Truex RC, Marshall J, et al. Spinal injury at the level of the third and fourth cervical vertebrae from football. J Bone Joint Surg 1977; 59A:1015–1019.

REHABILITATION OF THE POSTINJURED/POSTOPERATIVE CERVICAL SPINE

BENJAMIN SHAFFER, M.D.
MARY-BETH WALSH, P.T., Dip. M.P.T.

Rehabilitation has been essential in the management of virtually every sports injury, in both returning to activity and preventing reinjury. Perhaps in no other area of the body has rehabilitation been such a crucial part of the overall treatment plan as in injury of the cervical spine. In recreational level athletes, even deceptively "minor" sprains can recur, and hinder participation. At an elite level, even minimal postinjury or postoperative loss of normal strength, flexibility, or coordination threatens performance. This chapter reviews the principles and techniques by which rehabilitation can help the athlete return to pain-free, minimal-risk function after injury or surgery to the cervical spine.

PRINCIPLES OF REHABILITATION

Rehabilitation is not an adjunct but a mainstay of treatment. The specific program content, intensity, and duration depends on respecting the nature and extent of the injury or surgery, and the precautions of the treating physician. Although the specific indications for return to activity are beyond the scope of this chapter, such information in advance is important to the properly designed program, such that it is based on realistic and practical goals. Despite efforts to return the athlete to activity quickly, such a goal is not always possible; use of any "cookbook" program for expediting or assuring such return is untenable. The specific program of any athletes' rehabilitation is therefore effected through a "team" approach, under the mutual coordinated care of treating physician and therapist.

The goals of rehabilitation include avoidance of further injury, elimination of swelling and inflammation, promotion of healing, attainment of normal posture and flexibility, return of balanced strength, endurance and conditioning, and restoration of coordination and agility. These objectives are carried out in four philosophically discrete but practically overlapping phases:

Phase I— Minimize inflammation, swelling, further injury.
Phase II— Restore normal motion and strength.
Phase III— Improve strength, endurance and conditioning, posture and core strengthening.
Phase IV— Prepare for return to activity, emphasizing sport-specific exercises, coordination and agility drills, modification of activity as necessary, and instruction in injury prevention.

PHASE I: CONTROL FURTHER INJURY, RESOLVE INFLAMMATION

The goals of this phase are to minimize pain, swelling, inflammation, and promote healing. This phase is instituted immediately after injury or surgery, often with temporary immobilization of the cervical spine, which is thought to limit further injury and facilitate healing.

In stable injuries (sprains, strains, discs), such immobilization is most commonly achieved using a soft collar. Use is limited to 2 weeks to prevent patient dependency. In more severe injuries or after surgery, more secure immobilization such as with a Halo device may be necessary.

The use of a nonsteroidal anti-inflammatory drug (NSAID) for the first 2 to 3 weeks after injury has been empirically helpful. Various passive local techniques, known as modalities, are useful to minimize further injury and aid in the resolution of inflammation, swelling, and pain. Modalities include a variety of physical agents passively applied by the patient or therapist to an injured area in an attempt to decrease inflammation, swelling, and pain, and, when possible, to promote healing.

The most common modality used is cryotherapy, which includes the application of various cooling techniques such as ice, cold water, vaporizing liquids, or chemical packs to the skin, producing superficial local effects. There are several different techniques by which cryotherapy can be applied. The simplest and least expensive is ice, wrapped in towels or prepared in paper cups or popsicle sticks, applied directly over the areas of pain, tenderness, and spasm.

Cryotherapy techniques are most useful early on, with ice or cold compresses applied when possible at the time of injury or in the recovery room. Cold therapy is not as effective beyond the first 48 to 72 hours after injury, although it helps minimize pain during and after therapy treatments during subsequent phases. Pulsed ultrasound also proves effective in dispersing inflammation without increasing temperature.

PHASE II: PROMOTE HEALING, RESTORE MOTION AND STRENGTH

What most people think of as "rehabilitation" occurs during the next three phases, as efforts to restore motion and strength aim to return the patient to normal function. The first goal in phase II is to maintain or restore motion of the cervical spine. Motion is often restricted even after minor sprains and strains, and may be limited in more than one plane. Active and passive range of motion (ROM) is measured by the physical therapist in flexion, extension, lateral bending, lateral rotation, protraction, and retraction. Care is taken to observe any precautions against specific movements due to instability or neurologic complaint.

Efforts to restore ROM are initiated actively by the patient, who under supervision performs flexion, extension, lateral bending, and lateral rotation exercises, without resistance within the limits of their motion. Using adjunctive modalities, gentle passive assistance at the terminal range in each plane achieves a progressively increased amount of motion. Use of manipulative techniques at this stage can significantly improve motion. How much motion to expect depends on the patients' diagnosis, treatment, age, and overall flexibility.

As symptoms subside, active exercises incorporating resistance are added. Through exercise, the consequences of immobilization such as atrophy, adaptive shortening, and muscle hypertonicity are minimized. Exercises are first carried out within the pain-free range, and progressed as this range is extended. Initially such exercises should be isometric, in which contraction neither lengthens nor shortens the muscle. Resistance is increased slowly, minimizing compressive loads on the cervical spine.

Specifically, with the neck in extension, the patient attempts flexion against the resistance of either his or her own hand, or that of the therapist. This is repeated through intermittent arcs from full extension to full flexion, stopping each 10 degrees to repeat the exercise. The exercise is held for 5 seconds and repeated three times prior to continuing to the next arc. Similar exercises are continued in lateral bending and rotation (Fig. 1).

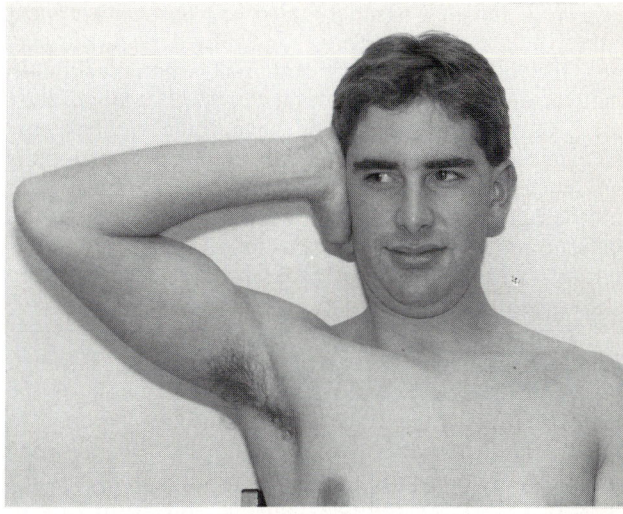

Figure 1 Isometric strengthening exercise in lateral bending is performed by the patient against the resistance generated by his own hand.

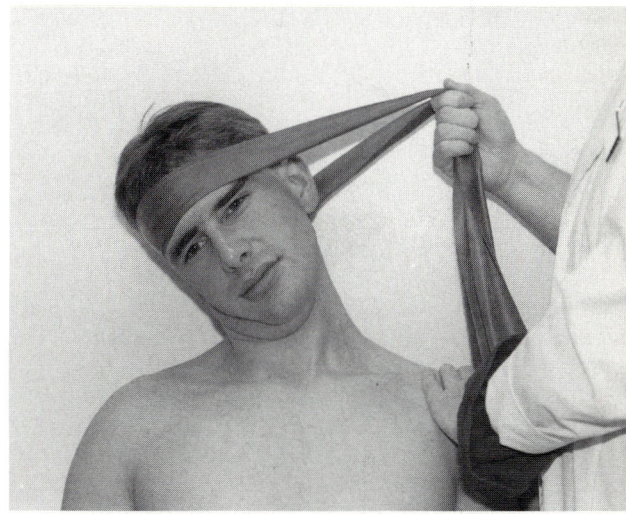

Figure 2 Exercise against resistance such as with elastic tubing allows progressive isotonic strengthening.

Isotonic exercises are added to the patients' program as strength increases. This can be achieved in a variety of ways, usually beginning with use of a simple bicycle innertube or elastic cord (Theraband) (Fig. 2), or more complicated (and expensive) machinery such as that designed by Nautilus.

PHASE III: IMPROVE STRENGTH, CONDITIONING, ENDURANCE, AND POSTURE

The focus of phase III is to amplify the motion and strength gains achieved earlier, increase endurance and conditioning, and correct and maintain proper posture. One of the keys of this phase is the concept that the best long-term stabilization of the cervical spine is ultimately achieved through strengthening of the paracervical spinal muscles. Improperly conditioned neck muscles put the athlete at significant risk when sustaining inadvertent or intentional blows to the head and neck area. Out of this perception have come what is now considered routine neck strengthening programs amongst most training programs for wrestlers and football players. Such specific exercises are added to the patient/athletes' regimen according to their sport. Repetition with light resistance promotes endurance strengthening.

Posture emphasis is critical in proper performance of exercises and eventual return to activity. Through injury or learned behavior, anterior positioning of the head relative to the trunk is common and can lead to neck pain or perpetuate symptoms in the rehabilitating athlete (Fig. 3, A). Such altered posture may actually lead to nerve root impingement and the formation of traction spurs.

Specific exercises to correct and maintain proper posture are taught to and performed by the patient five times a day until the patient demonstrates sound independent posture (Fig. 3, B). In addition, the "chest out position" has been promoted as important in preventing and treating cervical symptoms. In theory, the chest-out position achieves three benefits, including opening of the intervertebral foramina, reducing the effect of the weight of the head, and opening of the thoracic outlet. Both the neck posture and chest out position are emphasized during all phases of the rehabilitation program.

Proprioceptive Neuromuscular Facilitation (PNF) is a recently developed strategy in improving motion and strength based on known neurophysiologic principles. In the most common technique of application, known as autogenic inhibition, ROM is increased by having the patient hold a contraction of the agonist muscle in the fully elongated position, followed by instruction by the therapist to relax. Upon relaxation the therapist passively elongates the muscle further, combined with antagonistic muscle contraction.

Finally, a general conditioning program is important in the rehabilitation program of the injured or postoperative athlete. We find useful the stationary bicycle, stair-step machine, or treadmill for aerobic conditioning (Fig. 4). Although swimming, running, and rowing also provide good cardiovascular fitness, they place the neck in a biomechanically disadvantaged position, and are not recommended. Attention to proper spine mechanics and posture are instructed during this phase. Specific exercises, including those recommended by Watkins and McKenzie, seem effective at maintaining proper alignment during these strengthening and conditioning exer-

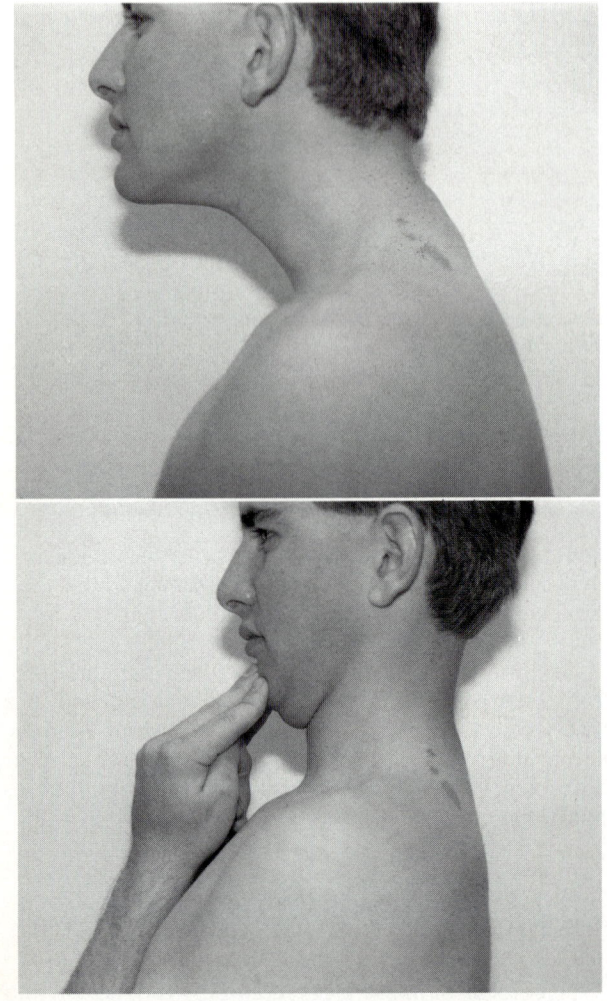

A

B

Figure 3 *A,* Anteior neck positioning is a common postural adaptation in athletes, which compromises function. *B,* Instruction in proper posture maintains advantageous biomechanics, here achieved by the patient under direct supervision.

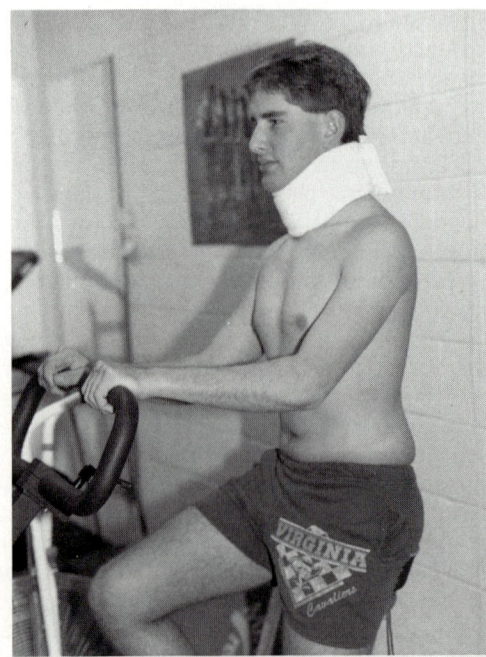

Figure 4 General conditioning to maintain fitness is instituted early, with stationary cycling providing a good aerobic work-out without undue cervical stress.

cises and will hopefully prevent set-backs as the program proceeds into the fourth final phase.

PHASE IV: EXERCISES IN PREPARATION FOR RETURN TO ACTIVITY

Without agility, proprioception, and proper posture, even the strong "bull-necked" athlete will be unsuccessful. Therefore, as motion and strength continue to improve, other exercises specific to the athletes' sport are incorporated (Fig. 5). The focus of this phase is on returning the athlete to his or her activity, incorporating the rehabilitation concept of Specific Adaptation to Imposed Demands (SAID). Although strengthening may lead to a pain-free mobile cervical spine, this in no way ensures preparation specific for the particular activity of that individual athlete. Anticipating return means to prepare for possible injury and prevent such an occurrence. Equipment modification or sometimes a change in the players' position is worthy of consideration. For example, in a football player who has had several "stingers" or "burners," modification of his shoulder pads or addition of a neck roll may be helpful. Following successful return to activity, continuing warm-up, strength, and conditioning exercises into a "prehabilitation" injury prevention program is worthwhile.

REHABILITATION OF COMMON SPORTS-RELATED CERVICAL SPINE INJURIES

We present here a brief overview of the basic principles and techniques used in caring for some common athletic injuries of the cervical spine.

Strain/Sprain

Sprain or strain of the muscles and/or ligaments is the most common athletic injury affecting the cervical

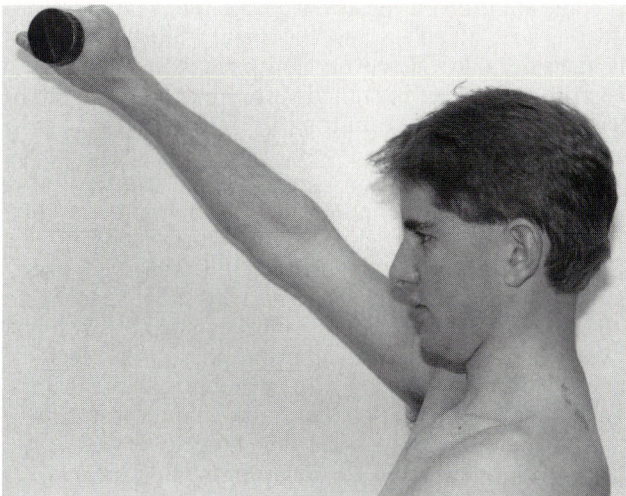

Figure 5 Exercises specific to the athlete's sport are carried out with attention to proper posture control.

spine, varying from mild to severe, and occasionally accompanied by more severe disc or nerve damage. The pain may be incapacitating with inability to even turn the head slightly or there may be pain only at the extreme of motion, which stretches the involved muscle/ligament. Pain and stiffness may be pronounced and occasionally accompanied by headache.

Treatment begins with use of moist heat and soft tissue massage. As pain subsides, restoration of motion is emphasized, using gentle active and passive stretching. Isometric strengthening is subsequently initiated. The patient is counseled to avoid active neck motion that causes him/her pain. Light resistance exercises using elastic tubing is begun as symptoms resolve and motion returns to near normal. Contact stress is avoided until normal motion and strength have completely returned.

In more severe sprains/strains, temporary immobilization using a soft collar may be necessary. Moist heat, gentle massage, and, when necessary, use of a Transcutaneous electrical stimulation machine (TENS) unit are helpful at decreasing, and sometimes breaking, the pain cycle. Occasionally, use of ultrasound, traction, massage, or rhythmic stabilization are effective techniques in restoring pain-free motion.

Neurogenic Pain (Stinger, Burner)

Burning sensation down the arm and occasionally the fingers has been described as a "stinger" or "burner," a usually reversible neurapraxia of the brachial plexus. In mild cases, sensation and strength are usually normal. However, in cases of persistent pain and sometimes weakness, emphasis on rehabilitation is important. This includes emphasis on ROM, strengthening, and postural re-education. Particularly helpful are equipment modifications, which have been shown effective at decreasing the risk of reinjury by absorbing shock, protecting the shoulders, fitting the chest, and fixing the mid-cervical spine to the trunk.

Cervical Disc Herniation

Herniation of a cervical disc is relatively common, presenting with radicular neck pain. This symptom complex usually responds to conservative modalities and manual techniques, and in severe cases is helped by the use of traction. Occasionally, persistence of symptoms or neurologic compromise leads to surgery, most commonly an anterior cervical discectomy accompanied by fusion at the same level. The duration of postoperative immobilization varies. Upon discontinuation of immobilization, gradual motion, stretching, postural, and strengthening exercises are encouraged.

Spondylosis

Common in older athletes, spondylosis refers to compressive neuropathy of the cervical spine nerve roots due to degenerative pathology, usually of the apophyseal joints, discs, or both. Rehabilitation is the mainstay of treatment, involving reduction of pain, maintenance or restoration of flexibility, use of traction intermittently, posture correction, and core strengthening.

Stable Fractures

"Stable" injuries such as "tear-drop" or "clay shoveler's" fractures may be treated much as sprains/strains. While allowing healing, which may or may not require temporary immobilization, motion, strengthening, and a general conditioning program are instituted.

Unstable Fractures

Fractures involving the arches of C1 or C2, the odontoid, or C3-7 accompanied by subluxation or dislocation, with or without associated neurologic deficit, are often unstable. The most important principle in rehabilitation for these types of injuries is to ensure healing without instability or risk of neurologic compromise prior to allowing motion exercises. Some limited isometric exercises may be acceptable to restore tone, but this decision should be made with the treating physician.

Serious Ligament Injury with Facet Subluxation/Dislocation

Subluxation or dislocation of the facet joint(s) implies significant force and usually requires manipulative reduction, surgical intervention, or both. Immobilization post-injury or surgery depends on the treatment method and the confidence of the surgeon. As the Halo vest or firm collar is weaned, passive modalities and massage to restore tone are initiated. Progressive restoration of function including increased motion and strength continues under the care of the treating physician.

SUGGESTED READING

Greenfield J, Ilfeld FW. Acute cervical strain. Clin Orthop 1977; 122:196-200.
Guyer RD, Ohnmeiss DD, Triano John J, Hyde T. Nonsurgical treatment of sports-related spine injuries. Spine 1990; 4(2).
Harris W. Cervical traction: Review of the literature and treatment guidelines. Phys Ther 1977; 57:8.
Knott M, Voss DE. Proprioceptive neuromuscular facilitation, patterns and techniques. Ed 2. New York: Harper and Row, 1968.
Marino M. Current concepts on rehabilitation in sports medicine: research and clinical interrelationships. In James A, Nicholas E, Hershman B, eds. The Lower Extremity and Spine in Sports Medicine. Vol. 2. St. Louis: CV Mosby, 1986.
Markey K, DiBenedetto M, Curl W. Upper trunk brachial plexopathy: The stinger syndrome. Am J Sports Med 1993; 21:650-655.
Mayer TG, Gatchel RJ. Functional restoration for spinal disorders: The sports medicine approach. Philadelphia: Lea & Febiger, 1988.
McKenzie R. Treat your own neck. New Zealand: Spinal Publications Ltd., 1983.
O'Leary P, Boiardo R. The diagnosis and treatment of injuries of the spine in athletes. In: James A, Nicholas E, Hershman B, eds. The lower extremity and spine in sports medicine. Vol. 2. St. Louis: CV Mosby, 1986.
Ragnarsson KT. Rehabilitation of patients with cervical spine disorders. In: Martin B, Camins P, O'Leary F, eds. Disorders of the cervical spine. Baltimore: Williams & Wilkins, 1992.
Tan JC, Nordin M. Role of physical therapy in the treatment of cervical disk disease. Orthop Clin North Am 1992; 23:435-449.
Teitz CC, Cook DM. Rehabilitation of neck and low back injuries. Clin Sports Med 1985; Vol 4.
Torg JS, Vegso JJ, Torg E. Rehabilitation of athletic injuries: An atlas of therapeutic exercise. Chicago: Year Book, 1987.
Watkins RG. Neck injuries in football players. Clin Sports Med 1986; Vol 5.
Welsh TM. Physical therapy, ergonomics, and rehabilitation. In Wiesel SW, Boden SD, Borenstein DG, Feffer HL, eds. Neck pain. 2nd Ed.
Wiens JJ, Saal JA. Rehabilitation of cervical spine and brachial plexus injuries. Phys Med Rehab 1987; Vol. 1.
Wilberger J, Maroon J. Athletic cervical spine injuries. In: Camins MB, O'Leary PF, eds. Disorders of the cervical spine. Baltimore: Williams & Wilkins, 1992.

CRITERIA FOR RETURN TO CONTACT ACTIVITIES AFTER CERVICAL SPINE INJURY

JOSEPH S. TORG, M.D.

Injury to the cervical spine and associated structures as a result of participation in competitive athletic and recreational activities is not uncommon. It appears that the frequency of these various injuries is inversely proportional to their severity. Whereas Albright has reported that 33% of college football recruits sustained "moderate" injuries while in high school, catastrophic injuries with associated quadriplegia occurs to less than 1 in 100,000 participants per season at the high-school level. The variety of possible injuries to the cervical spine is considerable and the severity variable. The literature dealing with diagnosis and treatment of these problems is considerable. However, conspicuously absent is a comprehensive set of standards or guidelines for establishing criteria for permitting or prohibiting return to contact sports (Boxing, Football, Ice Hockey, Lacrosse, Rugby, Wrestling) after injury to the cervical spinal structures. The explanation for this void appears to be twofold. First, the combination of a litigious society and the potential for great harm should things go wrong makes "no" the easiest, and perhaps most reasonable advice. Second and perhaps most important, with the exception of transient quadriplegia, is the lack of credible data pertaining to postinjury risk factors. Despite a lack of credible data, this chapter attempts to establish guidelines to assist the clinician as well as the patient and parents in the decision-making process.

Cervical spine conditions requiring a decision as to whether or not participation in contact activities is advisable and safe can be divided into two categories: (1)

congenital or developmental, and (2) post-traumatic. Each condition has been determined to present either: (1) no contraindication, (2) relative contraindication, or (3) an absolute contraindication on the basis of a variety of parameters. Information compiled from over 1,200 cervical spine injuries documented by the National Football Head and Neck Injury Registry has provided insight into whether various conditions may or may not predispose to more serious injury. A review of the literature in several instances provides significant data for a limited number of specific conditions. Analysis of many conditions predicated on an understanding of recognized injury mechanisms has permitted categorization on the basis of "educated" conjecture. And lastly, much reliance has been placed on personal experience that must be regarded as anecdotal.

The structure and mechanics of the cervical spine enables it to perform three important functions. First, it supports the head as well as the variety of soft tissue structures of the neck. Second, by virtue of segmentation and configuration, it permits multiplannar motion of the head. Third, and most important, it serves as a protective conduit for the spinal cord and cervical nerve roots. A situation that would impede or prevent the performance of any of the three functions in a pain-free manner either immediately or in the future is unacceptable and contraindicated.

The following proposed criteria for return to contact activities in the presence of cervical spine abnormalities or after injury are intended only as guidelines. It is fully acknowledged that for the most part they are, at best, predicated on the antidotal and no responsibility can be assumed for their implementation.

Critical to the application of these guidelines is the implementation of coaching and playing techniques that precluded the use of the head as the initial point of contact in a collision situation. Exposure of the cervical spine to axial loading is an invitation to disaster and relegates any and all safety standards as meaningless.

CRITERIA

Congenital Conditions

Odontoid Anomalies

Hensinger has stated that "patients with congenital anomalies of the odontoid are leading a precarious existence. The concern is that a trivial insult superimposed on already weakened or compromised structure may be catastrophic." This concern became a reality during the 1989 football season when an 18-year-old high-school player was rendered a respiratory dependent quadriplegic while making a head tackle that was vividly demonstrated on the game video. Postinjury roentgenograms revealed an os ondontoidium with marked C1-C2 instability (Fig. 1, *A* and *B*). Thus, the presence of odontoid agenesis, ondontoid hypoplasia, or os odontoidium are all absolute contraindications to participation in contact activities.

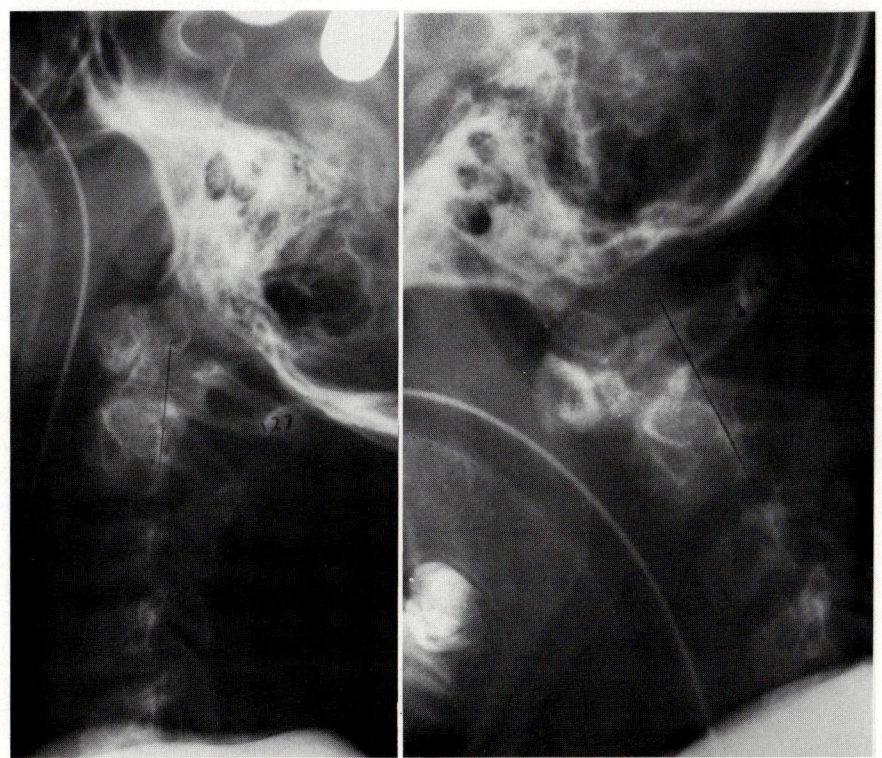

A   B

Figure 1 Inherent instability at C1 in a patient with an os odontoidium resulting in respiratory dependent quadriplegia after a spear tackle by this 18-year-old high-school football player. The reduction in the space available for the cord is vividly demonstrated by the lateral extension and flexion views postinjury.

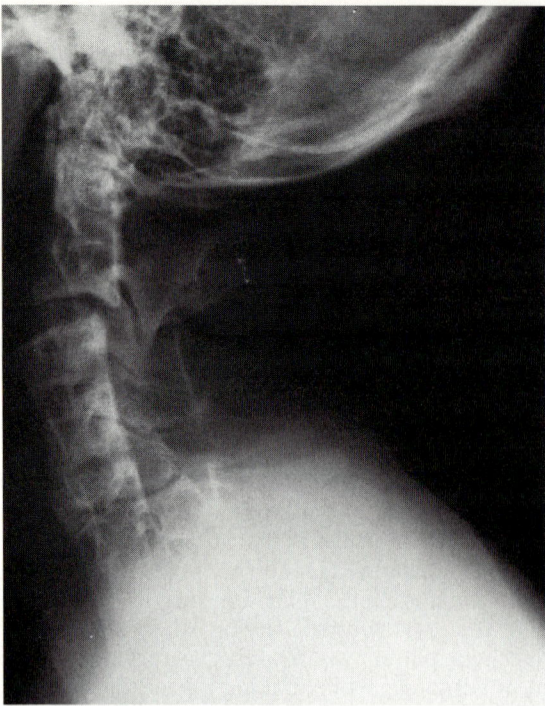

Figure 2 Type I Klippel-Feil deformity with multiple level fusions and deformities as demonstrated on the lateral roentgenogram.

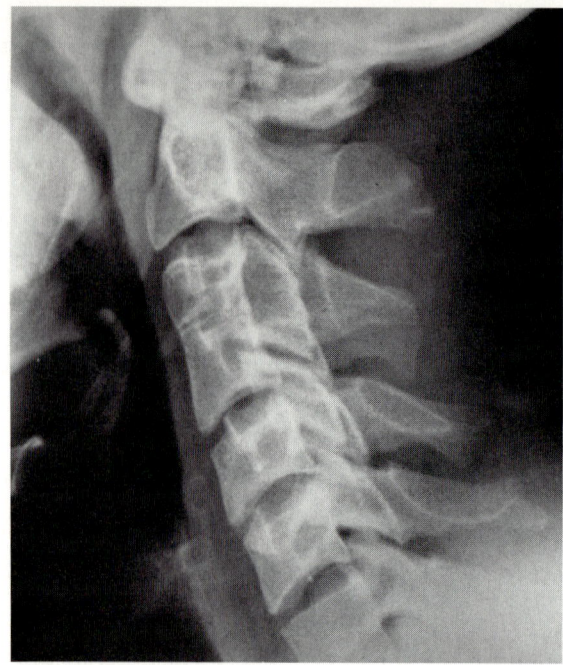

Figure 3 Type II Klippel-Feil deformity with a one level congenital fusion at C3-C4 involving both the vertebral bodies and the lateral masses.

Spina Bifida Oculta

This is a rare, incidental roentgenographic finding that presents no contraindication.

Atlantoccipital Fusion

This is a rare condition characterized by partial, or complete congenital fusion of the bony ring of the atlas to the base of the occiput. The onset of signs and symptoms are referable to the posterior columns due to cord compression by the posterior lip of the foramen magnum, unusually occur in the third or fourth decade. They usually begin insidiously and progress slowly, but sudden onset or instant death have been reported. Atlantoccipital fusion as an isolated entity or coexisting with other abnormalities constitute an absolute contraindication to participation into contact activities.

Klippel-Feil Anomaly

Klippel-Feil anomaly is the eponym applied to congenital fusion of two or more cervical vertebrae. For purposes of this discussion, the variety of abnormalities can be divided into two groups: Type I-mass fusion of the cervical and upper thoracic vertebrae (Fig. 2), and Type II-fusion of only one or two interspaces (Fig. 3). To be noted, the variety of associated congenital problems have been identified to be associated with congenital fusion of the cervical vertebrae and include pulmonary, cardiovascular, and urogenital.

Pizzutillo has pointed out that "children with congenital fusion of the cervical spine rarely develop neurologic problems or signs of instability." However, he further states that "the literature reveals more than 90 cases of neurologic problems. . .that developed as a consequence of occipital cervical anomalies, late instability, disc disease, or degenerative changes also constitutes absolute contraindication to participation. On the other hand, Type II lesion involving fusion of one or two interspaces at C3 and below in an individual with full cervical range of motion and an absence of occipital cervical anomalies, instability, disc disease, or degeneration changes should present no contraindication.

Developmental Conditions

Cervical Spinal Stenosis

Developmental narrowing (stenosis) of the cervical canal with cord neurapraxia and transient quadriplegia has been well defined. Defining narrowing or stenosis as a cervical segment with one or more vertebra having a canal/body ratio of 0.8 or less is predicated on the fact that 92% of all reported clinical cases have fallen below this value at one or more levels. To be noted, 12% of asymptomatic controls also fell below the 0.8 level as did 48% of asymptomatic professional and 45% of asymptomatic college players. In the group of reported symptomatic players, there was in every instance complete neurologic return and in those who continued with contact activities, reoccurrence was not predictable.

Clearly, the presence of developmental narrowing of the cervical spinal canal does not predispose permanent neurologic injury. Eisman et al have indicated, on the

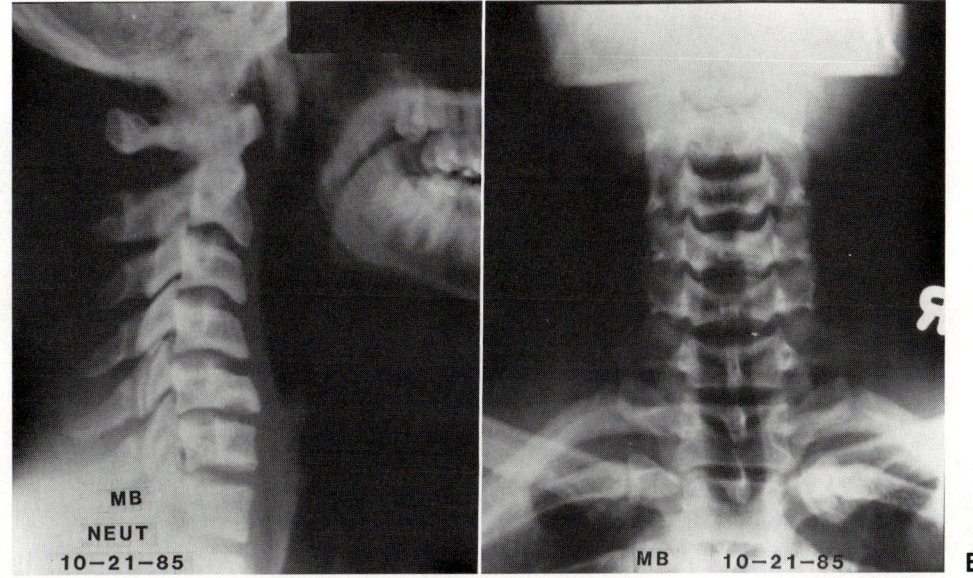

Figure 4 Radiographic characteristics of "Spear Tacklers' Spine" include developmental narrowing of the cervical canal, an old compression injury of C5, and reversal of the normal cervical lordosis in the erect, neutral position on the lateral view (*A*) and suggestion of a wry neck attitude with tilt of the cervical spine to the left on the anteroposterior view (*B*).

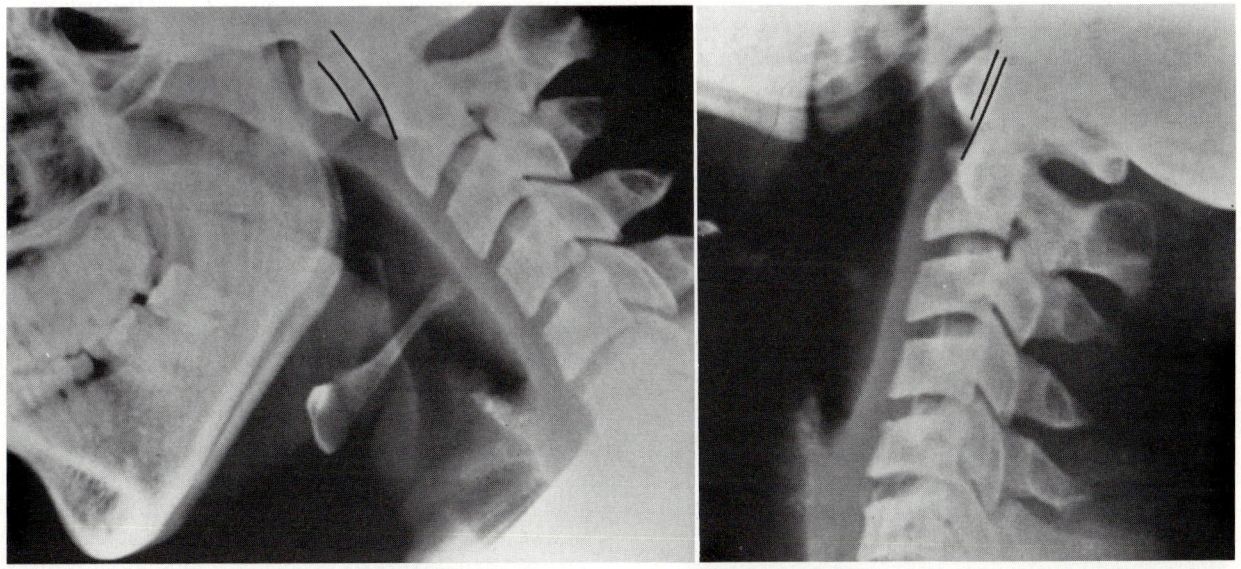

Figure 5 The atlas-dens interval ADI is the distance on the lateral roentgenogram between the anterior aspect of the dens and the posterior aspect of the anterior ring of the atlas. In children the ADI should not exceed 4.0 mm, whereas the upper limit in the normal adult is less than 3.0 mm. C1-C2 instability is vividly demonstrated in these extension and flexion views.

basis of experience with cervical fractures/dislocations resulting from automobile accidents, that the degree of neurologic impairment was inversely related to the anterio-posterior diameter of the canal. Due to the all or nothing pattern of axial load football spine injuries, this phenomena has not been observed in athletic related injuries.

The presence of a canal/vertebral body ratio of 0.8 or less is not a contraindication to participation in contact activities in asymptomatic individuals. We further recommend against preparticipation screening roentgeno-grams in asymptomatic players. Such studies will not contribute to safety, are not cost effective and will only contribute to the hysteria surrounding this issue.

In those individuals with a ratio of 0.8 or less who experience either motor and/or sensory manifestations of cervical cord neurapraxia there is a relative contraindication to return to contact activities. In these instances, each case must be determined on an individual basis depending on the understanding of the player and parents and their willingness to accept any presumed theoretical risk.

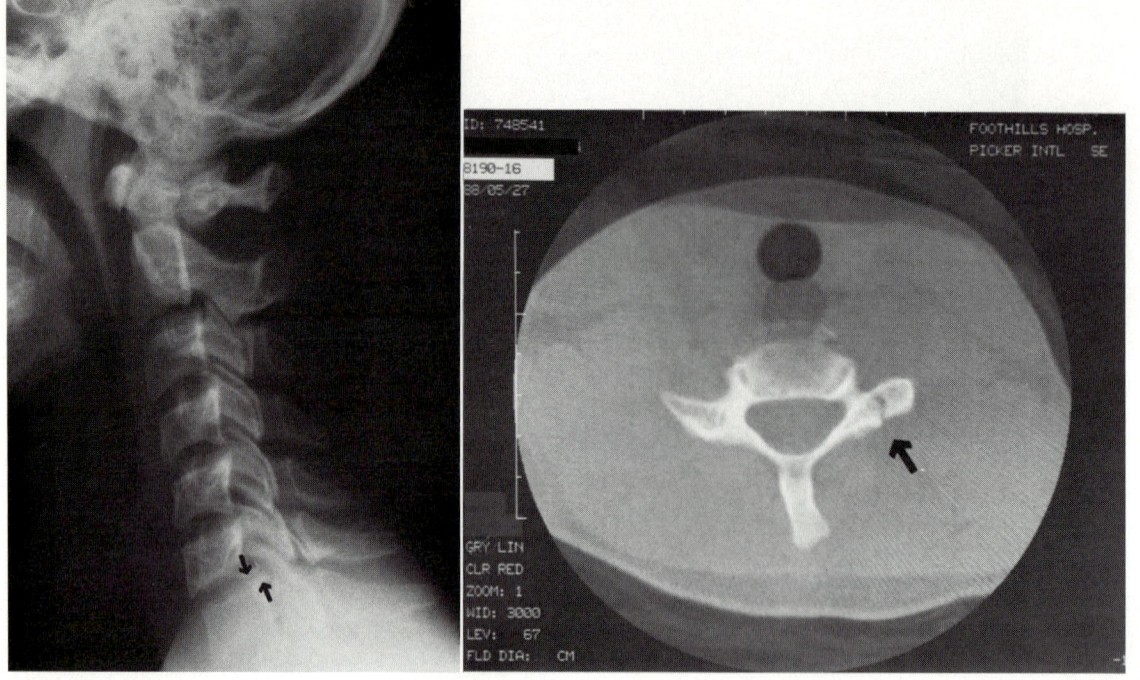

A   B

Figure 6 *A,* Lateral roentgenogram of the cervical spine in the erect neutral position of a 21-year-old college football player demonstrates anterior translation of C6 on C7 of greater than 3.5 mm *(dark arrows). B,* CT scan of C6 in the sagittal plane demonstrates a fracture through the lateral mass *(arrow).* Persistent displacement despite healing of the fracture is an absolute contraindication to further participation in contact sports.

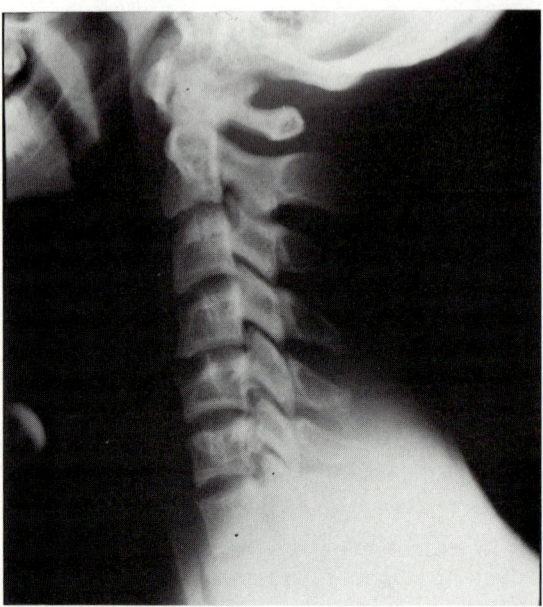

Figure 7 Lateral roentgenogram of the cervical spine taken in the erect neutral position demonstrates an anterosuperior compression defect in the vertebral body of C5 *(open arrow).* There is no evidence of angulation or displacement indicating the inherent stability of the spine. Such a radiographic finding would not constitute a contraindication to further participation.

Absolute contraindication to continued participation applies to those individuals who experience a documented episode of cervical cord neurapraxia associated with any of the following: (1) ligamentous instability, (2) intervertebral disc disease with cord compression, (3) degenerative changes with cord compression, (4) MRI evidence of cord defects or swelling, (5) symptoms or positive neurologic findings lasting more than 36 hours, or (6) more than one occurrence.

"Spear Tacklers' Spine"

Analysis of material recently received by the National Football Head and Neck Injury Registry has allowed for the description of "Spear Tacklers' Spine," an entity that consists of: (1) developmental narrowing, (2) reversal of normal cervical lordosis or kyphosis, (3) subtle torticollis, and (4) x-ray evidence of prior injury, in an individual who employs spear tackling techniques (Fig. 4, *A* and *B*). Two cases of preinjury roentgenograms as well as video documentation of axial loading of the spine due to spear tackling resulted in a bilateral C3-C4 facet dislocation, in one instance and C4-C5 fracture dislocation in the other instance with both being rendered quadriplegic. Whether the straightened "segmented column" alignment of the spine or the head first tackling technique, or a combination of the two predisposes those with "spear tacklers' spine" to catastrophic injury is not clear. However, this combination of factors constitutes an absolute contraindication to further participation in contact sports.

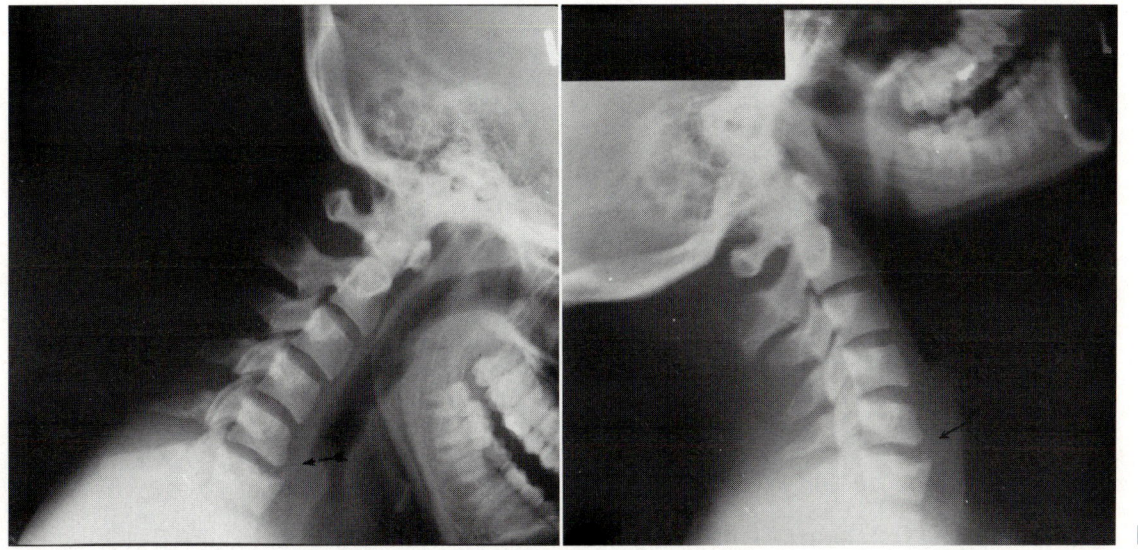

Figure 8 Lateral flexion and extension views of a healed, stable end-plate fracture involving the superior aspect of C6 in a 22-year-old intercollegiate football player. The injury had occurred 4 years prior while participating in high school. At that he relates having had a sore neck, missing two games but not having been radiographically evaluated. There were no subsequent problems despite participation in high-school and college varsity football.

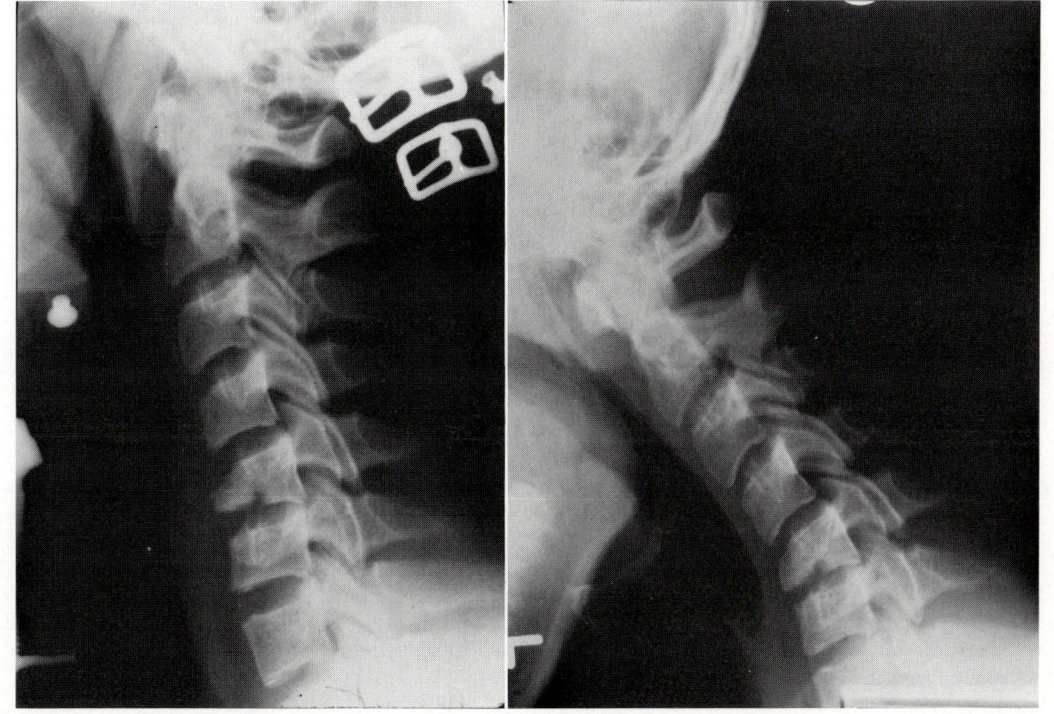

Figure 9 *A,* Lateral roentgenogram of the cervical spine taken while in a cervical brace demonstrate a displaced compression fracture of the vertebral body of C5. Of note is the fact that there is no associated angulation, displacement, intevertebral disc space narrowing, facet incongruity or fanning of the spinous processes. *B,* Lateral flexion view demonstrates pathologic angulation as defined by White et al. There is no translation, disc space narrowing, facet incongruity, or fanning of the spinous processes suggesting a stable lesion. The increased angulation is attributed to the deformity of the vertebral body. Assuming that there was no progression of the deformity, evidence of instability, and the patient had a pain-free neck with normal range of motion, this would constitute a relative contraindication to participation in contact activities depending on the player's level, position, and willingness to accept risk of reinjury.

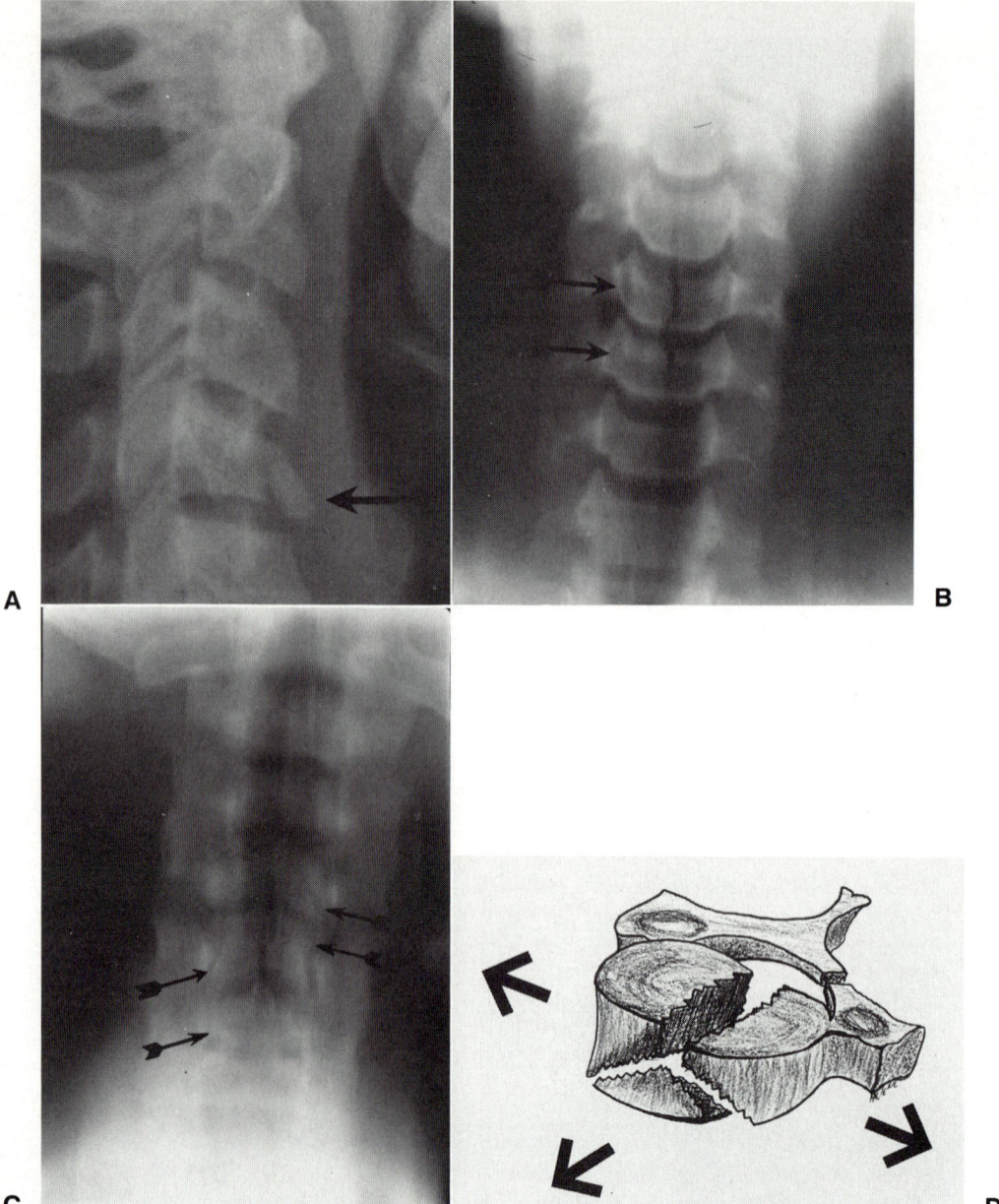

Figure 10 *A,* Lateral view of the cervical spine of a 17-year-old high-school football player who was struck on the top of his head with spring loaded tackling device demonstrates a so-called "teardrop" fracture C4. *B,* Anteroposterior views demonstrate sagittal fracture through the body of C4 and C5. *C,* Laminograms in the anteroposterior projection through the neural arch demonstrate concomitant fractures through the posterior structures. Although the youngster remained neurologically intact and went on to successful healing of the fractures, return to contact activities was absolutely contraindicated because of involvement of both anterior and posterior elements. In keeping with Steele's Rule of the Ring, a sagittal fracture through the vertebral body is associated with a disruption of the neural arch. *D,* A diagram of the axial load tear drop partial rupture demonstrates an anteroinferior corner fracture fragment and a sagittal fracture through the entire vertebral body. The posterior arch is fractured.

Traumatic Conditions of the Upper Cervical Spine (C1-C2)

The anatomy and mechanics of C1-C2 segment of the cervical spine differ markedly from the middle or lower segments. Lesions with any degree of occipital or atlantoaxial instability portend a potentially grave prognosis. Thus, most injuries involving the upper cervical segment that involve a fracture or ligamentous laxity are an absolute contraindication to further participation in contact activities (Fig. 5, *A* and *B*).

Healed, nondisplaced Jefferson fractures, healed Type I and Type II odontoid fractures, and healed lateral mass fractures of C2 constitute relative contraindications providing the patient is pain free, has a full range of cervical motion, and no neurologic findings.

Because of the uncertainty of the results of cervical

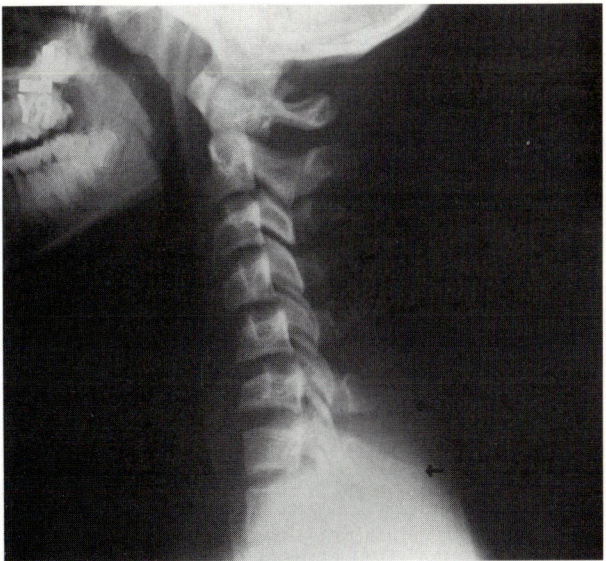

Figure 11 Lateral roentgenogram of the cervical spine in the erect neutral position demonstrates an anterosuperior compression defect in the vertebral body of C6 (*large arrow*). In addition, there is fanning of the C5-C6 spinous process indicating posterior instability due to disruption of the intraspinous and posterior longitudinal ligaments (*small arrows*). This situation constitutes an absolute contraindication to contact sports.

fusion, the gracile configuration of C1, and the importance of the alar and transverse odontoid ligaments, fusion for instability of the upper segment constitutes an absolute contraindication regardless of how successful the fusion appears roentgenographically.

Traumatic Conditions of the Middle and Lower Cervical Spine

Ligamentous Injuries

The criteria of White and Panjabi for determining clinical instability were intended to help establish indications for surgical stabilization. However, although the limits of displacement and angulation correlated with disruption of known structures, no one determinant was considered absolute. In view of the observations of Albright et al that 10% (7/75) of the college freshmen in his study demonstrated "abnormal motion" as well as on the basis of our own experience, it appears that in many instances some degree of "minor instability" exists in populations of both high school and college football players without apparent adverse effect. The question of course is what are the upper limits of "minor" instability? Unfortunately, there are no available data to relate this to the clinical situation that allow reliable standards. Clearly, however, where lateral roentgenograms demonstrate more than 3.5 m of relationship to another or more than 11 degrees rotation than either adjacent vertebra represent an absolute contraindication to further participation in contact activities (Fig. 6, *A* and *B*). With regard to lesser degrees of displacement and rotation,

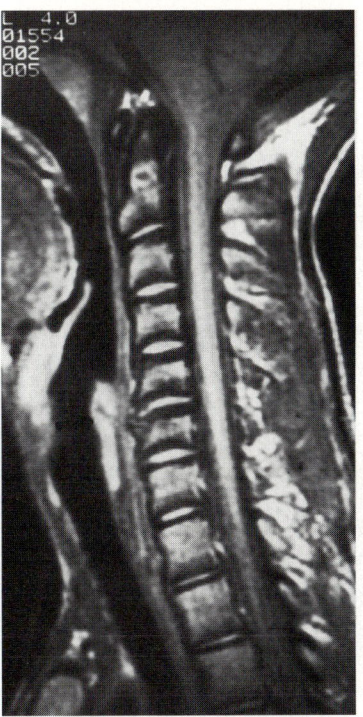

Figure 12 Magnetic resonance sagittal image of the cervical spine in a 17-year-old high-school football player with a history of prior neck injury. An anterior intervertebral disc herniation with disc space changes at the C5-C6 level is visualized (*arrow*). At the time of follow-up examination the youngster was asymptomatic, neurologically negative, and had a pain-free full range of cervical motion. He was permitted to return to contact activities.

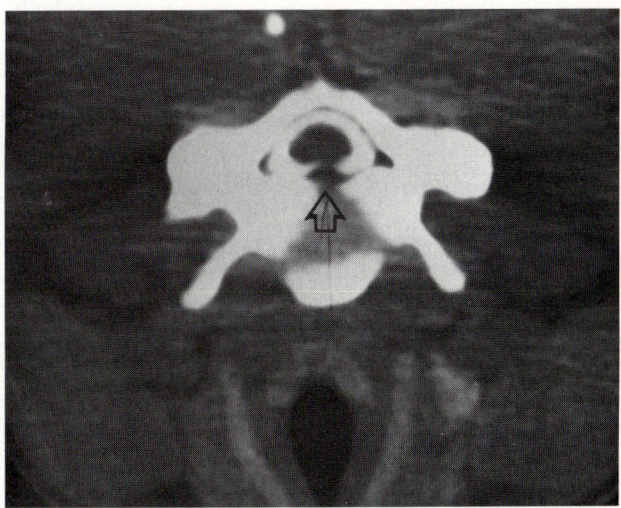

Figure 13 Coronal section of a CT myelogram through the C5-C6 interspace demonstrates a central herniation without pressure on the spinal cord. The patient, a high-school football player had had an episode of cervical cord neurapraxia associated with congenital narrowing (stenosis) of the cervical canal. Lateral roentgenograms demonstrated reversal of the normal cervical lordosis. In addition, he had a rye neck attitude and decreased neck motion. His situation represents an absolute contraindication to participation in contact activities.

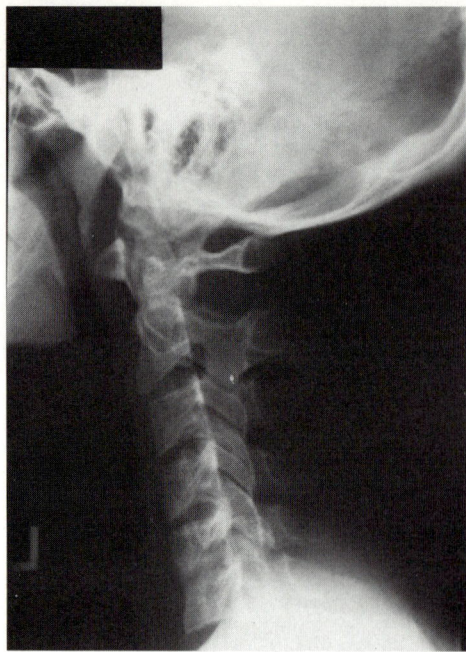

Figure 14 Lateral roentgenogram of a 28-year-old professional ice hockey player who underwent a successful one-level interbody fusion at C5-C6 for instability. He subsequently played 2 years without a problem.

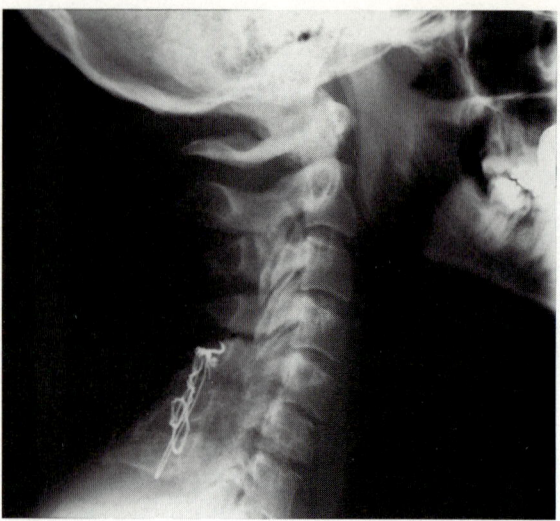

Figure 15 Lateral roentgenogram of the cervical spine of a 28-year-old former professional football player who had undergone a C4-C5-C6 posterior fusion of a post-traumatic instability. He subsequently returned to play football, however, he developed stiffness, neck discomfort, and limited motion. The individual who elects to return to contact activities following more than a two-level fusion must understand that the probability of symptoms resulting from degenerative changes at the articulations above and below the fusion must be considered.

further participation enters the realms of "trial by battle" and such situations can be considered a relative contraindication depending on such factors as level of performance, physical habitus, position played (i.e., interior lineman versus defensive backs), etc.

Fractures

An acute fracture of either the body or posterior elements with or without associated ligamentous laxity constitutes an absolute contraindication to participation. The following healed, stable fracture in an asymptomatic patient who is neurologically normal and has full range of cervical motion can be considered to have no contraindication to participation in contact activities.

1. Stable compression fractures of the vertebral body without a sagittal component on anterior/posterior roentgenogram and without involvement of either the ligaments or posterior bony structures (Fig. 7).
2. A healed stable endplate fracture without a sagittal component on anterior/posterior roentgenograms or involvement of the posterior or bony ligamentous structures (Fig. 8, *A* and *B*).
3. Healed spinous process "Clay Shoveler" fractures.

Relative contraindications apply to the following healed stable fractures in individuals who are asymptomatic, neurologically normal, and have a full pain-free range of cervical motion.

1. Stable displaced vertebral body compression fractures without a sagittal component on anterior/posterior roentgenograms. The propensity for these fractures to settle with increased deformity must be considered and carefully followed (Fig. 9, *A* and *B*).
2. Healed stable fractures involving the elements of the posterior neural ring in individuals who are asymptomatic, neurologically normal, have a full pain-free range of cervical motion. In evaluating radiographic and imaging studies to find the location and subsequent healing of posterior neural ring fractures it is important to understand that, as pointed out by Steel, a rigid ring cannot break in one location. Thus, healing of paired fractures of the ring must be demonstrated.

Absolute contraindication to further participation in contact activities exist in the presence of the following fractures.

1. Vertebral body fracture with a sagittal component (Figs. 10, *A* to *C*, and 11).
2. Fracture of the vertebral body with or without displacement with associated posterior arch fractures and/or ligamentous laxity (Fig. 11).
3. Comminuted fractures of the vertebral body with displacement into the spinal cord.
4. Any healed fracture of either the vertebral body or posterior components with associated pain,

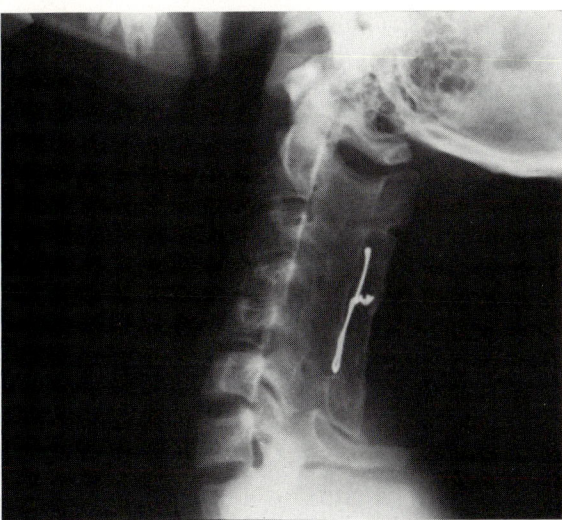

Figure 16 Lateral roentgenograms of an 18-year-old youngster who had injured his neck playing football when he was 13. At that time, a three-level posterior fusion and wiring was performed, however, it appears that periosteal stripping of adjacent vertebra above and below resulted in a five-level fusion. Such a situation is an absolute contraindication to participation in contact activities.

neurologic findings, limitation of normal cervical motion.

5. Healed displaced fractures involving the lateral masses with resulting facet incongruity.

Intervertebral Disc Injury

There is no contraindication to participation in contact activities in individuals with a healed anterior or lateral disc herniation treated conservatively (Fig. 12) or those requiring an intervertebral discectomy and interbody fusion for a lateral or central herniation who have a solid fusion are symptomatic, neurologically negative, and have a full pain-free range of motion.

A relative contraindication exists in those individuals with either conservatively or surgically treated disc disease with residual facet instability.

An absolute contraindication exists in the following situations: (1) acute central disc (Fig. 13); (2) acute or chronic "hard disc" herniation with associated neurologic findings, pain, and/or significant limitation of cervical motion; and (3) acute or chronic "hard disc" herniation with associated symptoms of cord neurapraxia due to concomitant congenital narrowing "stenosis" of the cervical canal.

Status Postcervical Spine Fusion

A stable one-level anterior or posterior fusion in a patient who is asymptomatic, neurologically negative, is pain free and a normal range of cervical motion presents no contraindication to continued participation in contact activities (Fig. 14).

Individuals with a stable two- or three-level fusion who are asymptomatic, neurologically negative, and have a pain-free full range of cervical motion present a relative contraindication (Fig. 15). Because of the presumed increased stresses at the articulations of the adjacent uninvolved vertebra and the propensity for the development of degenerative changes at these levels, it appears to be the rare exception who should be permitted to continue contact activities.

In those individuals with more than a three-level anterior or posterior fusion, continued participation in contact activities is absolutely contraindicated (Fig. 16).

SUGGESTED READING

Albright JP, Moses JM, Feldich HG, et al. Non-fatal cervical spine injuries in interscholastic football. JAMA 1976; 236:1243-1245.

Bailes JE, Hadley MN, Quigley MR. Management of athletic cervical spine and spinal cord injuries. J Neurosurg In Press.

Eismont FJ, Clifford S, Goldberg M, et al. Cervical sagittal spinal canal size in spine injuries. Spine 1984; 9:663-666.

Hensinger RN. Congenital anomalies of the odontoid: The cervical spine. 2nd Ed. The Cervical Spine Research Society Editorial Committee. Philadelphia: JB Lippincott, 1989:248.

Pizzutillo PD. Klippel-Feil syndrome: The cervical spine. 2nd Ed. The Cervical Spine Research Society Editorial Committee. Philadelphia: JB Lippincott, 1987:258.

Torg JS, Truex R, Quedenfeld TC. The national football head and neck injury registry: Report and conclusions. JAMA 1979; 241:1477-1479.

Torg JS, Vegso JJ, Sennett B. The national football head and neck injury registry; 14 year report on cervical quadriplegia, 1971 through 1985. JAMA 1985; 254:3439-3443.

Torg JS, Pavlov H, Genuario SE, et al. Neurapraxia of the cervical spinal cord with transient quadriplegia. J Bone Joint Surg 1988; 68A:1354-1370.

Torg JS, Vegso JJ, O'Neill J. The epidemiologic, pathologic, biomechanical and cinematographic analysis of football-induced cervical spine trauma. Am J Sports Med 1990; 18:50-57.

White AA, Johnson RM, Panjobi MM, et al. Biomechanical analysis of clinical stability in the cervical spine. Clin Orthop 1975; 109:85.

BACKACHE

IAN MacNAB, M.B., Ch.B., F.R.C.S., F.R.C.S.(C)

REFERRED PAIN

A major factor that has clouded and confused the diagnosis of soft tissue lesions of the back is the phenomenon of referred pain. When a deep structure is irritated, whether by trauma, disease, or the experimental injection of an irritating solution, the pain resulting may be experienced locally, referred distally, or experienced both locally and radiating to a distance. It is important to recognize that tenderness may also be referred to a distance, as has been shown by the injection of hypertonic saline into the lumbosacral supraspinous ligament. Under such circumstances, pain not only may radiate down the leg but also may be associated with tender points, which are commonly situated over the

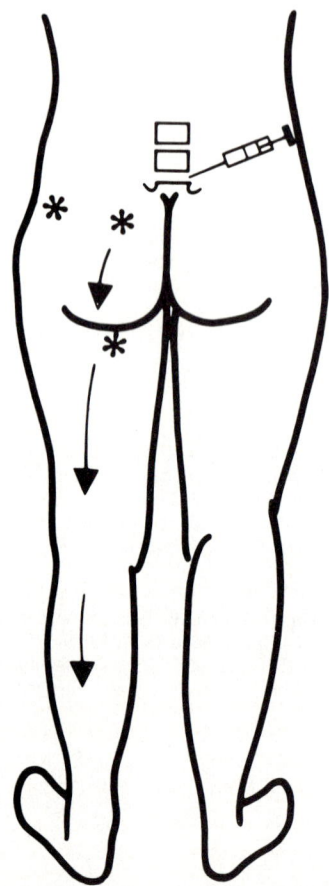

Figure 1 The injection of hypertonic saline into the supraspinous ligament between L5 and S1 gives rise to local pain and pain referred down the back of the leg in sciatic distribution. Usually, this does not extend below the knee, and there are points of tenderness in the lower limbs, most commonly noted at the sites marked by the asterisks.

sacroiliac joint and the upper outer quadrant of the buttock (Fig. 1).

The complaint of pain and the demonstration of local tenderness may obscure the fact that the offending lesion is centrally placed and may lead the clinician to believe erroneously that the disease process underlies the site of the patient's complaints. This false belief may apparently be confirmed by the temporary relief of pain on injection of a local anesthetic when in reality there is no local problem at all. These points must be borne in mind when considering the site and nature of soft tissue injuries giving rise to low back pain; a failure to do so will lead to diagnostic and therapeutic errors.

MYOFASCIAL SPRAINS OR STRAINS

Partial tears of the attachment of muscles may occur, giving rise to local tenderness and pain, generally of short duration. There is always a history of specific injury, either a blunt blow or a forceful movement, usually rotation. The pain and tenderness are always away from the midline. This is a young man's injury with strong muscles guarding a healthy spine. A similar injury sustained by an older man with weaker muscles and with degenerate discs is much more likely to result in a posterior joint strain.

These lesions heal with the passage of time despite, rather than because of, treatment.

Injections of local anesthetic (with or without the addition of local steroids) in and around the area of maximal tenderness certainly afford temporary relief of varying duration, but it is doubtful whether they speed the resolution of the underlying pathologic condition. The symptoms may persist for about 3 weeks in varying degree, during which time the patient is well advised to avoid provocative activity. If symptoms persist beyond this period, the problem should be carefully reassessed lest some more significant underlying lesion be overlooked.

TENDINITIS

Tendinitis by custom has come to be associated with athletic activities. However, it must be remembered that tendinitis is just a clinical syndrome, the pathologic basis of which is inadequately defined. Clinically, it is recognized that well-localized areas of tenderness may develop at the attachment of tendons, fascia, or ligaments to bone, anywhere in the body.

In the spine, breakdown changes of this nature may occur at the attachment of muscles to the sacrum or iliac crest, or the supraspinous ligaments may give rise to pain after having been subjected to moderate to mild trauma. On examination, the areas of breakdown present a small but well-localized area of tenderness. Pressure over the area not only elicits tenderness, but when maintained reproduces the symptoms.

The pathologic basis of this syndrome is probably a local area of tendon breakdown or degeneration, which invokes an inflammatory or autoimmune response. It is possibly the vascular reaction associated with localized edema that accounts for the pain and tenderness. Empirically, it has been found that gratifyingly rapid relief of pain can be obtained by the injection of steroids.

KISSING SPINES: SPRUNG BACK

Approximation of the spinous processes (kissing spines) and the development of a bursa between them have been indicated as a cause of low back pain after hyperextension injuries. "Sprung back" is a term coined by Newman to describe rupture of the supraspinous ligament following a sudden flexion strain applied to the spine with the pelvis fixed, as in falling on the buttocks with the legs outstretched. It is doubtful whether either of these entities is of itself a cause of low back pain (Fig. 2) in the absence of disc degeneration allowing excessive movement at the segment.

With a normal disc, extension of a segment is limited by the anterior fibers of the annulus, and at the limit of normal extension the spinous processes do not come into contact. Contact between the spinous processes is seen only with abnormal mobility associated with disc degeneration. Although apposition of the spinous processes and the development of a painful bursa may aggravate and intensify the symptoms derived from segmental instability associated with degenerative disc disease, these are never the sole source of symptoms. Tearing of the supraspinous ligament, thought to be the basis of "sprung back," can occur only in the presence of disc degeneration allowing an abnormal degree of flexion, or with an injury severe enough to disrupt the posterior fibers of the annulus and the capsule of the posterior joints.

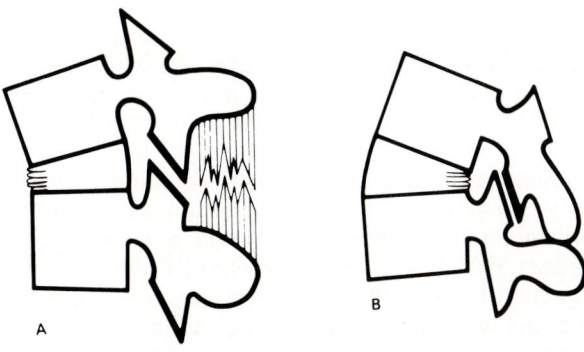

Figure 2 *A,* An acute flexion injury of the spine may produce a tear of the supraspinous ligament. This lesion has been referred to as a "sprung back." It is unlikely, however, that this lesion can occur in the absence of gross disc degeneration, which by itself is probably the source of the patient's complaint. *B,* The radiologic demonstration of apposition of the spinous processes has been referred to as "kissing spines." This anatomic disposition of the spinous processes cannot occur in the absence of an unstable disc segment. In the balance of probabilities, it is the associated disc degeneration rather than the bony apposition of the spinous processes that is the cause of the symptoms.

Separation and apposition of the spinous processes when symptomatic are indicative of segmental instability associated with disc degeneration, and the treatment of such lesions is therefore that of the associated disc degeneration.

DISC DEGENERATION

It is necessary to discuss briefly the changes associated with disc degeneration and the manner in which they predispose to symptoms after minor to moderate injury.

The intervertebral discs are composed of a combination of the annulus, the nucleus pulposus, and the hyaline cartilage plate, which makes for a very efficient coupling unit, provided that all the structures remain intact. Normally, the vertebral bodies roll over the incompressible gel of the nucleus pulposus, whose structural integrity is maintained by the annulus, with the posterior joints guiding and steadying the movement. Once degenerative changes involve any one of the components of the disc, such as inspissation of the nucleus pulposus, a tear in the annulus, or a rupture of the hyaline cartilage plate, the smooth roller action is lost and the movement between adjacent vertebral segments becomes uneven, excessive, and irregular. Although these changes occur most commonly at about the age of 40, they may affect younger age groups, especially when there is a family history of low back pain.

Normally, on flexion of the spine, the discal borders of the vertebral bodies become parallel above the level of L5. This is the maximal movement permitted. In the stage of segmental instability, excessive degrees of extension and flexion are permitted and a certain amount of backward and forward gliding movement also occurs (Fig. 3). This abnormal type of movement can be shown clinically by roentgenograms taken with the patient holding the spine in full extension and in full flexion. One problem posed by motion studies is the fact that when a patient is in pain, the associated muscle guarding does not permit adequate flexion and extension films to be taken. However, there are two radiologic changes that are indicative of instability, the Knuttson phenomenon of gas in the disc and the "traction spur."

The traction spur differs anatomically and radiologically from other spondylophytes in that it projects horizontally and develops about 2 mm above the vertebral body edge (Fig. 4). It owes its development to the manner of attachment of the annulus fibers. With abnormal movements, an excessive strain is applied to the outermost annulus fibers, and it is here that the traction spur develops. It is a small traction spur that is clinically significant in that it is probably indicative of present instability.

Segmental instability by itself is probably not painful, but the spine is vulnerable to trauma. A forced and unguarded movement may be concentrated on the wobbly segment and produce a posterior joint strain or a posterior joint subluxation. Repeated injuries may

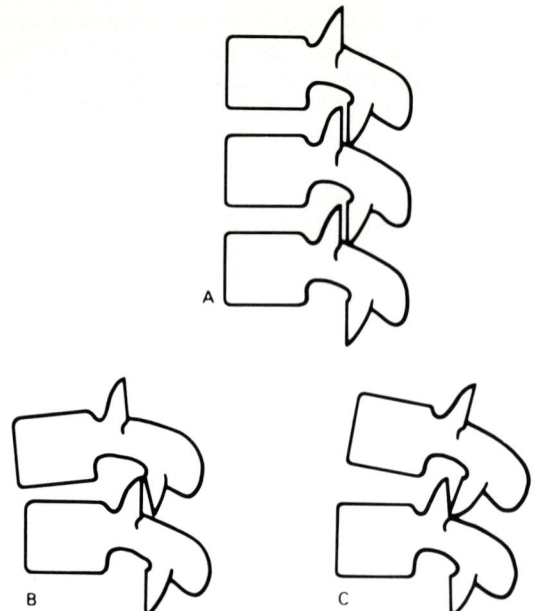

Figure 3 In the early stages of degenerative disc disease, excessive degrees of flexion and extension are permitted at the involved segment. This abnormal mobility is associated with rocking of the posterior joints (*B* and *C*).

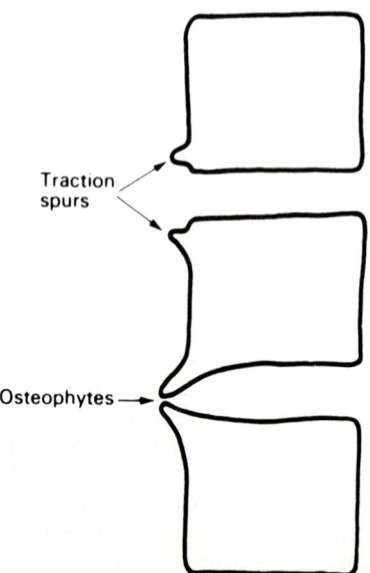

Figure 4 The traction spur projects horizontally from the vertebral body about 1 mm away from the discal border.

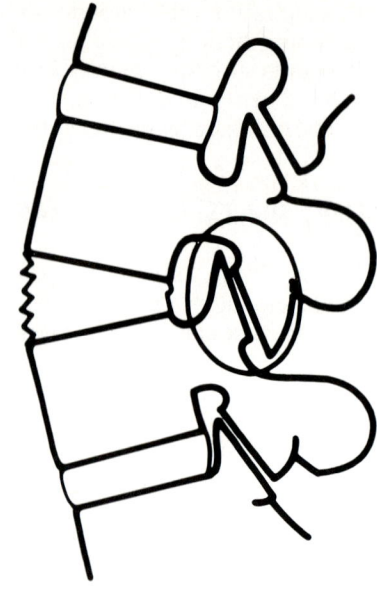

Figure 5 When the anterior fibers of the annulus lose their elasticity, the involved segment falls into hyperextension, permitting subluxation of the related posterior joint.

indeed produce osteochondral fractures and loose bodies in the posterior joints.

In the next stage of disc degeneration, segmental hyperextension occurs. Extension of the lumbar spine is limited by the anterior fibers of the annulus. When degenerative changes cause these fibers to lose their elasticity, the involved segment or segments may hyperextend (Fig. 5). A similar change may be seen in the next stage of disc degeneration, disc narrowing. As the intervertebral discs lose height, the posterior joints must override and subluxate (Fig. 6). In both segmental hyperextension and disc narrowing, the related posterior joints in normal posture are held in hyperextension, and this postural defect is exaggerated if the patient has weak abdominal muscles or tight tensors.

When the posterior joints are held at the extreme of their limit of extension, there is no safety factor of movement, and the extension strains of everyday living may push the joints past their physiologically permitted limits and thereby produce pain.

On the premise that most backaches occur before the age of 40, the roentgenograms of 300 40-year-old laborers, who had been engaged in heavy work all their lives, were reviewed. Of these, 150 denied any history of low back pain and 150 were under treatment for backache at the time of the review. A careful statistical analysis of the films showed no difference in the incidence of anatomic variants and the incidence of degenerative changes in the two groups studied. This is important because the mere demonstration of an anatomic anomaly or a minor pathologic change is no reason to prevent the athlete from continuing with sports activities.

With our present state of knowledge regarding disc degeneration, only the following may be stated: (1) disc degeneration may occur and may remain asymptomatic; (2) disc degeneration may be associated with changes within the disc itself, which may be productive of pain; and (3) disc degeneration may give rise to mechanical instability that renders the spine vulnerable to trauma, as a result of which pain may arise from ligamentous or posterior joint damage.

The pain experienced may remain localized to the

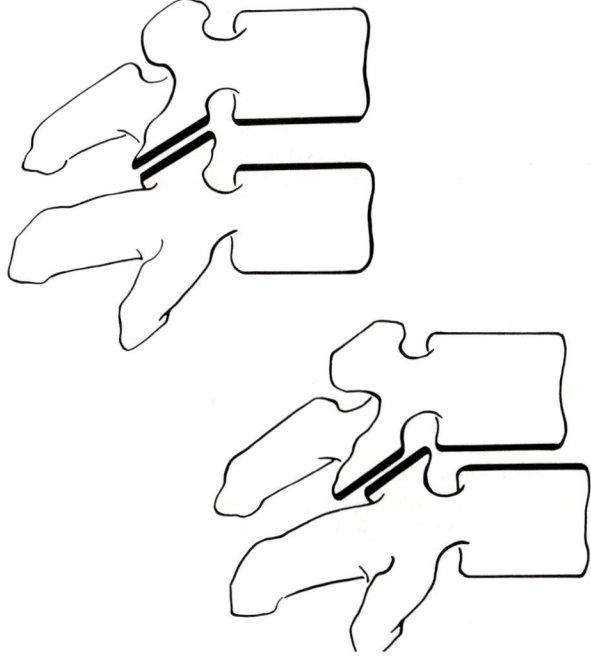

Figure 6 As the intervertebral discs lose height and the vertebral bodies approach one another, the posterior joints must override and assume the position normally held in hyperextension. It is to be noted that owing to the inclination of the posterior joints, as the upper vertebral body approaches the vertebral body beneath it, it is displaced backward, producing a retrospondylolisthesis. This posterior displacement of the vertebral body, indicative of posterior joint subluxation, is readily recognizable on routine x-ray examination of the lumbar spine.

back; there may be both local pain and referred pain; or there may be referred pain only.

DISC RUPTURES

An intervertebral disc separating two vertebral segments may be likened to the old-fashioned motorcar tire, with a hard, outer fibrous casing and an inner tube — in this case filled with jelly. A ruptured disc may occur in one of two forms: either similar to a blister in the motorcar tire with a weakening of the outer casing, or on occasion as a complete blowout (sequestration) of the inner tube through the hole in the outer fibers of the annulus.

In 1934 Mixter and Barr suggested that sciatic pain could result from irritation of a lumbar nerve root by a prolapsed intervertebral disc. Although skeptically received at first, this concept soon became universally accepted and founded the "dynasty of the disc," during which time the complaint of sciatic pain tended to become uncritically equated with a diagnosis of disc herniation. Surgical exploration of patients with evidence of lumbar nerve root irritation revealed that there are indeed several sources of nerve root compromise, of which a ruptured intervertebral disc is but one example.

A ruptured intervertebral disc produces nerve root

pressure and this presents as radicular pain, i.e., pain radiating from the buttock to the ankle, associated with paresthesia, associated with signs of root tension, and on occasion with evidence of impairment of root conduction. This lesion does not commonly result from a sports-related injury.

If the person has a mechanically insufficient spine and sustains a vigorous strain, the symptoms resulting, as stated previously, may be backache with pain *referred* down the leg in sciatic distribution. This referred pain rarely goes below the knee; it is not associated with paresthesia; it is not associated with signs of nerve root tension, such as limitation of straight leg raising; and it is never associated with any evidence of impairment of root conduction, as reflected by changes in reflex activity, sensory apppreciation, or motor power.

If patients are just about to suffer from a prolapsed disc, they may well sustain the prolapse while going down a ski slope, but the sport of skiing is not of itself commonly associated with the production of a ruptured disc. The back injuries associated with athletics are the injuries of joint sprains and associated muscle and fascial damage. The pain resulting from this varies in severity. Characteristically, while patients are carrying out normal activities in sports, they are suddenly seized with back pain and cannot move ("I was paralyzed with pain"). The lumbar spine is splinted rigidly, and patients can move only with painful caution, clutching their back and walking with the trunk leaning forward, keeping the hips and knees slightly bent.

Examination reveals that all movements of the spine are limited by pain and muscle spasm, but there is no evidence of nerve root tension. The clinical picture is explosively dramatic and threatening to the patient. Physicians must not overreact, but constantly remind themselves that even if they elected to treat the patient by rolling peanut butter on each buttock, in the balance of probabilities the patient would get well fairly quickly.

In most such cases the patient is suffering from a "sprain" of one of the zygoapophyseal joints. When trying to rationalize treatment, one should compare the lesion with a severely sprained ankle in a patient who has only one leg and who is unable to wear a prosthesis. There is only one way to treat a sprained ankle in such a patient — the patient has to be put to bed. Theoretically, the patient with an acute low back strain should also be treated by strict bed rest. However, theoretical treatment must be tempered by reason, and reasoning must be tempered by the patient's reaction to therapeutic suggestions.

Let me repeat: you are treating a patient and not a spine, and the experience of the lay world is that many (in fact, most) get better by just creeping around with the pain mollified by analgesics. Some patients, however, cannot cope; their pain is too severe. In such instances, if they cannot do their normal daily work, they should be sent to bed.

A patient with pneumonia is ill and defeated, and happy to go to bed. Patients with severe low back pain feel well in themselves and do not want to go to bed. They are mad at their affliction, and your insistence on bed rest will increase their frustration unless you take time to explain in detail the purpose of this apparently neglectful form of management. It is advisable to give patients some literature explaining in detail the probable underlying pathology and the rationale of treatment by bed rest. You must advise them about toilet facilities. Using a bedpan at home is an impractical acrobatic feat. Crutches make it easier for patients to get to the bathroom, and the purchase of a high toilet seat is essential.

To relieve the pain, local ice application has definite merit for the first 48 hours. Local application of ice over

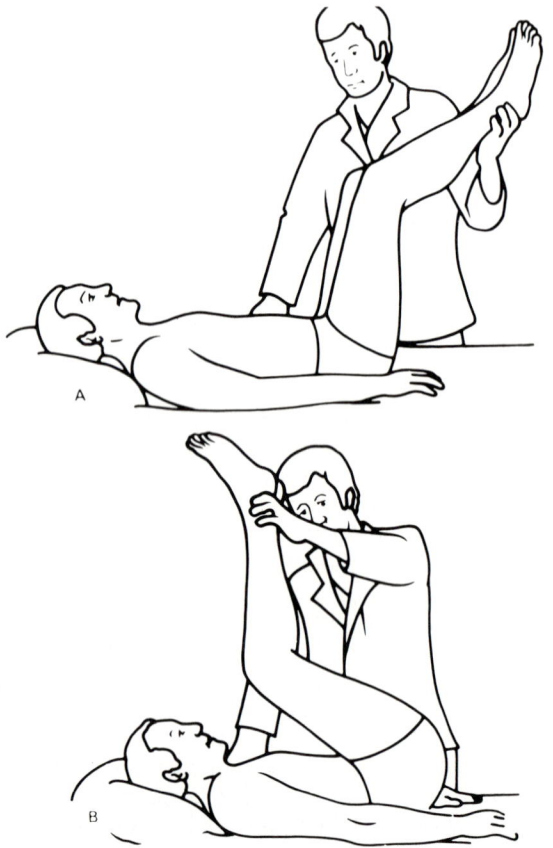

Figure 7 *A*, Flexion manipulation by the physician, who raises the patient's legs, maintaining the knees in flexion. *B*, By applying pressure to the heels, the physician then pushes the patient's knees toward the shoulders.

a muscle probably acts on the muscle's spindle system. A muscle that retains its extensibility through its normal resting length is usually pain free. When it does not retain its extensibility, it is considered to be in "spasm" and a source of pain. Ice applied to the overlying skin probably sends impulses to the cord that "compete" with the pain, producing impulses that are conveyed by much slower fibers. The ice-produced impulses temporarily cause a refractory period in the other impulses, and the muscle spasm is momentarily relieved. Stretch of the muscle is now possible, which decreases the spasm. If ice is applied for too long a period, the muscle may become literally chilled, and this increases muscle spasm and adds to the pain.

There are very few orally administered muscle "relaxants" that have any effect on skeletal muscles. If they were truly effective, the eye muscles would also be grossly relaxed, and the patient would develop nystagmus. Their major action is as a tranquilizer. Analgesics in sufficient doses can be given, but they must be given on a time-dependent basis and not on demand. These patients must not be allowed to pop pills for pain; otherwise the physician is just inducing a habituation. In the vast majority of patients, after 2 or 3 days the "smoke clears away" and they can get around each day with increasing comfort.

If on neurologic examination there is neither evidence of nerve root compression or irritation nor of impairment of root conduction, the resolution of symptoms may be speeded by a flexion manipulation (Fig. 7). The patient lies on the back and the physician raises the patient's legs, maintaining the knees in flexion. By applying pressure on the heels, the physician then pushes the patient's knees toward the shoulders; this is done very slowly. The degree of flexion obtained is determined by the discomfort the patient experiences. The movement is then repeated slowly and rhythmically over a period of 5 minutes. In most cases the range of movement that can be achieved by this passive manipulation gradually increases, and at the conclusion of the manipulation the patient is instructed to flex his knees fully and allow his feet to come down to the bed, soles first.

The patient then carries out a series of passive flexion manipulations of his spine once an hour. He does this by lying on his back and pulling his knees slowly up to his chest (Fig. 8). He should maintain this position for

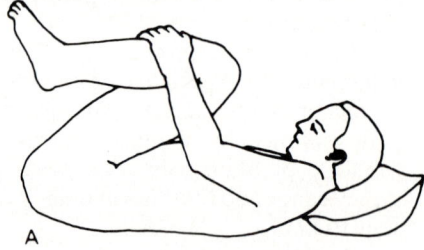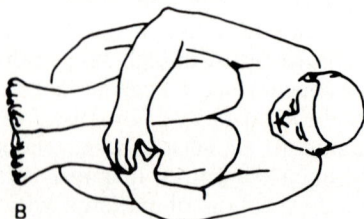

Figure 8 A patient may abort an acute episode of low back pain by lying on his back and pulling his knees slowly up to his chest. *A*, He should maintain this position for 5 minutes. If pain is severe, the patient may find it easier to assume the same position lying on his side *(B)*.

5 minutes. In very acute attacks with severe pain, the patient may find it easier to assume the same position lying on his side. By the second day the patient should be able to carry out the flexion manipulations of his back himself (Fig. 9).

Once the attack is over, the patient and the physician are now faced with the difficulty of trying to prevent recurrent episodes. Adequate trunk muscles are the major guardians against repeated attacks. It must be remembered that the spinal column is not a self-supporting structure. If the trunk and abdominal muscles are paralyzed, as in infantile paralysis, the spine collapses. The spine is supported by muscle action in much the same way the mast of a ship is supported by stays (Fig. 10). In addition to this, the abdominal cavity acts as a hydraulic sac, dissipating loads by pressing upward on the diaphragm and downward on the pelvic floor, thereby unweighting the spine (Fig. 11). Because of this, the tone and strength of the abdominal muscles are of vital importance in protecting the spine against weight bearing and extension strains.

The exercise program is started by pelvic tilting. This is best carried out with the patient lying supine on a firm surface. The patient lies in a comfortable position with the hips and knees flexed, keeping the soles of both feet flat on the bed or floor. The patient now presses the lower back down flat against the floor so that the lumbar lordosis is obliterated. This movement is achieved by a combined contraction of the abdominal muscles and the glutei. In order to help the patient get into this habit, it is often easier to ask him to put his hands behind his back and press his spine back onto his hands.

Once the lumbar spine is pressing against the floor,

the pelvis is rotated by raising the buttocks from the floor. As the buttocks are being raised, the lower back must not be permitted to leave the floor. Raising the buttocks away from the floor reverses the lumbar lordosis. Patients may find it easier if they put one hand on the symphysis pubis and the other on the xyphoid process and then try to bring their hands together while doing the exercises. As patients become more adept at this exercise, they should practice the movement rhythmically, initially with the hips and knees flexed before trying the same exercise with the hips and knees flat.

Pelvic tilting can also be practiced with the patient standing with his back flat against the wall and his feet about 2 feet away from the wall. Holding his lumbar spine flat against the wall (checking this with a hand placed between his spine and the wall), he then gradually brings his heels toward the wall and tries to straighten his knees. To begin with this is difficult, but when he can achieve this easily he has managed to learn the art of pelvic tilting in a manner that will overcome a tendency to hyperlordosis.

When flexion exercises are started, the patient should lie on his back with his hips and knees bent and his feet *supported*. He should put his hands forward to touch his thighs and then gradually crawl up his thighs until his hands are on the top of his knees. He should then take his hands away from his knees and let his back fall gently into the supine position. Flexion exercises should never be performed with the patient holding his knees fully extended. The only way it is possible to get up with the knees extended is to whip the back up, because the weight of the trunk is greater than the weight of the legs. A person has to put an extension strain on the lower

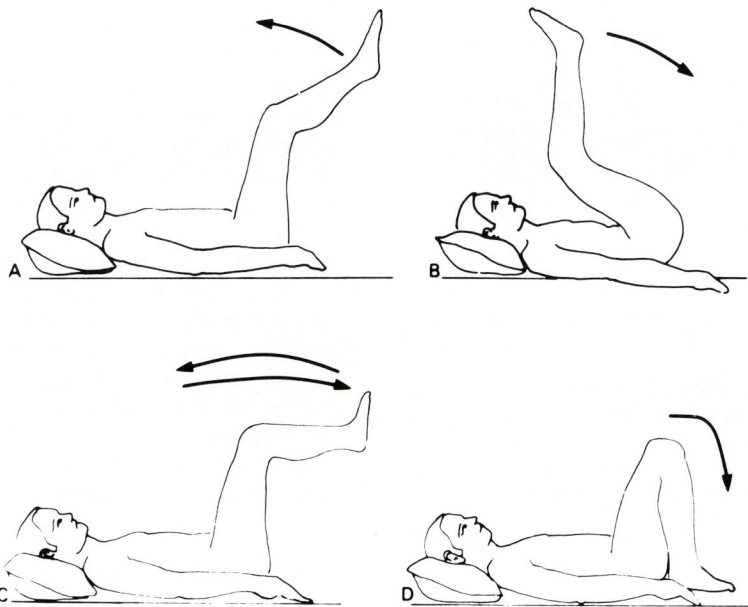

Figure 9 Flexion exercise-manipulation of the lumbar spine. The patient lies on the bed with his head supported by a pillow. *A,* The hips are flexed to 90 degrees and the knees slightly flexed. *B,* The patient now attempts to kick his feet over his head, raising the buttocks approximately 6 inches off the bed. *C,* After each "kick-up" the patient returns to the starting position. *D,* After five kick-ups, the patient rests by lowering his legs with the knees fully flexed, thereby putting his feet on the bed, soles first. It is very important not to lower the legs with the knees fully extended because this places a painful hyperextension strain on the spine.

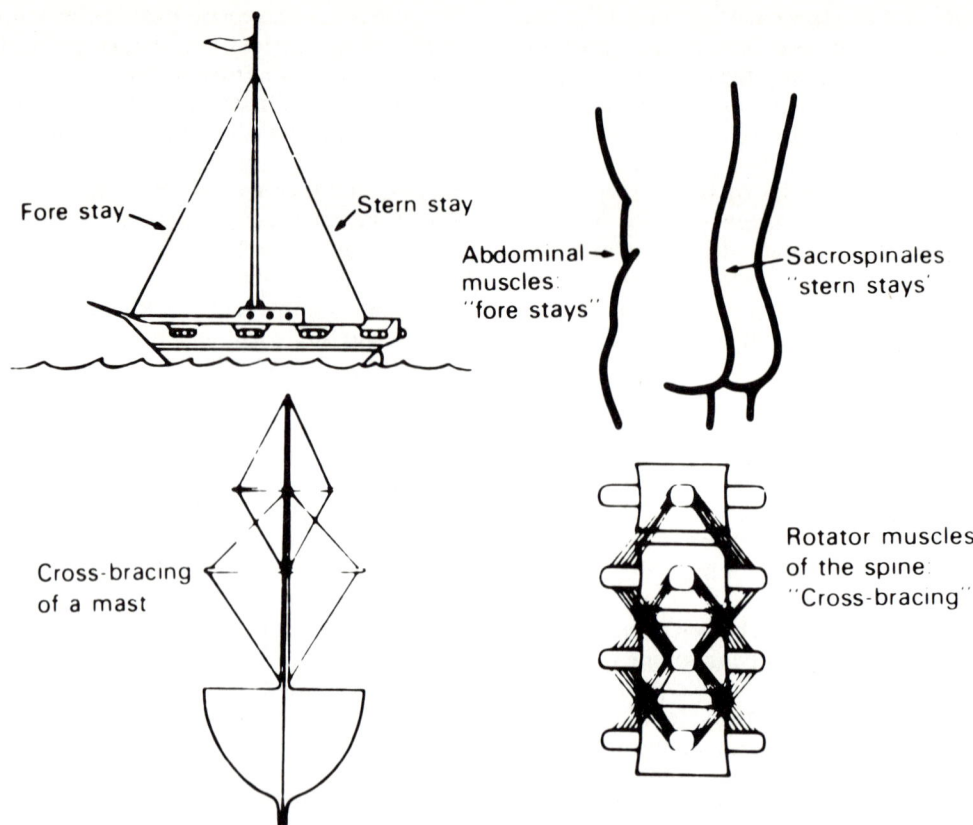

Figure 10 It is interesting to note the similarity between the bracing used to support the mast of a ship and the muscular bracing of the human spine.

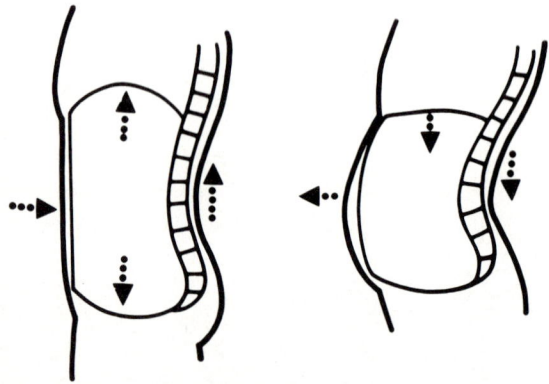

Figure 11 The abdominal cavity acts in a manner similar to a hydraulic sac. By increasing intra-abdominal pressure, the diaphragm is pushed up and the pelvic floor is pushed down. This tends to "elongate" the lumbar spine, thereby taking some of the weight off the discs and the posterior joints.

back to begin the movement and then the rest of the spine is flung forward, as with a whiplash.

At this stage it is necessary, in the prevention of recurrence of back pain, to test for the flexibility of the hamstrings and the heel cords. The supine position is again used. One leg is fully flexed at the hip with the knee and thigh against the chest. The leg undergoing the

stretching of the hamstrings is maintained in full extension. The patient now tries to sit up slowly and reach toward the toes of the extended leg. The fixed, flexed leg prevents the occurrence of hyperlordosis during the act of sitting up. If the heel cords are found to be tight, the extended leg should be placed in such a manner that the sole of the foot is flat against the wall. The heel cords can also be stretched by leaning forward against the wall, keeping the feet flat on the floor, and the force applied to the heel cords can be increased by getting the patient to squat down.

On occasion, a tight tensor fascia femoris causes anterior pelvic rotation, which increases the lumbar lordosis. This needs passive stretching by a physiotherapist.

As in all therapeutic exercises, a few specific exercises are initially directed toward the lesion being treated, but once the discomfort starts to subside it is of vital importance that the patient engage in a general controlled physical exercise program.

FURTHER INVESTIGATION

The question is often asked, "When should you take an x-ray?" Probably the following criteria are adequate:

1. Severe back pain following significant trauma.
2. Incapacitating back pain.

3. Excessively anxious patients. In such people, an x-ray examination is an essential part of treatment; they cannot be reassured by clinical examination alone.

4. Patients in whom the history and examination are suggestive of an early ankylosing spondylitis. A specific request should be made for oblique views of the sacroiliac joint.

5. Patients with clinically apparent spinal deformity.

6. Patients with significant root tension and patients presenting with evidence of impairment of root conduction. It must be remembered that being very athletically inclined does not prevent these young people from having a tumor of the cauda equina.

7. If severe pain persists for longer than 2 weeks despite treatment, an x-ray examination is indicated, not only to exclude the possibility of some obscure spinal abnormality, but also to reassure patients that they are not suffering from a serious progressive disease.

On occasion the radiograph reveals a spinal anomaly. Of the spinal anomalies once believed to cause back pain, such as sacralization of L5, spina bifida occulta, the ossicle of Oppenheimer, and a unilateral iliotransverse joint, all are now recognized as being incidental findings that have no influence on the development of low back pain.

There remains just one bone anomaly that gives rise to concern. If the radiograph reveals a spondylolysis of L5 with or without a listhesis, the question always arises whether this defect in the pars interarticularis developed as a result of repeated trauma on the football field or whether the patient had this defect before he started playing football.

It has been reported, and convincingly demonstrated radiographically, that linebackers may develop in the course of the season, as a result of the vigorous hyperextension strains they place on each other, a stress fracture through the pars interarticularis, giving rise to a spondylolysis. Without specific therapy and certainly without surgery, over the course of the next 6 months, these stress fractures heal by themselves and will not be the source of further disability.

In patients in whom a routine x-ray examination reveals a spondylolisthesis of grade I or more, the question is always raised whether it is safe to let the young athlete continue with contact sports. There is no evidence that vigorous physical contact will cause an increasing slip. These patients may have a pain derived either from the subjacent disc, from the syndesmosis at the site of the isthmic defect, or most probably from degenerative disc changes occurring at the level above the slip. Any one or all three of these factors may be responsible for repeated episodes of discomfort during play and may markedly interfere with the patient's competence.

In these patients, there are two choices. Either they must give up contact sports or, if this is going to be their profession, the question is raised whether they should be admitted to the hospital for more detailed analysis of the source of the discomfort, to see whether it is possible to stop abnormal movement at the level of the defect and stabilize the degenerative disc above the slip by a localized intertransverse fusion. It must always be remembered that it will take at least 9 months to 1 year before this young person returns to competitive sports.

In the diagnosis and management of a patient presenting with low back pain, orthopedic surgeons must play many roles: family practitioner, internist, radiologist, physiatrist, orthotist, psychiatrist, social worker, and friend. They should rarely find it necessary to play the role of their chosen avocation—orthopedic surgeon.

SPINAL DEFORMITIES

LYLE J. MICHELI, M.D.
ELLY TREPMAN, M.D.

The physician dealing with sports-related injuries must have a working knowledge of both normal spinal contour and structural spinal deformities. The importance of the spine in normal function cannot be overemphasized. It is the structural centrum from which extremity motion initiates, and it contains important elements of the central nervous system and the origin of the peripheral nerves. Spinal deformities may increase the potential for spinal injury or compromise spinal function during athletic activities.

The four major issues pertaining to spinal deformities are:

1. Detection of spinal abnormalities that may render sports participation ineffective or even dangerous for a child.

2. Early detection of spinal deformity in the child athlete, with the initiation of ongoing assessment or bracing.

3. Effective management of relatively mild spinal deformities with bracing or electrical stimulation techniques and directed exercises while a child continues to participate in sports.

4. Determination of the level of athletic participation that is safe and effective for a child who has required a spinal fusion.

THE NORMAL AND ABNORMAL SPINE

The spine consists of a series of seven cervical, 12 thoracic, and five lumbar vertebrae perched upon the sacrum, and is designed for both stability and movement. In the sagittal plane, this semirigid column has a normal thoracic kyphosis (convex posterior angulation) and lumbar lordosis (convex anterior angulation). The cervical spine is capable of a wide range of motion, but normally is postured in a position of slight lordosis (Fig. 1).

The degree of angulation of the spine is determined by the Cobb technique (Fig. 2). The angle subtended by the top of the most tilted vertebra above, and the bottom of the most tilted vertebra below, is defined as the angle of curvature.

The range of normal magnitude of these angulations is controversial. In general, when a person is standing, the normal range of thoracic kyphosis is 20 to 50 degrees; deviations outside these limits are either hypokyphosis (<20 degrees) or hyperkyphosis (>50 degrees). Similarly, the range of normal lumbar lordosis is 20 to 50 degrees (see Fig. 1).

The incidence of dorsal (thoracic) hyperkyphosis may be increased among athletically active adolescents, especially males. This condition, known as Scheuermann's kyphosis, is defined as a dorsal kyphosis of more than 50 degrees in which there is at least 15% wedging of at least three vertebral bodies, narrowing of the disc spaces, and irregularity of the vertebral body end plates. The condition may have a genetic predisposition, or it may be acquired, secondary to repetitive microtrauma on the anterior aspects of the vertebral bodies of the dorsal spine, with resultant wedging. A tight lumbar lordosis may contribute to the problem by preventing adequate forward flexion of the lumbar spine; as a result, with forward flexion, more flexion must occur in the thoracic spine, leading to injury of the anterior aspect of the vertebral bodies, with secondary structural changes and dorsal roundback deformity.

Any curvature of the spine in the coronal plane is defined as scoliosis. This condition is abnormal and is therefore considered a deformity, even though 10% of the population may have a mild scoliosis (up to 10 degrees) in some portion of the spine.

Scoliosis may be functional—the result of muscle spasm, postural angulation of the spine, or extraspinal factors such as limb length discrepancy or pelvic obliquity. In functional scoliosis, there is no fixed deformity of the spine, and when the causative factor is corrected the spine becomes straight.

In contrast, structural scoliosis is a fixed deformity of the spine, although it may be partially corrected with mechanical techniques such as pulsion pressure or traction. The causes of structural scoliosis include (1) paralytic disorders such as poliomyelitis or myelodysplasia, (2) congenital abnormalities of the spine, or (3) idiopathic scoliosis. Rotational deformity of the spine in the horizontal plane is associated with coronal plane deformity in structural scoliosis.

Idiopathic scoliosis, the most common type of scoliosis in North America, is often familial, with a

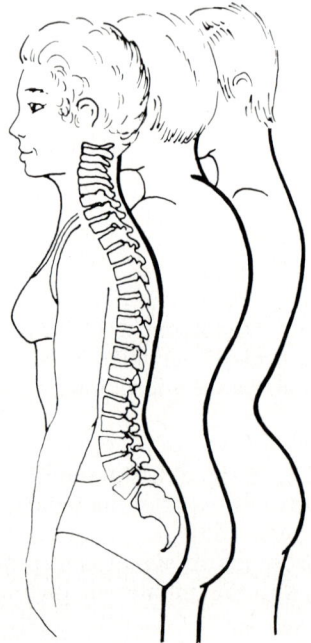

Figure 1 The normal range of thoracic kyphosis and lumbar lordosis is 20 to 50 degrees.

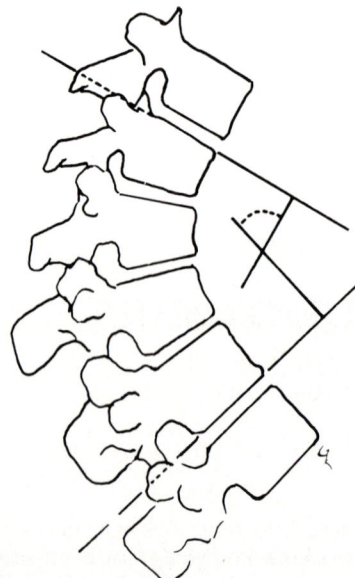

Figure 2 The Cobb angle, a quantitative measure of spinal curve, is the angle between the top of the most tilted vertebral body at the superior limit of the curve and the bottom of the most inferior vertebral body.

fivefold increased risk in family members. It may become apparent at a specific time in the growth and development of the child. The classification of idiopathic scoliosis includes (1) infantile-onset scoliosis, which is evident during the first year of life; (2) juvenile-onset scoliosis, which begins during the prepubescent period; and (3) adolescent-onset scoliosis, which can develop rapidly and progressively once adolescence begins.

Most conditions that cause scoliosis occur during childhood or adolescence. Therefore, it is important to consider the possibility of spinal deformity in childhood participation in sports, because (1) the deformity may influence the child's ability to engage in sports safely and effectively, and (2) the sports environment, particularly that of organized team sports, provides an excellent opportunity for early detection of a developing spinal deformity. The preparticipation physical examination, which should be performed annually for any child involved in organized sports, should include an assessment and careful measurement of the posture and contour of the body, with special attention to the spine, torso, and pelvis. The child who exhibits symmetric posture on examination may the following year show signs of progressive scoliosis or early kyphosis (dorsal roundback).

Abnormalities of posture and contour are carefully assessed in school screening programs, which are currently mandated in more than half of the United States as well as in Canada. These programs are at least 85% effective in the early detection of spinal abnormalities. In combination with an effective bracing or electrical stimulation program, they can often prevent the progression of spinal deformity and the need for surgery.

DIFFERENTIAL DIAGNOSIS

Spinal deformities or structural abnormalities, congenital or acquired, may significantly increase the risk of injury from sports participation.

Certain congenital conditions, such as Down or Morquio syndrome, are associated with an increased incidence of instability of the upper cervical spine. This is of particular concern for Special Olympics competition. In these children, lateral radiographs in flexion and extension are recommended to rule out measurable mechanical instability of the cervical spine. An excursion greater than 5 mm of C1 on C2 is a sign of ligamentous instability or laxity. In cases of detected instability, opinions vary regarding the indications for prophylactic fusion, but there is general agreement that contact sports and head-impact activities, such as heading the ball in soccer, are absolutely contraindicated.

Klippel-Feil syndrome, characterized by shortness of the neck or webbing, may be associated with congenital abnormalities of the cervical spine. In these cases, plain radiographs and, if indicated, lateral flexion and extension views of the cervical spine may also be necessary to confirm the mechanical stability of the spine before allowing such activity.

In the lumbar spine, spondylolysis or spondylolisthesis may result in postural deformity or scoliosis. An athlete with either of these conditions may have increased tightness of the hamstrings, relative flattening of the lumbar spine with posture, and pain on hyperextension of the spine. Radiographs of the lumbar spine, including oblique views, are usually diagnostic (Fig. 3).

If a frank lack of continuity of the neural arch is detected at the pars interarticularis, a standing lateral radiograph of the lumbar spine is recommended to determine the amount of instability at this site, if any, and the coexistence of spondylolisthesis. In our experience, symptomatic spondylolysis or grade I spondylolisthesis in young athletes appears to be a stress fracture of the lumbar spine, and rarely progresses to frank instability.

Spinal deformity may be the presenting sign of more significant disease, such as localized spinal infection, discitis, or spinal tumor. These conditions may be more common in the young athlete than in the adult, and may present initially with scoliosis. Any spinal deformity or scoliosis that persists beyond 3 weeks and is associated with muscle spasm and pain must be investigated

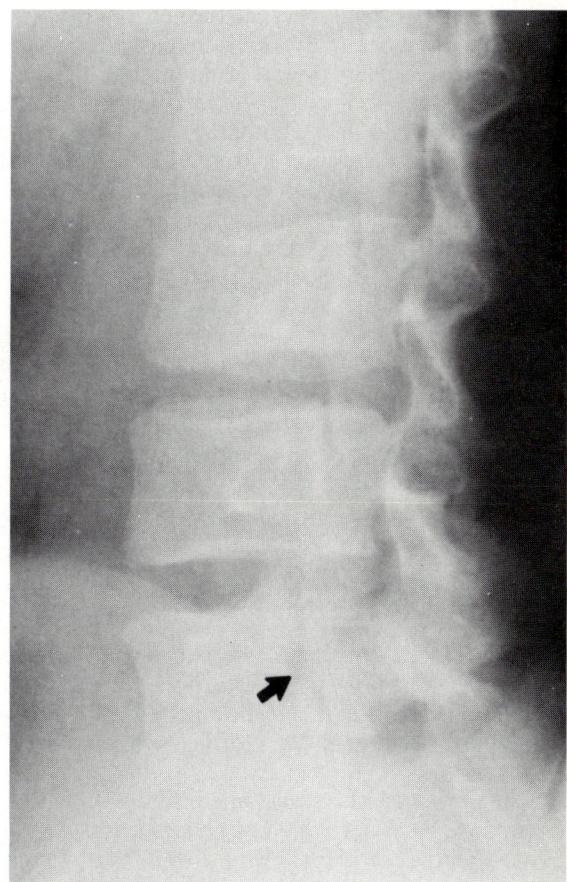

Figure 3 Spondylolysis, a defect in the pars interarticularis of the vertebra, is best visualized on the oblique radiograph.

thoroughly, and must not be ascribed to a minor back strain or sports injury.

EARLY DETECTION OF SPINAL DEFORMITY

The preparticipation evaluation provides an excellent opportunity for scoliosis screening. Symmetry of shoulder and pelvic heights, balance in the sagittal or coronal plane, and the symmetry of contour between the two sides of the back or lumbar spine are noted. On forward bending, asymmetry of the height of the torso may be a reflection of idiopathic scoliosis, due to the axial rotation of the spine and torso that occurs in addition to the curvature.

After limb length discrepancies or other causes of functional spinal curvature have been eliminated, cases of coronal or sagittal decompensation are further evaluated by obtaining standing posteroanterior (PA) and lateral radiographs of the thoracolumbar spine. If these reveal a scoliosis curvature of less than 15 degrees, or a dorsal kyphosis of more than 50 degrees, we recommend a program of directed exercises to increase the strength and flexibility of the spine and pelvis. Dorsal extension or asymmetric lateral bend exercises are also instituted for hyperkyphosis or scoliosis, respectively.

It is imperative to continue regular follow-up of any curvature, large or small, because of the risk of progression. The child is initially re-evaluated after 3 to 4 months with a repeat clinical examination. If Moiré topographic photography is available, comparison of the initial with the follow-up photograph may help determine any progression of torso asymmetry associated with scoliosis. If this is not available, the clinical examination can determine whether truncal asymmetry has progressed. If spinal asymmetry appears to have increased, a repeat radiograph is obtained; a single view (standing posteroanterior for scoliosis or lateral for kyphosis) is sufficient to evaluate for radiographic progression of the curvature of scoliosis. If this has progressed beyond 15 degrees, and at least 3 degrees since the previous radiograph, corrective bracing should be instituted.

NONOPERATIVE TREATMENT OF SPINAL DEFORMITY

Scoliosis

In most cases, spinal bracing is the most effective and the most readily available technique for preventing progression of scoliosis. The Milwaukee brace has been the standard treatment in North America for the management of progressive spinal disorders. However, during the past 15 years several different low-profile orthoses have been developed, which appear to manage scoliosis effectively while allowing a significant increase in function. In our experience, these orthoses can adequately prevent progression of a scoliosis curvature if the apex of the curvature is below T9.

Electrical muscle stimulation for scoliosis must be considered experimental. The techniques being used at present provide obvious advantages for the sports-active child. The treatment, which is applied at night, consists of intermittent pulses that stimulate the muscles in the convexity of the curve. During the day, full sports participation continues unhindered.

Full-time brace treatment has usually been required to prevent progression of the curvature. In our clinic, this consists of 23 hours per day of treatment, including use at night, with 1 hour out of the brace to permit bathing and exercising. The sports-active child is allowed to remove the brace during periods of sports participation or practice, for a maximum of 4 additional hours per day, and no ill effects such as increased rate of progression or brace failure have been noted. Most children can participate in sports while wearing the low-profile brace, and this includes physical education in school and most recreational sports activities such as bicycle riding, climbing, and running.

Most physicians treating juvenile-onset idiopathic scoliosis (in patients aged 6 to 10 years) report a dramatic mechanical response to brace treatment over a period of 3 to 6 months. After this, a part-time bracing regimen is adopted, usually 12 hours per day. Ongoing follow-up is mandatory to determine whether there is loss of correction with this program. We prescribe this part-time bracing program for younger patients with juvenile-onset scoliosis, who must wear the brace until skeletal maturity has been reached, sometimes for 5 to 6 years. This regimen has been successful in allowing an essentially normal lifestyle, while preventing progression of the curvature.

In the fully mature athlete, a scoliosis curve as great as 40 to 50 degrees is not a contraindication to full active sports or dance participation (Fig. 4). It is noted that as many as 25% to 30% of serious young amateur or professional dancers in modern dance or ballet have scoliosis curvatures. Despite this, there is no increased incidence of backache or long-term disability in these individuals. When a young, fully mature candidate for dance participation is noted to have a scoliosis curvature, we obtain a standing posteroanterior radiograph of the spine to document the degree of curvature before encouraging full dance or sports activity, in conjunction with a full back exercise program. A history of menstrual irregularity or menstrual disorder may be present in the young competitive dancer that may contribute to the development of scoliosis and stress fractures in these individuals.

Scheuermann's Kyphosis

Early detection of Scheuermann's kyphosis is imperative because of the dramatic reversal that may occur, if growth remains, as a result of prompt and early bracing techniques. Although scoliosis generally requires bracing until growth ceases, Scheuermann's kyphosis can be treated effectively for 9 to 12 months, with reconstitution of anterior vertebral height and restoration of a relatively normal contour of the spine. A disadvantage of the bracing regimen is that it usually requires a full brace

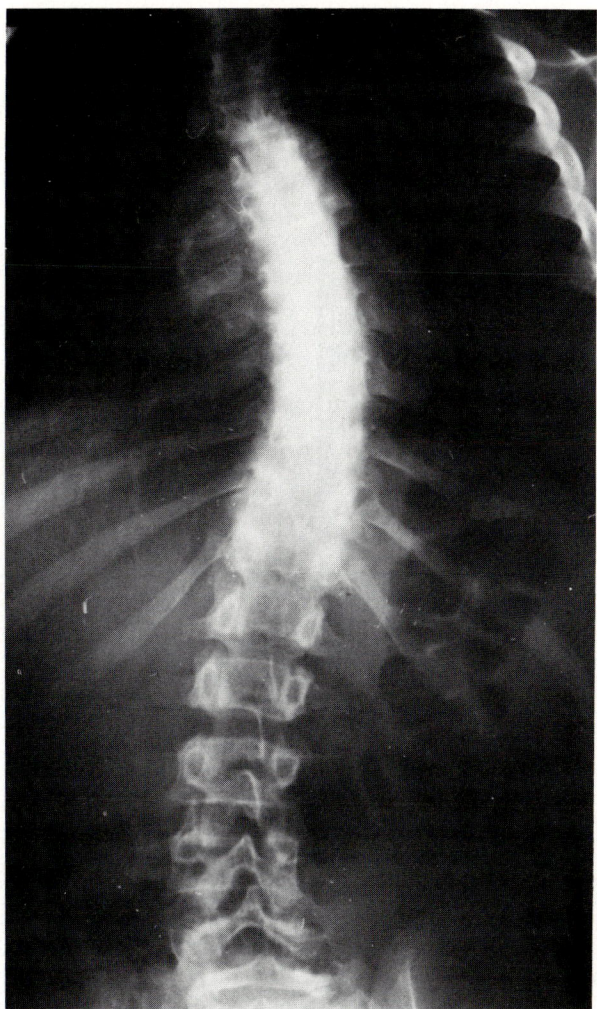

Figure 4 Mild scoliosis in a skeletally mature adolescent is not a contraindication to full sports participation.

with neck ring, especially in the young adult male. The treatment program should include an exercise regimen specifically directed at restoring strength and flexibility of the lumbar spine and hamstrings.

Lumbar Hyperlordosis

Hyperlordotic posturing ("swayback") of the low back may be flexible or fixed. With flexible lumbar hyperlordosis, forward bending causes the lumbar spine to flatten and reverse, and there may be no excessive tightness of the lumbodorsal fascia or hamstrings. The child with this posture is treated with an antilordotic exercise program and reassessed at regular intervals.

For fixed lumbar hyperlordosis, we institute a directed exercise program of antilordotic strengthening, with lumbodorsal fascia and hamstring flexibility exercises. If exercises alone are ineffective, an antilordotic bracing program is added.

Certain sports, such as figure skating, gymnastics, and ice hockey, appear to increase the tendency to develop lumbar hyperlordosis. Participants in these activities should perform prophylactic abdominal strengthening and lumbar flattening exercises, with particular emphasis on the pelvic tilt.

Lumbar hyperlordosis increases the risk of spondylolysis, and continuous or intermittent hyperlordotic posturing may also predispose to disc herniation. Therefore, young athletes who perform hyperlordotic maneuvers should also maintain a prophylactic antilordotic exercise program.

The young athlete with hyperlordosis and back pain should be completely evaluated for spondylolysis, disc problems, or other etiologic conditions, before the diagnosis of mechanical back pain is made. If exercises alone do not relieve the back pain, antilordotic bracing should be considered. The response to such bracing is often dramatic, with progressive reposturing of the lumbar spine, resolution of the pain, and concurrent full participation in sports activity. The young athlete initially wears the antilordotic, low-profile brace during sports activity; when the pain is relieved and the patient remains asymptomatic during sports participation, the brace can be safely removed for sports, but must be worn for the rest of the day. A minimum of 6 months of brace treatment is required to attain satisfactory realignment of the spine.

In contrast, brace treatment for spondylolysis is effective only with full-time wearing of the antilordotic, low-profile brace, which flattens and immobilizes the lumbar spine, and therefore relieves pain and promotes healing of the defect (Fig. 5). A concurrent antilordotic strengthening and flexibility exercise program should be maintained, and the bracing program is continued for a minimum of 6 months. Radiographic healing of the pars defect, in addition to resolution of pain, may be observed. When the child becomes asymptomatic and free of pain, and when hamstring flexibility is increased, participation in sports can be safely and effectively resumed, even while the brace is worn.

SPINAL FUSION

Fusion of the spine may be required in certain cases of severe or progressive spinal deformity such as dorsal roundback and scoliosis. Furthermore, localized fusion may be required for instability due to a previous spinal injury or deformity. The athlete will need recommendations regarding the safety and possibility of returning to sports participation after spinal fusion.

Spinal instrumentation, which is commonly used in conjunction with spinal fusion, has improved our ability to straighten the spine and may increase the rate of fusion from such a procedure (Fig. 6). In some situations, postoperative external casting or brace support may not be required. Nevertheless, it is generally agreed that establishment of a stable, solid spinal fusion takes approximately 12 months after surgery. Vigorous sports activities that involve twisting, turning, or potential impact to the spine should not be resumed earlier than this. We do allow swimming early in the postoperative period, occasionally as early as 6 to 8 weeks after spinal fusion, with a protective plastic brace.

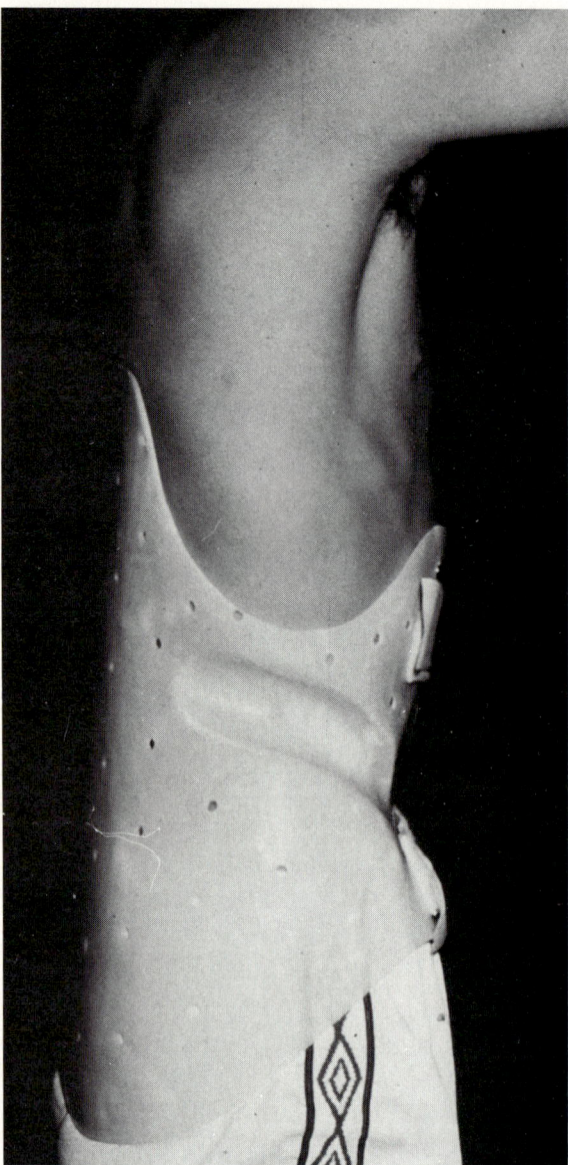

Figure 5 A thermoplastic low-profile brace used to treat spinal deformities or certain cases of low back pain in young athletes.

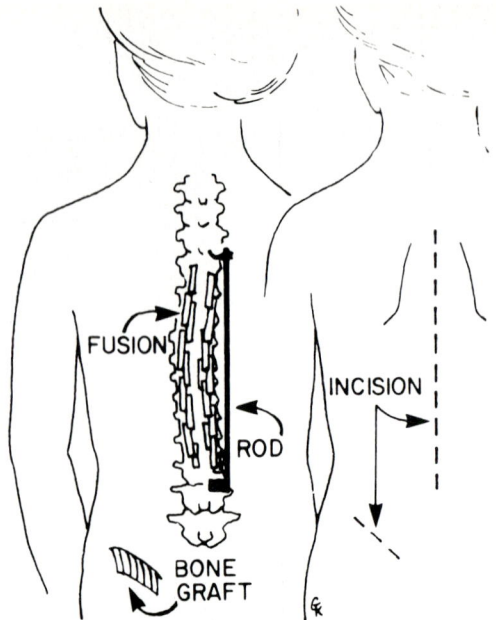

Figure 6 Extensive spinal fusion with instrumentation is a contraindication to contact sports, but many other sports and fitness activities are allowed.

vigorous sports participation, particularly if this includes active impacting or use of the head and neck.

The presence of associated neurologic symptoms or compromise at the time of the initial injury must also be a factor in the decision regarding continued participation in sports activity.

The athlete who has had lumbosacral fusion is generally allowed to return to full sports participation, including contact sports, after 1 year, if it is certain that a stable fusion has been attained and there is no neurologic compromise in the lower extremities. In some instances, with newer techniques of localized instrumentation of the fractured pars interarticularis, return to sports participation has been allowed as early as 3 months after fusion, but this is decided on an individual basis.

A child or adolescent who has had spinal instrumentation and fusion of more than two segments of the spine should be strongly counseled against participation in high-impact sports such as gridiron football or rugby, even after solid fusion has been established. However, moderate contact sports such as basketball, soccer, or field lacrosse are generally allowed.

In the case of more localized fusion, such as single-level fusion of the cervical spine for antecedent trauma, or fusion across the lumbosacral junction for spondylolysis, the return to sports participation must be individualized. With any spine fusion, there is an increased risk of long-term problems due to deterioration of the spinal elements immediately above or below the area of fusion. This deterioration may be hastened by

SUGGESTED READING

Micheli LJ. Low back pain in the adolescent: differential diagnosis. Am J Sports Med 1979; 7:362–364.

Micheli LJ. Back injuries in dancers. Clin Sports Med 1983; 2:473–484.

Micheli LJ. Sports following spinal surgery in the young athlete. Clin Orthop 1985; 198:152–157.

Micheli LJ. The use of the modified Boston brace system (B.O.B.) for back pain: clinical indications. Orthot Prosthet 1985; 39:41–46.

Micheli LJ, Hall JE, Miller ME. Use of modified Boston brace for back injuries in athletes. Am J Sports Med 1980; 8:351–356.

Stanish W. Low back pain in athletes: an overuse syndrome. Clin Sports Med 1987; 6:321–344.

Winter RB. Spinal problems in pediatric orthopaedics. In: Lovell WW, Winter RB, eds. Pediatric orthopaedics. 2nd Ed. Philadelphia: JB Lippincott, 1986:569.

RUPTURED LUMBAR DISCS (HERNIATED NUCLEUS PULPOSUS)

JOHN A. McCULLOCH, M.D., F.R.C.S.(C)

It is a simple matter to treat a ruptured disc. It is an altogether different matter to arrive at the correct diagnosis. Unfortunately, a ruptured lumbar disc is not an obvious diagnosis like a sprained ankle or a limb fracture. In fact, if someone could guarantee the diagnosis of a ruptured lumbar intervertebral disc, spine surgeons would strike a treatment "bonanza."

Problems arise when patient motivational factors are mixed in with the disability. Is someone consciously or unconsciously embellishing the illness to avoid competition? Are there hidden diseases that are fortuitously being brought to light at the moment that symptoms of the disc herniation are noted? An example might be a young male patient with referred buttock discomfort on one side who may appear on the surface to have a disc herniation, but upon closer scrutiny is found to have ankylosing spondylitis. Are we actually dealing with a disc herniation, or is this a problem of mechanical back pain with referred leg pain? If this is a ruptured disc, what is the level? Is it at L4-L5 or is it at L5-S1? Is there an asymptomatic structural lesion present such as spondylolisthesis that is deflecting the diagnosis away from the true cause of symptoms such as a herniated nucleus pulposus (HNP) at another level? So many factors go into the correct diagnosis of a ruptured lumbar disc that it is easy to miss the diagnosis when it is the cause of the leg pain, or to conclude that the diagnosis is a ruptured disc when there is another cause of radiating leg pain.

If this is not enough to confuse the issue, it is apparent to everyone dealing with low back pain that almost all patients with a mechanical low back condition get better with the passage of time. This well-known placebo effect can serve anyone's purpose when reporting expertise with treating low back problems. On the other hand, it is not unusual to read a series on a particular treatment for low back conditions and be told that a success rate of 70% to 80% is acceptable. This percentage of success, presented to total joint surgeons, would be a joke! The final common denominator in spine problems is that the aging process gets us all: if you live long enough you will eventually develop degenerative changes in your discs and may even rupture a lumbar disc. By now you have a handle on how difficult it is to make the diagnosis of a ruptured lumbar disc. Therein lies the juggernaut of spine surgery.

DEFINITION

A herniated nucleus pulposus causing sciatica fulfills the criteria listed in Table 1.

Table 1 Criteria for the Diagnosis of the Acute Radicular Syndrome (Sciatica Usually Due to an HNP)*

Two Symptoms
1. Leg pain, including buttock discomfort, dominating over the back pain
2. Presence of localizing neurologic symptoms (e.g., paresthesia in a dermatomal distribution)

Two Signs
1. Marked reduction in straight leg-raising ability and/or bowstring discomfort and/or cross-over pain
2. Two of four neurologic signs (wasting, weakness, sensory loss, reflex alteration)

*Three or four of these criteria are required for diagnosis. The exception is the young patient (<25 years) who may have no neurologic symptoms or signs.

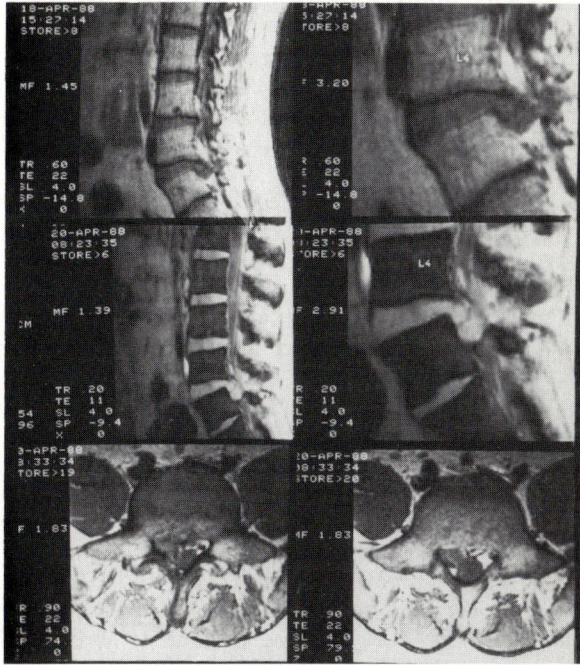

Figure 1 MRI showing a disc extrusion, L4-L5 right. *Top,* Axial T1 weighted images. *Middle,* Axial partial T2 weighted images. *Lower,* Axial views.

There are two different "breeds" of disc herniation. There is the kind that occurs in the young patient, usually in the form of a disc protrusion containing much proteoglycan or nuclear jelly. The second "breed," which occurs in the older patient (above 35), is more collagenous in nature and often is of the extruded or sequestered variety (Fig. 1). It is almost as if we were treating two separate conditions when disc ruptures are considered in age groupings. As with any general rule in medicine, there are exceptions: there are younger patients with older discs and older patients with young discs!

VERIFICATION OF STRUCTURAL LESION AND ANATOMIC LOCATION

History has declared that the gold standard for investigating a patient with a disc rupture is myelography. Times are changing and the standard of investigation today is quickly becoming magnetic resonance imaging (MRI). MRI provides all the information needed to verify the diagnosis of a disc rupture, to determine the anatomic level, and to allow for a "fine-tuned" treatment decision. It is unusual for myelography or even computed tomographic (CT) scanning to be required if good MRI facilities are available. Unfortunately, MRI is an easy test to order and has a reasonably high false-positive rate when interpreted in the vacuum of no clinical information. MRI should be carried out only if the patient fails to respond to conservative treatment and is being considered for surgical intervention.

ADEQUATE CONSERVATIVE CARE

If the diagnosis of a lumbar disc rupture has been made, what constitutes adequate conservative care? Remember that it is natural for the symptoms of a disc rupture to subside spontaneously. Even while waiting for this spontaneous cure, it is possible to allow patients to function at a reasonable level, provided that they understand that increasing symptoms with increasing activity represent hurt and not harm. Unless patients insist on pursuing a high level of repetitive bending or lifting activities, it is unlikely that effects detrimental to a disc herniation will occur with continuing light activities. Of course, if the sciatic discomfort is so severe that a patient cannot stand on the affected leg, this rule does not apply. This leads to the next consideration in conservative treatment: to match the proposed conservative treatment with the severity of the disability. If a patient cannot swing a nine iron without producing leg pain, it seems unreasonable to prescribe 2 weeks of bed rest to treat the problem. On the other hand, if a patient has severe leg pain and needs crutches to get around, it is absurd to propose exercise treatment intervention. Although these are two extreme examples, a lot of "fine tuning" is needed to determine what constitutes an adequate conservative treatment program.

There are only two useful forms of conservative treatment for a disc rupture. First is rest, which may include complete bed rest, a bed on the patient's back (a corset), weight reduction, job modification, or activity modification. Second is the passage of a reasonable amount of time before one pronounces failure. For the first occurrence of sciatica, it is reasonable to extend conservative treatment for not less than 6 weeks, provided that the symptom is not severely incapacitating. If bed rest is prescribed, how long is long enough? The duration of prescribed bed rest is undergoing dramatic modification in the past few years. In the past, it was not unusual to request 2 weeks of complete bed rest as a standard of care for an acute disc rupture. It is now evident that, at most, 5 days is all that is required, as long as the examiner notes two key parameters: (1) the relief of leg pain and (2) the degree of improvement in straight leg-raising ability. If after 5 days of complete bed rest the patient shows no improvement in leg pain or no improvement in straight leg-raising ability, it is likely that

continuing complete bed rest will be fruitless.

Antiinflammatory medicine, if tolerated, is a useful adjunct to bed rest. Many other therapies have been invoked to cure the so-called ruptured disc, including the various forms of exercises and other treatments such as manipulation, ultrasonography, massage, deep heat, and diathermy. There is no body of scientific evidence to support these forms of treatment as useful in the management of an acute disc rupture.

RESPONSE TO TREATMENT

There are three responses to conservative treatment: (1) the patient is cured; (2) the patient is not cured; or (3) although the patient is initially cured, there is a recurrence of symptoms.

INDICATIONS FOR SURGERY

If a patient fails to respond to conservative treatment or initially responds to such treatment only to have recurrent episodes of sciatica, surgical intervention is indicated. The two other classic indications for surgical intervention on an emergent basis are bladder and bowel involvement and an increasing neurologic deficit. Controversial indications for surgical intervention include a significant neurologic deficit and a significant structural lesion found on investigation. Perhaps the most controversial recommendation is that all patients below the age of 20 to 25 years will almost certainly fail to respond to conservative treatment for a ruptured disc, and should be treated much more aggressively than older patients.

CHOICES OF INVASIVE TREATMENT

There are three invasive options for treating patients who have failed to respond to conservative treatment: (1) chemonucleolysis, (2) surgery, and (3) percutaneous discectomy.

Basic Science Considerations

In trying to decide upon the best form of invasive surgical therapy for a patient with a disc rupture, it is important to determine the nature of the fragment of disc material pressing on the nerve root. There are two components in a ruptured disc fragment: proteoglycan and collagen. The younger the patient, the more likely it is that there is a high proteoglycan content to the disc rupture; the older the patient, the more likely there is to be a high collagen content in the ruptured disc material. Other changes such as calcification and air in the disc cavity or the ruptured disc material are also suggestive of a low proteoglycan content. Finally, a disc rupture that is extremely large, and a disc rupture that has migrated away from the disc space, either up behind the vertebral body above or down behind the vertebral body below, are suggestive of a low proteoglycan content and a higher collagen content. The significance of trying to determine the extent of proteoglycan content in the disc herniation becomes evident in the following section on chemonucleolysis.

Chemonucleolysis

Chymopapain is a proteolytic enzyme that is extracted from the papaya plant. It is a protein foreign to the body and capable of invoking a wide variety of allergic reactions, the most feared being anaphylaxis. When injected into a disc protrusion containing a lot of proteoglycan, the positively charged enzyme is attracted to the negatively charged proteoglycans. It splits off the mucopolysaccharide side chains, interfering with the proteoglycan's ability to hold onto water. In essence, the chemonucleolysis "deflates" a bulging disc, relieving pressure on the nerve root.

Chemonucleolysis should be seen as the last step in conservative care rather than the first step in surgical care. It is a nonsurgical procedure that is accomplished by placing a needle into the offending disc and injecting a small amount of enzyme to dissolve the disc rupture. Obviously, it only affects disc protrusions and only affects discs that have a high proteoglycan content. It does not affect any other conditions of the spine, such as bony root or canal encroachment. There are a number of contraindications to the use of chymopapain, including an allergy to the drug, previous surgery, a previous chymopapain injection, pregnancy, or an associated neurologic diagnosis of unknown etiology such as multiple sclerosis.

Chymopapain is a safe drug when injected into the intradiscal cavity. When injected in error into the subarachnoid space, it has a devastating effect on the basement membranes of the pia-arachnoid vessels. The result is a dissolution of these membranes and a subarachnoid hemorrhage, which can spread to include an intracerebral hemorrhage, a cauda equina syndrome, and a somewhat delayed sinister complication of transverse myelitis. These three severe neurologic complications have actually occurred in chymopapain-treated patients (fortunately not often), but it is my opinion that they are all due to technical errors and not related to any inherent problem with the drug.

The dreaded complication of anaphylaxis has been brought under control with preinjection skin testing. If a patient has a negative skin test, an anaphylactic reaction is highly unlikely, on the basis of my experience with over 1,000 cases.

The procedure is usually performed in the operating room under local neuroleptic anesthesia. Single levels should be injected, since disc ruptures occur at single levels and not multiple levels. The approach to the disc space must not violate the subarachnoid space, and thus the posterolateral approach is necessary (Fig. 2). Following the manufacturer's recommendation to reduce the dose of chymopapain injection to 0.75 to 1.0 ml, the incidence of postinjection back spasm has been reduced.

Patients may leave the hospital on the day of the procedure or a day or so afterward. They are best supported in a light canvas corset for approximately 4 to 6 weeks, after which time an x-ray film should be taken

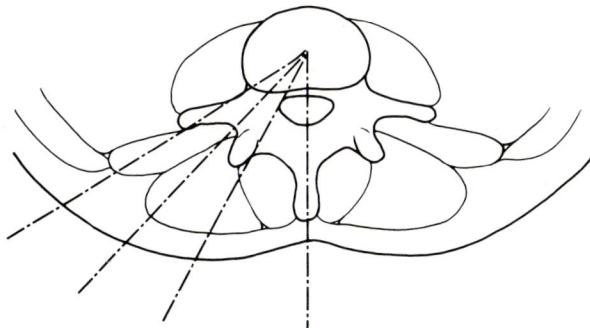

Figure 2 Posterolateral approach.

to decide whether there is disc space narrowing. A successful result at this stage is considered to be relief of leg pain, increased straight leg-raising ability, and disc space narrowing on x-ray examination. Success at 6 weeks allows for institution of a rehabilitation program that will get the patient back to athletic activities by 3 months. Failure represents a patient with persistent sciatica or persisting reduction in straight leg-raising ability, with or without disc space narrowing on plain radiograph. If patients fail to respond to a chymopapain injection, a determination should be made within 6 weeks to take them on to surgical intervention.

In young patients (below the age of 25 to 30) with a disc herniation, chemonucleolysis probably represents the best choice of treatment.

Surgical Intervention

It is my recommendation that the standard laminectomy-discectomy for surgical management of patients with disc rupture is no longer necessary. Instead, a microsurgical approach can be used, which reduces the size of the skin incision, the extent of the muscular dissection, the size of the postoperative hematoma, and finally the healing by secondary intention (i.e., the formation of scar). The smaller incision decreases the postoperative morbidity significantly, allowing for early ambulation on the day of surgery or the day after. This in turn has a very beneficial effect on the formation of collagen tissue.

The use of the microscope to assist in decompression of a nerve root compromised by a disc herniation represents nothing more than the technical advancement of using the magnification and illumination that are a part of the microscope. Whether or not the magnification and illumination are used to assist the surgeon is not important; what *is* important is that the nerve root is adequately decompressed. If a disc excision is "completed" but the nerve root is still compromised by residual disc material, or if there is another pathologic condition such as bony root encroachment, patients will not be relieved of the sciatic discomfort, regardless of whether or not the microscope was used.

After microsurgical excision of a disc herniation, patients are ambulated the day of surgery or the day after. As with chemonucleolysis, a canvas corset support is recommended for 4 to 6 weeks as a reminder to

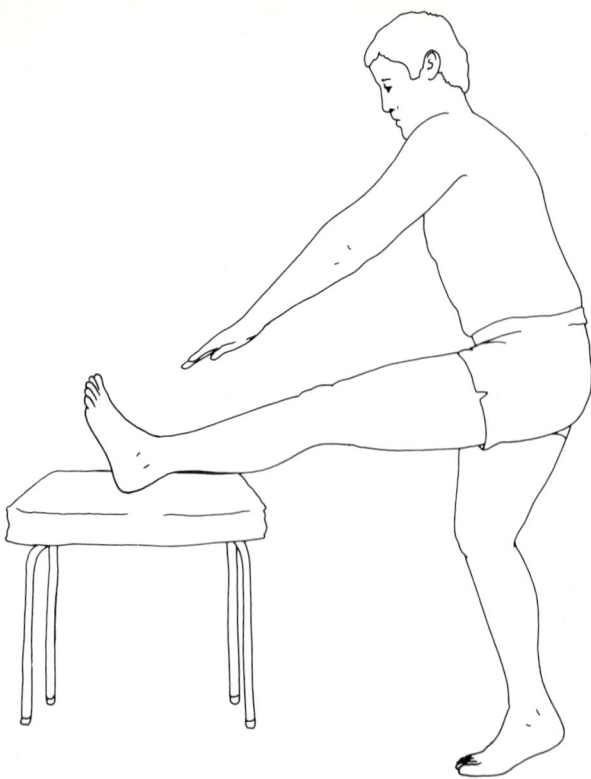

Figure 3 The postoperative stretching exercise.

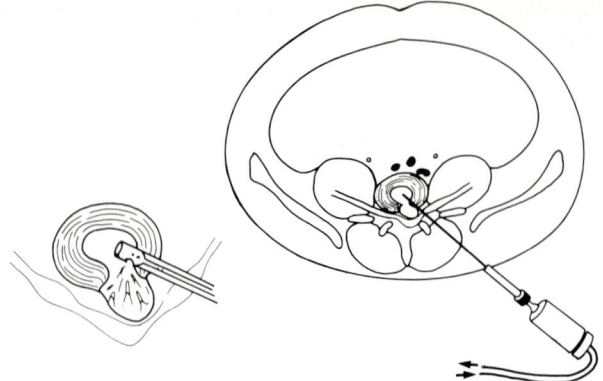

Figure 4 The percutaneous discectomy with the "suction" nucleotome.

patients that an operation has taken place. During that time, patients are on routine activity limitations and should perform a stretching exercise of the affected leg (Fig. 3). As with chemonucleolysis, success or failure is determined at 6 weeks and a physical therapy rehabilitation program is started to return the patient to full activity 3 to 6 months post-operatively.

There are many causes of failure to relieve sciatic discomfort when using a limited surgical exposure. The most common cause is exposing the wrong level, which is a constant threat to any surgeon performing microsurgery. In addition, if the radiographs have not been interpreted carefully with regard to the exact location and nature of the disc herniation or other root encroachment pathology, it is possible to leave behind fragments of disc material or other root encroachment. Minor complicating features of the limited surgical exposure include bleeding that obscures the field of vision, damage to neurologic structures because of the limited field of work, and finally a slightly increased incidence of disc space infection (because of the presence of some exposed parts of the microscope over the wound).

Percutaneous Discectomy

The technology of managing a disc rupture is in a state of evolution. The original modification to the standard laminectomy-discectomy was chemonucleolysis, which was first proposed in the early 1960s. Next came the microsurgical approach to root decompression, and now there are percutaneous approaches to the disc space with either a suction probe or grasping forceps. This approach is depicted in Figure 4 and is similar to the chemonucleolysis route. However, instead of injecting an enzyme into the disc space, a suction probe or a grasping instrument is used to remove the discal material.

The advantages of percutaneous discectomy are that it is a nonoperative procedure, and thus eliminates a number of complications attendant upon general anesthesia and a surgical wound. The procedure is minor enough to be done under local neuroleptic anesthesia on an out-patient basis. The disadvantages of the procedure are that (1) the technique is somewhat more difficult to learn than chemonucleolysis, (2) it is possible with a larger-bore cannula to injure the nerve root when attempting to enter the disc space, and (3) it is highly likely that if a disc fragment is extruded or sequestered outside the confines of the disc space, it will not be reached with a probe. If the surgeon is unfamiliar with the technique and is somewhat clumsy, the incidence of disc space infection is raised.

Perhaps the most serious concern with percutaneous discectomy is that not all the nuclear material can be reached with the approach and the recurrence rate is likely to be high. The technique is young in its development, and I predict that a higher than acceptable recurrence rate will detract from the advantages. To date there are few scientific studies to support its widespread use.

SUGGESTED READING

Bell GR, Rothman RH. The conservative treatment of sciatica. Spine 1984; 9:54-56.

McCulloch JA, Dolovich G, Canham W. Skin testing for chymopapain allergy: A preliminary report. Allergy 1985; 55:609-611.

VanRoyen BJ, O'Driscoll SW, Dhert WJA, Salter RB. A comparison of the effects of immobilization and continuous passive motion on surgical wound healing in mature rabbits. Plast Reconstr Surg 1986; 78:360-366.

SPONDYLOLYSIS AND SPONDYLOLISTHESIS

JOHN R. McCARROLL, M.D.
DANIEL E. KRAFT, M.D.

Low back pain in athletic adolescents has long been a concern to the medical community. Various studies have indicated that 15% to 38% of all adolescent athletes with significant episodes of low back pain will show evidence of spondylolysis on radiologic evaluation.

Spondylolysis is a stress defect in the pars interarticularis. Spondylolisthesis is the forward slippage of one vertebra in relation to the vertebrae below it. This forward slippage is thought to result from lack of support from the posterior neural arch secondary to spondylolysis.

Two distinct subsets of individuals are afflicted with lumbar spondylolytic defects. The first is the nonathlete or congenital subset. These individuals develop spondylolytic lesions mainly between the ages of five and eight years and are commonly asymptomatic. The general occurrence rate in the population appears to be 4% to 6% for this group. These children may have some congenital predisposition to the condition, which explains the increased familial incidence in some populations, such as the natives of northern Alaska. The second group consists of individuals with athletically acquired spondylolysis. These athletes normally develop their lesions between the ages of 10 and 18 years and often have associated low back pain. This chapter focuses on the diagnosis and treatment of spondylolysis and spondylolisthesis in athletes.

ETIOLOGY

Various mechanical activities expose athletes to repeated stress and shear force on the pars interarticularis, ultimately resulting in a pars stress fracture. Repetitive cycles of flexion-hyperextension movements in gymnastic maneuvers is thought to be an etiology of spondylolysis in young gymnasts. The drive upward and forward while extending the lumbar spine during blocking creates excessive anterior-posterior shear forces across the lumbar vertebrae leading to spondylolysis in football linemen. In addition, a small preliminary study on soccer players seems to indicate that a combination of large torque, shear, and side-bending forces produced while kicking a soccer ball may account for stress fractures in soccer players (Hosea TM, McCarroll JR, Kraft DE, presented at AMSSM Annual Meeting, Sun Valley, Idaho, July 1993). The higher incidence of spondylolysis in gymnasts and football linemen helps to reinforce the mechanical etiology of spondylolysis as a type of overuse injury in athletes.

CLINICAL EXAMINATION

Athletes with spondylolysis or spondylolisthesis typically complain of aching low back pain of a few weeks to months in duration. This pain may be unilateral or bilateral and is aggravated by sports activity. The pain is confined to the lumbosacral area with no radicular leg pain. By the time they seek medical attention, most athletes have begun limiting their sports activity secondary to pain.

Pain with extension of the low back is the hallmark of clinical diagnosis for spondylolysis. The single leg hyperextension test is a sensitive clinical diagnostic tool. The test is performed with the patient weight bearing on one leg and extending the back toward the same leg. A positive test is indicated by reproduction of pain on the extended side of the low back. Patients may have increased tightness in the hamstrings, but typically they do not elicit any neurologic symptoms or have any neurologic deficits on physical examination. In addition, patients usually have little pain and normal range of motion in forward flexion and side bending.

RADIOGRAPHIC EVALUATION

All athletic adolescents with low back pain of three or more weeks duration should have a radiologic evaluation. Initial evaluation with plain films of the lumbar spine including anteroposterior (AP), lateral, and lateral oblique views can be normal. Scintigraphy changes in stress fractures may precede radiographic changes by at least 2 or 4 weeks. Therefore, a bone scan or Single Photon Emission Computed Tomography (SPECT) scan may reveal a subradiographic spondylotic lesion in a patient who has normal plain films. The presence of biologic activity on scintigraphy testing indicates the need for brace treatment.

Recent studies have indicated that the SPECT scan is more sensitive in diagnosing pars stress fractures than planar bone scans. The SPECT scan algebraically reconstructs data from multiple projections to provide contrast enhancements that cannot be obtained by planar imaging. This allows the SPECT scan to more accurately localize the athlete's injury to the posterior neural arch as opposed to the vertebral body.

TREATMENT OF SPONDYLOLYSIS

A review of the sports medicine literature reveals a wide variation in treatment options that appear to be currently accepted across the country. Options range from activity modification with no brace treatment to treatment with a Boston overlap brace for 12 months.

Athletic adolescents with spondylolysis may have normal plain radiographs, a positive bone scan or SPECT scan, and routinely will have had symptoms for only a few weeks or months. These athletes can be offered two options for treatment. The first is complete activity modification with no sports activities for at least

3 months, which is not desirable for many in-season athletes. The second option of activity modification with bracing offers the athlete the best opportunity to become pain free and return to sports quickly. Athletes are withheld from practice or competition until they are asymptomatic after institution of treatment with the Boston overlap brace. This time period allows the athlete to become accustomed to wearing the brace and relieves some of the increased stress and irritation affecting the pars interarticularis. Athletes are instructed to wear their brace 23 hours per day, including during all athletic activities. Once the athlete is pain free in activities of daily living (ADLs), they can be progressed back to practice and competition through a functional progression program. Most adolescents become asymptomatic within 3 to 4 weeks of bracing and are able to return to play. Pain continues to be the patient's main guide throughout the entire brace treatment. Any activity that causes pretreatment type low back pain for more than a few days or is intolerable should be stopped or modified so the pain is relieved. Some athletes notice mild muscular trunk and back pain upon return to play that is not related to the stress fracture and is not an indication for withdrawal from activities. Adolescents may compete in any athletic activity, including contact sports, during brace treatment using the above pain guidelines. Our routine brace treatment lasts 3 months. Any athlete who is still having pain after 3 months is continued in brace treatment for an additional 3 months. Further diagnostic testing via a CT scan or magnetic resonance imaging may be indicated if pain persists after 3 months of bracing and activity modification. Athletes are referred to a spinal specialist if pain persists after 6 months of treatment.

After approximately 3 weeks of activity modification and bracing, most patients are generally asymptomatic and ready to start a rehabilitation program. This rehabilitation program is emphasized to be equally as important as the brace treatment itself. The spondylolysis rehabilitation program incorporates antilordotic exercises (William's flexion and posterior pelvic tilt exercises), abdominal strengthening, and trunk control exercises. Hamstring flexibility is addressed in the program, but is not overly stressed. Patients are expected to perform their rehabilitation exercises daily during the 3 month bracing period. Once the brace treatment has concluded, patients are encouraged to continue their exercise programs three to four times weekly throughout their competitive athletic careers. Thus, the rehabilitation program becomes a vital adjunct to bracing in our adolescent athletes with spondylolysis.

The athletic patient may also present with spondylolytic lesion on plain film in addition to a positive bone scan or SPECT scan. Theoretically, this athlete has a further advanced stress process than the previous group, but still has some possibility for bony healing since the bone scan shows continued biologic activity at the stress area. These patients are treated in an identical manner to the previous group.

Adolescent athletes with spondylolytic lesions on plain films and a negative bone scan and SPECT scan are believed to have a chronic injury and are treated in a more symptomatic manner than acute spondylolysis. These athletes do not have any active bone formation at their stress fracture site and have an extremely low possibility of undergoing bony healing, even with brace treatment. Therefore, a less rigid warm and form orthosis is used for symptomatic treatment and comfort. These patients are immediately started on the same spondylolysis rehabilitation program as noted above. Once the athlete is pain free in ADLs, they can be progressed back to practice and competition through a functional progression program. These athletes routinely recover quickly and are able to return to sporting activities in 3 to 4 weeks. The warm and form orthosis does not need to be continued once the adolescent returns to practice and is asymptomatic. However, the importance of continuing strengthening exercises throughout the athlete's competitive career should be stressed.

Though the vast majority of symptomatic spondylolysis patients are adolescents, occasionally we treat older recreational athletes who show evidence of a spondylolytic lesion on plain films. These older athletes are treated identically to adolescents with chronic spondylolytic lesions. We do not routinely pursue further diagnostic testing with a bone scan or SPECT scan since spondylolytic lesions are thought to develop prior to final maturity of the spine at age 18 to 20 years. Again, the treatment program of a warm and form orthosis and rehabilitation program appears to be effective in this group. These athletes often become asymptomatic clinically and are able to return to their recreational activities in 3 to 6 weeks.

TREATMENT OF SYMPTOMATIC SPONDYLOLISTHESIS

Most athletes with symptomatic spondylolisthesis can be treated effectively with conservative treatment. Studies have shown that the vast majority of athletes with spondylolisthesis are Grade I (< 25% slip) or Grade II (< 50% slip) upon presentation. Studies have also indicated that significant progression of Grade I or Grade II spondylolisthesis in the athletic population is rare. Thus, a conservative symptomatic approach to spondylolisthesis can be effective and safe for the patient. Athletes with symptomatic Grade I or Grade II spondylolisthesis are started immediately in the rehabilitation program and placed in a Boston overlap brace for comfort. Again, the rehabilitation program is stressed as a vital component to the athlete's treatment. As with chronic spondylolysis, adolescents may return to competition when they are pain free. Athletes with incidental spondylolisthesis may be started on a rehabilitation program, but do not require any further treatment. Grade I spondylolisthesis does not restrict an athlete from sports, including football and other contact sports. Varied opinions regarding athletic participation by adolescents with Grade II spondylolisthesis can be found in the literature. Most adolescents with Grade II spondylolisthesis can compete in sports, but should be discouraged from competing in gymnastics, football, and other contact sports. High-grade spondylolisthesis (> 50%), however, is an indication for withdrawal from these sports and referral to a spine specialist.

Frequent radiographic follow-up for patients with spondylolysis and spondylolisthesis should be continued even after the athlete is asymptomatic and has returned to sports. Initially a lateral plain film is repeated at 6 months and 1 year after initiation of brace treatment in all patients. In patients with symptomatic, asymptomatic, and incidental spondylolisthesis, more frequent radiographic studies are required. A lateral plain film is obtained at 3 months, 6 months, 1 year, and every year thereafter to check for progression of the slip. Plain films should continue to be obtained in both groups until the athletes reach 18 to 20 years, when the spine has matured and the risk of further progression of the lesion vanishes. Thus, continued radiographic evaluations are important in following these athletes for any further progression of their lesions.

SURGICAL REFERRALS

Although most athletes with spondylolysis and spondylolisthesis can be effectively treated by any sports medicine physician, occasionally athletes do not respond to conservative treatment and need evaluation by a spine specialist for possible surgical treatment. One indication for referral at our clinic is any Grade III or IV spondylolisthesis. Athletes who undergo comprehensive conservative treatment, including radiographic evaluation and brace treatment for 6 months and still complain of pain are also referred for further evaluation. The other indication is any progression of spondylolisthesis while undergoing brace treatment. Although most athletes are able to become asymptomatic and return to sports, a small group will fail conservative treatment and need evaluation for possible surgery.

COMMENTS

Most athletes with spondylolysis or spondylolisthesis can be treated conservatively and return to athletics without problems. In our clinic we combined short-term activity modification with Boston overlap bracing and a solid rehabilitation program as a main form of treatment. Routinely patients are able to return to practice when asymptomatic and progress quickly to competition.

Athletes are kept in a Boston overlap brace for 23 hours per day for 3 months. Though we have had success with this treatment plan, we, like many other authors, cannot provide scientific data to support this form of treatment. Therein lies the need for future research on spondylolysis and its treatment. The effectiveness of Boston overlap brace treatment in the acute management of spondylolysis needs to be confirmed with prospective studies. Finally, the natural outcome of acquired spondylolysis in athletic adolescents must be found through long-term follow-up to determine which factors, if any, may cause spinal problems later in life. All these questions must be answered if we are to develop the most appropriate treatment plan for athletes with spondylolysis.

SUGGESTED READING

Ammann W, Matheson GO. Radionuclide bone imaging in the detection of stress fractures. Clin J Sport Med 1991; 1:115–122.

Bell DF, Ehrlich MG, Zaleske DJ. Brace treatment for symptomatic spondylolisthesis. Clin Orthop 1988; 236:192–198.

Bellah RD, et al. Low-back pain in adolescent athletes: Detection of stress injury to the pars interarticularis with SPECT. Radiology 1991; 180:509–512.

Ciullo JV, Jackson DW. Pars interarticularis stress reaction, spondylolysis, and spondylolisthesis in gymnasts. Clin Sports Med 1985; 4:95–110.

Collier BD, et al. Painful spondylolysis or spondylolisthesis studied by radiography and single-photon emission computed tomography. Radiology 1985; 154:207–211.

Fredrickson BE, et al. The natural history of spondylolysis and spondylolisthesis. J Bone Joint Surg 1984; 66:699–707.

Jackson DW, Wiltse LL, Cirincione RJ. Spondylolysis in the female gymnast. Clin Orthop 1976; 117:68–73.

Johnson RJ. Low-back pain in sports: Managing spondylolysis in young patients. Physician Sports Med 1993; 21:53–59.

Kraus DR, Shapiro D. The symptomatic lumbar spine in the athlete. Clin Sports Med 1989; 8:59–66.

McCarroll JR, Miller JM, Ritter MA. Lumbar spondylolysis and spondylolisthesis in college football players: A prospective study. Am J Sports Med 1986; 14:404–406.

Micheli LJ. Back injuries in gymnastics. Clin Sports Med 1985; 4:85–91.

Papanicolaou N, et al. Bone scintigraphy and radiography in young athletes with low back pain. AJR 1985; 145:1039–1044.

Rossi F. Spondylolysis, spondylolisthesis and sports. J Sports Med 1978; 18:317–335.

Steiner ME, Micheli LJ. Treatment of symptomatic spondylolysis and spondylolisthesis with the modified Boston brace. Spine 1985; 10:937–943.

Stewart TD. The age incidence of neural arch defects in alaskan natives considered from the standpoint of etiology. J Bone Joint Surg 1953; 35:937–950.

Watkins RG, Dillin WH. Lumbar spine injury in the athlete, Clin Sports Med 1990; 9:419–448.

Weiker GG: Evaluation and treatment of common spine and trunk problems. Clin Sports Med 1989; 8:399–417.

LITTLE LEAGUE ELBOW

JOSEPH S. TORG, M.D.

MECHANICS OF PITCHING

The nature of the stresses are better understood by first analyzing the mechanics of the pitching act. To propel a basketball with speed and control requires a coordinated mobilization and spending of body forces from three sources: (1) trunk and lower extremities, (2) shoulder and arm, and (3) forearm and hand.

The role each of these forces plays are described in the four phases of the pitching act: (1) wind-up, (2) cocking, (3) acceleration, and (4) release and follow-through.

During the wind-up phase the trunk is rotated away from the direction of the throw, and the entire body weight is loaded upon the ipsilateral lower extremity. Lower extremities are coiled in preparation to initiate the release of muscular and subsequent potential energy of the body weight. This is accomplished with an explosive rotation and thrust of the truck in the direction of throw associated with ipsilateral hip, knee, and ankle extension. The shoulder, arm-forearm-hand component assumes an abducted and extended attitude in relation to the trunk. During this phase significant stresses are not yet exerted on the extremity.

The cocking phase is characterized by transfer of body weight to the contralateral lower extremity, with thrust of the trunk in the direction of throw. The throwing extremity lags behind, forcing the humerus into extreme abduction and external rotation. The elbow is flexed, thus enhancing the degree of torque exerted on the humeral shaft, glenohumeral capsule, and structures crossing the shoulder joint. Owing to the extreme external humeral rotation during this phase, extraordinary stresses are exerted on these structures.

During the acceleration phase the inertia of the trunk and leg is supplemented by contraction of intrinsic and extrinsic muscle of the shoulder. These combined forces whip the arm in the direction of throw with a violent force. During this phase the biceps and triceps as well as the forearm musculature support the stability of the elbow. However, the whip-like action tends to force the ulna and radius into a valgus attitude with respect to

the distal humerus. This generates a compressive force at the lateral radiohumeral capitellar articulation and a distracting force at the medial ulnohumeral articulation. This is the mechanism responsible for medial elbow overload and lateral elbow compression. With the olecranon forced into the humeral trochelea in a somewhat valgus attitude, aberration in the mechanics of this articulation may also result.

With release and subsequent follow-through control of the baseball is facilitated by a powerful flexion-pronation of the forearm and hand. This aspect of the pitch is responsible for avulsion stresses at the origin of the flexor-pronator musculature in the area of the medial humeral epicondyle.

TYPES OF INJURIES

Although the mechanics of pitching are similar for both child and adult, the injuries produced are quite different. In the child, the bony structures are characterized by the presence of the elements of enchondral ossification; that is, the epiphyses, apophyses, and epiphyseal, or growth plates. These structures represent the weakest link in the musculoskeletal chain and are easily injured. In the adult, these structures are no longer present and the stresses of pitching are exerted on the ligaments, tendons, and bone itself.

Further understanding of the effects of competitive pitching on the arm of the preadolescent requires insight into the nature of enchondral ossification and definition of its components.

Enchondral ossification is the mechanism by which longitudinal and configurational bone growth is effected by the orderly transformation of hyaline cartilage to mature cancellous bone. It can be best described in terms of specific areas of growth, each having its own peculiarities that make it susceptible to injury.

The epiphysis is the secondary center of ossification at either end of the long bones. It develops from a cartilage analog by enchondral ossification, but actually contributes little if anything to longitudinal growth. With a few exceptions, the epiphysis is bounded on one end by articular cartilage and on the other by the growth plate. From the standpoint of blood supply, it is isolated from the shaft of the bone by the growth plate. If the epiphyseal vessels are injured, the epiphysis undergoes avascular necrosis. Also, these relatively fragile secondary centers of ossification are prone to avascular changes from compressive forces. Such localized avascular changes are called osteochondrosis.

The growth plate is the component of enchondral ossification responsible for longitudinal growth. Siffer divided the plate into three functional zones: (1) growth zone, (2) zone of cartilage transformation, and (3) zone of ossification. It is recognized that the compression of the plate retards growth, probably at the growth zone. Conversely, distracting forces stimulate germinal cell proliferation. The zone of ossification is the area most susceptible to stress in the growth plate. Here shearing forces separate the plate between the last layer of cartilage cells and the zone of provisional calcification. This is the mechanism responsible for the vast majority of growth plate injuries.

Adjacent to the growth plate lies the metaphysis followed by the diaphysis. Aberrations in the growth plate may become manifest in these areas.

An apophysis is a secondary center of ossification responsible for configurational rather than longitudinal growth. Also, rather than being covered by articular cartilage and involved in a joint, it serves as a site for muscle attachment. Apophyses and their growth plates react to physiologic and pathologic stresses in the same manner as epiphyses.

"Little League elbow" actually encompasses a group of disorders affecting the growth elements about the pitching elbow. These lesions may be classified as follows:

A. Medial epicondylar apophysitis
  1. Accelerated apophyseal growth with delayed closure of the medial epicondylar growth plate.
  2. Traction apophysitis (fragmentation of medial epicondylar apophysis).
  3. Avulsion of the medial epicondylar apophysis.
B. Osteochondrosis of the head of the radius.
C. Osteochondrosis of the humeral capitellum.
D. Non-union of a stress fracture of the olecranon epiphysis.

The term *Little League elbow* is used to describe several different problems. Medial epicondylar apophysitis, itself a poor term, can manifest as one of three different clinical and roentgenographic entities.

Accelerated medial apophyseal growth with delayed closure of the medial epicondylar growth plate is seen in Little Leaguers who have been subjected to repetitious pitching. Generally, the symptoms are minimal and the diagnosis is made on the basis of the roentgenogram. In my experience, this condition does not cause significant disability. If symptoms warrant treatment, simply resting the arm is sufficient.

Traction apophysitis likewise has a classic roentgenographic picture. Again, the cause is repetitious pitching, which can result in pain, swelling, and tenderness over the medial humeral epicondylar apophysis. If symptoms are significant, the arm should be rested.

Complete avulsion of the medial epicondylar apophysis occurs acutely with attempts to throw as hard as possible. Pain, swelling, and tenderness are present over the apophysis. If separation of the apophysis is less than 5 mm, the extremity should be immobilized in plaster for 3 weeks. If the separation is 5 mm or more, open reduction and pin fixation are indicated.

Osteochondrosis of the radial head is a relatively rare lesion, although Ellman has documented five cases, Adams two, and Tullos and King one, all occurring in preadolescent pitchers. Characteristically, pain develops in the elbow of the pitching arm and increasing with throwing. Clinically, swelling and tenderness are localized over the radial head and there is limitation of extension. On the basis of roentgenographic and histologic evidence, Ellman found changes in the radial head similar to those seen in the capital femoral epiphysis in Legg-Calve-Perthes disease—this is, condensation, fragmentation, and bony restoration with deformity, articular incongruity, and subsequent arthritic changes. Initial treatment consists of immobilization until the acute symptoms subside. Any further pitching is prohibited. If the radial head becomes markedly deformed, excision may be considered after the healing phase has been completed.

Osteochondrosis of the humeral capitellum also occurs in preadolescents who have pitched in Little League. In all probability this also represents an osteochondritis dissecans of the involved area. Basically, this lesion can be divided into three types. Type I lesion demonstrates an area of radiolucency involving the capitellum but no evidence of bony displacement or involvement of the articular cartilage. Management consists of absolute restriction of vigorous activities. A Type II lesion, in addition to radiographic findings of bone involvement, is associated with fissuring and softening of the articular cartilage or an articular fracture associated with a partial detachment lesion. Arthroscopic in-situ pinning have been recommended, however, when this lesion progresses to involve both bone and articular cartilage the prognosis is generally poor. Type III lesions are completely detached, becoming a loose body in the joint. Arthroscopic removal of the fragments with curettage of the base of the lesion is indicated. The prognosis is poor and the patient should be advised to discontinue throwing activities.

Non-union of a stress fracture to the olecranon epiphyseal plate had been observed in adolescent baseball pitchers. The patients present with pain associated with pitching, a discernible flexion contracture of the involved elbow and tenderness over the olecranon. X-ray films demonstrate a transverse regular radiolucency with surrounding sclerotic margins involving the site of the former epiphyseal plate of the olecranon. Recent reports in the literature have documented healing with conservative management. Specifically, the elbow should be immobilized for 4 to 6 weeks. If subsequent roentgenographic examination reveals persistence of the lesion, then an operative procedure with curettage of the sclerotic margins and placement of an in-laid autogenous bone graft across the defect is recommended.

OVERUSE SYNDROMES

C. STEWART WRIGHT, M.D., F.R.C.S.(C)

TENNIS ELBOW

Lateral epicondylitis refers to an overload syndrome affecting the forearm extensor origin at the bone tendon junction. Most authors consider that the extensor carpi radialis brevis (ECRB) is the most responsible tendon. Problems in this area may be the result of a single overload episode such as a poorly hit backhand shot in tennis. Occasionally, local trauma may be the original cause. More commonly, however, it is a cumulative overload against the background of a poorly conditioned extensor mechanism. This underscores the importance of a preseason conditioning program and a pre-exercise warm-up with one of the various types of racquet sports.

The hallmark of this condition is pain at the origin of the extensor tendon, particularly on impact loading. In the chronic state there may be a background of nagging pain exacerbated by activities that use these muscles.

GOLFER'S ELBOW

A similar symptom complex may occur in relation to the medial epicondyle and common flexor origin. As with the lateral side, repeated microtrauma may lead to a mild degenerative reaction with an associated low-grade inflammatory response. Again, the importance of a pre-exercise stretching and strengthening program should be emphasized.

OLECRANON IMPACTION SYNDROME

This third entity involving the elbow is usually seen in the throwing sports. It refers to discomfort centered in the olecranon fossa at full extension of the elbow. It usually presents as an ache that occurs during release of the ball or during some other action that results in full elbow extension or hyperextension. This needs to be differentiated from a triceps tendinitis, which usually shows local tenderness over the insertion of the tendon.

NEUROLOGIC CONDITIONS

Medial epicondylitis should be differentiated from ulnar nerve neuritis. Local sensitivity over the nerve behind the epicondyle and distal sensory complaints usually distinguish the two conditions. Occasionally, the two coexist and may both require treatment.

Lateral epicondylitis may occasionally be confused with a radial nerve entrapment syndrome in the radial tunnel. The area of local tenderness is usually 2 to 3 cm distal to the lateral epicondyle. Clinically, this may present as an ache in the extensor mass with radiation both proximally and distally. Electromyographic (EMG) studies are usually not helpful. Resisted extension of the middle finger with the wrist in neutral (the middle finger test) may reproduce the typical distribution of pain. Pain with resisted wrist extension is more likely to be tennis elbow.

Four potential areas of compression in the radial tunnel are identified in the following locations:
1. By fibrous bands lying anterior to the radial head.
2. By the radial recurrent vessels (the leash of Henry).
3. At the tendinous margin of the extensor carpi radialis brevis.
4. At the arcade of Froshe, a ligamentous band over the deep branch of the nerve at its entrance into the supinator muscle. (This is the most common area of involvement.)

MANAGEMENT

Conservative

Some modification of the athlete's usual activity is required. This may involve a change in racquet head and grip size, string tension, and frequency of activity or may necessitate an evaluation of stroke mechanics. A lesson with the local club professional is often a good starting point.

Local icing, ultrasonography, and deep heat are also useful in the attempt to limit the inflammatory response. Stretching the involved muscle tendon groups is important both before and after exercise. Strengthening exercises are necessary both for conditioning and as part of a rehabilitative program. Flexor muscle bulk may be enhanced by squeezing a soft squash ball or doing wrist curls with light weights. Stretching a firm elastic band by spreading the fingers or doing reverse wrist curls will help to strengthen the extensor musculature.

Nonsteroidal anti-inflammatory agents are most useful in the acute stage of the condition and should probably be used for only 2 to 3 weeks. Steroid injections into the bone tendon junction should be used as a second-line treatment if the nonsteroidal agents fail. A suggested limit of three steroid injections over a 6 month interval should be effective for the vast majority of patients with epicondylitis. Beyond this, surgery should be considered.

Splints and braces designed to dissipate impact load through the forearm musculature may be useful for certain patients. These should not be applied too firmly; they should be positioned over the bulk of the musculature rather than over the point of tenderness. In this manner, they can share the impact load with the musculature.

Surgery

Most patients respond to a combination of conservative measures, but some require surgery.

Lateral epicondylitis is approached through a lateral incision over the epicondyle and radial head. The proximal tendon and extensor origin is exposed and released from the epicondyle. The tendon attachment to the annular ligament is released from the anterior neck of the radius. A portion of the epicondyle is removed with an osteotome and the bed drilled with a 2 mm drill bit. This enhances vascular supply and relieves venous hypertension in the bone. The fascia is then closed and a gentle stretching and strengthening program begun during the first week. Resolution of symptoms usually takes 3 months after surgery. Return to activity should be delayed until full flexibility has been achieved and all pain to local pressure or impact resolved.

Medial epicondylitis is treated in a similar fashion with release of the origin, excision of part of the epicondyle, drilling of the bone bed, and resuturing of the fascia.

In the ulnar impaction syndrome the triceps is split, the tip of the olecranon excised, and the olecranon fossa cleansed of loose body or fibrous tissue. Care is taken to ensure that no bone impingement occurs at full extension of the elbow.

For the radial tunnel syndrome, an anterolateral approach is made (after Henry). The nerve can be identified easily in the interval between the brachialis and the brachioradialis. It can then be traced distally through the potential areas of compression. Both the superficial and deep branches are explored, and care is taken to release the arcade of Froshe adequately, because this is the most common area of compression.

As in the management of other chronic tendonitides, early recognition of the entity and modification of the factors provoking it are the surest way to minimize the disability. Once chronically established, these conditions are difficult to resolve conservatively. The results of surgery are generally very satisfactory, but there may be a protracted period before a return to sporting activities is possible.

SUGGESTED READING

DeHaven KE, Evarts CM. Throwing injuries of the elbow in athletes. Orthop Clin North Am 1973; 4:801.

Eversmann WW. Entrapment and compression neuropathies. In: Green DP, ed. Operative hand surgery. New York: Churchill Livingstone, 1982.

Froimson AI. Tenosynovitis and tennis elbow. In: Green DP, ed. Operative hand surgery. New York: Churchill Livingstone, 1982.

Nirschl RP. The etiology and treatment of tennis elbow. J Sports Med 1974; 2:308.

MEDIAL EPICONDYLITIS

C. THOMAS VANGSNESS, Jr., M.D.

Medial epicondylitis is generally considered to be a rare injury. Lateral epicondylitis is a more common injury and both are seen together in the same elbow. Flexor overuse is the etiology with the basic pathology involving the tendon insertion of the common flexor at the medical epicondyle of the elbow.

Little has been written on this subject, and no prospective studies evaluating the outcome of this injury have been done to date. Only one study dealing specifically with medial epicondylitis has been published, although several studies have discussed it in conjunction with lateral epicondylitis.

This injury has been associated with occupations requiring flexing and extending, and pronation and supination. Generally, any repetitive activity involving active pronation of the wrist, or active flexion of the wrist tend to exacerbate this problem. In sports, this could include the throwing of a baseball, the serve and overhand strokes of tennis, as well as the pullthrough strokes of swimming. Both eccentric and concentric muscle contractions can aggravate this problem.

DIAGNOSIS

Diagnosis is made by history and physical examination. The patient history should be consistent with repetitive activities involving flexion of the wrist and/or pronation of the forearm. There may be pain with simple grasping motions.

The physical examination shows tenderness at the medial epicondyle. Resisted flexion and resisted pronation may exacerbate the pain. Associated involvement of the ulnar nerve with distal radiations is common. Motor weakness involving the ulnar nerve is generally not present. Magnetic resonance imaging and bone scan have been reported to aid in the diagnosis, however, these tests are generally not necessary. Injection of a pain relieving anesthetic helps to confirm the exact origin of this pain at the medial epicondyle.

This injury should be differentiated from cervical spine pathology, intra-articular loose bodies of the elbow, and focal elbow arthritis. Medial collateral ligament laxity can mimic and exacerbate this condition.

PATHOLOGY

Pathologic studies have confirmed the common flexor tendon as the origin of this problem. Involvement of the pronator teres and the flexor carpi radialis has

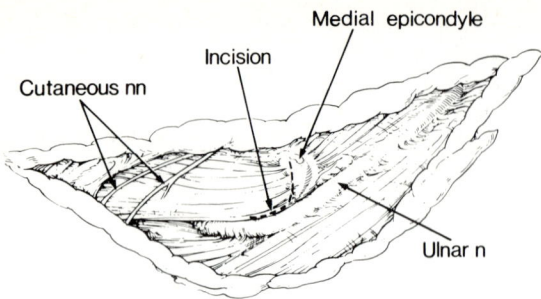

Figure 1 Medial skin incision with deep structures.

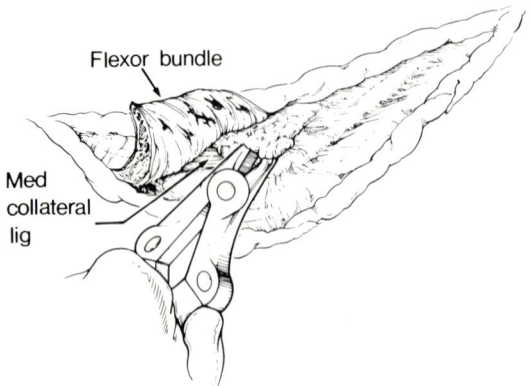

Figure 2 Reflection of common flexor origin and excision of degenerated tissue.

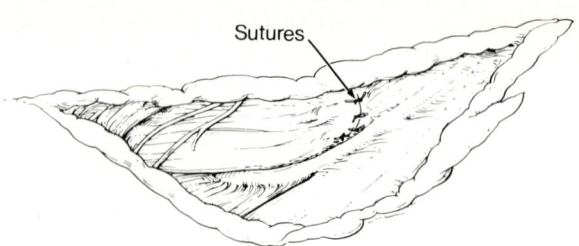

Figure 3 Reattachment of forearm flexors.

been noted. Abnormal healing of these tendons with calcification, vascular tissue and tendon degeneration have been noted. Generally, inflammatory changes are not seen in the histologic analysis of this area of the elbow. Pathologic changes under the surface of the flexor sublimis origin, the palmaris longus, and the flexor carpi ulnaris have been noted.

Calcification has been reported to be present in 15% to 40% of these cases, by pathology and roentgenograms. Ulnar nerve involvement has been present in 10% to 40% of cases. Medial collateral ligament strain or tear and intra-articular changes involving the cartilage surfaces have been noted at surgery.

TREATMENT

Treatment is generally conservative and similar to treatment for lateral epicondylitis. Rest, splinting, and decompression straps have been reported in the literature. Physical therapy modalities of stretching, strengthening, phonophoresis, and iontophoresis have been recommended. Contraforce bracing may also decrease symptoms. Injections of cortisone into the area have been reported to help, however, the exact type of cortisone, amount, and number of injections have never been established. Failure of a conservative regimen of 6 to 12 months is an acceptable reason for surgical intervention. Unrelenting pain, precluding simple activities of daily living, is an indication for surgical intervention.

SURGICAL TECHNIQUE

A 10 to 12 cm incision is centered on the medial epicondyle (Fig. 1), cutaneous nerves being exposed and protected. The common flexor origin is detached by sharp dissection and reflected without disturbing the deep medial collateral ligament. Any abnormal tissue is identified and excised (Fig. 2) before the medial epicondyle is stripped of soft tissue and drilled with multiple small holes. The common flexor origin is reattached to this bleeding bone, care being taken to preserve the normal resting length of the forearm flexors (Fig. 3) and avoid the ulnar nerve.

POSTOPERATIVE TREATMENT

Postoperatively the arm is placed in a 90 degree posterior splint with the wrist free. Sponge squeezing exercises and wrist movements start immediately, but care is taken to avoid resisted wrist flexion or pronation for 6 to 8 weeks. Exercises against light resistance should progress to active participation in sport after 4 to 6 months, as tolerated.

RESULTS

With so little published data available on this rare injury, a firm consensus of results from any treatment plan cannot be determined. Surgery can improve medial elbow function and strength with expectations similar to the 85% to 95% excellent and good results as published for lateral epicondylitis.

SUGGESTED READING

Baumgrad SH, Schwartz DR. Percutaneous release of the epicondylar muscles for humeral epicondylitis. Am J Sports Med 1982; 10: 233–236.

Boyd HB, McLeod AC. Tennis elbow. J Bone Joint Surg 1973; 55:1183–1187.

Coonrad RW, Hooper WR. Tennis elbow: Its course, natural history, conservative and surgical management. J Bone Joint Surg 1973; 55:1177–1182.

Doran A, Gresham GA, Rushton N, Watson C. Tennis elbow: A clinicopathologic study of 22 cases followed for 2 years. ACTA Orthop Scand 1990; 535–538.

Enzenauer RJ, Nordstrom DM. Anterior interosseous nerve syndrome associated with forearm band treatment of lateral epicondylitis. Orthopedics. 1991; 7:788–790.

Ernst E. Conservative therapy for tennis elbow. Br J Clin Prac 1992; 46:1:55–57.

Goldberg EJ, Abraham E, Siegel I. The surgical treatment of chronic lateral humeral epicondylitis by common extensor release. Clin Orthop 1988; 8:208–212.

Goldie I. Epicondylitis lateralis humeri (epicondylalgia or tennis elbow): A pathogenetical study. ACTA Chir Scand Suppl 1964:339.

Ilfeld FW. Can stroke modification relieve tennis elbow? Clin Orthop 1992; 276:182–186.

Johannsen F, Gam A, Hauschild B, et al. An adjunct in physical medicine? Arch Phys Med Rehab 1993; 4:438–440.

Labelle H, Guibert R, Joncas J, et al. Lack of scientific evidence for the treatment of lateral epicondylitis of the elbow: An attempted meta-analysis. J Bone Joint Surg 1992; 74:646–651.

Nirschl RP. Tennis elbow. Orthop Clin North Am 1973; 4:787.

Nirschl RP. Medial tennis elbow: Surgical treatment. Orthop Trans Am Acad Orthop Surg 1980; 7:298.

Nirschl RP, Pettron FA. Tennis elbow. J Bone Joint Surg 1979; 61:832–839.

Nirschl RP, Sobel J. Conservative treatment of tennis elbow. Physician Sports Med 1981; 9:42.

Posch JN, Goldberg VM, Larrey R. Extensor fasciotomy for tennis elbow: A long-term follow-up study. Clin Orthop 1978; 135:179–182.

Regan W, Wold LE, Coonrad R, Morrey BF. Microscopic histopathology of chronic refractory lateral epicondylitis. Am J Sports Med 1992;746–749.

Richards RR, Regan WD. Medical epicondylitis caused by injury to the medial antebrachial cutaneous nerve: A case report. Can J Surg 1989/9; 32:366–369.

Snyder-Macker L, Epler M. Effect of standard and Aircast tennis elbow bands on integrated electromyography of forearm extensor musculature proximal to the bands. Am J Sports Med 1989; 17:278–281.

Spencer GE, Herndon CH. Surgical treatment of epicondylitis. J Bone Joint Surg 1953; 35:421–424.

Vangsness CT, Jobe FW: Surgical treatment of medial epicondylitis. J Bone Joint Surg 1991; 73:409–411.

Verhaar J, Walenkamp G, Kester A, et al. Lateral extensor release for tennis elbow: A prospective long-term follow-up study. J Bone Joint Surg 1993A; 75:1034–1043.

Wittenberg RH, Schaal S, Muhr G: Surgical treatment of persistent elbow epicondylitis. Clin Orthop 1992;73–80.

VALGUS EXTENSION OVERLOAD IN THE PITCHING ELBOW

JAMES R. ANDREWS, M.D.
KEITH MEISTER, M.D.

Chronic changes in the elbow joint occurring secondary to the repetitive throwing motion have long been recognized as sequelae of the forceful overload nature of the act. Baetzner, in 1936, studied the common ailments and changes in the joints of athletes and discovered three kinds of radiographic articular changes: marginal articular projections, para-articular areas of ossification, and intra-articular loose bodies. Even before Baetzner, Heiss studied the elbow joints of 930 athletes and found radiographic changes in 30%. A subgroup of 41 javelin throwers had notable changes in greater than 50%, including loose fragments and ossifications at the tip of the olecranon and coronoid processes. In 1946, Waris in an additional study on javelin throwers, recognized similar persistent changes at the tip of the olecranon as well as para-articular ossification of particularly the medial soft tissues. However, George Bennett is to be credited as the first to draw our attention to the affects of pitching on the elbow. He commonly recognized osteochondritis and persistent loose body formation off the olecranon tip and coronoid in veteran throwers. Since then, much has been written to aid in furthering our understanding of the elbow in the throwing athlete. Slocum also recognized the predictable pattern of injury

and radiographic changes, but categorized injuries according to their pathophysiology: medial tension overload, lateral compression, and extension stress.

Pain is a common problem in the throwing elbow. Tullos and King noted that 50% of all professional pitchers experience sufficient elbow or shoulder joint symptoms to keep them from pitching at various times in their careers. One of the most common sources of pain occurs in the posterior compartment of the elbow as a result of abutment of the tip of the olecranon with forceful extension of the joint during the throwing motion. Waris in his observations on javelin throwers hypothesized, "When the elbow is suddenly straightened during the last stage of javelin-throwing, the tip of the olecranon strikes its fossa and stops the extension movement. This violent blow is no doubt the cause of the changes in the olecranon."

King et al pointed out that 50% of all pitchers have flexion contractures and 30% cubitus valgus deformity. In pitchers, he was the first to recognize that the combination of hypertrophy of the olecranon fossa and the humerus, with cubitus valgus deformation, leads to impingement of the tip of the olecranon tip on the medial aspect of the fossa. Some authors felt that players seldom returned to competitive pitching when these bony changes occurred. Indelicato et al recognized this area of pathology and felt that it was due primarily to stress in the acceleration phase of pitching. The senior author, however, was the first to recognize the treatable nature of this isolated lesion and that aggressive surgical management could predictably allow for the return of the athlete to the premorbid level of throwing. Since the original publication outlining indications and surgical treatment of the Valgus Extension Overload (VEO) syndrome, many more throwers have been similarly treated and successfully returned to their original level of function.

PATHOPHYSIOLOGY

The throwing motion is broken down into five phases: wind-up, cocking (early/late), acceleration, deceleration, and follow-through. Wind-up begins at the initiation of arm motion and ends as the ball is removed from the glove. Cocking begins at the completion of wind-up and is completed at the point of maximal shoulder external rotation. The acceleration phase commences as the arm begins to move forward from its point of maximal shoulder external rotation and ends as the ball is released. Deceleration begins at ball release and is completed as the shoulder reaches a point of maximal shoulder internal rotation. The follow-through phase is the remainder of the motion and allows for rebalancing of the body as the arm comes to a complete stop.

As a result of the development of techniques to better evaluate the throwing motion, a greater understanding of the kinetics and kinematics of the throwing motion has been attained. The normal throwing motion results in high speeds of movement, excessive ranges of motion, and the generation of tremendous forces that are concentrated on the shoulder and elbow during throwing. Thus, the elbow becomes particularly susceptible to injury during this act. During acceleration, elbow extension speeds as high as 3,000 degrees/second have been observed. The forces and torques producing these movements at the shoulder and elbow place tremendous tension on the soft tissues of the medial elbow and tend to compress the lateral side of the joint. More recent laboratory analysis of the throwing arm has shown that a maximum varus torque of approximately 122 N·m is produced at the medial side of the elbow at the earliest point of acceleration. Additionally, a significant compression force equal to about 400 N also occurs at the time of peak varus torque with concomitant firing of the triceps, wrist flexor/pronator group, and the anconeus.

Isolated primary impingement of the posterior tip of the olecranon during follow-through does not occur. Posterior impingement of the olecranon in to the olecranon fossa does not occur before full extension, with the elbow in throwing reaching a maximum extension of only about 15 degrees. Therefore there has to be additional explanation for the build-up of osteophyte posteriorly.

In the early phase of acceleration we have now been able to document the build-up of maximum valgus stress. This valgus load causes a wedging effect of the olecranon into the olecranon fossa (Fig. 1). This impingement leads to osteophyte production at the posterior and posteromedial aspect of the olecranon tip, causing chondromalacia and loose body formation. Secondarily, after early symptoms and osteophyte begin to appear, impingement during follow-through may begin to occur in maximum extension, resulting in further symptomatology.

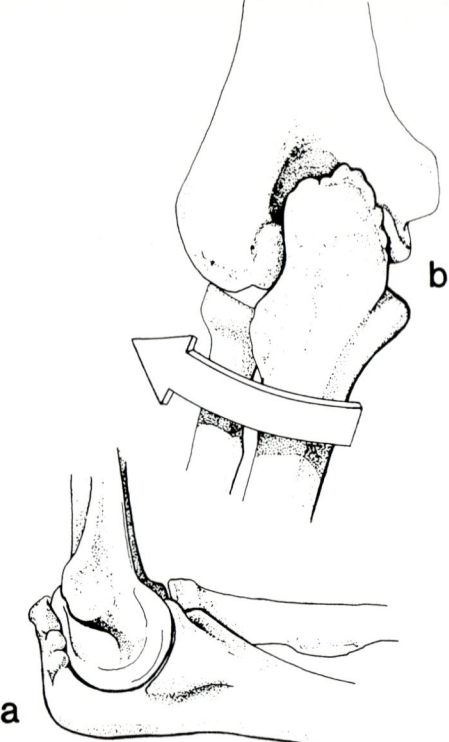

Figure 1 *a,* Lateral diagram of the elbow showing the extent of medial build-up of the posterior osteophyte. *b,* Posterior diagram of the elbow revealing posteromedial impingement and the mechanism for build-up of osteophyte. (From Wilson FD, Andrews JR, Blackburn TA, McCluskey G. Valgus extension overload in the pitching elbow. Am J Sports Med 1983; 11:84; with permission.)

A question remains as to the role of the ulnar collateral ligament (UCL) in contributing to or preventing the development of this lesion. The anterior bundle of the UCL is the primary stabilizer of the elbow when it is subjected to valgus stress. Thus, concomitant incompetence of the anterior bundle of the UCL with VEO, may result in increased symptoms, or may even be the initiating event in leading to an increase in posteromedial impingement. Clinically, although posterior osteophyte formation can occur as an isolated phenomenon, there appears to be an association of these two lesions. Empirically, we are in the process of evaluating this in a laboratory setting.

EVALUATION

History

The major complaint of pitchers with VEO syndrome is pain in the elbow. Pain is characteristically of insidious onset. The location of the pain may be vague and occur only during the act of throwing. Additionally, if not felt during early acceleration, it may be difficult for the pitcher to determine when in the throwing cycle maximum pain is occurring. Characteristically, the individual will be initially effective with the first signs of difficulty being a loss of control. After two or three innings, the pain gradually increases and the pitches tend to rise and sail high as ball release occurs earlier in the acceleration phase.

Increased pain causes an inhibition of movement that gradually causes the pitcher to tire easily and become ineffective. With fatigue, pain increases, as attempts to rely more on arm whip to add velocity results in further exacerbation of symptoms. Specific complaints about the medial elbow with regard to pain and popping, and complaints of sensory changes and deficit in the distribution of the ulnar nerve, should raise concerns of a concomitant medial side lesion (i.e., ligamentous, neurologic, or both).

Physical Examination

Thorough evaluation of the thrower involves complete evaluation of the neck and shoulder of the dominant extremity. Evaluation of the elbow begins with inspection of the extremity with characteristic findings of increased valgus and flexion contracture noted. Palpation of the joint often yields tenderness at the tip of the olecranon and within the posterior olecranon fossa. Both can best be felt with the elbow in approximately 45 degrees of flexion. Tenderness more proximal to the tip may occur secondary to a tricep tendinitis, and tenderness more distal may occur secondary to a stress fracture of the olecranon.

Careful palpation overlying the course of the anterior bundle of the UCL revealing tenderness may raise suspicion of concomitant ligament failure. Most commonly, tenderness is found at the distal insertion of the bundle at the base of the coronoid. With the elbow in 30 degrees of flexion, valgus stability should be assessed and compared to the opposite extremity. Subluxation and dislocation of the ulnar nerve with elbow flexion and extension, although common in many throwers, may or may not be symptomatic. The most significant finding on physical examination is re-creation of symptoms with the VEO maneuver; forced extension of the elbow with an applied valgus load resulting in posterior elbow pain.

Radiographic Evaluation

Standard radiographic evaluation involves five views of the elbow: anteroposterior (AP), lateral, medial and lateral obliques, and an axial view. Most importantly, the lateral and oblique views, taken at 45 degrees oblique to the AP, may reveal characteristic build-up of osteophyte at the tip of the olecranon. The axial view was first described in the original report and found to best show the articulation of the olecranon and the posteromedial osteophyte with the trochlea (Fig. 2). Purely cartilaginous lesions may not be revealed radiographically and may be seen only at the time of operative evaluation.

Routine evaluation now also includes stress evaluation of the elbow using the Telos device. A side-to-side difference of 2 mm or greater, or an absolute opening of greater than 3 mm has been found to be predictive of UCL incompetence (Fig. 3). If further suspicion exists concerning the intactness of the medial side structures work-up continues with a contrast magnetic resonance imaging (MRI). MRI can delineate the anterior bundle of the UCL and with added contrast reveal undersurface tearing predicted by the "T sign" (Fig. 4). This sign has been arthroscopically correlated to prove with high sensitivity the incompetency of the anterior bundle of the UCL.

Occasionally, videoanalysis is used to detect alterations in the throwing motion. Abnormal mechanics are corrected in the treatment phase while returning an individual to full function. Such analysis is particularly useful if the individual has been recorded prior to injury, allowing for postinjury comparison.

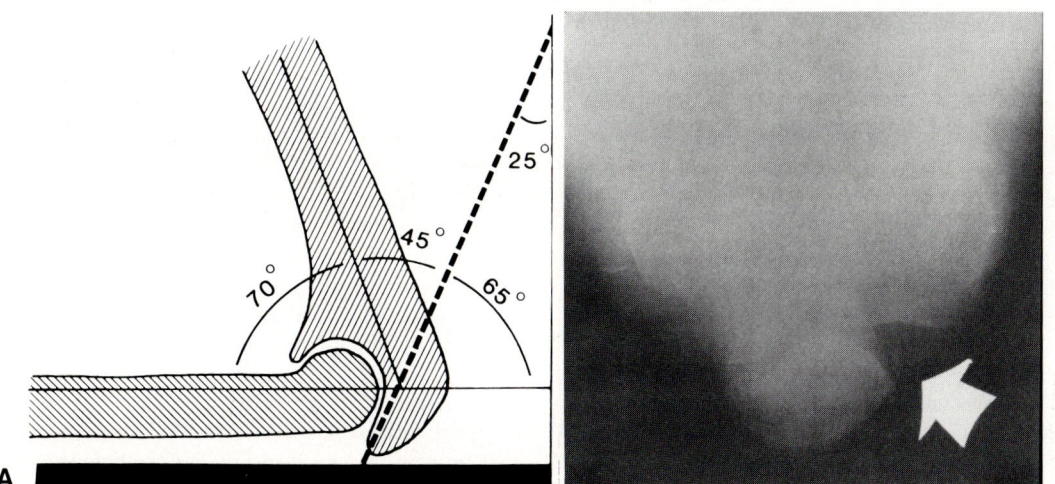

Figure 2 *A,* Diagram showing the radiographic technique for the axial view of the elbow. *B,* Axial view revealing the posteromedial osteophyte and profile of the trochlear articulation. (From Wilson FD, Andrews JR, Blackburn TA, McCluskey G. Valgus extension overload in the pitching elbow. Am J Sports Med 1983; 11:85; with permission.)

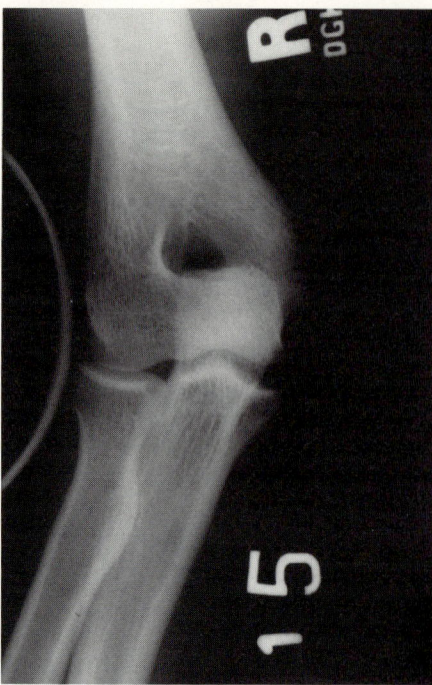

Figure 3 Telos stress examination revealing medial opening of the elbow.

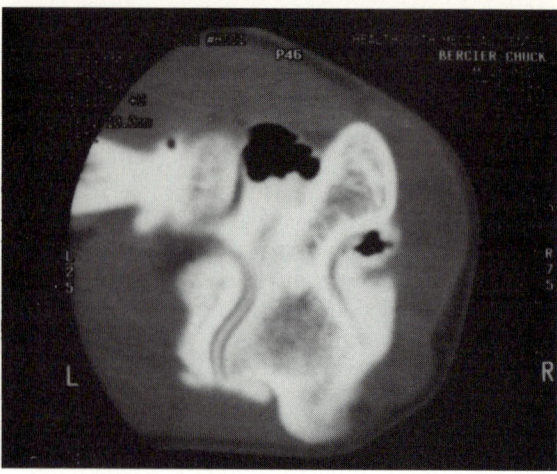

Figure 4 Contrast CT scan revealing the capsular "T sign."

TREATMENT

Conservative

After an adequate work-up and determination of an accurate diagnosis, attempts are made at resolution of symptoms with a conservative management program. The goals of this program are twofold; elimination of pain and restoration of strength and endurance. For reduction of pain routine administration of nonsteroidal anti-inflammatory drugs as well as physical therapy modalities (i.e., heat, ultrasound, massage, and phonophoresis) are employed. Strengthening and flexibility are achieved through a routine series of exercises designed for both the shoulder and elbow. During the initial phases, the individual is kept from throwing, but continues to condition.

Once pain is reduced and strength and endurance are regained, an interval throwing program is begun. If after 3 to 6 months of nonoperative management successful return to throwing is not achieved and the diagnosis is well established, surgical management is recommended.

Surgical

Surgical management of VEO was initially obtained via an open technique. However, as techniques and skill with the arthroscope have advanced, rarely is an isolated lesion now addressed through an arthrotomy.

The open approach involves a straight skin incision overlying the lateral epicondylar ridge of the humerus and extending 4 to 5 cm distally. The edge of the triceps

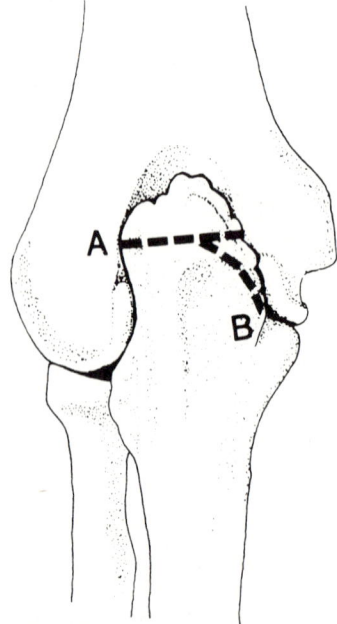

Figure 5 Diagram showing the level of olecranon resection. (From Wilson FD, Andrews JR, Blackburn TA, McCluskey G. Valgus extension overload in the pitching elbow. Am J Sports Med 1983; 11:86; with permission.)

tendon and anconeus fibers are identified and sharply elevated off the ridge. With retraction, the posterior compartment of the elbow may now be visualized. Sharp dissection of some of the synovial tissue and flexion and extension of the elbow may be required for complete visualization of the olecranon tip. A one-quarter inch osteotome is then used to osteotomize the distal 1 cm tip of the olecranon process. A one-quarter inch curved osteotome may then be used to take off the medial edge of the olecranon process with the remainder of the posteromedial osteophyte (Fig. 5). A rongeur may be used to complete any further required debridement.

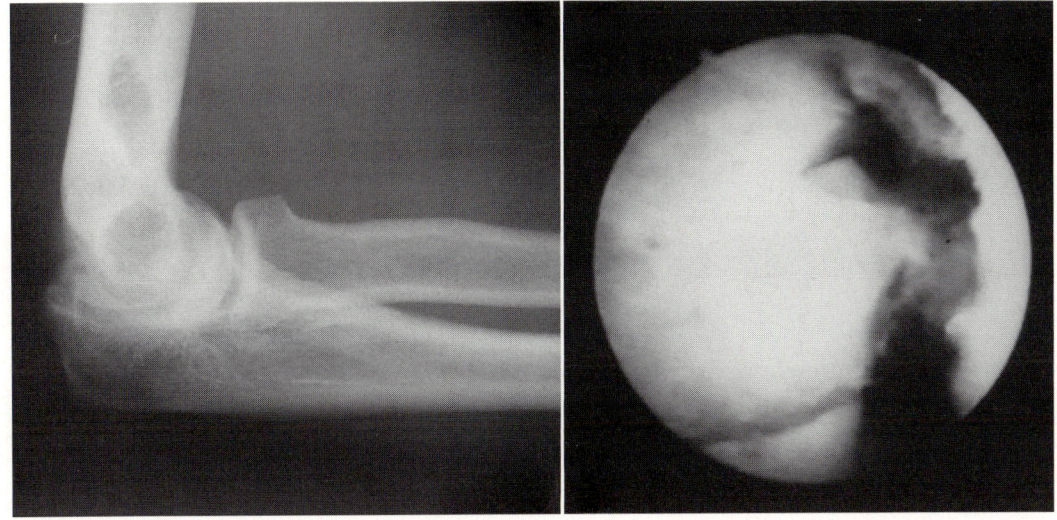

Figure 6 *A,* Lateral radiograph revealing the posterior osteophyte in a pitcher. *B,* Arthroscopic view through the posterolateral portal showing resection of the olecranon tip.

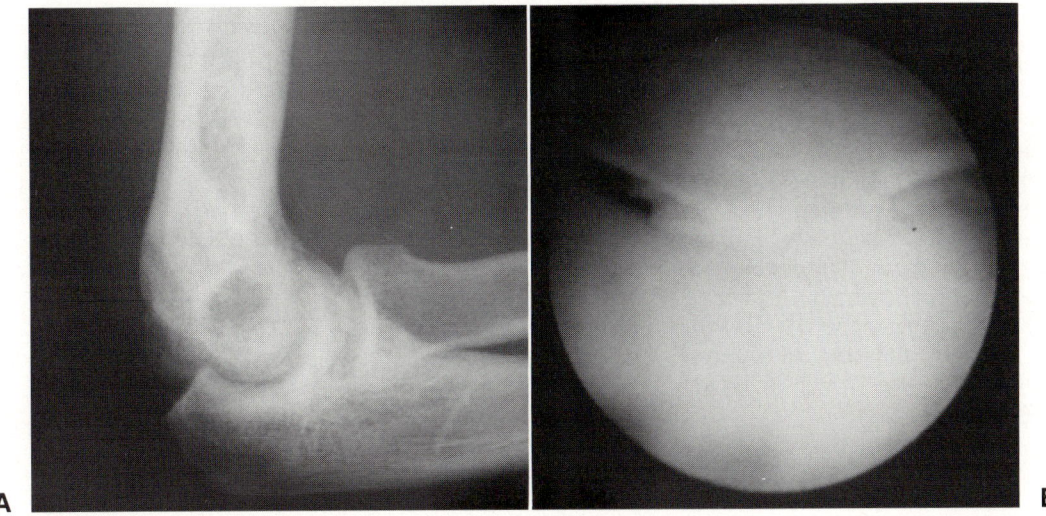

Figure 7 *A,* Postoperative lateral radiograph revealing the level of adequate resection. *B,* Arthroscopic posterolateral portal view following completion of the resection.

Adequate irrigation of the elbow should follow prior to wound closure.

If the lesion occurs in conjunction with UCL instability or isolated ulnar neuritis, a similar open technique is used through a small posteromedial arthrotomy. Once transposition of the ulnar nerve has been performed, access to the posterior compartment of the elbow is easily achieved with a small capsular incision.

Our preferred method for an isolated lesion is with the use of the arthroscope. Elbow arthroscopy is routinely performed in the supine patient with the elbow suspended with about 5 pounds of traction. Complete examination of the joint is carried out before treatment of the posterior lesion. The anterolateral portal is established first for visualization of the anterior com-

partment. If improved visualization of the radiocapitellar joint is needed the arthroscope may be placed through a standard anteromedial portal.

A third portal, the direct lateral portal, is then established through the lateral soft spot for visualization of the ulnotrochlear articulation. By looking posterior beyond the olecranon articular surface, the posterolateral portal may be established under direct visualization. The arthroscope is then reintroduced into the back of the elbow and through the posterolateral portal the entire posterior compartment of the elbow can be visualized.

In order to excise the olecranon osteophyte a direct posterior portal is established 2 to 3 cm proximal to the tip of the olecranon. Through this access the 3.5 mm shaver is used to clean the soft tissue off the tip of the olecranon to improve viewing. Then using a 4.0 mm round arthroscopic burr and a one-quarter inch straight osteotome, the debridement is performed (Fig. 6). Upon completion, with the elbow flexed to approximately 45 degrees, the trochlear articulation should come into view (Fig. 7). Wounds are closed with Steri-strips, a medium Hemovac drain is placed into the joint, and a soft bulky dressing is applied to the elbow. The drain is removed in the out-patient recovery area prior to discharge of the patient.

Postoperative Course

The postoperative rehabilitation of the elbow is divided into three phases; phase I, the immediate motion phase; phase II, the intermediate phase; and phase III, the advanced strengthening phase.

The goals of phase I are to regain full range of motion (ROM), decrease pain, and retard muscular atrophy. Motion is begun immediately after surgery with active and mild passive assistance in order to quickly regain motion. Strengthening is begun first with isometrics of the flexors and extensors of both the wrist and elbow. By about day 11 at least 10 to 100 degrees of motion has been obtained, and a light resistive exercise program is begun.

At about 2 weeks postsurgery, the intermediate phase is begun to complete restoration of ROM and improve strength and endurance. ROM emphasis is therefore continued as are the resistive exercises for the elbow and wrist. Shoulder exercises for the rotator cuff are added and at week 4 a light upper body conditioning program is added to the regimen.

By week 8 with a full nonpainful ROM established and 75% of strength present, an interval throwing program may be initiated with a gradual return to full activity. This basic program may be accelerated as progress dictates. Most throwers are returning to full activity by 8 to 10 weeks postdecompression.

SUGGESTED READING

Andrews JR, St. Pierre RK, Carson WG. Arthroscopy of the elbow. Clin Sports Med 1986; 5:653–662.

Andrews JR, Craven WM. Lesions of the posterior compartment of the elbow. Clin Sports Med 1991; 10:637–651.

Bennett GE. Shoulder and elbow lesions of the professional baseball pitcher. JAMA 1941; 117:510–514.

Conway JE, Jobe FW, Glousman RE, Pink M. Medial instability of the elbow in throwing athletes. J Bone Joint Surg 1992; 74-A:67–83.

DeHaven KE, Evarts CM. Throwing injuries of the elbow in athletes. Orthop Clin North Am 1973; 4:301–808.

Indelicato PA, Jobe FW, Kerlan RK, Carter US. Correctable elbow lesions in professional baseball players: A review of 25 cases. Am J Sports Med 1979; 7:72–75.

King JW, Brelsford HJ, Tullos HS. Analysis of the pitching arm of the professional baseball pitcher. Clin Orthop 1969; 67:116–123.

Morrey BF, An KN. Articular and ligamentous contributions to the stability of the elbow. Am J Sports Med 1983; 11:315–319.

Slocum DB. Classification of elbow injuries from baseball pitching. Tex Med 1968; 64:48–53.

Sojbjerg JO, Oveson J, Nielson S. Experimental and elbow instability after transection of the medial collateral ligament. Clin Orthop 1987; 281:186–190.

Timmerman LA, Schwartz ML, Andrews JR. Ulnar collateral ligament: Preoperative evaluation by MRI and CT arthrogram in 25 baseball players with surgical confirmation. Presented at AOSSM annual meeting. Sun Valley, Idaho, June, 1993.

Waris W. Elbow injuries of javelin throwers. Acta Chir Scand 1946; 93:563–574.

Wilson FD, Andrews JR, Blackburn TA, McCluskey G. Valgus extension overload in the pitching elbow. Am J Sports Med 1983; 11:83–88.

Wisleder D, Fleisig GS, Dillman CJ, et al. Biomechanics—Development of a biomechanical analysis of throwing with clinical applications for pitchers. Sports Med Update 1989; 4:28–31.

OLECRANON STRESS FRACTURES IN THROWING ATHLETES

GORDON W. NUBER, M.D.
MARK K. BOWEN, M.D.

Upper extremity injuries in throwing athletes are common. The act of throwing places significant stress on the elbow joint. Occurring repetitively, these stresses lead to both physiologic and pathologic changes. Physiologic changes include hypertrophy of bone and soft tissues, along with development of flexion contractures and valgus inclination of the joint. Pathologic changes include development of osseous spurs, propagation of loose bodies, disruption of ligamentous structure, and ulnar nerve compression.

While stress fractures in weight-bearing bones are well documented, a stress fracture of the olecranon in the throwing athlete is an uncommon injury. This chapter describes the relevant literature, etiology, diagnosis, and treatment of this rare problem.

HISTORY

Breithaupt, a Prussian military physician, is credited with the first description of stress fractures of the foot in military recruits. Since his description in 1855, various authors have written about the significance of stress

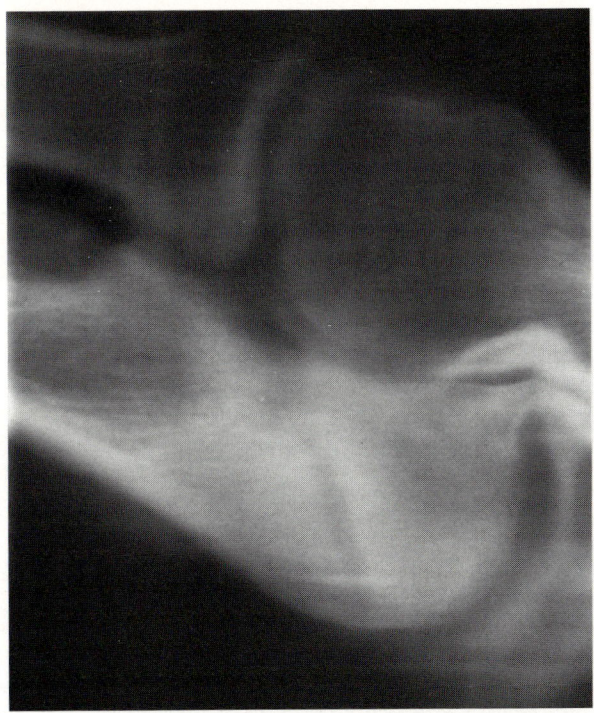

Figure 3 Tomographic evidence of stress fracture in professional pitcher.

TREATMENT

Our experience has shown that these fractures will do well treated by restriction of throwing. We have allowed return to throwing only after documented evidence of healing. In addition, initial mobilization may be warranted. We have found it helpful to splint these athletes for a brief period. This ensures restriction of activity in an individual who may have minimal or no pain when not throwing.

Olecranon stress fracture is primarily a tension type of fracture, and nonunions are a potential complication. If delayed union, nonunion, or displacement of the fracture is noted, open reduction and bone grafting is warranted. We prefer the tension band type of fixation. Unfortunately, without a larger series of patients, definitive conclusions and recommendations are difficult to make.

Olecranon tip fractures, a different entity, frequently go on to nonunion, and form loose bodies. These should be excised surgically, either arthroscopically or through a posterolateral approach.

SUGGESTED READING

Bennett GE. Elbow and shoulder lesions of baseball players. Am J Surg 1959; 98:484–492.

Breithaupt MD. Zur pathologie des mensch lichen fussess. Medizin Zeitung 1855; 24:169–177.

Dafner RH, Pavlov H. Stress fractures: Current concepts. AJR 1992; 159:245–252.

Hershman EB, Mailly T. Stress fractures. Clin Sports Med 1990; 9:183–214.

Hullko A, Orava S, Nikula P. Stress fractures of the olecranon in javelin throwers. Int J Sports Med 1986; 7:210–213.

Jones BH, Harris J, Vinh TN, Rubin C. Exercise-induced stress fractures and stress reactions of bone: Epidemiology, etiology and classification. Exercise Sports Sci Rev 1989; 17:379–422.

King JW, Brelsford HJ, Tullos HS. Analysis of the pitching arm of the professional baseball pitcher. Clin Orthop 1969; 67:116–123.

Kvidera DJ, Pedegana LR. Stress fracture of the olecranon: Report of two cases and review of literature. Orthop Rev 1983; 12:113–116.

Malffulli N, Chan D, Aldridge MJ. Overuse injuries of the olecranon in young gymnasts. J Bone Joint Surg 1992; 74:305–308.

Miller JE. Javelin thrower's elbow. J Bone Joint Surg 1960; 42:788–792.

Nuber GW, Diment MT. Olecranon stress fracture in throwers: A report of two cases and a review of the literature. Clin Orthop 1992; 278:58–61.

Pavlov H, Torg JS, Jacobs B, Vigorita V. Nonunion of olecranon epiphysis: Two cases in adolescent baseball pitchers. AJR 1981; 136:819–820.

Slocum DB. Classification of elbow injuries from baseball pitching. Texas Med 1968; 64:48–53.

Torg JS, Moyer RA. Non-union of stress fracture through the olecranon epiphyseal plate observed in an adolescent baseball pitcher. J Bone Joint Surg 1977; 59:264–265.

Tullos HS, Erwin WD, Woods GW, et al. Unusual lesions of the pitching arm. Clin Orthop 1972; 88:169–182.

Waris W. Elbow injuries of javelin-throwers. Acta Chir Scand 1946; 93:563–575.

Wilkerson RD, Johns JC. Nonunion of an olecranon stress fracture in an adolescent gymnast. Am J Sports Med 1990; 18:432–434.

ULNAR NEURITIS AND MEDIAL ELBOW INSTABILITY

FRANK W. JOBE, M.D.
JOHN E. CONWAY, M.D.
JAMES P. BRADLEY, M.D.

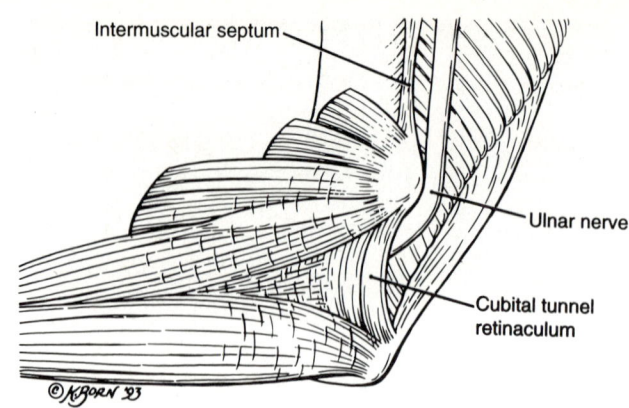

Figure 1 The ulnar nerve passes behind the intermuscular septum and medial epicondyle where it enters the cubital tunnel beneath the cubital tunnel retinaculum.

Overhead throwing creates potentially destructive forces acting on the elbow joint and adjacent structures. These forces are classified as medial tension overload, lateral compression overload, and posterior valgus extension overload. Ulnar collateral ligament (UCL) injuries and ulnar neuritis are two of several pathologic conditions that occur as a result of overuse and harmful tensile forces acting on the medial elbow.

ULNAR NEURITIS

Etiology

After entering the anterior compartment of the upper arm, the ulnar nerve passes into the posterior compartment by penetrating the dense fibrous arcade of Struthers. Coursing distally behind the septum, the nerve runs posterior to the medial epicondyle and enters the cubital tunnel. The borders of the cubital tunnel are the posterior fossa of the medial epicondyle, the capsule of the elbow, the posterior and transverse bundles of the UCL, and the medial edge of the trochlea. The roof of the cubital tunnel is formed by the cubital tunnel retinaculum, previously described as the arcuate ligament, which extends from the medial epicondyle to the olecranon process (Fig. 1). Beyond the cubital tunnel, the ulnar nerve travels underneath the aponeurosis and the muscle fibers of the flexor carpi ulnaris (FCU) until it exits beneath the deep flexor pronator aponeurosis. Articular branches and the first motor branches to the FCU may arise proximal to, within, or distal to the cubital tunnel. Potential sites of compression along the course of the nerve occur at the arcade of Struthers, the proximal edge of the cubital tunnel retinaculum, the cubital tunnel, and the deep flexor pronator aponeurosis.

Ulnar neuritis is observed in athletes participating in a wide variety of sports. Due to the repetitive valgus stress on the medial elbow and the rapid change in elbow position involved in the overhead throwing motion, baseball pitchers and athletes in sports that require a similar use of the arm are most at risk for this condition. Adaptive and physiologic factors (hypertrophy of the muscle and bone, valgus deformity of the elbow, mobility of the ulnar nerve, and reduction in the cubital tunnel volume during elbow flexion), pathologic mechanical factors (compression from changes in the adjacent soft tissues, friction due to hypermobility of the nerve, and traction secondary to tethering of the nerve or valgus instability of the elbow), and direct local trauma contribute to the pathogenesis, and each must be considered to determine appropriate management.

The act of repetitive throwing overhead creates enormous stress on the entire arm in addition to tensile stress on the medial elbow structures. Adaptive changes that occur in response to this stress include hypertrophy of the triceps and FCU muscles, enlargement of the humerus and olecranon, valgus deformity of the elbow joint, and fixed flexion contracture of the elbow joint. These changes may predispose the ulnar nerve to injury from compressive and tensile forces. Rarely hypertrophy of an anomalous anconeus epitrochlearis muscle may cause local compression on the nerve.

As the elbow flexes beyond 90 degrees, the posterior bundle of the UCL tightens, the proximal edge of the cubital tunnel retinaculum becomes taut, and the volume of the cubital tunnel is reduced. These physiologic changes result in transient focal compression on the ulnar nerve. Pathologic hypertrophy or contracture of the cubital tunnel retinaculum causes chronic compression with indentation and swelling of the nerve. Further, the ulnar nerve elongates an average of 4.7 mm during elbow flexion and the medial head of the triceps may push the nerve up to 7 mm medially. Adhesions occurring within the cubital tunnel, tether the nerve and compromise its normal function by impairing normal longitudinal and transverse mobility.

During the acceleration phase of throwing, the elbow is flexed beyond 90 degrees with the shoulder in abduction and the wrist in flexion. In this position, the intraneural pressure within the ulnar nerve has been demonstrated to reach six times the pressure of that noted in the relaxed nerve near extension. When valgus stress is additionally applied during throwing motion, the pressures may be higher, particularly in the face of UCL laxity. Repetitive local compression and transient ischemia may eventually result in intraneural fibrosis and ulnar neuritis.

Hypertrophy, calcification, attenuation, or rupture of the UCL jeopardizes normal ulnar nerve function by indirectly compromising the volume of the cubital tunnel and by creating local adhesions from inflammation or hemorrhage. Valgus instability from ligament laxity demands greater than normal elongation of the nerve and ulnar neuritis results from the combined stress of compression and traction.

Ulnar nerve hypermobility has been documented to occur in 16.2 percent of the population and results from laxity in the soft tissue restraints. During elbow flexion, the subluxated or dislocated ulnar nerve becomes progressively elongated as it passes over the prominent medial epicondyle until it slides free. When "popping" of the nerve is noted during the throwing motion, injury to the ulnar nerve occurs primarily from tension forces; however, compression and friction forces against the medial epicondyle also contribute. Incompletely dislocated nerves (Type A) are more prone to direct trauma while chronically dislocated nerves (Type B) are more likely to develop neuritis as a result of traction and friction stresses.

Clinical Presentation

In the throwing athlete, the physical findings of ulnar neuritis are often subtle and the diagnosis relies on a complete history and a strong clinical suspicion. Symptoms are usually elicited or aggravated by throwing, and rest may afford complete relief. Dull pain over the medial elbow radiating into the forearm and hands is the most frequent symptom. Mild numbness and tingling in the ring and small fingers are common. Weakness, heaviness, and clumsiness of the hand may be appreciated after throwing. Abrupt lancing pain during rapid elbow motion that radiates to the forearm or hand suggests either recurrent subluxation of the nerve onto the epicondyle or tethering of the nerve within the cubital tunnel. Painful snapping or popping implies recurrent ulnar nerve dislocation.

The percussion test, performed by tapping over the ulnar nerve at the elbow, is the most common physical finding and may help to localize the site of pathology. Local tenderness may be present but is not specific for ulnar neuritis. Hypermobility of the nerve is easily recognized and the nerve will often have a thickened, doughy texture. Mildly diminished light touch is commonly noted. Interossei muscle atrophy, clawing, and decreased two-point discrimination are rare but may be seen late. Proximal muscle atrophy is almost never seen.

Cervical radiculopathy, thoracic outlet syndrome, superior sulcus tumor, cubital tunnel mass or ganglion, UCL injury, flexor pronator muscle tear, medial epicondylitis, posterior olecranon fossa osteophytes, chronic forearm compartment syndrome, and entrapment of the nerve in Guyon's canal must be considered.

Standard radiographs, including a cubital tunnel view, are required. Routine nerve conduction velocity studies may localize the area of involvement to the region of the elbow and are often positive when symptoms become persistent. The focal site of compression is more accurately identified utilizing short segment incremental nerve conduction studies, but the application of this study is unclear. Possibly, this study will allow for the selection of those athletes who would reliably respond to simple decompression. Electromyography is usually normal but the documentation of fibrillation potentials predicts a less satisfactory recovery.

Treatment

McGowan has graded the severity of ulnar neuropathy as follows: stage 1 has minor subjective paresthesia or hypesthesia; stage 2 additionally has atrophy of the interossei muscles; and stage 3 represents severe involvement with complete or partial anesthesia, marked atrophy of the interossei and hypothenar muscles, and clawing. Nonoperative care of athletes with McGowan stage 1 ulnar nerve findings provides good results in 50% of patients. The conservative program includes relative rest, ice, nonsteroidal anti-inflammatory drugs (NSAIDs), and an elbow splint at 30 degrees of flexion for 2 weeks. Steroid injections are not recommended.

When conservative care fails or when muscle atrophy exists, surgical management is indicated. Subcutaneous transposition and medial epicondylectomy are not recommended because of the lack of protection for the nerve. Simple decompression is a viable option in McGowan stage 1 when associated conditions are absent and the site of compression can be documented well distal to the medial epicondyle using short segment incremental nerve conduction studies. If the ulnar nerve is unstable after decompression, transposition is necessary. Anterior submuscular ulnar nerve transposition is most commonly indicated and provides adequate protection for the nerve and yields reliably good results.

Surgical Management

Anterior submuscular ulnar nerve transposition is performed under general endotracheal anesthesia with the use of a pneumatic tourniquet and the arm abducted to the side on an arm board. A 10 cm incision based over the medial epicondyle is carried through the subcutaneous tissues preserving the crossing branches of the medial antebrachial cutaneous nerve. The ulnar nerve is exposed beneath the investing fascia of the upper arm, mobilized proximally, and released from the arcade of Struthers. The cubital tunnel retinaculum is divided, the aponeurosis and muscle fibers of the FCU are split, and the deep flexor pronator aponeurosis is bisected. The ulnar nerve is mobilized along with accompanying blood vessels and protected with a Penrose drain. Motor branches of the nerve to the FCU are routinely preserved, and articular branches are spared when possible. External neurolysis is performed when focal constriction is encountered. Internal neurolysis is not recommended.

The flexor pronator muscles are divided from the medial epicondyle leaving a cuff of tissue for later repair and then elevated from the underlying capsule and ulnar collateral ligament. Dissection distally is adequate when the nerve can be transposed without creating a secondary site of impingement on the nerve. Similarly, 5 cm of the medial intermuscular septum is resected from above the medial epicondyle to avoid proximal impingement

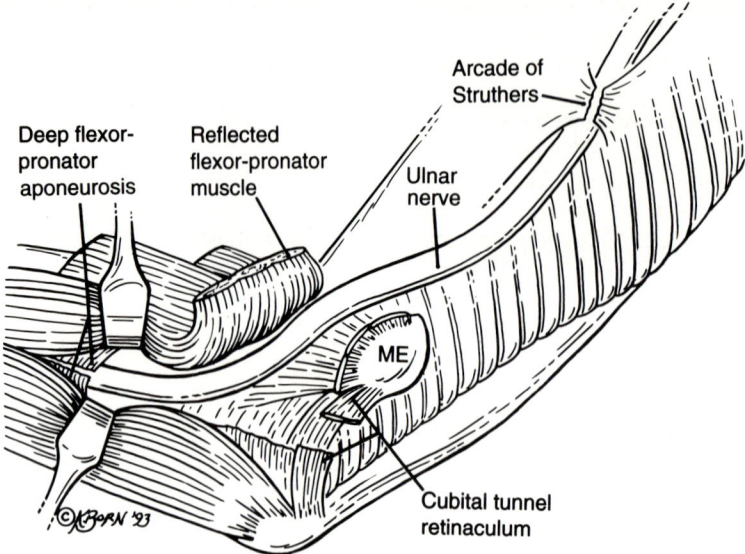

Figure 2 The ulnar nerve is transposed anteriorly. Potential sites of secondary impingement have been released including the arcade of Struthers, the medial intermuscular septum, and the deep flexor-pronator aponeurosis.

after transposition. The UCL and the posterior olecranon fossa may be inspected for associated pathology and addressed when indicated.

The mobilized ulnar nerve is transposed over the medial epicondyle (ME) to pass along a course similar to the median nerve and rest on the anterior elbow capsule and the UCL (Fig. 2). Interrupted absorbable sutures through a cuff of tendon on the epicondyle or through drill holes in the epicondyle are placed to repair the detached flexor pronator muscles. The tourniquet is released, hemostasis is obtained, and the wound is closed.

Rehabilitation

The elbow is immobilized in a posterior splint for 10 days at 90 degrees of flexion with the wrist free. Active elbow range of motion begins at 10 days and light forearm muscle strengthening exercises are allowed at 3 to 4 weeks. Shoulder and elbow strengthening exercises begin as early as comfortably possible and combine with the use of the upper body ergometer at 6 weeks for overall upper extremity conditioning. In preparation for throwing, rotator cuff conditioning begins at 8 weeks and adding an interval throwing program is allowed at 10 to 12 weeks. Return to full competition is permitted 6 months after surgery.

ULNAR COLLATERAL LIGAMENTOUS INSTABILITY

Etiology

The medial ligament of the elbow, termed the ulnar collateral ligament complex, includes three parts: an

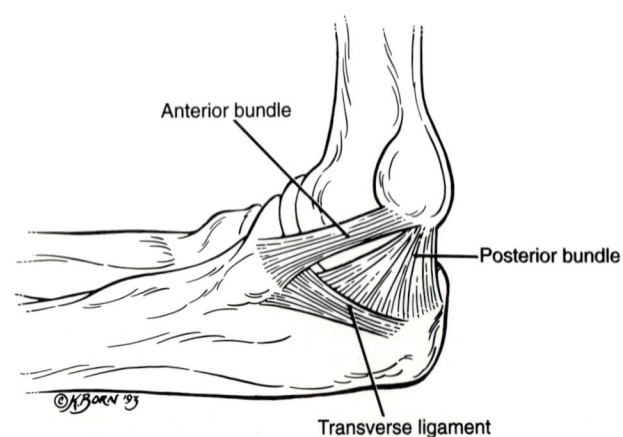

Figure 3 The medial ligaments of the elbow.

anterior oblique bundle, a posterior fan-shaped bundle, and a relatively nonfunctional transverse segment (Fig. 3). The anterior bundle remains taut throughout the elbow range of motion and is the primary constraint resisting valgus stress applied to the elbow joint. When the anterior bundle is divided, the greatest valgus instability occurs at 70 degrees of flexion.

During the acceleration phase of the overhead throwing motion, the elbow flexes progressively from 90 to 120 degrees of flexion and then rapidly extends over a period of 30 to 40 ms to 25 degrees of flexion. The forearm lags behind the upper arm, generating immense valgus forces on the medial elbow structures, while the joint is in a position that is almost solely dependent on the anterior bundle of the UCL for valgus stability. These forces can exceed the tensile strength of the ligament and cause microscopic tears within the ligament. Continued throwing in the presence of injury (and probably altered throwing mechanics) may lead to ligament attenuation or rupture. When this occurs, a throwing athlete can no longer compete at his or her previous level.

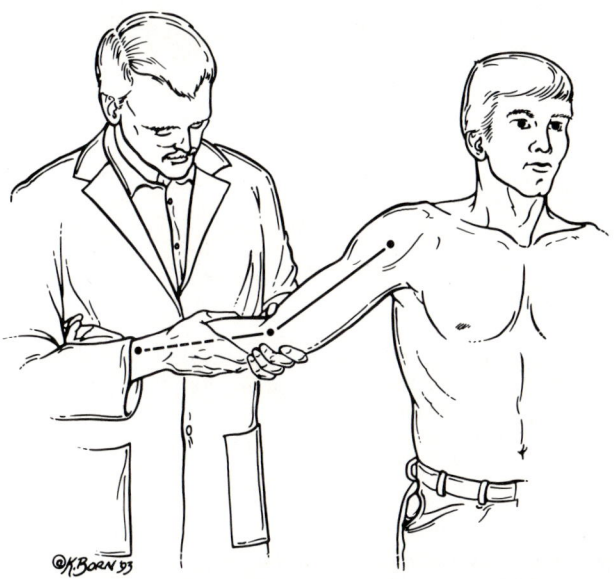

Figure 4 Examination for evaluating medial instability of the elbow. See text for description.

Clinical Presentation

The diagnosis of a torn or incompetent UCL is primarily based on the history and clinical findings from routine physical examination. Conventional plain radiographs, stress radiographs, and magnetic resonance imaging (MRI) may be used to confirm clinical impressions.

The most common complaint from a throwing athlete with an injured UCL is pain over the medial aspect of the elbow during the acceleration phase of throwing. About one third will note that the greatest pain occurs at ball release and a history of elbow pain in previous seasons is common. The pain may be gradual or intermittent in onset. More than one half the athletes who eventually require ligament reconstruction will recall a single throw accompanied by an acute "pop" or sudden sharp pain over the medial elbow, after which they are unable to continue throwing effectively. For reasons previously discussed, symptoms of ulnar neuritis are common. Pain during the follow through phase of throwing or with forced hyperextension on examination suggests coexisting valgus extension overload in the posterior olecranon fossa.

Physical findings may include focal tenderness over the UCL, swelling over the medial aspect of the elbow, or loss of elbow range of motion. Pain occurs over the ulnar collateral ligament with valgus stress. Asymmetric valgus laxity is best revealed in the following manner. The arm of the standing patient is held with the shoulder in abduction, extension, and external rotation. The elbow is flexed 30 degrees and the forearm is supinated.

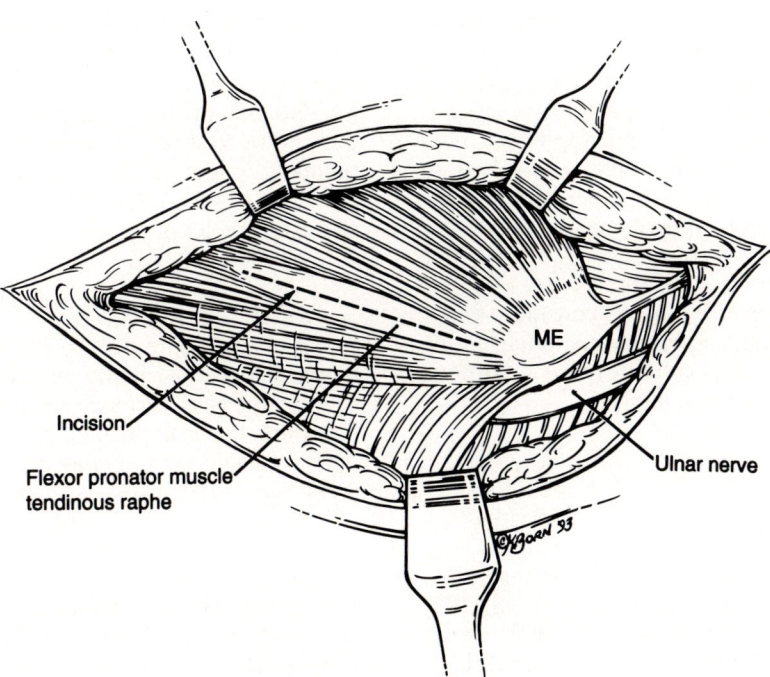

Figure 5 Exposure of the medial epicondyle (ME) and flexor pronator muscles allows identification of the posterior tendinous raphe through which the ulnar collateral ligament can be exposed.

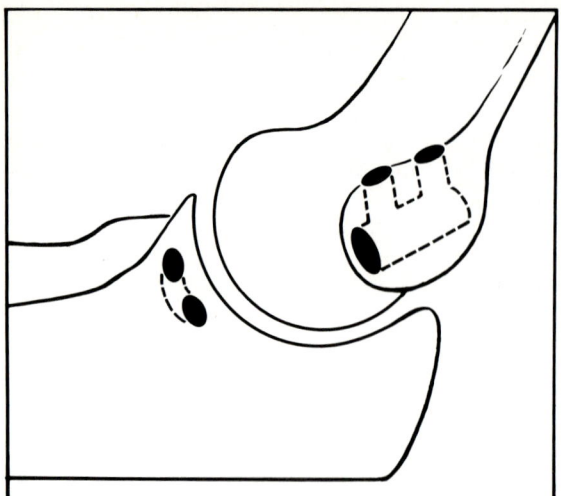

Figure 6 Diagram representing appropriate placement of drill holes for ligament isometry.

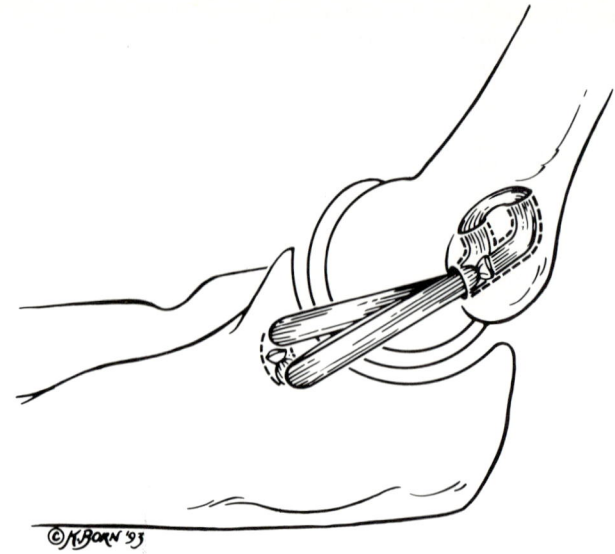

©KBORN '93

Figure 7 Diagram illustrating the proper figure-of-eight placement of the palmaris longus tendon graft to reconstruct the ulnar collateral ligament.

Valgus stress is applied to the elbow while palpating over the medial joint line beneath the UCL (Fig. 4). Be aware that occasionally throwing athletes will have asymptomatic UCL attenuation and valgus laxity while others with a significant ligament injury may have no palpable laxity at all.

Although routine radiographs are obtained to document ligament calcification, epitrochlear marginal osteophytes, posterior olecranon fossa loose bodies or osteophytes, and capitellar osteochondrotic lesions, a normal radiograph does not exclude UCL injury. Valgus stress radiographs, which may be obtained using manual stress or a graded pressure instrumented device, can document excessive medial joint opening and confirm ligament laxity. In our experience, manual stress radiographs are adequate.

Arthrography and computed tomography (CT) arthrography have not been reliable studies for evaluating UCL injuries. MRI, particularly when performed after elbow joint saline injection, is becoming increasingly recognized as a valuable diagnostic tool, but further experience is necessary.

The differential diagnosis must consider flexor pronator muscle tear, medial epicondylitis, ulnar neuritis, and valgus extension overload, but these conditions may exist along with the UCL injury.

Treatment

Nonoperative management for up to 6 months may arrest the progression of instability and functional impairment when begun soon after onset of symptoms. The nonoperative program includes relative rest, NSAIDs, local physical therapy modalities, strengthening, and a thorough assessment of the athlete's throwing mechanics. Steroid injections are not recommended. Two attempts to progress in an interval throwing program are allowed. Successful progress in a conservative program is unlikely when the athlete reports either a long unremit-

ting history of medial elbow pain with throwing or a painful "pop" over the medial elbow during a single throw preventing further effective throwing.

Surgery is indicated for a motivated athlete who has an incompetent UCL based on history and clinical exam, has failed to improve with nonoperative treatment, and wishes to return to competitive overhead throwing. Direct repair of the ligament is rarely indicated because reconstruction more reliably returns the athlete to throwing. A modification of the reconstructive procedure by one of us (FWJ) avoids the need for routine anterior submuscular ulnar nerve transposition. A 15 cm long portion of the ipsilateral palmaris longus tendon is our choice for graft material; however, the contralateral palmaris longus tendon, the plantaris tendon, a 3 to 5 mm strip of the Achilles' tendon, and the third or forth toe extensor tendons are acceptable.

Surgical Management

When ulnar neuritis exists concomitantly with UCL injury, the reconstructive procedure may be performed as previously described, transposing the ulnar nerve anteriorly beneath the flexor pronator muscle. When the ulnar nerve does not appear to be involved, the new technique is performed as follows.

Reconstruction of the UCL is performed under general endotracheal anesthesia with a pneumatic tourniquet on the arm. The patient is supine with the arm abducted to the side on an arm board. A 10 cm incision centered over the medial epicondyle is carried down through the subcutaneous tissues protecting the crossing branches of the medial antebrachial cutaneous nerve. There are two to three tendinous raphe dividing the flexor pronator muscle mass, and the most posterior of these raphe lies directly over the UCL.

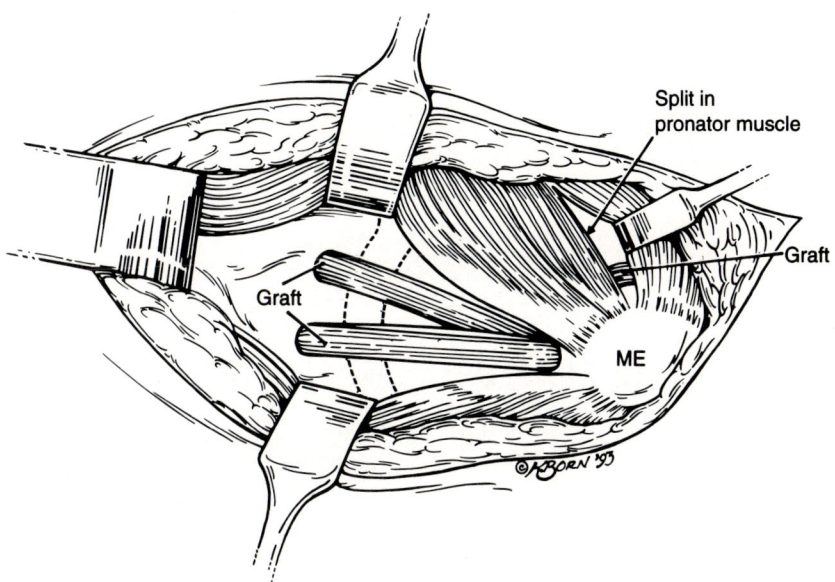

Figure 8 The ulnar collateral ligament may be reconstructed with appropriate graft tissue without requiring detachment of the flexor pronator muscles or transposition of the ulnar nerve.

For exposure of the UCL, a longitudinal split is made in the tendinous raphe and the underlying muscles in line with the fibers as they arise from the epicondyle (Fig. 5). Retractors are placed and care is taken to avoid injury to the ulnar nerve, which lies 5 to 10 mm posterior to the split in the tendinous raphe. The overlying muscle is then reflected off the ligament with a key elevator. An incision dividing the anterior and posterior portion of the anterior UCL in line with its fibers is made, exposing the articular surfaces. The quality of the remaining ligament is determined and valgus stress is applied to evaluate laxity.

The anatomic sites of ligament attachment on the ulna and humerus are identified. A 3.2 mm drill bit is used with a slow speed drill and drill guide to make converging tunnels in the proximal ulna. A 4.5 mm drill bit is used to create a tunnel in the medial epicondyle, beginning at the origin of the ligament, extending back to the posterior cortex of the medial epicondyle (Fig. 6). Care is taken not to pass through the posterior cortex because of the close proximity of the ulnar nerve. An incision is made in line with the fibers of the pronator teres muscle and carried down to the anterior cortical surface of the epicondyle. An elevator is used for exposure. A 3.2 mm drill bit is used to create two tunnels connecting with the previously drilled 4.5 mm tunnel, preserving an anterior bone bridge.

The tendon graft is obtained and passed through the bony tunnels in a figure-of-eight, creating a functional substitute for the anterior bundle in the UCL (Fig. 7). The elbow is supported to prevent valgus stress, and the graft is pulled taut and sutured to itself (Fig. 8). Remnants of the original ligament are then sutured into the graft for additional strength and the flexor pronator muscle tendinous raphe is repaired side-to-side. Hemostasis is confirmed after the tourniquet is released.

Rehabilitation

The elbow is immobilized in a posterior splint for 10 days at 90 degrees of flexion with the wrist free. Active elbow range of motion begins at 10 days and light forearm muscle strengthening exercises are initiated at 3 to 4 weeks. Shoulder and elbow exercises begin as soon as comfortably possible, but valgus stress on the elbow is avoided until 4 months postoperative. At 4 months the athlete begins an interval throwing program designed to allow return to competition by 12 months after surgery. Competitive throwing is permitted when the following criteria are met: there is no pain while throwing, strength of the forearm muscles has returned to normal, the elbow and shoulder have normal range of motion and strength, and overall normal throwing balance, rhythm, and coordination have been re-established.

SUGGESTED READING

Amadio PC, Beckenbaugh RD. Entrapment of the ulnar nerve by the deep flexor-pronator aponeurosis. J Hand Surg 1986; 11A(1):83.

Campbell WW, Pridgeon RM, Sahni KS. Short segment incremental studies in the evaluation of ulnar neuropathy at the elbow. Muscle Nerve 1992; 15:1050–1054.

Conway JE, Jobe FW, Glousman RE, Pink M. Medial instability of the elbow in throwing athletes. J Bone Joint Surg 1992; 74A:67.

Dellon AL. Review of treatment results for ulnar nerve entrapment at the elbow. J Hand Surg 1989; 14A:688.

Jobe FW, Fanton GS, Elattrache NS. Ulnar nerve injury. In: Morrey BF, ed. The elbow and its disorders. Philadelphia: WB Saunders, 1993:560.

Morrey BF. Applied anatomy and biomechanics of the elbow joint. Instructional Course Lectures 1986; 23:59–68.

O'Driscoll SW, Horii E, Carmichael SW, Morrey BF. The cubital tunnel and ulnar neuropathy. J Bone Joint Surg 1991; 73B:613.

Pappas AM, Zawacki RM, Sullivan TJ. Biomechanics of baseball pitching: a preliminary report. Am J Sports Med 1985; 13:216–222.

Regan WD, Korinek SL, Morrey BF, An K. Biomechanical study of ligaments around the elbow joint. CORR 1991; 271:170–179.

Sojbjerg JO, Ovesen J, Nielsen S. Experimental elbow instability after transection of the medial collateral ligament. CORR 1987; 218: 186–190.

Tullos HS, Schwab G, Bennett JB, Woods GW. Factors influencing elbow instability. Instructional Course Lectures 1981; 30:185–199.

ARTHROSCOPY OF THE ELBOW

WILLIAM G. CARSON, Jr., M.D.

Arthroscopy is most commonly utilized to treat various disorders of the knee; however, it now is also being applied to smaller joints such as the shoulder, the ankle, and even the elbow. Arthroscopic procedures on these smaller joints require meticulous attention to detail, since the arthroscopic instruments must be placed through deeper muscle layers and close to important neurovascular structures. This is unlike the situation in the knee, where instruments pass through a thin retinacular layer only and maintain generous distances from neurovascular structures. Thus, the need for attention to detail when performing surgical procedures such as arthroscopy of the elbow become readily apparent.

INDICATIONS

Arthroscopy of the elbow is a relatively new advancement in the field of arthroscopy, and the indications for its use are still being determined. The following indications appear to be appropriate:

1. Removal of loose bodies.
2. Evaluation and debridement of osteochondritis dissecans of the capitellum.
3. Evaluation and/or debridement of chondral or osteochondral lesions of the radial head.
4. Debridement and lysis of adhesions of post-traumatic origin or arising from certain degenerative processes about the elbow.
5. Partial synovectomy in rheumatoid disease.
6. Partial excision of humeral or olecranal osteophytes.
7. Flexion contracture release.
8. Evaluation for medial elbow instability.

Contraindications for elbow arthroscopy include bony ankylosis or severe fibrous ankylosis that would prevent the introduction of the arthroscopic instruments into the elbow joint. Further contraindications include certain surgical procedures such as anterior transposition of the ulnar nerve or other procedures that have altered the anatomy around the elbow so that placement of the usual arthroscopic portals might jeopardize the neurovascular structures.

SURGICAL TECHNIQUE

I prefer general anesthesia for elbow arthroscopy as I feel it affords complete relaxation and comfort for the patient. I do not recommend interscalene or axillary block anesthesia as this interferes with the immediate postoperative neurovascular evaluation in the recovery room. A tourniquet is routinely used: care should be taken to use a cuff of the proper size with proper padding, and in most cases to limit tourniquet time to no longer than 2 hours.

The patient is placed on the operating table in the supine position with the affected scapula just to the edge of the operating table, to allow the upper arm and forearm to hang free over the edge of the table. The hand and forearm are placed in a prefabricated forearm gauntlet that is connected to an overhead suspension device so that the elbow is flexed to 90 degrees (Fig. 1). Only enough traction is applied to the arm to allow the arm to suspend and keep the elbow flexed 90 degrees. This position provides excellent access to both the medial and lateral aspects of the elbow, and the forearm may be freely pronated and supinated throughout the surgical procedure. It is important to maintain the elbow in this 90 degree flexed position at all times when examining the anterior structures of the elbow arthroscopically, so as to completely relax the neurovascular structures in the antecubital fossa. An alternative position is the prone position.

The bony anatomic landmarks are now outlined with a marking pen before the procedure is begun. As there can be a large amount of extravasation of fluid during the arthroscopic procedure, this previous marking allows one to maintain identifiable landmarks throughout the surgery. The bony landmarks that are usually marked are the radial head and the lateral humeral epicondyle on the lateral side of the elbow, and the medial humeral epicondyle on the medial aspect of the elbow. Posteriorly the olecranon is identified.

The three arthroscopic portals used most commonly for elbow arthroscopy include the anterolateral, anteromedial, and posterolateral portals. Before the insertion of the arthroscope into any of the portals, however, the

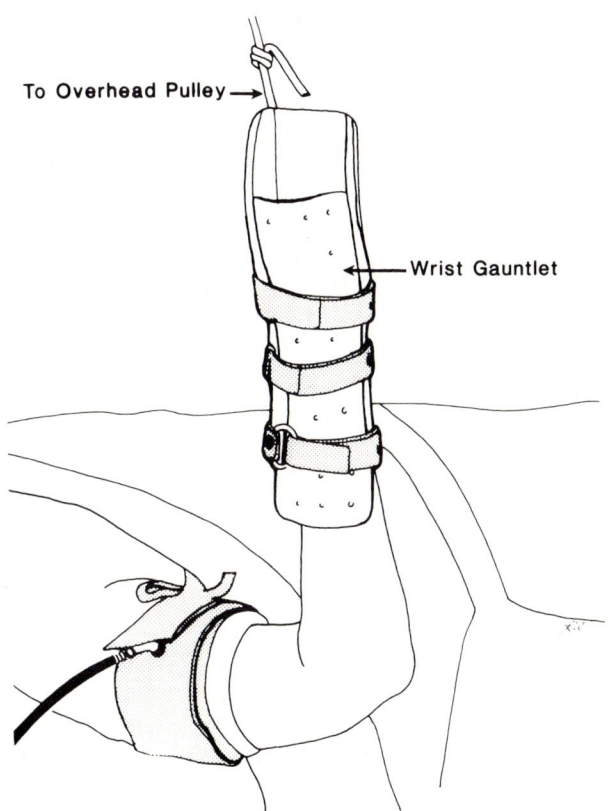

Figure 1 Position of the arm for arthroscopy of the elbow. (From Andrews JR, Carson WG. Arthroscopy of the elbow. Arthroscopy 1985; 1:98; with permission.)

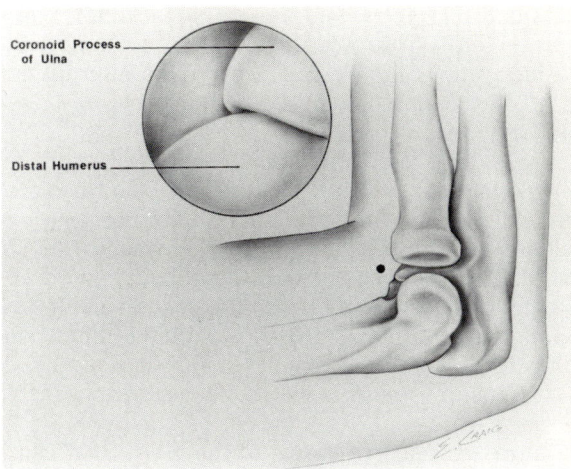

Figure 2 The anterolateral portal is located approximately 3 cm distal and 2 cm anterior to the lateral humeral epicondyle. Arthroscopic anatomy as seen through this portal includes the distal humerus and coronoid process of the ulna. (From Andrews JR, Carson WG. Arthroscopy of the elbow. Arthroscopy 1985; 1:99; with permission.)

elbow should be maximally distended with fluid through an 18 gauge spinal needle. I prefer to inject this needle into the triangular area over the lateral aspect of the elbow bordered by the radial head, the lateral humeral epicondyle, and the tip of the olecranon. This area is often used to aspirate the elbow for a hemarthrosis, such as would occur with a radial head fracture, and through this area the needle traverses only skin, a thin subcutaneous layer, the anconeus muscle, and the capsule. Thus, with the elbow flexed 90 degrees, the needle is placed into the elbow joint through this area and the elbow maximally distended with the use of a 50 ml syringe connected to an intravenous tubing. Proper placement into the elbow joint is verified by brisk backflow from the needle. Once verification of entry into the elbow is made, the needle is removed and the elbow is left maximally distended. The anterolateral portal is now established.

Anterolateral Portal

The anterolateral portal is usually the one first used for elbow arthroscopy, primarily for diagnostic purposes. The anteromedial portal is usually established only under direct visualization after the anterolateral portal is already in place. With the elbow flexed 90 degrees and maximally distended with fluid, the 18 gauge spinal needle is now placed approximately 3 cm distal and 2 cm anterior to the lateral humeral epicondyle (Fig. 2). It is

important to realize that this is an *approximate* location and changes in each elbow. The needle is aimed directly toward the center of the joint. The needle course is just anterior and proximal to the radial head, which can be verified by pronating and supinating the forearm. Verification of entry into the elbow joint is confirmed by free backflow provided by the fluid previously placed into the elbow joint. Once proper needle placement is confirmed and the elbow is maximally distended, the larger arthroscopic instruments can be introduced. At this point a small skin incision is made, taking care to avoid injury to the underlying subcutaneous nerves. The superficial nerves to be avoided during the establishment of the anterolateral portal include the lateral and posterior antebrachial cutaneous nerves. At this point, rather than using the sharp trocar and cannula as is usually the case in the shoulder or the knee, the blunt cannula is used initially. This can often be readily inserted through the subcutaneous fat and the muscles; then, once resistance is noted, the sharp trocar can be inserted to pass through the deeper fascial and capsule layers, and the blunt trocar can be introduced again as the elbow joint is entered. By using the blunt trocar as much as possible, damage to nearby neurovascular structures is minimized, and superficial or deeper nerves may be less injured than with the sharp trocar. Use of the blunt trocar also reduces damage to the articular cartilage in this small joint. As the trocar and cannula system is inserted, great care must be taken to direct the instruments toward the center to the elbow joint as the elbow is kept flexed 90 degrees at all times. Once the elbow capsule is entered, free backflow of fluid will be noted through the cannula, and at this point the arthroscope is inserted and diagnostic arthroscopy begun. Continuous distention of the elbow is maintained by the use of overhead bags of normal saline attached to the arthroscope. Occasionally, more pressure is required to distend the elbow, and an additional inflow can be attached to the arthroscopic sleeve with a 50 ml syringe and intravenous tubing. Suction may be intermittently placed on the arthroscopic sleeve to remove any cloudy fluid or debris.

I use the 4 mm, 30 degree angled arthroscope as I feel this provides optimal visualization of the elbow joint. This is the same arthroscope that is used in larger joints such as the shoulder or knee. The smaller 2.7 mm "needle" arthroscope has been described; however, the difference in diameter between this smaller arthroscope and the larger 4 mm arthroscope is only 1.3 mm. Thus, the rationale of using smaller arthroscopes to avoid injury to neurovascular structures does not appear to be valid.

Intra-articular structures of the elbow that can be visualized from the anterolateral portal are the distal humerus and trochlear ridges as well as the coronoid process of the ulna (see Fig. 2). Flexion and extension of the elbow allows one to see the coronoid process of the elbow, and extension of the elbow provides a better view of the medial and lateral trochlear ridges and the trochlear notch of the distal humerus. By slowly retracting and angling the 30 degree arthroscope toward the radial head, a small portion of this may be seen from the anterolateral portal.

Cadaveric dissections of the arthroscopic portals of the elbow have revealed that during the establishment of the anterolateral portal, the arthroscope passes anterior to the radial head and through the extensor carpi radialis brevis muscle. The arthroscope passes 4 to 7 mm from the radial nerve. Studies have demonstrated that the arthroscope passes within a mean distance of 4 mm from the radial nerve regardless of the flexion or extension of the elbow, with no distention in the capsule with fluid. However, studies have demonstrated that when 35 to 40 ml of fluid is inserted into the elbow capsule, the radial nerve moves an additional 7 mm anteriorly. Thus, maximal distention of the elbow should be maintained at all times when establishing the arthroscopic portals.

Anteromedial Portal

After the anterolateral portal has been established, the anteromedial portal can now be safely established by direct visualization intra-articularly. The anteromedial portal is located approximately 2 cm distal and 2 cm anterior to the medial humeral epicondyle (Fig. 3). With the arthroscope in the anterolateral portal, an 18 gauge spinal needle is inserted at the above-described entry point with the elbow flexed 90 degrees and the elbow maximally distended with fluid. The needle is aimed directly toward the center of the joint. Confirmation of the needle's entry is provided by direct visualization through the arthroscope in the anterolateral portal. The needle passes just anterior to the medial humeral epicondyle and inferior to the antecubital structures. A small skin incision is made and the arthroscopic cannula and trocar system are introduced. An interchangeable cannula system should be used so that one may freely change from the anterolateral to the anteromedial portal.

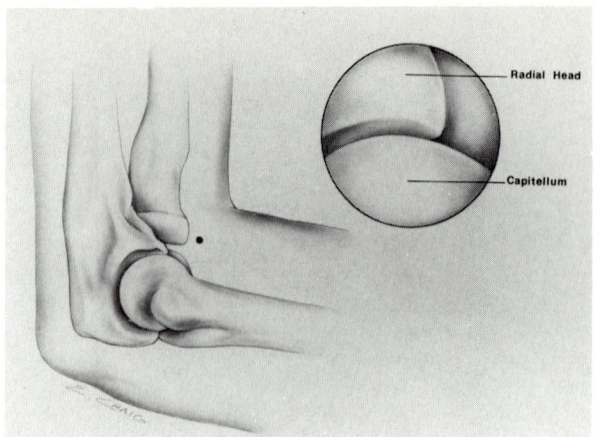

Figure 3 The anteromedial portal is located approximately 2 cm distal and 2 cm anterior to the medial humeral epicondyle. The radial head and capitellum are well visualized from this portal. (From Andrews JR, Carson WG. Arthroscopy of the elbow. Arthroscopy 1985; 1:100; with permission.)

The capitellum and radial head are best visualized from the anteromedial portal, with examination of the radial head facilitated by pronation and supination of the forearm. One can occasionally visualize the annular ligament coursing across the radial neck, and by slowly retracting the arthroscope and directing it toward the ulna, the coronoid process is visible through this anteromedial portal.

Most arthroscopic surgical procedures in the elbow are performed for processes located over the lateral aspect of the elbow, such as loose bodies or osteochondritis dissecans of the capitellum. The anteromedial portal provides superior visualization of these structures as compared with the anterolateral portal, and thus it is necessary to be technically proficient at establishing both portals.

Cadaveric dissections have revealed that in establishing the anteromedial portals, the arthroscope enters through the tendinous portion of the pronator teres and penetrates the radial aspect of the flexor digitorum superficialis. As these muscles are penetrated, the median nerve is approximately 1 cm lateral to the arthroscope and the brachial artery is just lateral to the median nerve. As the arthroscope passes deeper and closer to the joint capsule, it comes to within 6 mm of these same neurovascular structures. If 35 to 40 ml of fluid is injected into the elbow, however, the median nerve and brachial artery move 10 mm and 8 mm, respectively, farther anterior from the entering arthroscopic instruments. Thus, again one should keep the elbow in 90 degrees of flexion at all times and provide maximal distention as the arthroscopic instruments are inserted from this anteromedial portal.

Posterolateral Portal

The posterolateral portal is established approximately 3 cm proximal to the tip of the olecranon, just superior and posterior to the lateral humeral epicondyle. This portal is placed just off the lateral border of the triceps muscle (Fig. 4). This portal is established with the elbow in 20 to 30 degrees of flexion, and the 18 gauge spinal needle is directed toward the olecranon fossa. Structures that may be visualized from this portal are the olecranon fossa located over the posterior aspect of the distal humerus and the tip of the olecranon. Flexion and extension of the elbow help to delineate various portions of the distal humerus. Neurovascular structures to be avoided when establishing this portal include the posterior antebrachial cutaneous nerve, which courses over the posterolateral distal humerus, and the ulnar nerve, which lies approximately 2.5 cm medial to the center of the joint.

Accessory Portals

When pathology is encountered that is not amenable to the arthroscopic portals mentioned above, three accessory portals—the straight lateral portal, the accessory lateral portal, and the straight posterior portal—may be used. The straight lateral portal is located in the triangular area bordered by the lateral humeral epicondyle, the radial head, and the olecranon. Through this portal the trocar system passes through the anconeus muscle and the posterior capsule, the same area in which the 18 gauge spinal needle is inserted for initial distention of the elbow joint. This portal may be established without direct visualization by using an 18 gauge spinal needle and the sharp and blunt trocar system. When this portal is established, the posterior antebrachial cutaneous nerve should be avoided. Occasionally a small 2.7 mm arthroscope is placed through this portal and has the advantage of being smaller in this tight area of the elbow joint. Alternatively, one may use the 4 mm arthroscope.

The radial ulnar joint and the inferior surface of the radial head can be seen through the straight lateral portal. In addition, the under surface of the capitellum can be followed posteriorly. At times the arthroscope will slip directly into the posterior compartment, providing a view of this area as well.

Lateral Accessory Portal

An accessory lateral portal can be made at this point if needed. The 18 gauge spinal needle is inserted through the skin approximately 2 cm distal to the lateral portal. The needle is aimed toward the tip of the arthroscope. Once the needle is visualized the portal is made with a knife and blunt trocar or a shaver may be placed through it. This area of the elbow is usually a small space, and it is not uncommon to inadvertently pull the arthroscope or shaver out of the joint. Rotation of the arthroscope at 30 degrees rather than moving the arthroscope to change the view will help prevent this. If the accessory portal and lateral portals are made too close to each other, "crowding" will occur and triangulation will be awkward.

Straight Posterior (Transtriceps) Portal

The straight posterior or transtriceps portal is located approximately 2 cm medial to the posterolateral

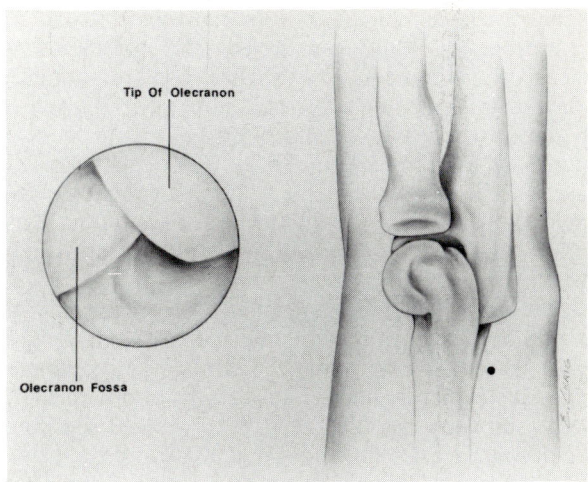

Figure 4 The posterolateral portal is located 3 cm proximal to the tip of the olecranon, just posterior and superior to the lateral epicondyle. This portal is established with the elbow extended to visualize the tip of the olecranon fossa. (From Andrews JR, Carson WG. Arthroscopy of the elbow. Arthroscopy 1985; 1:101; with permission.)

portal and directly traverses the triceps tendon. The elbow is flexed 20 to 30 degrees. This portal is established by placing the 18 gauge spinal needle through the area under direct visualization. With the arthroscope in the posterolateral portal, the skin over the needle is incised in the direction of the triceps fibers. The straight posterior portal is the "working" portal posteriorly and is useful for removing loose bodies from the posterior aspect of the elbow and the occasional resection of an impinging olecranon osteophyte.

Proximal Medial Portal—Prone Position

Some surgeons have proposed placing the patient in a prone position for elbow arthroscopy. This position provides ready access to both the anterior and posterior aspects of the elbow and allows gravity to help move the neurovascular structures in the antecubital fossa away from the entering instruments. Poehling et al believes this position improves mobility because it does not require a traction suspension system. They assert that the prone position of the arm is more stable than the supine suspension with the arm suspended in an overhead traction apparatus. When used in conjunction with a proximal medial portal as the initial arthroscopic portal, the instruments enter more parallel to the neurovascular structures and possibly may protect these structures in initiation of the arthroscopic portal. An improved view of the anterior joint with use of this portal has also been reported.

Instrumentation

Surgical techniques for arthroscopy of the elbow do not differ significantly from other joints with the exception that greater care is appropriate to avoid causing articular cartilage damage by scuffing of the articular surfaces. The elbow joint has inherent stability and there is less room to maneuver the various instruments in the elbow joint. Arthroscopic instrumentation in the elbow should be slow and deliberate so as not to slip out of the elbow capsule and cause unnecessary re-entry of the various cannulas back into the joint. This causes further risk of damage to the articular cartilage, and in addition these repeated passes in and out of the capsule cause fluid extravasation and further risk of neurovascular compromise.

Motorized instruments should be used as much as possible to avoid having to make repeated passes with simple hand-held instruments. All hand-held and motorized instruments should be carefully used within this small joint and should never be wedged between articular surfaces, otherwise breakage could occur. As with arthroscopic surgery of the other joints, the instrument being used should be kept in full visualization at all times.

Basic arthroscopic equipment includes:

- 18 gauge spinal needles
- Marking pen
- 50 ml syringe
- Intravenous connecting tubing
- #11 knife blade
- Hemostat
- Probe
- Punches
- Graspers with teeth
- Ruler
- Blunt and sharp trocars
- 4 mm, 30 degree angled arthroscope
- 2.7 mm, 30 degree angled arthroscope
- Interchangeable cannula systems for 4 and 2.5 mm arthroscopes
- Motorized shavers, trimmers, and burrs
- Pump system (optional)

POSTOPERATIVE ROUTINE

At the completion of the arthroscopic procedure, the joint is thoroughly irrigated to remove all debris. The arthroscopic portals may be either left open or closed with suture material, depending on the preference of the surgeon and the amount of subcutaneous swelling. A soft dressing is applied to the elbow, and in most instances immobilization is not necessary. Active range of motion of the elbow is begun as pain and swelling permit, and then flexibility and strengthening exercises are usually initiated.

COMPLICATIONS

Complications of elbow arthroscopy are similar to those encountered with any arthroscopic procedure such as infection, problems associated with the use of a tourniquet, instrument breakage, iatrogenic scuffing of articular surfaces, and neurovascular complications.

Infection is infrequent with elbow arthroscopy because of the large amount of fluid passed through the joint during the surgical procedure as well as the small incisions required for arthroscopic instrumentation.

More serious neurovascular complications, however, have been reported. In a series of 21 elbow arthroscopies, Lynch et al reported one transient low radial nerve palsy, a transient low median nerve palsy, and formation of a neuroma of the medial antebrachial cutaneous nerve. It was believed that the transient low radial nerve palsy was a result of overdistention of the joint and the condition resolved in 8 hours. The transient low median nerve palsy was believed to be secondary to the use of a local anesthetic. The neuroma of the medial antebrachial cutaneous nerve ultimately required resection.

Casscells described a case of irreparable damage to the ulnar nerve during abrasion arthroplasty of the elbow. Thomas et al described a radial nerve injury and Papilion described compression neuropathy of the radial nerve during elbow arthroscopy. In a series of 45 patients, Guhl reported one injury to the sensory branch of the radial nerve, and Morrey reported a transient radial nerve palsy secondary to fluid extravasation. In a series of 24 arthroscopies reported by Andrews and Carson, one patient experienced a transient median nerve palsy. This transient nerve palsy was believed to be secondary to leakage of local anesthetic from the capsule causing a temporary nerve block.

In a survey of members of the Arthroscopy Association of North America, 395,556 surgical arthroscopic procedures were evaluated, 569 of these being elbow arthroscopies. The respondents were performing an average of 0.74 elbow arthroscopies per month and had been performing surgical elbow arthroscopy on an average of 3.9 years. Of this entire group, only one reported a neurovascular complication, a radial nerve injury. I am also aware of undocumented cases of compartment syndrome of the forearm, complete transection of the median nerve, and complete transection of the radial nerve secondary to elbow arthroscopy.

DISCUSSION

Arthroscopy of the elbow is a demanding surgical technique that requires significant attention to detail in order to perform a safe and reproducible surgical procedure. Unlike the knee, where the arthroscopic portals are readily and safely initiated over the anterior aspects of the knee and the most technically difficult part of knee arthroscopy appears to be dealing with the intra-articular pathology, the most demanding part of elbow arthroscopy is the initiation of the arthroscopic portals.

Several technical points warrant further discussion. As previously mentioned, various studies have demonstrated the necessity of maintaining maximal distention of the elbow in order to move neurovascular structures farther away from the arthroscopic instruments, to provide better visualization of the elbow, and to give more room in which to manipulate the various instruments. The distention of the elbow can usually be obtained by using 3 liter bags elevated above the patient, thus allowing gravity to distend the elbow. However, at times additional inflow is required and one can use a 50 ml syringe connected to the arthroscopic cannula to provide further distention manually. I have had no experience with the infusion pump method of distention of the elbow, and feel that this requires further study before its use can be recommended on a routine basis. Because one is trying to maintain maximal distention of the elbow at all times, the extracapsular extravasation can be impressive and needs to be monitored closely. This extracapsular extravasation is most often seen when one has made repeated attempts at establishing the arthroscopic portals, thus making multiple holes in the capsule with resultant fluid leakage. When using an inflow cannula, one needs to be sure that the cannula has an opening at the end only and does not have any "side vents"; if the inflow cannula slips back during the arthroscopic procedure, the side vents will then be outside the joint capsule and fluid will go directly into the subcutaneous tissues.

Because of the obvious risks of damage to nearby neurovascular structures and because fluid extravasation can be significant, it is recommended that the bony landmarks be identified with a marking pen before initiation of the procedure. Thus, the bony landmarks will stay in constant relationship during the arthroscopic procedure and one can maintain proper orientation at all times.

Another technical consideration is the exacting detail required and the actual maneuvering of instruments inside the elbow joint. There is usually a very short distance between the articular surface of the elbow and the joint capsule, and thus it is quite easy to slip out of the capsule when performing elbow arthroscopy. Once the arthroscope does come out of the joint capsule or the cannula slips back, there is further extravasation and one has to reintroduce the arthroscope, with further risk of damage to neurovascular structures or to the articular cartilage. Thus, when performing elbow arthroscopy, one needs to move the arthroscope quite slowly about the elbow, particularly when retracting the arthroscope, and stabilize the cannula sleeve with the opposite hand next to the skin so that one can be sure not to slip out of the elbow joint.

Although elbow arthroscopy involves many technical considerations and the risks of neurovascular injury are real, this procedure has been used effectively to treat various disorders of the elbow and appears to have the best surgical results when extracting simple loose bodies. In addition, certain easily accessible osteophytes about the elbow can be removed. In other instances degenerative processes such as chondroplasties of the articular surface or intra-articular lysis of adhesions can be performed. However, these latter arthroscopic surgical procedures are less rewarding than simply removing a loose body.

SUGGESTED READING

Andrews JR, Carson WG. Arthroscopy of the elbow. Arthroscopy 1985; 1:97–107.

Carson WG. Arthroscopy of the elbow. In: Zarins B, Andrews J, Carson WG, eds. Injuries to the throwing arm. Philadelphia: WB Saunders, 1985:221.

Carson WG. Arthroscopy of the elbow. In: Bassett F, ed. American Academy Orthopaedic Surgery Instructional Course Lecture. Vol. 37. St. Louis: CV Mosby, 1988:195.

Carson WG, Meyers JF. Diagnostic arthroscopy of the elbow: Surgical techniques and arthroscopic portal anatomy. In: McGinty JB, ed. Operative arthroscopy. New York: Raven Press, 1991:583.

Lynch GJ, Meyers JF, Whipple TL, et al. Neurovascular anatomy and elbow arthroscopy: inherent risks. Arthroscopy 1986; 2:191–197.

Meyers JF. Elbow arthroscopy. In: Shahriaree H, ed. O'Connor's textbook of arthroscopic surgery. Philadelphia: JB Lippincott, 1992:641.

Verhan J, Van Mameren H, Brondsma A. Risks of neurovascular injury in elbow arthroscopy: Starting anteromedially or anterolaterally? Arthroscopy 1991; 7:287–290.

DISTAL BICEPS TENDON RUPTURES: SURGICAL MANAGEMENT

DONALD F. D'ALESSANDRO, M.D.

Disruption of the distal biceps tendon is relatively uncommon, yet the physician treating an active athletic population probably encounters this injury several times in his or her career. Approximately 200 cases have been reported in the literature, with the majority being individual surgeon's accounts of two or three cases. Only recently have series been published that contain at least 10 cases where the treatment outcomes have been critically analyzed with isokinetic and functional testing. The uniformly excellent results obtained with anatomic repair compel the surgeon to adopt this approach for the active individual with high functional demands.

This chapter presents the clinical presentation, rationale for operative treatment, and surgical technique for performing repair of distal biceps tendon ruptures. Full functional recovery and return to unrestricted athletic participation can be anticipated with prompt diagnosis and treatment.

CLINICAL PRESENTATION

Distal biceps tendon ruptures usually occur in well-muscled males who average 40 to 50 years of age.

However, recently a report that consisted of bodybuilders and weight lifters averaged only 40 years. A casual relationship between the use of anabolic steroids and distal biceps tendon ruptures could not be demonstrated in these athletes. Perhaps their ability to generate such large tensile forces with their hypertrophied biceps muscles predisposed them to this injury. Most ruptures occur from a single traumatic event and involve the dominant extremity. The mechanism of injury most often occurs with the elbow flexed at 90 degrees when a biceps contraction is overwhelmed by a sudden extension force. Scenarios found in the literature that exemplify this mechanism include spotting a falling gymnast, striking the back of an opponent while playing handball, an accidental single arm grip on a ring apparatus, and not releasing while being thrown rodeo riding.

Although there have been rare reports of partial tearing and attenuation of the distal biceps tendon, complete avulsion from the radial tuberosity is the usual finding. The pathophysiology leading to this lesion is thought to be repetitive stress failure from pronation and supination against a local bony excrescence at the radial tuberosity. Occasional radiographic findings of slight irregularity and enlargement of the radial tuberosity lend credence to this concept. Morrey has suggested that chronic inflammation of the deep bicipital radial bursa at the radial tuberosity may contribute to the degeneration of the biceps tendon and subsequent rupture.

At the time of injury, the patient experiences acute tearing-like pain often associated with an audible pop. Most patients will seek medical attention after the acute injury. Antecubital swelling and ecchymosis may disguise the altered biceps contour. Palpation should reveal the absence of a biceps tendon and proximal retraction of the muscle belly (Fig. 1). Occasionally the overlying lacertus fibrosus may remain intact and this can be misinterpreted as the biceps tendon. Comparison of this structure to the normally substantial and discrete biceps tendon on the opposite arm can be helpful. Demonstration of strength deficits of both elbow flexion and forearm supination is necessary to confirm the diagnosis. In acute cases, decreased elbow flexion strength can be readily appreciated. However, in the chronic setting, the brachialis and brachioradialis muscles may have had time to hypertrophy and compensate for the loss of the biceps, making residual flexion weakness clinically insignificant. Weakness in supination can always be found owing to the dominant role that the biceps plays in this function. It is this loss of supination strength and endurance that commonly causes fatigue pain and diminished performance in high demand patients such as laborers and athletes. Activities such as using a screwdriver or hammer precipitates symptoms.

A lateral radiograph of the elbow in supination may reveal subtle hypertrophic changes at the radial tuberosity but usually these abnormalities are not present. In cases of a partial tear or if the diagnosis is in question, magnetic resonance imaging may clarify the patho-anatomy.

RATIONALE FOR OPERATIVE TREATMENT

Considerable debate existed in the early literature concerning the recommended treatment for distal biceps tendon ruptures. Only within the last decade has acute anatomic repair been universally considered the treatment of choice in the active patient.

Those patients who elect nonoperative treatment can expect restoration of full pain-free range of motion within 4 to 6 weeks after the injury. Elbow flexion weakness is present initially but improves with time as

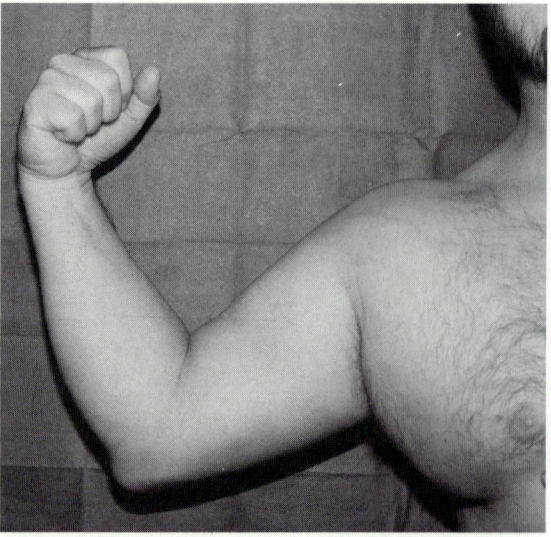

Figure 1   Clinical photograph of patient with 5-week-old distal biceps tendon rupture. Note the ecchymosis has resolved but the abnormal biceps contour from the proximal retraction of the muscle belly can be appreciated.

described above. On the other hand, the supinator does not appear capable of adequately compensating for the loss of the biceps supination function. The clinical significance of this supination strength deficit depends on the individual's need to do supination activities. Isokinetic muscle testing has documented elbow flexion strength deficits of 30% to 36% and supination strength deficits of 40% to 55% after nonoperative treatment. One could argue that nonoperative treatment is appropriate when the nondominant arm has been injured in a relatively low demand patient. Otherwise persistent complaints of weakness and fatigue pain coupled with permanent strength deficits and an alteration of the shape and size of the arm support the recommendation of surgical treatment in those patients requiring optimal function.

Two operative approaches advocating different sites of reattachment of the tendon have been offered in the literature for the treatment of this injury. Early reports claimed good results with suturing the tendon to the brachialis muscle even though this ignores the contribution of the biceps to forearm supination. In fact, isokinetic assessment of a patient whose tendon was repaired back to the brachialis confirmed a permanent supination strength deficit.

Anatomic repair back to the radial tuberosity restores both biceps functions. Trying to accomplish this repair solely through an anterior approach can place the radial nerve at risk for injury. Anatomic repair to the radial tuberosity can be done safely using the double incision technique of Boyd and Anderson. Excellent clinical results have been reported both with regard to patient satisfaction and restoration of essentially normal supination and flexion strength. For example, in a study evaluating the results in weight lifters and bodybuilders, all the athletes were satisfied with their functional and aesthetic outcome, returning to full unrestricted activity. In those athletes with the repaired dominant extremity, supination strength and endurance as well as elbow flexion strength were normal. While isokinetic testing did reveal an average loss of 20% less endurance with elbow flexion, subjective complaints were not found in this group. Only three patients injured their nondominant extremity. While elbow flexion strength and endurance were essentially normal in this group, two of the three still had approximately 40% supination strength deficits. Interestingly these athletes chose to pursue dominant arm oriented sports after their injury, namely racquetball and handball, sports that do not condition the nondominant extremity. The one patient who had full recovery of his operated nondominant arm returned to weight training regularly, a bilateral activity. Thus rehabilitation of the operated arm is essential for complete recovery, especially in those cases involving the nondominant extremity.

There may be a delay in diagnosis because the patient does not come immediately to the physician after the injury or because the significance of the injury is not appreciated upon the first evaluation. In these cases, primary repair can still be accomplished up to 6 weeks after the injury without compromising the results. The

dissection may be slightly more extensible as mobilization of the retracted tendon is necessary and delineation of the bicipital tunnel leading to the radial tuberosity is more difficult. When a patient presents very late after a distal biceps rupture, their complaints must be carefully assessed before contemplating surgical intervention. Primary repair is not possible in this group. Late reconstruction using either a ligament augmentation device or fascia lata graft to reattach the retracted biceps tendon may be necessary. While these techniques have been proposed for the salvage situation, no clinical results are available in the literature. Only in those cases where the patient's occupation or life-style is significantly hampered and where the patient has reasonable expectations should late reconstruction be considered.

SURGICAL PROCEDURE

The recommended surgical technique involves reinserting the biceps tendon into the radial tuberosity using a modification of the two-incision approach described by Boyd and Anderson. The patient is placed in the supine position with the elbow extended and the forearm supinated on an arm board. An oblique curvilinear incision is made beginning medially and proximal to the elbow crease and extending distally and laterally (Fig. 2). We have found this incision to lie in the crease along the distal edge of the biceps muscle after repair and is often unnoticeable in the flexed posture. The lacertus fibrosus may still be intact. It should be released to reveal the underlying biceps tendon. Care must be taken to protect the lateral antebrachial cutaneous nerve, which lies just lateral to the biceps tendon and on top of the brachialis muscle. The end of the tendon is localized and debrided. In Bunnell fashion, two nonabsorbable No. 1 sutures are placed in the tendon (Fig. 3). In acute cases a tunnel leading directly

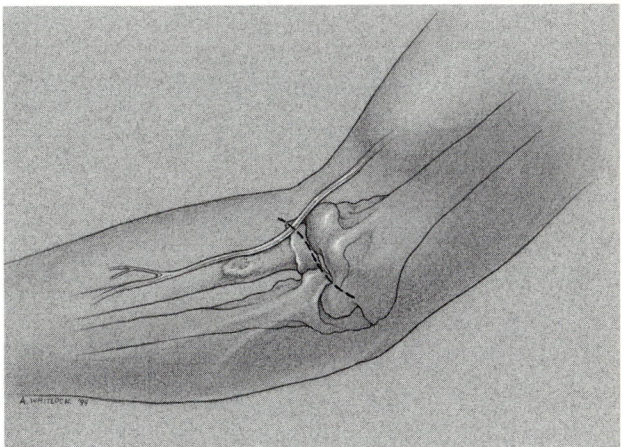

Figure 2 Cosmetic curvilinear incision across the elbow crease. Care must be taken to identify and protect the lateral antebrachial cutaneous nerve with this approach. (Adapted from Shields CL, ed. Manual of sports surgery. New York: Springer-Verlag, 1987; with permission.)

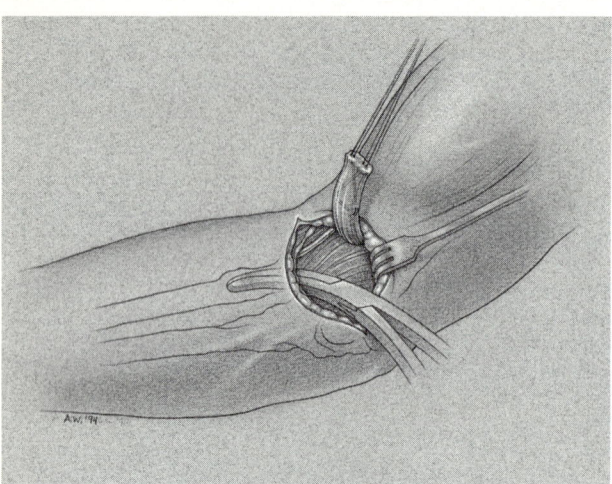

Figure 3 The distal biceps tendon stump is identified proximally and the bicipital tunnel leading to the radial tuberosity is found distally. See text for details. (Adapted from Shields CL, ed. Manual of sports surgery. New York: Springer-Verlag, 1987; with permission.)

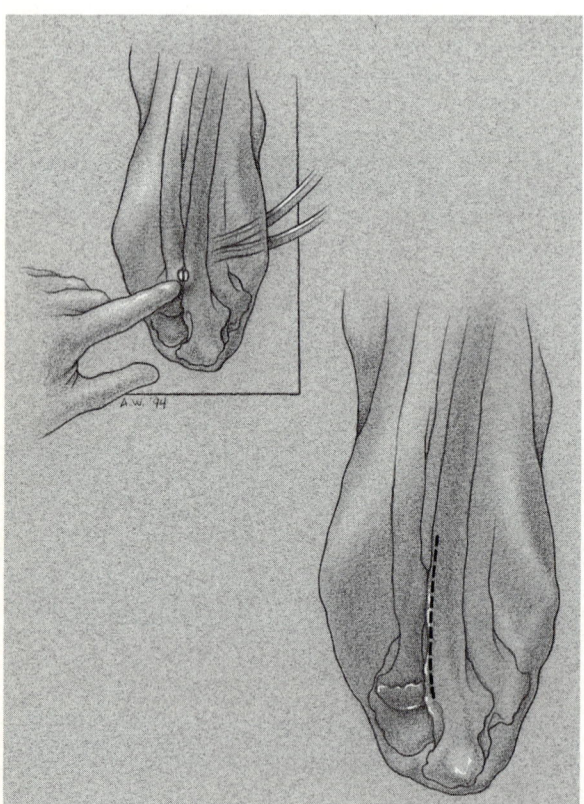

Figure 4 The site for the posterior incision is localized by passing a curved clamp between the radius and ulna through the anterior incision and tenting the skin of the proximal forearm on the radial aspect of the ulna. Approximately an 8 cm incision paralleling the radial border of the ulna is necessary to gain adequate exposure. (Adapted from Shields CL, ed. Manual of sports surgery. New York: Springer-Verlag, 1987; with permission.)

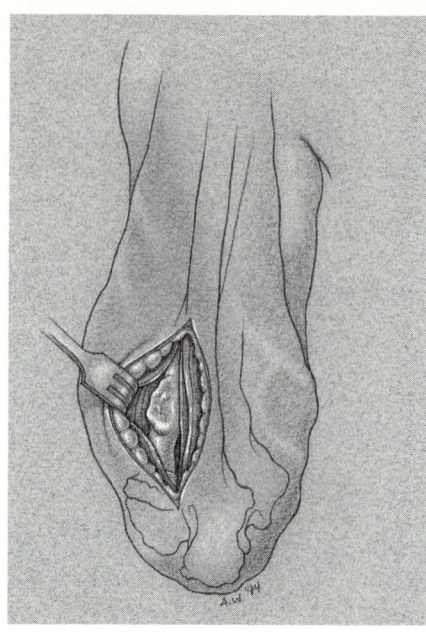

Figure 5 A limited muscle splitting approach through the extensor muscle mass without elevating the periosteum from the ulna is used. The forearm is pronated to visualize the radial tuberosity. (Adapted from Shields CL, ed. Manual of sports surgery. New York: Springer-Verlag, 1987; with permission.)

to the radial tuberosity can be readily identified. Invariably the tendon is cleanly avulsed from the tuberosity.

A curved clamp is then inserted through the anterior incision, passed between the radius and ulna, and directed posterolaterally, tenting the skin of the forearm (Fig. 4). The elbow is flexed and a posterior longitudinal incision is made of approximately 8 cm in length paralleling the radial border of the ulna. A limited muscle splitting approach through the extensor muscle mass without elevating the periosteum of the ulna is used to visualize the radial tuberosity (Fig. 5). Morrey has recommended this approach in an effort to decrease the chance of radioulnar synostosis, an uncommon yet serious complication of this procedure. Full pronation of the forearm is necessary to direct the radial tuberosity towards the posterior wound. The radial tuberosity is then cleared of soft tissue and a ⅛ inch drill used to make a pilot hole in the center of the tuberosity. The hole is enlarged with a ¼ inch drill and then the cavity excavated with a high speed burr if necessary (Fig. 6). The wound is promptly irrigated to remove bone dust. Two smaller holes are then drilled through the opposite cortex of the proximal radius using a ⁵⁄₆₄ inch drill bit. The tendon is now inserted from anterior to posterior through the soft tissue tunnel between the radius and ulna. The nonabsorbable sutures are passed through the large drill hole into the radial tuberosity and out through the smaller holes using a 24 gauge wire as a suture passer. The arm is supinated and the sutures pulled firmly making sure by direct palpation through the anterior incision that the tendon can be well seated into the excavated radial tuberosity (Fig. 7).

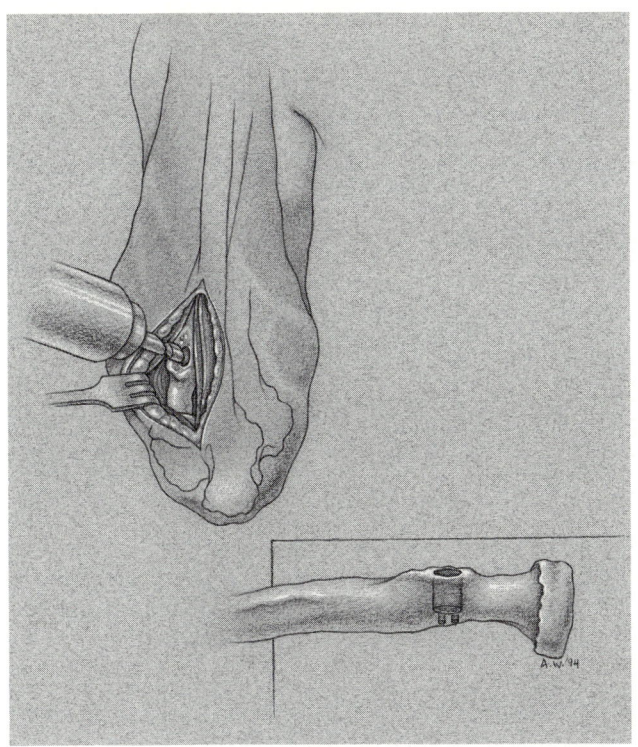

Figure 6 A cylindrical tunnel is placed in the radial tuberosity in preparation for accepting the distal stump of the biceps tendon. See text for details. (Adapted from Shields CL, ed. Manual of sports surgery. New York: Springer-Verlag, 1987; with permission.)

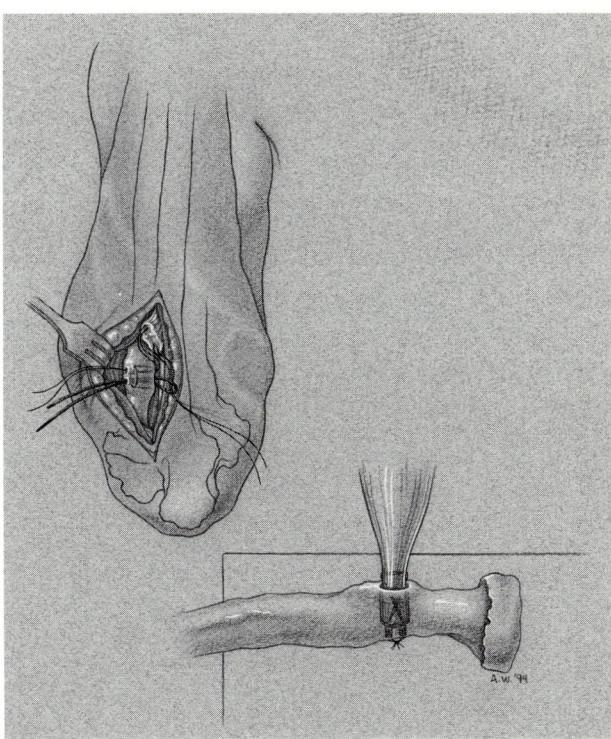

Figure 7 The sutures are passed through the excavated tuberosity and the holes in the opposite cortex of the radius. The forearm is supinated and the tendon seated into the bone tunnel. (Adapted from Shields CL, ed. Manual of sports surgery. New York: Springer-Verlag, 1987; with permission.)

Before tying the sutures the tourniquet is deflated, hemostasis obtained, and the anterior incision is closed over a drain. The elbow is flexed 90 degrees and the forearm supinated as the sutures are tied securely. The posterior wound is then closed over a drain.

POSTOPERATIVE MANAGEMENT

For the initial 3 weeks postoperatively, a long arm splint is used to hold the forearm in supination and the elbow in 90 degrees of flexion. Gentle active range of motion in both flexion-extension and pronation-supination planes is then begun. Passive extension exercises must be avoided. Progressive resisted strengthening is begun at 6 weeks postoperatively with isokinetic exercises instituted at 12 weeks. Unrestricted activities such as weight training and returning to a vigorous labor job are not permitted until 6 months postoperatively. The patient is encouraged to continue rehabilitation for up to a year to obtain full restoration of strength and endurance.

COMPLICATIONS

Complications with this procedure are uncommon. To date not a single case of a recurrent rupture after operative repair has been reported.

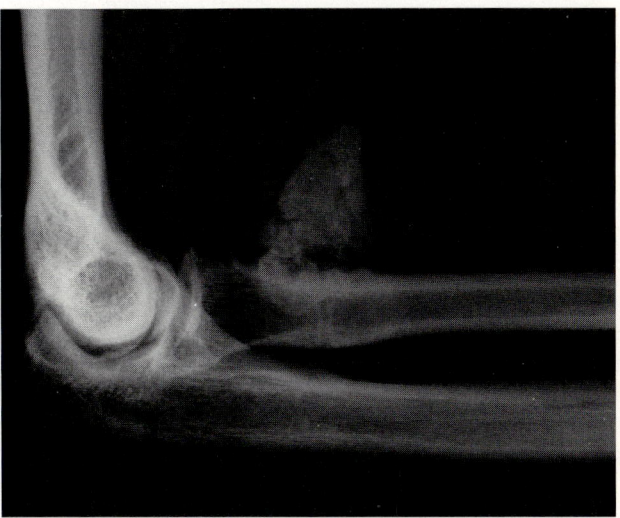

Figure 8 Radiograph after distal biceps tendon repair shows an unusually large calcification of the tendon as it inserts into the radial tuberosity.

The two-incision technique has been successful in essentially eliminating the risk of radial nerve injury when performing anatomic repair of the biceps to the radial tuberosity. Only a single case of transient radial neurapraxia which resolved entirely by three months postoperatively has been reported. Although rare, the most significant complication following this procedure is proximal radioulnar synostosis. Failla et al collected four cases of synostosis following the use of the two-incision technique. Subperiosteal elevation of the anconeus and extensor muscles from the ulna and perforation of the proximal portion of the interosseous membrane were considered to be responsible for the synostosis formation. Resection of synostosis with interposition of a silastic sheath was successful in only half the patients. The small posterior muscle splitting approach is recommended in an effort to avoid this complication.

Limitations of range of motion particularly in the pronation-supination arc were occasionally seen if the arm was immobilized for 6 weeks postoperatively. Earlier range of motion exercises beginning 3 weeks after surgery have solved this problem. Calcification of the tendon at the site of its reinsertion to the radial tuberosity can occur but surprisingly its presence has not adversely affected the range of motion or clinical results (Fig. 8).

Baker BD, Bierwagen D. Rupture of the distal tendon of the biceps brachii: Operative versus non-operative treatment. J Bone Joint Surg 1985; 67A:414–417.

Boyd JB, Anderson LD. A method for reinsertion of the distal biceps brachii tendon. J Bone Joint Surg 1961; 43A:1041–1043.

D'Alessandro DF, Shields CL. Biceps rupture and triceps avulsion about the elbow. In: Jobe FW, ed. Operative techniques in upper extremity sports injuries. Philadelphia: Mosby–Year Book, 1994.

D'Alessandro DF, Shields CL, Tibone JE, Chandler, RW. Repair of distal biceps tendon ruptures in athletes. Am J Sports Med 1993; 21:114–119.

Failla JM, Amadio PC, Morrey BF, et al. Proximal radioulnar synostosis after repair of distal biceps brachii rupture by the two-incision technique: Report of four cases. Clin Orthop 1990; 253:133–136.

Morrey BF. Tendon injuries about the elbow. In: Morrey BF, ed. The elbow and its disorders. Philadelphia: WB Saunders, 1985.

Morrey BF, Askew LJ, An KN, et al. Rupture of distal tendon of the biceps brachii: A biomechanical study. J Bone Joint Surg 1985; 67A:418–421.

Norman WH. Repair of avulsion of insertion of biceps brachii tendon. Clin Orthop 1985; 193:189–194.

Tibone JE. Repair of distal biceps tendon rupture. In: Shields CL, ed. Manual of sports surgery. New York: Springer-Verlag, 1987.

SUGGESTED READING

Aging HJ, Chess JL, Goekstra DV, et al. Rupture of the distal insertion of the biceps brachii tendon. Clin Orthop 1988; 234:34–38.

ISOLATED FRACTURE OF THE ULNAR SHAFT

I.W.D. DYMOND, M.B.B.Ch., F.R.C.S.(Ed), F.C.S.(SA) Ortho, M. Med Ortho

Isolated fracture of the ulnar shaft is a common injury caused by direct trauma. The fracture occurs most frequently in the distal forearm, where it is known as the "paree fracture." It is an injury often seen in those who practice the martial arts, where the forearm is used in defensive action.

The diagnosis of the fracture itself presents little problem. The difficulty is in establishing whether it is an isolated injury. Two factors that help in making this decision are (1) the mechanism of injury: direct trauma usually results in isolated fractures, whereas indirect or rotatory injuries generally cause complex fractures with involvement of the radiohumeral articulation (Monteggia's fracture), and (2) the location: isolated fractures usually occur in the distal forearm, whereas those that occur proximally are usually complex.

The management of these fractures seems to be simple, yet there is considerable controversy. Immobilization in an above-elbow cast is probably the most

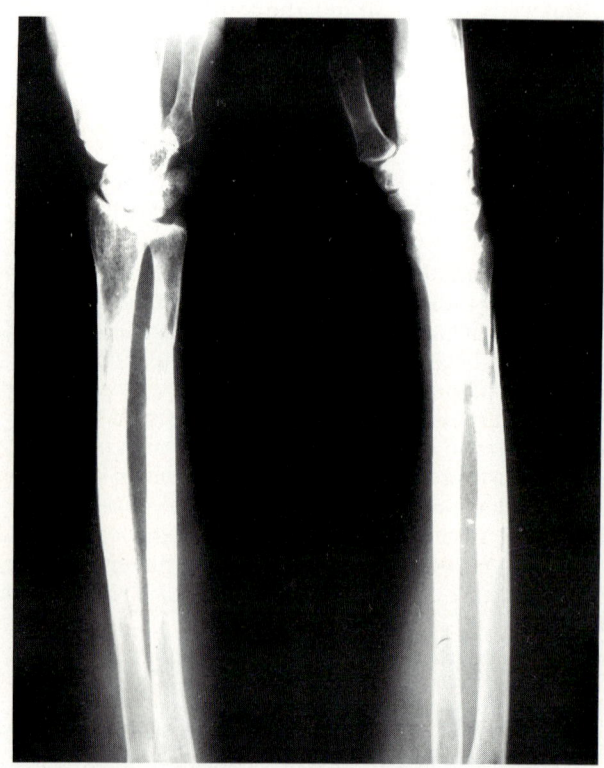

Figure 1 Type I fracture. There is less than 50% displacement, which indicates minimal loss of soft tissue integrity.

frequently used treatment for undisplaced fractures, and open reduction with internal fixation the most common for displaced fractures. Unorthodox methods such as simple bandaging are also known to be used with apparently no adverse results. Modification of the

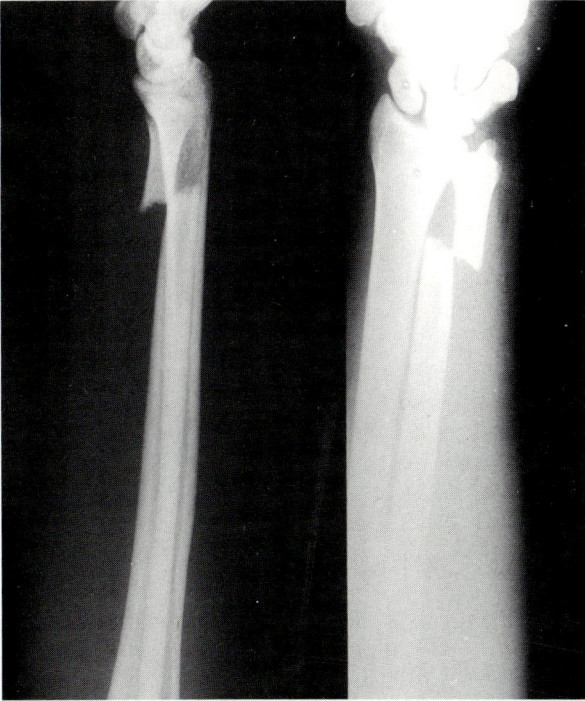

Figure 2 Type II fracture. There is more than 50% displacement, indicating disruption of the periosteal sleeve and interosseous membrane.

treatment by the patient himself is also not uncommon. Despite these variations in management, the fractures unite with few complications.

According to principles, protection of the fracture and prevention of rotational forces acting upon its fragments require immobilization of the joint above and below the fracture.

Mechanically the ulna participates in flexion and extension of the elbow and wrist, but acts as an immobile support during rotatory movements of the forearm. During pronation and supination of the forearm, the radius rotates around the ulna (the ulna cannot rotate because of its articulation with the trochlea of the humerus). The radius pivots at the radiohumeral joint, and hinges at the interosseous membrane and distal radioulnar joint, during these movements. The interosseous membrane not only unites the two forearm bones, but also acts as a restraint to rotational movement of the forearm. Isolated undisplaced fractures behave in a different manner from displaced fractures. This is due to the disruption of the interosseous membrane and periosteal sleeve that occurs with displacement. Experimental studies performed on cadavers revealed that in a fracture that is displaced less than 50% of the ulnar diameter, the interosseous membrane is largely intact and the periosteum is minimally disrupted. These fractures are stable throughout a full range of movement. However, in fractures displaced more than 50%, marked separation of the interosseous membrane and tearing of the periosteal sleeve occurs. The fracture under these circumstances is unstable during pronation and supination.

From these observations, I classified isolated fractures of the distal ulna into two categories: type

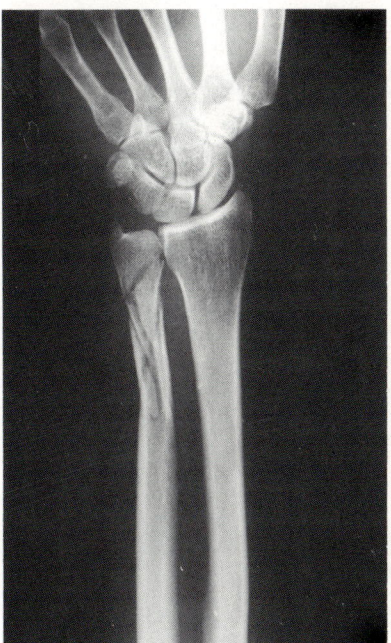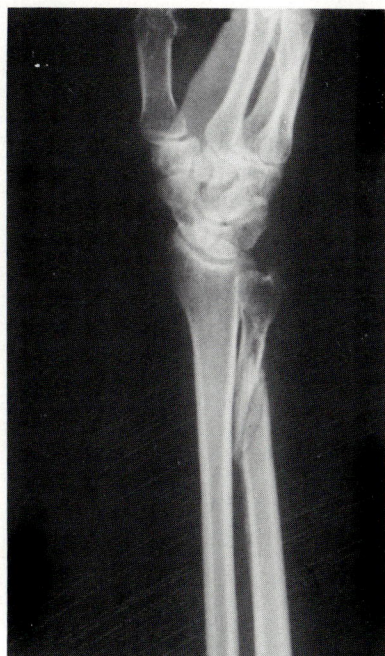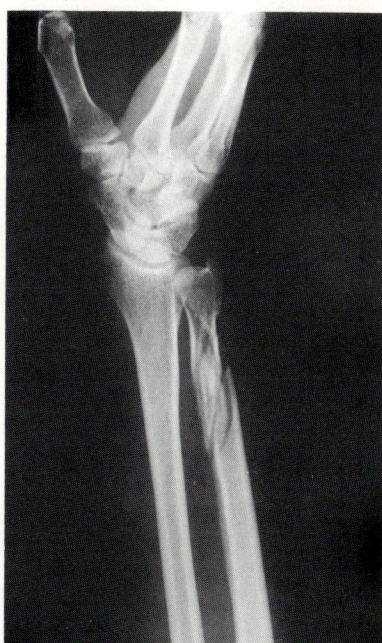

A　　　　　　B　　　　　　C

Figure 3 Type I fracture in *(A)* supination, *(B)* neutral, and *(C)* pronation, demonstrating stability of the ulna throughout the range of movement.

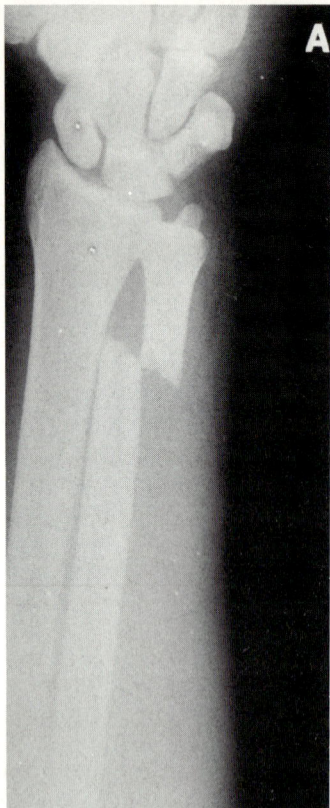
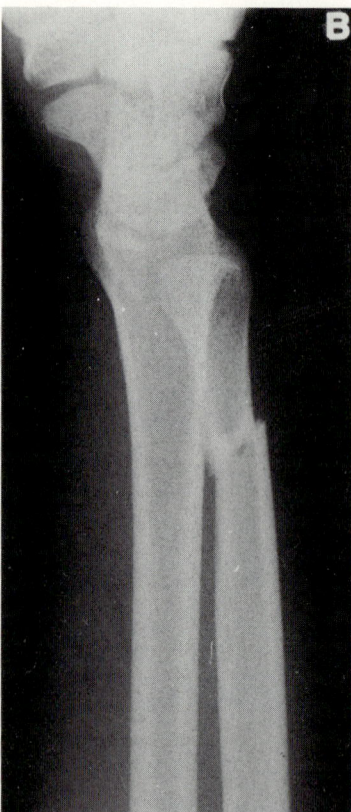
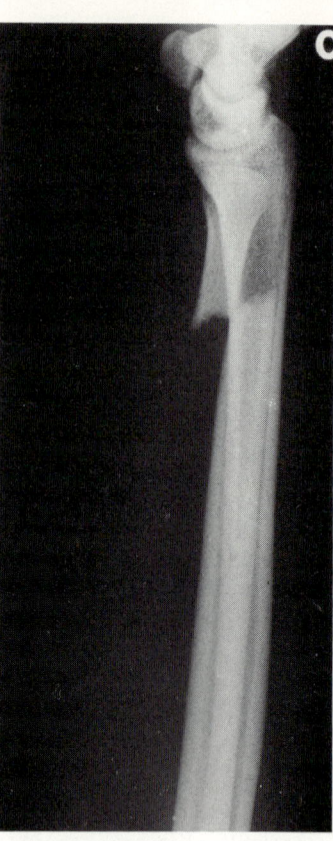

Figure 4 Type II fracture in *(A)* supination, *(B)* neutral, and *(C)* pronation, demonstrating instability of the ulna with movement.

I—fractures with less than 50% displacement, which are stable (Fig. 1); and type II—fractures with more than 50% displacement, which are unstable (Fig. 2).

Dynamic radiographs taken of acute fractures, under regional anesthesia before immobilization, supported these experimental findings. The injured forearm was rotated from pronation to supination and back again, while the stability of the fracture was observed. In type I fractures no significant displacement occurred, whereas in type II fractures considerable movement at the fracture site took place (Figs. 3 and 4).

These observations were used in a prospective clinical trial in which treatment was determined by the classification described above. Type I fractures in which, because of their less than 50% displacement, there was assumed to be a largely intact interosseous membrane and periosteum to help stabilize the fracture, were treated in a below-elbow cast for 6 weeks. During this time the patients were able to continue their daily activities. When the cast was removed, all had a full range of pronation and supination and were generally symptom free. Radiographic union was complete by 9 weeks (Fig. 5).

Patients with type II fractures were assumed to have lost the stabilizing effect of the interosseous membrane and periosteum, and were treated with an above-elbow cast for 6 weeks. Daily activities were severely restricted during this period, and it took 2 to 3 weeks for patients to regain full movement. Radiographic union was complete by 12 weeks.

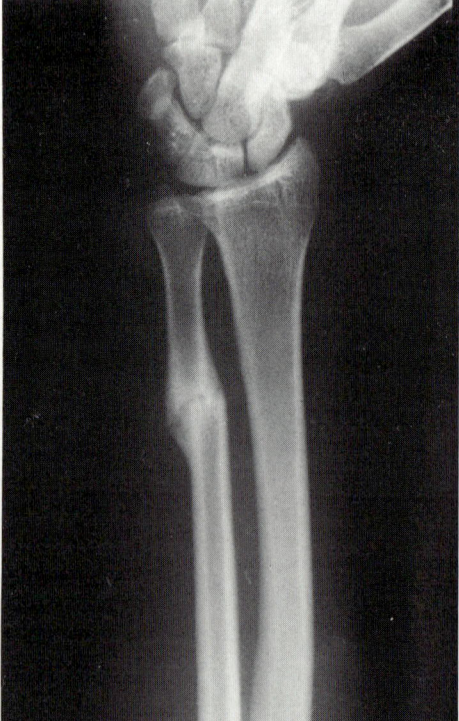

Figure 5 Type I fracture after 6 weeks in a below-elbow cast. The cast was not molded as is done in functional bracing. It was used more for protection than for immobilization.

In my experience, most isolated fractures of the ulna are in the distal half of the bone, are caused by direct trauma, and are less than 50% displaced (type I fractures). Treatment consists of a simple below-elbow cast to protect the fracture, since it is inherently stable. This allows considerably more freedom for the activities of daily living than an above-elbow cast.

This simple classification allows for the rational management of ulnar fractures, obviates the unnecessary use of above-elbow casting for fractures that are inherently stable, and identifies accurately those that require additional immobilization.

SUGGESTED READING

Anderson LD, Sisk TD, Tooms RE, Parks WI III. Compression plate fixation in acute diaphyseal fractures of the radius and ulna. J Bone Joint Surg 1975; 57A:287–297.

Boyd HB, Boals JC. The Monteggia lesion. A review of 159 cases. Clin Orthop 1969; 66:94–100.
Crenshaw AH Jr. Fractures of shaft of radius and ulna in adults. In: Crenshaw AH, ed. Campbell's operative orthopaedics. 8th Ed. Vol 2. 1992; 1035–1046.
Du Toit FP, Grabe RP. Isolated fractures of the ulna shaft. S Afr Med J 1979; 56:21–25.
Dymond IWD. The treatment of isolated fractures of the distal ulna. J Bone Joint Surg 1984; 66B:408–410.
Pollock FH, Pankovich AM, Prieto JJ, Lorenz M. The isolated fracture of the ulna shaft. Treatment without immobilization. J Bone Joint Surg 1983; 65A:339–342.
Sarmiento A, Kinman PB, Murphy RB, Phillips JG. Treatment of ulna fractures by functional bracing. J Bone Joint Surg 1976; 58A: 1105–1107.

TENNIS ELBOW TENDINOSIS: NONOPERATIVE MANAGEMENT

ROBERT P. NIRSCHL, M.D., M.S.

The understanding of the pathoanatomy of tennis elbow has been aided significantly by surgical experience over the past decade. Many concepts advanced by investigators of prior decades have proven flawed including the terminology. Although this discussion is dedicated to tennis elbow tendinosis it should be appreciated that tendinosis in other body parts (rotator cuff, patellar tendon achilles tendon, and plantar fascia) share the same principles of treatment.

NOMENCLATURE AND PATHOANATOMY

The histologic evaluation of tennis elbow tendinosis identifies a noninflammatory response in tendon. This histopathology has been named angio-fibroblastic tendinosis (Fig. 1) and is likely the result of a degenerative and avascular process. The histologic appearance is characterized by disorganized immature collagen formation in association with immature fibroblastic and vascular elements. In view of the histopathology, such names as epicondylitis and tendinitis are misnomers.

The gross pathologic presentation of surgical specimens of medial and lateral elbow tendinosis reveal a grayish edematous friable material. The location of tendinosis is classically in the extensor carpi radialis brevis (ECRB) tendon (100%) and the extensor com-

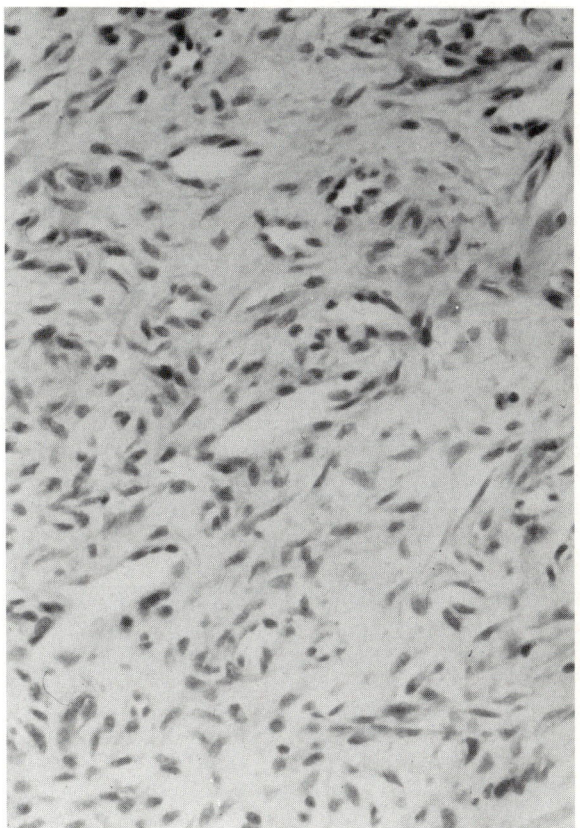

Figure 1 Photomicrograph of angio-fibroblastic tendinosis. These changes consist of young vascular and fibroblastic elements without evidence of inflammatory cells.

munis (EC) tendon (35%) laterally and in the pronator teres (PT) and the flexor carpi radialis (FCR) (95%) medially. Twenty percent of lateral elbow cases have associated bony exostosis at the lateral epicondyle.

Approximately 35% of surgical cases of medial elbow tendinosis also have associated clinical symptoms of ulnar nerve neurapraxia.

ETIOLOGY

Tennis elbow tendinosis issues are varied but most factors are focused on age, systemic factors, and repetitive overuse. The male-female ratio has been essentially equal.

Age. The usual range is 30 to 55 years old with median 42.5 years. Highly active forearm activity such as competitive tennis may result in younger age groups (age 12 is the youngest in my experience).

Systemic Factors (Mesenchymal Syndrome). Observation has identified an important subset (approximately 15%) of patients who present with multiple areas of tendon abnormality including combination problems of shoulder tendinosis, medial and lateral elbow tendinosis, neurapraxia of ulnar and median nerves (carpal tunnel syndrome), trigger fingers, and de Quervain's syndrome (all often bilateral). I have termed this clinical presentation the Mesenchymal syndrome and have theorized a systemic factor (perhaps an alteration of the cross linkage of collagen). An important subset of the Mesenchymal syndrome may include estrogen deficiency in women as this subset is often associated with premature hysterectomy (e.g., before 35 years) and low estrogen levels.

Repetitive Overuse. Most elbow tendinosis patients have a clear association with repetitive overuse of the dominant arm secondary to performance activities (e.g., sports, occupational, and performing arts). Common activities include racquet and throwing sports, occupational computer keyboard and hand shaking (politicians), and manual activities (e.g., dentistry, carpentry, electrical work). Musical performing arts (piano, string instruments, drums) are common elbow tendinosis producers. In addition, a broader pathoanatomy of inflammatory myositis may be present in the injuries to musicians.

It is theorized that multiple repetition overuse (often eccentric loading, especially in racquet sports) results in tension loading with secondary anoxic and degenerative consequences ("heart attack of tendon"). In those patients with Mesenchymal syndrome, it is theorized that a pre-existent vulnerability is present that is highly susceptible to overuse exposure.

INCIDENCE

The incidence of elbow tendinosis varies dependent upon etiologic exposure both hereditary and environmental. A study of adult tennis players revealed that 50% will experience symptoms of elbow tendinosis during their playing years. Lateral elbow tendinosis is five times more common than medical elbow tendinosis in my overall series. Posterior elbow tendinosis (triceps) also occurs on occasion but is most likely to occur in

association with olecranon fossa chondromalacia (most commonly competitive baseball pitchers and javelin throwers).

ASSOCIATED MYOSITIS

My clinical observations support the consideration of an associated muscular problem in a minority of cases of medial and lateral elbow tendinosis. This clinical presentation is most common in the extensor muscle groups particularly in computer keyboard and musical activities (piano and bow hand of string instruments). The symptoms are more diffuse with tenderness over the muscle mass (usually wrist extensors) in contradistinction to the more classical presentation of tenderness and provocative stress testing at tendon origin. It is theorized that muscle overuse especially in association with fine finger movement results in a form of inflammatory myositis.

RADIAL NERVE NEURAPRAXIA

It has been widely circulated, especially among hand surgeons, that compression and malfunction of the posterior interosseous branch of the radial nerve is a major contributor to the etiology of lateral elbow tendinosis. In my experience, this malady is rare. The symptoms, like those associated with extensor muscle myositis are more diffuse in the muscle mass. Provocation with forearm supination is most common. I believe that confirmation by electromyelogram (EMG) is mandatory to confirm the diagnosis. My experience with elbow tendinosis is now approaching 1,000 cases. Only two cases of objectively identifiable radial nerve neurapraxia have been noted in this series.

CLINICAL PRESENTATION

The typical presentation of lateral elbow tendinosis is a history of increased wrist extensor activity related to gradual onset of pain over the origin of the ECRB tendon and proximal forearm extensor muscle mass.

Palpable tenderness is classical over the ECRB tendon origin. Less palpable tenderness may be noted over the finger extensor (EC) tendon origin. Provocative signs include pain with manual wrist and finger extension stress testing with the elbow flexed and extended. Finger extension pain to provocation suggests involvement in the EC tendon. Pain at the ECRB origin is also common with provocative pronation stress testing. Radiograms may reveal bony exostosis at the lateral epicondyle in 20% of cases.

The onset of medial elbow tendinosis is similar. Wrist flexor and pronation activity results in pain in the common flexor origin close to the medial epicondyle. Medial tendinosis pain is exaggerated by provocative stress testing (e.g., wrist flexion and forearm pronation). Associated ulnar nerve problems may include a positive

Table 1 Treatment Algorithm

A. Relief of pain (comfort potential)
  1. Relative rest (e.g., absence from abuse)
  2. PRICEMM (*Protection, Rest, Ice, Elevation, Medication, Modalities*)
     a. Rest and anti-inflammatory medications do not heal
     b. Medication (usually anti-inflammatory pain relief) is utilized to free the patient from pain to allow compliance with the rehabilitation program.
B. Rehabilitation exercise (curative potential)
  1. Goals
     a. Transformation of devitalized unhealthy tendinosis tissue to healthy tissue (e.g., painful tissue to painless tissue)
     b. Neovascularization with production and maturation of collagen via fibroblastic proliferation
     c. Restoration of strength, endurance, and flexibility
  2. Methods
     a. Resistance exercise
     b. Multiple resistance systems (isometric, isotonic, isoflex, isokinetic, aqua, calisthenic and plyometric) and modes (eccentric and concentric)
C. Restore general fitness
D. Control abusive overload
  1. Alter activity technique
  2. Alter equipment or work place
  3. Alter frequency and duration of activity
  4. Counter-force bracing
E. Transition exercise
  1. Work hardening
  2. Plyometrics
  3. Higher speeds to reduplicate performance activity
F. Surgical intervention — failure of conservative prescription
  1. Goal of surgery: resection of pathoanatomy (*not tendon release*)
  2. Tend to associated problems (e.g., ulnar nerve, bony exostosis, collateral ligament, and intra-articular problems)
  3. Incidence of surgery (author's experience)
     a. 10% previously untreated
     b. 20% of previously treated
  4. Surgical success rate for tendinosis — 97%

Table 2 Basic Forearm Exercise Program

WRIST CURL (FLEXORS — MEDIAL ELBOW)

A. Exercise Benefit:	Forearm flexors
B. Starting Position:	Sit in chair forearm resting on table, wrist and hand extending past edge of table. Hold weight with palm up and wrist stretch down.
C. Exercise Action:	
Phase 1.	Lift hand (flex wrist as high as possible) hold: then return to starting position.

WRIST CURL (EXTENSORS — LATERAL ELBOW)

A. Exercise Benefit:	Forearm extensors
B. Starting Position:	Sit in chair forearm resting on table, wrist and hand extending past edge of table. Hold weight with palm down and wrist stretch down.
C. Exercise Action:	
Phase 1.	Lift hand as high as possible. Hold, then return to starting position.

FOREARM ROTATION

A. Exercise Benefit:	Forearm pronators and supinators
B. Starting Position:	Sit in chair. Hold dumbbell at weight end (not in the middle) with elbow bent to 90°. Forearm supinated (palm up).
C. Exercise Action:	Slowly roll forearm to full pronated (palm down) position. Hold, then return to starting position.

FINGER EXTENSION

A. Exercise Benefit:	Strengthens forearm and finger extensors.
B. Starting Position:	Place thick rubber band around thumb and fingers between end finger knuckle joint.
C. Exercise Action:	
Phase 1.	Actively pull finger and wrist into fully straightened position. Hold for three seconds.
Phase 2.	Release hand and return to starting position. Repeat until fatigue occurs.

HAND SQUEEZE

A. Exercise Benefit:	Strengthens forearm flexors and extensors muscles.
B. Starting Position:	Holding a tennis ball.
C. Exercise Action:	
Phase 1.	Squeeze ball firmly and hold for three seconds.
Phase 2.	Release ball and repeat until fatigue occurs.
D. Speed:	Moderate
E. Note: You may need to start with a nerf ball or racquet ball and progress to a tennis ball.	

Courtesy of Virginia Sportsmedicine Institute and Nirschl Orthopedic & Sportsmedicine Clinic — Arlington, Virginia.

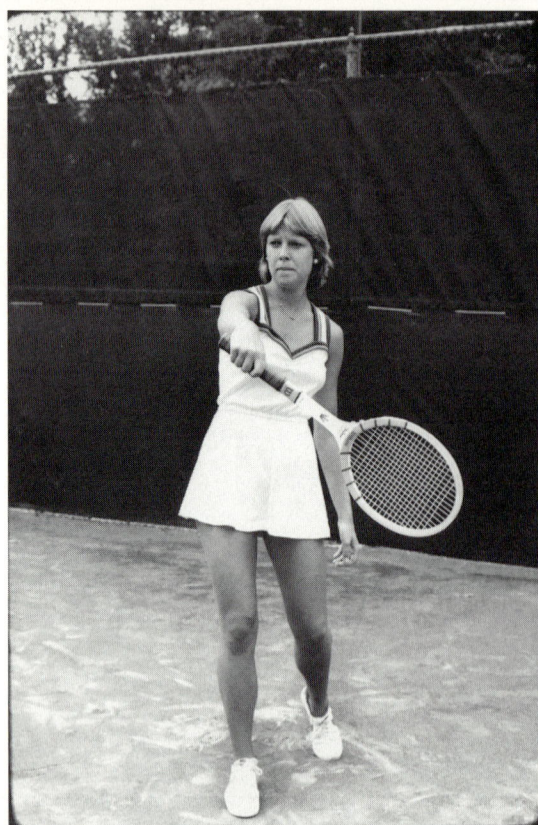

Figure 2 Performance technique such as the illustrated poor quality backhand in tennis is a significant factor in overuse injuries.

Tinel's sign at the zone 3 level of the medial epicondylar groove.

TREATMENT PROGRAM

The treatment protocol for tennis elbow tendinosis follows a pattern implemented and utilized at our institution for the past 15 years. The basics of treatment fall into two broad categories: comfort and cure (Table 1). The comfort aspect of the program usually progresses in 1 to 2 weeks to a point when the curative aspect of the program can be implemented. The key to the curative aspect of the program resides in rehabilitative exercise. The goals of rehabilitation are to revascularize and recollagenize tendinosis tissue as well as restore strength, endurance, and flexibility. It should be noted that the entire extremity including the shoulder and upper back are often weak and the exercise programs must be dedicated to all these regions. On average the rehabilitative process takes 4 months. The program is initiated in our Sportsmedicine rehabilitation facility (usually two times per week for 3 weeks) and proceeds thereafter on a home exercise program (Table 2) with occasional re-evaluation as needed.

As a companion to the rehabilitation program control of overuse is always appropriate particularly

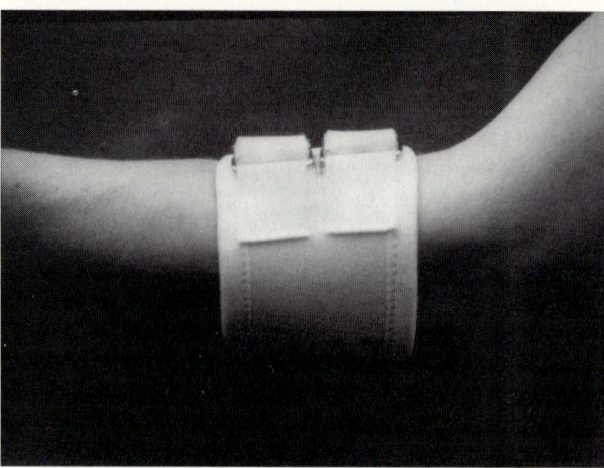

Figure 3 Lateral elbow counter-force brace. Brace design, which allows balanced muscular activity, supports the rehabilitation goals, and is highly effective in pain control. (Courtesy Medical Sports, Inc., Arlington, Va.)

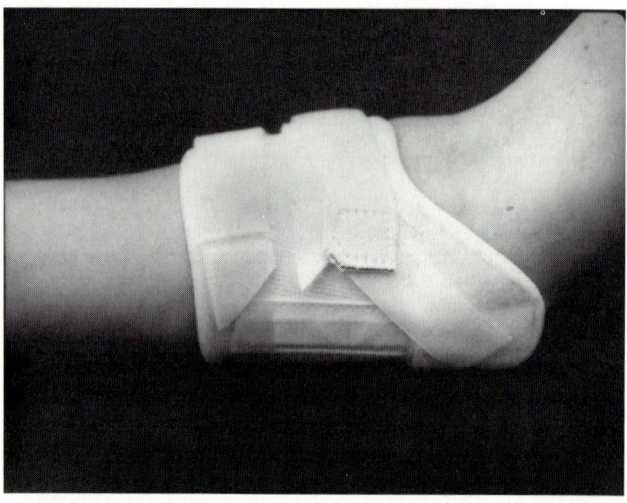

Figure 4 Medial elbow counter-force brace. (Courtesy Medical Sports, Inc., Arlington, Va.)

upon return to performance activities. Alteration of the intensity, duration, and frequency of activity is relatively easy to attain. Beneficial technique and equipment changes may be more difficult but should always be addressed (Fig. 2). Counter-force bracing, which maintains even a muscular balance, is important and offers helpful pain diminution in the majority of cases (Figs. 3 and 4).

RESULTS

The program as presented is basic to all tendinosis (cumulative overuse) problems. Ninety percent of my previously untreated patients have returned to full activity after the nonsurgical treatment program. This success is somewhat predicated upon patient activity level and it might be noted that the patient population at our institution is highly active. Patients who have had prior treatment focused on comfort (especially with iatrogenic damage secondary to multiple cortisone injections) have less success with the conservative effort, but it is still worthwhile to pursue if a meaningful rehabilitative effort has not been previously attempted. Those patients who have unacceptable pain and compromised activity level in spite of a quality rehabilitative effort can usually benefit from surgical intervention.

SUGGESTED READING

Groppel J, Nirschl RP. A biomechanical and electromyographical analysis of the effects of counter-force braces on the tennis player. Am J Sports Med 1986; 14:1986.

Gruchow HW, Pelltier D. An epidemiological study of tennis elbow: Incidence, recurrence and effectiveness of prevention strategies. Am J Sports Med 7: 234-238.

Nirschl RP, Sobel JR. Arm care. The prevention and treatment of tennis elbow. Arlington, Va, Medical Sports Publishing, 1994.

Nirschl RP. Elbow tendinosis/tennis elbow. Clin Sports Med 1992; 11:851-870.

Nirschl RP. Mesenchymal syndrome. Virginia Medical 1969; 96:659.

O'Connor FG, Sobel JR, Nirschl RP. Five step treatment for overuse injuries. Phys Sports Med 1992; 20:128-142.

O'Connor FG, Wilder RP, Sobel JR. Overuse injuries of the elbow. J Back Musculoskel Rehabil 1994;4(1), 17-30.

Priest JD, Braden V, Gerbierich JG. The elbow and tennis. Phys Sports Med 1980; 8(4):80.

TENNIS ELBOW TENDINOSIS: OPERATIVE MANAGEMENT

ROBERT P. NIRSCHL, M.D., M.S.

Most tennis elbow tendinosis patients respond to a quality rehabilitation program. The goals of rehabilitation in such a program are based upon the principles of revascularization and collagenization of the devitalized angio-fibroblastic tendinosis tissue. A minority of high activity level patients fail the rehabilitative process (10% to 20% dependent upon variables) and surgical intervention may be indicated. In the case of lateral tennis elbow, the extensor carpi radialis brevis (ECRB) tendon is the most common involved. The extensor communis (EC) (30%) and to a lesser degree the extensor carpi radialis longus (ECRL) and extensor carpi ulnaris may also demonstrate abnormality. In medial tennis elbow ("golfer's elbow"), tendinosis changes are primarily in the pronator teres (PT) and flexor carpi radialis (FCR) with occasional additional charges noted in the palmaris longus, flexor carpi ulnaris (5%), and rarely the origin of the flexor digitorum sublimis.

INDICATIONS FOR SURGERY

The ultimate final decision for surgery is made by the patient dependent upon the magnitude of symptoms and the alteration of quality of life. Indications for surgery (Table 1) include unacceptable pain with decreased function following an appropriate rehabilitation program. Pain is usually present even with light activities of daily living. It should be noted that a quality rehab program requires active patient participation and generally takes 4 months. In general, it is rare to seek

Table 1 Surgical Indications

Failure of quality rehabilitation program
   3 or 4 months of supervised resistance exercise
   Properly sequenced exercises
   Quality effort by patient
Presence of persistent pain (generally exceeding 1 year)
   Requiring sport or occupational activity change
   Persisting with activities of daily living
   Rest pain (note: rule out other potential factors for rest pain, including malignancy)
Requirement of high activity level

Table 2 Predictors for Failed Rehabilitation

Iatrogenic atrophy from multiple cortisone injection
Initiation of symptoms by direct trauma
Mesenchymal syndrome (history of widespread tendinosis)
Presence of epicondylar bony exostosis

surgical solutions before 1 year of symptoms. In our series the average time from the onset of symptoms to surgical intervention is 2 years. Certain patients are unlikely to experience a favorable result with rehabilitative management and are, therefore, more likely to require surgical intervention (Table 2).

REASONS FOR FAILED SURGERY (TABLES 3 AND 4)

My experience with salvage procedures for failed medial and lateral elbow tendinosis surgery is extensive. The overwhelming reason for the lack of primary surgical success is failure to address the tendinosis pathoanatomy (e.g., the tendinosis pathology has not been resected). The failed operative intervention is always some form of tendon release. On the lateral side the finger extensors have been released and on the medial side the common flexor origin. Salvage surgery is dedicated to reidentifying and excising the true patho-

Table 3 Failed Lateral Elbow Surgery

Failure to address tendinosis pathology
  Tendon release of extensor aponeurosis when pathology is in
    extensor brevis
Iatrogenic harm
  Failure of extensor aponeurosis reattachment
  Postero-lateral elbow instability secondary to disruption of
    lateral collateral ligament
  Scar impingement about radial head
Wrong diagnosis—problems of secondary gain

Table 4 Failed Medial Elbow Surgery

Failure to address tendinosis pathology
  Release of common flexor origin without resection of
    pathoanatomy
Iatrogenic harm (valgus instability)
  Failure of reattachment of common flexor origin
  Distortion of ulnar collateral ligament
Iatrogenic harm
  Causalgic neuroma medial antebrachial cutaneous nerve
Ulnar Nerve
  Failure to address compression of nerve at intial surgery
  Post-surgical iatrogenic scar about nerve
Wrong diagnosis—problems of secondary gain

---

anatomy. Iatrogenic surgical harm is also commonplace. On the lateral side, this includes the failure of finger extensor reattachment, postero-lateral elbow instability secondary to lateral collateral ligament disruption and scar entrapment in the area of the radial head. On the medial side, valgus instability, ulnar nerve symptoms, and neuroma causalgia of the medial antebrachial cutaneous nerve are typical presenting iatrogenic problems. The most common problem both medially and laterally is, however, failure to achieve the preoperative goals of pain relief and functional improvement.

SURGICAL PRINCIPLES

The surgical management of tennis elbow has undergone several developments. Early surgical techniques focused on tension release such as the common extensor aponeurosis lateral or the common flexor origin medial. In 1979, Nirschl and Pettrone introduced a new procedure for the surgical treatment of tennis elbow. The key to this technique is identification and removal of the pathologic tissue (angiofibroblastic tendinosis). In contrast to previous techniques, normal tendon origins are not released. It is emphasized again that the goal of surgery is not tendon release but an actual identification and removal of the painful pathological angiofibroblastic tendinosis tissue. Further clarification of this important principle may best be presented in the form of a question: Who would release an achilles tendon from its insertion in the treatment of achilles tendinosis?

Lateral Elbow Surgery

The described technique (my preferred technique) is for the classic case and represents the majority of cases (Fig. 1). The tissues most commonly involved are the ECRB (100%) and the anterior edge of the EC (30%). A bony exostosis of the lateral epicondyle is present in 20% of cases and posterolateral synovitis in 5%. Such associated pathology is also addressed at the time of surgery, as needed.

The incision extends from 1 inch proximal and just anterior to the lateral epicondyle to the level of the radial head. The interface between the extensor longus and extensor aponeurosis is identified, and a splitting incision is made between. The extensor longus is retracted anteriorly, bringing the extensor brevis origin into view. A technique note is worth emphasizing at this stage in the operation. A common error is to penetrate with a vertical dissection too deeply, thereby failing to clearly identify the entire ECRB origin at its attachment points (the extensor aponeurosis and lateral epicondyle). The ECRL at this level is thin (2 to 3 mm) and should be carefully elevated and retracted in a horizontal antero-medial direction. This technical subtlety is important to avoid premature distortion of the extensor brevis origin, which can result in difficulty in identifying the pathologic areas. The brevis origin normally attaches to the underside anterior edge of the aponeurosis distal to the epicondyle and to the distal humeral ridge at the epicondyle. In the properly selected case, the pathologic change of dull-grayish edematous tissue will be noticed replacing normal glistening tendon.

This pathologic tissue often encompasses the entire origin of the extensor brevis to the level of the joint line. In approximately 35% of cases, pathologic change will be noticed in the anterior underside of the extensor aponeurosis, and this is also removed. In 20% of cases, calcific exostosis of the lateral epicondyle is present and is removed after partially peeling away the anterior aspect of the extensor aponeurosis.

A small longitudinal opening may be made in the synovium anterior to the radial collateral ligament for inspection of the lateral compartment. In the classic case, it is rare to have any lateral joint compartment, synovial fringe, or orbicular ligament changes and we no longer do an arthrotomy as a routine.

The wounds are irrigated and two or three drill-holes are placed through the exposed cortical bone of the lateral condyle to cancellous depth to enhance vascular supply. The extensor brevis maintains some soft tissue attachments at the level of the radial head; thus, minimal brevis retraction takes place. It is, therefore, unnecessary to suture the remaining brevis to obtain proper mechanical length. This concept is pertinent to retaining normal strength after healing has occurred.

Medial Elbow Surgery

The principles for medial elbow surgery (my preferred technique) are similar to those for the lateral elbow (Fig. 2). The goal again is to resect pathologic tissue without harm to normal tissue. Pathologic tissue is noted at the interface of the PT and the FCR (70%),

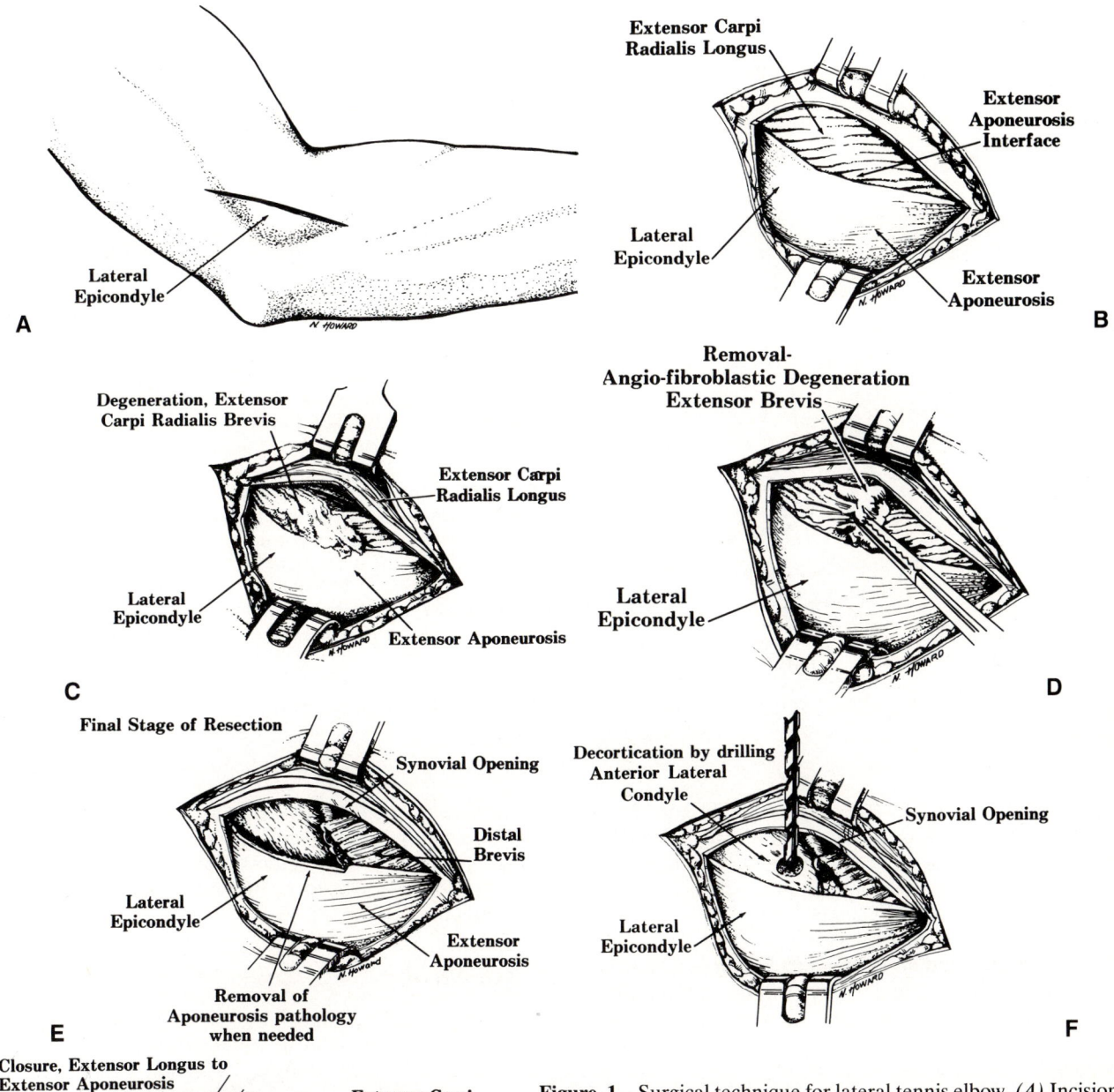

A Lateral Epicondyle

B Extensor Carpi Radialis Longus / Extensor Aponeurosis Interface / Lateral Epicondyle / Extensor Aponeurosis

C Degeneration, Extensor Carpi Radialis Brevis / Extensor Carpi Radialis Longus / Lateral Epicondyle / Extensor Aponeurosis

D Removal- Angio-fibroblastic Degeneration Extensor Brevis / Lateral Epicondyle

E Final Stage of Resection / Synovial Opening / Distal Brevis / Lateral Epicondyle / Extensor Aponeurosis / Removal of Aponeurosis pathology when needed

F Decortication by drilling Anterior Lateral Condyle / Synovial Opening / Lateral Epicondyle

G Closure, Extensor Longus to Extensor Aponeurosis / Extensor Carpi Radialis Longus / Lateral Epicondyle / Extensor Aponeurosis

Figure 1 Surgical technique for lateral tennis elbow. *(A)* Incision is slightly anterior to the lateral epicondyle and extends from the level of the joint to 1 inch proximal to the lateral epicondyle. *(B)* Interface between extensor carpi radialis longus and extensor aponeurosis is identified. *(C)* Incision is made in the extensor longus-aponeurosis interface. The extensor longus is 2 to 3 mm thick in this area. Do not make the incision too deep, as the origin of the extensor brevis will be distorted, thereby compromising the identification of the pathologic areas. The extensor carpi radialis longus is retracted anteromedially and the origin of the extensor carpi radialis brevis comes into view. The normal brevis origin includes some attachment to the anterior edge of the extensor aponeurosis. The typical changes of grayish edematous tendon alteration should also be visible without the use of optical assistance if the operative slection is correct. *(D)* Removal of angiofibroblastic degeneration of the extensor brevis. In the typical case, the extensor aponeurosis and lateral epicondyle are not disturbed. *(E)* Final stage of resection. All pathologic tissue is removed. In approximately 35% of cases, some alteration is noted in the anterior edge of the extensor aponeurosis. This pathologic change is removed if present. In 20% of cases, some lateral epicondylar exostosis is also noted. If exostosis is encountered, a small section of the aponeurosis is peeled back and the exostosis removed. *(F)* To enhance vascular supply, three holes are drilled through the cortical bone of the anterior lateral condyl to cancellous bone level. *(G)* The extensor longus is firmly repaired to the anterior margin of the extensor aponeurosis. Because the extensor brevis is still attached to the underside of the extensor longus, it is unnecessary to suture the distal brevis. Note that a firm attachment of the extensor aponeurosis to the lateral epicondyle is maintained at all times. (From Nirschl RP. Elbow tendinosis/tennis elbow. Clin Sports Med 1992; 11:851-870.)

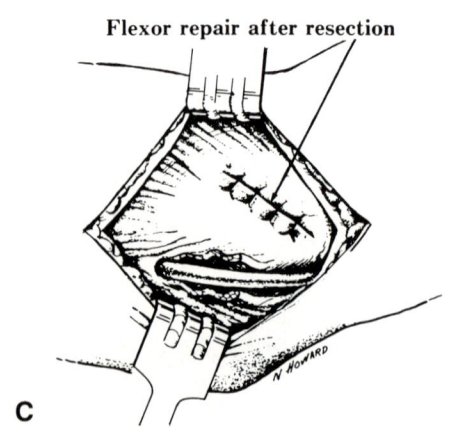

A

Medial
Epicondyle

B

Angio-fibroblastic
degeneration
Flexor origin

Medial
Epicondyle

Zone 3
Medial
Epicondylar
Groove

C

Flexor repair after resection

Figure 2 Surgical technique for medial tennis elbow and compression neurapraxia of the ulnar nerve. *(A)* Incision is made as shown. Care is taken to avoid harm to the sensory cutaneous nerve (medial antebrachial) just anterior to the medial epicondyle. *(B)* Angiofibroblastic changes are usually in the origin of the pronator teres and flexor carpi radialis. The pathologic tissue is removed by longitudinal and elliptic fashion, leaving attachments of normal tissue intact. In 60% of cases, dysfunction of the ulnar nerve has been noted clinically; decompression of the ulnar nerve in zone 3 of the medial epicondylar groove is performed if indicated. *(C)* Repair of the common flexor origin is undertaken. Note that the medial epicondylar attachments of normal tissue are not disturbed. (From Nirschl RP. Elbow tendinosis/tennis elbow. Clin Sports Med 1992; 11:851-870.)

more extensively in the PT (25%), and in the flexor carpi ulnaris (5%). Associated problems include ulnar nerve compression at zone 3 of the medial epicondylar groove (35%), congenital subluxation of the ulnar nerve (5%), medial collateral ligament laxity (5%), and olecranon fossa chondromalacia (5%).

For classic medial tennis elbow, the incision is longitudinal, approximately 3 inches long, and parallels the medial epicondylar groove, starting approximately 1 inch proximal and just posterior to the medial epicondyle. Care is taken to avoid a sensory branch (medial antebrachial cutaneous nerve) just distal and anterior to the medial epicondyle. A thin muscle layer may mask the pathologic changes underneath, so it is important to precisely locate the patient's primary area of tenderness prior to the administration of anesthesia, as the area of tenderness focuses to the area of pathologic change.

A longitudinal incision is made in the tendon origins at the prime area of patient tenderness, extending from the medial epicondyle distally for about 2 inches. The tendons are spread, and the lesion will come clearly into view if the surgical indications are correct. All excision of pathologic tissue is done longitudinally and elliptically, including resection to the joint in the occasionally indicated case. All normal tissue attachments to the medial epicondyle are left intact. This is a key principle as the common flexor origin is a key medial stabilizer, and indiscriminate release of normal tendon attachment

may lead to medial instability as well as the common problem of increased and unnecessary postoperative scar morbidity. After removal of tissue, the resulting elliptic space is closed firmly with absorbable sutures (usually 0 to 1 in size).

Ulnar Nerve

The medial epicondylar groove is divided into three zones: zone 1 proximal to the medial epicondyle, zone 2 at the medial epicondyle, and zone 3 distal to the medial epicondyle (Fig. 3). Most ulnar nerve symptoms are the result of compression in zone 3. Decompression of this zone by release of the flexor ulnaris arcade generally resolves the symptoms. Compression from osteophytic spurs, loose bodies, or rheumatoid synovitis can also occur in zone 2, and compression in zone 1 may be caused by a tight medial intermuscular septum.

Anterior transfer of the ulnar nerve is occasionally indicated, primarily when ulnar nerve symptoms are related to tension. Indications include (1) nerve subluxation or dislocation from epicondylar groove; (2) skeletal valgus; (3) dynamic valgus ligamentous instability; and (4) need for surgical exposure to the medial elbow compartment. When ulnar nerve transfer is indicated, my preference is subcuticular with a small fascial sling for buttress. The keys to ulnar nerve transfer success are relaxed angles in zones 1 and 3.

POSTOPERATIVE CARE

The postoperative protocols for lateral and medial elbow are similar (Table 5). The elbow is protected at 90 degrees for 1 week in a lightweight elbow immobilizer (Fig. 4). The immobilizer allows active use of the wrist, hand, and shoulder as the patient's tolerance permits. The immobilizer is removed for active and active-assisted range of motion exercise starting on postoperative day 3, but is worn at other times for up to 1 week. Most patients tolerate normal activities of daily living by day 10. Rehabilitative exercises, as described in the chapter on nonoperative treatment, commence 3 weeks after surgery. A counterforce elbow brace is worn during rehabilitative exercises as well as during higher forearm activity (including return to sport). Although full racquet and throwing sport competitive activity is not recommended until full strength returns, modified sport technique patterns are often initiated starting 6 to 8 weeks after lateral elbow surgery, and 10 to 12 weeks after medial elbow surgery. Full strength and thus clearance for competitive play is typically restored by 6 months provided that a quality rehabilitative exercise program has been adhered to.

RESULTS

My experience with the described surgical techniques has been highly consistent and rewarding. Overall improvement to a level of activity that existed prior to the onset of symptoms has been observed in 90% of cases. Significant relief of pain for all activities has been observed in 97% of cases. It is emphasized that a positive result also depends on quality rehabilitation following surgery. A number of variables may play a role in those

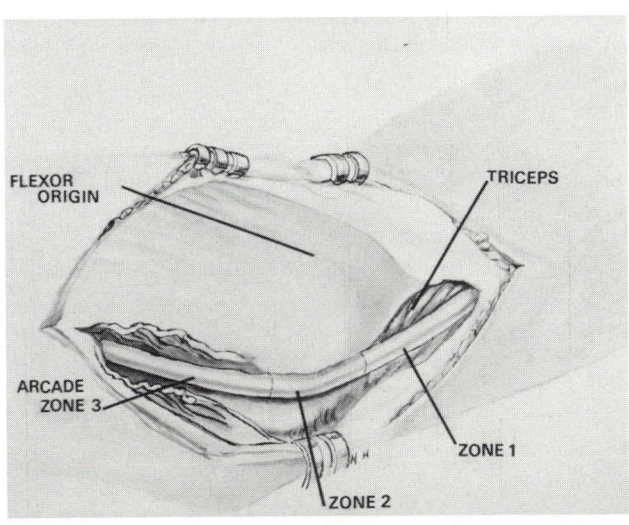

Figure 3 Medial epicondylar groove—ulnar nerve zones.

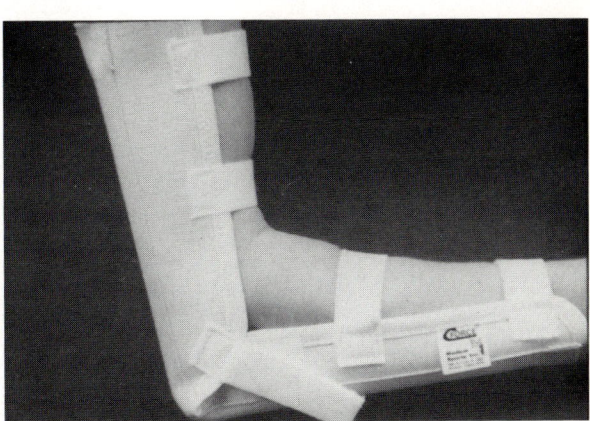

Figure 4 Elbow immobilizer. Lightweight velcro fastening elbow immobilizer provides marked improvement over a plaster splint in patient comfort and rehabilitative enhancement. (Courtesy Medical Sports, Inc., Arlington, Va.)

Table 5 Tennis Elbow Postoperative Protocol

Days 1 to 7:	Ice 3 to 4 times per day for 20 min at a time. Medication: Anti-inflammatory or pain medications as per physician's instructions. Maintain full shoulder motion with active ranging several times per day.
Days 1 to 3:	Keep elbow bandaged and in immobilizer at all times.
Day 2:	Start ranging fingers and wrist for 2 minutes, 3 to 5 times per day.
Day 3:	May shower; remove bandage and gently range elbow in shower. Cleanse wound with alcohol.
Days 3 to 6:	Wear immobilizer except for showering and gently limbering the elbow.
Days 7 to 17:	Continue elbow ranging activities with bending and straightening motions (80% of normal motion by day 17 is normal). Continue active motion of shoulder, wrist, and fingers. Add active pronation and supination. May use arm for light activity only. Immobilizer is used for protection only. Leave immobilizer off the majority of the time.
Days 17 to 21:	Begin tennis elbow exercise program without weights Begin squeezing a Nerf ball. Use counterforce brace when exercising.
Day 21:	Progress tennis elbow exercise program to include resistance exercises. Increase use of arm to include normal activities of daily living.
6 to 8 Weeks:	Begin modified return to sport activity following lateral tennis elbow surgery.
10 to 12 Weeks:	Begin modified return to sport activity following medial tennis elbow surgery.
6 Months:	Return to competitive play.

Adapted from the Virginia Sportsmedicine Institute and Nirschl Orthopedic Clinic instruction manual. Used with permission.

patients with unsuccessful results. These variables include the presence of multiple pathologic issues beyond tendinosis (e.g., associated nerve and ligament injury and osteoarthritis), emotional aspects of pain, and secondary gain issues such as the hidden agenda of the worker's compensation system.

SUGGESTED READING

Coonrad RW, Hooper WR. Tennis elbow: Its course, natural history. Conservative and surgical management. J Bone Joint Surg 1973; 55A:1177.

Goldie I. Epicondylitis lateralis humeri (epicondylagia or tennis elbow): A pathologic study. ACTA Chir Scand 1964; (Suppl):339.

Hohmann G. Das wesen und die dehand lung des sogenannten tennis—Ellen Bagens. Muchen Med Wochenschr 1933; 80:250-252.

Morrey B: The elbow and its disorders. Philadelphia, W.B. Saunders, 1985.

Nirschl RP, Pettrone FA. The surgical treatment of lateral epicondylitis. J Bone Joint Surg 1979; 61A:832-839.

Nirschl RP. Medial tennis elbow: Surgical treatment. Orthop Trans 1980; 4:298.

Nirschl RP. Elbow tendinosis/ tennis elbow. Clin Sports Med 1992; 11:851-870.

COACH'S FINGER

FRANK C. McCUE III, M.D.
MICHAEL R. REDLER, M.D.

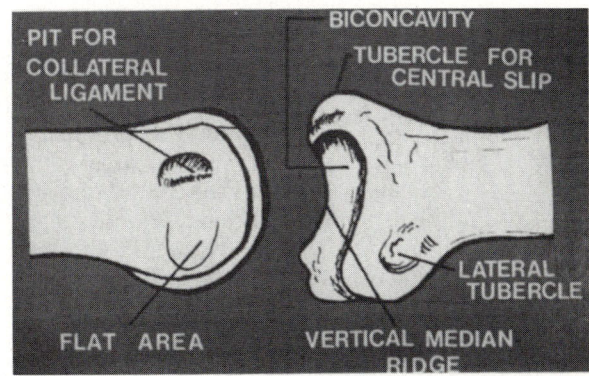

Figure 1 Proximal interphalangeal joint bony anatomy.

Injuries to the proximal interphalangeal (PIP) joint of the finger are exceedingly common in athletic competition. The exact frequency of the injury is not completely known, as many are treated on the sideline by the coach, the trainer, or the player himself. Very often, the injured finger is splinted with tape to the adjacent finger and the player is allowed to re-enter the game. This sideline treatment may represent the only therapeutic intervention for the injury. The poorly supervised athlete tends to return to competition with unprotected use of the finger long before adequate healing has taken place. The result, 2 to 3 months later, is a painful, stiff, and deformed finger that we have previously termed "coach's finger."

The coach's finger problem is further complicated by inadequate diagnosis, lack of radiographic studies, and improper splinting. Proper treatment of injuries to the PIP joint is particularly important because any fixed flexion or extension deformity is extremely disabling. The PIP joint is especially vulnerable to injury because of the relatively long proximal and distal lever arms that transmit lateral and torque stress to this hinge type of joint, which has minimal lateral mobility.

Accurate diagnosis requires a knowledge of the anatomy of the PIP joint and also of the mechanisms of the stress applied in the various injuries. The PIP joint has a range of motion of 0 to 120 degrees in a plane perpendicular to the palm. All the lateral ligaments and the volar plate are thick and strong and, in conjunction with the central slip of the extensor tendon and the volar sheath of the flexor tendons, form a firm soft tissue enclosure. The head of the proximal phalanx is bicondylar. The dorsolateral aspect of the head has a concavity for the proximal attachment of the collateral ligament. As the finger flexes, the ligament glides volarly over a smooth flat area on the head of the phalanx (Fig. 1).

The base of the middle phalanx has a biconcavity with a vertical medial ridge. These concavities articulate with the condyles of the proximal phalanx. The volar lip of the middle phalanx has a roughened area for the thick distal attachment of the volar plate (Fig. 2). The volar plate, with its additional lateral attachments, functions to resist dorsal displacement. The proximal membranous portion of the volar plate attaches to the distal portion of the proximal phalanx. There is a central accordion portion to allow flexion, and lateral thickened attachments to help prevent hyperextension.

The oblique retinacular ligament arises from the flexor tendon sheath about the proximal phalanx, and runs obliquely and distally to insert into the extensor apparatus. It functions as an extensor of the distal interphalangeal (DIP) joint through a tenodesis effect when the PIP joint is flexed. The transverse retinacular ligament lies superficial to the oblique ligament and runs from the flexor tendon sheath to insert on the lateral extensor band. Cleland's ligament arises from the joint capsule deep to the transverse retinacular ligament, and runs dorsal to the neurovascular bundle to insert on the skin. Grayson's thin transparent ligament has an origin off the flexor tendon sheath, and passes volar to the neurovascular bundle.

All these ligaments must move and glide freely to allow proper motion. The volar cul-de-sac must also be free of scar tissue to allow the base of the middle phalanx to glide into the sac during flexion. The synovial pouch that lines this cul-de-sac lies deep to the flexor sheath. Injuries or scarring in any of these regions cause a painful stiff finger that loses much of the necessary motion or stability needed by athletes to compete in their sport.

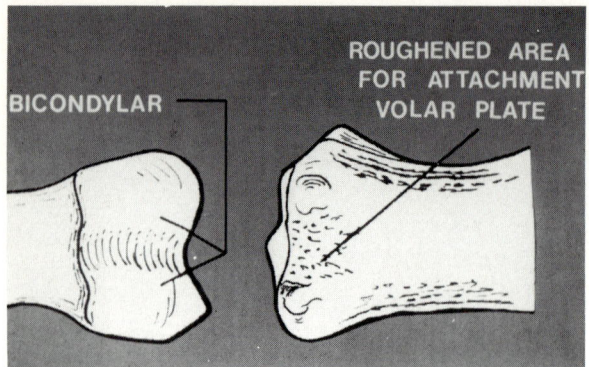

Figure 2 Attachment site of the volar plate.

The coach's finger injuries include collateral ligament injuries, articular fractures, fracture-dislocations, and boutonnière and pseudoboutonnière deformities. We believe that these are all potentially serious injuries. Early recognition and proper treatment is paramount in returning the athlete to competition.

COLLATERAL LIGAMENT INJURIES

Collateral ligament injuries to the PIP joint represent the most common type of coach's finger injury. A swollen, jammed finger is frequently the presenting complaint. The radial and ulnar collateral ligaments are the chief restraints to lateral stress in the initial 20 degrees of flexion. The volar plate aids in lateral stability at this point. The collateral ligament consists of the stronger proper component and a volar accessory component, which may be a factor in flexion contractures with shortening that occurs in the flexed position. The radial side collateral ligament is more commonly injured with avulsion of the proximal attachment. This is usually associated with partial or complete rupture of the volar plate.

The acute injury is often caused by a ball or other dull object striking the extended finger. This is accompanied by pain and localized swelling on the side of the injured ligament. It is important to ascertain whether this injury represents a strain, the more common injury, or a complete disruption of the ligament. Complete rupture creates lateral instability. This can be demonstrated radiographically with stress films or with the finding of a small bone fragment associated with the ligament rupture (Fig. 3). We routinely perform examination under digital nerve block. It is important to remember, however, that too rigorous stress may convert a partial collateral ligament strain into a complete rupture.

The treatment for a mild strain of the collateral ligament consists of splinting the finger in a functional position. The finger is protected until full pain-free motion can be achieved. Protection often consists of molding a polypropylene splint to be used in competition. For a mildly injured finger, we often tape it to the adjacent finger during competition; this provides some support as well as mobility. It must be stressed, however,

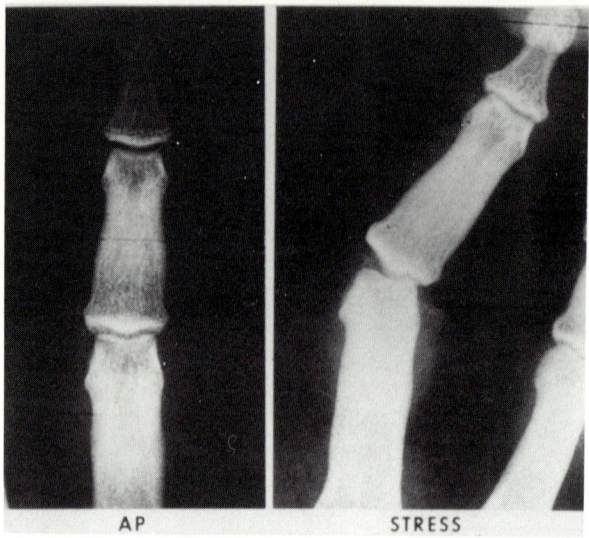

Figure 3 Stress films of a complete tear of the collateral ligament.

that taping is not appropriate protection for the acutely injured, swollen, painful finger.

For injuries in which there is joint laxity and incomplete tearing of the ligament, the finger should be splinted in 30 degrees of flexion. Active motion exercises should be started in 10 to 14 days. Protective splinting is continued for at least 3 weeks. Active sports participation is then allowed, with the finger protected with a molded splint. Again, protection is continued until complete pain-free motion is possible. Discontinuation of protection too early can lead to further injury, including a complete tearing of the ligament.

Although there is controversy regarding the treatment of complete tears of the collateral ligament of the PIP joint, we believe that optimal treatment of these injuries includes open inspection and repair of the torn ligament. Operative treatment is performed in order to restore stability and decrease subsequent pain, swelling, and functional loss. Nonoperative treatment is prone to leave the patient with a swollen, tender joint that is unstable and susceptible to additional injury, as well as to subsequent degenerative changes.

Acute complete ruptures are approached surgically, using a long midlateral incision. The collateral ligament is exposed by an oblique incision through the transverse retinacular ligament. Most of these ruptures occur from the proximal attachment of the ligament. The acute collateral ligament may be repaired using a Bunnell-type suture of No. 34 wire passed through drill holes in the bone and then tied over a button. In certain cases when an adequate proximal stump remains, a mattress stitch with a nonabsorbable suture may be used. The associated tear of the volar plate is repaired with interrupted absorbable suture. In reconstruction of chronic tears, repair is accomplished by transferring the adjacent sublimis slip to augment the proximal end of the collateral ligament and associated soft tissue. The finger is splinted for 3 weeks, at which point protected motion exercises are employed. Generally, splinting is continued for an additional 5 weeks, or until full pain-free motion is possible.

ARTICULAR FRACTURES

If neglected or improperly treated, fractures of the articular surfaces of the PIP joint have the potential for loss of motion or early degenerative changes. The most common PIP joint fracture involves one condyle of the head of the proximal phalanx. Long and short oblique fractures, T-type fractures, avulsion fractures, comminuted fractures, and fractures of the base of the middle phalanx are also seen.

Stable fractures with minimal disruption of the articular surface and little or no ligamentous instability can be treated nonoperatively. This includes small chip fractures or avulsion fractures. These fractures are splinted with aluminum volar splints lined with moleskin, with the PIP joint in 30 degrees of flexion for approximately 3 weeks. After this initial period, early protected motion is allowed. Splinting is continued during competition and practice until full pain-free motion has been regained.

Indications for open reduction and internal fixation include displaced articular fractures involving more than one-fourth of the articular surface; comminuted or displaced fractures; volar lip fractures, which can cause subsequent subluxation or block flexion; and dorsal avulsion fractures, which include the insertion of the central slip into the base of the middle phalanx. An accurate, anatomic reduction is imperative for maximal return of function and motion of this tight-fitting hinged joint. Reduction may not be possible in massively comminuted fractures; in these cases, nonoperative treatment with early motion is encouraged.

The PIP joint is exposed through a long midlateral incision or through a dorsal curved incision centered at the flexion crease of the PIP joint laterally. The incision should curve in an arc proximally and distally to allow dorsal exposure, which gives optimal visualization of the fragments. The collateral ligament is exposed by making an oblique fiber-splitting incision anterior to the oblique retinacular ligament. The collateral ligament is then divided near its distal attachment. The articular surface is inspected and anatomically reduced. Pinning is done with one or two small, smooth Kirschner wires (Fig. 4). The collateral ligament, joint capsule, and oblique fibers are repaired using 4-0 Tycron sutures.

Postoperatively the finger is splinted in the fashion described for nonoperative treatment. Active isolated motion is initiated 3 weeks after surgery. Return to competition is allowed after 3 to 4 weeks, with a protected molded splint.

FRACTURE-DISLOCATIONS

Hyperextension of the PIP joint, often after a fall, is the most common method of dislocating this joint. The middle phalanx dislocates dorsally, rupturing the volar

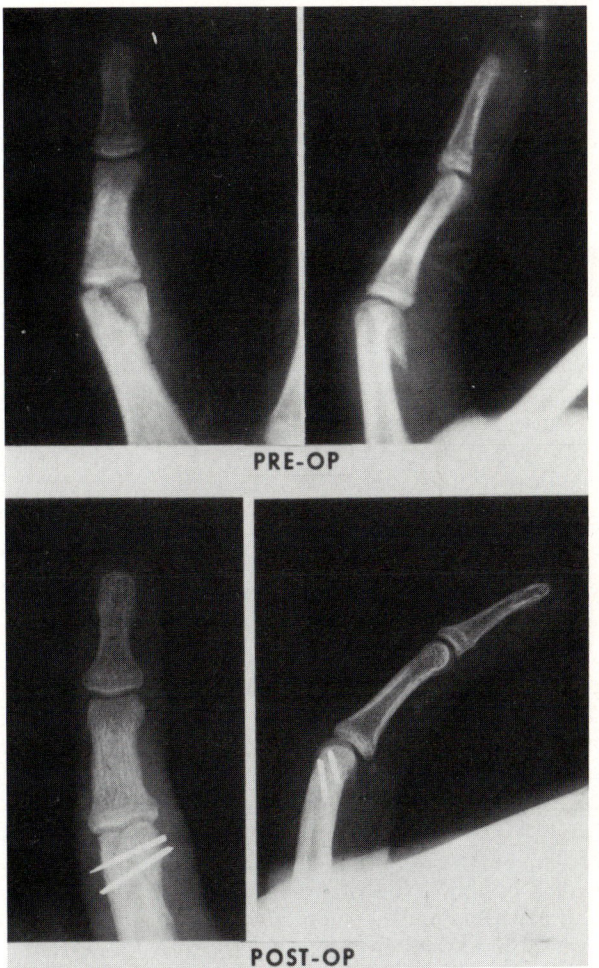

Figure 4 Open reduction and internal fixation of an intra-articular fracture of the proximal interphalangeal joint.

plate at its distal attachment. This occurs with or without a fracture of the volar lip at the base of the middle phalanx (Fig. 5).

Closed reduction of a dorsal dislocation without a concomitant fracture is usually quite stable. Occasionally, a volar subluxation with avulsion of the central slip of the extensor mechanism occurs. This injury usually requires open reduction, since the head of the proximal phalanx can be entrapped by the lateral band. Postoperatively the finger has to be held in extension to allow for healing of the repaired extensor mechanism.

When a fracture of the volar lip of the middle phalanx does occur, the buttressing effect of this fragment is lost. The volar fragment can vary widely in size and comminution. When the fragment is small enough not to impair stability of the joint, the finger may be splinted in 25 degrees of flexion with an extension block. Early active flexion exercises help prevent the onset of stiffness.

The stability of the joint may not be ascertained from the x-ray film alone. Once closed reduction has been accomplished, examination of the joint, under digital block, is necessary to determine stability. The collateral

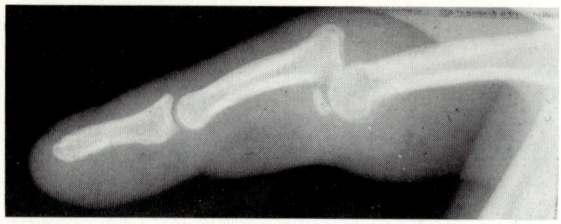

Figure 5 Dorsal dislocation of the proximal interphalangeal joint with a volar lip fracture.

ligaments must be tested to make certain they are intact and that the injury was not a lateral dislocation. In lateral dislocations, the collateral ligaments and volar plate are both torn. Treatment of these injuries depends on the stability of the joint after reduction. This may be accomplished in conjunction with stress radiography. Instability is an indication for open reduction, as is a large volar lip fragment. The volar lip fragment most often is larger at surgery than it appears on the radiograph.

A long midlateral approach is used, and the reticular portion of the fibrous flexor sheath, as well as part of the annular pulley, are excised to allow retraction of the flexor tendons. The volar plate is then detached to give maximal exposure to the volar lip fragments. Single fragments are pinned with a small, smooth K-wire. Multiple comminuted fragments are reduced with a loop of No. 34 wire, which is brought out dorsally and tied over a button. Even fragments that are devoid of soft tissue attachments are pinned when there is no significant evidence of avascular necrosis. A transarticular K-wire is used with the PIP joint flexed to 30 degrees, and the finger is then protected by a splint. Exercise is begun 3 weeks after open reduction, with the finger protected during athletics until complete pain-free motion is possible. In significantly comminuted and unstable fractures with associated dorsal dislocation, treatment by closed means may be best. A posterior flexion block is applied at the angle that prevents dorsal subluxation. When the acute reaction has abated, active flexion under close radiographic control can be carried out. Although the x-ray film may not show an anatomic positioning of the fragment, the functional result often is superior despite joint incongruity. Dorsal protection and early active exercises are also effective treatment in stable volar fractures to allow early return of motion.

BOUTONNIÈRE DEFORMITY

The classic boutonnière deformity consists of hyperextension of the metacarpophalangeal (MCP) joint, flexion of the PIP joint, and hyperextension of the DIP joint. The lesion is a disruption of the central slip from the dorsal lip of the middle phalanx. This disruption is most often due to a closed rupture of the extensor mechanism, and is the second most common closed tendon injury in athletes, after the jersey finger deformity.

The initial injury is usually due to blunt trauma, leaving a buttonhole-like split in the dorsal covering of the middle phalanx. The PIP joint herniates dorsally through the tear in the supporting central slip. The resulting deformity develops over time, especially in fingers in which the diagnosis is not made and that are either not splinted or splinted in flexion.

Early diagnosis is difficult after an acute injury with swelling, because the PIP joint naturally goes into 15 to 30 degrees of flexion. The inability to extend the joint is improperly attributed to pain and swelling, while in reality it is due to disruption of the extensor tendon. If the injury is truly a boutonnière deformity, there will be point tenderness over the dorsal lip of the middle phalanx.

If the finger is incorrectly splinted in flexion, there will be continued separation of the disrupted ends of the central slip and healing will be prevented. The natural course of the untreated boutonnière deformity is flexion of the PIP joint due to unopposed flexors, and contraction of the volarly displaced lateral bands and of the oblique retinacular ligaments.

Any PIP joint injury with an extension lag of more than 30 degrees and tenderness directly over the base of the middle phalanx should be treated as an acute extensor tendon rupture. The PIP joint is immobilized in full extension for at least 6 to 8 weeks, using a splint short enough to allow continued active and passive motion of the DIP joint. Splinting is continued during athletic competition until full pain-free flexion and maximal extension are possible. In injuries with restricted passive extension, correction with a safety pin splint is necessary before surgical reconstruction.

Surgical repair is indicated when an adequate trial of splinting does not control the deformity. Advancement of the central slip with reattachment to the dorsal lip of the middle phalanx is accomplished by direct repair through an S-shaped dorsal skin incision. A transarticular wire across the extended joint is used for 3 weeks in conjunction with an external splint. Additional protective splinting is used for competition until full pain-free motion is possible. Chronic boutonnière deformities have been corrected by a variety of methods, but results are not uniformly predictable.

PSEUDOBOUTONNIÈRE DEFORMITY

A hyperextension injury to the PIP joint can result in a disruption of the volar plate at its thin membranous proximal portion, leading to the formation of a pseudoboutonnière deformity. The volar plate is composed of a thin membranous proximal portion and a thick cartilaginous distal portion attached to the base of the middle phalanx. The volar plate can be injured when an extended finger is hyperextended, as when struck by a baseball, basketball, or football. The patient experiences acute onset of pain and swelling, with point tenderness over the volar aspect of the joint. X-ray films may reveal a small bony avulsion.

A pseudoboutonnière deformity can resemble a true

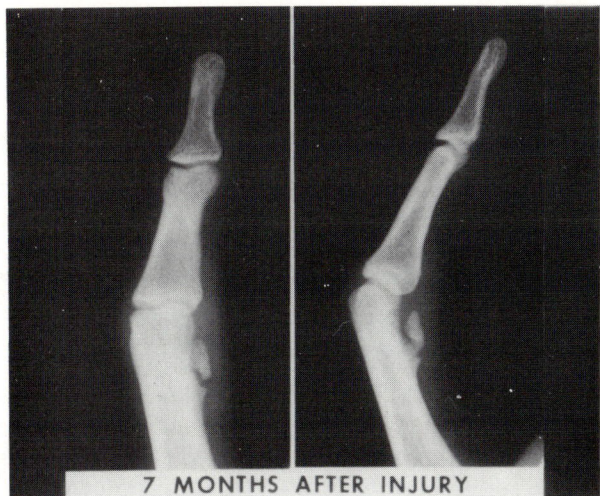

Figure 6 Pseudoboutonnière development with calcification at the distal end of the proximal phalanx.

boutonnière deformity, except that there is no disruption of the central slip. The diagnostic features of a pseudoboutonnière deformity include a flexion contracture of the PIP joint that is often resistant to passive flexion, slight hyperextension of the DIP joint, radiologic evidence of calcification at the distal end of the proximal phalanx, and a history of a hyperextension or twisting injury to the PIP joint. The little finger seems to be most commonly involved.

Initially after injury the flexion contracture of the PIP joint is less than 30 degrees, but when left untreated it slowly progresses. Radiographic evidence reveals that calcification often develops after 3 to 6 months. Calcification can progress to an osteophyte or a spur with an associated increase in flexion deformity, especially along the radial border (Fig. 6).

A mild deformity, less than 40 degrees of contracture, usually responds to safety pin splinting, used in conjunction with active and passive range-of-motion finger exercises. The points of pressure of the splint on the volar surface are the base of the distal phalanx and the distal palm. Progressive and continuous traction splinting is applied for 30 to 60 minutes, at least three times a day.

For injuries with a flexion contracture of greater than 45 degrees, surgical correction is usually necessary. Repair is accomplished through a midlateral incision,

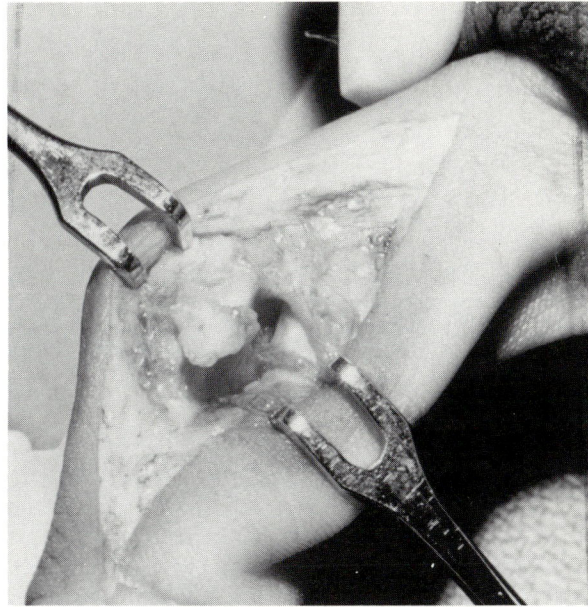

Figure 7 Operative findings in a pseudoboutonnière deformity including scarred volar plate and calcification.

and consists of release and distal advancement of the scarred proximal volar plate, excision of the bone spur or calcification, and release of the accessory collateral ligament (Fig. 7). The PIP joint is maintained in extension for 3 weeks by use of a transarticular K-wire in conjunction with an external splint.

SUGGESTED READING

McCue FC III, Andrew WF, Oh WY. Athletic injuries of the proximal interphalangeal joint: coach's finger. Contemp Orthop 1981; 6:516–525.

McCue FC III, Andrews JR, Gieck JH. The coach's finger. Sports Med 1974; 2:270–276.

McCue FC III, Hakala MW, Andrews JR, Gieck JH. Fractures and soft tissue injuries of the PIP joint. Contemp Surg 1974; 5:57–64.

McCue FC III, Honner R, Gieck JH, Andrews JR, Hakala M. A pseudo-boutonnière deformity. Hand J Br Soc Surg Hand 1975; 7:166–170.

McCue FC III, Honner R, Johnson MC, Gieck JH. Athletic injuries of the proximal interphalangeal joint requiring surgical treatment. J Bone Joint Surg 1970; 52A:937–956.

Schneider RC, Kennedy JC, Plant ML. Sports injuries: mechanisms, prevention and treatment. Baltimore: Williams & Wilkins, 1985:743.

METACARPAL FRACTURES

ARTHUR C. RETTIG, M.D.
GREGORY A. ROWDON, M.D.

The hand is particularly prone to injury during athletic endeavors and metacarpal (MC) fractures are one of the most common significant hand injuries seen in sports. In a 1 year period at the Methodist Sports Medicine Center, MC fractures represented 18% of all hand injuries and two-thirds of all hand injuries in basketball and football players.

Because energy absorption by the hand is usually low in athletic injuries, the fracture patterns are often relatively simple. Nonetheless, significant playing time can be lost and even a simple fracture may lead to permanent impairment of the digital performance due to malunion, joint stiffness, tendon adhesions, or other complications.

The primary goal of treatment is to achieve the most predictable complication-free method for fracture union, and to allow for the earliest safe return to play. The treating physician must be aware of the methods of managing each fracture pattern as well as the sport-specific needs of the athlete. This ensures that the proper course of treatment is chosen for both the patient's athletic career and future hand performance.

MECHANISM OF INJURY

Metacarpal fractures may occur through torque, angular, or compressive forces or a direct blow. A direct blow to the MC, such as a crush injury in football or hockey, usually results in a transverse fracture pattern in the mid-third of the MC. When a single MC is involved, support by adjacent tissue including metacarpals, interosseous muscles, and intermetacarpal ligaments provide stability. When a direct force is applied over a larger area, multiple metacarpals may be fractured, resulting in greater instability.

Indirect force to the MC head or the proximal phalanx may result in MC fractures. The most common indirect force injury is the axial loading injury, which occurs when the fist impacts an object, resulting in a MC neck fracture. Although this is termed the "boxer's fracture," the more common fracture in this situation involves the MC shaft.

Torsional forces applied to the proximal phalanx may result in spiral fractures of the MC. Malrotation may occur in spiral fractures due to shortening caused by extrinsic and intrinsic muscle tendon units. Oblique fractures of the MC may occur with simultaneous axial and torsional loading.

Attempts to prevent MC injuries in various sports have been made. The use of gloves in lacrosse and hockey and protective padding in football linemen help prevent direct-force injuries. Indirect forces with resulting fractures may still occur despite protective device wear.

PHYSICAL EXAMINATION

When examining the athlete with a suspected MC injury, the physician should look for points of maximum tenderness, any localized edema or crepitus over the MC area, and/or motion at the suspected fracture site. Each individual MC should be axially loaded to localize significant discomfort. Passive movement will ascertain range of motion (ROM) as well as any malrotation. Neurocirculatory status should be assessed including two point discrimination of each digit. If the examiner feels that the injury is in acceptable position and stable following initial assessment, a protective pad may be applied and the athlete returned to competition (if he or she desires). If malrotation, obvious crepitation, or instability exists, then a splint should be applied and x-ray films obtained. Ice and elevation should also be applied to the hand, although care must be taken not to compromise digital circulation with the application of ice.

RADIOGRAPHIC EXAMINATION

Minimal radiographs to adequately evaluate the hand for MC fractures include posteroanterior, lateral, and oblique views. Oblique views frequently enable the examiner to better visualize a long oblique fracture and assess its displacement. Specialized views are occasionally indicated. The Brewerton view provides better visualization of MC head and neck avulsion fractures. Magnification views are used in epiphyseal injuries in the very young athlete.

TREATMENT

Metacarpal Neck Fractures

Fractures of the MC neck are most commonly seen in axial loading injuries in which an object is struck with a clenched fist. The metacarpals have concave palmar surfaces that contribute to the longitudinal arch of the hand. Compressive loads to the MC head result in a fracture through its weakest point, the subcapital region proximal to the head. Dorsal angulation invariably occurs in these fractures due to the shape of the MC and the pull of the intrinsic musculature.

In MC neck fractures, the dorsal cortex fails in tension. The volar cortex fails in compression, usually accompanied by volar comminution. For this reason, closed reduction is frequently unsuccessful and the fracture tends to settle back to its original presentation.

Important considerations in the treatment of MC neck fractures include: (1) the MC involved, (2) the degree of angulation and/or rotation of the fracture, and (3) the prominence of the MC head in the palm.

A significant difference exists between the amount

of angulation acceptable in the ring and small finger and the amount that is acceptable in the index and long fingers. It is generally considered that an angulation of 40 to 50 degrees in the ring and small metacarpals is acceptable. Some authors, however, recommend reduction in the ring finger and small finger if the angulation is greater than 20 and 30 degrees, respectively. Angulation greater than 10 to 15 degrees in the index and long metacarpals is unacceptable. This discrepancy is due to the fact that there is more mobility in the carpometacarpal (CMC) joints in the fourth and fifth rays as opposed to that in the second and third.

Angulation may result in "clawing." The metacarpophalangeal (MCP) joint appears to be in neutral, but is actually hyperextended. This causes the central slip of the extensor mechanism to be inefficient in extending the proximal interphalangeal (PIP) joint, resulting in extensor lag at the PIP joint. Excessive volar prominence of the MC head in the palm may also result from a MC neck fracture. The greater the distance of the fracture site from the MCP the greater is the prominence in the palm.

Treatment of MC neck fractures, therefore, may be determined by the initial examination and x-ray film. If the clinical examination and x-ray criteria are acceptable (full digital ROM without evidence of clawing, malrotation, or prominence of the MC head in the palm), the fracture may be treated conservatively.

Conservative treatment involves the use of a short arm cast or simple hand-based orthoplast splint and buddy taping to the adjacent digit. Return to play is allowed when the athlete is comfortable and can perform the sport without significant difficulty. If the sport allows use of a playing cast or splint, return may be as early as 5 to 10 days (Fig. 1).

If the fracture is deemed unacceptable, attempts must be made to correct and maintain alignment. These options include closed reduction as recommended by Jahss, closed reduction and percutaneous pin fixation, or open reduction and internal fixation using K-wires, tension band wiring, or, in certain situations, a mini blade plate or intermedullary K-wire fixation.

In our experience closed reduction without fixation is very difficult to maintain due to the volar comminution that frequently accompanies these fractures. Our preferred method of treatment is closed reduction and percutaneous pin fixation involving either fixation to the adjacent MC or crossed K-wire fixation (Fig. 2). The pins may be buried deep into the skin and, in certain situations, the athlete may participate with the pins in place. In other cases, the patient must remain out of the sport until the pins are removed.

When closed reduction cannot be achieved, open reduction and internal fixation (ORIF) is indicated. Soft tissue interposition, usually involving periosteum and occasionally extensor tendon, may occur, and is an absolute indication for ORIF. When this occurs, particularly with accompanying volar comminution, tension band wiring is our treatment of choice (Fig. 3).

Fractures of the Metacarpal Shaft

Shaft fractures of the MC may be divided into transverse, oblique or spiral oblique, and comminuted. Usually the forces involved in athletic trauma are not great enough to produce comminuted fractures. Treatment of shaft fractures of the MC in the athlete depends upon: (1) fracture location and configuration, (2) degree of displacement, and (3) the number of metacarpals involved.

Transverse shaft fractures result from either a direct blow (as from a helmet) or an indirect axial load (as seen

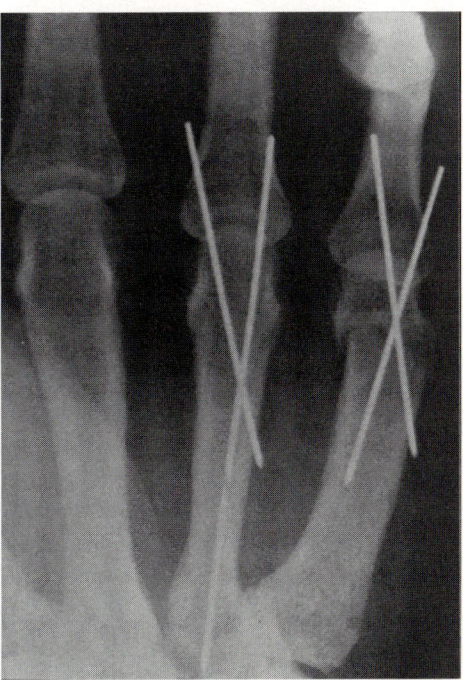

Figure 2 Closed reduction using Jahss maneuver and percutaneous crossed pins. (From Stern PJ. Fractures of the metacarpals and phalanges. In: Green DP, ed. Operative hand surgery, ed. 3, New York, 1993, Churchill Livingstone; with permission.)

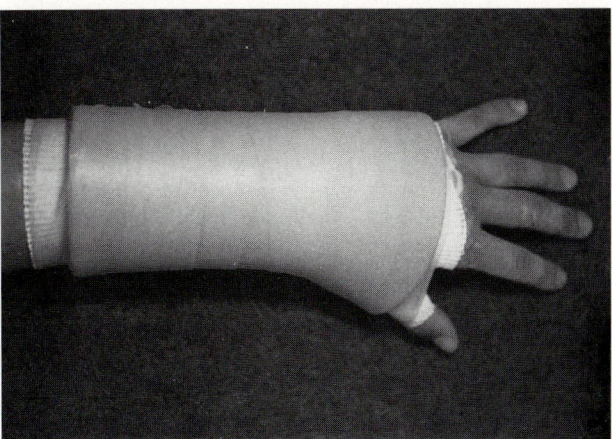

Figure 1 RTV11 Playing cast.

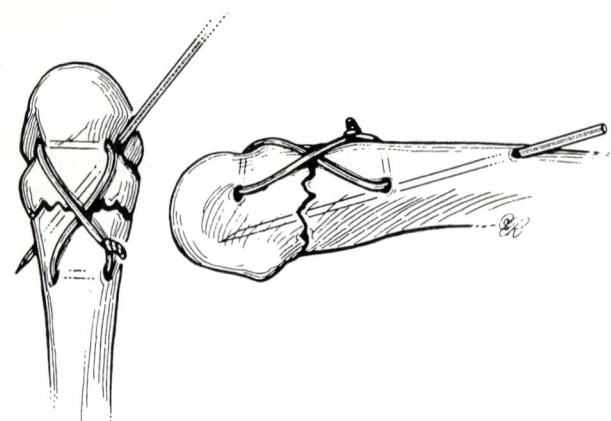

Figure 3 Tension band wiring and single Kirschner pin fixation of a metacarpal neck fracture. (From Stern PJ. Fractures of the metacarpals and phalanges. In: Green DP, ed. Operative hand surgery, ed. 3, New York, 1993, Churchill Livingstone; with permission.)

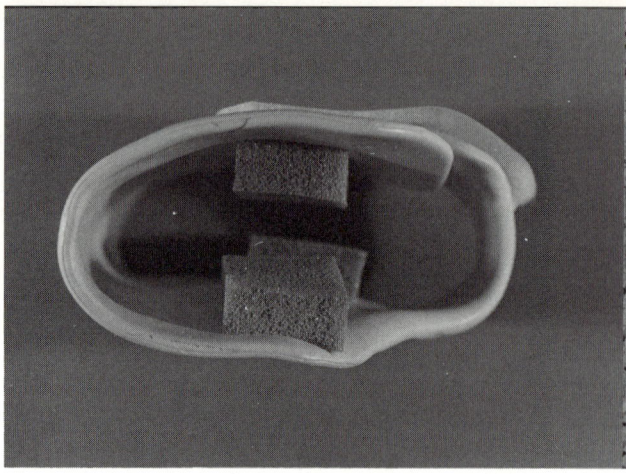

Figure 4 Hand-based orthoplast splint with 3-point fixation.

in a boxer). Angulation considerations are similar to MC neck fractures. However, generally less angulation is acceptable due to the greater distance of the fracture from the MCP joint. Stern states that angulation in excess of 30 degrees and 20 degrees in the small and ring fingers, respectively, and any angulation in the long and index fingers should be considered for reduction.

Oblique and spiral shaft fractures frequently result in malrotation of the digit. Five degrees of malrotation in the MC fracture may cause 1.5 cm of digital overlap. Opgrande and Westphal have stated that 1 degree of MC shaft rotation may produce 5 degrees of rotation at the tip of the digit. Malrotation is best judged clinically and should be assessed by having the patient simultaneously flex all his digits.

Fracture shortening of up to 5 mm is acceptable according to Burkhalter. Freeland et al state that a shortening greater than 3 to 4 mm leads to clawing due to weakening of the intrinsic musculature and should be corrected. If no significant clawing or extensor lag exists on clinical examination, the amount of shortening is probably acceptable.

Treatment decisions depend on the physical examination and presenting x-rays. If the patient has no clawing, minimal shortening or malrotation, and x-ray films show satisfactory alignment, conservative treatment is recommended.

Conservative treatment for MC shaft fractures involves initial use of a short arm cast or hand-based orthoplast splint attempting to incorporate three point fixation into the splint (Fig. 4). The digit involved is buddy taped to the adjacent digit to enhance stability during the early period of treatment. The Galveston brace has been proposed for use in stable MC fractures. Complications of skin necrosis with its use have been reported, although a similar splint incorporating the three point fixation concept is frequently used.

Rettig et al found that 82% of MC shaft fractures occurring in athletic trauma were stable and amenable to conservative treatment. Overall time lost from sport in these stable fractures was 12.3 days. Average time lost in football was 10.6 days and from basketball was 19.8 days.

In sports where playing casts are permitted and do not significantly interfere with performance, the athlete may return to practice and competition when comfortable. In college and professional football, any type of cast covered with closed cell foam padding is allowed. In high-school athletics, rigid devices are not permitted. We have utilized semi-rigid (silicone rubber) playing casts (Fig. 1). These have protected the injury well, allowed no change in the fracture position, and caused no injury.

In transverse fractures in which the angulation or physical examination is unacceptable, operative treatment is indicated. Closed reduction and percutaneous pinning, either to the adjacent MC or by cross pinning, may be utilized. In situations where rapid return to play is desired and unsplinted hand function is necessary, more rigid internal fixation using a dorsal 2.7 mm Dynamic Compression Plate or neutralization plate may be utilized.

It is well documented in the literature that internal fixation using plate and screws is superior to other forms of fixation with regard to bending and rotational stresses. Black et al have shown that plate and screw fixation with satisfactory volar cortical apposition results in stability approaching that of normal bone.

Spiral oblique fractures are common in sports and occur secondary to indirect loading of the metacarpals either through the proximal phalanx or MC head. A twisting or torsional mechanism is usually present. Spiral oblique fractures often present with shortening and malrotation and should be evaluated similarly to transverse fractures.

If the initial presentation of the spiral oblique fracture is acceptable, functional treatment is employed similar to that with transverse fractures. If excessive shortening or malrotation is present, we proceed with ORIF. If the fracture surface is greater than twice the diameter of the shaft of the MC, then 2.0 or 2.7 mm interfragmentary screws may be utilized. If the fracture surface is less than two times the diameter, an interfragmentary screw and dorsal neutralization plate is recommended. Once rigid fixation is employed, early ROM may be instituted and a return to play is possible as tolerated. In our 1989 series, 9% of fractures underwent ORIF using plates and screws. All healed primarily and the average return to play was 13.6 days.

Stability in multiple MC fractures is directly related to the number of metacarpals involved. This is due in part to the lack of support of an adjacent intact MC. In cases where fractures of the central two (long and ring) metacarpals are minimally displaced, treatment may be conservative. Except in the above case, multiple MC fractures are frequently unstable and require internal fixation.

Metacarpal Fractures of the Thumb

Metacarpal fractures of the thumb occur in the shaft, base, and proximal articular surface. Shaft fractures are uncommon because of the lack of firm fixation of the proximal portion of the MC. Also, stress is usually well tolerated by the strong cortical MC shaft and dissipated by the soft cancellous bone at its base. Proximal shaft fractures or fractures through the MC base are usually transverse or oblique. Deforming forces include the abductor pollicis longus, the flexor pollicis brevis distally, and the adductor pollicis proximally. These forces result in fracture angulation with the apex pointing dorsally and the distal fracture fragment being adducted, flexed, and, according to Burton and Eaton, supinated.

Due to the abundant motion of the trapezium MC-joint, angulation up to 30 degrees is acceptable. If the angulation is greater than 30 degrees a compensatory hyperextension at the MCP joint will be present and correction of the deformity should be attempted. If angulation is acceptable, conservative treatment may be employed, and a short arm thumb spica cast applied. A playing splint or cast may be utilized, and return to play is possible when comfortable. If angulation is unacceptable, the fracture is usually amenable to closed reduction and percutaneous pin fixation. This is our treatment of choice. Again, with adequate protection, return to play is possible within 2 to 3 weeks.

Intra-articular fractures at the base of the thumb are common in sports. Bennett's fracture is due to an adduction stress of the first MC and is frequently seen in the throwing hand of a quarterback as it strikes a helmet during follow through. This injury is actually a fracture/subluxation of the basilar joint of the thumb. A volar lip fragment that is attached to the trapezium by means of the beak ligament is usually present. The remaining MC base displaces and subluxes radially, proximally, and dorsally.

Physical examination findings consist of swelling and tenderness at the base of the first MC joint, and frequently, subluxation of the joint is demonstrated on examination. Radiographs as described by Billing and Gedda are obtained to get a true lateral view of the joint. Goals of treatment in Bennett's fracture/subluxation

are to restore stability of the CMC joint and to restore articular congruity of the thumb MC base. Closed reduction is usually possible in these fractures by abducting and pronating the thumb. When possible, closed reduction with percutaneous pin fixation is the treatment of choice, particularly when the fragment is less than 15% to 20% of the articular surface. In larger fragments, ORIF utilizing a 2.7 mm interfragmentory 4.0 cancellous screw has been advocated.

Return to play after a Bennett's fracture depends on the sport, position played, and the method of treatment. Return to play in a protective playing cast may be possible as early as 2 to 3 weeks if percutaneous pinning is performed. Cancellous bone generally takes approximately 3 weeks for healing to occur, and after this period it is probably safe. If rigid internal fixation is utilized, return to play may be sooner, particularly if protective splinting is possible. In the throwing arm of a quarterback or in other sports requiring full use of the hand, a minimum of 6 to 8 weeks out of play is necessary so healing can occur followed by hand rehabilitation.

Metacarpal Fractures in Boxers

Shaft fractures of the MC are common injuries in boxing. Melone has studied this injury in over 100 professional fighters and recommends that no shortening should be accepted in these fractures. He recommends fixing the fracture in anatomic position with percutaneous pinning to the adjacent MC. This percutaneous technique eliminates the dorsal scarring, which may be a significant problem in boxers who incur repetitive trauma to the dorsum of the hand.

Melone recommends that no return to pugilistic activities be permitted until the pins are removed and solid union has occurred. The average return to boxing in his experience is greater than 3 months after injury.

RECOMMENDATIONS

Our approach to the athlete with a MC fracture is to decide if the fracture position is acceptable and stable at the initial examination. If this occurs, the treatment is conservative using a resting splint or cast and a return to sport allowed in a playing cast where possible. This results in a return to play at an average of 12 to 13 days from the time of injury. In football where a protective splint may be utilized, the average return is 10 days whereas in basketball the average is 19 days.

If the fracture is felt to be unstable and the position unacceptable, we recommend fixation with as rigid a device as possible to permit early ROM and rehabilitation. The average return to sport in patients fixed by this technique is 14 days.

SUGGESTED READING

Amadio PC, et al. Fractures of the hand and wrist. In: Jupiter JB, ed: Flynn's hand surgery. ed 4, Baltimore, 1991, Williams & Wilkins.

Belsole RJ, Greene TL. Comparative strengths of internal fixation. Hand Surg 1985; 10A:315.

Billing L, Gedda KO. Roentgen examination of Bennett's fracture. ACTA Radiol 1952; 28:471-476.

Black D, et al. Comparison of internal fixation techniques in metacarpal fractures. J Hand Surgery 1985; 10A:466-472.

Burkhalter WE. Hand fractures instructional course lectures, 1990; 34:249-253.

De Carlo M, et al. Perfecting a playing cast for hand and wrist injuries. Phys Sports Med 1992; 20:7.

Freeland AE, Jabaley ME, Hughes CL. Stable fixation of the hand and wrist. New York, 1986, Springer-Verlag.

Hastings H II. Management of extraarticular fractures of the phalanges and metacarpals. In Strickland JW, Rettig AC, eds: Hand injuries in athletes. Philadelphia, 1992, WB Saunders.

Hastings H II. Unstable metacarpal and phalangeal fracture treatment with screws and plates. Clin Orthop 1987; 214:37.

Jahss SA. Fractures of the metacarpals: A new method of reduction and immobilization. J Bone Joint Surg 1938; 20:178.

Melone CP, ed. Hand injuries in boxing. New York, 1993, CRC Press.

Opgrande JD, Westphal SA. Fractures of the hand. Orthop Clin North Amer 1983; 14:779-792.

Posner MA. Injuries to the hand and wrist in athletes. Orthop Clin North Am 1977; 8:593-618.

Rettig AC, Ryan RO, Stone JA. Epidemiology of hand injuries in sports. In: Strickland JW, Rettig AC, eds. Hand injuries in athletes. Philadelphia, 1992, WB Saunders.

Rettig AC, et al. Metacarpal fractures in the athlete. Am J Sports Med 1989; 17:567-572.

Stern PJ. Fractures of the metacarpals and phalanges. In: Green DP, ed. Operative hand surgery. ed 3. New York, 1993, Churchill Livingstone.

ACUTE ULNAR COLLATERAL LIGAMENT RUPTURE OF THE METACARPOPHALANGEAL JOINT OF THE THUMB

LEWIS B. LANE, M.D.

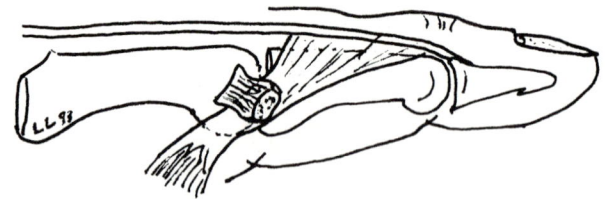

Figure 1 *A,* In the normal, uninjured, state the ulnar collateral ligament lies deep to the adductor expansion and the extensor hood. *B,* With a complete rupture the ulnar collateral ligament can lie outside of the adductor expansion and the extensor hood creating a Stener lesion, diagrammed here.

Injury to the ulnar collateral ligament (UCL) of the metacarpophalangeal (MCP) joint of the thumb is extremely common in sports. This is due, in large part, to the vulnerability of the UCL at the base of the unprotected lever arm of the proximal phalanx. The degree of injury depends on the magnitude and direction of the injuring force and the unique anatomy of the ulnar aspect of the MCP joint of the thumb.

ANATOMICAL CONSIDERATIONS

The thumb MCP joint is similar to other hand ginglymus (hinge) joints in that it has a palmar plate, dorsal capsule, flexor and extensor tendons, and two collateral ligaments. It is unique in that one ligament, the UCL, when completely avulsed, usually lies proximal to and/or outside of the adductor pollicis expansion and the extensor hood (Fig. 1). This phenomenon, called a *Stener lesion*, prevents the UCL from healing spontaneously, and requires surgical treatment. Conversely, when the UCL is not fully avulsed or outside the extensor hood, nonoperative treatment is usually successful.

DIAGNOSIS

Two factors are crucial in accurately diagnosing and subsequently treating UCL injuries. First, the degree of injury must be determined, and then an acute injury must be distinguished from a chronic or an acute-on-chronic injury.

Like other collateral ligament injuries, there are three grades of injury. Grade I is defined as no change in ligamentous stability, Grade II as some loss of stability but not gross instability, and Grade III as complete rupture of the UCL. Dorsal capsular tears and/or palmar plate tears may be present but usually do not require specific and separate treatment.

An accurate diagnosis of UCL injury usually can be based on physical examination alone. The degree of swelling, discoloration, ecchymosis, tenderness, and deformity should be assessed and recorded. The severity of injury generally correlates with the degree of these physical findings. A Grade I injury may have significant tenderness, but usually has minimal swelling or ecchymosis. A Grade II injury may have more, while in a Grade III injury ecchymosis often extends into the thenar eminence and first web space while swelling may extend over the dorsum of the hand. When the avulsed stump of the UCL is palpable on the ulnar side of the metacarpal head it usually is diagnostic of a Stener lesion, a Grade III rupture.

Stress testing of the UCL, the most important part of the exam, is done to measure the degree of opening of the UCL and to assess the amount of associated pain. First, the MCP joint must be flexed 30 degrees to relax the palmar plate. Otherwise, the palmar plate, tight in extension, would stabilize the joint and mask a UCL rupture. The ulnar side of the thumb MCP joint is cautiously stressed and the amount of angulation, in degrees, is recorded. (The examiner must measure from directly dorsally, not obliquely, otherwise the amount of ulnar deviation would be increased artificially by misinterpreting flexion as ulnar deviation.) The injured thumb is compared to the contralateral side. The radial collateral ligament (RCL) of each thumb is also stress tested and results recorded.

When findings are unclear to the examiner, or if the exam is too painful, the exam should be repeated under median and radial nerve wrist block. A note of caution: the stress test must be done carefully and under control so as not to increase the degree of injury. Further caution: nondisplaced avulsion fractures should not be stress tested at all, or with extreme care, so as not to convert a nondisplaced fracture, treated by casting, into a displaced one needing surgery.

If uncertainty still exists, stress x-rays should be obtained. It is important to have a knowledgeable professional stress the thumb when the x-rays are taken as patient-performed studies leave much to chance. The two sides are compared and angulation measured. Radial subluxation of the proximal phalanx across the metacarpal head, measured and compared to the opposite side, also correlates with the degree of injury.

Routine x-rays must be taken to determine if a fracture is present. The common types of fracture are large avulsion fractures (often Salter III epiphyseal injuries), either displaced or nondisplaced, and comminuted fractures. When fracture fragments are seen widely displaced from the base of the proximal phalanx, they are almost always indicative of a Stener lesion. Severely comminuted or large shear fractures at the base of the proximal phalanx also occur, but they are outside the scope of this chapter and will not be addressed here.

X-rays are also of value if they show a palmar subluxation of the proximal phalanx on the metacarpal head. Since the UCL arises from the dorsal portion of the metacarpal head and inserts on the mid and palmar portion of the proximal phalanx, it has the additional function of preventing palmar subluxation and supination of the proximal phalanx. The dorsal capsule also contributes to dorsal stability. Thus, if there has been a rupture of the dorsal capsule and the UCL, the x-rays may show palmar subluxation of the proximal phalanx. This finding may help in formulating the correct diagnosis.

The diagnosis is then made based on all the findings. If the injured UCL is as stable as the contralateral one,

if there is a definite end-point to stress testing, and if there is limited swelling and ecchymosis, then a Grade I injury is diagnosed. If the hand is ecchymotic and swollen, if there is much pain, and if the stress test is markedly positive with no solid end-point, then a Grade III injury is present. The difficulty arises with the in-between cases when the findings are more subtle and less clearly discernible. In these situations, the most important single factor is the stress test with x-ray documentation, if necessary.

Though the criteria for grading UCL injuries are somewhat controversial, the following is fairly well accepted. A Grade III rupture is defined as laxity of the UCL in excess of 35 degrees and/or 15 degrees greater than the contralateral thumb. Certainly if there is also an identifiable Stener lesion, and/or no solid end-point to the stress testing, and/or a widely displaced fracture, the injury is classified as Grade III. A Grade I injury is one in which the UCL remains stable. A Grade II injury is, by default, everything in-between.

It is very important to distinguish between Grade II and Grade III, as the treatment for Grade II injuries is nonoperative, while that for Grade III is surgical. Great care, therefore, must be taken when performing the physical examination and reviewing x-rays to make the correct diagnosis. Attention must be paid to the subtleties of the laxity on one side compared to the other. The examiner should repeat the stress test several times on each side so as to discern even a few degrees difference and the quality of the end-point. With the correct diagnosis made, the patient can then be properly advised and the optimal treatment appropriately undertaken.

A note about chronic and acute-on-chronic UCL instability is needed. Here again, an accurate diagnosis is crucial as the treatment for chronic and acute-on-chronic Grade III instability is quite different from that for acute instability. The most significant distinction in chronic and acute-on-chronic cases is the paucity or unimpressive nature of physical findings. Typically, an individual not recalling any previous injury will describe a recent injury, a fall while skiing for example, and have gross instability but remarkably little tenderness or swelling. One should not be mislead by the history of recent injury into treating this patient as an acute Grade III rupture.

TREATMENT

Grade I and II

Grade I and II injuries are best treated nonoperatively. Immediately after injury both should be treated with cold application and elevation to control the initial pain and swelling. Immobilization in a thumb spica splint should be instituted as soon as possible for pain control while allowing other activities of daily living (ADL).

A Grade I injury can be mobilized as soon as the patient is comfortable. In the mildest cases a splint may not be needed at all, but for most injuries 1 to 3 weeks in a splint, weaned as ADLs are increased, is best.

Occasionally, pain lingers for an extended period, and patients are reluctant to remove their splints. In these cases it is not unusual to continue the splint for 6 weeks and then to require an aggressive hand rehabilitation program.

For sports, figure-of-eight taping allows protected use, as does a flexible orthosis. A rigid orthosis is required for high energy or impact sports. Certainly, the needs of and demands on the patient must be carefully considered. The orthosis must support the MCP joint and protect the UCL. Many different orthoses are used. I prefer a dorsal, hand based orthosis that is mounted from the ulnar side of the palm, across the dorsum, and around the thenar eminence. Distally the orthosis extends to the interphalangeal (IP) joint of the thumb yet leaves the fingers free for full motion (Fig. 2). A thenar/thumb cone can also be used, but its smaller size often provides less support of the UCL and MCP joint.

A Grade II injury has increased instability but not a complete rupture. Immobilization for 3 to 4 weeks is needed for ligament healing. Although thumb spica casting traditionally has been recommended, recent reports encourage using a removable orthosis. When the pain is great, however, it may be better to cast in a thumb spica for 2 to 4 weeks and then convert to an orthosis. About 4 weeks after injury, depending on symptoms, a progressive mobilization program should be started. Strengthening is needed but the ulnar side of the thumb must not be overstressed in order to protect the healing UCL. Continued use of the orthosis up to 12 weeks after injury is prudent for impact sports/high energy thumb uses. As some ligament instability often remains after Grade II injuries, regardless of the duration of immobilization, the patient needs to be fully advised of the lasting nature of the instability and the possibility of lingering symptoms.

Grade III

Complete rupture of the UCL is best treated by surgical repair, especially if there is a Stener lesion, because the extensor hood becomes a barrier between the ligament and the proximal phalanx and obstructs direct healing. Although cast treatment has been advocated in the past for this injury, its proponents are becoming fewer and fewer. This is especially so as patients more frequently undergo surgery under regional anesthesia on an ambulatory basis and have better results with a more rapid return to their previous activity level.

Surgery should be undertaken as soon as feasible, although immediate repair is not mandatory. If there is a great deal of swelling, elevation, cold application, and splinting may be employed until the swelling subsides. Furthermore, even late treatment delayed weeks or months after injury has been reported with good results, as long as the UCL can be identified, preserved, and utilized for repair.

At surgery, the patient is positioned supine with the injured arm abducted on a surgical armboard. Regional block anesthesia is often sufficient, but in young or

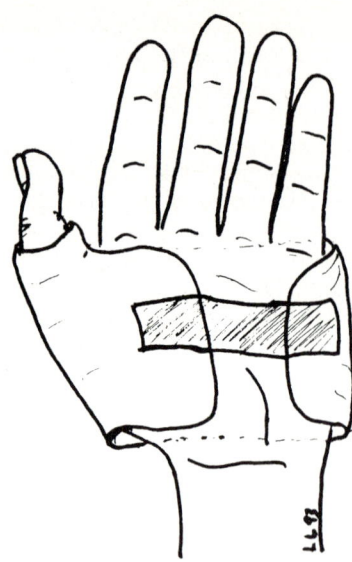

Figure 2 A hand-mounted thumb spica orthosis protects the ulnar collateral ligament by immobilizing the metacarpophalangeal joint, but is small enough to allow motion of the wrist, fingers, and thumb interphalangeal joint.

unsettled patients, general anesthesia may be more advisable. The surgeon should sit on the "dorsal" side of the arm. The incision is drawn along the ulnar mid-axis of the proximal phalanx and, at the UCL, extends obliquely in a dorsal, proximal, and radial direction to the radial edge of the extensor pollicis longus (EPL) tendon. Just before making the incision, the pneumatic tourniquet should be inflated.

After making the incision, dissection is carried down to the layer of the extensor hood. It is best to spread with scissors, in order to identify the dorsal branch(es) of the radial nerve. Small twigs may be divided, but one or two 1.0 mm to 2.0 mm branches are frequently encountered, usually at the deep aspect of the subcutaneous layer. These branches should be preserved and treated gently because, if cut or vigorously retracted, they may develop painful neuromas or become annoyingly dysesthetic.

The extensor hood is exposed and the area of injury examined. The proximal edge of the extensor hood is usually distinct. If the injury is quite recent, the UCL should be readily indentifiable just under or proximal to the hood. If surgery is delayed, organizing reactive tissue will obscure the UCL and the proximal edge of the hood. To expose this area and the ulnar side of the MCP joint, the extensor hood should be incised just palmar to the EPL tendon. Be sure to leave a 1.0 mm cuff of tissue to which to repair the hood at closure. Also, the most distal 1.0 cm of the hood should not be incised, but, rather, left intact. The hood should be sharply dissected off the underlying tissue and reflected palmarly. This layer is paper thin and is easily perforated; particular care is required. The ulnar side of the metacarpal head, MCP joint, and proximal phalanx is now exposed. The surgeon must first identify the proximal portion of the UCL, any remaining ligament cuff distally, any fracture fragments, and the joint capsule, and then inspect the joint, bone margin, palmar plate, and soft tissues. Debris should be removed, but strong organizing connective tissue on the proximal phalanx must be preserved as often it is the tissue to which the UCL is sutured.

At this point the decision must be made about which repair method to employ. Obviously, the type of repair is dependent on the type of rupture. The simplest rupture is one in which there is a healthy remant of UCL cuff remaining on the base of the proximal phalanx. If so, the UCL is sutured directly with several interrupted sutures. I prefer three or four 2-0 braided polyester sutures. A small, stout cutting needle makes suture placement straightforward. If the repair is secure, and it usually is, no transfixing wire is inserted across the joint.

If there is a single large avulsed bone fragment, anatomic reduction and internal fixation is best. After clearing debris, the fragment is reduced, and then pinned with one or two 0.035 inch smooth K-wire(s) (my preference) or tension banded with 26 gauge wire. Placement of a temporary transfixtion wire across the joint can be justified in this situation as the security of the fixation of the fragment is often unpredictable.

The most difficult rupture to repair is one in which there is no soft tissue on the proximal phalax to which to suture. This occurs either after a comminuted avulsion fracture that leaves a sizable bony defect or after the ligament is totally stripped off the proximal phalanx. The problem is solved by securely attaching the avulsed UCL to the proximal phalanx. There are many techniques described in the literature, and each, of course, has its own rationale. I will describe the four techniques that I favor and explain the weaknesses I see in the traditional pull-out suture method (Fig. 3).

The goal of treatment is to achieve the most secure and reliable repair that will most safely and rapidly return the patient to full activities. When there is no ligament cuff to suture to directly, the surgeon either must "find" some tissue to which to suture or must somehow attach the ligament to the bone. The first and simplest substitute is the periosteum of the proximal phalanx. Usually it will not hold sutures and can not be used. However, if sufficient time has elapsed since the injury, a robust layer of organizing fibrous tissue may develop that is strong enough to accept and hold sutures, thus permitting direct reattachment.

The second method (my preferred method) is suturing the UCL to the tendinous insertion of the adductor pollicis onto the proximal phalanx. Anatomically this structure lies immediately palmar to the normal point of attachment of the UCL. The adductor pollicis is robust and will hold several sutures. Before suturing, the UCL must be mobilized from its recoiled and often fibrosed bed alongside the metacarpal head, pulled out to length, and tested to see if it reaches the proximal phalanx. If not, gentle dissection on the undersurface of the ligament usually frees it up enough so that it will reach the proximal phalanx. Care must be taken not to suture the ligament too far palmarly; therefore, the placement of the sutures is done with close attention to the three-dimensional relationships of the various structures. The sutures are not tied until they are all inserted.

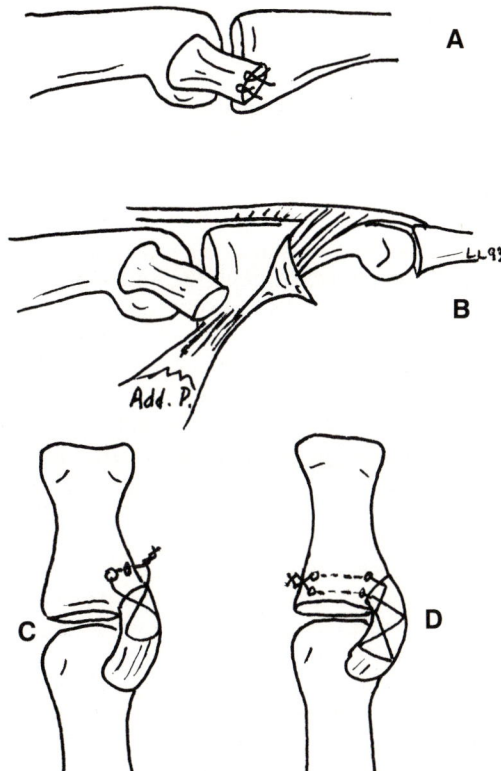

Figure 3 *A,* The ulnar collateral ligament can be sutured to fibrous tissue on the ulnar side of the proximal phalanx if it is strong enough to hold the sutures and provide stability. *B,* The tendinous insertion of the adductor pollicis into the proximal phalanx is immediately distal and palmar to the normal ulnar collateral ligament insertion. The ulnar collateral ligament can be reattached with several interrupted sutures. *C,* The ulnar collateral ligament can be reattached with a figure-of-eight suture or wire. This technique is particularly useful for a large single bone avulsion fragment. *D,* The traditional "pull-out" suture technique can be modified into a "pull-through" technique that securely fixes the ligament to bone, thus allowing an early mobilization program.

(Most often I use three or four 2-0 braided polyester sutures.) The thumb is then ulnarly deviated to reduce the ligament and the sutures tied beginning with the most palmar one. Once the sutures are tied, dramatic restoration of stability should be noted. If not, the surgeon must determine why it hasn't and must correct the problem.

The main theoretical flaw in this method is that the UCL might be shifted too far palmarly. Ways to avoid this include splaying out the dorsal portion of the ligament when placing the most dorsal suture, and suturing the dorsal edge of the UCL to the palmar edge of the dorsal capsule. This latter technique should always be employed during closure as capsular repair with light reabsorbable sutures is recommended for all cases. The greatest value of the adductor pollicis technique is that it gives immediate and reliable fixation with several sutures, does not require temporary K-wire fixation, and allows early mobilization.

The other two techniques I recommend are both variants of the traditional pull-out method. In the first method, two drill holes are made (0.035 or 0.045 inch smooth K-wires work well for this) in the metaphysis at the upper and lower margins of the UCL insertion. A wire or nonreabsorbable suture is weaved in a figure-of-eight through the ligament and beneath the bone bridge, and then tied securing the ligament to the bone. The second technique starts by weaving a modified Bunnell pull-out suture through the ligament. Two drill holes are made across the proximal phalanx from the UCL insertion to the opposite cortex. A small incision is made on the radial side of the proximal phalanx and the exiting drill holes are exposed by blunt dissection. The suture tails are passed through the proximal phalanx and tied snugly against the radial cortex as the ligament is held against the bone.

The greatest disadvantage of these latter two techniques is that each relies on a single suture. Obviously, if the single suture or wire breaks, postoperative mobilization must be slowed to prevent recurrence of laxity, and ligament stability must be carefully monitored. Their greatest theoretical advantage is that the ligament is replaced anatomically, although my experience has not shown the bone suture technique to be superior to the adductor pollicis technique.

In the traditional pull-out suture method, a single Bunnell pull-out suture in the UCL is passed through the proximal phalanx and tied over a button on the radial side of the thumb while the joint is held with a transfixing K-wire for 4 weeks. There are several disadvantages with this technique. First, the suture is tied over a button outside the skin, and this permits some laxity due to the compressibility of the soft tissues. Second, a K-wire is needed to hold the joint to protect the pull-out suture, and this delays mobilization. The K-wire may also become infected, back out or advance too deeply, or be difficult to remove. Third, the pull-out suture can break, and fixation would be lost. Fourth, the pull-out suture can be tied too tightly, and this would cause compression necrosis of the underlying skin. Fifth, if a synthetic monofilament pull-out suture is used and if mobilization is initiated with the suture still in place, the suture can stretch causing fixation to become less secure.

Regardless of the repair technique chosen, the capsule and extensor hood are closed with reabsorbable suture. After the skin is closed and the wound dressed, a light thumb spica cast is applied. It must protect the ulnar side of the MCP joint. The cast should be short both proximally to allow some wrist motion and distally so thumb IP joint flexion and extension can be begun immediately.

AFTERCARE

If direct suture was performed, the cast should be removed 10 to 14 days postoperatively and a rehabilitation program initiated. Until 4 weeks postoperatively, rehabilitation should concentrate mainly on flexion/extension of the thumb ray and cautious circumduction.

If an avulsion fracture was pinned, the cast should be maintained for 4 weeks. At 4 weeks a more aggressive program is undertaken with strengthening and passive flexion/extension, if necessary. As has been reported, patients treated by this surgical and rehabilitation protocol have returned to their previous level of sport activity faster than those treated by traditional methods.

As soon as the cast is removed, the patient must use a hand-mounted thumb spica orthosis. This both protects the healing ligament and allows the patient to begin ADLs immediately. While low stress use of the hand out of the splint can be initiated after cast removal, increasing ADLs must be customized for each patient based on the clinical picture and on the demands of activities and sports. For example, running, swimming, tennis (if the injured hand is used only for the toss), skating, and soccer usually can be begun immediately with the hand in the splint. For some athletes skiing, football (offensive line), and sailing with the hand in the splint might be permissible early on. However, high stress/impact sports (paticularly those involving the injured hand) may need to be postponed for up to 6 to 12 weeks even when the patient wears the protective orthosis. Above all, patients must be cautioned that ligament rerupture can occur, especially in the first 3 months postoperatively, and that a protective splint must be worn appropriately during this period. If the patient wishes to return to high impact sports sooner, a warning about the risk of rerupture must be clearly stated.

OUTCOME

The results of treatment of UCL injuries reported in the literature are consistently good. If stability is restored, most patients return to their original level of function and regain all, or nearly all, of their strength. Some motion is often lost, but since there is such a wide range of thumb motion in different individuals, it is probably not significant. Strength and ligament stability are better prognosticators of overall result. Functional success and the rapidity of return to sports appear to correlate with initiating rehabilitation early in the postinjury course.

PREVENTION

Since the hand in general and the thumb in particular are so exposed during sports, it is not at all surprising that UCL injuries occur frequently. There has been an increasing awareness of the vulnerability of the UCL of the thumb MCP joint among players, trainers, coaches, parents, and even the sports industry as a whole. New ski gloves and a range of ski poles have been designed with the goal of reducing the frequency of UCL injury. Recent reports indicate that little headway has been made, however. It would seem, therefore, that the primary burden falls on physicians, therapists, trainers, coaches, and others to promptly recognize and treat UCL injuries, to provide close follow-up, and to wisely counsel patients in rehabilitation and the return to sports and ADLs.

SUGGESTED READING

Bostock S, Morris MA. The range of motion of the MP joint of the thumb following operative repair of the UCL. J Hand Surg 1993; 18B:710–711.

Jupiter JB, Shephard JE. Tension wire fixation of avulsion fractures in the hand. Clin Orthop 1987; 214:113–120.

Lane LB. Acute grade III ulnar collateral ligament injuries of the thumb. Orthop Trans 1990; 14:245.

Lane LB. Acute grade III ulnar collateral ligament injuries: a new surgical and rehabilitation protocol. Am J Sports Med 1991; 19:234–238.

Mc Cue FC, Mayer V, Moran DJ. Gamekeeper's thumb: ulnar collateral ligament rupture. J Musculoskel Med 1988; 5:53–63.

Melone CP. Joint injuries of the fingers and thumb. Emerg Med Clin North Am 1985; 3:319–333.

Miller RJ. Dislocations and fracture dislocations of the metacarpophalangeal joint of the thumb. Hand Clin 1988; 4:45–65.

Posner MA, Retaillaud J-L. Metacarpophalangeal joint injuries of the thumb. Hand Clin 1992; 8:713–732.

Rettig AC, Wright HH. Skier's thumb. Phys Sports Med 1989; 17:65–75.

Smith RJ. Post-traumatic instability of the metacarpophalangeal joint of the thumb. J Bone Joint Surg 1977; 59A:14–21.

Stener B. Displacement of the ruptured ulnar collateral ligament of the metacarpophalangeal joint of the thumb. A clinical and anatomic study. J Bone Joint Surg 1962; 44B:869–879.

PROTECTIVE DEVICES FOR HAND INJURIES

BRIAN J. SENNETT, M.D.

Injuries to the hand and wrist account for approximately 8% to 20% of all athletic injuries, with rates approaching 50% to 70% in football, basketball, baseball, and gymnastics. Lost days of athletic participation could be enormous if injuries are allowed to completely heal before athletes return to competition. An individual's (1) understanding of the protective devices available, (2) knowledge of the rules regulating the use of sports equipment in the involved sport, (3) ability to determine whether an injury is stable or not, and (4) comprehension of the mechanics of the particular sport will enable athletes to resume play sooner without causing further damage to the injured extremity.

PROTECTIVE DEVICES

There are a wide variety of materials and prefabricated devices available to serve as protective devices for the wrist and hand. Knowledge of these materials, their applications, and fabrication when necessary will assist an individual in protecting an injured hand. These devices can be categorized as semi-rigid splints, rigid splints, and casts.

Semi-rigid Splints

Semi-rigid materials can be utilized when complete immobilization is not necessary such as in the management of simple sprains and contusions. These materials include athletic taping, manufactured devices such as the "lion's paw" used in gymnastics, silicone rubber splints, foam, and wrap materials. Athletic taping is cheap, commonly used, and highly effective when applied properly. The lion's paw is utilized in gymnastics and limits wrist dorsiflexion and provides protection against wrist injuries. Silicone rubber splints require time-consuming fabrication but are durable, are widely accepted by officials, and provide excellent shock absorption. The fabrication process is described below. Foam and wrap materials (Plastizote and Scotchwrap, respectively) allow excellent padding with minimal effort with foam being applied locally and wrap materials applied circumferentially.

Rigid Splints

These splints provide greater protection and limitation of motion than semi-rigid splints and are often utilized when treating fractures or ligamentous injuries. The devices available include alumiform splints, stack splints, Kombi Thumb Saver ski gloves, and thermoplastics. Alumiform splints are composed of an aluminum splint with foam padding attached and are commonly used to splint isolated finger injuries. Stack splints are premanufactured plastic splints utilized in the treatment of mallet fingers, and Kombi Thumb Saver gloves provide protection to the thumb through a built in steel guard. Thermoplastics, available in different thicknesses, can be cut and contoured to various shapes and allow excellent rigid protection to the injured hand and wrist (Fig. 1, A).

Thermoplastic splints should be fabricated as follows: (1) utilizing a hot water bath, heat the thermoplastic material to 150° F to 160° F until soft, (2) trace the region to be splinted onto the softened thermoplast, (3) apply a cloth stockinette to the injured wrist or hand, (4) cut the splint out of the thermoplast, pad where necessary and apply it smoothly to the wrist or hand, and (5) secure the splint to the hand with self-securing nylon tapes while it hardens.

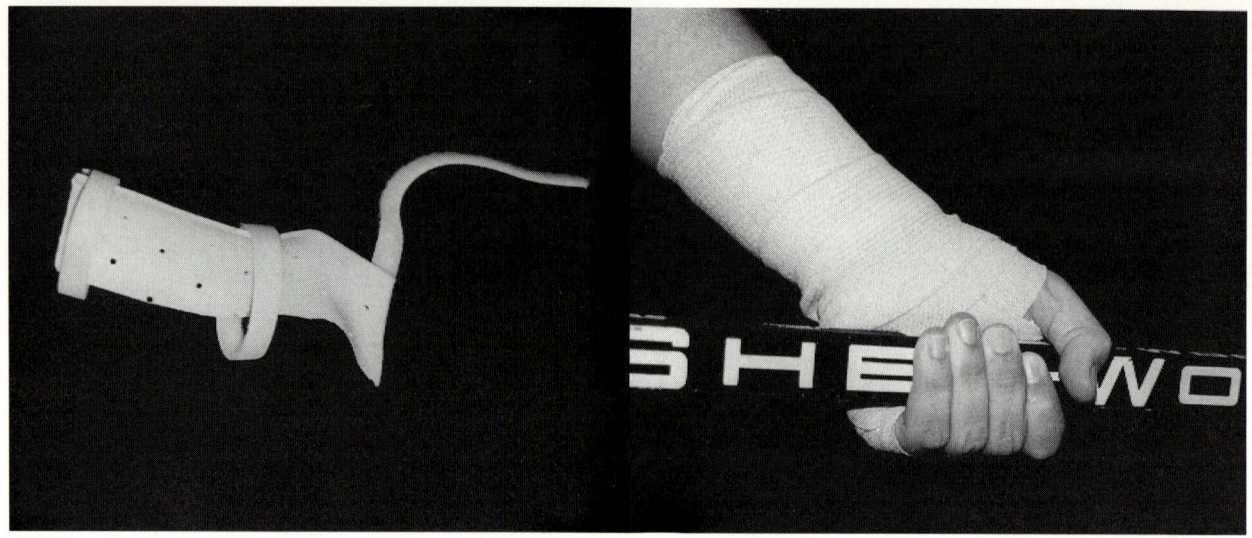

Figure 1 *A*, Thermoplastic splints are useful in the management of wrist and hand injuries and are easily contoured and applied with Velcro straps. *B*, Equipment to be used during competition should be grasped while the thermoplast hardens to provide a better contour to the splint.

Basic principles of splinting should be adhered to including positioning of joints and padding over bony prominences. When splinting, the wrist should be placed in 30 degrees of dorsiflexion, the metacarpophalangeal (MCP) joints placed in 70 degrees of flexion, and the interphalangeal (IP) joints placed at 30 degrees of flexion when possible. Adaptations for equipment use should be performed while the thermoplast is soft. While the splint is malleable, the piece of equipment is grasped and the thermoplast is allowed to harden in this position (Fig. 1, *B*). Any adapted splint that promotes joint contractures by inappropriate joint positioning should be alternated with a conventional splint. If the splint is to be worn inside a glove, the glove is placed over the splint after fabrication and customized at that time. With respect to pressure, the most troublesome regions include the distal radius and ulna, metacarpal heads, and the dorsal aspect of the IP joints if placed in flexion. Padding inside the splint should be applied when necessary prior to contouring and hardening. Tape or Coban can be used to secure the splint during participation.

Casts

Casts provide the greatest protection and are available in plaster, fiberglass, and silicone rubber. While plaster and fiberglass are more durable and provide stronger support, they are not allowed in most high school athletic competitions. For this reason silicone rubber has become widely used and accepted in the treatment of the high school athlete. This material must be approved by both the treating physician and officials prior to use in competition. The soft cast has been used extensively and shown to have no ill-effect on the management of injuries and has not been linked to any injuries of opposing players in numerous studies.

Fabrication of fiberglass and plaster casts is common and straightforward. However, the application of a RTV silicone cast deserves discussion. RTV, usually available in 1 or 12 lb containers, can be divided and frozen in 4 oz containers to increase the half-life. Three to four containers can be thawed for application as the average cast requires approximately 12 to 16 oz of material. A catalyst, also supplied by the manufacturer, is added in a 1:10 proportion (catalyst:silicone) immediately prior to cast application. Fabrication of the RTV silicone cast should be performed as follows: (1) Apply vaseline liberally to the skin over which the cast is to be applied, followed by one layer of stockinette or rubber glove (Fig. 2, *A*), (2) apply alternating layers of double thickness plastic wrap and activated RTV silicone (Fig. 2, *B*), (3) continue alternating applications until the appropriate thickness is obtained (thumb immobilization—three layers; wrist immobilization—five layers) (Fig. 2, *C*), (4) wrap cast with plastic followed by an Ace wrap and allow to cure for approximately 3 hours (time may vary depending on the compound used), and (5) split cast along the uninjured border, trim where necessary, and reapply when needed with an elastic wrap. Silicone casts should be alternated with a conventional bivalved cast as they are nonporous and will result in macerated skin with extended use.

RULES AND REGULATIONS

A thorough knowledge of the rules governing the involved sports is necessary when prescribing protective devices for the injured athlete. As rules vary between states, between sports, and between competitive levels, local officials and rules committees must be consulted to ensure compliance with regulations. As an example, rigid casts with three-quarter inch thick closed-cell padding are allowed in collegiate football while the use of rigid casts at the high school level is prohibited. The News-

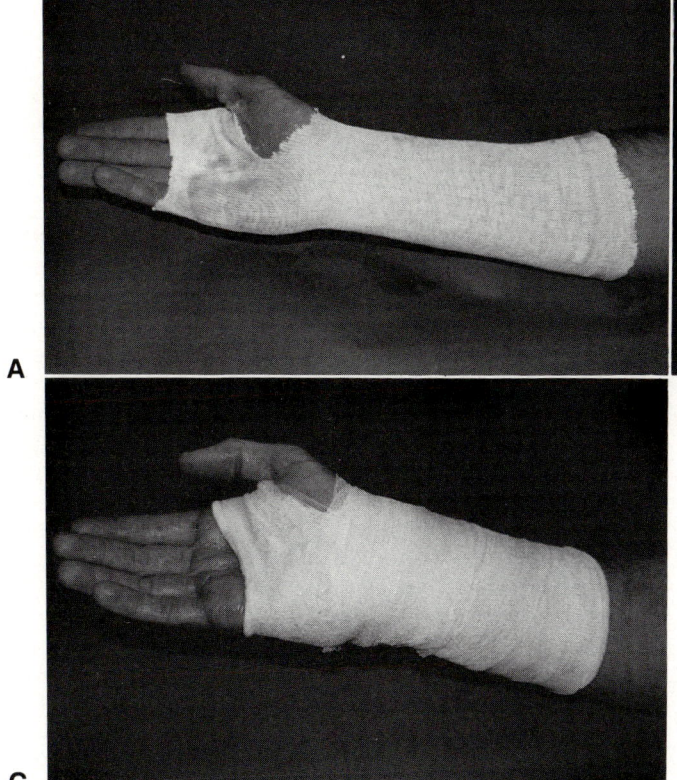

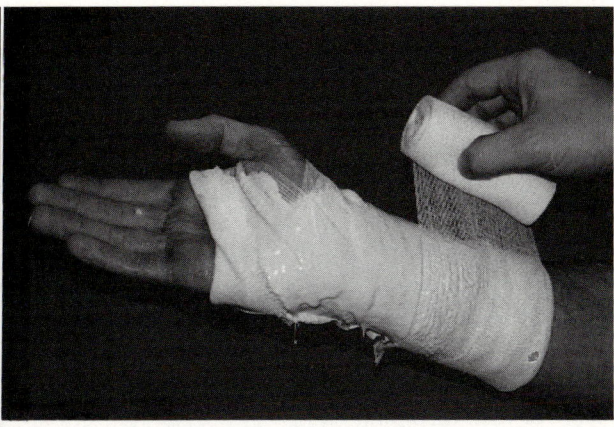

Figure 2 Fabrication of a silicone cast includes *(A)* application of vaseline followed by a stockinette and/or surgical glove depending on what region the cast is being applied to, *(B)* alternating layers of double thickness kling and activated RTV silicone, until *(C)* the appropriate thickness is obtained (three layers — thumb; five layers — wrist). Curing takes approximately 3 hours and is facilitated by wrapping the cast with plastic wrap. The cast is then split and reapplied with an elastic wrap for competition.

letter of the National Association of Sports Officials provides rule interpretation (1-414-632-5949) or will respond to mail inquires (2017 Lathrop Avenue, Racine, WI 53405) when local consultation is unavailable.

PROTECTION OF COMMON HAND AND WRIST INJURIES

Distal Phalangeal Fractures

Fractures of the distal phalanx account for more than one half of all hand fractures and fortunately are usually stable injuries. Protection of these stable injuries involves the application of an aluminum, orthoplast, or stack splint with the distal interphalangeal (DIP) joint in extension for approximately 4 weeks. Intra-articular fractures must be assessed for "step-off" with mallet finger injuries being protected as discussed below. Evaluation of concomitant nail bed injuries must be performed with repair of the nail bed when necessary. Protection of nail bed injuries involves replacement of the nail along with the application of a splint.

Mallet Finger Injuries

Mallet finger injuries result from a blow to the extended digit forcing the DIP joint into flexion. These injuries are categorized as (1) fractures, (2) extensor tendon avulsions or ruptures, and (3) extensor tendon stretching. All of these injuries can be managed with continuous immobilization of the DIP joint in extension

with an aluminum, stack, or orthoplast splint for 6 weeks followed by night splinting. Operative treatment is reserved for injuries with concomitant subluxation of the DIP joint. Athletes may compete immediately with continuous immobilization.

Middle and Proximal Phalangeal Fractures

Phalangeal fractures are treated according to their stability. Stable fractures involving the base and shaft of the proximal phalanx should be immobilized with the MCP joint at 70 degrees of flexion and the IP joints in extension. Fractures involving the head or neck can often be managed with the IP joint in extension in a cylinder cast, leaving the MCP joint free. Unstable injuries require reduction and fixation, and the athlete cannot return to participation until adequate healing has occurred. With rigid internal fixation, an athlete may return to competition as early as 3 weeks with adequate protection. When adequate healing has occurred, cast immobilization can be replaced by splinting or buddy taping.

Proximal Interphalangeal Ligamentous Injuries

Ligamentous injuries to the proximal interphalangeal (PIP) joints can occur with or without concomitant dislocations of the joint. Volar plate injuries usually result from dorsal dislocations of the PIP joint and can be protected with volar splinting of the joint in 30 degrees of flexion for 3 weeks with an orthoplast or aluminum splint followed by "buddy-taping" until a full pain-free range of motion is obtained. Protection of this injury while healing allows immediate return to athletics.

Injuries to the central slip, which can occur with the rarer volar dislocation, should be immobilized with the PIP joint in extension and the DIP joint free for 6 weeks, followed by night splinting for an additional 4 weeks. Orthoplast or aluminum splints can be utilized for protection of this injury with immediate return to competition.

Collateral ligament injuries with or without associated dislocations are managed with respect to the laxity present. Mild sprains are "buddy-taped" continuously to the digit on the side of the involved ligament for at least 3 weeks. Protective buddy-taping during competition is continued for approximately 3 months. Management of complete tears is controversial, with some advocating open repair. However, conservative care can be utilized with extension and lateral splint of the PIP joint for 2 weeks followed by continuous "buddy-taping" for an additional 4 weeks. An individual may return to competition immediately with appropriate protection.

Metacarpal Fractures

Fractures of the metacarpals are common in contact athletics due to the tremendous forces encountered by the hand. Fortunately, due to the soft tissue attachments, many of these fractures are stable and allow participation once initial pain levels subside. The hand should be initially casted with the wrist in 20 degrees of dorsiflexion and the MCP joint of the involved and adjacent rays in 70 degrees of flexion. Buddy-taping of the involved and adjacent digits should be performed at the time of immobilization to control rotation at the fracture site. Cast immobilization can often be replaced by splinting at 4 weeks to increase mobility of the hand. Fractures of the distal shaft, neck, and head can often be protected with a hand-based splint, while metacarpal base fractures require wrist immobilization when stable.

Ulnar Collateral Ligament Injuries

Injuries to the ulnar collateral ligament (UCL) of the thumb are common in ball-handling sports as well as contact athletics. These ligamentous injuries are divided into partial and complete tears, which are treated quite differently. Complete ruptures of the UCL often requires surgical repair and healing prior to return to participation. Partial ligamentous tears are managed with thumb spica immobilization with the MCP joint in an adducted position for a duration proportional to the severity of the injury, with the maximum being 3 weeks. The form of immobilization, casting or orthoplast splinting, should be determined as a result of future anticipated stresses to this joint.

Wrist Injuries

Ligamentous and capsular injuries to the wrist are treated according to their severity. Disorders of the wrist that often can be treated with protective splinting and allow for return to competition include mild ligamentous sprains, tendinitis, ganglions, and dorsal impaction syndrome. Major ligamentous injuries and unstable fractures involving the scaphoid often require operative treatment and healing prior to return to competition.

Mild ligamentous injuries can often be protected with a combination of a resting orthoplast splint and casting during participation. Return to competition is allowed once the athlete is comfortable. Tendinitis, usually occurring in sports requiring repetitive motions, can often be managed with a resting orthoplast splint with the wrist in 30 degrees of dorsiflexion. Once again, the athlete is able to return to competition when comfortable.

Ganglions, which most commonly arise from the dorsal scapholunate ligament, can be managed symptomatically. Orthoplast splint immobilization of the wrist in 30 degrees of dorsiflexion will often reduce the athletes' level of discomfort and allow them to complete the season prior to removal of the ganglion. Surgical treatment is only necessary if symptoms persist or if there is any doubt as to the diagnosis.

Dorsal impaction syndrome of the wrist is commonly seen in gymnastics due to the combined dorsiflexion and weightbearing involved in this sport. The wrist can be protected from injuries with a "lion's paw" brace. This is a semi-rigid device that limits dorsiflexion while competing in gymnastics and reduces load transmission across the dorsal aspect of the wrist.

Stable scaphoid fractures are amenable to thumb spica cast immobilization at the collegiate and professional levels. However, rigid casts are not allowed at the high school level and only nondisplaced middle-third scaphoid fractures can be managed with silicone casts during competition, alternating with continuous conventional casting. Individuals with unstable scaphoid fractures treated with open reduction and internal fixation may return to play once healing has occurred. At that time, a playing cast is usually fabricated for protection during return to competition.

Major ligamentous injuries generally require operative treatment and 6 to 8 weeks of healing prior to return to athletics. The wrist is then protected with either a playing cast or protective splint upon return to competition.

SUGGESTED READING

Bergfeld JA, Weiker GG, Andrish JT. Soft playing splint for protection of significant hand and wrist injuries in sports. Am J Sports Med 1982; 10:293–296.

DeCarlo M, Darmelio J, Rettig AC. Perfecting a playing cast for hand and wrist injuries. Physician Sportsmed 1992; 20:95–104.

Hilfrank BC. Protecting the injured hand for sports. J Hand Therapy 1991; 4:51–55.

Rettig A, Alexy C, Malone K. Protective devices for hand and wrist injuries. J Musculoskeletal Med 1992; 9:62–75.

Sadler J, Koepfer J. Rehabilitation and splinting of the injured hand. In: Strickland J, Rettig A, eds. Hand injuries in athletics. Philadelphia: WB Saunders, 1991:235.

WRIST ARTHROSCOPY

A. LEE OSTERMAN, M.D.
DAVID J. BOZENTKA, M.D.

Surgical and diagnostic wrist arthroscopy has become a well-established procedure that continues to evolve. The anatomic complexity of the wrist, with its eight carpal bones, their intrinsic and extrinsic restraining ligaments surrounded by numerous tendons and neurovascular structures, offer innumerable pathologic possibilities. The proximity of these structures often make precise diagnosis elusive and chronic wrist pain a diagnostic dilemma. The development of smaller diameter arthroscopes and more precise instrumentation has made wrist arthroscopy a valuable adjunct not only in the assessment of wrist pain, but also in the treatment of many of its causes.

Physical examination does not always indicate a specific diagnosis. It can, however, provide an index of suspicion. The examiner should search diligently for various clicks and clunks. Table 1 lists the current provocative tests used in examining a wrist. It should be emphasized that in order for a "click" to be considered pathologic it should reproduce the patient's pain and should not be present in the asymptomatic contralateral wrist. The examination should also include a measurement of grip strength and its quantitation by a Jamar dynamometer. Grip strength requires a stable, pain-free wrist, and therefore significant wrist disorders usually weaken grip strength. Finally, well-placed anesthetic injections may help localize and define the anatomic source of the tenderness.

Even if the physical examination seems conclusive, routine four-view studies of the wrist are usually needed. These views may reveal an unsuspected avulsion fracture or static ligamentous deformity. Active studies such as a clenched-fist view or cineradiography may be needed to define a dynamic instability. Triple-phase bone scanning may highlight wrist synovitis or lunate avascular necrosis.

For tears of the triangular fibrocartilage and intrinsic ligament tears, wrist arthrography has become the benchmark. However, radiocarpal arthrography alone may not fully confirm tears of the triangular fibrocartilage. In a study by Roth, arthroscopy was found to be more sensitive than radiocarpal arthrography in diagnosing perforations at the triangular fibrocartilage. Furthermore, unlike arthroscopy, arthrography does not allow the determination of the size and type of triangular fibrocartilage complex (TFCC) tear. We are currently performing triple-compartment injections. A radiocarpal injection is followed 1 hour later by injections of the midcarpal and distal radial ulnar joint. This has lowered the false-negative rate to almost zero for tears of the TFCC and the intrinsic ligaments.

We use a specialized wrist coil for magnetic resonance imaging (MRI) to define wrist pathology. Its accuracy is extremely high in defining intra-articular fluid, avascular necrosis of the lunate, TFCC tears, and scapholunate tears. It is less accurate in defining lunatotriquetral tears.

None of the above mentioned studies, including MRI, allow visualization of the volar wrist ligaments, or the evaluation of chondral defects of the carpal bones. By allowing direct visualization of the articular surfaces and palpation of the ligaments, wrist arthroscopy approaches these problems directly. Wrist arthroscopy therefore has several advantages over other means of evaluating wrist pathology. It provides direct visualization of cartilage surfaces and ligamentous structures. The examiner can probe the ligaments and evaluate their

Table 1 Provocative Wrist Maneuvers

Test	Technique
Radial stress test (for scapholunate stability)	Fingers on Lister's tubercle, thumb on distal scaphoid tuberosity. Causes radial and ulnar deviation of the wrist, both actively and passively.
Shear test (for pisitriquetral problems)	Fingers dorsal to triquetrum, thumb "rocks" or pushes pisiform into triquetrum.
Shuck test (for lunatotriquetral stability)	Fingers dorsal to lunate while thumb is on the pisitriquetral joint. Causes radial and ulnar deviation of the wrist, both actively and passively.
Lunatotriquetral ballottement test (for lunatotriquetral stability)	Fix lunate with thumb and index of one hand, while other hand displaces the triquetrum and pisiform both volarly and dorsally.
Piano-key test (for distal radioulnar joint)	Volar-dorsal stability of distal ulnar tested at different rotatory positions.
Triangular fibrocartilage load test (for wrist ulnar deviation)	With passive manipulation of carpus against the ulna will produce painful crepitus.
ECU subluxation test	Examine dorsum of wrist with forearm supinated and ulnar deviation against resistance. A visible and palpable subluxation of the ECU is noted, often with a snap.
Grip strength	The jamar curve from intrinsic to extrinsic grasp should generate a bell shaped curve. A flat-line plot often indicates voluntary submaximal performance.
Rapid exchange grip test	Patient grasps dynomometer strongly at optimal grasp position and is asked to alternate rapidly from one hand to the other. Normally with rapid exchange, grip strength decreases slightly. Voluntary weakness of grip cannot be controlled and often grip strength is elevated.

tensile strength directly. In intra-articular fractures of the distal radius, the surgeon can confirm the congruency of the reduction, or in scaphoid nonunions, the degree of coexistent arthritic change. Also, wrist arthroscopy can be therapeutic. The surgeon can remove loose bodies, perform synovectomies and chondroplasties, and debride frayed ligaments. If there is damage to the triangular fibrocartilage, he can debride central tears and repair peripheral tears. Finally, he can perform arthroscopic reductions and percutaneous fixation for carpal instabilities. Wrist arthroscopy is a safe and valuable diagnostic and therapeutic procedure.

BASIC SET-UP AND PORTAL PLACEMENT

The patient is placed supine on the operating table. Either axillary regional block or general anesthesia is administered and a pneumatic tourniquet is applied. Most operations are done on an out-patient basis. One of the various commercially available traction towers is ideal for suspending and distracting the radiocarpal and midcarpal joints. The hand and forearm are prepped and freely draped. All four fingers are then placed in sterile nylon fingertraps to minimize the risk of digital nerve neuropraxia. Ten to 15 pounds of traction are applied and can be regulated by the strain gauge on the traction tower. If a traction tower is not available the fingertraps can be suspended from a trapeze connected to the opposite side of the table. A sling is then placed over the arm with a 7 to 12 pound weight attached to the sling. At the beginning of the procedure, the tourniquet is applied and inflated only if bleeding hinders visualization. The surgeon may be sitting or standing with the monitor, light source, and video recorder directly opposite on the contralateral side of the patient.

For evaluation of the radiocarpal joint, we prefer a short-barrel (50 to 60 mm) scope with an outside diameter of 2 to 3 mm and an angle of 25 to 30 degrees. For midcarpal and distal radial ulnar joint arthroscopy, the smaller videoscopes measuring 1.5 to 2 mm are more easily maneuvered. A light-weight chip camera is attached to the arthroscope. When the larger radiocarpal scopes are used, irrigation is connected directly to the scope, with the flow maintained by gravity feed. Several instruments are now available to help define and modify wrist joint disease. A small hook-probe is essential for palpating the ligaments and also serves as a reference probe for magnification. Shutt baskets, grasping forceps, and suction punches ranging from 2 to 3 mm are also desirable. Small diameter shavers with disposable cutting blades and burrs are available.

Arthroscopy is performed from the dorsum of the wrist, and portal sites are defined by the extensor tendons (Fig. 1). There are 11 arthroscopic portals: five for the radiocarpal, four for the midcarpal, and two for the distal radial ulnar joints.

It is also important to keep in mind the neurovas-

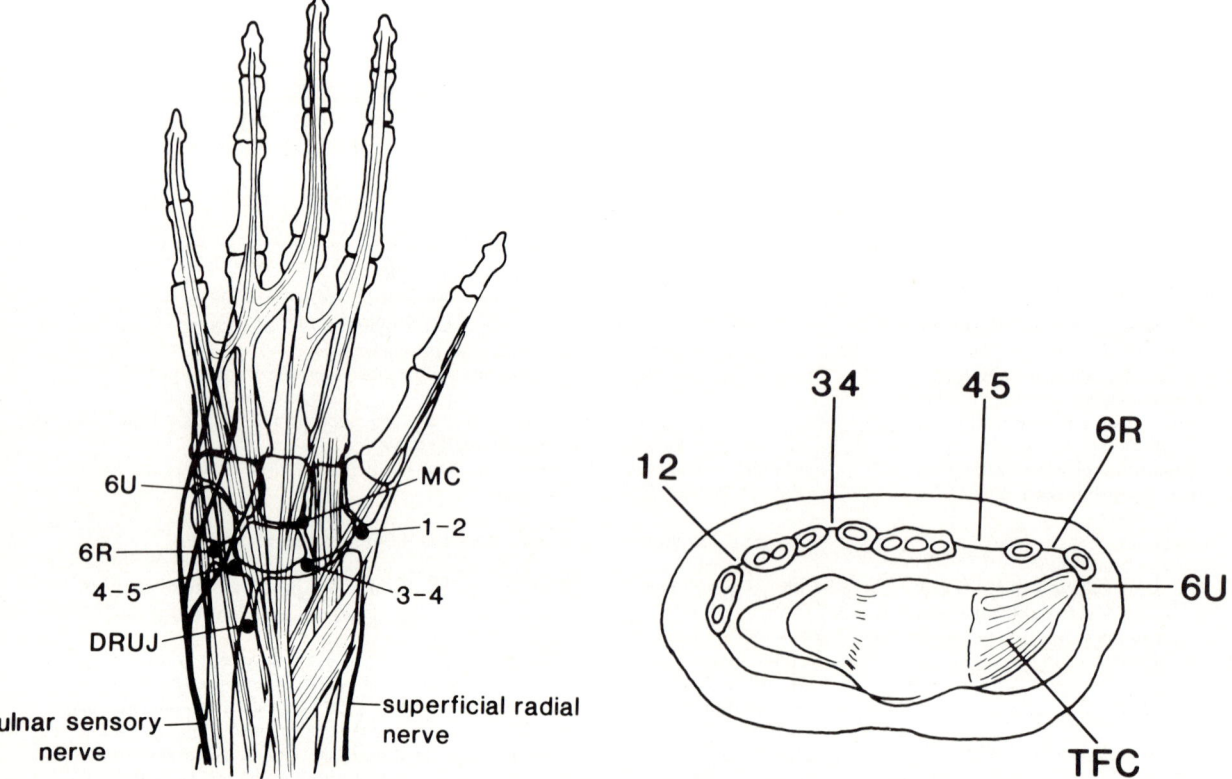

Figure 1 Arthroscopic portals are named for the extensor intervals they define. Care should be taken to avoid the dorsal sensory structures and radial artery.

cular structures on the dorsum of the wrist. These include the deep branch of the radial artery and the superficial dorsal sensory branches of the radial and ulnar nerves. All other major neurovascular structures run on the volar aspect of the wrist; this is the main reason that dorsal portals are used. The deep branch of the radial artery lies in the anatomic snuffbox entering under the tendons of the first extensor compartment. The superficial radial nerve sweeps across the snuff-box and supplies sensation to the thumb and index and long fingers dorsally. The dorsal branch of the ulnar nerve passes along the medial aspect of the distal forearm. At the level of the distal ulna it runs dorsally to supply sensation to the dorsum of the small and ring fingers.

It should be emphasized that the portal sites are named for their relationships to the extensor compartments (see Fig. 1). Portal 1-2 lies between the first and second extensor compartments. It is just radial to the extensor carpi radialis longus tendon, distal to the radial styloid, and special care should be taken to avoid the extensor pollicis longus (EPL) tendon as it turns obliquely across to the thumb. Branches of the superficial radial nerve and dorsal radial artery lie across the entrance of this portal, so care must be taken to spread with a mosquito to the level of the capsule before entering the joint. This portal is used to visualize the scaphoid fossa, radial volar ligaments, and proximal pole of the scaphoid.

Portal 3-4 is the main working portal and the preferred site for the initial examination of the radiocarpal joint. Its central location allows examination of the radiocarpal joint in both its radial and ulnar aspects. It is located by palpating the radial margin of the extensor digitorum communis tendons and lies 1 cm distal to Lister's tubercle.

Portal 4-5 enters the radiocarpal joint directly over the midportion of the triangular fibrocartilage. It is found by palpating the ulnar side of the extensor digitorum communis. It is most useful for evaluation of the triangular fibrocartilage, and also serves as a portal for arthroscopic debridement.

Portal 6R (radial to the extensor carpi ulnaris [ECU]) is the main ulnar working portal. Portal 6U (ulnar to the ECU) is useful for joint distension and outflow, but the dorsal ulnar sensory nerve runs in this area and is at risk for injury. Through the 6R portal, one has a direct approach to the triangular fibrocartilage as well as good visualization of the ulnaluno and ulnatriquetral ligaments. One also can assess the intrinsic lunatotriquetral ligament.

There are four portals for the midcarpal joint. The radial midcarpal portal is most commonly used. It is located 1 cm distal to the 3-4 portal in line with the radial margin of the third metacarpal. The site is palpable as a small depression just radial to the extensor digitorum communis tendon to the index finger. This portal allows entry between the capitate and the concave surface of the scaphoid. It is suitable for visualization of both carpal rows as well as the triscaphe joint. The ulnar midcarpal portal is in line with the fourth metacarpal shaft and is useful for insertion of instruments and shaving. There

are two accessory portals that are less frequently used. The STT portal is placed just ulnar to the EPL tendon and is located at the distal pole of the scaphoid. Care must be taken not to injure the dorsal radial sensory nerve, and if the portal is placed too radially, the radial artery is at risk. The second accessory midcarpal portal is located at the triquetral hamate articulation and may be useful for inflow or outflow canula.

Two portals are present at the distal radial ulnar joint (DRUJ). With supination of the wrist, the dorsal capsule is relaxed and the scope sheath enters proximal to the DRUJ. A second portal can be made under the TFCC. This is useful for visualizing the articular surface of the ulna and the underside of the triangular fibrocartilage. It is not an accessible portal in all patients.

We have found that before initiating the arthroscopic procedure, it is helpful to use a marking pen to mark Lister's tubercle, the radial and ulnar borders of the extensor digitorum communis, the ECU, the EPL, and the radial border of the extensor carpi radialis longus. Once the structures have been distorted by swelling, these landmarks may be more difficult to locate. After inflation of the tourniquet, a needle is placed in the 3-4 compartment to distend the radiocarpal joint. It should be remembered that the surface of the radius has a volar and radial tilt, and the needle and arthroscopic sheath should therefore be inserted in this direction. A short, longitudinal skin incision is made with a No. 11 scalpel. Because of the proximity of the extensor tendons care must be taken not to stab. A hemostat is used to bluntly dissect to the wrist capsule. The wrist joint is then entered with the blunt probe.

Postoperatively, a single nylon stitch is used to close each portal incision. The patient's wrist is wrapped in a sterile dressing and immobilized in a volar plaster splint, supporting the wrist and metacarpal phalangeal joints for 1 week unless other arthroscopic procedures have been performed.

VIEWING SEQUENCE

The arthroscopic examination of the wrist should be carried out in an orderly and sequential manner. Intimate familiarity with wrist anatomy is necessary (Figs. 2 and 3).

Inspection of the radiocarpal joint is begun through the 3-4 portal. Immediately upon entering the wrist, the physician will note the synovial fat pad overlying the radioscapholunate ligament (Fig. 4). This not only provides a useful landmark for the underlying ligament, but is directly opposite and intimate with the intrinsic scapholunate ligament. It lies volar to the interfacet ridge of the radius and serves as a convenient dividing point between the radial and ulnar sides of the joint.

After this landmark has been identified, the scope is advanced toward the ulnar side of the wrist until the prestyloid recess is seen. A large-gauge needle is then inserted just ulnar to the ECU tendon through the 6U portal. The outflow needle can then be observed in the joint.

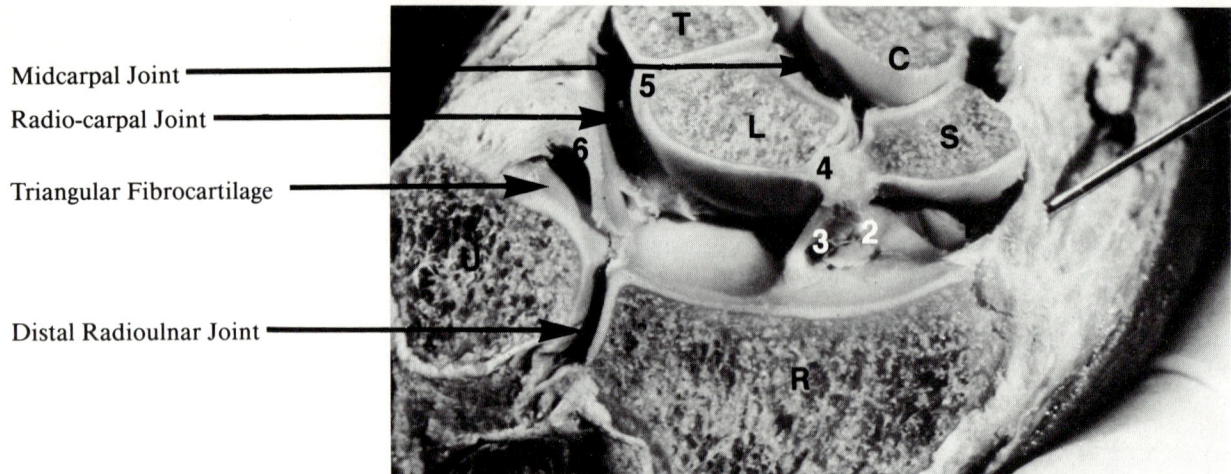

Figure 2 Coronal section of a wrist viewed from the dorsum. R = radius; U = ulna; T = triquetrum, L = lunate, S = scaphoid; C = capitate. 1 = radioscaphocapitate ligament; 2 = radiolunatotriquetral ligament; 3 = fat pad and radioscapholunate ligament; 4 = intrinsic scapholunate ligament; 5 = intrinsic lunatotriquetral ligament; 6 = ulnocarpal ligaments.

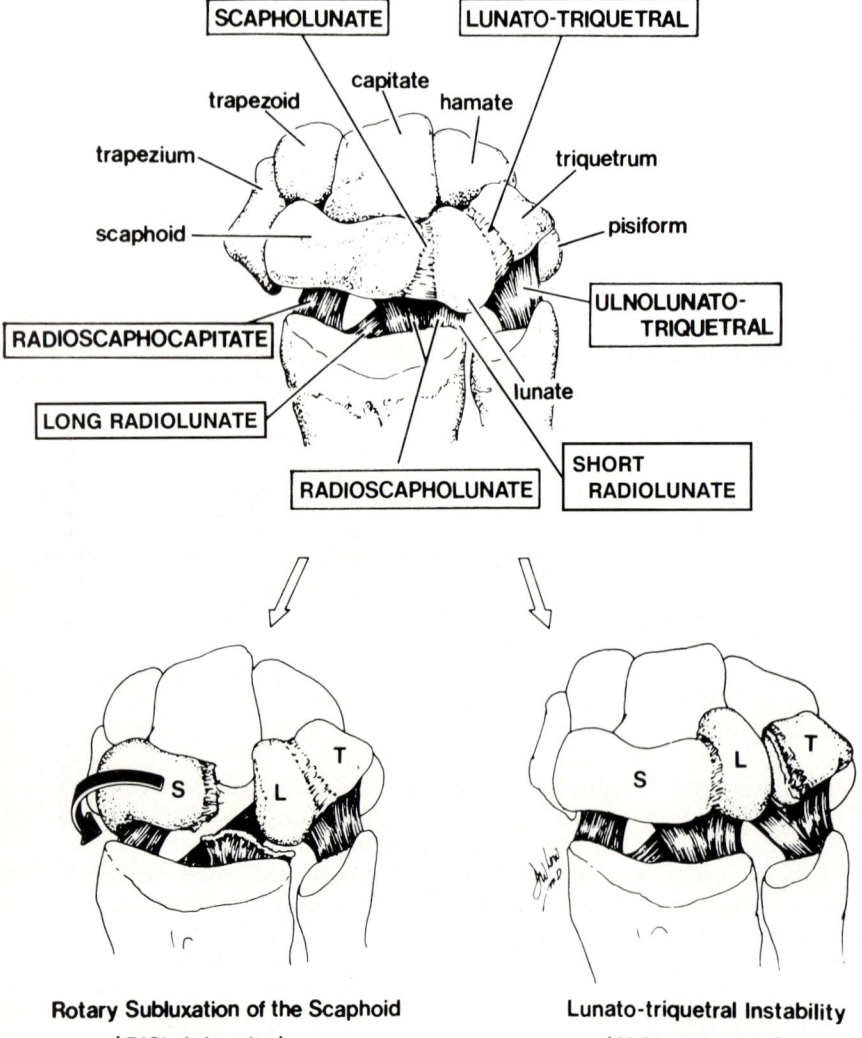

Rotary Subluxation of the Scaphoid
(DISI deformity)

Lunato-triquetral Instability
(VISI deformity)

Figure 3 Diagram of the intrinsic carpal instabilities: rotary subluxation of the scaphoid and lunatotriquetral instability.

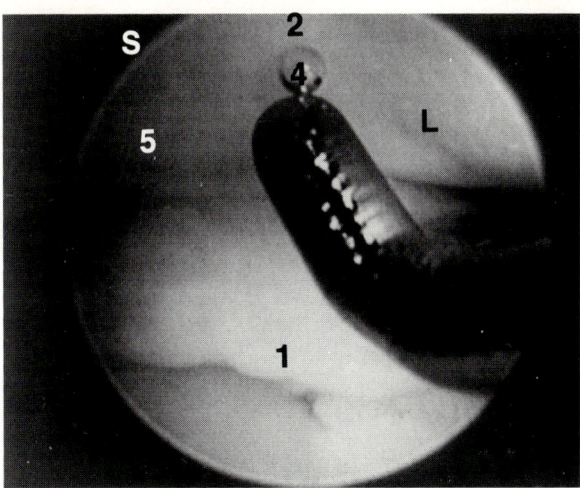

Figure 4 Arthroscopic view on entering the 3-4 portal. 1 = fat pad synovium overlying the radioscapholunate ligament; 2 = intrinsic scapholunate ligament. Probe lies against it and small air bubble (4). S = proximal pole scaphoid; L = lunate.

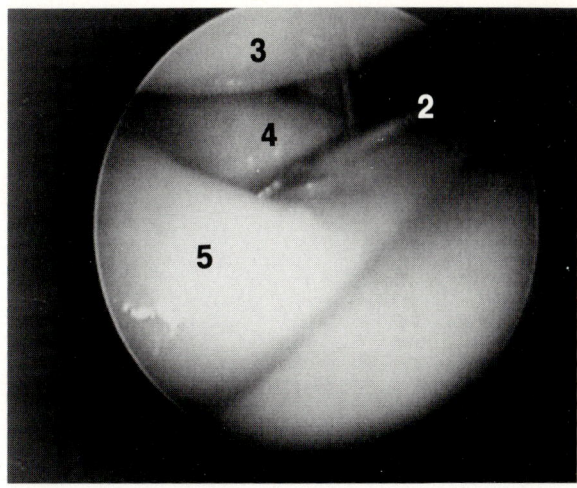

Figure 5 Arthroscopic view from 3-4 portal toward radial side of the wrist. Probe (1) is in the 1-2 portal; 2 = articular surface scaphoid facet of radius; 3 = proximal pole scaphoid; 4 = radioscaphocapitate ligament; 5 = radiolunatotriquetral ligament.

Next, the 6R portal is established through direct arthroscopic observation just radial to the ECU tendon. Aside from palpation, the arthroscopic light itself can provide a guide to establishing this portal. Initially, this portal is used to insert the probe. The probe is used as a palpating "finger" to determine the structural integrity and help define both normal and pathologic anatomy. If there is a great deal of active synovitis in the wrist, a small shaver can be inserted through the 6R portal and the joint cleaned of the obscuring synovium before the observation.

Once these portals have been established, the examiner returns to the fat pad overlying the radioscapholunate ligament. As stated previously, this is in intimate contact with the scapholunate intrinsic ligament (Fig. 4).

When it is intact, the fat pad overlying the radioscapholunate ligament is often indistinguishable from the cartilage of the scaphoid and lunate because of its convex surface. The probe helps distinguish between the articular cartilage and the ligament. When it is disrupted, the probe will pass into the midcarpal joint, and in the case of gross disruption, the scope can easily be passed into the midcarpal joint.

As one advances radially, the scaphoid facet of the radius is obvious, as is the proximal pole of the scaphoid. The radioscaphocapitate ligament is the most radial ligament and acts as a fulcrum around which the scaphoid flexes and extends (Fig. 5). The broader ligament ulnar to it is the long radiolunate ligament, previously called the radiolunatotriquetral ligament. These fibers are directed from the radius toward the triquetrum. Finally, the radioscapholunate ligament, often called the ligament of Testut, is usually hidden by the fat pad, but can be visualized by moving the fat pad aside with the probe.

Moving ulnar to the fat pad and across the sagittal

ridge, one enters the ulnar side of the wrist joint. The short radiolunate ligament that is palmar to the lunate facet of the radius is visualized. One can also visualize the main portions of the triangular fibrocartilage as it originates from the radius and proceeds in an ulnar direction. Here again the probe is helpful in palpating the transition between the radius and the central cartilaginous portion of the triangular fibrocartilage. One can continue to visualize the ulnocarpal ligaments, the lunatotriquetral interval, and the prestyloid recess through the 3-4 portal, but it is most convenient to switch viewing and working portals at this time. The scope is therefore transferred to the 6R portal and the probe to the 3-4 portal. Through the 6R portal, one can fully appreciate the extent of the triangular fibrocartilage as well as the ulnoluno and ulnotriquetral ligaments (Fig. 6). One can also visualize the prestyloid recess and the lunatotriquetral ligament (see Fig. 2).

Midcarpal examination should be performed routinely. Arthroscopy of the midcarpal joint is particularly helpful in evaluating carpal instability since the concave surfaces on the distal aspects of the scaphoid, lunate, and triquetrum provide for more accurate anatomic alignment than do the convex surfaces that are visualized through the radiocarpal portals. Also this view allows visualization of the distal pole of the scaphoid, the scaphoid trapezial area, and the evaluation of the hamate triquetral interface, a common source of early arthritic change. The scope is inserted through the radial midcarpal portal, and the ulnar midcarpal portal is used for outflow and/or probes. The proximal surface of the capitate is a useful source of alignment against which one can visualize the concave surfaces of the scaphoid, lunate, and triquetrum (Fig. 7). Two variations of the lunate distal articular surface can be seen. A type I lunate articulates distally only with the capitate. A type II lunate has a separate medial facet that additionally

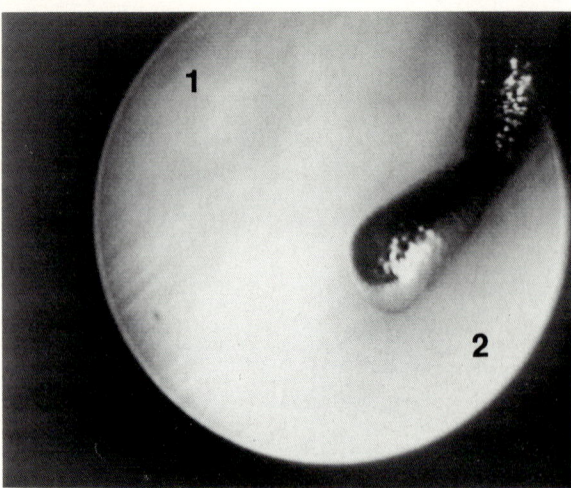

Figure 6 Arthroscopic view of the triangular fibrocartilage and its juncture with the lunate facet of the radius. When the TFCC is intact, the probe may be useful in differentiating the spongy area of the transection from bone. 1 = intact TFCC; 2 = lunate facet of radius.

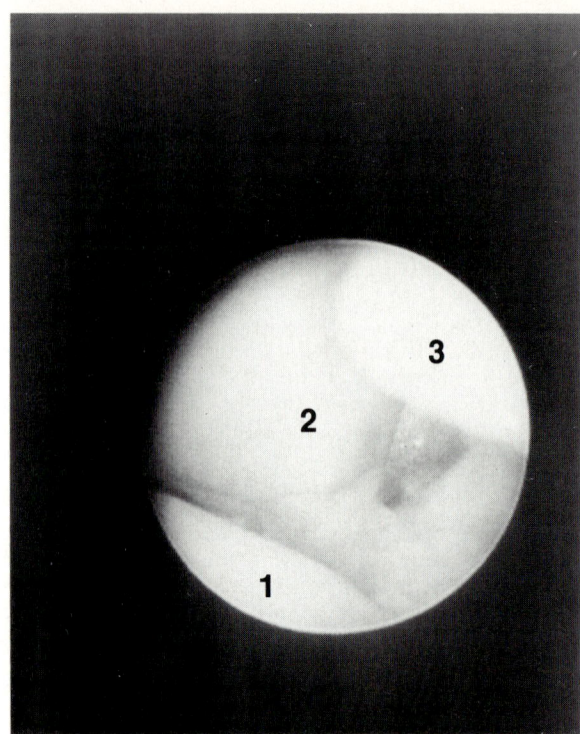

Figure 8 Arthroscopic view of the midcarpal joint. 1 = distal pole scaphoid; 2 = trapezium; 3 = trapezoid.

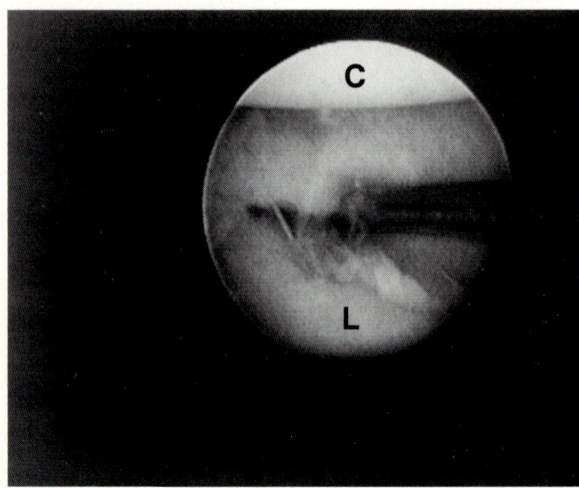

Figure 7 Arthroscopic view of the midcarpal joint. C = capitate; L = lunate distal surface and probe area of tear in volar midcarpal capsule.

articulates with the proximal pole of the hamate. In the type II lunate, chondral changes can be visualized on the proximal pole of the hamate, which are not evident on plain radiographs. Note that the probe can pass freely between the scapholunate and lunatotriquetral joint since on the midcarpal surface of these bones there is no intrinsic ligament. One can direct the scope radially and observe the scaphotrapezial joint (Fig. 8). One can also observe the volar intercarpal ligaments, such as the triquetrohamate and deltoid ligaments. Generally, however, the midcarpal joint is an extremely tight joint, and if these structures are easily seen, it implies either significant ligamentous laxity or ligament damage.

Once a thorough examination has been conducted, the examiner can consider certain treatment alterna-

tives. The therapeutic benefits of wrist arthroscopy must be integrated with open surgical procedures in the treatment of wrist disorders. Merely modifying the anatomy by shaving or trimming is not likely to produce a lasting result if a coexisting ligamentous problem is not also addressed. The best therapeutic results occur when arthroscopy can be used in lieu of open procedures with their higher morbidity and achieve a similar result. When this can be done, the patient has less postoperative pain and an earlier return to function. In most patients, this arthroscopic intervention can be performed on an out-patient basis and in a more economic fashion.

TRIANGULAR FIBROCARTILAGE LESIONS

The triangular fibrocartilage is a unique structure and differs from the classic knee meniscus. Wrist investigations have clarified its role both as a stabilizer of the DRUJ through its volar and dorsal radial ulnar ligaments and as an axial load-bearing role in transmitting forces across the wrist. In a wrist with neutral ulnar variance, approximately 20% of the applied load across the wrist is transmitted to the ulna. If less than two-thirds of the central portion of the triangular fibrocartilage is excised, this physiologic load transmission is relatively undisturbed. Excising more than two-thirds of the central portion and disturbing the continuity of the volar and dorsal ligaments as well as the attachments to the base of the ulnar styloid and ulnar carpal ligaments can seriously compromise DRUJ stability.

Isolated TFCC perforations are frequently implicated as the cause of chronic wrist pain. Because asymptomatic age-related perforations are common, symptoms related to such perforations are not fully understood and often reflect other mechanical derangements. Although tears or perforations of the central cartilaginous portion will not heal, many will become asymptomatic. Thus, most patients should have a trial of conservative treatment involving restriction of activities, splinting, and anti-inflammatories administered either locally or systemically.

Currently TFCC lesions should be suspected in a patient who has sustained a rotatory injury and presents with pain over the ulnar side of the wrist. Often there is a secondary ECU tendonitis, and it is therefore important to rule out instability of the ECU tendon. The patient may have symptoms of clicking, which was the case in more than half of our patients, and "catching" or locking was seen in approximately one-fifth of our patients. Pain, when present, is usually intermittent and increases with use of the wrist. Ulnar deviation of the wrist with passive manipulation of the carpus against the ulna may reproduce a click or painful crepitus. The clinical diagnosis can be confirmed by radiocarpal and/or DRUJ arthrography, and by high-resolution MRI.

Tears can be classified in two broad categories: traumatic or degenerative. Traumatic tears are usually associated with a defined rotatory event and are more common when the ulnar variance pattern of the wrist is neutral or slightly negative. When the ulna is long in relation to the distal radius, the force across the triangular fibrocartilage is increased, and in this situation attritional or degenerative lesions of the TFCC are common. Over time, a progressive wear phenomenon occurs with the central cartilaginous portion perforated first, followed by erosions of the lunate, triquetrum, and distal ulna, and in some cases, by lunatotriquetral ligament perforations. In such cases, arthroscopic debridement of the central portion of the triangular fibrocartilage should also include a chondroplasty of the distal ulna. One can shorten the ulna approximately 1 to 4 mm using a burr through the radiocarpal portal, termed the Arthroscopic Wafer Procedure. When coexistent lunotriquetral perforations are present the joint should be assessed for stability manually or by using a probe. Instability of the lunotriquetral joint can be treated by percutaneous pin fixation, ligament reconstruction, ulnar shortening osteotomy, or limited intercarpal arthrodesis. Peripheral tears of the TFCC have sufficient vascularity and thus potential for healing.

These injuries can be repaired arthroscopically using a variety of techniques. We most frequently perform the outside-in repair, which is similar to the technique used for meniscal injuries. Two or three nonabsorbable sutures are placed in the disc peripherally and tied over the capsule subcutaneously.

In 1990, we reported a prospective series of 52 patients with isolated TFCC tears who were treated by arthroscopic debridement. The average duration of symptoms before arthroscopy was 11 months. All patients had failed a trial of splinting and injection.

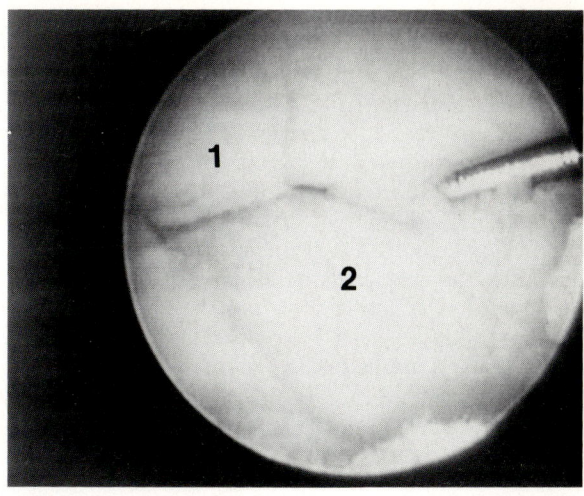

Figure 9 Arthroscopic view of the torn triangular fibrocartilage after debridement. 1 = edge of TFCC tear; 2 = distal ulna.

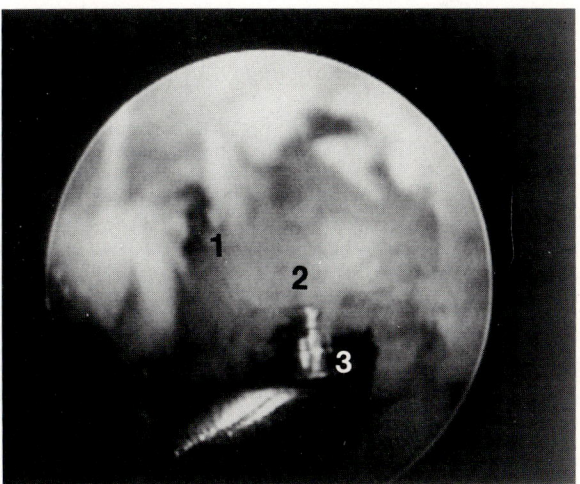

Figure 10 Arthroscopic debridement of chondromalacic distal ulna through a degenerative tear of the TFCC in a patient with positive ulnar variance. 1 = distal ulna, 2 = edge TFCC; 3 = curette.

Preoperative physical examination showed that two-thirds had some degree of ulnarly based tendonitis. There was mild limitation of extremes of rotatory motion in one-third. A click could be elicited in 60% of the patients. In 70%, it was unilateral, and in 29%, the click was bilateral. In three-fourths of those patients in whom a click could be elicited this maneuver reproduced their symptoms.

A radiocarpal arthrogram showing an isolated tear of the TFCC was a criterion for entry in the study. Ulnar variance was positive in 29% of the patients, neutral in 39%, and negative in 32%. It should be emphasized that those wrists with positive ulnar variance were believed to have attritional tears, and in these cases, a resection of the distal portion of the ulna was also performed. In most patients (96%), surgery was performed on an out-patient basis with the patient under regional anesthesia. The operative time averaged 75 minutes (Fig. 9). Follow-up on this series exceeded 3 years. Postoperatively, three-fourths of the patients felt that their pain was fully improved, 12% continued to have intermittent but milder symptoms, 10% felt no change from the preoperative symptoms, and 5% experienced worse pain. In those with preoperative clicking and "catching," the clicking resolved within 2 weeks, although in one-fourth, the click remained (but was not painful). Of importance on follow-up, no clinical or radiographic ulnar instability was noted. No infections were noted. A mild extensor tendon derangement was noted in one patient who had a persistent extensor digiti quinti minimi lage of 30 degrees. No unresolved neurovascular problems such as reflex sympathetic dystrophy or neuropraxias occurred. Two patients did have transient dorsal ulnar sensory symptoms that cleared within 3 months. Those patients with injury of a sports-related nature returned to unrestricted activity at an average of 6 weeks. Patients receiving worker's compensation were unable to work for an average of 3.2 months (a range of 1 week to 6.2 months). Patient satisfaction was high, with 88% considering the surgery worthwhile. Two of the three patients with bilateral tears had the opposite wrist operated on.

Arthroscopic debridement of an isolated TFCC perforation is not only technically feasible, but in the short term, is of benefit in reducing symptoms without increasing ulnar instability. It is associated with less morbidity than the other options, which involve either open resection of the triangular fibrocartilage, or procedures addressing the distal ulna. It should be emphasized that if significant positive ulnar variance was noted radiographically or if chondromalacia changes were seen at surgery, a limited resection of the distal ulna was performed (Fig. 10).

OTHER THERAPEUTIC USES FOR WRIST ARTHROSCOPY

Carpal Instability

Instabilities of the scapholunate and lunatotriquetral joint can be treated arthroscopically (see Fig. 3). The torn and frayed ligament and the accompanying synovitis are debrided. An accurate reduction is then performed. The adequacy of the reduction is best visualized by keeping the scope in the midcarpal joint where the concavity of the surface allows more accurate alignment. Particularly in patients with scapholunate instability, the use of joy-stick pins placed percutaneously in the lunate and scaphoid may provide further control in positioning the carpal bones. This technique cannot be used when the deformities are fixed. Once anatomic reduction has been achieved, pins are placed percutaneously across the intercarpal areas. In patients with scapholunate instability, a pin is usually placed across the scapholunate joint and across the scaphocapitate joint. In lunatotriquetral instability, pins are placed across the lunatotri-

quetra interval. The radiocarpal joint is almost never pinned. The 0.045 Kirschner (K-) wires are buried subcutaneously and do not substitute for cast immobilization. At approximately 8 weeks, the pins are removed and motion is begun. The short-term results of these arthroscopic reductions and internal fixations have been rewarding.

Intra-articular Fracture Reduction

Arthroscopy may be beneficial in achieving and confirming congruent reduction of distal radial and carpal fractures. For comminuted distal radius fractures an external fixator is applied after a closed reduction. The wrist arthroscope is then inserted through the 3-4 portal. Small loose fragments and clot are debrided. The large chondral fragments are elevated into an anatomic position under direct visualization. Smooth pins are placed subchondrally to support the fragments. The external fixator and percutaneous pins are generally left in place for 6 weeks. Certain precautions must be observed in scoping acute injury situations. We use Coband or an Esmarch bandage around the forearm along with elevation of the tourniquet to avoid extravasation of excessive fluid into the soft tissue with its potential for neurovascular compromise. We are also cognizant of the amount of fluid instilled.

Nondisplaced scaphoid fractures may be considered for arthroscopic reduction and internal fixation with the cannulated Herbert screw. The advantage of this technique is early mobilization, which will prevent wrist stiffness. The arthroscope is placed in the radial midcarpal portal and the scaphoid is reduced. The target hook of the jig is placed in the 1-2 portal. The barrel is placed on the distal scaphoid through a volar incision. The guide wire is driven through the barrel across the fracture site, and the position is verified fluoroscopically. A second guide wire is placed to control rotation. The cannulated Herbert screw is inserted after the scaphoid has been drilled and tapped.

Synovectomy, Particulate Body Removal, and Release Arthrofibrosis

Through the arthroscope, one can perform a relatively complete synovectomy of the wrist of both the radiocarpal and midcarpal joints. One can also remove foreign bodies or loose bodies arthroscopically. Wrist stiffness due to arthrofibrosis can be treated with arthroscopic release of the intra-articular adhesions. The debridement of the adhesions requires the use of a suction punch, full radius resector and various basket forceps.

Chondroplasties

Abrasion arthroplasty and debridement of articular defects in the wrist are similar to those done in the knee, but because it is not a weight-bearing joint, the results are often better. When the chondral lesion is secondary to an underlying ligament derangement, however, the benefit derived is temporary unless the primary problem is addressed.

Carpal Bone Excision

Ectomy surgery of the carpal bones through the scope is also possible. Procedures that we have performed include excision of small proximal pole fragments of the scaphoid, lunate excision in late-stage Kienbock's disease, and proximal row carpectomy. It should be emphasized, however, that such carpal bone excisions tend to destabilize the wrist, and one should consider the possibility of some type of concurrent carpal stabilization, which requires an open procedure.

Ganglion Resection

The dorsal ganglion most commonly arises from the dorsal capsule in the region of the scapholunate joint. This position allows visualization of the stalk for arthroscopic resection. The arthroscope is first placed in the 6R portal and the stalk is visualized by viewing dorsally. The 3-4 portal is then established and the ganglion is ruptured. The stalk is resected using a shaver and suction punch to create a 1 cm defect in the dorsal capsule. Due to the proximity of the neurovascular structures, resection of the volar ganglion is not performed.

Modified Darrach Procedures and Radiostyloidectomies

Both modified Darrach procedures and radiostyloidectomies procedures can be performed arthroscopically. Debridement of the distal ulna or arthroscopic water procedure has already been addressed in the discussion of traingular fibrocartilage tears associated with ulnar positive variance and chondromalacia of the distal ulna. Approximately 3 to 4 mm can easily be excised. If the triangular fibrocartilage is intact, one must perform an arthroscopic shortening through the distal radial ulnar joint.

In a chronic scaphoid nonunion with degenerative changes, the patient may symptomatically benefit by radiostyloidectomy. When the plain radiographs show early arthritic changes, arthroscopy may allow staging of the amount of change before a definite approach to scaphoid union. If excessive arthritis is present, a radial radiostyloidectomy can be performed arthroscopically. This should be considered a salvage procedure to be used when achieving scaphoid union is not likely to improve the patient symptomatically because of the arthritic change.

COMPLICATIONS

Significant complications in wrist arthroscopy are uncommon. Injury to the sensory nerves can occur while establishing portals. This can be avoided by incising the skin only and using a blunt hemostat on dissecting to the wrist capsule. Due to this complication we have abandoned the 6U portal as a working portal, and it is now used mainly as an outflow portal. Sensory nerves can also be injured while placing percutaneous pins; therefore, a protective guide should be used for K-wire placement. Nylon finger traps are used instead of wire finger traps to prevent digital nerve or soft tissue injury. Iatrogenic cartilage and ligament injury can be prevented by precise portal placement and knowledge of instrument position at all times. Other potential complications include anesthesia, equipment failure, infection, and reflex sympathetic dystrophy.

SUGGESTED READING

Bednar MS, Arnoczky SP, Weiland AJ. The microvasculature of the triangular fibrocartilage complex: Its clinical significance. J Hand Surg 1991; 16A:1101–1105.

Bora FW, Osterman AL, Maitin E, Bednar J. The role of arthroscopy in the treatment of disorders of the wrist. Contemp Orthop 1986; 12:28–36.

Brown DE, Lichtman DN. The evaluation of chronic wrist pain. Clin Orthop 1984; 15:183–191.

Green DP. The sore wrist without a fracture. Instructional course lectures. Am Acad Orthop Surgeons 1985; 34:300–313.

Mikik Z. Age changes in the triangular fibrocartilage of the wrist joint. J Anat 1978; 126:367.

North ER, Thomas S. An anatomic guide for arthroscopic visualization of the wrist capsular ligaments. J Hand Surg 1988:13A:815.

Osterman AL. Arthroscopic debridement of triangular fibrocartilage complex tears. Arthroscopy: The Journal of Arthroscopic and Related Surgery 1990; 6:120–124.

Palmer AK, Werner FW. Biomechanics of the distal radioulnar joint. Clin Orthop 1984: 187:26.

Palmer AK, Werner FW. The triangular fibrocartilage complex of the wrist: Anatomy and function. J Hand Surg 1981; 6:153–162.

Palmer AK, Werner FW, Glisson RR, Murphy DJ. Partial excision of the triangular fibrocartilage complex. J Hand Surg 1988; 13A: 391–394.

Poehling GG. Wrist arthroscopy. In: Illustrated guide to small joint arthroscopy. Dyonics Company, 1989.

Roth J. Radiocarpal arthroscopy: Operative technique. Orthopedics 1988; 11:1309–1313.

Roth JH, Haddad NG. Radiograph arthroscopy and arthrography in the diagnosis of ulnar wrist pain. Arthroscopy 1986; 2:234–243.

Roth JH, Poehling GG, Whipple TL. Arthroscopic surgery of the wrist. Instructional Course Lectures. Am Acad Orthop Surgery 1988; 37:183–194.

Viegas SF. Technical note midcarpal arthroscopy: Anatomy and technique. Arthroscopy: The Journal of Arthroscopic and Related Surgery 1992; 8:385–390.

Viegas SF, Ballantyne G. Attritional lesions of the wrist joint. J Hand Surg 1987; 12A:1025.

Whipple TC. Arthroscopic surgery — the wrist. Philadelphia: JB Lippincott, 1992.

Whipple TC, Marotta JJ, Powell JH. Techniques of wrist arthroscopy. Arthroscopy 1986; 2:244.

I SHOULDER

INJURIES TO THE ACROMIOCLAVICULAR JOINT

EDWARD P. FINK, M.D.

Injuries to the acromioclavicular joint are among the more common disorders of the shoulder incurred by athletic participants. Frequently sustained through a direct force imparted to the shoulder upon impact during a fall, these ligamentous injuries are well described and often easily recognized. The early medical writings of Hippocrates describe the salient features of this disorder. Yet since that time there has evolved no common consensus of opinion regarding treatment, as innumerable imaginative immobilization techniques and surgical procedures have been proposed in an attempt to restore anatomic alignment. Even today there remains considerable controversy over optimal management. This dilemma derives, in part, from an incomplete understanding of the functional anatomy of the acromioclavicular joint, the pathomechanics of ligamentous disruption, and the natural history of complete acromioclavicular separations. Insight into these principles can assist the practioner in implementing appropriate treatment to obtain predictable results in athletes with these injuries.

ANATOMY

Knowledge of the anatomy of the shoulder girdle is imperative in understanding the normal biomechanics of the shoulder, and conceptualizing the altered function that may occur with injuries to the acromioclavicular joint. The acromioclavicular joint is similar to many diarthrodial joints, with a fibrocartilaginous meniscus separating the articular cartilage, which invests the ends of both the clavicle and the acromion. The acromioclavicular ligaments encapsule the joint, yet are thin and weak, providing little inherent structural stability. The contribution of the surrounding soft tissues helps to maintain the integrity of the joint. The aponeuroses of the anterior deltoid and lateral trapezius blend in with the superior portion of the acromioclavicular ligaments to help strengthen the articulation. This anatomic configuration provides stability in the transverse plane, preventing anterior or posterior translation of the clavicle in relation to the acromion.

The coracoclavicular ligaments are the primary suspensory ligaments of the upper extremity and help to maintain the anatomic relationship of the acromioclavicular joint. Comprised of the conoid and trapezoid ligaments, the coracoclavicular ligaments provide vertical stability of the shoulder girdle, suspending the scapula and arm from the clavicle. A breech of these ligaments causes the arm to droop inferiorly due to its weight, creating incongruity of the acromioclavicular joint in the coronal plane.

The sternoclavicular joint is classically not discussed in treatises on acromioclavicular joint injuries, although its role in shoulder function and stability is most important. The sternoclavicular ligaments not only stabilize the clavicle by counteracting the weight of the upper extremity acting through a long lever arm on the lateral clavicle, they also accommodate the majority of clavicular motion. Clavicular motion occurs primarily through the sternoclavicular joint, with little movement evidenced through the acromioclavicular joint. The clavicle moves like a hinge on the sternum with shoulder abduction and adduction, while forward flexion and extension causes the clavicle to rotate as much as 40 to 50 degrees on the sternum as the scapula glides over the dorsal ribs.

MECHANISM OF INJURY

Injuries to the acromioclavicular joint are usually sustained from a fall, resulting in a direct blow to the lateral aspect of the shoulder with the arm adducted. With an appropriately directed force, the shoulder and the clavicle are suddenly forced inferiorly. The ultimate descent of the clavicle is blocked by the first rib upon which the clavicle impinges. More significant forces create more severe injuries that occur sequentially. Initially the acromioclavicular ligaments are strained, and then may rupture. As distraction forces increasingly develop between the clavicle and the shoulder girdle, stress is placed across the coracoclavicular ligaments, ultimately resulting in their failure. The trapezial attachments to the clavicle tear with further descent of the shoulder, while the deltoid muscle origins may be torn with forceful separation of the acromioclavicular joint. Most acromioclavicular derangements are produced by a direct blow to the shoulder. Much less commonly, a fall onto the outstretched arm forces the humeral head against the undersurface of the acromion. The acromioclavicular ligaments may be disrupted, and with increasing force, the coracoclavicular ligaments may be torn sequentially as well. As a result of these injuries, the upper extremity loses its ligamentous support and sags inferiorly. Clinical and radiographic evaluations reveal downward drooping of the scapula and arm, not a true superior displacement of the clavicle. The clavicle actually deviates little from its anatomic position due to the stabilizing sternoclavicular ligaments.

CLASSIFICATION OF INJURY

The classification system of acromioclavicular joint injuries is based on the degree of disruption of the acromioclavicular ligament, the coracoclavicular ligaments, and the surrounding soft tissues. Anatomically these injuries should be referred to as scapuloclavicular dislocations, because ligaments other than those at the acromioclavicular joint may be disrupted. Joint incongruence, however, is seen primarily at the acromioclavicular joint, and by convention this nomenclature has been adopted.

Classically, three types of injury to the acromioclavicular joint are recognized, and three additional injury variants have been described. The progression of injury from one type to the next is determined primarily by the amount of force imparted to the shoulder. The direction of transmitted forces produce the less common types of acromioclavicular displacements.

In type I injuries, a mild force to the lateral aspect of the shoulder produces a strain to the fibers of the acromioclavicular ligament. The ligaments are stretched but there is no significant soft tissue disruption and the joint is stable.

In type II injuries, a stronger force onto the shoulder is propagated, completely rupturing the acromioclavicular ligaments. The coracoclavicular ligaments are stretched yet remain intact. Instability of the acromioclavicular joint is produced in the horizontal plane with possible anterior and posterior translation of the clavicle. Stability in the vertical plane is maintained by the intact coracoclavicular ligaments.

As the force continues, the coracoclavicular ligaments are ruptured, producing a type III acromioclavicular injury. With disruption of both the acromioclavicular and coracoclavicular ligaments, the scapula and arm droop inferiorly. The origin of the deltoid muscle becomes detached from the distal end of the clavicle. Occasionally a variant of a type III acromioclavicular separation is noted as the coracoclavicular ligament remains intact, avulsing a fragment of the coracoid process.

In the uncommon types IV, V, and VI injuries, further forces produce clavicle displacement in addition to disruption of the acromioclavicular and coracoclavicular ligaments. In type IV the clavicle is driven posteriorly, oftentimes becoming incarcerated through a rent in the trapezius muscle. Type V injuries are created by an accentuation of forces from type III injuries, causing disruption of deltoid and trapezial attachments to the clavicle. Greater vertical instability develops, revealed as a greater distance between the clavicle and coracoid process, often tenting the overlying skin. In the rare type VI injury, inferior displacement of the clavicle beneath the coracoid process occurs posterior to the conjoined biceps and coracobrachialis tendon origins.

CLINICAL EXAMINATION

The examination of a patient with a suspected acromioclavicular joint injury should be performed with the patient in the standing position. The weight of the arm in a dependant position may accentuate a deformity that may not otherwise be apparent in the sitting or the supine positions. In type I injuries, pain is often present with palpation over the acromioclavicular joint, with no detectable instability. Type II injuries engender pain over the acromioclavicular joint, and at times may result in increased motion in the transverse plane with attempts at anterior or posterior displacement of the clavicle. In type III injuries the weight of the arm produces an impression of superior displacement of the clavicle. Pain is elicited over the acromioclavicular joint and coracoclavicular ligaments, and the incongruence of the acromioclavicular joint may be easily palpated.

RADIOGRAPHIC STUDIES

Most commonly a routine anteroposterior (AP) radiograph of the shoulder is taken to assess injuries to the shoulder girdle. While abnormalities of the acromioclavicular joint may be detected, this radiograph is exposed for the glenohumeral joint, and often the acromioclavicular joint is overexposed or not well visualized. The ideal radiographic views are an AP view centered over the acromioclavicular joint, directed 15 degrees cephalad, and a lateral view of the acromioclavicular joint. These views require approximately one-third the radiation exposure of a radiograph of the shoulder joint.

Stress views of the shoulder are often recommended to detect the presence of injuries that may have been sustained yet do not produce readily discernable deformities on clinical or radiographic evaluations. Ten to 15 pounds of weight are suspended from the wrists of the patient, not held in the hands. AP views of both acromioclavicular joints are taken simultaneously. The distance between the coracoid process and the clavicle is measured, comparing the injured and uninjured sides. Normal coracoid to clavicle distance is approximately 1.3 cm, and an increase of 40% to 50% of the distance compared to the uninjured shoulder is diagnostic of a type III acromioclavicular joint disruption.

MANAGEMENT

The treatment of athletes and individuals at all levels of activities should attempt to restore function and allow prompt return to sports with predictable results. Management of acromioclavicular joint injuries is predicated on the degree of ligamentous and soft tissue disruption.

Grade I sprains usually create no treatment dilemmas or complications. Ice may be applied to the injured shoulder for 24 hours, while a sling provides immobilization for pain relief. Within 7 to 10 days, pain diminishes sufficiently to allow the implementation of exercises and gradual return to normal levels of activity. Heavy lifting and contact sports should be delayed until a full active range of motion of the shoulder has been restored with no pain, not uncommonly requiring up to 2 weeks.

Nonoperative treatment for type II acromioclavicular injuries similarly produces excellent results. Owing to the greater soft tissue disruption, immobilization is employed for 1 to 2 weeks to allow resolution of pain. Gentle range of motion (ROM) exercises may be instituted during this period. Contact sports and heavy lifting activities should be proscribed for 6 weeks due to concerns with creating a type III disruption through a second similar injury.

Considerable controversy surrounds the treatment of acute type III acromioclavicular dislocations. This derives in part from the principles of treatment of other joint dislocations, namely anatomic reduction and maintenance of the reduction while early protective ROM exercises are instituted. The critical issue appears to be whether a complete anatomic reduction is essential for the restoration of normal shoulder function.

Clinical studies have repeatedly demonstrated little correlation between maintenance of an anatomic reduction and the functional result. Nonoperative treatment in which an acromioclavicular joint subluxation or dislocation persists produces excellent clinical results. However, there is often a compelling urge to restore anatomic alignment through surgical reconstruction in an attempt to gain shoulder stability. Many studies have documented the subjective reports of patients treated conservatively without surgery, noting that they return to work and sporting activities more quickly, and are more satisfied with the results of their treatment. Objective strength testing with a Cybex dynamometer showed strength of the shoulder was not significantly diminished with chronic subluxation or dislocation of the acromioclavicular joint.

Most individuals sustaining a type III acromioclavicular dislocation should be managed nonoperatively. Immobilization should be employed until discomfort has diminished sufficiently to allow pain-free movement of the shoulder. Physical therapy and rehabilitation are utilized to re-establish full active ROM of the shoulder, often requiring 3 to 4 weeks. Progressive strengthening exercises should be performed concurrent with increasing activities. Full return to sports participation should be prohibited until the athlete regains a full active ROM of the shoulder, experiences no pain, displays normal strength, and has confidence in the use of the extremity in sports participation.

The treatment of the more uncommon types IV, V, and VI acromioclavicular injuries may require surgical intervention. The principles of treatment of a type IV injury are to reduce the posterior displacement of the clavicle from within the trapezius, creating a type III injury. Conservative treatment should then be employed, with surgical intervention only if the clavicle cannot be reduced by manipulation. Type V injuries require more prolonged immobilization, to allow healing of the extensive soft tissue injury. Treatment should reduce the amount of displacement between the coracoid process and the clavicle equal to that of a type III dislocation. This can easily be obtained with sling immobilization to support the weight of the arm. The treatment of type VI injuries often requires surgical extraction of the clavicle from its position inferior to the coracoid process.

Surgical intervention should be considered for two types of individuals whose unique demands of shoulder function may cause discomfort or restrict athletic activities without an anatomic reduction. Individuals involved in heavy labor at times experience fatigue and a dull aching sensation in the shoulder after 4 to 6 hours of work if the shoulder girdle remains unsupported. In addition, certain young athletes, often under 30 years of age, experience discomfort in the shoulder with repetitive overhead activities after a type III acromioclavicular injury. The motions of the shoulder employed in tennis, swimming, and throwing activities are provocative. In these situations, reduction of the acromioclavicular joint, repair of the ruptured ligaments and avulsed tendons, and stabilization of the clavicle to the coracoid process produce superior functional results.

The importance of a complete history at the time of injury cannot be overemphasized. The functional needs and demands of each athlete must be determined to allow proper individualization of care. Heavy laborers and patients requiring repetitive overhead use of their arms who wish to return to their preinjury level of activities should be identified, and surgical options should be discussed with them. A more protracted rehabilitation time to return to heavy manual labor or sports should be envisioned.

COMPLICATIONS

Individuals with an acromioclavicular joint injury may develop degenerative changes within the joint. This is more frequently seen following types I and II injuries either due to initial injuries to the articular cartilage and disc, or secondary to chronic subluxation and progressive degenerative changes. Radiographic incongruence of the acromioclavicular joint is not usually seen. Pain may become manifest within the first 6 months after injury, occurring with activities requiring flexion and adduction of the shoulder. Radiographs often reveal joint space narrowing and osteophytic proliferation indicative of degenerative joint changes. Conservative management should initially be employed with a steroid injection into the acromioclavicular joint. This may be effective in diminishing the inflammatory component associated with degenerative changes. If pain persists, a resection of the lateral clavicle should be performed, either arthroscopically or through an open surgical procedure. A resection arthroplasty is produced, removing approximately 1 cm of the lateral clavicle, preventing abutment of the clavicle on the acromion with flexion and adduction of the shoulder.

Occasionally in heavy laborers, persistent fatigue and discomfort develops in chronically unreduced type III dislocations due to inferior droop of the shoulder and lack of support. These individuals often benefit through surgical reapproximation of the shoulder girdle to the clavicle. However, because the acromioclavicular joint has been chronically dislocated, the joint must be resected due to degenerative changes. This is achieved by resection of the lateral clavicle, reconstruction of the coracoclavicular ligament, and stabilization of the clavicle to the coracoid to allow ligamentous and soft tissue reapproximation. In this late reconstruction,

surgical intervention can decrease pain and achieve shoulder stabilization allowing increased functional results.

Post-traumatic osteolysis of the outer end of the clavicle occurs infrequently after subluxation or dislocation of the acromioclavicular joint. The etiology is unknown, although autonomic nerve dysfunction affecting blood supply to the clavicle is thought to cause resorption of bone from the outer end of the clavicle. Pain and weakness occur with adduction and flexion of the arm. Although symptoms may be self-limiting after 1 year, resection of the outer 1 cm of the clavicle and joint debridement may be required to alleviate the pain and allow restoration of shoulder motion. Calcification and ossification of the coracoclavicular ligament may also be seen after injuries around the acromioclavicular joint. These findings are primarily radiographic and do not produce pain nor compromise shoulder function. An acromioclavicular injury with a coracoid process fracture is optimally managed conservatively, as the fracture heals uneventfully.

ATRAUMATIC OSTEOLYSIS OF THE DISTAL CLAVICLE

BERNARD R. CAHILL, M.D.
MICHAEL T. LEE, M.D.

According to Strauch, Dupas in 1936 first reported a case of traumatic osteolysis of the distal part of the clavicle. In 1963 Madsen summarized the findings in eight patients of his own and reviewed eight other cases reported in the literature, although he did not review the two patients reported by Stahl. From 1963 through 1982, 20 additional cases were reported, making a total of 38 cases described in the world literature. Thirty-four of these 38 patients had a history of acute trauma to the shoulder or acromioclavicular (AC) joint.

Atraumatic osteolysis was first reported by Ehricht in 1959, when he described the occurrence of osteolysis of the distal clavicle in an air hammer operator. This report was followed by descriptions of osteolysis in a patient who practiced judo, a delivery man, and a handball player. None of these four patients had a history of injury to the shoulder. In 1982 Cahill reported 46 cases of atraumatic osteolysis, all in males, 45 of whom were weight lifters.

Although pathologic changes in the AC joint subsequent to trauma, resulting in osteolysis of the distal part of the clavicle, are common and usually recognized, the same sequence of events in a patient without a

history of shoulder trauma continues to be a diagnostic problem for many orthopedists.

This chapter reviews the clinical course and presentation, radiographic findings, and treatment of atraumatic osteolysis of the distal clavicle (AODC), and describes the frequent association of this entity with other shoulder conditions producing dysfunction and pain in the athlete.

CASE MATERIAL

Since 1982, when 46 patients with AODC were reported, 76 other patients have been treated by the senior author. None of these 122 patients had a significant history of injury and none had an acute injury. With the exception of two patients, all were athletes or exercisers. However, it is notable that the two nonathletes were involved in occupations requiring heavy manual labor and overhead lifting.

Strength training exercise as practiced by body builders and competitive weight lifters remains the leading feature of the history of AODC, followed by football and swimming. During the past 30 years, strength training has become an integral part of the training regimen of all sports, and the development of AODC has followed.

Bilateral symptoms are common, representing nearly 37% of this series, and joint scintigraphy indicates a 50% bilateral involvement of the distal clavicle. In fact long-term follow-up shows bilateral involvement approaching 70% in the most recent review.

The throwing athlete is no longer immune to

AODC. Seven baseball pitchers, four tennis players, and two racquetball players are included in this post-1982 material. Eleven of these athletes had a significant history of strength training.

No cases of AODC in females were reported in 1982. Since then, 12 female athletes, all with strength training as a part of their programs, have been treated. Their sports were weight events in track and field (four), volleyball (two), basketball (three), and body building (three).

The average age of patients with AODC reported in 1982 was 23.3 years. This presenting age has dropped to 21 years in the reports from 1982 to 1991 and is presumed to be a result of the cumulative stresses on the AC joint generated by earlier entry of the athlete into sports, the addition of strength training, and the intensity of the training programs.

CLINICAL PICTURE

Symptoms begin with a slow onset of pain in the area of the AC joint. It is usually described as a dull ache and occurs several hours after the exercise bout. There may be some radiation to the adjacent deltoid muscle or proximally along the superior border of the trapezius. As AODC progresses, the athlete describes the onset of pain at the beginning of exercise, and the pain eventually prevents or interferes with performance.

When strength training is a significant aspect of the training program, the athlete characteristically describes pain at the AC joint with bench pressing, dips, or push-ups.

When uncomplicated by other conditions, the range of motion of the glenohumeral joint is normal and muscle atrophy of the shoulder joint has not been noted.

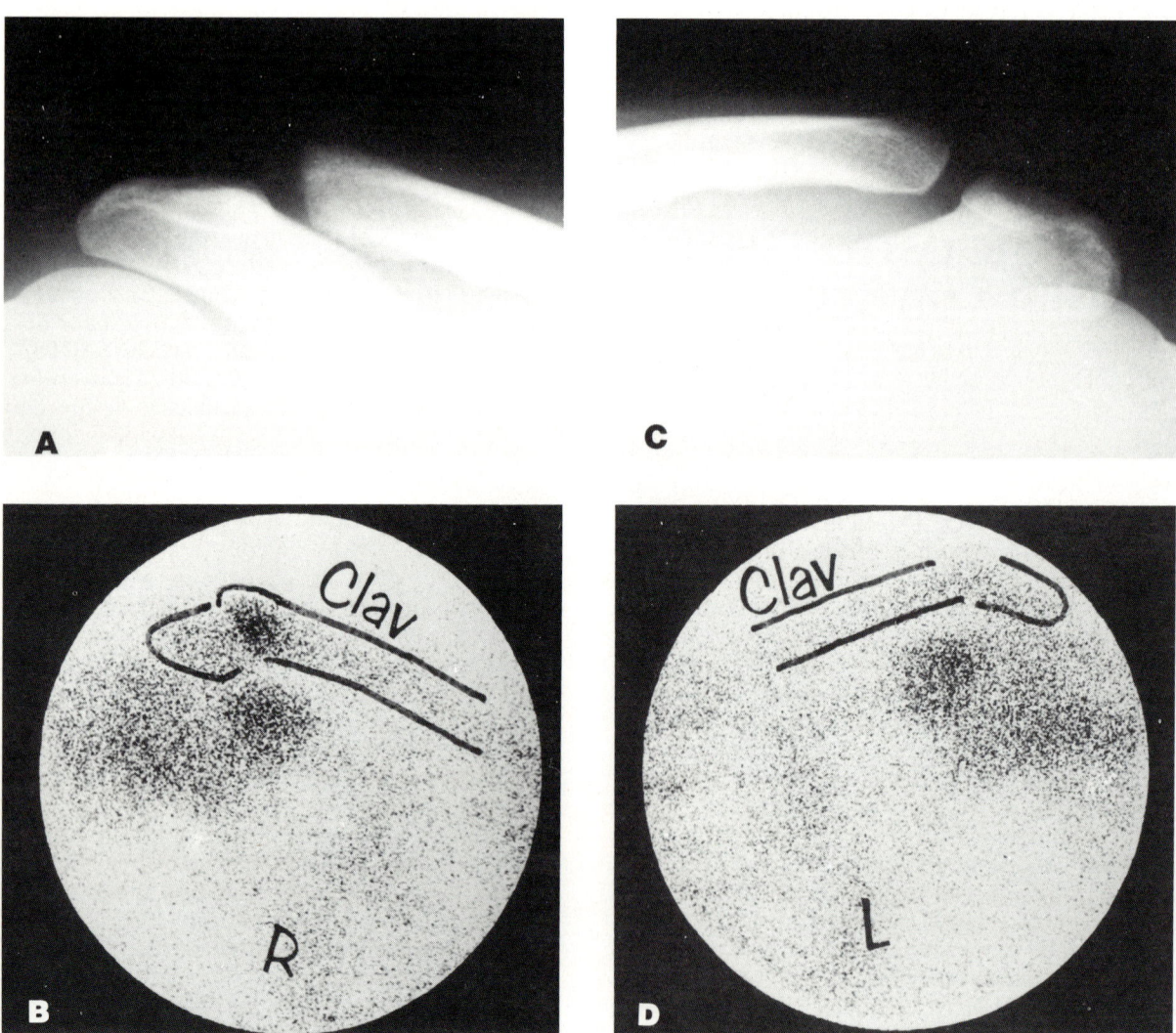

Figure 1 Radiograph of the symptomatic right shoulder of a 17-year-old football player with AODC and the asymptomatic normal left shoulder. *A,* Early microcystic changes and loss of the subchondral line are seen. View taken with the 15 degree cephalad technique. *B,* Scintigram shows that the distal clavicle is involved but not the acromion process. *C,* Radiograph of the asymptomatic left shoulder is normal. Note the intact subchondral line. *D,* Normal joint scintigraphy of the left shoulder.

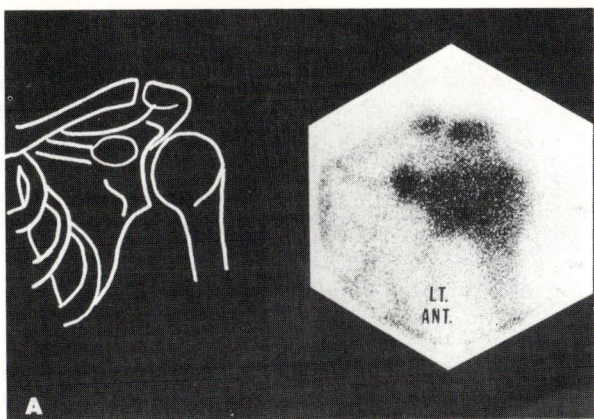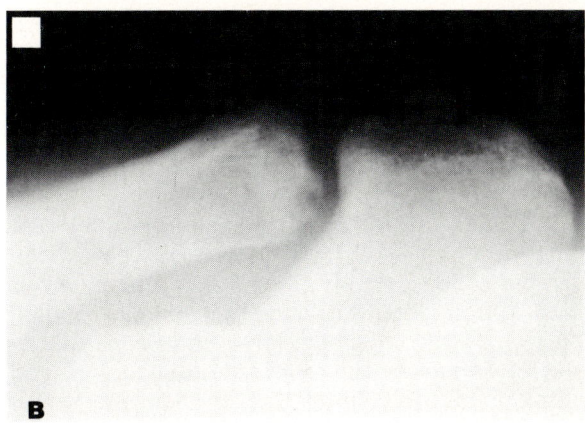

Figure 2 The left shoulder of a college football player. *A,* The asymptomatic left shoulder. The scintigram shows involvement of both the distal clavicle and the acromion process. *B,* Three years later the radiograph of the now symptomatic left shoulder shows microcystic changes and loss of the subchondral line. This patient underwent bilateral resections of the distal clavicle, and 14 years after surgery on the right and 5 years after surgery on the left shoulder, considers his shoulders to be normal. (From Cahill BR. Osteolysis of the distal part of the clavicle in male athletes. J Bone Joint Surg 1982; 64A:1053-1058; with permission.)

There may be mild prominence of the AC joint, although in the common bilateral presentation this may be difficult to evaluate. Tenderness is always present at the AC joint. Instability of this joint is not a feature of AODC, but crepitation may be. As AODC progresses, all throwing motions become painful and the activities of daily living may be affected.

The dominant extremity has a slightly higher incidence of symptomatic AODC. There is a higher correlation than dominance that is related to the architecture of the AC joint as discribed by DePalma. The highest incidence is seen in Type III followed by Type II.

RADIOGRAPHIC FINDINGS

Zanca made the most comprehensive radiographic study of the AC joint and pointed out the quotidian occurrence of degeneration of that joint, which was usually asymptomatic. He did not compare his data with scintigraphic activity in the AC joint.

The radiographic finding in traumatic osteolysis of the distal clavicle, described by Madsen and Levine and colleagues as tapering of the distal part of the clavicle, is not seen in AODC. Murphy and colleagues and Jacobs stated that the earliest radiographic changes of osteolysis after trauma may ensure in 4 weeks. In our experience with AODC, radiographic changes as recorded by standard x-ray techniques are subtle and late manifestations.

These radiographically revealed alterations consist of a loss of subchondral bone detail and microcystic appearances in the subchondral area of the distal clavicle (Figs. 1, *A,* and 2, *B*). Osteoporosis of the latcral third of the clavicle may occur. To evaluate the AC joint adequately, the 15 degree cephalad technique as well as joint scintigraphy must be performed. Neither nuclear magnetic resonance imaging (MRI) nor computed tomographic (CT) scans have been helpful in the diagnosis of AODC.

JOINT SCINTIGRAPHY

Technetium-99m-labeled phosphate scintigraphy is essential to confirm the diagnosis of AODC. Joint scintigraphy demonstrating increased uptake of the radiotracer was positive in one or both shoulders in all 113 patients in this series. It is the sine qua non of AODC.

Approximately 50% of the patients with AODC have increased scintigraphic activity of the adjacent acromion.

Pathologic material from 14 patients operated on was examined microscopically. This was histologically represented by articular degeneration, chronic inflammation, fibrosis, loss of trabecular structure, and osteoblastic activity. Numerous areas of subchondral microfractures were also noted and these together represent attempts at chronic fracture repair.

The increased scintigraphic activity seen in patients with AODC is due to increased osteoblastic activity and not entirely to an increased regional blood flow.

The sensitivity of joint scintigraphy in detecting pathology in patients with radiographically normal joints is well known. Scintigraphy was found to be positive in 17% of AODC patients with contralateral asymptomatic and radiographic normal shoulders. Symptomatic shoulders with normal x-rays were scintigraphically positive in over 70% of the patients.

DIAGNOSIS

The diagnosis of AODC must be considered in any athlete or exerciser with pain in the epaulet area (point of shoulder) who also has a history of strength training. The differential diagnosis must consider cervical, glenohumeral, coracoacromial arch, and other sources of shoulder pain. The diagnosis is probable if there is a history of epaulet pain later localizing at the AC joint and local tenderness at this joint. Radiography may be contributory to the diagnosis. See Figure 3.

The final diagnosis is confirmed only by positive joint scintigraphy of the AC joint. MRI scans have been utilized but at this time afford no significant benefit or additional information warranted by the relatively high cost. They may prove helpful, however, in early identification of asymptomatic contralateral shoulders and furthermore in the confirmation or identification of etiology.

ETIOLOGY

The cumulative stresses applied to the shoulder joint over an ever-lengthening athletic career and the additional stresses of strength training must eventually become physiologically intolerable to some peculiarly susceptible weak link in some athletes. This physiologic intolerance to cumulative stress is a stress failure syndrome, now poorly termed an "overuse syndrome."

In the shoulder, as with stress failure syndromes elsewhere in the musculoskeletal system, several anatomic areas may become simultaneously or sequentially symptomatic. There may be a cause and effect as in foot dysfunction contributing to patellar stresses and the anterior knee pain syndrome. Alternatively, the stress failure syndrome may be a simultaneous development, as when multiple stress fractures are present in the lower extremity of a runner.

ASSOCIATION OF AODC WITH OTHER SHOULDER SYNDROMES

In the shoulder, AODC is frequently associated with the impingement syndrome and glenohumeral instability. It is usually both a contributor to impingement and simultaneously a distinct entity when associated with glenohumeral instability.

Impingement Syndrome

Neer and colleagues pointed out the frequent contribution that the AC joint makes to the overall pathology of the impingement syndrome. They further emphasized the importance of resection of the distal clavicle in order to decompress the coracoacromial arch adequately in some patients with impingement. Neer considers the AC joint to be an integral part of the arch.

The association of AODC in athletes with the impingement syndrome is probable if there is localized tenderness at the AC joint, and this may be confirmed by joint scintigraphy. The latter is not positive in uncomplicated athletic impingement syndromes. In Cahill's series of patients with athletic impingement syndromes,

the incidence of AODC as demonstrated by positive AC joint scintigraphy may be as high as 15%. Therefore, all patients with athletic impingement who are potential surgical candidates should undergo a scintigraphic evaluation, and excision of the distal clavicle as a potential adjunctive procedure to the standard coracoacromial arch decompression when scintigraphy is positive.

Glenohumeral Instability

In any athlete with glenohumeral instability, a careful history must be taken for shoulder pain during periods of glenohumeral stability. If there is shoulder pain during periods of stability, the clinician should be suspicious of an additional pathologic condition. An additional tocsin of combined pathology is AC joint tenderness in the athlete with shoulder instability. If there is a history of pain between episodes of instability, or AC joint tenderness in the absence of pain, joint scintigraphy should be performed and can confirm the association of AODC. In such patients, resection of the distal clavicle should be considered when reconstructing the glenohumeral joint.

There has been no alteration in the rehabilitative pattern or results in the 11 patients Cahill (1992) identified with glenohumeral instability and AODC (seven with dislocations, four with subluxation) who underwent combined reconstruction and resection of the distal clavicle.

TREATMENT

Conservative treatment of AODC should be directed toward eliminating the most symptom-provocative aspect of the training program. This is usually discovered to be strength training routines. It is often beneficial to eliminate or alter provocative strength training exercises or decrease their intensity. Nonsteroidal anti-inflammatory drugs or intra-articular injections are temporizing and pernicious methods of therapy. They should not be employed in the young athlete.

AODC is inexorably progressive if the implied stresses are not reduced or altered. Even temporary cessation of provocative activity has failed if that activity is once again resumed. Since Cahill's 1982 report on AODC, it has become increasingly difficult to counsel the athlete to accept a lower level of stress to the shoulder. The reasons are both philosophic and socioeconomic and are a separate topic. As a result, fewer athletes or exercisers are willing to accept conservative recommendations.

The indications for surgical management of AODC are unchanged from the 1982 report and are (1) a confirmed diagnosis of AODC and (2) an unwillingness on the part of the athlete to accept a lower level of performance.

Gurd and Mumford, while they both reported resection of the distal clavicle in 1941, were not the discoverers of this procedure. The poor results of this

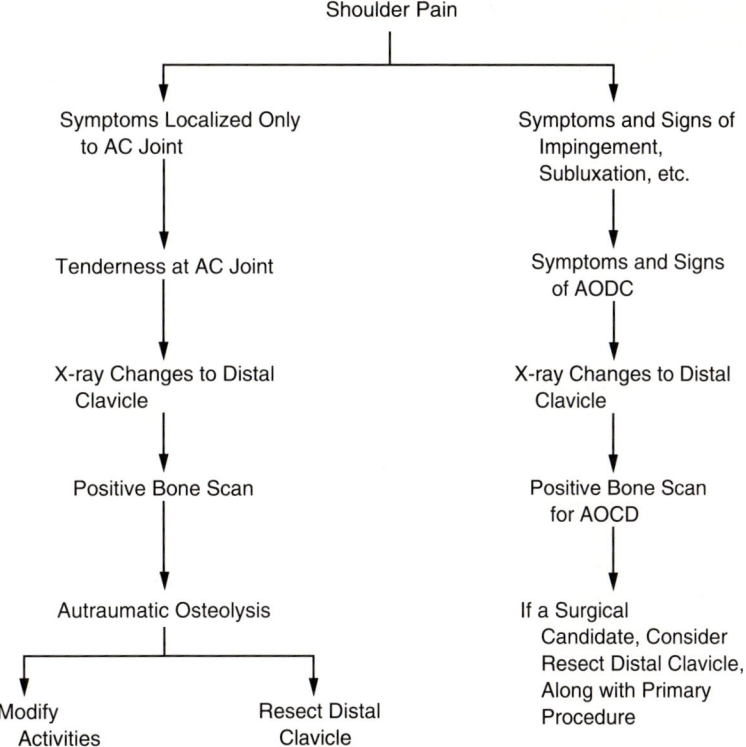

Figure 3 Algorithm for atraumatic osteolysis of the distal clavicle (From Cahill BR. Atraumatic osteolysis of the distal clavicle. Sports Med 1992; 13:214-222; with permission.)

procedure as reported are usually due to the pathologic process for which the excision was chosen. Resection of the distal clavicle for acute or chronic AC instability has a poor to dismal success rate.

Since the Cahill report in 1982, 36 of the 67 AODC patients have undergone resection of the distal clavicles. The results have been consistently good or excellent in 94% of patients. A recent review by Slawski and Cahill with average follow-up of 25 months showed full return to work or sports at an average of 9 weeks, at or exceeding the previously achieved activity level before onset of the symptoms that led to their surgery.

A recent arthroscopic alternative to open resection has been described and has been found to be equally as efficacious with lower morbidity and even a more rapid return to normal activity.

With the increasing numbers of athletes participating in strength training programs and a recent prospective matched study showing radiographic AODC prevalence among weight lifters at 28% and symptomatic prevalence at 44% this will be a common presentation to many sports medicine physicians. We do not hesitate to recommend surgical resection of the distal clavicle in well-motivated mature patients.

SUGGESTED READING

Cahill BR. Osteolysis of the distal part of the clavicle in male athletes. J Bone Joint Surg 1982; 64A:1053-1058.

Cahill BR. Atraumatic osteolysis of the distal clavicle. Sports Med 1992; 13:214-222.

Flatow EL, Cordasco FA, Bighani LU. Arthroscopic resection of the outer end of the clavicle from a superior approach: A critical quantitative radiographic assessment of bone removal. J Arthroscopic Rel Surg 1992; 8(1):55-64.

Gurd F. The treatment of complete dislocation of the outer end of the clavicle; An hitherto undescribed operation. Ann Surg 1941; 113:1094-1098.

Lamont MK. Osteolysis of the outer end of the clavicle. NZ Med J 1982; 95:241-242.

Levine AH, Pais MJ, Schwartz EE. Posttraumatic osteolysis of the distal clavicle with emphasis on early radiologic changes. Am J Roentgenol 1976; 127:781-784.

Madsen B. Osteolysis of the acromial end of the clavicle following trauma. Br J Radiol 1963; 36:822-828.

Mumford E. Acromioclavicular dislocation. J Bone Joint Surg 1941; 23:799-802.

Murphy OB, Bellamy R, Wheeler W, Brower TD. Post-traumatic osteolysis of the distal clavicle. Clin Orthop 1975; 109:108-114.

Scavenius M, Iverson BF. Nontraumatic clavicular osteolysis in weight lifters. Am J Sports Med 1992; 20(4):463-467.

Seymore EQ. Osteolysis of the clavicular tip associated with repeated minor trauma to the shoulder. Radiology 1977; 123:56.

Slawski DP, Cahill BR. Atraumatic osteolysis of the distal clavicle: results of surgical excision. Am J Sports Med 1994; 22(2):267-271.

Stahl F. Considerations on post-traumatic absorption of the outer end of the clavicle. Acta Orthop Scand 1954; 23:9-13.

Zanca P. Shoulder pain: involvement of the acromioclavicular joint (analysis of 1,000 cases). Am J Roentgenol 1971; 112:493-506.

ARTHROSCOPIC RESECTION OF THE ACROMIOCLAVICULAR JOINT

GARY M. GARTSMAN, M.D.

Shoulder pain is a common cause for presentation to the orthopedist. While the exact incidence of acromio-clavicular (AC) joint pathology is not known, patient complaints of pain around the AC joint frequently occur either as an isolated entity or in combination with rotator cuff disease.

Arthroscopic resection of the AC joint is a natural outgrowth of our increased knowledge and expertise in shoulder arthroscopy. The most common shoulder arthroscopic procedure is the arthroscopic subacromial decompression. This procedure involves an inferior acromioplasty and resection of inferior AC joint osteophytes as necessary. As surgeons have become more familiar with shoulder arthroscopy, arthroscopic techniques are employed to accomplish a resection of the AC joint.

ETIOLOGY

Arthritis of the AC joint can be found as a result of a single injury such as a fall on the superior or lateral aspect of the shoulder or can result from repetitive microtrauma. Osteolysis of the distal clavicle can occur in weight lifters, but in my experience post-traumatic arthritis without osteolysis is much more common.

It is important to differentiate pain due to arthritis from pain due to an AC joint separation (Fig. 1). Type III, IV, V, and VI separations produce symptoms due to the disconnection of the arm to the axial skeleton (Type III, V) or due to extreme displacement of the distal clavicle, causing mechanical irritation to the surrounding soft tissues (Type IV, VI). When pain is due to disconnection the arm feels "heavy" and the patient notes "fatigue" with carrying or lifting. The surgical correction of this condition requires establishment of the anatomy such that the connection exists. Common methods include coracoclavicular ligament repair or substitution with a transferred coracoacromial ligament. The reduction may be temporarily maintained with a screw from the clavicle to the coracoid. At present such AC joint reconstruction is an open surgical procedure. When extreme displacement of the distal clavicle occurs in type IV or VI separations distal clavicle resection is combined with reconstruction.

Pathology of the AC joint that is amenable to arthroscopic resection requires that the only lesion involve the joint surface. Loss of articular cartilage with preservation of the bone architecture is the ideal situation.

CLINICAL PRESENTATION

The patient complains of pain in the AC joint area. Some complain of pain in the superior or anterior aspect of the joint. Such complaints are very well localized by the patient. Pain in the posterior aspect of the joint is often reported to be more diffuse with the patient often pointing to the trapezius muscle. Common complaints include pain while washing the opposite axilla or posterior aspect of the contralateral shoulder, attaching the chest portion of a seatbelt, reaching behind the back to fasten a brassiere, or reaching for a wallet. Sporting activities causing pain include bench press weight lifting, the backswing in golf, and the follow-through in tennis.

The physical examination begins with inspection of the joint. Obvious swelling or prominence may be noted. Tenderness to palpation is common. Maneuvers designed to evoke pain include both cross-body adduction and horizontal extension. Due to the overlap of AC joint disease and rotator cuff lesions the examiner must be certain that the above maneuvers cause pain *in the region of the AC joint* and not in the subacromial area. This distinction is often not clear in the clinical setting as altered shoulder mechanics due to rotator cuff pain can result in increased stress on the AC joint. Similarly, inflammation of the AC joint can irritate the rotator cuff tendons that pass immediately inferior to the joint during arm elevation. If the diagnosis is difficult I advise local anesthetic injection into the AC joint. If the injection eliminates the pain the diagnosis of AC joint arthritis is more certain.

IINJECTION TECHNIQUE

Injection of the AC joint requires some care. Though the joint is subcutaneous the joint space is small. Study the orientation of the joint on the anteroposterior (AP) radiograph to gain some appreciation of the joint inclination. I use a short barrel 25 g needle and a 3 cc syringe. The small needle diameter allows for easier joint entry. The short barrel guards against inadvertent penetration of the inferior joint capsule and erroneous infiltration of the subacromial space. The small syringe increases the sensitivity of the examiner to the pressure change that occurs upon joint entry. After the injection the maneuvers that produced joint pain (cross-body adduction or horizontal extension of the 90 degree abducted arm) are then repeated and the diminution or elimination of pain is noted. The injection test is positive if the pain is eliminated or markedly reduced.

RADIOGRAPHS

An axillary and AP view are required. Common findings include a loss of joint space, sclerosis of the bone ends, cystic formation in the distal clavicle, and hypertrophic spur formation. The axillary view can demonstrate loss of the joint space and also confirms that the joint is located. A type IV or posterior distal clavicle

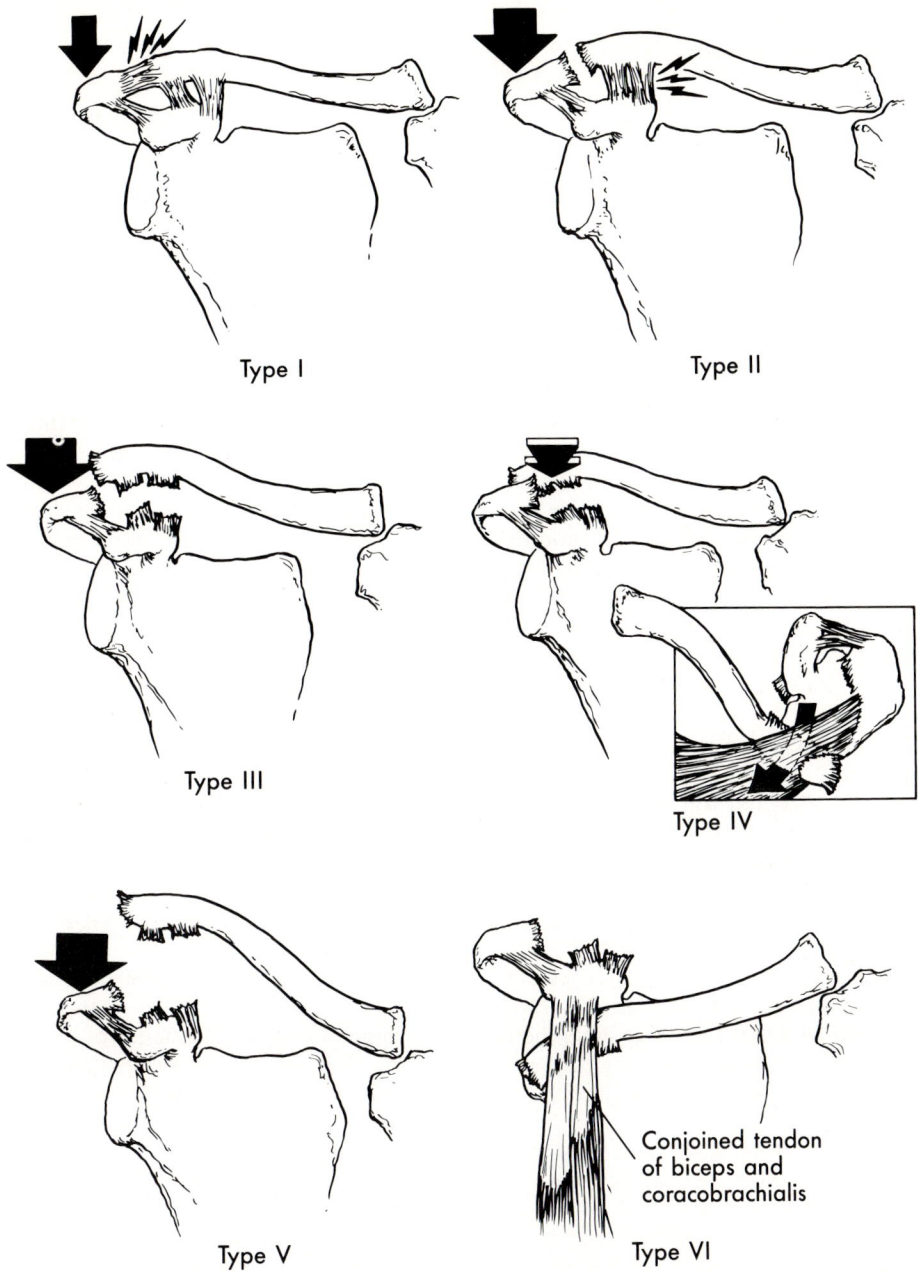

Figure 1 Classification of acromioclavicular (AC) injuries. Type I: neither AC nor coracoclavicular ligaments are disrupted. Type II: AC ligament is disrupted, and coracoclavicular ligament is intact. Type III: both ligaments are disrupted. Type IV: ligaments are disrupted, and distal end of clavicle is displaced posteriorly into or through trapezius muscle. Type V: ligaments and muscle attachments are disrupted, and clavicle and acromion are widely separated. Type VI: ligaments are disrupted, and distal clavicle is dislocated inferior to coracoid process and posterior to biceps and coracobrachialis tendons. (Redrawn from Rockwood CA Jr: Subluxations and dislocations about the shoulder. In: Rockwood CA Jr, Green DP, eds. Fractures in adults, ed 2, Philadelphia: JB Lippincott, 1984; with permission.)

dislocation can appear normal when viewed from single anterior projection. The AP projection will demonstrate any superior distal clavicle displacement and alert the orthopedic surgeon to the joint inclination. An appreciation of joint inclination is of value during joint injection or arthroscopic resection.

OTHER IMAGING MODALITIES

Magnetic resonance imaging (MRI) is used frequently to help in the diagnosis of soft tissue disorders around the shoulder. Currently the MRI seems overly sensitive to AC joint arthritis in that many asymptomatic individuals demonstrate impressive changes on the MRI films. Bone scans have similar strengths and weaknesses. While the bone scan often demonstrates increased uptake in the region of the AC joint, symptom-free patients often demonstrate the same findings. At present neither MRI nor bone scan is necessary to make the diagnosis of AC joint arthritis.

CONSERVATIVE TREATMENT

My impression is that the vast majority of individuals with symptomatic AC joint arthritis can be treated nonoperatively if they are willing to allow sufficient time to pass and to modify their activities.

The most important part of the conservative treatment program we employ is selective rest. By this I mean that the individual should avoid those activities and positions that cause pain in the AC joint. The shoulder should rest, not the patient. The weight lifter may continue to pursue that sport but should modify hand position on the bar so that the pain is eliminated. Alternatives include decreasing the amount of weight involved or the startlingly simple concept of abandoning the exercise altogether.

Patient education is also helpful. Even today many patients and trainers want to "work through the pain" thinking that the muscle soreness will go away. I have found that 6 to 12 months may lapse before the symptoms disappear. Usually patients balk at such a time period but when they are confronted with the surgical option, a waiting period can suddenly seem more attractive.

It is also helpful to explain to the patient that waiting will not increase the complexity of the surgery. I tell patients that it is the same procedure now as it will be in 1 year. Since the pain of AC arthritis is rarely disabling the conservative care program is continued for a minimum of 6 months. If the patient is improving but not cured after that time more waiting is advised. If the pain is not improved or if the pain worsens, surgical options are discussed.

SURGICAL TREATMENT

Indications and Contraindications

The surgical indications for arthroscopic resection of the AC joint are pain interfering with activities of daily living, work, or sports and failure to respond to appropriate conservative care for a minimum of 6 months. The pain should be localized to the AC joint by history and physical examination. A positive injection test is helpful.

Type III, IV, V, and VI joint dislocations are not amenable to arthroscopic correction. Type II injuries are relative contraindications as there are instances where the patient's pain is due to joint incongruity (and can be treated with arthroscopic resection) and instances in which the pain is due to joint instability and should be treated with open reconstruction.

Technique

Open resection of the distal clavicle or Mumford procedure for AC joint arthritis accomplishes two goals: the abnormal clavicle articular surface is removed and bone is resected to create enough space between the medial acromion and distal clavicle to eliminate painful contact between the two bones during shoulder movements. The arthroscopic approach removes the clavicular articular surface but also creates space by removing a small amount of bone from the medial acromion and correspondingly less bone from the distal clavicle (Fig. 2). I have termed this procedure *arthroscopic resection of the AC joint.*

Patient preparation, set-up, and instrumentation is identical to that of glenohumeral joint arthroscopy and subacromial decompression. I prefer the lateral decubitus position while others may prefer the sitting or beach chair position. I currently use an arthroscopic pump for fluid inflow.

The cannula and trocar are introduced into the subacromial space through an incision 1 cm medial and 1 cm inferior to the posterolateral corner of the acromion. I find it helpful to move the rod laterally and medially to release thick adhesions between the rotator cuff and the acromion. I also palpate the anterior and lateral aspects of the acromion. The cannula should be placed so that the tip is immediately posterior to the anterior acromial edge. The arthroscope is inserted and the pump connected.

I generally start with the pressure set around 80 mm. The subacromial space is inspected and the anterior acromial margin identified. I press with my fingertip at a

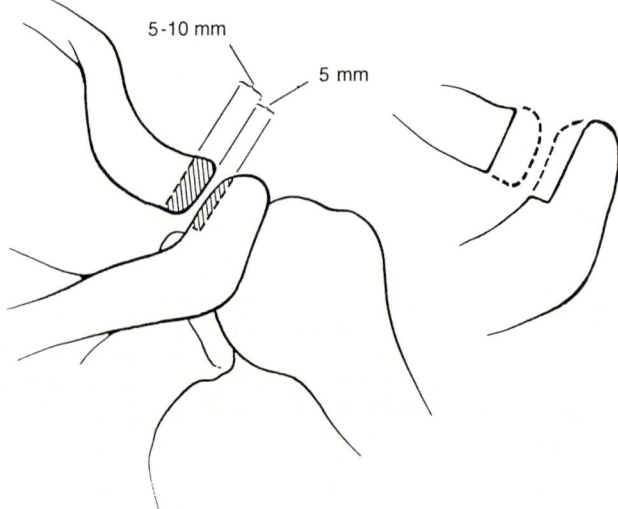

Figure 2 Hatched area represents desired bone removal. (From Ellman H, Gartsman GM. Arthroscopic shoulder surgery and related procedures. Malvern, Pa: Lea & Febiger, 1993; with permission.)

spot on the skin 2 to 3 cm distal to the anterior margin, directly inferior to the acromioclavicular joint. The movement can be appreciated in the subacromial space. A spinal needle is then introduced at this spot to enter the space parallel to the acromial undersurface to the AC joint. A small incision is made and the cannula and trocar inserted under direct vision.

The soft tissue resector is then used to remove any fibrous tissue that prevents an adequate examination of the superior rotator cuff surface. The undersurface of the acromion is palpated and fibrous tissue removed from the anterior medial surface of the acromion until cortical bone is visualized (Fig. 3). Once bone is observed directly orientation is simplified. The area underneath the AC joint is extremely vascular and before any bone or soft tissue resection commences the

area should be cauterized. The soft tissue resector should remove all fibrous tissue from the medial acromion bordering the AC joint.

The acromionizer burr is then introduced through the anterior cannula. The burr should be parallel to the joint (Fig. 4). Superior pressure is applied and acromion is removed from the anterior medial margin to the posterior medial margin. I attempt to remove the full thickness of the acromion. Often it is hard to see the superior surface to ensure that adequate bone has been removed. The arthroscope often must be advanced medially and rotated superiorly. Once a burr width (5.5 mm) of medial acromion has been removed the distal clavicle is clearly visualized (Figs. 5 and 6).

Remove any fragments of soft tissue covering the distal clavicle until bone is seen. Begin the distal clavicle resection at the anterior margin and resect medially until 1 burr width is excised. Continue in a superior and inferior direction until the resected surface is flat. Move the burr posteriorly and remove bone until the anterior and posterior aspects of the clavicle are level (Fig. 7). Once this has been achieved a 1 cm space should exist between the clavicle and the medial acromion. Additional bone is resected as necessary.

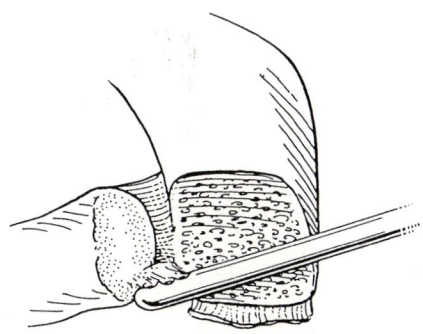

Figure 3 Acromioplasty and acromioclavicular joint resection combined. Inferior acromioclavicular joint ligaments removed to expose acromioclavicular joint. (From Ellman H, Gartsman GM. Arthroscopic shoulder surgery and related procedures. Malvern, Pa: Lea & Febiger, 1993; with permission.)

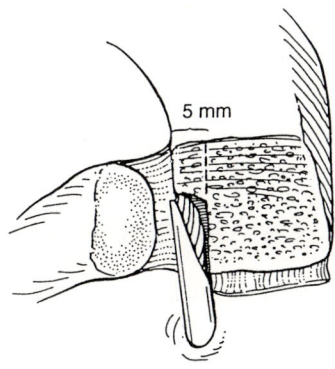

Figure 5 Burr removes 5.5 mm strip of medial acromion. (From Ellman H, Gartsman GM. Arthroscopic shoulder surgery and related procedures. Malvern, Pa: Lea & Febiger, 1993; with permission.)

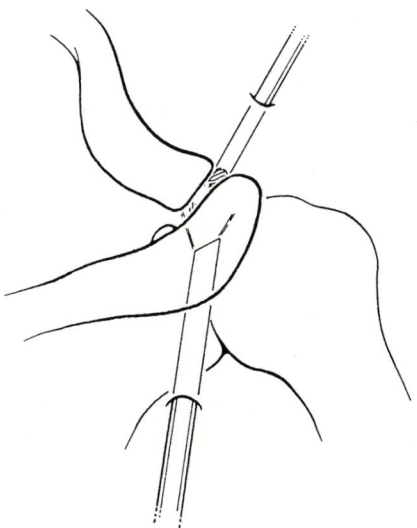

Figure 4 Burr placement anterior to acromioclavicular joint and parallel to joint surfaces. (From Ellman H, Gartsman GM. Arthroscopic shoulder surgery and related procedures. Malvern, Pa: Lea & Febiger, 1993; with permission.)

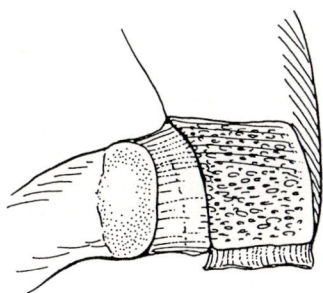

Figure 6 Wide joint exposure after removal of medial acromion. (From Ellman H, Gartsman GM. Arthroscopic shoulder surgery and related procedures. Malvern, Pa: Lea & Febiger, 1993; with permission.)

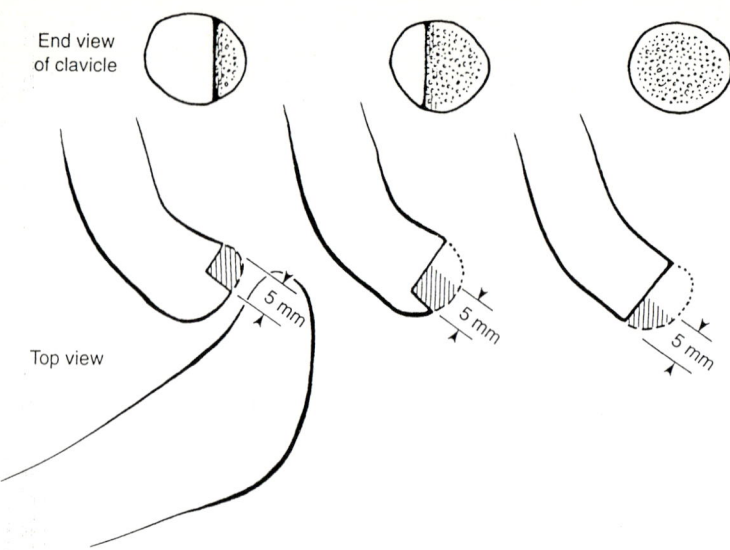

End view
of clavicle

Top view

5 mm

5 mm

5 mm

Figure 7 End view of the distal clavicle demonstrating the sequential removal of bone from anterior to posterior. (From Ellman H, Gartsman GM. Arthroscopic shoulder surgery and related procedures. Malvern, Pa: Lea & Febiger, 1993; with permission.)

Arthroscopic resection of the AC joint is complete when five criteria have been met:

1. 5 mm of the distal clavicle has been removed.
2. 5 mm of the medial acromion has been removed.
3. No sharp edges remain on the anterior, posterior, superior, or inferior clavicle surfaces.
4. The superior clavicle surface is clearly visualized and the superior AC joint fibers identified but not excised.
5. A 5 to 10 mm space exists between the medial acromion and the distal clavicle and no contact between the two bones occurs when the arm is guided through a range of motion (ROM).

The arthroscope and the cannulas are removed and the incisions are closed with single sutures. A sterile dressing is applied.

The surgery is performed on an out-patient basis unless medical conditions warrant in-patient admission.

POSTOPERATIVE MANAGEMENT

Patients begin rehabilitation the afternoon after surgery on a home program of passive and active ROM. A sling is worn for 1 day. Patients are encouraged to use the arm as normally as possible but to refrain from overhead work or sports until discomfort is minimal. They are seen in the office 1 to 2 weeks after surgery and instructed in a home program of isometric and isokinetic exercises. Return to work and sports is rapid and limited

more by accompanying rotator cuff disease than the actual joint resection.

RESULTS

Good results (85%) have been reported in the few literature references. Common areas of failure are technical and patient selection.

Failure to achieve adequate amount of bone removal and smooth resected bone surfaces is associated with continued patient complaints. If excess bone is removed and the AC joint destabilized further complaints of shoulder pain and fatigue will occur.

Probably the most common source of misdiagnosis involves failure to address rotator cuff disease associated with impingement or glenohumeral instability causing posterior superior shoulder pain. A thorough history, physical examination, examination under anesthesia, and glenohumeral arthroscopy should all be performed to reliably localize the AC joint as the lesion requiring surgical treatment.

SUGGESTED READING

Cook F, Tibone J. The Mumford procedure in athletes: an objective analysis of function. Am J Sports Med 1988; 16:97–100.
Ellman H, Gartsman GM. Arthroscopic shoulder surgery and related procedures. Malvern, Pa: Lea & Febiger, 1993.
Flatow EL, Cordasco FA, Bigliani LU. Arthroscopic resection of the clavicle from a superior approach. Arthroscopy 1992; 8:55–64.
Gartsman GM. Arthroscopic resection of the acromioclavicular joint. Am J Sports Med 1993; 21:71–77.

ARTHROSCOPIC RESECTION OF THE DISTAL CLAVICLE FROM A SUPERIOR APPROACH

EVAN L. FLATOW, M.D.

HISTORY

The acromioclavicular (AC) joint is a common source of shoulder pain. Most patients respond to conservative management, generally consisting of non-steroidal anti-inflammatory medication, heat, activity modification, and a steroid injection. For refractory cases, resection of the distal clavicle has been a reliable treatment.

Open resection of the distal clavicle for painful conditions of the AC joint was described by Gurd and Mumford in 1941, and subsequent authors have reported good results after open treatment. Arthroscopic approaches to the AC joint were first described in conjunction with arthroscopic subacromial decompression, when inferior clavicular osteophytes encroached upon the subacromial space and contributed to the impingement pathology. Although debridement of these osteophytes is usually all that is needed for impingement, patients who have concomitant AC joint pain and tenderness require complete resection of the distal clavicle. In these cases, arthroscopic resection may be performed through this same approach, in which the distal clavicle is viewed from below in the bursa. When pathology is limited to the AC joint, as in osteolysis of the distal clavicle, an isolated procedure of the AC joint can successfully relieve symptoms. Johnson described a superior approach to the AC joint in which the arthroscope and instruments are inserted directly into the AC joint, allowing direct visualization of the joint surfaces.

The technical ability to remove distal clavicular bone both through the bursal approach and the superior approach has been shown to be comparable to the amount removed by open methods. Clinical evaluation of arthroscopic distal clavicle resection and open resection is difficult when they are part of more extensive procedures. A comparison between arthroscopic and open distal clavicle resection as an isolated procedure for a single diagnosis, AC pain from osteolysis of the distal clavicle, was performed by Flatow and co-workers. Bone removal and pain relief were found to be comparable, but return to full activity occurred an average of 3 to 4 months sooner in the arthroscopic group than in the open resection group.

CLINICAL PRESENTATION, EVALUATION, AND INDICATIONS FOR SURGERY

Simple excision of the distal clavicle is not appropriate for unstable AC joints, such as those that are chronically dislocated. These cases are better treated with fixation to the coracoid and ligament reconstruction. Most chronic AC disorders, for which resection of the distal clavicle might be considered, are due to osteolysis of the distal clavicle or to AC arthritis.

AC joint arthritis can develop after trauma, including type III intra-articular distal clavicle fractures and grade II AC joint separations, but more commonly the etiology is idiopathic. DePalma reported that degeneration of the AC joint was an age-related process. Symptoms at the AC joint do not necessarily correlate with the radiographic appearance of the joint, and treatment should be directed towards specific symptoms and signs of AC joint pathology.

Osteolysis of the distal clavicle was first reported in conjunction with acute trauma. Intra-articular distal clavicle fractures and AC separations can lead to osteolysis. Other etiologies include rheumatoid arthritis and hyperparathyroidism. However, the most common etiology of osteolysis of the distal clavicle is repetitive microtrauma, especially weight-lifting. The small area of the AC joint and the large forces transmitted along the clavicle (acting as a strut) by muscles such as the pectoralis major result in large joint stresses, and compressive failure with microfractures may be a factor in initiating osteolysis.

Patients usually complain of anterosuperior shoulder pain, often radiating to the trapezius and the base of the neck. The cardinal physical finding is tenderness to direct palpation of the AC joint. Pain may generally be produced with provocative maneuvers that twist or compress the AC joint, such as extreme internal rotation or horizontal adduction of the arm. An injection test with a local anesthetic can be extremely helpful in confirming that the AC joint is the source of the pain, and in demonstrating to a patient with other problems (e.g., cervical disease) how much relief may be reasonably expected with resection of the distal clavicle.

A standard radiographic evaluation includes an anteroposterior (AP) view in the scapular plane, a trans-scapular lateral, and an axillary view. In addition, AP radiographs of the AC joint with and without cephalic tilt using "soft tissue" technique (reduced penetration) are taken to detect subtle changes in the distal clavicle. These x-rays also helped determine inclination of the joint. Radiographic findings indicative of osteolysis are loss of subchondral bone detail, cystic reabsorption of the distal clavicle, and a generalized osteopenia of the distal clavicle. These findings may be subtle. Magnetic resonance imaging is usually not necessary, but can detect soft tissue enlargement and synovitis in the AC joint, as well as any encroachment of distal clavicular osteophytes on the underlying bursa and rotator cuff tendons. Technetium bone scans may show increased activity at the distal clavicle in osteolysis, but this finding may not be specific.

Most patients respond to conservative treatment as noted above. If not, surgical treatment should be considered.

TECHNIQUE

Bursal versus Superior Approach

The bursal approach for resection of the distal clavicle requires resection of soft tissue and the fat pad from under the AC joint for adequate visualization of this joint. This results in bleeding and inflammation in the subacromial space, which is generally not involved in isolated AC disorders (e.g., osteolysis, post-traumatic arthritis). For this reason I prefer the direct superior approach for isolated AC pathology. This is especially so in young, athletic patients such as weight-lifters and gymnasts, who, in my experience, recover use much faster after a procedure limited to the AC joint than after one that results in bursal swelling and deltoid soreness.

When a bursal procedure such as an acromioplasty is also indicated, resection of the distal clavicle may be initiated from the same bursal approach. However, I then reposition the arthroscope into a direct AC portal to allow final, precise bone contouring. The ability to clearly see the margins of the clavicle will reduce the risk of an uneven resection.

Direct Superior Approach

In the direct superior approach, the arthroscope and instruments are placed through anterosuperior and posterosuperior portals into the AC joint, and the pathology is visualized directly without violating the glenohumeral joint or subacromial bursa (Fig. 1). Regional interscalene anesthesia is routinely used, and arthroscopy is performed in the beach-chair position. De Palma and Petersson have demonstrated that there is an age-related narrowing to the AC joint, and that there is variability to the inclination of the joint line. It is thus important to determine the joint position and inclination exactly. This is done with three 22 gauge needles. The joint is then insufflated with normal saline. The antero-superior portal is placed in line with the AC joint and ¾ cm anterior to it, and the posterosuperior portal is in line with the joint and ¾ cm posterior. The portals are injected with 1% lidocaine with epinephrine to decrease skin bleeding.

An 11-blade scalpel is used to incise the skin and pierce the capsule of the AC joint for each portal. Initially the 2.7 mm wrist arthroscopy unit is utilized from the posterior superior portal. Normal saline with a 1:300,000 dilution of epinephrine is used for irrigation. A motorized 2.0 mm resector from the anterior portal can then, under direct vision, debride the meniscal remnant and joint debris. This exposes the articular surfaces. The acromial side is usually avoided, and small burrs, beginning with the 2.0 mm burr, are used to resect distal clavicular bone to widen the joint space. The standard 4.0 mm arthroscopic unit can then be utilized.

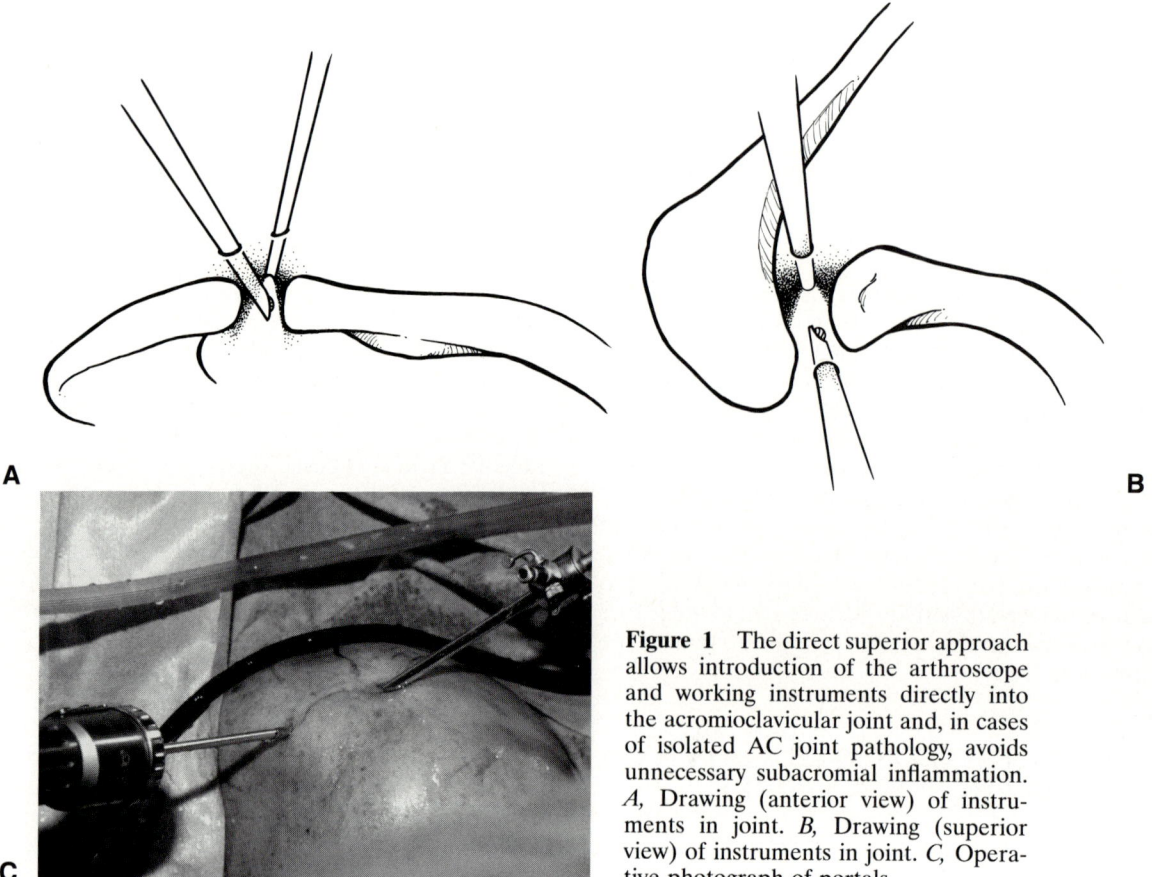

A

B

C

Figure 1 The direct superior approach allows introduction of the arthroscope and working instruments directly into the acromioclavicular joint and, in cases of isolated AC joint pathology, avoids unnecessary subacromial inflammation. *A,* Drawing (anterior view) of instruments in joint. *B,* Drawing (superior view) of instruments in joint. *C,* Operative photograph of portals.

Electrocautery is used to "shell-out" the distal clavicle from the surrounding soft tissues (Fig. 2). The capsule and ligaments are not incised, but are subperiosteally elevated to expose the bone. This provides visualization of the distal clavicle and allows precise resection. Now a larger burr can be used to complete the resection of the distal clavicle (Fig. 3). The burr is switched from the anterior superior to the posterior superior portal, and the arthroscope from posterior superior to anterior superior, to facilitate uniform resection of bone. It is important not to leave retained ridges or edges that might abut the acromion. Burring must be performed in a sequential fashion across the surface of the distal clavicle to avoid retained peripheral ridges (Fig. 4). Final beveling of the bone surface can be done with an arthroscopic rasp. The joint is then examined to remove any debris or remaining soft tissue. The joint is insufflated with a long-acting local anesthetic and skin closure is obtained.

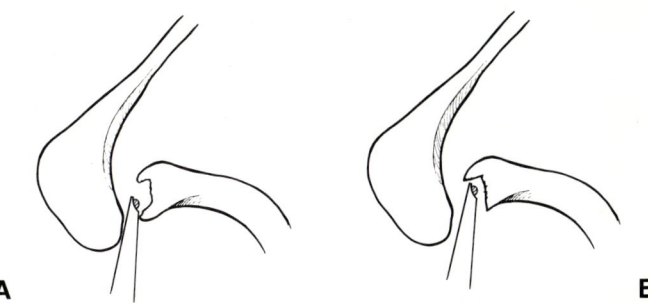

Figure 4 A common pitfall of arthroscopic distal clavicle resection is uneven bone resection. *A,* A retained anterior bone margin prevents maneuvering of the burr and limits further resection. *B,* Sequential burring affords the technical ability to evenly resect an adequate amount of distal clavicle.

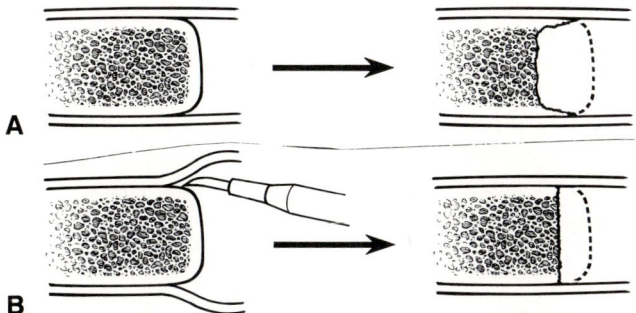

Figure 2 *A,* Uneven resection of the distal clavicle may leave bone peripherally, which can lead to continued pain. *B,* This can be avoided if the electrocautery is used to "shell out" the distal clavicle from the intact AC joint capsule, thereby allowing an even resection of bone.

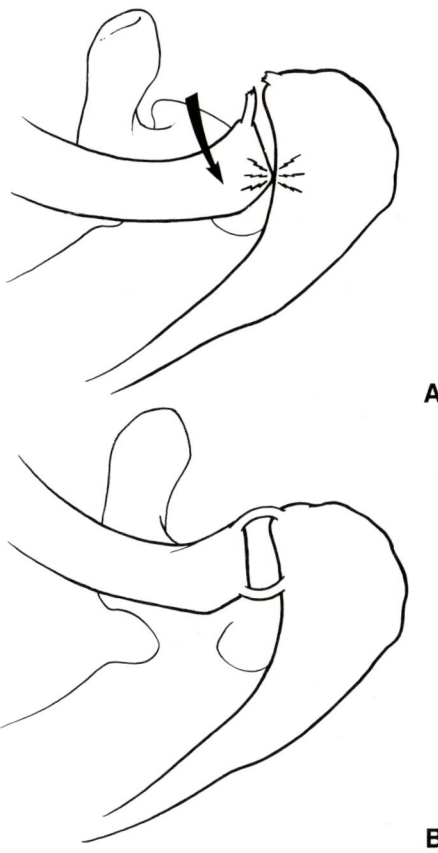

Figure 5 *A,* Incompetence of the AC joint ligamentous complex can lead to excessive posterior translation of the distal clavicular stump and painful abutment against the acromion. *B,* Arthroscopic resection of the distal clavicle preserves the AC joint ligamentous complex, thereby avoiding abutment. (From Flatow EL. The biomechanics of the acromioclavicular, sternoclavicular, and scapulothoracic joints. In: Heckman JD, ed. Instructional course lectures. Vol. 42. Rosemont, Ill: American Academy of Orthopaedic Surgeons, 1993:237; with permission.)

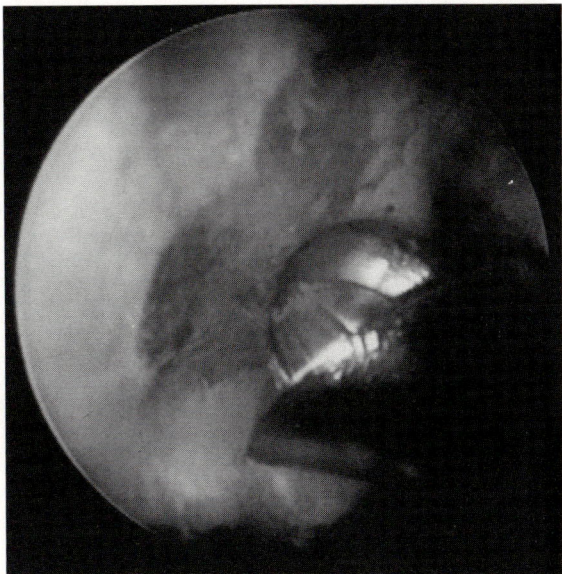

Figure 3 The direct superior approach allows visualization of the distal clavicle and precise burring.

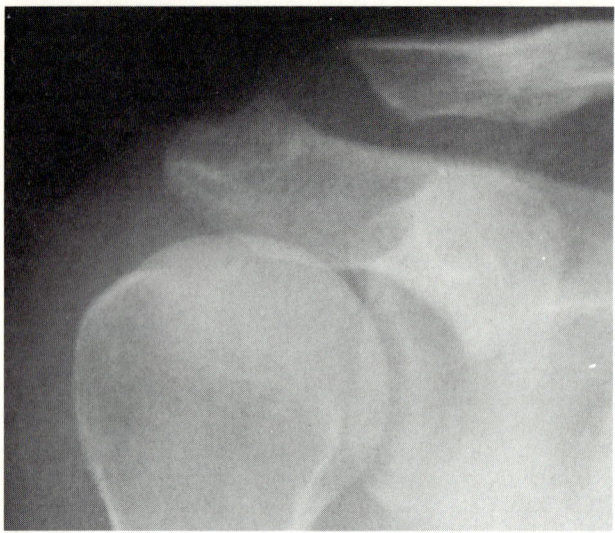

Figure 6 A postoperative x-ray demonstrating an even arthroscopic distal clavicle resection.

The deltoid origin has not been violated and motion can begin immediately. The pain and swelling subside quickly, and active motion is started, usually 3 to 5 days postsurgery. A sling is required for comfort and may be used for several days.

Amount of Bone Removal

Most authors have recommended excision of up to 2 or even 2.5 cm of distal clavicle. Failure of distal clavicle resection when less bone is removed has been reported to be due to abutment of the distal clavicle against the acromion with arm motion. This would suggest significant relative motion between the clavicle and acromion. However, studies by Kennedy and Cameron and by Rockwood employing percutaneous pins into the scapulae and clavicles of "volunteers," found that only minimal relative motion could be detected. I believe that abutment of the clavicle against the acromion results more from destabilization of the AC joint from trauma (grade II injury) or surgery (open resection of the distal clavicle) than from inadequate bone removal.

I and others have noted failure of open distal clavicle resection due to posterior translation of the distal clavicle so that it abuts against the curved base of the acromion. Biomechanical studies have shown that the AC capsule and ligaments represent 90% of the restraint to posterior translation of the clavicle at both small and large displacements. These structures may be damaged during exposure of the distal clavicle for open resection, and are ruptured in grade II AC injuries. Arthroscopic resection of the distal clavicle preserves the ligamentous envelope of the AC joint (Fig. 5). Under direct arthroscopic visualization I have noted very little change in the joint space as the arm is manipulated. I now remove only 5 to 7 mm of bone and have seen no diminution of results if the AC joint is stable and if the resection is even (Fig. 6).

I have noted a high failure rate after arthroscopic resection of the distal clavicle in patients with grade II AC separations, and even in patients with palpable AC hypermobility in the setting of generalized ligamentous laxity. These degrees of subtle instability have not previously been considered contraindications to simple resection of the distal clavicle. Indeed, most authors recommend excision of the distal clavicle for grade II injuries resistant to nonoperative treatment. However, the high failure rate in these patients has led me to reconsider this approach. Although it is possible that removal of more bone in this subgroup might improve results, I have seen failure even when large amounts of distal clavicle have been resected. For this reason I now consider open resection with ligament reconstruction in such cases.

SUGGESTED READING

Bigliani LU, Flatow EL, Weiss RA, et al. Interscalene block for shoulder arthroscopy: Comparison with general anesthesia. Arthroscopy 1991; 7:323.

Cahill BR. Osteolysis of the distal part of the clavicle in male athletes. J Bone Joint Surg 1982; 64A:1053–1058.

Cook FF, Tibone JE. The Mumford procedure in athletes: An objective analysis of function. Am J Sports Med 1988; 16:97–100.

Flatow EL. The biomechanics of the acromioclavicular, sternoclavicular, and scapulothoracic joints. In: Heckman JD, ed. Instructional course lectures. Vol. 42. Rosemont, Ill: American Academy of Orthopaedic Surgeons, 1993:237–245.

Flatow EL, Bigliani LU. Arthroscopic acromioclavicular joint debridement and distal clavicle resection. Op Techniques Orthop 1991; 1:240–247.

Flatow EL, Cordasco FA, Bigliani LU. Arthroscopic resection of the outer end of the clavicle from a superior approach: A critical, quantitative, radiographic assessment of bone removal. Arthroscopy 1992; 8:55–64.

Fukuda K, Craig EV, An K, et al. Biomechanical study of the ligamentous system of the acromioclavicular joint. J Bone Joint Surg 1986; 68A:434–439.

Gartsman GM. Arthroscopic resection of the acromioclavicular joint. Am J Sports Med 1993; 21:71–77.

Gartsman GM, Combs AH, Davis PF, Tullos HS. Arthroscopic acromioclavicular joint resection: an anatomical study. Am J Sports Med 1991; 19:2–5.

Gurd FB. The treatment of complete dislocation of the outer end of the clavicle: a hitherto undescribed operation. Ann Surg 1941; 63:1094–1098.

Johnson LL. Diagnostic and surgical arthroscopy. St. Louis: CV Mosby, 1981.

Meyers JF. Arthroscopic debridement of the acromioclavicular joint and distal clavicle resection. In: McGinty JB, Caspari RB, Jackson RW, et al, eds. Operative arthroscopy. New York: Raven, 1991:557.

Mumford EB. Acromioclavicular dislocation: a new operative treatment. J Bone Joint Surg 1941; 23:799–801.

Snyder SJ. Arthroscopic acromioclavicular joint debridement and distal clavicle resection. Techniques Orthop 1988; 3(1):41–45.

Weaver JK, Dunn HK. Treatment of acromioclavicular injuries, especially complete acromioclavicular separation. J Bone Joint Surg 1972; 54A:1187–1194.

PRINCIPLES OF SHOULDER ARTHROSCOPY

JAMES R. ANDREWS, M.D.
SCOTT P. SCHEMMEL, M.D.
SCOTT DAVID MARTIN, M.D.

Advances in equipment, techniques, and individual expertise have resulted in expanded use of arthroscopy in the diagnosis and treatment of intraarticular pathologic conditions.

Initially, the use of shoulder arthroscopy was limited to the evaluation of the glenohumeral joint with simple, limited interventional techniques for shoulder pathology. Currently, more complex and technically demanding arthroscopic surgical procedures can be applied to shoulder joint disorders. These include arthroscopic shoulder stabilization, rotator cuff repair, subacromial decompression, and acromioclavicular joint resection in selected patients. These advances have greatly expanded the indications for and use of arthroscopy for the shoulder and have necessitated a redefinition of the term "shoulder arthroscopy."

Arthroscopic evaluation of the shoulder is not complete until the glenohumeral joint and the subacromial space have been inspected. When indicated, the acromioclavicular joint should be evaluated either via the subacromial space or by direct transcutaneous entrance into the joint from above.

The purpose of this chapter is to discuss the principles of shoulder arthroscopy, as employed in the evaluation of glenohumeral, subacromial, and acromioclavicular pathology. Treatment of the various other pathologic entities encountered is discussed elsewhere in this volume.

GLENOHUMERAL JOINT ARTHROSCOPY

Arthroscopic investigation of any joint is an equipment-intense endeavor that must be carried out in a systematic and reproducible manner with minimal variation, while still allowing for adaptive maneuvers when necessary. Before the procedure is begun, the following equipment should be available: one 30 degree and one 70 degree 4.0 mm arthroscope, an 18 or 20 gauge spinal needle, an interchangeable interlocking 4.5 and 5.5 mm cannula system without "side ports," a full-radius synovial resector, a meniscal resector, a burr, and a fluid pump or 3 liter bags of normal saline for joint distention.

Surgical Technique

With the patient under anesthesia, an examination is made to determine shoulder instability and document range of motion. The patient is placed in the lateral decubitus position with the torso supported by a vacuum bean bag. The arm is suspended in a prefabricated wrist gauntlet or a soft wrap secured by Velcro straps. We prefer the arm to be suspended at 70 degrees of abduction and 15 degrees of forward flexion by means of a rope and pulley system attached to the surgical table. Approximately 15 (never more than 20) pounds are necessary for adequate distraction and subsequent visualization. It is important to ensure that the patient's torso does not drift anteriorly as the procedure is carried out, because this would make the procedure technically more difficult and might cause the arm to become extended. The extended arm position should always be avoided, since it results in traction being applied to the brachial plexus. Once adequately and securely positioned, the patient's exposed arm and shoulder region is prepared and draped, and the wrist gauntlet is covered with a sterile towel and a plastic drape.

The surgeon is positioned behind the patient with the surgical technician and necessary equipment toward the patient's feet. Optimally, the video monitor should be placed immediately anterior to the patient and directly across from the surgeon.

Bone landmarks about the shoulder are palpated and outlined with a surgical marking pen. These landmarks include (1) the anterolateral and posterolateral borders of the acromion, (2) the acromioclavicular joint, and (3) the coracoid process. They serve to orient the surgeon in establishing initial portals and additional portals as needed during the procedure. Without such markings, extravasation of fluid can make the later points of entry difficult to identify.

Diagnostic arthroscopy is begun through a posterior portal approximately 2.5 to 3 cm distal and slightly medial to the posterolateral tip of the acromion. This area should correspond to the interval between the infraspinatus and teres minor muscles, which is a palpable "soft spot." An 18 gauge spinal needle is inserted through this soft spot and is directed anteriorly toward the coracoid process. A common error is to direct the needle too horizontally, thus entering into the subacromial space rather than the glenohumeral joint itself. Ten to 15 ml of saline solution is injected into the joint, and free backflow confirms proper needle placement. A total of 40 to 50 ml of saline is then injected into the joint, and the needle is removed. A small skin incision is made at the point of needle entry, and a sharp 4.5 mm trocar and sleeve are inserted, following the same path as the needle. Once the subcutaneous tissues and muscle interval are penetrated, a blunt trocar replaces the sharp one, and the posterior glenoid rim and humeral head are palpated through the capsule with the trocar. The glenohumeral interval is thus identified, and with anterior pressure the trocar penetrates the joint capsule. It is important to "step off" the posterior glenoid rim and to enter the joint as close to the posterior rim as possible, thus avoiding penetration of the infraspinatus tendinous contribution to the rotator cuff. The arthroscope is introduced through the posterior sheath, and inflow is provided through the scope.

It is possible to inspect the glenohumeral joint

through a one-portal technique; however, for complete evaluation of the rotator cuff and posterior shoulder structures we routinely establish an anterior portal. This portal also serves as a "utility" portal for the passage of instruments, including motorized shavers if intraarticular pathology is noted. With the arthroscope in the posterior portal, an 18 gauge spinal needle is inserted into the glenohumeral joint from a point midway between the coracoid process and the anterolateral tip of the acromion. The needle is observed to penetrate the anterior capsule just inferior to the biceps tendon but superior to the subscapularis tendon, in the area referred to as the "safe triangle." Once correct placement of the needle is confirmed by direct arthroscopic visualization, a 5 mm skin incision is made at the needle entry point. A 4.5 mm trocar and sleeve are directed into the joint parallel to the path of the needle.

Once established, the anterior portal may serve as both an inflow portal and a "utility" portal. Alternatively, an infusion pump which flows through the scope cannula may be used to facilitate distention of the joint. Suction can be placed on the arthroscope, shaver, or a side portal of the anterior cannula if needed to enhance flow and/or remove debris.

Some arthroscopists will utilize a supraclavicular portal when scoping the glenohumeral joint. This portal is established at the junction of the lateral clavicle and scapular spine where it penetrates the supraspinatus near its musculotendinous portion. This portal may be quite functional and harmless in many cases. However, it should be avoided in throwing athletes, who frequently have a propensity for rotator cuff pathology secondary to the biomechanical stresses of throwing.

Arthroscopic Anatomy of Glenohumeral Joint

Arthroscopic evaluation should be conducted in a systematic fashion, identifying and inspecting all structures regardless of the preoperative diagnosis. The biceps tendon is the first structure identified. With the patient positioned as previously described, this structure is orientated approximately 15 degrees away from an imaginary vertical line. The tendon should be visualized from the bicipital groove anteriorly to its insertion into the supraglenoid tubercle at the superoposterior aspect of the glenoid where it is continuous with the glenoid labrum.

Next, the glenoid labrum is inspected. The "12 o'clock" position on the glenoid that corresponds to the biceps tendon labrum continuum is identified. From here the labrum is followed anteriorly; with momentarily increased traction of the arm, the anteroinferior labrum can be seen. With slight retraction of the arthroscope the posterior labrum can be followed inferiorly to superiorly back to the "12 o'clock" position.

The humeral head and glenoid articulation are visualized next. By internally and externally rotating the humerus, the entire articular surface of the humeral head can be inspected. The smaller, pear-shaped glenoid can be seen clearly at this point.

The glenohumeral ligaments, consisting of superior, middle, and inferior structures, are next scrutinized. These ligaments may have capsular origins or sometimes arise distinctly from the labrum itself.

The superior glenohumeral ligament is sometimes hidden behind the biceps tendon and not well seen. However, when identified, it courses from the anatomic neck of the humerus up to the superoanterior glenoid and also sends an attachment to the coracoid process. Although the middle glenohumeral ligament is broad, its middle portion is that which is most identifiable arthroscopically. This portion of the ligament can be seen arising just posterior to the subscapularis tendon and sweeping posteriorly to insert into the anterior border of the glenoid at its middle and inferior third. Occasionally, the middle glenohumeral ligament fuses with the subscapularis tendon. The anterior band of the inferior glenohumeral ligament arises from the inferior aspect of the surgical neck of the humerus and sweeps back to insert into the anteroinferior glenoid.

Subscapularis Tendon and Recess

With the patient's arm in the 70 degree abducted position, the subscapularis tendon can be seen in the anterior aspect of the glenohumeral joint. Arthroscopically, the posterosuperior edge of the subscapularis tendon is visualized. This structure is usually well defined and easily identifiable. However, in some shoulders this tendon may be obscured or may appear to blend with the middle glenohumeral ligament. The subscapularis recess can be found also in the anterior aspect of the shoulder, usually superior but occasionally inferior to the middle glenohumeral ligament.

Rotator Cuff

Examination of the rotator cuff begins by returning to the biceps tendon landmark. The supraspinatus tendon can be seen directly superior to the biceps tendon. The tendinous fibers of the rotator cuff structures can be seen to insert along the articular margin of the humeral head. After visualization of the supraspinatus contribution to the rotator cuff, the arthroscope is retracted slightly and is swept down along the posterior margin of the glenoid. With the arthroscope lens rotated superiorly, the infraspinatus and the teres minor contributions to the rotator cuff can be visualized. It is important to observe these more posterior contributions to the cuff closely for any signs of fraying or obvious tearing.

Superior Recess

The superior recess is located superior and slightly anterior to the superior aspect of the glenoid and to the insertion of the biceps tendon. This recess should be routinely examined for any abnormalities, specifically loose bodies.

Once a systematic evaluation of the glenohumeral joint has been completed from the posterior portal, the arthroscope is switched to the anterior portal while maintaining the posterior portal with a cannula. This allows for further evaluation of any previously identified pathology and may reveal abnormalities not noted through the posterior portal. This is particularly important in regard to the posterior rotator cuff structures.

Subacromial Space

Subacromial space pathology can occur either in conjunction with glenohumeral joint pathology or independent of it. Evaluation of the subacromial space as part of a general arthroscopic shoulder examination helps to ensure that concomitant subacromial space pathology is identified and appropriately treated, and that it does not later have a less than satisfactory result when more obvious glenohumeral joint pathology has been corrected. Subacromial pathology, as in the spectrum of the impingement syndrome, should be recognized and treated.

Surgical Technique

After completion of the glenohumeral joint evaluation and treatment, the arthroscope is redirected into the subacromial space. The 4.5 mm cannula with a blunt trocar is introduced through the posterior skin portal and redirected toward the posterolateral aspect of the acromion. The undersurface of the posterolateral tip of the acromion is palpated with the trocar, and the cannula with trocar is then advanced into the subacromial space. The trocar is removed, and the arthroscope is reinserted.

If a separate inflow portal is needed, it can be established utilizing the anterior skin portal to introduce a 5.5 mm cannula and trocar anterolateral into the subacromial space. Ideal placement of the cannula is through the coracoacromial ligament. Placement of the trocar and cannula medial to the coracoacromial ligament inhibits inflow and limits visualization, making diagnosis and any operative procedure difficult. In addition, medial placement of either the anterior or posterior cannula may cause bleeding from branches of the thoracoacromial artery, leading to impaired visualization and significant operative delays. If an anterior portal is required, the posterior cannula and trocar can be invaginated into the anterior cannula. This step ensures that both the inflow cannula and the arthroscopy cannula are within the same plane as the subacromial space and are not separated by bursal tissue planes. Such separation by soft tissue makes flow within the subacromial space difficult and hinders any further attempts at visualization or instrumentation. The trocar is removed from the 4.5 mm cannula, and the arthroscope is introduced through the sheath. The anterior cannula is then slowly retracted anteriorly until the arthroscope is freed from the 5.5 mm sheath. The inflow portal is then immediately assessed to determine adequate placement through the coracoacromial ligament; once this is confirmed, diagnostic arthroscopy of the subacromial space can continue.

Quite often, especially when bursitis and tendinitis associated with the impingement syndrome are present, visualization of the rotator cuff and the undersurface of the acromion is difficult initially. The bursal tissue may need to be removed with a full-radius synovial resector, which is introduced through a lateral portal. This portal is established through triangulation after introduction of an 18 gauge spinal needle approximately 2 to 3 cm directly lateral from the acromion. This needle passes through the muscle and fascia of the deltoid and into the subacromial space. Once the needle is visualized, a 6 mm skin incision is made at the point of its insertion, and a 5.5 mm blunt trocar and sheath are introduced into the subacromial space. The trocar is removed and, with a full-radius synovial resector, the subacromial bursa is removed and adequate visualization of the important structures is possible. Alternatively, the full radius resector and other instruments can be inserted directly through the lateral skin portal.

It is important that continuous flow through the subacromial space be established and subsequently maintained throughout the course of the diagnostic or operative procedure. Because bleeding may be encountered with instrumentation of this space, particularly around the acromioclavicular joint, 1 ml of a 1:1,000 epinephrine solution is added to each 3 liter bag of fluid. Over the last several years, the senior author has utilized an arthroscopic infusion pump which has greatly enhanced visibility in the subacromial space by fine tuning pressure and inflow. Ideally, the patient's systolic blood pressure should not exceed 50 mm Hg over the infusion pump pressure for proper control of capillary bleeding.

The normal subacromial space is usually well defined, with a thin layer of bursal tissue overlying the rotator cuff tendons. If the bursal tissue is hypertrophic or shows evidence of abrasions, it will be necessary to resect it carefully with a synovial resector from the underlying tendons so that they can be fully inspected for partial-thickness tears or abrasions. By internally and externally rotating the arm, a significant portion of the rotator cuff—particularly the supraspinatus and infraspinatus—can be visualized clearly. The undersurface of the acromion is covered with a relatively thick and continuous layer of fibrous tissue, which should be smooth in appearance. By palpation with a blunt instrument, the anatomic borders of the acromion can be established laterally, anteriorly, and posteriorly. An 18 gauge spinal needle passed through the acromioclavicular joint from above serves to identify the medial border of the acromion. Any fraying of the fibrous tissue on the undersurface of the acromion, particularly when this is combined with inflammation, erythema, or hypertrophy of the subacromial bursa or underlying rotator cuff, indicates an impingement phenomenon. By abducting the arm under direct visualization, an area of fraying on the undersurface of the acromion often corresponds with an area of erythema on the rotator cuff, as these two surfaces are approximated. By removing the soft tissue about the acromioclavicular joint, the undersurface of the clavicle can be identified. The acromioclavicular joint serves as an important landmark in subacromial decompression, delineating the medial extent of the decompression. In addition, this area should be explored to rule out the existence of spurs arising from the inferior surface of the distal clavicle. The coracoacromial ligament is easily identified, particularly if the anterior cannula was placed appropriately as it pierces directly through this white ligamentous structure. The coracoacromial ligament itself may be frayed, but only rarely are changes within the substance of the ligament indicative of any specific pathologic condition. It is not within the realm of this chapter to discuss fully the technique of subacromial decompression, although by using the lateral portal, a full-radius synovial resector, and a large high-speed burr, it is possible to carry out this procedure systematically and reproducibly.

The acromioclavicular joint can be evaluated through the subacromial space. If necessary, acromioclavicular joint decompression with removal of the joint meniscus and resection of the distal clavicle can be completed. If acromioclavicular joint resection is done concomitantly with subacromial decompression, a bursal (indirect) arthroscopic approach is carried out utilizing routine anterior, posterior, and lateral portals. Upon completion of the subacromial decompression, the 30 degree scope is left in the posterior portal and electrocautery is used through the lateral skin portal to remove the inferior capsule of the AC joint. Next, a 5.5 mm burr is introduced through the lateral portal to begin the resection. Ideally, 8 mm of bone is resected from the distal clavicle, which is approximately the diameter of the burr. The undersurface of the distal clavicle is burred level with the subacromial decompression. At this point, the burr is introduced into the anterior portal and the 30 degree scope is switched with a 70 degree scope for better upward visualization of the distal clavicle. Visualization is further enhanced by manually depressing the distal clavicle during resection. Great care is taken to remove all bone within the resection area, especially over the posterior superior aspect of the AC joint where bone is often missed and may continue to cause painful symptoms.

When the acromioclavicular joint is identified preoperatively as the source of the patient's complaints and when no glenohumeral or subacromial pathology is otherwise identified at the time of arthroscopy, we prefer to perform direct acromioclavicular joint debridement and distal clavicle resection. For this we use an arthroscopic technique that involves the transcutaneous introduction of the arthroscope and necessary equipment directly into the acromioclavicular joint from above.

The acromioclavicular joint is identified by direct palpation, and two 18 gauge spinal needles are introduced into the joint. One needle is introduced approximately 5 mm anterior to the anterosuperior edge of the AC joint, and the other is introduced about 5 mm posterior to the posterosuperior edge of the joint. This allows the proper inclination for easy passage of scope and instruments into the AC joint. Saline is injected through the posterior spinal needle with a 40 ml syringe, and flow through the joint is confirmed by the presence of saline from the anterior spinal needle. At the beginning of this procedure, a third spinal needle should also be introduced directly through the center of the acromioclavicular joint. Outflow should be confirmed through this third spinal needle as fluid is injected through the posterior spinal needle. Once all three needles are determined to be within the acromioclavicular joint, the posterior spinal needle is removed. A small skin incision is made, and a 4.5 mm cannula and trocar (or in a tight joint, a 2.7 mm cannula and trocar) are introduced. An arthroscope of the appropriate size is placed into the joint, and the central and anterior spinal needles are identified. Flow is then established through both the arthroscope and the central spinal needle, and instrumentation is brought in anteriorly once the anterior spinal needle has been removed and a 2.7 mm or 4.5 mm cannula and trocar have been placed. When there is adequate visualization and instrumentation within the joint, debridement of the acromioclavicular joint meniscus and distal clavicular resection, using full-radius synovial resectors and high-speed burrs, can be accomplished. Care must be taken to avoid directing the instrumentation too far inferiorly, thus entering the subacromial space and inadvertently injuring the underlying rotator cuff structures.

SUGGESTED READING

Andrews JR, Carson WG. Arthroscopic anatomy of the shoulder. In: McGinty JB, ed. Shoulder surgery in the athlete: techniques in orthopaedics. Rockville, MD: Aspen Systems Corp, 1985:25.

Andrews JR, Carson WG. Arthroscopy of the shoulder. Orthopedics 1983; 6:1157.

Andrews JR, Carson WG, Ortega K. Arthroscopy of the shoulder: technique and normal anatomy. Am J Sports Med 1984; 12:1.

Caspari RB. Anatomy and portals for arthroscopic surgery of the shoulder. In: Jackson DW, ed. Shoulder surgery in the athlete: techniques in orthopaedics. Rockville, MD: Aspen Systems Corp, 1985:15.

Johnson LL. Diagnostic and surgical arthroscopy of the shoulder. St. Louis: Mosby-Year Book 1993.

Lombardo SJ. Arthroscopy of the shoulder. Clin Sports Med 1983; 2:209.

Matthews LS, Terry HL, Vetter WL. Shoulder anatomy for the arthroscopist. Arthroscopy 1985; 1:83.

Matthews LS, Vetter WL, Helfet DL. Arthroscopic surgery of the shoulder. Adv Orthop Surg 1984; 8:203.

Matthews LS, Zarins B, Michael RH. Anterior portal selection for shoulder arthroscopy. Arthroscopy 1985; 1:33.

McGinty JB. Operative arthroscopy. New York: Raven Press, 1991: 425.

McGlynn FF, Caspari RB. Arthroscopic findings in the subluxating shoulder. Clin Orthop 1984; 183:173.

ARTHROSCOPIC SUBACROMIAL DECOMPRESSION

HARVARD ELLMAN, M.D.

A method of performing arthroscopic subacromial decompression (anterior acromioplasty) using arthroscopic surgical techniques is described here. The operative goal is to (1) release the coracoacromial ligament, (2) resect the anterior undersurface of the acromion, and (3) when indicated, debride the bursa or cuff and relieve calcareous deposits with a needle technique.

INDICATIONS

The procedure is indicated for

1. Stage II impingement syndrome unresponsive to conservative treatment for at least 6 to 12 months.
2. Selected irreparable rotator cuff tears with intractable pain.
3. Superficial calcareous deposits with chronic impingement.

It is not recommended as a substitute for open repair of routine full-thickness rotator cuff tears.

EQUIPMENT

The procedure involves the use of basic arthroscopic instruments that are readily available, including the following:
Thirty-degree arthroscope.
Powered shaver system.
Synovial resector shaver blade.
Meniscal trimmer shaver blade.
Large arthroplasty burr.
Small open bone curette.
Electrosurgical generator.
Meniscal electrode with plastic coated tip.
Plastic cannula with diaphragm.

The patient is placed in a lateral recumbent position, and after routine preparation and draping, the extremity is maintained in 15 to 20 pounds of "sky-hook" traction with the arm abducted about 20 degrees. The bone landmarks of the acromion, acromioclavicular (AC) joint, and coracoid are outlined (Fig. 1).

The course of the coracoacromial ligament is indicated traveling from the coracoid to insert on the anterior edge of the undersurface of the acromion. The arm should be placed in traction before these landmarks are outlined. The posterior angle of the acromion is identified and two portals are marked. First, the arthroscopic portal (a) is marked 1 cm below and 1 cm

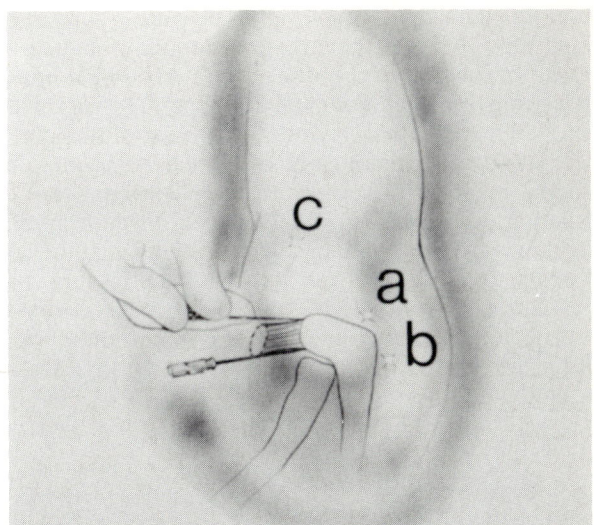

Figure 1 Bone landmarks drawn. Orientation pins outline the coracoacromial ligament attachment. Portals are marked (a) arthroscope, (b) accessory fluid inflow, and (c) operative cannula. (Republished with permission from Takagishi NT. The shoulder. 4th Ed. Tokyo: Professional Postgraduate Services, 1987:192-194.)

anterior to the posterior angle of the acromion. A second portal for an accessory fluid ingress cannula (b) is marked 1 cm inferior and medial to the posterior angle. Portals are infiltrated with a few milliliters of 0.25 percent bupivacaine with epinephrine, and the subacromial space is distended with 20 ml of normal saline.

Orientation pins are next placed to outline the acromial attachment of the coracoacromial ligament; 18 guage lumbar puncture needles are used with the stylet left in position. The medial needle is introduced just anterior to the AC joint. The more lateral needle is located at the anterolateral angle of the acromion. The arthroscope is introduced to lie directly under the anterior edge of the acromion. When properly positioned, both medial and lateral needles can be visualized. The needles can be wiggled to aid in their identification.

INSERTION OF OPERATIVE CANNULA

A 5 mm plastic cannula with rubber diaphragm is introduced (Fig. 2) into the subacromial space at this point (c) 3 to 4 cm from the acromion and in a direct line with the marker pins. A blunt-nosed powered shaver is introduced and the subacromial space is thoroughly debrided to enhance visualization. Both the floor and roof of the bursa should be cleared; this debridement will allow good visualization of the marker pins.

The coracoacromial ligament is then cut with a plastic coated or right-angled electrosurgical instrument (Fig. 3). The electrosurgical pencil is introduced through the operating cannula and visualized in a trial passage from one pin to the other. The plastic coating on the tip of the electrode permits it to work effectively while using normal saline irrigation solution. The cutting current on a specially designed generator is gradually increased until it begins to cut the thickened subacromial bursa, underlying the coracoacromial ligaments. The cut travels from the medial pin in a straight line toward the lateral pin. A surprising amount of thickened bursa must be divided in some cases before the ligament itself is actually cut. The cut is placed adjacent to the acromial attachment of the ligament, thereby minimizing the risk of injury to a branch of the coracoacromial artery. The coagulation current can be utilized when necessary to control bleeding from this artery. It is important to avoid prolonged instillation of distilled water; 15 minutes should be sufficient.

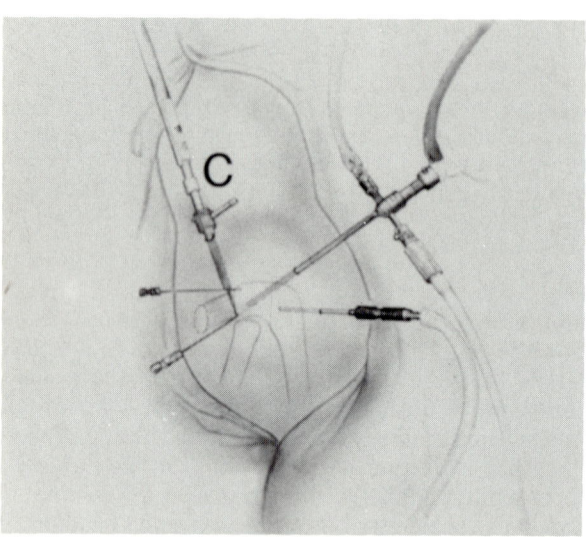

Figure 2 Surgical cannula (*c*) introduced 3 to 4 cm from the acromion in direct line with marker pins. An electrosurgical pencil passes through the cannula. All other instruments are in place. (Republished with permission from Takagishi NT. The shoulder. 4th Ed. Tokyo: Professional Postgraduate Services, 1987:192-194.)

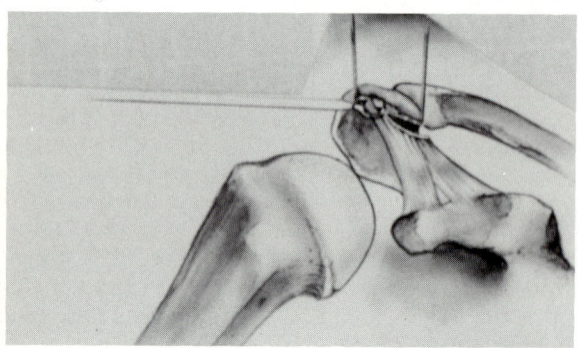

Figure 3 Cut coracoacromial ligament with an electrosurgical pencil from the medial marker pin toward the lateral pin. Distilled water irrigation is required temporarily for electrocautery to function. (Republished with permission from Takagishi NT. The shoulder. 4th Ed. Tokyo: Professional Postgraduate Services, 1987:192-194.)

ANTERIOR ACROMIOPLASTY

The anterior undersurface of the acromion is visualized and the thickened subacromial bursa attached to this area is removed, initially with a small open curet and subsequently with an angled synovial resector. This tissue must be removed for effective use of the burr. The large arthroplasty burr is then placed under the anterior acromion (Fig. 4) and applied to an area where the bone has been exposed. The burr is then used to thin the anterior edge of the acromion to a degree desired by the surgeon. The full width of the acromion should be reduced from the anterior edge to a point about 2 cm posteriorly. Any spurs projecting from the undersurface of the outer end of the clavicle should also be removed (Fig. 5). Bleeding from cancellous bone and resected synovium may make visualization difficult. Copious irrigation and distention will permit inspection to confirm the amount of bone removed. Distilled water

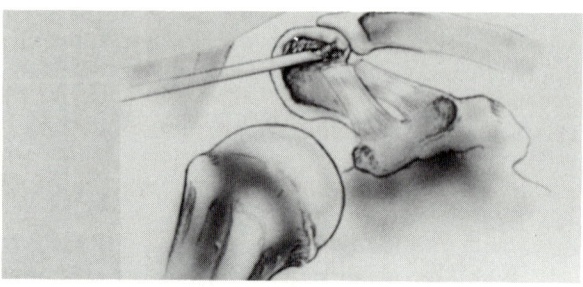

Figure 4 Open curet is used to resect the undersurface of the anterior acromion. (Republished with permission from Takagishi NT. The shoulder. 4th Ed. Tokyo: Professional Postgraduate Services, 1987:192-194.)

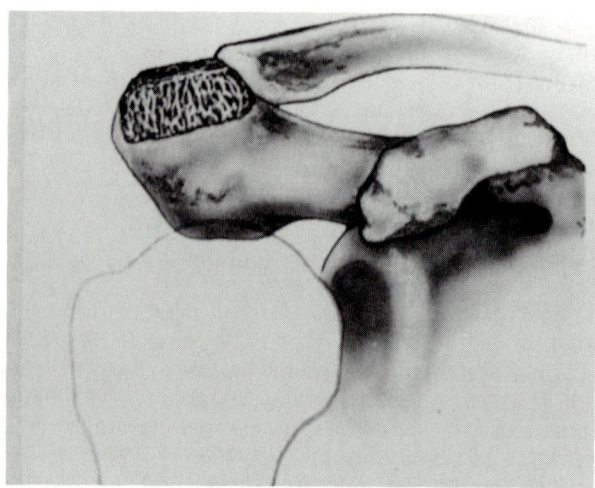

Figure 5 Burring completed. The acromion is thinned across the full width from the anterior edge to at least 2 cm posteriorly. Any spurs beneath the outer end of the clavicle are also resected. (Republished with permission from Takagishi NT. The shoulder. 4th Ed. Tokyo: Professional Postgraduate Services, 1987:192-194.)

may be introduced for a short time and the electrocautery unit used to obtain hemostasis. This will facilitate final burring and debridement. Fifteen milliliters of 0.25 percent bupivacaine with epinephrine is instilled at the conclusion of the procedure, and the portals are closed with 4-0 nylon sutures.

POSTOPERATIVE MANAGEMENT

Patients are encouraged to resume full active range of motion on the evening of surgery. They are instructed to stretch the arm overhead while supine and perform pendulum exercises every morning and evening for 1 minute in order to prevent adhesion formation. No sling is used, and there is no restriction on daily living activities, including driving and reaching overhead. Strenuous repetitive overhead activity, however, is avoided for at least 4 to 6 weeks; this includes tennis and throwing. Strengthening exercises utilizing surgical tubing are begun at 4 to 6 weeks, and the patient gradually resumes all normal activities as tolerated.

DECOMPRESSION AND DEBRIDEMENT OF ROTATOR CUFF TEARS

The treatment of irreparable or recurrent full-thickness rotator cuff tears with arthroscopic decompression and debridement is carried out in selected patients. The procedure is not performed as a substitute for open repair of the routine cuff tear. Debridement and decompression are reserved for patients in whom an extensive tear has been present for several years, and whose preoperative evaluation suggests that at best a "limited goals result" will be achieved.

CALCIFIED TENDINITIS

Large calcareous deposits in the supraspinatus tendon can be relieved arthroscopically. Calcification generally develops within the tendon, and unfortunately many small and medium-sized calcifications cannot be seen when the cuff is viewed from the surface. An inflamed hypertrophic bursa further tends to obscure

visualization. A needle is used to explore the rotator cuff in search of a calcific deposit; probing with the needle into a bed of calcium will liberate "snowflakes" of calcium into the bursa. Further needling, or a small incision in line with the fibers of the tendon, will permit the introduction of a curet, and large calcifications can be subsequently removed. Radiographic control assists in localization of the calcific deposit. The need for decompression in association with removal of calcific deposits is controversial.

RESULTS

This procedure has now been performed in over 750 patients during the past 10 years. The initial 82 patients in this series have been followed for 2 to 5 years and the results noted as 89% satisfactory and 11% unsatisfactory in patients without full-thickness rotator cuff tears.

The results of arthroscopic decompression are comparable with those of open anterior acromioplasty. The procedure is technically challenging. It can be performed as an out-patient procedure and there is minimal morbidity. Patients return to activities of daily living within a few days. Arthroscopic subacromial decompression is an alternative to open anterior acromioplasty in selected cases of advanced stage II or III impingement syndromes.

SUGGESTED READING

Ellman H. Arthroscopic subacromial decompression. Orthop Trans 1985; 9:48.

Ellman H. Arthroscopic subacromial decompression: analysis of 1-3 year results. Arthroscopy 1987; 3:173.

Hawkins RF, Kennedy JC. Impingement syndrome in athletes. Am J Sports Med 1980; 8:151.

Neer CS II. Anterior acromioplasty for the chronic impingement syndrome in the shoulder. A preliminary report. J Bone Joint Surg 1972; 54A:41.

Neer CS II. Impingement lesions. Clin Orthop 1983; 173;70.

Post M, Cohen J. Impingement syndrome — a review of late stage II and early stage III lesions. Orthop Trans 1985; 9:48.

Pujadas GM. Coracoacromial ligament syndrome. J Bone Joint Surg 1970; 52A:1361.

Raggio CL, Warren RF, Sculco T. Surgical treatment of impingement syndrome: 4-year follow-up. Orthop Trans 1985; 9:48.

ROTATOR CUFF TEARS: SURGICAL MANAGEMENT

JAMES P. BRADLEY, M.D.
JAMES E. TIBONE, M.D.

The appropriate surgical management of rotator cuff tears in athletes is dependent on many factors. Precise evaluation of age, etiology, competitive level, location, size, and goals may all play a role in the final decision. Typically, rotator cuff tears in athletes can be divided into three groups: (1) acute high-velocity trauma (partial or full-thickness tears), (2) chronic low-velocity microtrauma, and (3) repetitive microtrauma with secondary instability and associated rotator cuff tears. It is helpful to initially consider the age of the athlete as a prime determinant. In the younger population (18 to 35 years of age) of overhand throwing athletes, rotator cuff pathology often is secondary to glenohumeral instability or the new concept of internal impingement. In the older athlete (over 35 years of age), degenerative cuff pathology associated with spur formation, compromise of the subacromial space, and decreased vascular supply tends to be the antecedent. Excluding violent trauma, age is a very helpful initial determinant of the nature of the pathology. Similarly, competitive level, whether it be recreational, competitive, or elite, tends to have a predominant pattern of cuff pathology, although overlap does occur. The decision of the most appropriate techniques of prevention and treatment is contingent on a thorough analysis and understanding of the above factors.

BASIC CONCEPTS AND PATHOLOGY

Rotator cuff tears are defined as partial or complete and sometimes may be coupled with biceps tendon, acromioclavicular joint, and glenohumeral ligament involvement. Partial rotator cuff tears are further subdivided by length (i.e., 1 cm) and a percentage of the total tendon width that is torn, (i.e., 50% tear in the supraspinatus). The etiology of the cuff pathology can be divided into four basic groups: (1) the eccentric overload mechanism, (2) Jobe's concept of anterior instability with secondary impingement, (3) the classic Neer impingement process, and (4) internal impingement.

Eccentric Overload

Rotator cuff tears secondary to eccentric overload usually present in high-caliber overhand athletes. They are at risk due to the chronic, repetitive, high-velocity mechanical stress placed on the rotator cuff. During pitching, for example, the humeral internal rotation torque reaches 14,000 inch-pounds of force, which must first be generated and then subsequently dissipated.

Initially, partial degenerative cuff tears appear, which may progress to full thickness tears. An early presentation of this mechanism may be the rotator cuffitis or impingement tendinitis commonly noted in throwing athletes.

Impingement and Anterior Instability

Rotator cuff pathology is sometimes manifested in athletes with impingement secondary to anterior instability of the glenohumeral joint. Elite overhand athletes, especially pitchers, seem to be at the greatest risk. The chronology of events is described by Jobe as an "Instability Complex." This complex is a cascade of initial instability secondary to repetitive microtrauma, followed by subluxation that leads to impingement and terminally, rotator cuff tears. The essential pathology requires repetitive overhand throwing, thereby subjecting the glenohumeral ligaments and rotator cuff to repetitive microtrauma and eccentric overload. The anterior capsuloligamentous complex during late-cocking and acceleration and the posterior ligament complex during the follow-through stage of throwing must dissipate the tremendous forces generated. Over time, this leads to stretching and attenuation of the ligaments producing relative subluxation. Subluxation permits superior migration of the humeral head, thereby predisposing the rotator cuff to an impingement process beneath the coracoacromial arch. Typically, degenerative articular side partial-thickness tears of the rotator cuff evolve, however, complete tears are rarely evident. It must be emphasized that this mode of pathology is dependent on the specific population described above, other more common causes of rotator cuff tears is the rule.

Classic Impingement

Neer initially described the impingement process of the rotator cuff against the anterior acromion, and other authors expanded this concept to include the lateral acromion in overhand athletes. Microinjection dye investigation has demonstrated vascular compromise of the supraspinatus and biceps tendon adjacent to the insertion of the supraspinatus at the greater tuberosity of the humerus with the arm at the side. Variations of the geometry (shape, size, angle) of the acromion in other studies have theorized a predisposition to impingement and ensuing rotator cuff tears. Most authors summarize the impingement process as initial bouts of rotator cuff tendinitis succeeded by wear of the cuff, fibrosis, and scarring of the subacromial bursa, bony spurring, partial cuff tears, and finally resulting in full-thickness rotator cuff tears.

Neer classified the impingement process into three stages and Jobe modified the third stage in athletes and divided it into a third and fourth stage.

Stage I: Edema and hemorrhage (any age)
Stage II: Fibrosis and tendinitis (usually in patients over 25 years of age)
Stage III: Degeneration, bone changes, and tendon

ruptures (usually in subjects over 40 years of age)

Stage IV: Rotator cuff tears greater than 1 cm in length (tears less than 1 cm are placed in Stage III, by Jobe)

Internal Impingement

Internal impingement is a new concept described as intra-articular impingement located between the posterosuperior border of the glenoid and the deep tendinous insertions of the supraspinatus and infraspinatus. Walch demonstrated arthroscopically and Jobe noted in cadaveric studies that the tendinous insertion of the rotator cuff became jammed between the humeral head and the glenoid when the arm was placed in the throwing position (90 to 150 degrees abduction and full external rotation). Typically, the patient is a throwing athlete between 15 and 30 years of age complaining of diffuse shoulder pain that is worse in the posterior part of the shoulder. Clinical, radiographic, and arthroscopic evaluations do not demonstrate anterior instability. Partial undersurface rotator cuff tears are demonstrated on arthrogram or arthroscopically usually in the supraspinatus. Associated lesions noted arthroscopically can include degenerative posterosuperior labral lesions with irregular scuffing and small flap tears behind the biceps insertion, and osteochondral lesions of the humeral head higher than the classic Hill-Sach's Lesion. It appears that internal impingement is probably physiologic, however, throwing athletes are at risk because of the repetitive high-velocity microtrauma that leads to attritional cuff damage.

DIAGNOSIS

The etiology of the rotator cuff tear can generally be assigned to one of the three groups discussed. The most common scenario is the weekend recreational athlete who presents with a classic Neer impingement process. Typically, the patient has endured multiple episodes of shoulder pain and limited function, which resolves with rest. Initially, postactivity pain is noted; subsequently, the pain hinders activities and becomes so intense at times that it precludes any overhead sports activity. Night pain becomes evident and a chronic dull ache intensifies enough to limit some daily activities. Symptoms may range from minimal to significant. Occasionally, an insignificant traumatic incident has resulted in inability to raise the arm overhead. Full thickness rotator cuff tears in this population demonstrate an inconsistent pattern of pain, range-of-motion (ROM), and strength. During the examination, palpation of the greater tuberosity and acromion elicit pain, there is a painful arch of abduction typically greatest between 80 and 90 degrees, and resistance at this level increases the pain or sometimes, causes the arm to drop. Although weakness of abduction and sometimes, external rotation, is very helpful in the diagnosis, pain may obviate any true appraisal of strength. Neer, Hawkins, and Jobe have described impingement signs that aid in the evaluation, basically each test is designed to impale the greater tuberosity and rotator cuff against the coracoacromial arch, thereby producing pain about the anterolateral acromion. Classically, long-standing rotator cuff tears illustrate atrophy in the supraspinatus fossa, weakness in abduction and external rotation, and chronic dull ache pain often increasing at night. Standard radiographs may aid in the diagnosis by demonstrating superior translation of the humerus decreasing the humeral acromial internal to less than 6 mm, notching of the insertion site of the supraspinatus on the greater tuberosity, eburnation of the greater tuberosity, and under surface of the acromion. Associated findings include anterior acromial spurs, distal clavicular spurring, and calcific degeneration at the supraspinatus insertion site. Nonetheless, a positive arthrogram continues to be the most sensitive.

The diagnosis of complete rotator cuff tears in high-level overhand athletes remains difficult. Generally, their symptom complex is not as conspicuous as classic rotator cuff tears. Activity and mild postactivity shoulder pain is the dominant complaint. Activity related weakness is variable, however, endurance problems may be more pronounced. Night pain and rest pain are not typically present. Pain related to one specific phase of throwing is not a common complaint. The physical examination usually does not demonstrate specific cuff weakness, probably because of the youthful well-conditioned state of the remaining shoulder musculature. Normally, one of the impingement signs (Neer's, Hawkins', Jobe's) is positive. Temporally, high-level athletes may display an accelerated symptom complex with progression of their cuff tears compared with the weekend athletes because their demand is higher.

The diagnosis of partial rotator cuff tears in these athletes is even more problematic. Pain continues to be the primary complaint with atypical activity-related "tiredness," but typically this does not prevent them from continuing the activity. The physical findings are tenuous and difficult to evoke. Impingement signs may be positive but are often inconsistent. In this situation, when the athlete has already failed a rehabilitation protocol, the integrity of the cuff is best delineated by double contrast arthrography, high resolution MRI, or arthroscopy.

In high-caliber overhand athletes that present with signs and symptoms of impingement and/or a partial rotator cuff tear, it is important to investigate the possibility of "silent subluxation" as the primary etiology of the shoulder pain. Basically, shoulder pain in high-profile throwers is instability related to anterior subluxation with secondary cuff pathology until proven otherwise. The pain is usually described in one of two ways, classic impingement pain or pain related to the late-cocking and acceleration phases of throwing. It is not uncommon for the athletes to complain of a migrating pain localized to the posterior shoulder and scapular rotators, because of the altered biomechanics. The physical finding of rotator cuff tendinitis or impingement are predominant.

Experience and sensitive fingers are the best tools to

uncover silent subluxation. The best test for this type of shoulder instability is to have the patient supine with the arm off the table at 90 degrees of abduction and external rotation. The humeral head is grasped and pushed anteriorly. Anterior pain is considered abnormal. The examiner then pushes the humeral head posteriorly and uses his palm as a buttress across the anterior shoulder. The pain typically subsides; however, once the buttress is released, the pain reappears. Importantly, the athlete complains of pain, not classic apprehension during this maneuver. If these tests are positive and a compatible history is present, the pathology is secondary to anterior inferior instability and the impingement findings are secondary. No one test is pathognomonic for anterior instability, but rather a constellation of historical and physical findings.

In high-caliber throwing athletes that present with diffuse shoulder pain, worse posteriorly and no signs of instability, it is helpful to investigate internal impingement as the possible cause of the rotator cuff pathology. The pain usually is relieved by stopping the sport and returns when play is resumed. In some cases, the pain becomes permanent, affecting activities of daily living and sleep. Impingement signs and supraspinatus weakness typically are apparent. Pain is evident when the arm is held in full external rotation and moved between 90 and 150 degrees of abduction. Atrophy of the supraspinatus or infraspinatus and tests for instability are not present. However, a positive relocation test is usually demonstrated, possibly because pushing the humeral head posteriorly stops it from impinging on the posterior glenoid. Arthroscopic clarification is very helpful by observing the posterior impingement in 90 to 150 degrees of abduction and full external rotation.

SURGICAL TREATMENT

Surgical management is dependent on etiology, competitive level, and morphology of the rotator cuff tear. Etiologic presentations include: (1) impingement related (classic or internal), (2) eccentric overload, and (3) anterior instability with secondary impingement. Competitive level is divided into recreational weekend athletes, competitive organized, or collegiate athletes and high-performance elite athletes. The tear morphology encompasses size, location, and partial versus complete rotator cuff tears. Management is a cognitive decision-making process that should entail all of the above factors.

High-Performance Athletes

The treatment of high-performance athletes is initially conservative in most cases, because this group usually presents with articular side partial rotator cuff tears localized to the under surface of the supraspinatus. Lohr has demonstrated that the vascular supply of the supraspinatus is much better on the acromial surface versus the articular surface. The etiology of the tear is either eccentric loading, anterior instability, or internal

impingement. Fortunately, these entities respond to nonoperative treatment in most cases. Investigations by Jobe have demonstrated, in the instability group, that upwards of 70% of pitchers will improve with nonoperative management. Physical therapy goals are symptomatic control, maintenance of ROM, strengthening, and progression to functional activities. Symptomatic control includes the use of nonsteroidal anti-inflammatory drugs (NSAIDs), rest from competition, ultrasound to improve blood flow, interferential stimulation, and sometimes a local steroid injection into the subacromial bursa. Steroid injections are used judiciously only after other modalities have proved ineffective. Athletes are protected from high-intensity activity for 2 weeks due to the steroids' effects on strength to failure of the cuff. ROM is maintained during the rehabilitation period and all deficits are addressed. Due to the delicate balance and synergistic activity of the shoulder musculature in this group of athletes, strengthening is advanced in a systematic progression based on the "3Es and 4Ps" concept of Pink and Jobe. Simply stated, for effective and efficient exercise program (3E), attention must focus on the 4Ps: glenohumeral "protectors" (rotation cuff), the scapulohumeral "pivoters" (scapular rotators), the humeral "positioners" (three heads of deltoid), and the "power drivers" (pectoralis major and latissimus dorsi). The sequence of strengthening starts with the protectors and pivoters first to provide stability, followed by the positioners to improve synchronous motion. The power drivers are addressed last. If the power drivers are strengthened too early, they may overpower the balance of the protectors and pivoters and asynchronous motion may occur. Once adequate strength and synchronous motion are apparent, functional activities are initiated. During this rehabilitation period, trunk and back strengthening and overall aerobic conditioning should be addressed. Surgery is sometimes indicated when failure of a formalized rehabilitation protocol is evident.

The purpose of surgical intervention is to alleviate pain primarily with functional improvement as a secondary objective. Shoulder arthroscopy plays a major role in evaluating and treating rotator cuff pathology in this group of athletes. Hurley reviewed 100 shoulder arthroscopies in athletes and noted a high percentage of concomitant pathology, which included labral tears (both superior and anterior inferior), biceps tendon lesions, and partial-thickness cuff tears that were unexpected. Initially, shoulder arthroscopy is utilized to identify unexpected pathology (i.e., instability), define the morphology of the tear (complete versus partial, length, width, location), and facilitate a rational surgical approach. Partial articular or bursal tears that are less than 1 cm in length and involving 50% of the width of the tendon or less, undergo debridement of the tear and an arthroscopic subacromial decompression. The width of the tear is sometimes hard to determine, however, a tear of 3 mm or greater is felt to be significant. Arthroscopic decompression includes subdeltoid bursa section, coracoacromial ligament resection, anterior and lateral acromioplasty, and excision of a distal clavicular spur if present. Tears greater than 1 cm in length and 50% of the width of the tendon are treated as complete tears. Complete tears are divided into four groups: (1) small (less than 1 cm), (2) moderate (1 to 3 cm), (3) large (3 to 5 cm), and (4) massive (greater than 5 cm).

Complete tears in groups one and two undergo an arthroscopic subacromial decompression and a rotator cuff repair through a mini-deltoid splitting incision. Recent investigations addressing arthroscopic subacromial decompression and arthroscopic rotator cuff repair using absorbable tacks, suture anchors, or nonabsorbable suture anchors are considered experimental at this point. However, the indications appear to be a young subject with a small (1 to 2 cm) mobile supraspinatus tear, with excellent bone and tendon.

High performance athletes seldom have large or massive tears unless a high-velocity injury causes an acute avulsion of the rotator cuff from its insertion on the greater tuberosity. In such cases, an open subacromial decompression, secure rotator cuff repair back to bone, and restoration of the deltoid is advocated. Rarely, superior labral anterior and posterior (SLAP) lesions present as associated pathology and are graded I-IV dependent on the fixation of the biceps insertion. Generally, they are arthroscopically debrided and the superior glenoid is burred to provide a vascular bed for healing. Recently, some investigators are reattaching the superior labrum with arthroscopic bioabsorbable fixation devices specifically if the biceps anchor is detached.

During examination under anesthesia and arthroscopic examination, it sometimes becomes apparent that the partial articular rotator cuff tear is secondary to anterior glenohumeral instability. Helpful arthroscopic findings include (1) attenuated anterior inferior glenohumeral ligament (AIGHL), (2) multiple small tears along the AIGHL, (3) positive "drive-thru sign" as described by Warren, (4) posterior scuff marks on humeral head medial to the normal bone area, and (5) arthroscopically observed anterior inferior subluxation as the arm is brought into 90 degrees of abduction and 90 degrees of external rotation. The surgical approach for this condition is an anterior capsulolabral reconstruction that stabilizes the anterior capsuloligamentous complex and allows maximal ROM so important in this athlete population. Subacromial decompressions in the face of anterior instability has been disappointing, and is not recommended. It should be emphasized that surgeons who deal with high-performance throwing athletes proportionally note a much larger incidence of eccentric overload and anterior subluxation versus those who handle recreational athletes, who have greater incidence of pure impingement syndrome.

Recreational Athletes

Treatment of weekend athletes with full-thickness rotator cuff tears is equivalent to that of the general population. Impingement is the overriding pathology and partial articular-sided surface tears are rare. Generally, symptoms are controlled with NSAIDs, rest, and physical therapy modalities. Physical therapy is instituted to regain ROM and strength of the shoulder. The program is similar to that described for elite athletes. Subjects usually respond to a rehabilitation protocol; however, return to sports, especially overhead sports, is limited. Operative treatment is indicated in those patients who have continuing symptoms, especially pain after a course of conservative treatment. The prime indication for surgery is pain relief; improvement in function is secondary, although with good surgical technique, it is often attainable. Successful outcomes of full-thickness rotator cuff repairs involves four principles: (1) adequate subacromial decompression, this may include the distal clavicle if symptoms warrant, (2) secure rotator cuff repair with nonabsorbable sutures (No. 2 silky Polydec, or 1 mm cottony Dacron) preferably to a bony trough, if at all possible, (3) meticulous reattachment of the deltoid to the acromion through bone, and (4) completion of a rotator cuff rehabilitation program.

Significant partial and small full-thickness tears (less than 1 cm) usually require an open subacromial decompression and either side-to-side or end-to-bone repair. Because this population is usually over 40 years of age and the pathologic process is caused by hypertrophic lesions in the coracoacromial arch with supraspinatus outlet narrowing (impingement) and the cuff tissue histologically shows degeneration, arthroscopic decompression and repair is not recommended.

There are five commonly recognized reasons for failure of an attempted rotator cuff repair: (1) bone failure over the greater tuberosity or cuff suture failure at the suture tendon junction, (2) suture failure, (3) postoperative adhesions, (4) inadequate subacromial decompression, and (5) failure of the reattached deltoid to the acromion. Fastidious surgical technique is the key to alleviate many of these problems.

REHABILITATION

Preventative rehabilitation based on shoulder biomechanics in athletes has proven helpful in protection and prevention tears of the rotator cuff and anterior stabilizers. Biomechanical studies by Jobe, Pink, and Tibone have provided a basis for normal and abnormal kinematics in overhand athletes. Studies by Moseley on scapular rotator rehabilitation, and Townsend on glenohumeral stabilizer rehabilitation has provided a group of core exercises for the athletic shoulder. This program consists of the six best exercises, documented by EMG and motion analysis, for strengthening the humeral protectors/positions and scapular pivoters. The three best exercises for the humeral protectors/positions are (1) elevation in the plane of the scapula in internal rotation, (2) horizontal abduction in external rotation, and (3) press-up. The four best exercises for the scapular pivoters are (1) press-up, (2) elevation in the scapular plane in external rotation, (3) rowing and, (4) push-up plus. Assimilation of these data by Jobe and Pink was developed into the concept of "3Es and

4Ps," which delineate the timing of each segment of the program (see previous section).

Postoperative rehabilitation after an open repair of a full-thickness rotator cuff tear consists of immediate passive ROM in the first postoperative week. In the third week, active assisted ROM is initiated. Active ROM exercises are started when healing of the cuff is evident, usually about the sixth week. When active ROM is comfortable, typically around the eighth week, terminal stretching and resistance exercises are initiated. If the repair was difficult and excessive tension was noted, the use of an abduction pillow has been helpful. Generally, the patient is held in the pillow between 3 and 6 weeks but timely passive ROM is started above the level of the pillow in the first week. The physical therapy program should be continued for at least 8 months to 1 year after surgery. After 6 months, recreational athletes may begin functional training for their sport. High-performance athletes will have a longer rehabilitation course primarily because of the biomechanic demands placed on the shoulder. Competitive and elite pitchers commonly are unable to pitch competitively for at least 1 year due to the problems of regaining external rotation, velocity, endurance, and synchronous throwing mechanics.

The rehabilitation following arthroscopic subacromial decompression and cuff debridement progresses quickly with immediate active ROM and stretching. Subsequently, within the first couple of weeks after surgery, concentric and eccentric exercises are added. The usual course requires 6 weeks of ROM and stretching followed by 6 weeks of strengthening and functional athletic exercises. Throwing athletes tend to require more time in resuming competitive activities.

SUGGESTED READING

Bradley JP, Tibone JE. Electromyographic analysis of muscle action about the shoulder. Clin Sports Med 1991; 10:789–805.

Burkhart SS. Arthroscopic treatment of massive rotator cuff tears: Clinical results and biomechanical rationale. Clin Orthop 1991; 267:45–56.

Ellman H, Hanker G, Bayer M. Repair of the rotator cuff: End-result study of factors influencing reconstruction. J Bone Joint Surg 1986; 68A:1136–1144.

Gartman GM. Arthroscopic acromioplasty for lesions of the rotator cuff, J Bone Joint Surg 1990; 72A:169–180.

Harryman DT, Mack LA, Wang KY, et al. Repairs of the rotator cuff. J Bone Joint Surg 1991; 73A:982–989.

Hawkins RJ, Kennedy JC. The impingement syndrome in athletes. Am J Sports Med 1980; 8:57.

Hawkins RJ, Misamore MD, Hobeika PE. Surgery for full-thickness rotator cuff tears. J Bone Joint Surg 1985; 77A:1349–1355.

Iannotti JP. Lesions of the rotator cuff: Pathology and pathogenesis. In Matsen FA, Fu FH, Hawkins RJ, eds. The shoulder: A balance of mobility and stability. Park Ridge, Ill.: American Academy of Orthopaedic Surgeons, 1992; 239.

Jobe FW, Bradley JP. Rotator cuff injuries in baseball: Prevention and rehabilitation. Sports Med 1988; 6:377–386.

Jobe FW, Bradley JP. The diagnosis and nonoperative treatment of shoulder injuries in athletes. Clin Sports Med 1989; 8:419–438.

Lohr JF, Uhthoff AK. The microvascular pattern of the supraspinatus tendon. Clin Orthrop 1990; 254:35–38.

Morrison DS, Bigliani LU. The clinical significance of variations in acromial morphology. Orthop Trans 1987; 11:234.

Moseley JB, Jobe FW, Pink M, et al. EMG analysis of the scapular rotator muscles during a shoulder rehabilitation program. Am J Sports Med.

Neer CS II. Anterior acromioplasty for chronic impingement syndrome in the shoulder: A preliminary report. J Bone Joint Surg 1972; 54A:41–50.

Neer CS II. Impingement lesions. Clin Orthop 1983; 173:70–77.

Norwood LA, Barrack R, Jacobson KE. Clinical presentation of complete tears of the rotator cuff. J Bone Joint Surg 1989; 71A:499–505.

Tibone JE, Elrod B, Jobe FW, et al. Surgical treatment of tears of the rotator cuff in athletes. J Bone Joint Surg 1986; 68A:887.

Townsend H, Jobe FW, Pink M, et al. EMG analysis of the glenohumeral muscles during a baseball rehabilitation program. Am J Sports Med 1991; 19:264–271.

Walch G, Boileau P, Noel E, et al. Impingement of the deep surface of the supraspinatus tendon on the posterosuperior glenoid rim: An arthroscopic study. J Shoulder and Elbow Surgery 1992; 1:238–245.

Wasilewski SA, Frankl U. Rotator cuff pathology: Arthroscopic assessment and treatment. Clin Orthop 1991; 267:65–70.

RUPTURE OF THE PECTORALIS MAJOR

SCOTT W. WOLFE, M.D.

Rupture of the pectoralis major is an uncommon event. Approximately 85 cases have been reported in the literature since the first report by Patissier in 1822. In that report, a butcher boy was said to have sustained the injury while trying to unhook an enormous side of beef. Subsequent early reports documented similar mechanisms, usually involving a sudden traumatic load on the extended, abducted arm; or rarely, a direct crushing blow to the chest wall. Recent series described the injury most frequently in athletes, and over one-half of recently reported cases involved bench pressing. Surgical treatment of acute ruptures in athletes is advocated by most authors for restoration of full strength, contour, and athletic performance. Conservative treatment is recommended for partial tears or tears in older or less active individuals.

ANATOMY AND FUNCTION

The pectoralis major is a broad, thick muscle that has an extensive origin from the clavicle, upper ribs, and the fascia of the abdominal musculature. The fibers converge like a fan (Fig. 1) into three laminae, which twist upon each other 90 degrees before coalescing into

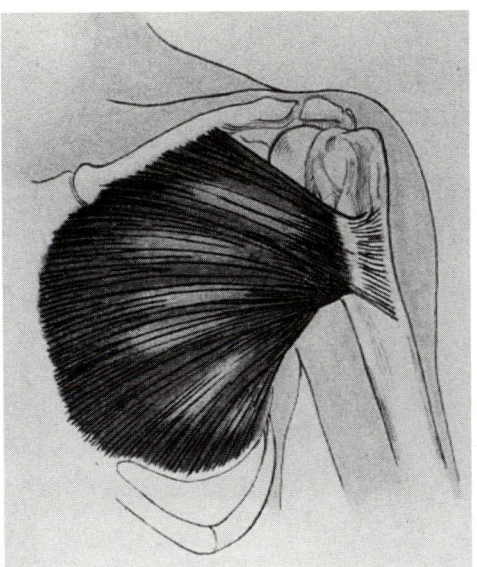

Figure 1 The pectoralis fibers converge like a fan onto their humeral insertion. The inferior fibers insert superiorly and posterior to the superior fibers, producing a 90 degree twist in the tendon at its insertion site. (From Wolfe SW, Wickiewicz TL, Cavanaugh JT. Ruptures of the pectoralis major. An anatomical and clinical analysis. Am J Sports Med 1992; 20:587-593; with permission.)

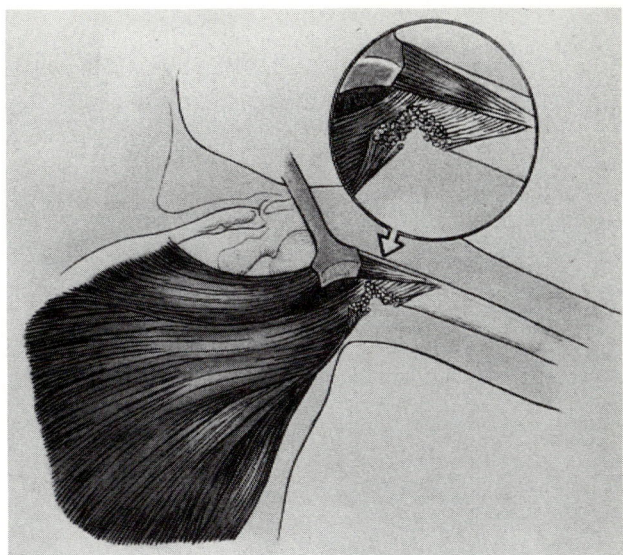

Figure 2 Disproportionate stretching of the inferior fibers during humeral extension and application of high load causes failure of these fibers. The tear propagates as tension increases on the remaining fibers.

a single tendon of insertion. The fibers of the clavicular head form the anterior lamina, which inserts anteriorly and distally on the humerus, while the sternal and abdominal heads form the middle and posterior lamina, which insert progressively more posteriorly and proximally, giving the tendon a coiled appearance. The tendon measures 5 cm in length and 5 mm in width, and inserts on the intertubercular groove of the humerus just lateral to the biceps tendon. The muscle is innervated by the medial and lateral pectoral nerves, and its vascular pedicle is the pectoral branch of the thoracoacromial trunk. The main function of the pectoralis major is in adduction of the humerus, and to a lesser extent, internal rotation and forward flexion.

PATIENT PROFILE

Pectoralis ruptures have been reported exclusively in males. The average age in the 67 reports in which age was recorded is 32; 80% of these injuries were in men between the ages of 20 and 35. The injury occurred most commonly during performance of the bench press. While many patients were bodybuilders, only five admitted use of anabolic steroids. Pectoralis ruptures have also been reported in football, wrestling, rugby, boxing, basketball, skiing, sailboarding, and ice hockey.

PATHOMECHANICS

The most common mechanism for pectoralis rupture involves application of maximal voluntary contraction at

a time when the muscle is passively stretched. In most early reports, the injuries were sustained while attempting to break a fall from a height or while being dragged behind a moving vehicle. Weightlifters classically describe the rupture occurring with the bar on or near the chest, usually during maximum or near-maximum load. Just after initiating a bench press maneuver, athletes consistently describe a "sticking point," where little incremental gain is made despite maximal contracture. A biomechanical analysis of this region by Elliot and co-workers suggests that the pectoralis is at a mechanical disadvantage at this point in the lift. A cadaveric study at our institution documented disproportionate stretching of the shorter, abdominal fibers of the pectoralis sternal head during the initial phase of the lift. We hypothesize that the application of high external loads to the pectoralis while the humerii are extended behind the thorax and the inferior fibers are stretched to an extreme mechanical disadvantage, produces rupture of these fibers. Continued loading increases the tension on the remaining fibers of the sternal head, and the rupture propagates through the remaining tendon (Fig. 2).

Most ruptures occur at the distal tendon, at or close to the musculotendinous junction. Approximately 20 cases of complete avulsion of the tendon from the humeral insertion have been reported. Intermuscular tears are quite rare, and usually result from a direct blow or crushing injury.

PHYSICAL EXAMINATION

The patient usually describes a history of forceful abduction and extension of the arm, frequently against active resistance. The patient may describe a sudden

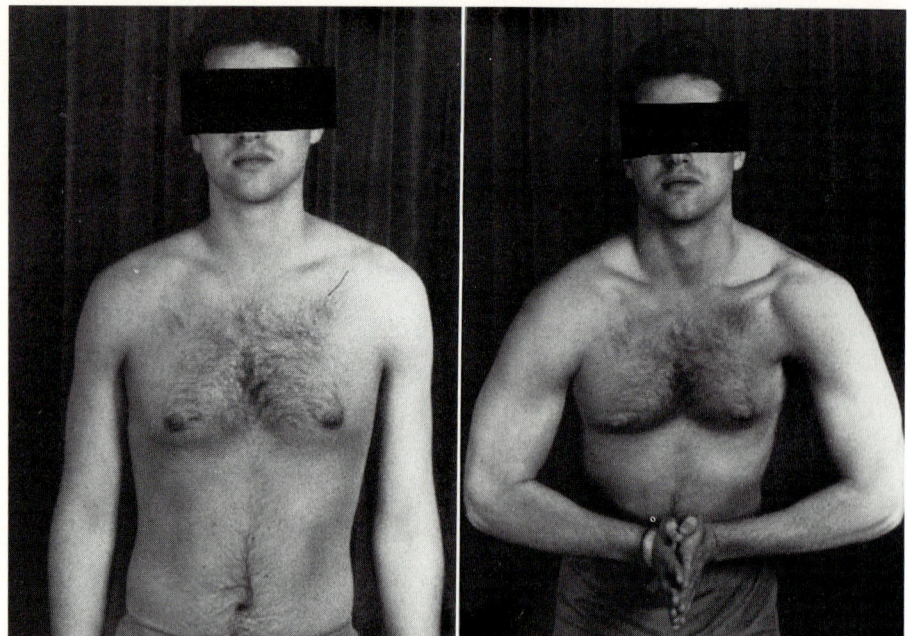

Figure 3 Characteristic contour defect following pectoralis rupture. *A,* No defect is recognized with the arms at the side. *B,* Adduction against resistance accentuates the axillary hollowing.

giving way, or audible "snap" during the injury, associated with intense, searing pain across the chest wall. Initial examination is limited by pain and swelling, but the patient will usually demonstrate weakness in adduction against resistance. Physical findings include marked swelling and tenderness in the deltopectoral groove. Within a week of the injury, there may be extensive ecchymosis of the axilla, chest wall, and upper arm. A defect in the axillary contour is not usually evident for 3 or 4 weeks, at which time atrophy and retraction of the torn muscle have occurred. While no defect may be apparent with the arms at the side, abduction will demonstrate a hollowing of the anterior axillary fold, with accentuation of the inferior border of the deltoid, and "webbing" of the axillary contour. The defect is most pronounced with adduction and internal rotation against resistance (Fig. 3). Occasionally the retracted muscle belly can be palpated on the anterior chest wall.

Physical findings may be deceptive, however, and the examiner may easily mistake a complete sternal head rupture for a partial tear. The clavicular head usually remains intact, accounting for an incomplete defect of the axillary fold. The torn tendon often retains attachments to the investing fascia of the arm, preventing further retraction. With resistance, the fascial attachment becomes a prominent band extending midway down the humerus along the medial border of the biceps, and may appear to represent an incomplete avulsion. Distal ruptures are usually complete, however, and the examiner should not be misled by what may appear to be only a mild deformity. Serial examinations over the first 4 weeks may help to establish the diagnosis of complete rupture when in doubt.

DIAGNOSTIC TESTS

Standard radiographs are usually normal, but may show an absence of the pectoralis soft tissue shadow, felt to be pathognomonic of complete rupture by some authors. Magnetic resonance imaging (MRI) has been helpful in some centers in defining the location and extent of the tear. A surface coil is recommended to decrease signal-to-noise ratio, and a fast-spin echo sequence to increase the contrast between fluid in the torn muscle fibers and the surrounding subcutaneous fat. MRI at this point should be considered a confirmatory test only, as there are insufficient data to compare the accuracy of this modality with physical examination in the diagnosis of a complete rupture.

Some authors have found dynamometry useful in evaluating chronic injuries to aid in patient selection for surgical repair. Dynamometry can objectively and independently assess strength in adduction, internal rotation, and forward flexion, and contrast the data with the uninjured side. Compensation by the anterior deltoid and latissimus dorsi may reveal no deficit on the injured side. Lack of significant strength deficit would mitigate against surgical intervention in these cases.

TREATMENT

Nonoperative treatment of pectoralis tears is associated with maintenance of normal motion and function in most daily activities. Patients complain of weakness in sports and activities requiring maximal strength, and demonstrate a moderate deformity of the axillary fold and chest contour. In 26 patients with subacute or

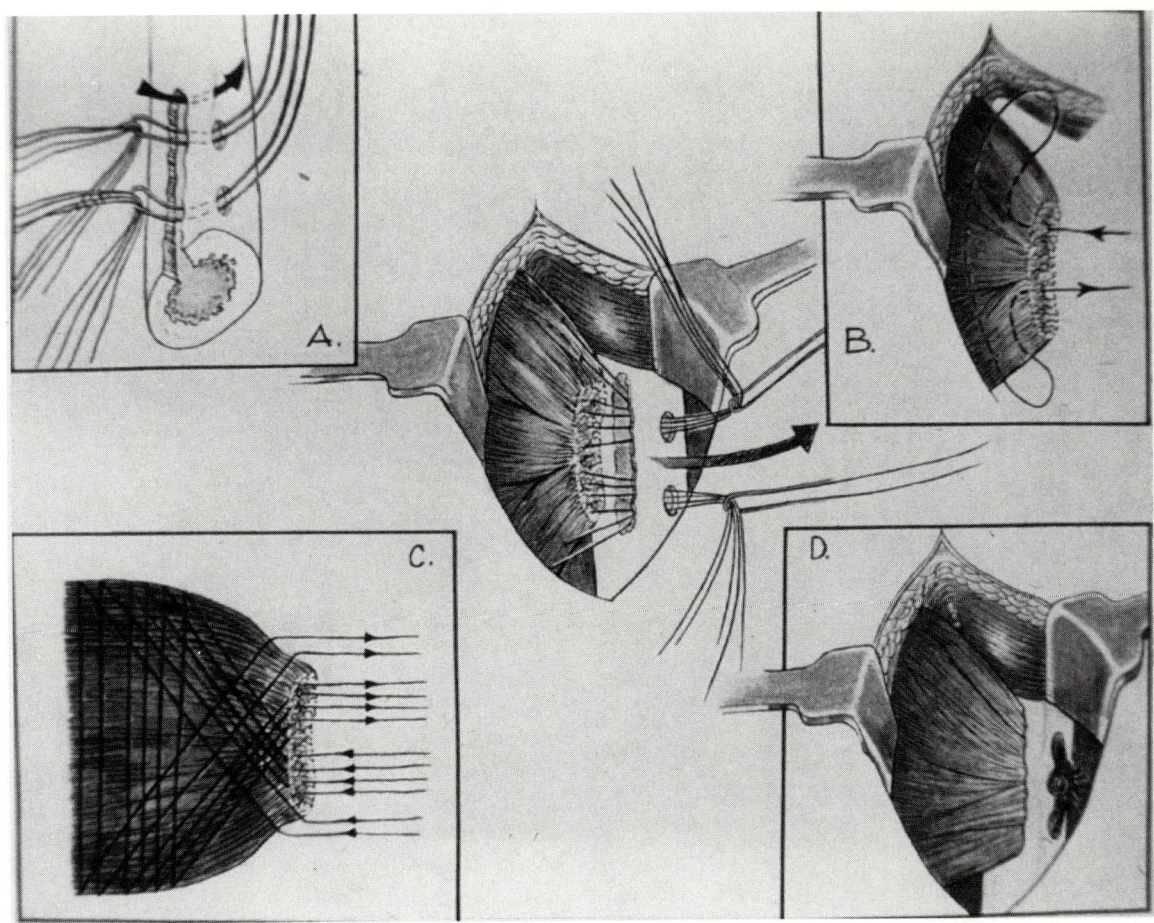

Figure 4 Technique of surgical repair. *A,* A trough is created at the pectoralis insertion site, and two one-eighth inch drill holes made lateral to the trough. Wire loops are threaded through the trough and drill holes, so that sutures may be passed. *B* and *C,* Multiple nonabsorbable sutures are woven through the fascia, muscle, and tendon remnant at different depths. *D,* The sutures are grouped into two bundles, which are threaded through the wire loops and pulled onto the trough. The tendon is firmly secured in place. (From Wolfe SW, Wickiewicz TL, Cavanaugh JT. Ruptures of the pectoralis major: An anatomical and clinical analysis. Am J Sports Med 1992; 20:587-593; with permission.)

chronic tears, weakness was the most frequent presenting complaint (66%), followed by cosmetic deformity (27%). Moderate or severe pain was uncommon with this injury, but was the presenting complaint in four patients. Objective testing of four patients with chronic complete ruptures using isokinetic dynamometry demonstrated peak torque deficits of 60% to 75% of their opposite, uninjured side.

Surgical treatment has been demonstrated by a number of authors to restore excellent strength, function, and contour with few reported complications. In three recent series 23 of 27 patients treated operatively obtained good to excellent restoration of strength, function, and contour, and returned to professional or vigorous recreational sporting activities, including body building. Three patients treated for chronic tears, at an average of 4 years from injury, did not regain full strength, but had marked improvement over preoperative status as measured by dynamometry. One patient, who was noncompliant with postoperative splint wear,

was dissatisfied because of a widened scar and subjective weakness. In 11 patients tested pre- and postoperatively with dynamometry in horizontal adduction at high speed, a 60% preoperative deficit was improved to a 108% postoperative measurement, when compared to the uninjured side.

SURGICAL TECHNIQUE

The patient is placed in a beach chair position after induction of general endotracheal tube anesthesia. The arm is draped free and the anterior thorax prepped to the mid-sternum. A long delto-pectoral incision is employed, and careful dissection along the inferior border of the deltoid performed to identify the conjoined tendon of the biceps and coracobrachialis. Scarring may make the initial dissection difficult. The dissection should not stray medial to the conjoined tendon, as the cords and peripheral nerves of the brachial plexus lie in

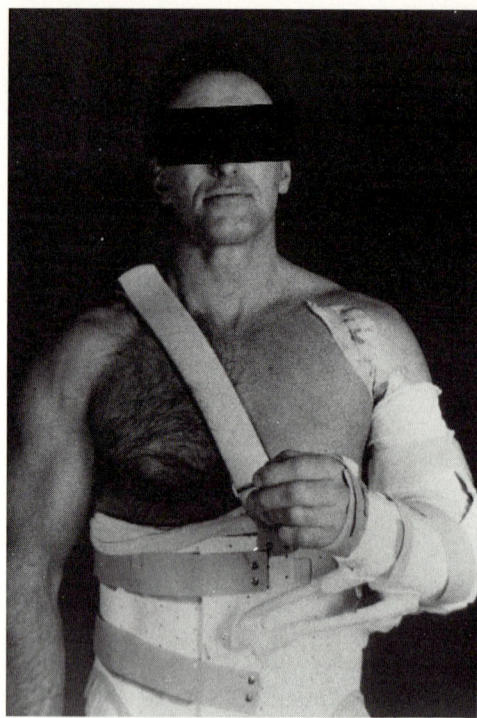

Figure 5 The patient is maintained in a passive position of forward flexion, adduction and internal rotation in a custom thermoplast splint for 4 weeks.

this interval. Usually a cuff of the ruptured tendon remains attached at the pectoralis insertion site, just lateral to the tendon of the long head of the biceps.

Subcutaneous dissection is carried out along the chest wall to identify the ruptured and retracted muscle. Remaining attachments to the investing fascia of the arm may create an illusion of an intact tendon, and need to be taken down to help identify the true proximal ruptured tendon border. Depending on the timing of the injury, a significant amount of mobilization of the muscle from the chest wall and overlying skin may be necessary. The pectoralis has a rich innervation from multiple branches of the medial and lateral pectoral nerves, so that dissection and identification of the pedicle is not usually necessary or warranted. Most of the branches course through the pectoralis minor and clavi-pectoral fascia, and are located near the superior border of the muscle.

Multiple grasping sutures of #2 nonabsorbable material are woven through the fascia and muscle at different depths and brought out through the remaining tendon. Traction should be applied to the suture groups to ensure that adequate mobilization of the muscle has been performed. With the muscle well mobilized and sutures anchored in the pectoralis fascia and remaining tendon, attention is redirected to the proximal humerus.

Subperiosteal elevation is performed about the insertion site at the intertubercular groove, and Bennett retractors placed about the humerus. A 4 cm trough is created at the original insertion site and two drill holes placed laterally in the humerus with a one-eighth inch drill.

The woven sutures are split into two groups and pulled into the humeral groove by wires threaded through each drill hole (Fig. 4). The two groups of sutures are tied with the arm adducted 20 degrees and internally rotated. The wound is closed in layers over suction drains and the arm placed in a custom prefabricated orthoplast splint in 20 degrees of internal rotation, 20 degrees forward flexion, and 20 degrees of abduction (Fig. 5).

REHABILITATION

Immobilization in the custom orthosis is maintained for 6 weeks. Passive external rotation, adduction, and overhead exercises are begun at 6 weeks. Gentle active resistance exercises are begun at 12 weeks. Return to weight lifting or competitive sports is delayed for 6 months.

PREVENTION

Many pectoralis ruptures are the result of random athletic injuries and cannot be prevented. It may be possible, however, to prevent those injuries that occur during bench pressing by modifying lifting technique. When the humerus is extended behind the thorax, our cadaveric analysis documented extreme stretching of the short fibers of the abdominal head, beyond the point where they can effectively contract. Application of high loads to the muscle with these fibers disproptionately stretched may produce failure. A modification of the technique that would eliminate this portion of the lift, perhaps by mechanically blocking the elbows from extending behind the thorax, may effectively prevent pectoralis ruptures.

PREFERRED TREATMENT

Acute complete ruptures of the pectoralis major from the humeral insertion should be surgically repaired in competitive athletes and young, active individuals to prevent the sequelae of weakness, deformity, and occasional pain. Nonoperative treatment is recommended for older or less active patients. Nonoperative treatment predictably results in a moderate deformity, but will not result in a significant functional loss. Chronic repairs, while somewhat more technically difficult due to shortening and scarring, can be performed with expectation of improved strength and contour.

Acknowledgement. The author would like to thank Dr. Jack Kelley for his contributions to this chapter.

SUGGESTED READING

Elliot BC, Wilson GJ, Kerr GK. A biomechanical analysis of the sticking region in the bench press. Med Sci Sports Ex 1989; 21:450–461.

Kretzler HH, Richardson AB. Rupture of the pectoralis major muscle. Am J Sports Med 1989; 17:453–458.

McEntire JE, Hess WE, Coleman SS. Rupture of the pectoralis major muscle. J Bone Joint Surg 1972; 54A:1040–1046.

Miller MD, Johnson DL, Fu FH, et al. Rupture of the pectoralis major muscle in a collegiate football player: Use of magnetic resonance imaging in early diagnosis. Am J Sports Med 1993; 21:475–477.

Wolfe SW, Wickiewicz TL, Cavanaugh JT. Ruptures of the pectoralis major muscle: An anatomic and clinical analysis. Am J Sports Med 1992; 20:587–593.

Zeman SC, Rosenfeld RT, Lipscomb PR. Tears of the pectoralis major muscle. Am J Sports Med 1979; 7:343–347.

SURGICAL MANAGEMENT OF POSTERIOR OSSIFICATIONS OF THE GLENOID IN THROWING ATHLETES

JIRO OZAKI, M.D.

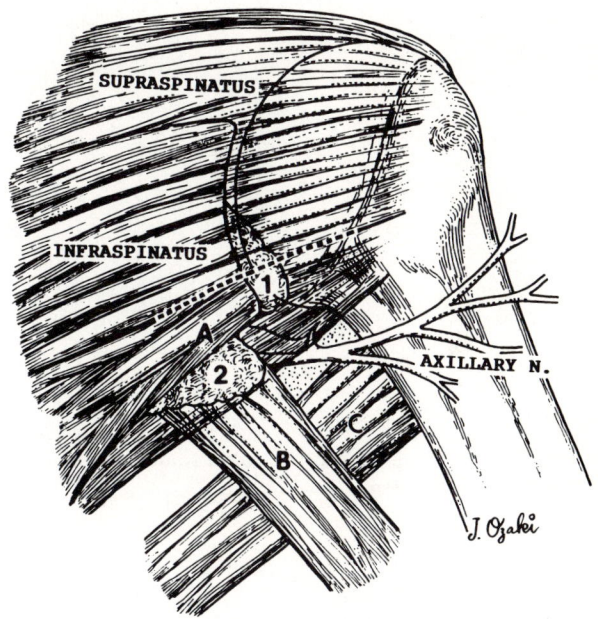

Figure 1 Anatomy of two types of posterior ossifications of glenoid. (1) Ossifications on posterior glenoid rim. (2) Ossifications on infraglenoid tubercle. *A,* Teres minor. *B,* Triceps long head. *C,* Teres major. (From Ozaki J. Surgical treatment for posterior ossifications of the glenoid in baseball players. J Shoulder Elbow Surg 1992; 1:91-97; with permission.)

In the throwing athlete with prolonged posterior shoulder pain, the pathologic findings of the posteroinferior glenoid osteophytes associated with axillary neuropathy are extremely important. A method of surgical management and a rationale of posterior ossifications of the glenoid are described here.

SURGICAL ANATOMY

The posteroinferior glenoid region lies under the posterior portion of the deltoid muscle. The quadrilateral space is formed by the posteroinferior glenoid rim and teres minor muscle above, the teres major muscle below, the long head of the triceps muscle medially, and the inner aspect of the upper end of the humerus laterally. This space is traversed by the axillary nerve and is clinically important.

There are two types of posterior ossifications of the glenoid. Ossifications on the posteroinferior glenoid rim are associated with posterior glenohumeral impingement, posterior glenoid labrum tears, and axillary neuropathy. Ossifications on the infraglenoid tubercle are associated with axillary nerve entrapment by the osteophytes and the thickened long head of the triceps muscle. Figure 1 shows the anatomy of this lesion.

INDICATIONS AND CLINICAL MANIFESTATIONS

The specific indications for surgical release of this lesion are prolonged throwing dysfunction with posterior shoulder pain and the presence of posteroinferior glenoid ossifications associated with axillary neuropathy. The muscle strength of the involved shoulder is less than one-half that of the contralateral shoulder. There is minimum atrophy of the deltoid muscle, but sensory examination reveals slight sensory loss in the outer aspect of the upper arm. Tenderness is present at the posteroinferior glenoid region including the quadrilateral space. Pain is elicited in the posterior aspect of the shoulder when the arm is placed in the abducted and externally rotated position behind the head. Roentgenogram of the overhead view of the shoulder is essential to detect this lesion (Fig. 2).

OPERATIVE PROCEDURE

The patient is placed in a lateral position on the edge of the operating table, with the affected side uppermost, and is draped to allow independent movement of the arm. The skin incision extends from the spine of the scapula to the axillary crease (Fig. 3). The fascia of the posterior deltoid muscle is incised, the posterior deltoid muscle is incised, and the posterior deltoid muscle is split vertically in the line of its fibers 5 to 7 cm in length

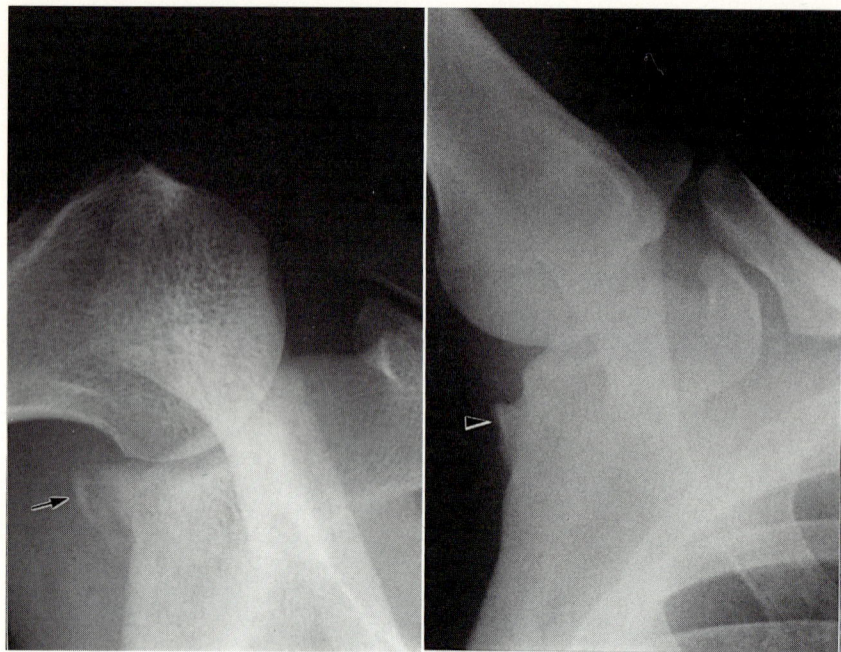

A

B

Figure 2 Radiographs of overhead view of shoulder show osteophytes *(arrow)* on posteroinferior glenoid margin *(A)* and osteophytes *(arrowhead)* on attachment of triceps long head *(B)*.

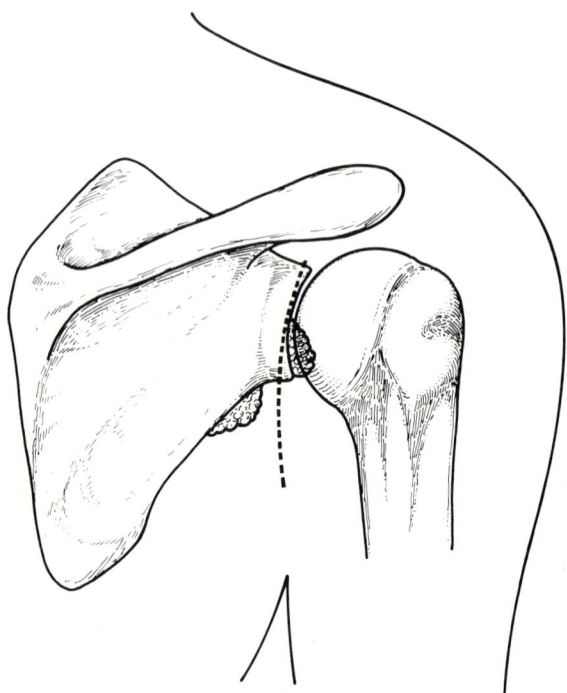

Figure 3 Skin incision (dashed line).

with individual variations toward the posterior axillary crease. The infraspinatus, the teres minor, and the quadrilateral space are exposed, with care taken not to injure the axillary nerve.

In the shoulders with posteroinferior glenoid rim osteophytes, an impingement occurs between the posterior greater tubercle of the humerus and the posterior glenoid osteophytes when the arm is placed in the abducted and externally rotated position. The axillary nerve is entrapped between the osteophytes and the teres major and is touched anterosuperiorly against the osteophytes at the overhead position. The capsule is exposed and incised transversely after the infraspinatus and the teres minor are separated, and the osteophytes are excised with a chisel (Fig. 4). As an additional operative manipulation, the axillary nerve that adheres at the superior border of the quadrilateral space should be released until the nerve moves freely in the quadrilateral space.

In shoulders with ossifications on the infraglenoid tubercle, when the quadrilateral space and the attachment of the long head of the triceps are exposed with retraction of the teres minor superiorly, the axillary nerve is entrapped by the osteophytes and by the thickened long head of the triceps. The axillary nerve is more likely to entrap at the abducted and externally rotated position or the overhead position. The osteophytes should be removed after the long head of the triceps is partially detached and after the nerve is released at the quadrilateral space (Fig. 5).

After the osteophyte is resected and the axillary nerve is released, it is essential to confirm that the axillary nerve can move freely and is not entrapped during any shoulder motion. The divided posterior part of the deltoid muscle is then reapproximated with interrupted sutures, and the skin is closed.

The involved arm is placed in a sling for 2 to 3 days after surgery. Pendulum and passive motion by the therapist is started within 3 days. The initial emphasis is on passive exercises for range of motion, which are soon advanced to the full self-assistive exercise regimen. Progressive active motion exercise is performed for 2 to 5 months. Pitching can be resumed at 3 to 6 months.

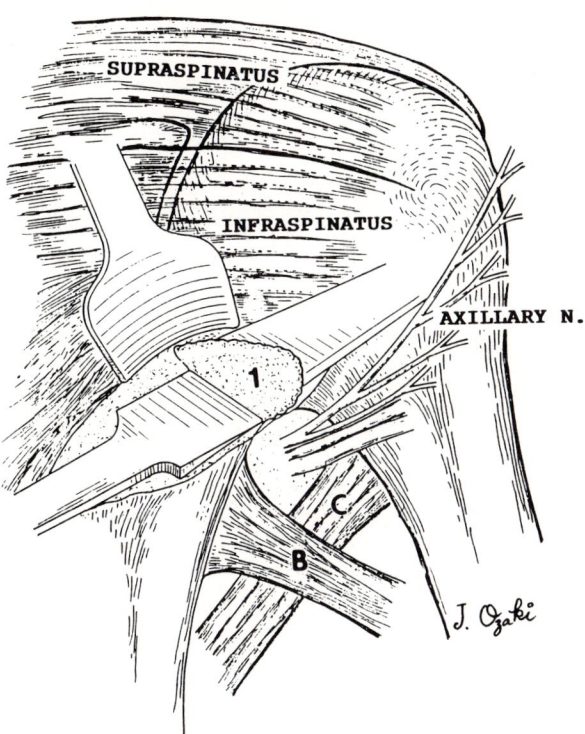

Figure 4 Operative procedure for shoulders with posterior glenoid rim ossifications (1). After posterior capsule is reached between interval of infraspinatus and teres minor, osteophyte (1) is removed with chisel. *B*, Triceps long head. *C*, Teres major. (From Ozaki J. Surgical treatment for posterior ossifications of the glenoid in baseball players. J Shoulder Elbow Surg 1992; 1:91-97; with permission.)

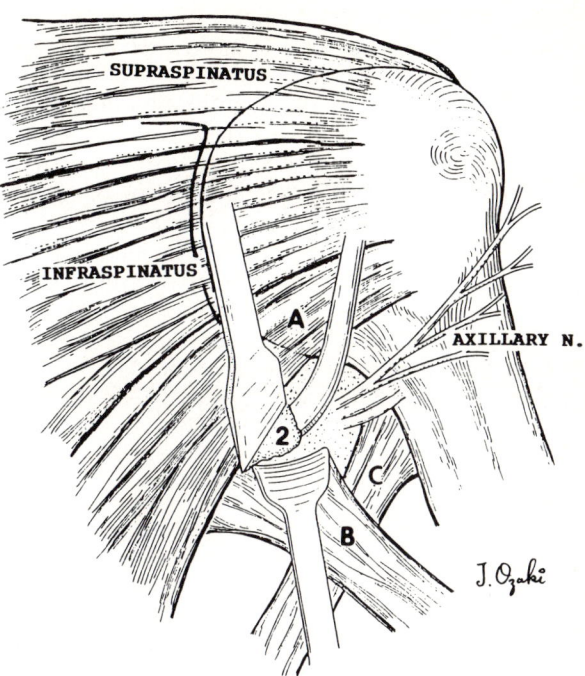

Figure 5 Operative procedure for shoulders with ossifications on infraglenoid tubercle (2). Osteophytes are removed after partial detachment of triceps long head (*B*). *A*, Teres minor. *C*, Teres major. (From Ozaki J. Surgical treatment for posterior ossifications of the glenoid in baseball players. J Shoulder Elbow Surg 1992; 1:91-97; with permission.)

RATIONALE FOR AND RESULTS OF OPERATIVE PROCEDURE

Posterior shoulder pain in throwing athletes can be caused by several lesions. Bennett studied athletes with hypertrophy of the capsule and ossifications at the posteroinferior glenoid region and noted that these lesions did not respond well to surgery. Beside Bennett's early report, reports on operated cases are very rare and the pathomechanisms and operative effects are still speculative. The repeated cocking and wringing action of throwing may cause the posterior glenohumeral impingement and posterior glenoid labrum tears, which may in turn initiate the process of osteophyte formation of the posteroinferior glenoid. Repetitive episodes of acceleration and follow-through with extreme traction may induce the stress fractures of the posterior glenoid margin of the infraglenoid tubercle, and may account for the development or the axillary nerve entrapment of osteophytes. Since our patients with osteophytes of the infraglenoid tubercle were adolescents, this lesion may be a traction epiphysitis that results when the powerful long head of the triceps muscle that inserts into a small area of infraglenoid tubercle exerts a contraction sufficiently powerful to cause tubercle avulsion and separation in an area of developing bone.

The axillary nerve traverses the quadrilateral space

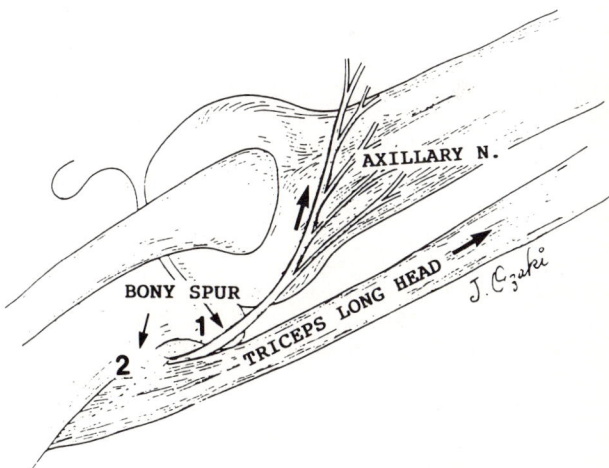

Figure 6 Pathologic mechanism of throwing in shoulders with posterior glenoid ossifications. (1): Osteophytes on posteroinferior glenoid rim. (2): Osteophytes on infraglenoid tubercle. (From Ozaki J. Surgical treatment for posterior ossifications of the glenoid in baseball players. J Shoulder Elbow Surg 1992; 1:91-97; with permission.)

and this space changes according to the shoulder motion. This space becomes more narrowed the more the arm is raised. When osteophytes are present at the posteroinferior glenoid rim or the infraglenoid tubercle, the quadrilateral space is more stenosed at the extreme overhand position. In the shoulders of extreme overhand throwers, the axillary nerve is more entrapped by the stenosed quadrilateral space and may be struck by the ossified lesions during the acceleration and follow-through phases (Fig. 6). Once the vicious cycle of the ossifications associated with axillary nerve entrapment has been established at the posteroinferior shoulder region, conservative treatment is rarely helpful. When conservative measures fail, operative treatment is indicated based on pathologic mechanisms, as previously described.

This procedure has now been performed in a total of 14 patients during the past 11 years. The initial 10 patients have been followed for an average of 5 years and the results noted as 90% satisfactory.

SUGGESTED READING

Barnes DA, Tullos HS. An analysis of 100 symptomatic baseball players. Am J Sport Med 1978; 6:62–66.
Bennett GE. Shoulder and elbow lesions distinctive of baseball players. Ann Surg 1947; 126:107–110.
Bennett GE. Shoulder and elbow lesions of the professional baseball pitcher. JAMA 1941; 117:510–514.
Lombardo SL, Jobe FW, Kerlan RK, et al. Posterior shoulder lesions in throwing athletes. Am J Sports Med 1977; 5:106–110.
Ozaki J. Surgical treatment for posterior ossifications of the glenoid in baseball players. J Shoulder Elbow Surg 1992; 1:91–97.

ANTERIOR CAPSULOLABRAL RECONSTRUCTION OF THE GLENOHUMERAL JOINT

RONALD S. KVITNE, M.D.
FRANK W. JOBE, M.D.

The shoulder joint in an overhand or throwing athlete is extremely vulnerable to injury due to high-energy repetitive forces. Over time, these repetitive activities may lead to tendinitis, impingement syndromes, and joint instability. In the young, overhand-throwing athlete with shoulder pain, it is important to recognize that glenohumeral joint instability or occult subluxation, rather than impingement, is the primary underlying pathology. Fortunately, conservative management is effective in most chronic overuse injuries and includes an initial period of relative rest, oral nonsteroidal anti-inflammatory drugs (NSAIDs), and a physical therapy program structured to provide local modalities to reduce inflammation and a strengthening program for the rotator cuff and scapular rotator musculature. For those athletes with continued symptoms, surgical intervention may become necessary. The anterior capsulolabral reconstruction addresses the problem of glenohumeral joint instability by correcting the capsular redundancy, labral damage, or both. When performed in the manner described, muscle attachments and proprioceptive muscle fibers are not disturbed and full shoulder range of motion can consistently be achieved, allowing these athletes to return to their prior competitive level.

PATHOPHYSIOLOGY

Throughout a full range of shoulder motion, there is a delicate balance between functional mobility and joint stability. The chronic stress from repetitive overhand or throwing activities may, over time, lead to attenuation of the static restraints (anterior joint capsule, glenohumeral ligaments, or glenoid labrum). Mild anterior translation of the humeral head may occur, but is usually compensated for by increased muscle activity of the dynamic stabilizers (rotator cuff and scapular rotator musculature). With continued throwing, however, fatigue of these muscles can lead to further anterior humeral head subluxation and secondary impingement.

Recent investigations have shown that in a throwing position (i.e., maximum humeral abduction and external humeral rotation), a normal shoulder allows 4 mm posterior humeral head translation with respect to the glenoid articular surface. The presumed mechanism is through selective tightening of the anterior joint capsule, which leads to this slightly posterior position. However, experimental evidence and arthroscopic observations in patients with joint laxity or anterior glenohumeral joint instability, reveal that this posterior translation does not occur. Rather, the humeral head is observed to translate anteriorly, producing a secondary "internal" impingement phenomena between the undersurface of the tendinous portions of the supraspinatus and infraspinatus muscles and the posterior-superior aspect of the glenoid rim. Thus, shoulder pathology can progress along a continuum from mild laxity to anterior subluxation, secondary impingement and subsequent rotator cuff tearing. This injury pattern that has been observed is now identified as the "instability complex."

DIAGNOSIS

A carefully obtained history and detailed physical examination is essential in establishing the diagnosis in the overhand or throwing athlete. Unfortunately, symptoms are often vague and the physical findings are subtle. As the shoulder is often the site of referred pain, cervical spine problems and potential sites of neurovascular compromise should routinely be evaluated and excluded.

Among throwers, shoulder pain is the most common complaint. Pain that is associated with a specific phase of throwing (i.e., late cocking or acceleration) is most likely due to mild anterior instability with secondary "internal" impingement.

In the throwing athlete, an evaluation of shoulder stability is crucial in determining the cause of shoulder pain. Unfortunately, the information gathered during classic stability testing may be confusing. Impingement signs and apprehension signs are relatively straightforward. Signs of mild instability, however, are often subtle and must not be overlooked. Glenohumeral translation may be assessed with the "load and shift" test. This maneuver is best performed with the patient relaxed and lying supine. The uninvolved arm is evaluated first, followed by the symptomatic side. The arm to be tested is positioned off the edge of the examining table and placed in a position of approximately 20 degrees abduction and forward flexion. The humerus is then loaded axially as anterior and posterior forces are applied to the humeral head, noting the degree of posterior and anterior humeral head translation. By comparing the "load and shift" test in varying degrees of internal and external humeral rotation on both shoulders, the competency of the glenohumeral ligaments and capsule may be assessed and subtle underlying laxity patterns may be identified.

We have found that the most sensitive means of eliciting occult anterior glenohumeral joint instability is achieved through the use of the "classic" apprehension sign followed by the "relocation" test. These maneuvers are also performed supine and involve testing the uninvolved, followed by the symptomatic side. The arm to be tested is positioned off the edge of the examining

table in 90 degrees abduction and maximum external rotation. In this position, the apprehension test is performed first by gently applying an anteriorly directed force to the posterior aspect of the proximal humerus (Fig. 1). Apprehension, or apprehension and pain, in this setting, indicates gross instability, as seen with recurrent dislocations. The sensation of pain without apprehension may denote either primary "subacromial" impingement or mild anterior instability with secondary "internal" impingement of the undersurface of the rotator cuff along the posterior, superior glenoid rim (Fig. 2). To differentiate primary subacromial impingement from primary instability (subluxation) with secondary internal impingement, the relocation test is performed. With the arm maintained in a position of 90 degrees shoulder abduction and maximum external humeral rotation, a posteriorly directed force is now applied to the anterior aspect of the proximal humerus (Fig. 3). Those patients with primary subacromial impingement have no change in their perception of pain. Those patients with primary anterior instability and secondary internal impingement, however, experience a reduction of their pain. This occurs as the humeral head is reduced posteriorly, thereby relieving the undersurface rotator cuff impingement along the posterior, superior glenoid rim (Fig. 4).

Radiographic evaluation of overhand or throwing athletes includes standard anteroposterior (AP), axillary, and outlet views. Unfortunately, these standard films add very little diagnostic information for a throwing athlete. They must be included, however, in the investigation of persistent shoulder pain to rule out infection, fracture, or an unsuspected neoplasm. Additional diagnostic procedures, including arthro-computed tomogra-

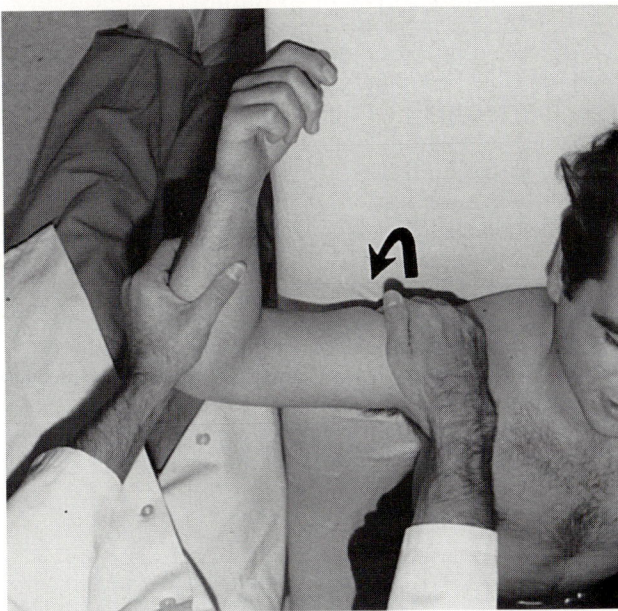

Figure 1 Apprehension test: shoulder held in 90 degree abduction and maximum external humeral rotation. An anteriorly directed force is applied with gentle fingertip pressure to the posterior aspect of the proximal humerus.

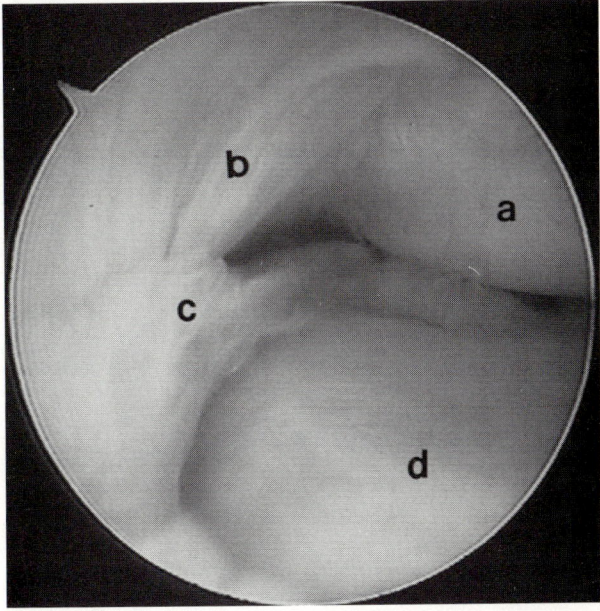

Figure 2 Posterosuperior glenoid impingement. *a*, Anteriorly translated humeral head. *b*, Undersurface rotator cuff fraying. *c*, Site of impingement along the posterosuperior glenoid labrum/rim. *d*, Glenoid fossa.

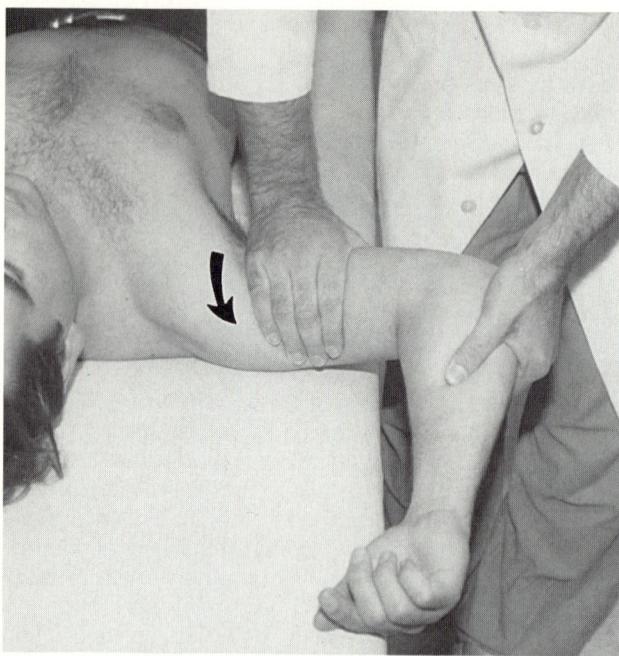

Figure 3 Relocation test: a posteriorly directed force is applied to the anterior aspect of the proximal humerus maintaining the head in a reduced position allowing further external humeral rotation.

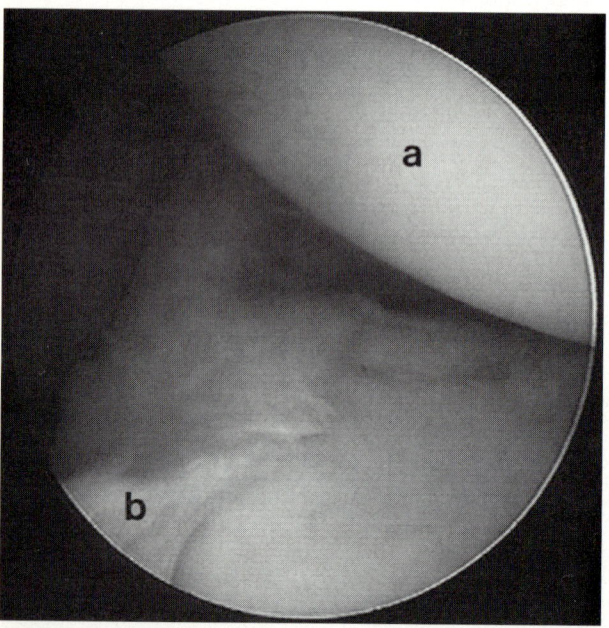

Figure 4 Reduced position of glenohumeral joint. *a,* Humeral head "reduced". *b,* Posterosuperior labral "fraying".

phy or magnetic resonance imaging with contrast (i.e., gadolinium), may provide additional information regarding the status of the glenoid labrum, glenohumeral ligaments, and/or rotator cuff. However, for those patients with suspected underlying occult instability and secondary impingement, an examination under anesthesia and diagnostic arthroscopy have been most helpful in confirming the diagnosis.

TREATMENT

As most shoulder injuries in the throwing athlete are the result of chronic repetitive microtrauma, an initial period of relative rest (avoidance of throwing) is indicated. Oral NSAIDs are recommended to reduce inflammation about the involved shoulder. Cortisone preparations, when injected about the shoulder joint, should be used judiciously. We advise against using more than three injections over 3 to 6 months for any condition.

Various physical therapy modalities are also employed, including cryotherapy, contrast baths, phonophoresis, iontophoresis, and electrical stimulation. These techniques help create an environment about the inflamed tissues that reduces swelling and facilitates the body's own healing response.

As pain and swelling subside, a supervised muscle strengthening program can be undertaken to re-establish "muscle synchrony" about the shoulder joint. Special emphasis is placed on regaining flexibility, as well as strength, power, and endurance of the rotator cuff muscles, scapular rotators, deltoid, trapezius, pectoralis major, coracobrachialis, and biceps and triceps muscles. Strengthening may begin with isometric exercises and subsequently utilize progressive resistive exercises, isotonic exercises, and finally isokinetic training. Those patients with underlying glenohumeral joint instability must be protected from further injury by avoiding shoulder hyperextension or abduction and external humeral rotation. This precaution applies throughout the rehabilitation, regardless of the exercise being performed.

An aggressive conservative rehabilitation program is continued for 3 to 6 months. If symptoms persist and the athlete is unable to return to throwing, surgical intervention must be considered.

An examination under anesthesia and preliminary diagnostic arthroscopy allow confirmation of the presumptive diagnosis and direct surgical treatment. Recently, glenohumeral joint stabilization has been accomplished using an anterior capsulolabral reconstruction, which is a modification of the procedure originally described by Bankart and Rowe. The capsular shift, which is fashioned on the glenoid side of the joint, tightens the attenuated or redundant capsule and, when present, corrects any lesions (i.e., Bankart) along the anterior, inferior glenoid rim. The most recent modification of this procedure utilizes the Mitek instrumentation system (Fig. 5). These "suture-anchors" allow secure reattachment of the capsular flaps to the anterior neck of the scapula, immediately adjacent to the glenoid margin.

SURGICAL TECHNIQUE

Existing surgical instruments have been modified to facilitate the operative technique (Fig. 6). The patient is positioned supine with the involved extremity supported by an arm board. Two folded surgical towels are placed

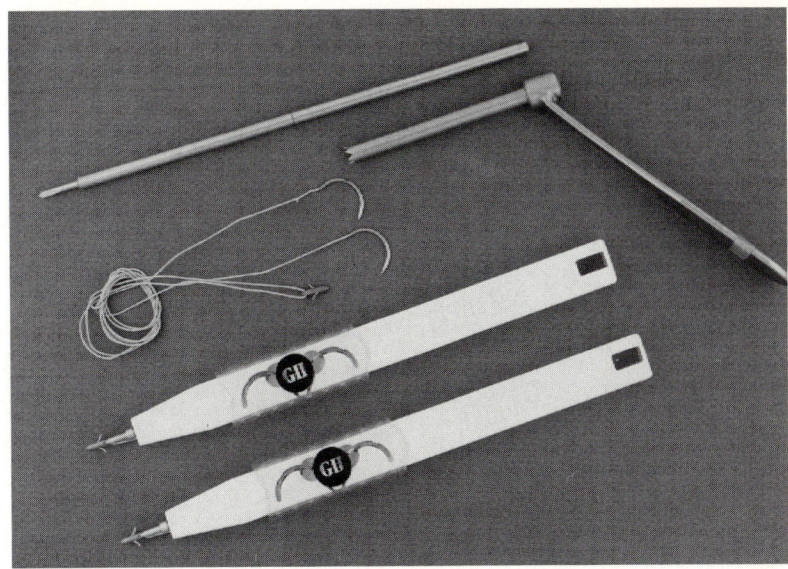

Figure 5 MITEK instrumentation: #1 Ethibond sutures preloaded onto G-2 MITEK anchors.

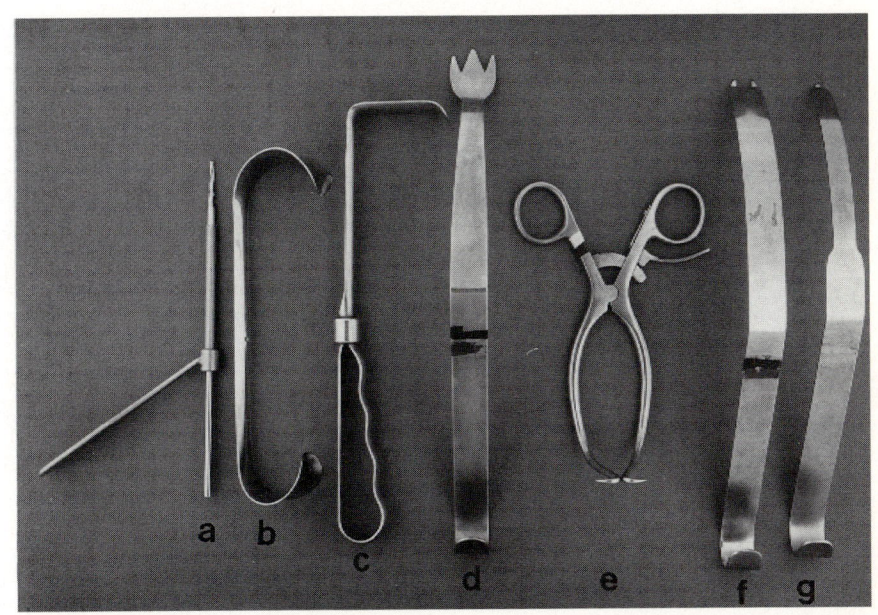

Figure 6 ANSPACH shoulder instruments: *a,* Mitek drill guide and drill bit. *b,* Modified Goulet retractors. *c,* Long narrow Richardson retractor. *d,* Pitchfork retractor. *e,* Modified gelpi retractor. *f,* Double-pronged humeral head retractor. *g,* Single-pronged humeral head retractors.

beneath the body of the scapula to provide additional stability for the shoulder girdle. An anterior axillary skin incision is then made and the deltopectoral interval is divided, retracting the cephalic vein laterally with the deltoid muscle (Fig. 7). Modified Goulet retractors are used to keep this interval open, allowing exposure of the underlying conjoined tendon (Fig. 8). A long, narrow Richardson retractor is used to retract the conjoined tendon medially, allowing exposure of the underlying subscapularis muscle (Fig. 9). The arm is now externally rotated to provide improved exposure of the subscapularis muscle and position the long head of the biceps laterally "out of harms way." Electrocautery is then used to split the subscapularis horizontally, along the direction of its fibers at the junction of the upper two-thirds and lower one-third (Fig. 10). Blunt dissection, begin-

ning medially and progressing laterally, facilitates the dissection of the overlying subscapularis from the closely adherent underlying joint capsule. A modified Gelpi retractor is then used to maintain this interval. A blunt-tipped 3-pronged "pitchfork" retractor is then carefully positioned along the anterior scapular neck, just medial to the glenoid rim, allowing exposure of the entire anterior glenohumeral joint capsule (Fig. 11). A capsular incision is then created horizontally at the level of the upper two-thirds and lower one-third (Fig. 12). Manual distraction of the glenohumeral joint allows placement of a narrow single- or double-pronged humeral head retractor across the joint to retract the humeral head laterally. This allows better visualization of the glenohumeral joint and exposure of the anterior glenoid rim. Stay sutures are placed in the superior and

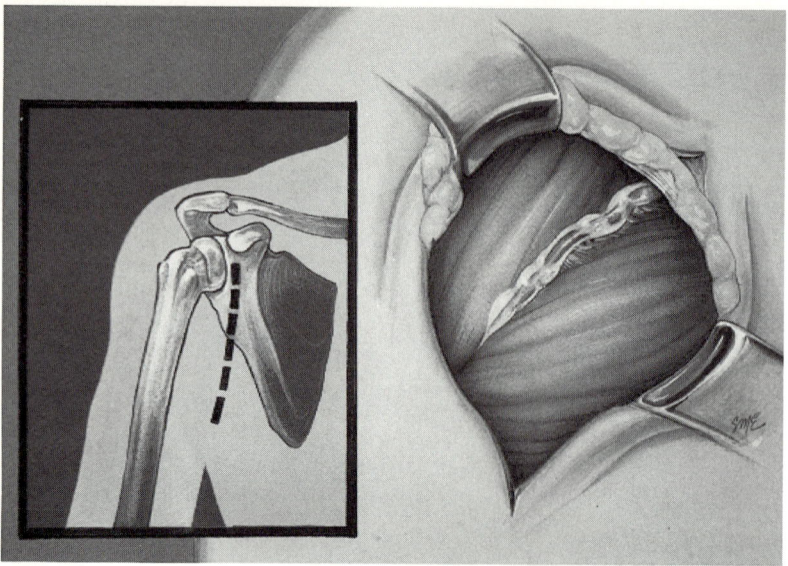

Figure 7 Anterior axillary skin incision and deltopectoral interval.

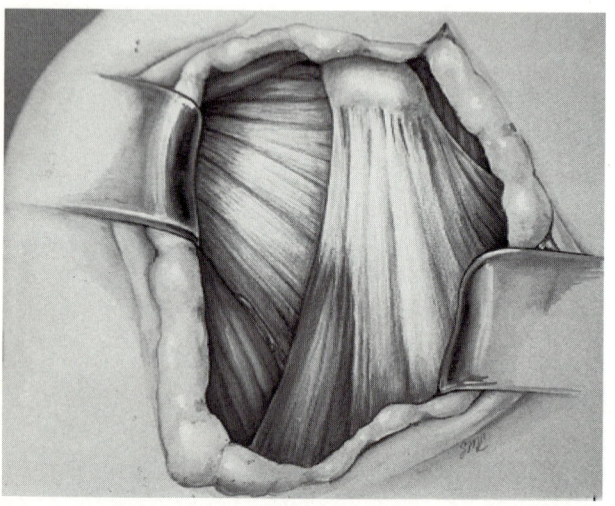

Figure 8 Exposure of conjoined tendon.

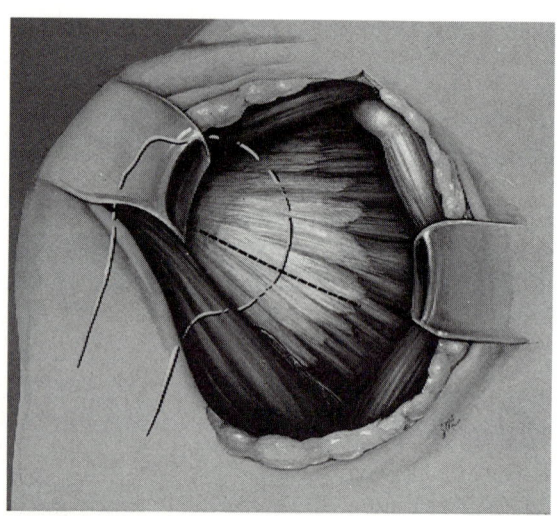

Figure 9 Exposure of subscapularis muscle.

inferior capsular flaps at the level of the glenoid rim to facilitate handling of these capsular tissues. With sharp dissection, the capsule and periosteum are elevated from the anterior scapular neck. The inferior flap must be dissected inferiorly to the 6 o'clock position to allow sufficient superior advancement and completely eliminate the redundant inferior capsular pouch. If the labrum is intact but the capsule lax and redundant, the capsulotomy (when carried out medially) must be carefully performed to avoid cutting the intact labrum. If a Bankart lesion is encountered, the damaged labrum is incised and elevated along with the capsular flaps and incorporated into the capsular reconstruction.

Using the #2 Mitek drill bit, drill sleeve, and power drill, three separate drill holes are created along the anterior, inferior glenoid rim 2 to 3 mm medial the articular margin (Fig. 13). These drill holes are approximately located at the 2, 4, and 5 o'clock positions for the right shoulder and 10, 8, and 7 o'clock positions for the

left shoulder (Fig. 14). The Mitek drill bit has been marked to indicate the correct tunnel depth that will accommodate the Mitek anchor and its attached suture. A single, #1 Ethibond suture is "loaded" onto each anchor, creating a double stranded "suture-anchor." These are then inserted sequentially into each drill hole.

By applying tension along the inferior stay suture, the inferior flap is advanced superiorly and secured into position using the double stranded #1 Ethibond sutures (Fig. 15). Each anchoring suture must be placed within the capsule at the level of the glenoid margin, as indicated by the previously placed stay suture. Placement of the sutures laterally will excessively tighten the capsule and limit postoperative range of motion (ROM). The superior capsular flap is then shifted inferiorly, overlying the inferior capsular flap and is secured into position using the same double-limbed sutures (Fig. 16). To relieve undue tension on the capsular flaps while tying the sutures, the humeral head retractor may be

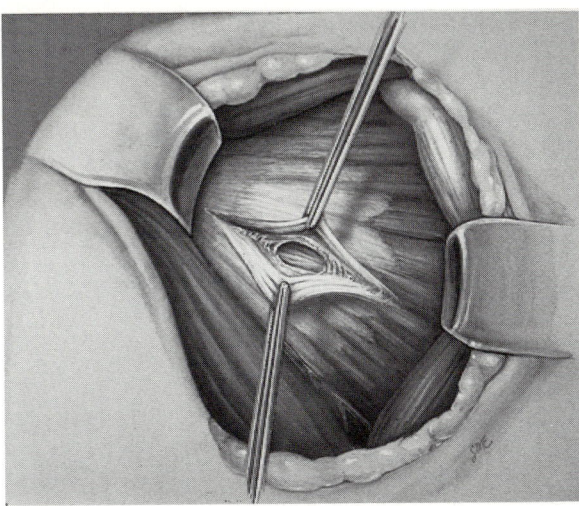

Figure 10 Subscapularis muscle split at junction of upper two-thirds and lower one-third.

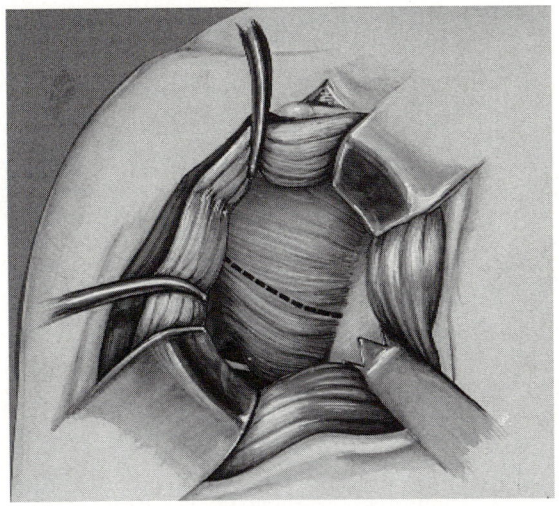

Figure 11 Glenohumeral joint capsule exposure. Dotted line indicates site of capsulotomy.

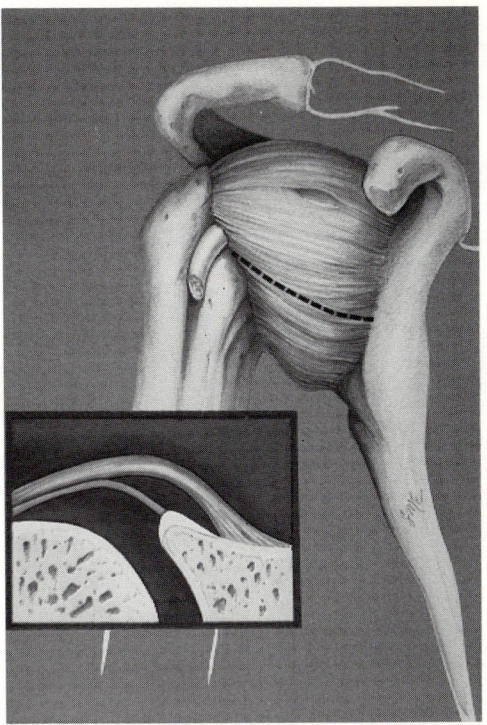

Figure 12 Capsular incision located at junction of upper two-thirds and lower one-third. Inset: Redundant anterior capsule with underlying synovial lining and intact glenoid labrum.

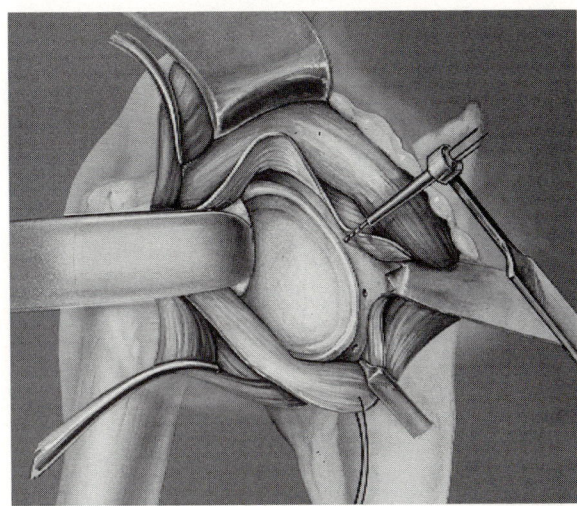

Figure 13 Mitek system used to drill anchoring holes for Mitek sutures.

removed. The arm is then positioned in 90 degrees abduction and 80 to 90 degrees external humeral rotation (to prevent overtightening), and the remaining capsulotomy is closed in a "pants-over-vest" fashion with nonabsorbable sutures (Fig. 17). This "capsular shift" procedure eliminates the capsular redundancy, reinforces the glenohumeral joint at the site of previous instability along the anterior glenoid margin, and provides secure fixation of these soft tissues to the anterior scapular neck. The patient is then placed in a shoulder-arm-system postoperative orthosis that maintains the arm in 90 degrees humeral abduction, 45 degrees external humeral rotation, and 30 degrees forward flexion. This position allows for capsular healing and a position of function that facilitates the rehabilitation and allows for an earlier return to full range of shoulder motion. The splint is worn full-time except during rehabilitative exercises and is discontinued when the patient can actively abduct and forward flex the arm to 90 degrees (usually within 2 weeks).

REHABILITATION

The rehabilitation program begins on the first postoperative day and continues for approximately 6 to 12 months. Each session lasts approximately 45 minutes

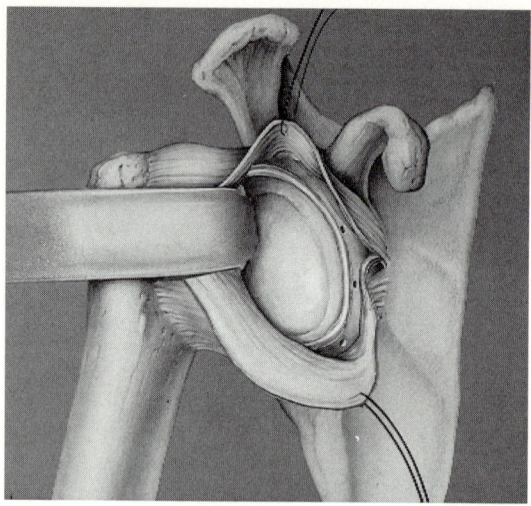

Figure 14 Drill holes located along anterior glenoid rim.

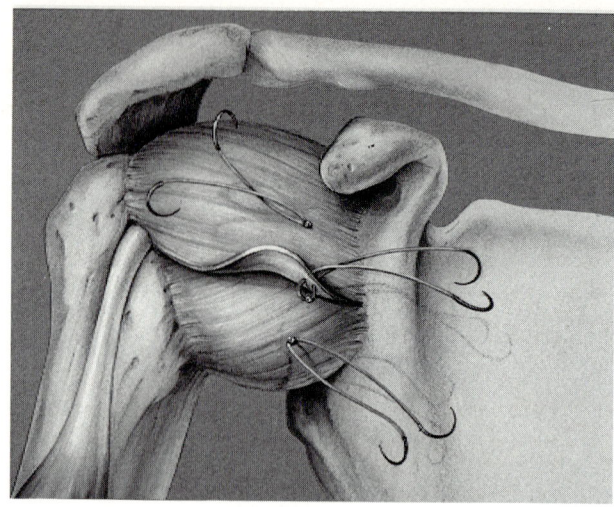

Figure 16 Superior capsular flap shifted inferiorly, overlying the inferior flap.

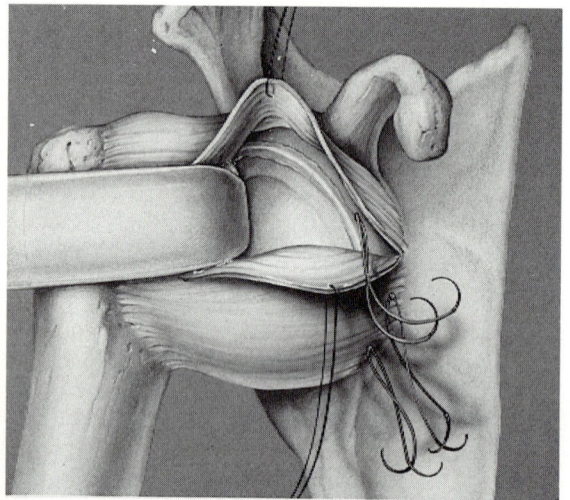

Figure 15 Inferior capsular flap shifted superiorly and anchored into position.

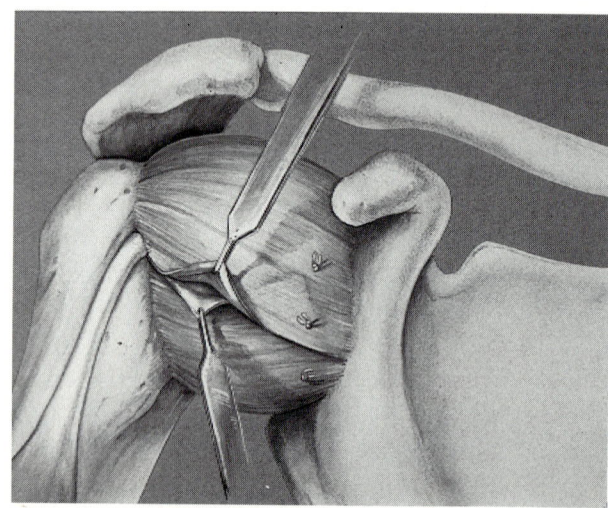

Figure 17 Closure of capsulotomy in "pants over vest" fashion.

to 1 hour. The shoulder is passively ranged in abduction, flexion, and external rotation as tolerated. This is done in the scapular plane with no forced motion. Active-assisted shoulder ROM as well as isometric abduction strengthening exercises are begun as tolerated.

Within 2 weeks most patients can actively abduct the arm from 0 to 90 degrees. Active internal rotation exercises with the arm at the side along with external rotation to neutral are begun with the use of rubber tubing to provide gentle resistance. As the patient progresses, shoulder extension exercises in the prone position, and external rotation to tolerance in the side lying position are added. Shoulder shrugs and active shoulder abduction exercises to 90 degrees are also begun.

For the first 2 months after surgery, strengthening exercises are continued with emphasis on rotator cuff muscles. Strengthening exercises and horizontal abduc-

tion and shoulder flexion are added, and upper body endurance training with an Ergometer at low resistance is instituted. Within 8 to 12 weeks, most patients have regained full forward flexion and abduction with some minor restriction of full external rotation. This is acceptable early during the rehabilitation phase as care is taken to protect the anterior capsule from being stretched too vigorously until all soft tissue healing is complete. As all postoperative pain resolves, a vigorous strengthening program is undertaken using isokinetic training machines with three different speeds to increase the strength, power, and endurance of the rotator cuff muscles. Strengthening of the scapular rotators, biceps, triceps, pectoralis, and deltoid muscles are also added and continued for a minimum of 1 year.

At 6 months, an isokinetic strength and endurance test can be performed to evaluate internal and external rotation, flexion/extension and abduction/adduction. If the patient has at least 80% strength of the contralateral shoulder, a progressive throwing program is begun. By 9 months, these patients are throwing for 30 minutes each day while continuing a total body conditioning program. Within 8 to 12 months most patients reach a point where strength and power is restored, muscle synchrony returns to normal, and performance is maximized. At this point, the athlete is allowed to return to all activities but is encouraged to maintain an ongoing home maintenance program of shoulder flexibility and strengthening exercises.

RESULTS

From December 1989 through July 1990, 35 consecutive athletes (including 18 baseball players, 13 of whom were pitchers) with shoulder pain secondary to anterior glenohumeral joint instability that failed to improve with conservative management, underwent an anterior capsulolabral reconstruction. There were 12 professional, 11 collegiate, and eight recreational athletes. The results were graded as excellent in 24 (71%), good in nine (26%), and poor in one (3%) at a minimum 2 year follow-up. Overall, 25 (75%) of the 35 athletes returned to their prior competitive level and competed in their sport for at least one complete season. Twelve (67%) of the 18 baseball players, including nine (69%) of 13 baseball pitchers and six (86%) of seven professional baseball pitchers returned to their prior level of competition. These athletes required an average of 12 months to return to full competition. The average loss of

postoperative range of motion was 2 degrees. There were no intraoperative or postoperative complications in patients involved in this study. Radiographs obtained at follow-up also demonstrated that all Mitek suture anchors had remained well seated within the anterior, inferior glenoid neck in all patients.

SUGGESTED READING

Bankart SAB. The pathology and treatment of recurrent, dislocations of the shoulder joint. Br J Surg 1938; 26:23–29.

Harryman DT, Sidles JA, Clark JM, et al. Translation of the humeral head on the glenoid with passive glenohumeral motion. J Bone Joint Surg 1990; 71A:1334.

Howell SM, Galinat BJ, Renzi AJ, Marone PJ: Normal and abnormal mechanics of the glenohumeral joint in the horizontal plane. J Bone Joint Surg 1988; 70A:227.

Jobe FW, Giangarra CE, Kvitne RS, Glousman RE: Anterior capsulolabral reconstruction of the shoulder in athletes in overhand sports. Am J Sports Med 1991; 19:428–434.

Jobe FW, Glousman RE: Anterior capsulolabral reconstruction. Techniques in Orthop 1989; 3:29–35.

Kvitne RS, Jobe FW: The diagnosis and treatment of anterior instability in the throwing athlete. Clin Orthop 1993; 291:107–123.

Montgomery WH, Jobe FW: Functional outcomes in athletes following modified anterior capsulolabral reconstruction. Accepted for publication. Am J Sports Med.

Rowe CR, Patel D, Southmayd WW: The Bankart procedure: A long-term end-result study. J Bone Joint Surg 1978; 60A:1–16.

Rubenstein DL, Jobe FW, Glousman RE, et al. Anterior capsulolabral reconstruction of the shoulder in athletes. J Shoulder Elbow Surg 1992; 1:229–237.

Walch G, Bioleau P, Noel E, Donnell ST: Impingement of the deep surface of the supraspinatus tendon on the posterosuperior glenoid rim: An arthroscopic study. J Shoulder Elbow Surg 1992; 1:238–245.

INFERIOR CAPSULAR SHIFT FOR GLENOHUMERAL INSTABILITY

MICHELE GLASGOW, M.D.

Many shoulder procedures have been popularized to address recurrent anterior shoulder dislocation. These include the Putti-Platt, Magnuson-Stack, Nicola, Bankart, and Bristow procedures, among others. No surgical approach, however, appears better suited to address the anatomic pathology of shoulder instability than the capsular shift procedure. This is especially true for the patient with multidirectional instability. The capsular shift procedure can also be adapted to treat anterior traumatic dislocators as well by limiting the amount of capsular dissection and performing an anatomic repair of the Bankart lesion when present. Therefore, the capsular shift and its modifications treat the spectrum of pathologies found in anterior shoulder instability.

INDICATIONS

The classic procedure described by Neer and Foster is indicated for anterior instabilities associated with significant capsular laxity, i.e., multidirectional instability. This patient may have recurrent dislocations or subluxations. The decision to proceed with surgery is predicated upon recurrent disabling episodes of instability or symptoms associated with instability such as pain and/or dead arm syndrome that have been unresponsive to physical therapy. Patients with capsular laxity may have a history of traumatic or atraumatic onset of instability.

The capsular shift procedure may be modified to address pathology in a population without ligamentous laxity. Surgical indications in this setting are similar to those used for the classic capsular shift procedure. These include symptoms related to shoulder instability that are recurrent and unresponsive to therapy. More aggressive operative management in young athletes should be determined on an individual basis. Surgical risk should be weighed against the risk of recurrent instability. Generally, the onset of instability in this group is associated with a traumatic event. Commonly, this patient has a Bankart lesion with a variable amount of intracapsular injury. Typically, a modified capsulorrhaphy and anatomic repair of the Bankart lesion will address the patient's pathology.

The strength of the capsular shift procedure rests in its ability to address a spectrum of pathology. Capsular tightening can be "fine tuned" to the individual patient. The procedure allows the surgeon to restore normal anatomy.

SURGICAL EQUIPMENT AND SET-UP

A diagnostic arthroscopy may precede the open shoulder reconstruction. A 30 degree arthroscope, cannula with diaphragm, and arthroscopy hooks or spinal needles may be useful in performing an intra-articular examination prior to the open procedure. The surgeon is cautioned here because lengthy arthroscopy or utilization of a pump can result in extravasation of fluid into the soft tissue, distorting the tissue planes and making subsequent dissection difficult.

The standard open procedure equipment tray includes a selection of Richardson retractors and Darrah retractors (George Tiemann). Specialized instruments include a small right angle curette, dental burr with small dental head, Bankart clamp or large towel clip, and Fukuda (humeral head) retractor.

The patient is examined under anesthesia in the supine position following the administration of a general anesthetic or scalene regional block. The direction of instability is noted and compared with the opposite normal shoulder. The arm is tested sequentially in anterior, inferior, and posterior directions. Anterior testing is performed with the arm at the side, in the plane of the scapula, and with the arm in 90 degrees of abduction and external rotation. Posterior instability is examined with the arm in 90 degrees of abduction and external rotation, in the scapula plane, and with the arm at the side in neutral rotation and internal rotation. Commonly this examination merely confirms the office evaluation but occasionally it contributes valuable information concerning the degree and/or direction of instability.

The patient is then placed in a semi-reclined beach chair position with approximately 20 to 30 degrees of torso and head elevation. This can easily be implemented by flexing the table and lowering the legs slightly. The shoulder and arm to the wrist are then sterilely prepped and draped. The use of a McConnell arm holder is helpful as it decreases the number of surgical assistants needed.

OPERATIVE PROCEDURE

Anterior skin folds are noted and the most prominent axillary fold is delineated with a marking pen. This outlines the incision measuring approximately 8 to 10 cm. This may be shifted inferiorly into the axilla to provide maximal cosmesis. The incision is made sharply without penetrating the deep dermis. At this time, a needle tip bovie is used to complete the incision. Subcutaneous flaps are elevated at the level of the deltoid fascia and dissected up to the acromion and along the clavicle over to the coracoid. Richardson retractors are used to facilitate exposure. The development of medial, lateral, superior, and inferior subcutaneous flaps allows the skin to shift as deeper dissection is performed. This permits excellent visualization even in the most inferior of incisions. The deltopectoral interval is opened with the cephalic vein taken laterally. Most of the vessels feeding into the vein enter laterally and are not disturbed. The clavipectoral fascia is incised up to the coracoacromial ligament. Strap muscles (coracobrachialis and short head of biceps) descending from the coracoid are identified and retracted medially to provide visualization of the subscapularis. The strap muscles shield the brachial plexus. Gentle retraction on these muscles reduces the potential of postoperative neuropraxia. A broad Richardson is placed under the deltoid, exposing the underlying bursa and rotator cuff. The coracoacromial ligament is identified and a small window can be excised from its most anterior aspect to facilitate exposure of the supraspinatus and rotator interval.

The bursa is excised widely by positioning the arm in internal and external rotation and in flexion and extension. At this stage, a Darrah may be useful if adhesions are present in the subacromial space. The Darrah, inserted into the subacromial space, may be swept to bluntly break up any subacromial scar.

The arm is positioned at the side in slight external rotation to visualize the subscapularis. The most inferior border of the subscapularis is generally muscular. Anterior circumflex vessels are closely opposed to the inferior margin. If the patient has a ligamentously lax shoulder, the surgeon may select to bovie these vessels to improve inferior exposure needed for the capsular shift. If the surgeon anticipates doing a capsular-labral repair for a Bankart lesion, which necessitates limited inferior exposure, these vessels may be retracted inferiorly.

At this juncture, the subscapularis is dissected off of the capsule. The landmarks for this dissection include the rotator interval superiorly, the leash of anterior circumflex vessels inferiorly, and an imaginary line running across the subscapularis tendon approximately 1 cm medial to the lesser tuberosity. The axillary nerve may be appreciated at this time at the lower border of the subscapularis muscle. It may be palpated by running an index finger from superior to inferior, along the subscapularis; the nerve feels like a cord at the lower margin of the subscapularis and it can be followed as it turns posteriorly to lie adjacent to the inferior capsular pouch (Fig. 1).

The subscapularis is elevated as a layer using the needle tip bovie; the bovie assists with hemostasis. Laterally, near the lesser tuberosity, the subscapularis tendon is adherent to the capsule, and they are difficult to separate. Careful inspection will guide the dissection; the subscapularis tendon fibers run longitudinally, me-

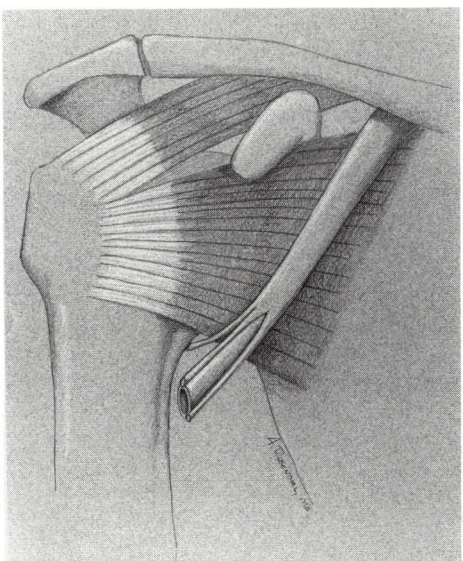

Figure 1 Relationship of axillary nerve to inferior capsule.

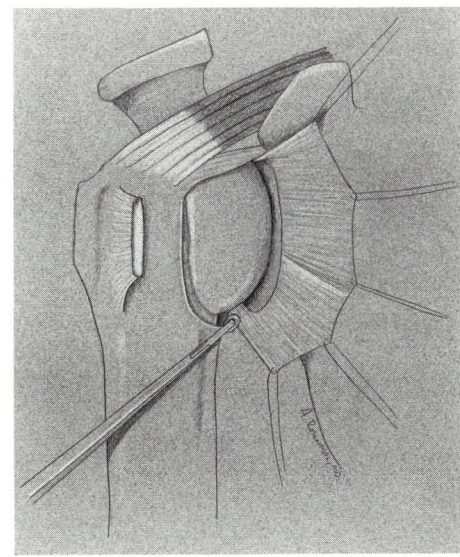

Figure 2 Dissection proceeds, hugging the humeral neck inferiorly, freeing the inferior capsular pouch. Cautious dissection averts axillary nerve injury.

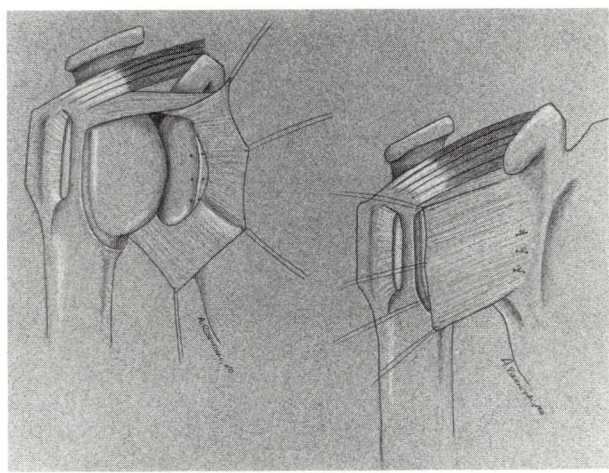

Figure 3 Bony drill holes are placed in the glenoid rim. Sutures placed through these holes are tied on the outside capsule. This secures the capsule to scapular neck, repairing the Bankart lesion.

dial to lateral. When the capsule is reached, the fiber pattern disappears. The subscapularis is developed as a sheet from the rotator interval to its most inferior border. Externally rotating the humerus and tagging the medial tendon edge with suture to improve retraction will assist the dissection. As the subscapularis dissection proceeds medially, the tissue planes become clearer. Near the musculotendinous junction, the subscapularis separates from the capsule. When this occurs, a Richardson may be placed to retract the subscapularis medially and expose the capsule.

The capsule is incised beginning at the rotator interval using a needle tip bovie. A 0.5 centimeter tag of capsule is left laterally so that the surgeon can reapproximate the capsule at the time of closure. The medial capsule edge is tagged every centimeter as the dissection proceeds. The arm is progressively externally rotated as the dissection moves inferiorly. In the most inferior aspect of the dissection, the axillary nerve is at risk. Gentle dissection with a "peanut" to separate the soft tissue inferior to the capsular pouch assures safety of the nerve (Fig. 2).

As the dissection approaches 5 to 6 o'clock on the humerus, the capsule is incised very close to the humeral neck with Metzenbaum scissors. If the inferior capsular dissection deviates medially, the capsular pouch can be easily cut in half. This would limit the ability of the surgeon to perform an extensive shift of the capsule if needed.

If the pathology appears to be due to a Bankart lesion, then capsular dissection beyond 6 o'clock on the humeral neck is generally not required. A Fukuda retractor is placed in the glenohumeral joint to reflect the humeral head. A Bankart lesion will be well visualized at this time. A Darrah or Bankart retractor may be placed along the scapula neck within the labral or capsular lesion. This provides excellent visualization of the scapula neck. The scapula neck is roughened using

either curette or motorized burr. I find it most helpful to use a motorized burr and remove the most anterior portion of the scapular neck cortex to facilitate placement of bony drill holes. At this time a small dental burr is used to place the bony drill holes, generally three in number. A number one cottony dacron with a KHC-4 needle has an excellent curve to accommodate the tight space along the glenoid rim. Sutures may be tied inside or outside the capsule (Fig. 3). I prefer tying mattress type sutures on the outside of the capsule. The objective of tightly opposing the labrum and stripped capsule to the glenoid rim can be achieved by both techniques.

If no Bankart lesion is found and the pathology appears to be a patulous capsule, the dissection is carried inferiorly and may proceed posteriorly along the hu-

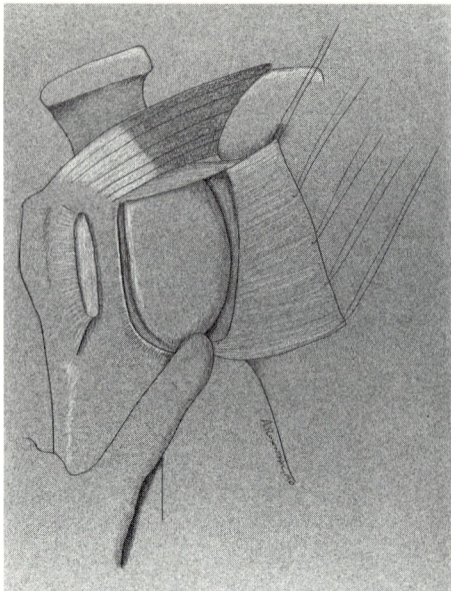

Figure 4 The surgeon can assess capsular tightening by placing a finger in the pouch. Sufficient inferior dissection has been performed when the capsular pouch is obliterated by pulling up on the tag sutures.

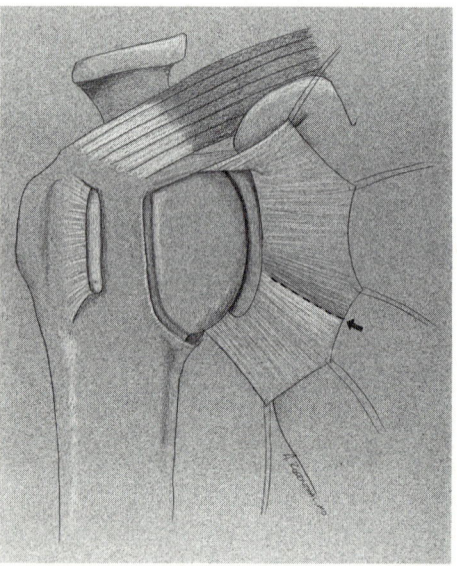

Figure 5 Incision between the middle and inferior glenohumeral ligaments is performed to within a few millimeters of the labrum.

meral neck. The dissection inferiorly is performed carefully because of the proximity of the axillary nerve. Placing the arm in progressively greater and greater external rotation presents the inferior and posterior capsule for further dissection. The free capsular edge is tagged every centimeter as the dissection proceeds. When the surgeon appreciates inferior and posterior capsular tightening and obliteration of the capsular pouch when pulling forward on the capsular tag sutures, sufficient dissection has been performed (Fig. 4). The

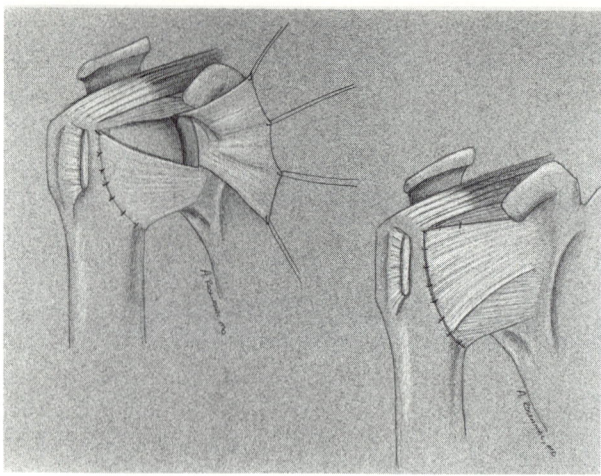

Figure 6 The shift is performed by advancing the inferior flap superiorly and securing this to the humerus. The superior flap is then drawn down to create a double layer of capsule anteriorly.

capsule is then reflected medially. Frequently, the intra-articular capsular anatomy can be appreciated, including the thickenings of the glenohumeral ligaments.

A patient with ligamentous laxity and multidirectional instability will have a patulous capsule. Generally, a split can be made between the middle and inferior glenohumeral ligaments using a Metzenbaum scissors. The incision is carried down to within a few millimeters of the labrum (Fig. 5). The inferior flap is now advanced superiorly to the rotator interval. During this process, there should be tightening of the posterior-inferior capsule that will prevent posterior subluxation postoperatively. Occasionally there is capsule in excess of what is needed to reach the rotator interval, and this may be excised. The free capsular edge is then repaired to the capsular stump remaining on the humerus; the repair proceeds from inferior to superior. During repair of capsule, the arm is maintained in the position of approximately 30 degrees of abduction, 30 degrees of external rotation, and slight-forward flexion. The superior flap is now drawn over the already superiorly positioned inferior flap (Fig. 6). This provides double-layer anterior reinforcement to the shoulder. The superior flap is repaired to the humeral capsular stump, laterally securing the reconstruction. The rotator interval is closed by suturing the superior aspect of the capsular reconstruction directly to the capsule at the most anterior border of the supraspinatus tendon.

Occasionally, the surgeon may encounter a patient with shoulder instability who has a lesser degree of capsular laxity. A "T" capsulorrhaphy in this patient will address his or her pathology. The capsular dissection is similar to the capsular shift though it does not generally proceed as far posteriorly. Incising the capsule near the interval between the middle and inferior glenohumeral ligaments allows the inferior flap to be drawn upward. This is secured to the lateral capsular stump with the arm positioned in slight flexion, 30 degrees of external rotation, and 30 degrees of abduction. The superior flap is drawn down and sutured laterally and, as with the capsular shift, the rotator interval is closed. This modified capsulorrhaphy is used when the degree of capsular laxity does not demand an extensive capsular shift. It is also useful in addressing the mild capsular redundancy that occasionally follows a repair of a Bankart lesion. Combining techniques of capsular-labral repair and capsulorrhaphy, addresses the Bankart lesion and any plastic deformation of the soft tissues resulting from the instability event(s).

After the capsule has been closed, the subscapularis is repaired anatomically. The arm is held at the elbow and the surgeon gently allows the arm to passively externally rotate. The shoulder generally rests at 30 degrees of external rotation as determined by the repair. The arm is then brought to rest against the chest, and the wound is closed. Sling and swathe are applied before transporting the patient to the recovery room.

REHABILITATION

Pendulums are begun in the first week and the arm is brought to neutral rotation. The sling is worn at all times except during these exercises, which are performed three or four times each day. During the second week, the patient is permitted to add passive forward elevation to 90 degrees. Exercises are done with and coordinated by a physical therapist. The patient is gradually progressed to 30 degrees of external rotation and 120 degrees of forward elevation during weeks two through six. This is done passively at first and progressed to active wand exercises. The sling is discarded during the day at the third or fourth week and at 6 weeks the patient is instructed to discard it for sleeping.

The patient is progressed from 120 to 180 degrees of forward flexion by the twelfth week. External rotation is increased gradually after 6 weeks and approaches the normal side by 3 months.

Shoulder isometrics are begun at 4 weeks and may be progressed to light isotonics. Weights are increased gradually to tolerance. Isokinetics are added at 6 weeks as tolerated. Throwing athletes begin a structured throwing program at 5 to 6 months. Gradual return to normal athletics is encouraged after 6 months.

The rehabilitation program is adjusted to the individual. Patients with true multidirectional laxity are rehabilitated more slowly than those who are ligamentously tight. Upper body ergometer (UBE) exercises are generally added at 6 weeks. In patients who have had extensive capsular shifts, UBE is held until 10 to 12 weeks. Restoration of motion is imperative. The rehabilitation is adjusted with the goal of achieving near normal motion by 12 weeks postsurgery. Strengthening is progressed to achieve normal function at 5 to 6 months.

RESULTS

Neer and Foster reported a 98% satisfactory result in 40 shoulders that underwent an anterior inferior capsular shift procedure. Follow-up in this group was short with only 17 shoulders being longer than 2 years from surgery at the time of the report. Cooper and Brems reported on 43 shoulders undergoing the capsular shift procedure. At greater than 2 years of follow-up, 89% achieved satisfactory results. Similarly, Pollock et al reported a 90% satisfaction rate in 151 shoulders followed for an average of 4.6 years (range = 2 to 11.5 years).

Recurrent instability following this procedure has been reported to be between 2% and 11%. At 4.6 years average follow-up, Pollock et al reported only 5% recurrence of instability.

SUGGESTED READING

Altchek DW, Warren RF, Skyhar MJ, Ortiz G. T-plasty modification of the Bankart procedure for multidirectional instability of the anterior and inferior types. J Bone Joint Surg 1991; 73:105.

Cooper RA, Brems JJ. The inferior capsular-shift procedure for multidirectional instability of the shoulder. J Bone Joint Surg 1992; 74A:1516–1522.

Kvitne RS, Jobe FW. The diagnosis and treatment of anterior instability in the throwing athlete. Clin Orthop 1993; 291:107-123.

Neer CS, Foster CR. Inferior capsular shift for involuntary and multidirectional instability of the shoulder. J Bone Joint Surg 1980; 897-908.

Pollock RG, Owens, JM, Nicholson, GP, et al. The anterior inferior capsular shift procedure for anterior glenohumeral instability: Long term results, presented American Academy of Orthopedic Surgery 1993 Meeting, San Francisco.

Silliman JF, Hawkins RJ. Classification and physical diagnosis of instability of the shoulder. Clin Orthop 1993; 291:7-19.

Zarins B, McMahon MS, Rowe CR. Diagnosis and treatment of traumatic anterior instability of the shoulder. Clin Orthop 1993; 291:75-84.

ANTERIOR GLENOHUMERAL SUBLUXATION/DISLOCATION: THE BANKART PROCEDURE

CARTER R. ROWE, M.D.

Recurrent instability of the shoulder in an athlete can be a very disabling condition, as the athlete's requirements are strength of the shoulder in all positions of motion, whether in football or ice hockey, which expose the shoulder to maximal body contact, or throwing or racquet sports, in which the need is for rapid and rhythmic coordination of the shoulder. Table 1 lists the different types of shoulder instability. This chapter discusses the traumatic and the transient subluxation (Types I and II).

Many advances in the pathology and in modifications of treatment of traumatic recurrent anterior dislocation and subluxation of the shoulder have evolved over the past decade.

In addition to the pathological lesions noted in Table 2, trauma to the subscapularis muscle, such as rupture, overstretching, and, at times, avulsion of its attachment to the lesser tuberosity, should be added. Also, traumatic widening of the seam between the subscapularis and supraspinatus muscles over the head of the humerus should be identified and repaired. Unfortunately, this lesion is frequently not recognized.

Technical alterations of the standard Bankart procedure have consisted chiefly in reattaching the avulsed capsule to the neck of the scapula, rather than back to the glenoid rim, by means of soft tissue anchors, a number of which have recently been produced. These can be inserted either by open surgery or by arthroscopy. The advantage and risks of these procedures have been discussed by recent orthopaedic panels. Although the insertion of the capsule anchors is an easier procedure than the standard Bankart procedure, it has not proved to be as strong.

Weber in 1994 concluded that "the Bankart repair remains the gold standard for instability surgery." We present the Bankart procedure, which we have used over the years with consistently satisfactory results, with options and improvements.

DIAGNOSIS

The diagnosis of a complete traumatic anterior dislocation can be accurately made if there is a subacromial defect, the arm is held in external rotation, and roentgenograms clearly reveal the dislocated head. Diagnosis of a transient subluxation, however, is more difficult, as radiographs do not reveal the diagnosis, but the history and physical findings are consistent. The patient is usually a young adult athlete whose shoulder has been injured by forceful overextension of the arm in elevation, and who on examination shows the typical "apprehension" test results (Fig. 1). Blazina and Satzman first reported their experience with transient subluxation of the shoulder in the athlete in 1969. In 1981 Rowe and Zarins identified two types of transient subluxation. In one group, patients were aware of the shoulder momentarily slipping out when the arm was in elevation, such as in throwing or swimming. In the other group, patients were *not* aware of the shoulder slipping out in those motions, but only of a sudden severe pain, which left the shoulder momentarily weak, or "dead." Quarterbacks are unable to throw the "long bomb," baseball players cannot throw out a base runner, and tennis players lose their ace serve. Roentgenogram results are usually normal. Often, patients are confused and depressed, because their problem has not been diagnosed and treatment has not been effective. The "apprehension" test is a consistent physical finding. In this position, the patient's symptoms are reproduced. The arm is elevated and externally rotated, usually in the throwing position. This test can also be carried out with the patient supine. Care must be taken, however, to rule out other conditions such as impingement syndrome, rotator cuff tears, instability of the biceps tendon, or thoracic outlet syndromes, all of which may mimic transient subluxation.

PATHOLOGY

It is generally agreed that there is no one essential lesion in shoulder instability. However, the Bankart lesion (avulsion of the capsule and labrum from the anterior glenoid rim) is the most common causative factor (Table 2). The Bankart lesion is found most frequently in complete traumatic dislocation of the shoulder, whereas the lesion in the subluxating shoulder is usually increased laxity or redundancy of the capsule. Damage to the glenoid rim and Hill-Sachs lesions are also more frequently found in complete traumatic dislocation, since added trauma is experienced in this group. A frequently missed lesion is the increased spread between the supraspinatus and subscapularis muscles over the head of the humerus.

Table 1 Types of Shoulder Instability

Traumatic
  Complete dislocation
    Most common
Subgroup
  Transient subluxation ("dead arm" syndrome)
    Forceful overextension of arm in elevation and external rotation
Atraumatic
  Incurred by functional use of arm
Voluntary
  Incurred by muscle control
Involuntary Subluxation
  Instability due to chronic laxity of tissues
  May be multidirectional

TREATMENT

Many patients wish to know whether there is any treatment other than surgery for recurrent instability of the shoulder. This is a logical question. Considering the overall classification of shoulder instabilities (see Table 1), specific resistive exercises are more effective in the atraumatic, voluntary, involuntary, and especially in the multidirectional groups than in complete traumatic dislocations or traumatic transient subluxations. Of the 50 traumatic transient subluxations in the series of Rowe and Zarins, only 10 responded to exercises; five were graded excellent, three good, and two fair. The remainder were treated surgically.

Surgical Treatment

For the athlete who requires maximal strength of the arm in all positions and in forceful contact, we prefer the Bankart procedure for the following reasons:

1. The exposure is anatomic, layer by layer down to the glenoid rim. In this way the various anatomic causative lesions may be identified and corrected. The muscle layers are then returned anatomically to their origins.
2. No muscles are compromised by transplantation. No muscles are traumatized by division or perforation.
3. No metal is used, such as screws and staples, which in contact sports may break or loosen and sometimes travel into the joint or toward the chest wall.
4. The approach is adjustable, so that when a Bankart lesion *is* present, the capsule can be reattached to the entire anterior glenoid rim, where the focus of strength is needed.
5. When a Bankart lesion is *not* present, the cause of the instability is usually a redundant or lax capsule. Since the anterior capsule has been exposed by this procedure, no change in the surgical exposure and no additional incision are necessary. A capsulorrhaphy can be carried out by taking up the laxity of the capsule, and double-breasting the repair along the anterior and inferior glenoid. If the patient also has

Table 2 Causative Lesions

	Traumatic Complete Dislocations (%)	Transient Subluxations (%)
Bankart lesions	85	64
Redundancy of capsule	15	26
Damage to glenoid rim	73	45
Hill-Sachs lesions	77	40

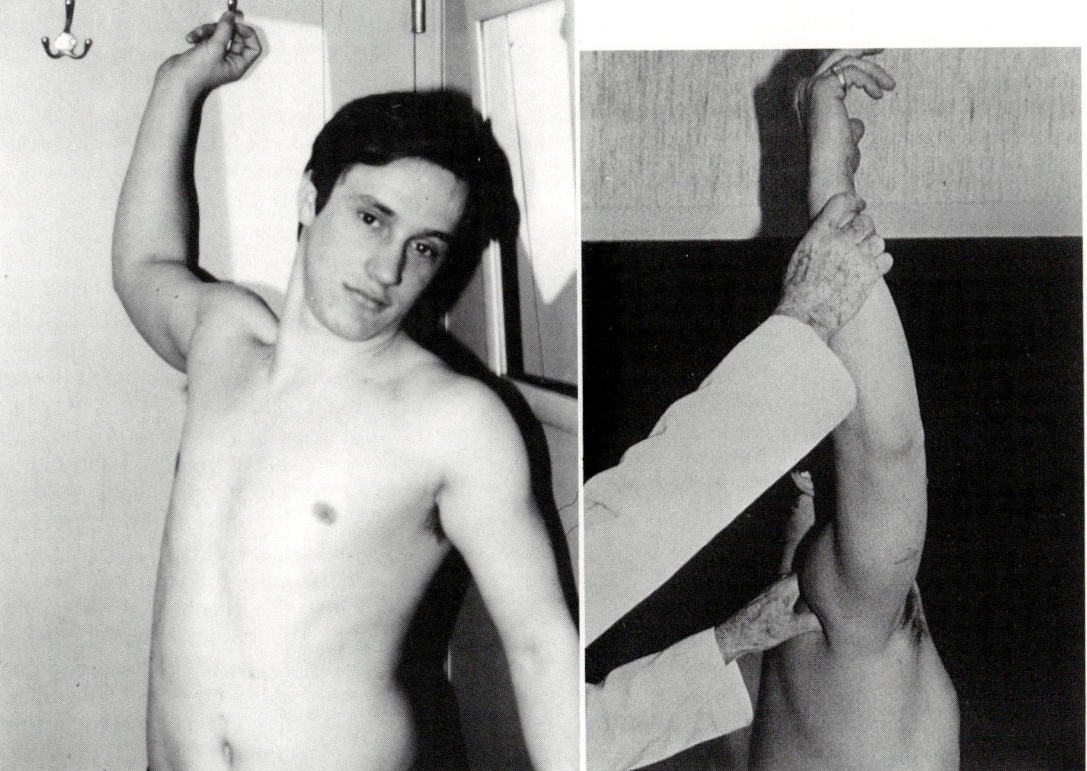

A   B

Figure 1 The "dead arm" syndrome. *A,* The patient's sudden shoulder pain is reproduced when the arm is in elevation and external rotation in the throwing position. This is referred to as the "apprehension" position. *B,* Arm is in elevation and pressure is applied to posterior humeral head.

evidence of multidirectional instability, the posterior capsule can be tightened from this exposure, eliminating the necessity of making a second posterior exposure.

6. Although holes (usually three in the Bankart procedure) are made through the rim of the glenoid (high, mid, and low), the perforations are covered by the smooth capsule, eliminating postoperative traumatic changes of the joint. No traumatic changes have been noted in our follow-up study over a 30 year period.

7. One of the most desirable features of the Bankart procedure is that, in cases of recurrent postoperative dislocations from subsequent injury, the muscle layers are not a mass of scar tissue or in poor condition for reuse, but are preserved and can be safely and effectively used again.

Surgical Technique

For a complete review and follow-up of the Bankart procedure, the reader is referred to Rowe's textbook, *The Shoulder*. This chapter discusses the high points and adjustability of the Bankart procedure.

1. The shoulder is exposed through the deltopectoral plane. The deltoid is not removed. The cephalic vein is not ligated, but turned back with the deltoid muscle.

2. Osteotomy of the coracoid process is optional (Fig. 2). The advantages of osteotomy include less traction on the attached tendons to the coracoid and to the musculocutaneous nerve, as well as greater exposure of the rotator cuff muscles and the joint. The advantages of not osteotomizing the coracoid include earlier use and function of the shoulder, and less chance of nonunion (although we have had only one nonunion in 40 years). In a heavy-muscled football player who wants as early a return of function as possible, one may proceed without osteotomizing the coracoid. However, if better exposure is needed during surgery, osteotomy of the coracoid will prove most helpful to the surgeon. At this point one should carry out complete examination of the top of the shoulder for injury to the rotator cuff.

3. We recommend removal of the subscapularis muscle from the anterior and inferior capsule in order to evaluate properly the laxity of the capsule. In this way, if a Bankart lesion is not present, a capsulorrhaphy can easily be performed. As a rule, we ligate the anterior circumflex vessels. This allows better exposure of the axillary fold of the capsule and less oozing during surgery. It also lessens the chance of injury to the axillary nerve, because the nerve is *turned back with the intact muscle*. To substantiate this, we have never encountered operative injury to the axillary nerve in the past 40 years. One should also avoid cauterizing oozing circumflex vessels,

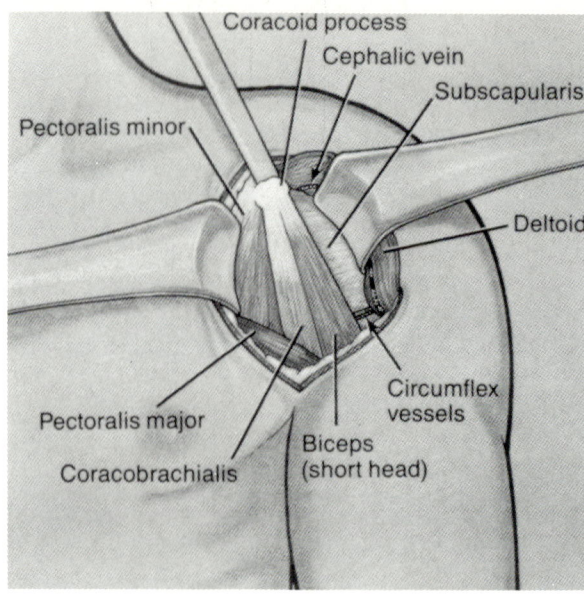

Figure 2 Osteotomy of the coracoid is optional. (From Rowe CR. The shoulder. New York: Churchill Livingstone, 1988:196. Reproduced by permission of Churchill Livingstone.)

because the axillary nerve might be injured.
Options
A. Rockwood prefers not to ligate circumflex vessels by leaving the lower portion of the subscapularis attached, and retracting the vessels inferiorly (Fig. 3).
B. Matsen, on the other hand, does not separate the subscapularis muscle from the capsule, but explores the joint by separating the subscapularis attachment from the lesser tuberosity, and working within the joint.
C. Montgomery and Jobe divide the subscapularis muscle horizontally.

4. With the capsule exposed, its laxity is tested with the arm in complete external rotation. The joint is then opened vertically 0.5 cm lateral to the glenoid rim (Fig. 4). By opening the capsule with the arm in external rotation, maximal external rotation will be obtained postoperatively. The vertical opening of the capsule into the joint is the same for a Bankart procedure as for a capsulorrhaphy. No alteration of the incision is necessary.

5. A special shoulder retractor is necessary to displace the humeral head and provide adequate exposure of the rim and the joint. The glenoid neck should be freshened with a small osteotome. Perforating the cortex of the glenoid neck with a small scaphoid gouge, or drill, facilitates the passage of the curved spike and lessens the chance of breaking or fracturing the anterior glenoid rim.

6. This part of the operation is *easier* with the coracoid osteotomized. Three holes are made through the rim at 10, 8, and 6 o'clock (for a left

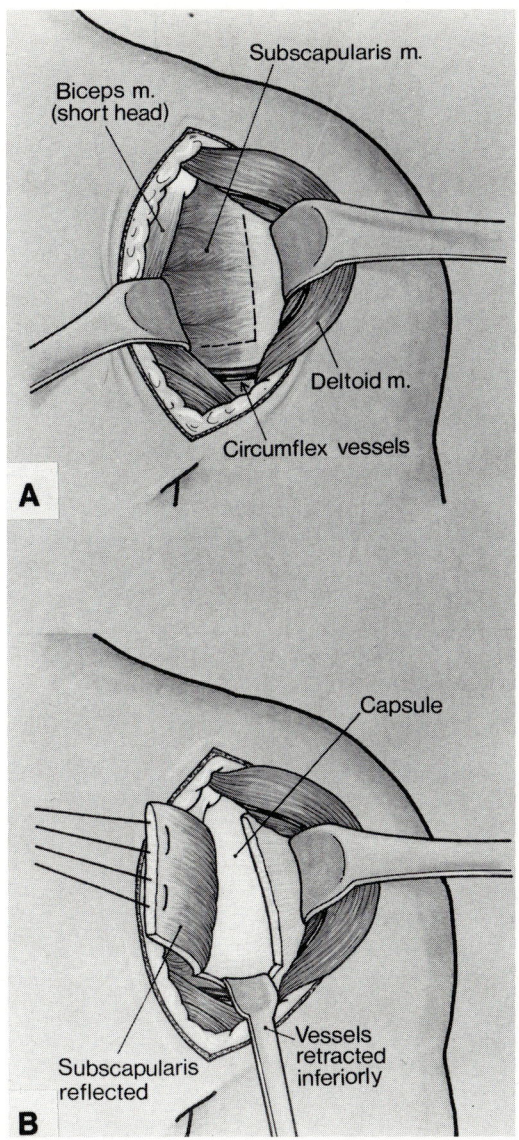

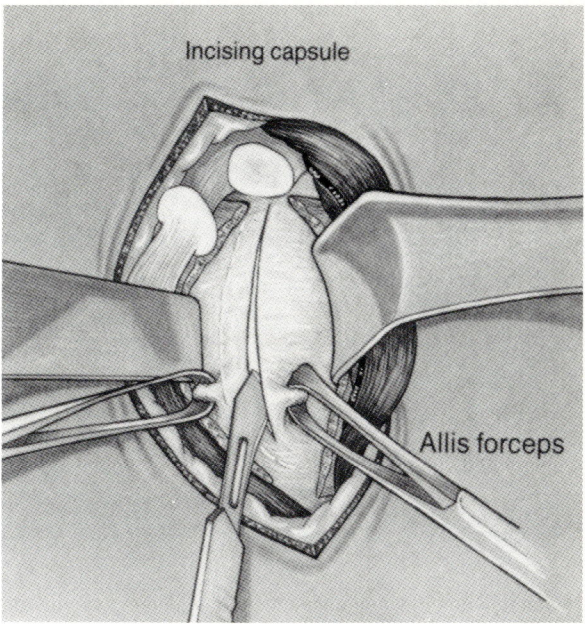

Figure 4 The joint is opened by a vertical incision 0.5 cm lateral to the glenoid rim with the arm in complete external rotation. This ensures maximal return of external rotation. (From Rowe CR. The shoulder. New York: Churchill Livingstone, 1988:198. Reproduced by permission of Churchill Livingstone.)

Figure 3 *A* and *B,* Rockwood retracts the circumflex vessels along with an inferior slip of subscapularis muscle.

shoulder) with the curved spike and the cutting forceps (Fig. 5).

7. One's favorite suture is then passed through the holes either with a No. 5 Mayo taper needle or with a barbed hook, and the lateral capsule is sutured to the glenoid rim (Fig. 6A) with over-lapping or double-breasting of the medial capsule (Fig. 6B); this gives added strength along the entire glenoid, where it is needed, especially at 6 o'clock.

8. The muscles are then returned to their original origins.

Capsulorrhaphy

When a Bankart lesion is *not* present, the instability of the joint is due usually to a redundant or overstretched capsule. Without altering the incision, the capsule can be

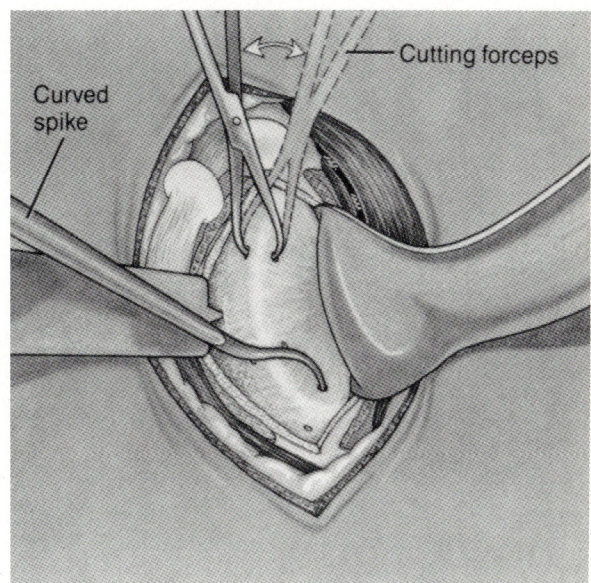

Figure 5 Holes are made through the glenoid rim high, mid, and low with the curved spike and cutting forceps. (From Rowe CR. The shoulder. New York: Churchill Livingstone, 1988: 200. Reproduced by permission of Churchill Livingstone.)

taken up as necessary and double-breasted along the anterior glenoid rim (Fig. 7). It is best to test the amount of take-up of the capsule to allow at least 35 degrees of external rotation of the arm, before suturing. With 35 degrees of external rotation at the time of closure, the patient will safely regain the remainder of rotation

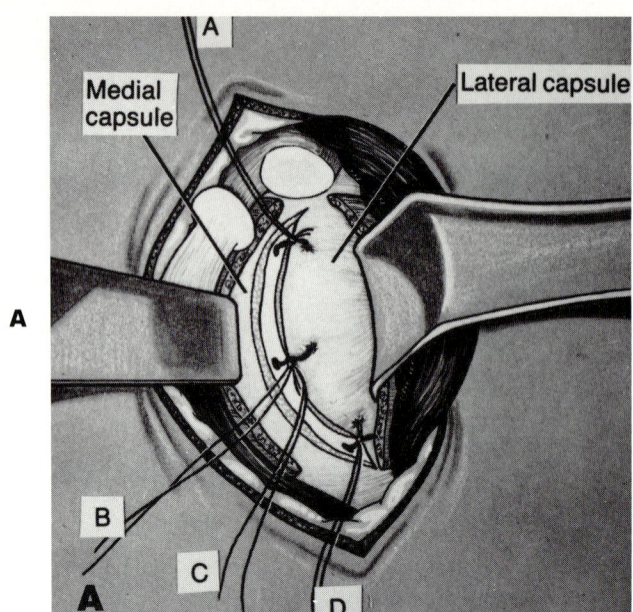
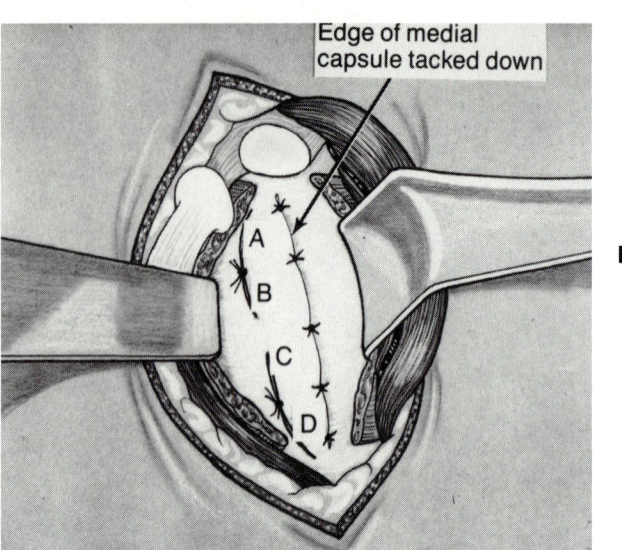

Figure 6 *A,* The lateral capsule is sutured to the anterior glenoid rim through the three holes, and the sutures are passed through the medial capsule flap. *B,* The medial capsule is then double-breasted over the lateral capsule for added strength. (From Rowe CR. The shoulder. New York: Churchill Livingstone, 1988:201. Reproduced by permission of Churchill Livingstone.)

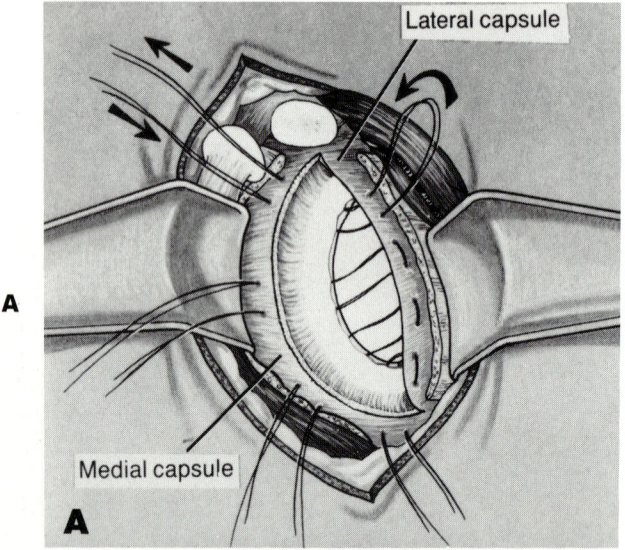
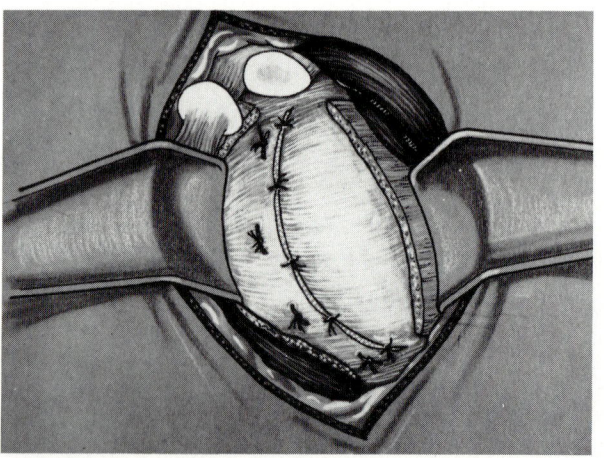

Figure 7 Capsulorrhaphy technique. *A,* When a Bankart lesion is *not* present, the capsule is taken up and double-breasted along the anterior glenoid. The suture is passed under the labrum, out through the lateral capsule, and back under the labrum. *B,* The medial capsule is then double-breasted over the repair, adding extra strength. (From Rowe CR. The shoulder. New York: Churchill Livingstone, 1988:236. Reproduced by permission of Churchill Livingstone.)

postoperatively. As pointed out previously, in the case of multidirectional instability the posterior capsule can be tightened through the anterior approach by drawing the capsule forward at 7 or 8 o'clock (for a left shoulder).

POSTOPERATIVE REGIMEN

This type of repair is sufficient to allow patients to use the arm as tolerated, immediately after surgery. The sling is omitted, usually on the second day, and the patient is begun on gentle pendulum exercises and encouraged to use the hand and arm within the range of tolerated motion. This is greatly appreciated by the patient. Forceful use of the arm is discouraged for 3 months, but during this time the patient increases the range of motion of the arm. We have not found specific physical therapy to be indicated. This is the period of healing and motion, not of regaining strength. At 3 months, activities are increased with wall weights, forearm weights, adjusted rowing, and so forth. Elevation of the arm is encouraged in the scapular plane (forward flexion) and not in abduction. By 6 months, with the return of motion and strength, patients are usually able to return to contact sports. Racquet sports may take a while longer for full use in serving. Pitchers must be on a special schedule, also with graduated tossing to throwing on schedule. Full rhythmic body motions, coordinated with the arm motion, are essential.

RESULTS

Our aim with the Bankart procedure is to avoid trauma to the muscle layers at surgery; avoid the use of metal, such as staples and screws; and return all tissues to their natural origins. In this way, a functional range of motion with full strength and agility can be obtained. We do not, at any stage, attempt to restrict the functional range of motion, such as external rotation, because the athlete needs as much stable motion as possible, particularly in throwing, serving in tennis, basketball, and free-style swimming. For further follow-up results, see Rowe's textbook *The Shoulder*. Seventy percent of our patients regained 100% of motion in every phase. Twenty-five percent regained 75% of motion, and only 5% gained less than this. Our recurrence rate has remained at 3.5% up to the present time in college and professional athletes in football, ice hockey, baseball, wrestling, combat, and basketball. Only one patient with a dominant arm and one with a recessive arm failed to return to previous sports activities.

SUGGESTED READING

Blazina ME, Satzman JS. Recurrent anterior subluxation of the shoulder in athletes—a distinct entity. J Bone Joint Surg 1969; 51A:1037.

Geiger DF, Hurley JA, Torey JA, Rao JP. Results of arthroscopic versus open Bankart suture repair, Paper read before 9th Open Meeting of the American Shoulder and Elbow Surgeons, San Francisco, Feb. 21, 1993.

Glasgow SG, Craythorne CB, Glasgow MT, Selder R, Torg JS. A long term evaluation of the modified Bristow procedure for anterior glenohumeral instability, Paper read before 9th Open Meeting of the American Shoulder and Elbow Surgeons, San Francisco, Feb. 21, 1993.

Kamft JF, Merrison D, Bonnomet P, Vogt F. Recurrent anterior instability of the shoulder treated by arthroscopic staple capsulorrhophy, Paper read before 9th Open Meeting of the American Shoulder and Elbow Surgeons, San Francisco, Feb. 21, 1993.

Konig DP, Rutt J, Treml O. A high rate of osteoarthritis and recurrent shoulder dislocation following Putti-Platt and Eden-Hybinette procedure, Paper read before 7th Congress of the European Society for Surgery of the Shoulder and Elbow, Aarhus, Denmark, June 10-12, 1993.

Matsen FA. Instructional course on the shoulder. San Francisco: American Academy of Orthopaedic Surgery, 1987.

Montgomery WH, Jobe FW. Functional outcomes in athletes after modified anterior capsulolabral reconstruction. Amer Jour Sports Med 1994; 22(3):352-357.

Neer CS II, Foster CR. Inferior capsular shift for involuntary inferior and multidirectional instability of the shoulder. J Bone Joint Surg 1980; 62A:897-908.

Resch H, Geiser K, Thoeni J, Sperner G. Arthroscopic repair of superior labral detachment. J Bone Joint Surg 1993; 12(3):147-153.

Rockwood CA Jr. Subluxation of the shoulder—the classification, diagnosis, and treatment. Orthop Trans 1979; 4:306.

Rockwood CA Jr, Matsen FA. The shoulder. Philadelphia: WB Saunders, 1990:594.

Rowe CR, Zarins B. Recurrent transient subluxation of the shoulder J Bone Joint Surg 1981; 63A:863-872.

Rowe CR, Southmayde WW, Patel D. The Bankart procedure. J Bone Joint Surg 1981; 1:1-16.

Rowe CR. The shoulder. New York: Churchill Livingstone, 1988:165.

Schippinger G, Shobi GE, Wallace WA. Strength of different suture anchors for reattaching the shoulder capsule. Paper read before 7th Congress of the European Society for Surgery of the Shoulder and Elbow, Aarhus, Denmark, June 10-12, 1993.

Tamai K, Sawezaki U, Hara I. Efficacy and pitfalls of Statak soft tissue attachment for Bankart repair. J Shoulder Elbow Surg 1993; 2(4):216-220.

Warner JP, Miller MD. Center for Sports Med. Univ. Pittsburgh. Arthroscopic Bankart repair with Suretac device: Clinical and experimental observations. Paper read before 3rd Scandinavian-Japanese Congress on Shoulder Surgery, Aarhus, Denmark, June 7-9, 1993.

Weber SC. The gold standard revisited: Recent experience with the open Bankart repair for recurrent anterior glenohumeral dislocation. Paper read before the American Orthopaedic Society for Sports Medicine, New Orleans, Feb. 27, 1994.

Zarins B, McMahon MS, Rowe CR. Diagnosis and treatment of traumatic anterior instability of the shoulder. Clin Orth 1993; Vol. 291.

Zarins B. Bankart repair of anterior shoulder instability. Tech Orthop 1989; 3(4).

GLENOHUMERAL STABILIZATION: ARTHROSCOPIC SURETAC TECHNIQUE

MICHAEL J. PAGNANI, M.D.
RUSSELL F. WARREN, M.D.
KEVIN P. SPEER, M.D.

Many operative procedures have been described for the treatment of shoulder instability. Until recently, the only available methods of surgical stabilization of the shoulder required an extensive anatomical dissection in order to address the pathologic process. These open techniques result in a significant amount of perioperative pain and morbidity and require in-patient hospitalization. In addition, overhead athletes and throwers are often unable to return to their premorbid level of function after such a procedure.

Arthroscopic shoulder stabilization procedures were developed in the early 1980s. These arthroscopic techniques can be performed on an out-patient basis and offer the potential advantages of reduced perioperative pain and morbidity. Because of minimal surgical trauma, there is hope that these techniques will better maintain function in overhead athletes.

Bankart called attention to the significance of anterior labral and capsular disruption in the pathogenesis of anterior instability. Anteroinferior labral detachment is usually associated with some degree of capsular disruption from the glenoid neck. The term *Bankart lesion* has evolved to refer to capsular-periosteal separation at the glenoid neck. This capsular-periosteal separation creates laxity in an important stabilizer, the inferior glenohumeral ligament complex (IGHLC), which is closely connected to the labrum. The IGHLC has been shown to be the primary check against anterior instability with the arm abducted between 45 and 90 degrees.

Rowe has noted that the Bankart lesion is present in approximately 85% of recurrent anterior dislocators. Arthroscopic techniques allow reattachment of the anterior capsule and labrum in those patients who have a demonstrated Bankart lesion.

Patients with capsular laxity, atraumatic dislocations, or enlargement of the "rotator interval" frequently do not have a Bankart lesion. Arthroscopic stabilization techniques utilizing an implant do not appear to be appropriate for these patients at present. Multidirectional instability and voluntary instability are absolute contraindications to an arthroscopic stabilization procedure. The finding of a poorly formed IGHLC or the lack of a Bankart lesion on arthroscopic examination are also contraindications. Some surgeons feel that an arthroscopic method should not be used in the presence of a large bony defect in the humeral head. Morgan recom-mended against using an arthroscopic technique in collision athletes.

The role of operative stabilization of acute dislocations in young, scholastic athletes is controversial. These patients appear to be at extremely high risk for recurrence. The acute dislocation often curtails sports activity for the current year, and the development of recurrent instability results in an extended period away from athletics and other activities. The treatment of these patients should be individualized on a case-by-case basis. The risk of recurrence should be explained as well as the potential risks of a surgical procedure. In some young athletes engaged in throwing or contact sports, early restoration of the disrupted anatomy would appear to provide the best opportunity to continue in their sport without losing a significant period of the following season.

Our basic approach is to perform an arthroscopic examination in all traumatic types of anterior instability, since the likelihood of capsular-periosteal disruption of the anterior glenoid is high in these patients. Patients with an atraumatic etiology are less likely to demonstrate a Bankart lesion, therefore an open technique is generally used in these patients. The presence of inferior laxity indicates multidirectional instability; patients who demonstrate inferior instability are treated with open stabilization methods.

We perform shoulder arthroscopy with the patient in the modified "beach-chair" position. The patient's back is placed at an angle of approximately 75 degrees from the floor, the hips are flexed to 90 degrees, and the knees are set in 30 degrees of flexion. The thorax is rotated slightly toward the nonoperative shoulder to expose the medial border of the scapula on the operative side. The position is fixed by molding a beanbag to the body and then deflating the beanbag to make it firm.

We feel that there are several advantages to the beach-chair position. We perform the vast majority of our shoulder procedures under interscalene block anesthesia. The patients are more comfortable in the semi-sitting position than in the lateral decubitus position and are able to observe the procedure on the arthroscopic monitor. The beach-chair position allows the surgeon to examine the shoulder in various positions of abduction and rotation since there is no traction on the arm. There is also a lower risk of neurapraxia from traction, and the anterior structures are not placed in a stretched, nonanatomical orientation. The beach-chair position allows easier access to the anterior shoulder during an arthroscopic stabilization. In addition, an arthroscopic procedure can be simply converted to an open procedure without the need for extensive repositioning and redraping. The beanbag is simply deflated, and the head of the operating table is lowered to the appropriate level.

After placement of the arthroscope within the glenohumeral joint, the labrum is probed for evidence of detachment or tearing. The presence and quality of the IGHLC is ascertained. Next, the joint is inspected to assess excess volume and to search for loose bodies. Translatory forces may be delivered in both anterior and posterior directions to assess the relationship between the head and the glenoid.

Pathologic findings during the arthroscopic examination include detachment of the anteroinferior capsulolabral structures, stretching of the IGHLC, and fraying or tearing of the anteroinferior labrum. Laxity of the pouch is present when the arthroscope is easily passed into the anteroinferior joint cavity without the normal restraint of the capsular tissues. This phenomenon is referred to as the *drive-through* sign.

Anteroinferior labral flaps are often associated with instability. Large labral flaps that appear nonfunctional can be debrided, but the surgeon must not destabilize the IGHLC. Altchek et al recently reported poor long-term results in patients who underwent arthroscopic debridement of labral flaps at all sites. This treatment provided temporary pain relief, but symptoms generally recurred by 3 year follow-up when the patients resumed normal activities and sports. Patients with evidence of labral detachment and instability did especially poorly. We do not recommend debridement of anteroinferior labral insufficiency as an isolated treatment.

The concept of repairing the capsular-periosteal separation at the anterior glenoid neck was first proposed by Perthes and later expounded on by Bankart. This technique attacks the pathology at its most common site and is directed at reconstitution of the primary static stabilizer of the shoulder, the IGHLC. When properly performed, the procedure results in a superior functional outcome compared to noncapsular operations. Arthroscopic stabilization techniques are generally modifications of the Perthes-Bankart concept.

In an effort to avoid tying sutures in proximity to the suprascapular nerve, the technical difficulty of transglenoid drilling, and problems related to the use of metal fixation devices, we have used an absorbable tac as a

fixation device for arthroscopic stabilizations. The tac is cannulated and is made of polyglyconate (Fig. 1). Its strength diminishes over a 4 week period. Ribs on the shaft of the tac increase its pullout strength to approximately 100 N. The tac's broad, flat head allows it to capture soft tissue.

OPERATIVE TECHNIQUE

A standard arthroscopic examination is performed. The labrum and anteroinferior capsule are carefully assessed to determine the quality of the tissue. If there is neither a functional labrum nor a robust IGHLC, the arthroscopic technique is likely to fail, and an open procedure would be performed.

If the labrum is functional but detached, it is grasped from the anterosuperior portal and brought toward the anterior glenoid neck. When tension is applied the labral-IGHLC complex should tighten. If the labrum is absent or nonfunctional, the anterior band of the IGHLC is advanced with the grasper and a similar observation is made to assess the quality and tension within the system. The axillary pouch should diminish in size when these tissues are advanced superomedially. In some cases, the electrocautery is used to extend the separation from the anterior glenoid neck in order to allow sufficient advancement of the capsulolabral system. The capsule should be detached from 1 o'clock to 6 o'clock in a right shoulder. If the tissue is somewhat attenuated, sutures may be placed in the capsule and labrum to permit superior traction prior to insertion of the Suretac.

If the tissue quality is felt to permit the performance of an arthroscopic stabilization, the anterior glenoid neck is carefully debrided to bleeding bone using a combination of a rasp, an arthroscopic shaver, and an arthroscopic burr (Fig. 2). Adequate preparation of the neck is an important part of the procedure.

A cannulated drill bit that contains a guide wire is placed through the anterior portal. The wire is locked so that it protrudes a few millimeters from the end of the drill bit (Fig. 3). The wire is used to pierce the capsulolabral tissue, and the tissue is then brought to the "4 o'clock" position on the glenoid neck (Fig. 4). The drill bit is advanced to a depth of approximately 12 mm into the bony glenoid (Fig. 5). The wire is then unlocked from the drill bit, and gently tapped to free it from the drill bit. The drill bit is removed, leaving the wire in place (Fig. 6). A tac is then placed over the wire and impacted into place using a cannulated pusher (Fig. 7). We generally attempt to place a second tac at the "2 o'clock" position. The key to success with this technique is superior advancement of the middle glenohumeral ligament and the IGHLC.

POSTOPERATIVE CARE

Patients treated arthroscopically may require a longer period of postoperative immobilization than

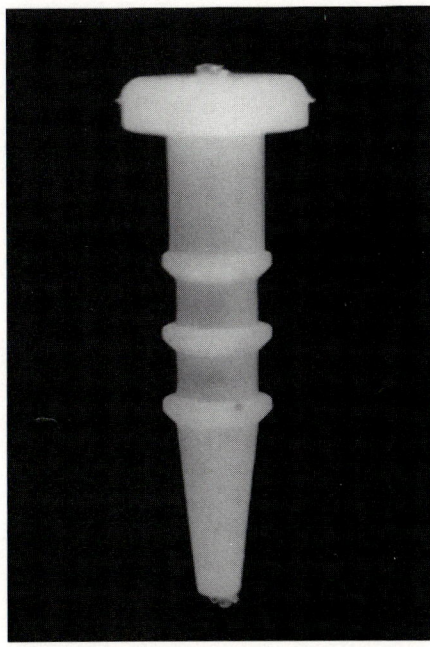

Figure 1   Enlarged photograph of the Suretac.

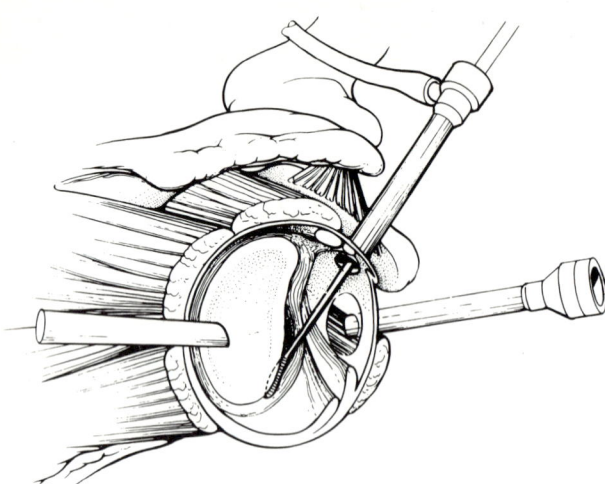

Figure 2 Preparation of the glenoid neck using a arthroscopic rasp.

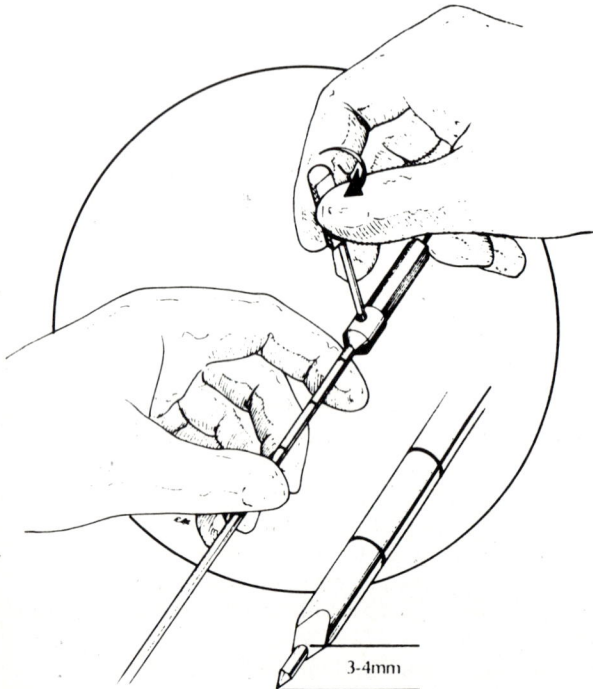

Figure 3 The guide wire is set within the cannulated drill bit so that a few millimeters of the wire protrudes from the end of the drill bit.

patients treated by open techniques. After an arthroscopic stabilization, patients are maintained in internal rotation in a shoulder immobilizer for 4 weeks. Pendulum and elbow range-of-motion exercises are encouraged during this period. Shoulder motion is increased at 4 weeks using active-assisted and passive techniques. When full range of motion (ROM) is obtained, resistance exercises are instituted. At 4 months, the patient may resume light throwing and underhand racquet sports. After 6 months, contact sports and unrestricted activity are permitted.

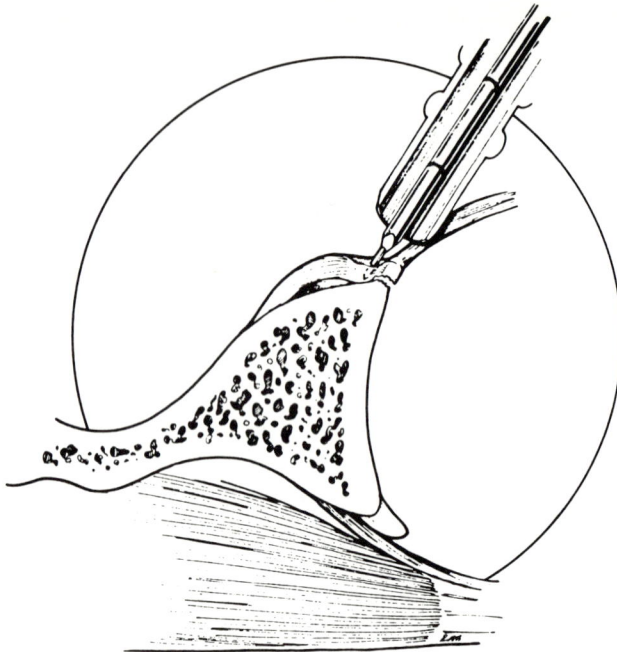

Figure 4 The drill bit and guide wire are used to advance the capsulolabral tissues superomedially on the glenoid neck.

CLINICAL RESULTS OF ARTHROSCOPIC SURETAC STABILIZATIONS

Acute Instability

Arciero et al recently presented the results of arthroscopic Suretac stabilization in army cadets after acute, first-time, traumatic dislocations. Eighteen patients were followed an average of 10 months after the procedure. None of the patients developed postoperative instability. This figure compares to an 80% recurrence rate noted in a similar group of patients who were treated with immobilization followed by rehabilitation. Sixteen of the 18 patients, including two intercollegiate football players, were able to return to full activity. There were no perioperative complications. The average loss of external rotation with the arm in 90 degrees of elevation was 3 degrees (range, 0 to 18 degrees).

Recurrent Instability

The clinical results of the initial group of patients whom we treated for recurrent anterior instability with the Suretac are now available. Fifty-two patients were followed for a minimum of 2 years after the procedure. Thirty-six of the patients had a preoperative diagnosis of recurrent anterior dislocation and 16 had recurrent anterior subluxation. There were no perioperative complications. All of the patients regained full ROM, and nearly three-fourths of the patients returned to full athletic activity.

However, 27% of the patients developed some degree of recurrent instability in the postoperative period. Three patients suffered traumatic injuries after

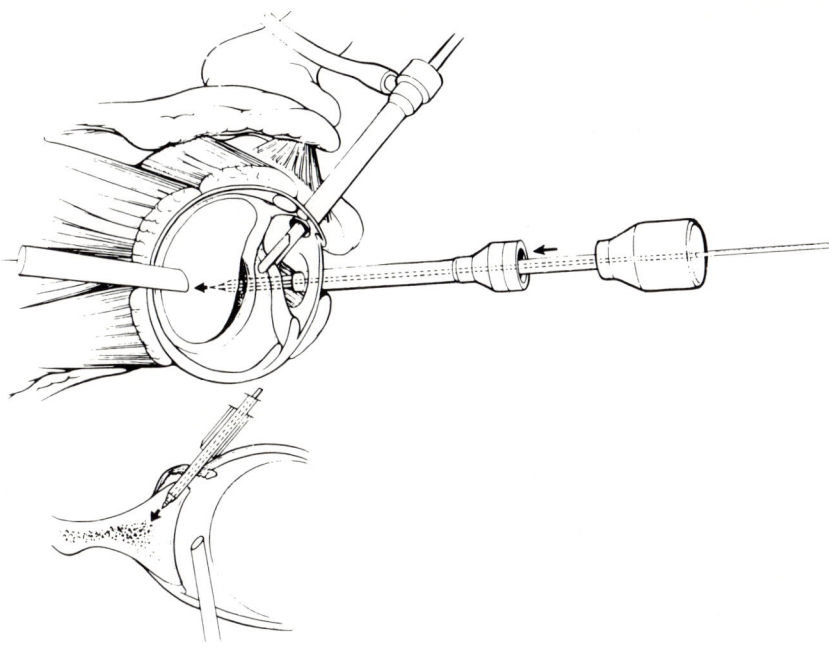

Figure 5 A hole is drilled in the anterior glenoid neck.

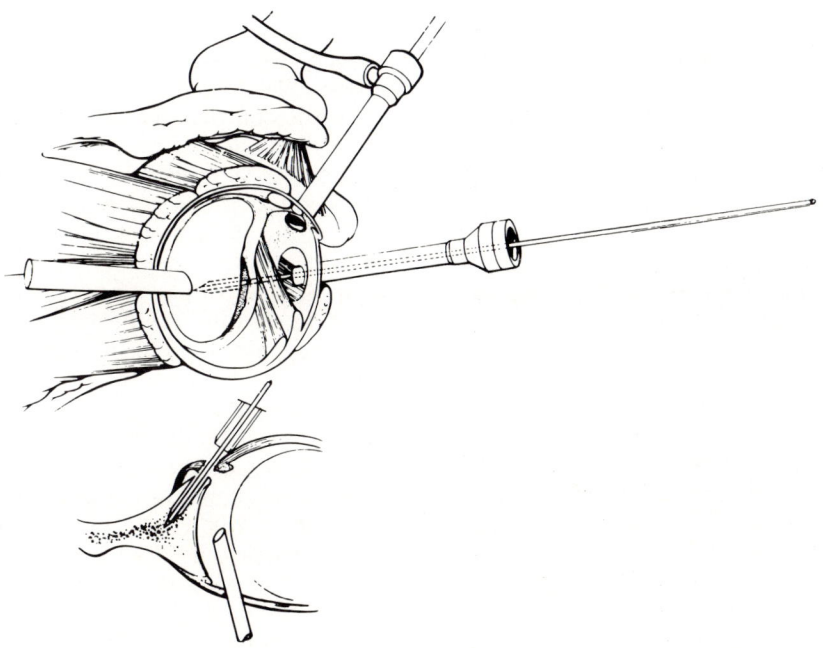

Figure 6 The drill bit is removed, and the guide wire is left in place.

they returned to contact sports. Each of the three was managed conservatively without further instability. Three other patients had subluxation that was associated with vigorous overhead activity. These patients modified their activities and had no subsequent problems. The eight remaining patients required reoperation with open stabilization. Seven of the eight patients were noted to have healed Bankart lesions, and residual capsular laxity was implicated in their postoperative recurrence. In the final patient, the Bankart lesion failed to heal. We have gradually modified our technique to include greater tightening of the capsule as well as repair of the Bankart lesion. Hopefully, this will lower our recurrence rate.

SURETAC FIXATION OF SUPERIOR LABRAL LESIONS

Recently, Snyder et al have coined the term *SLAP lesion* to describe "an injury to the superior aspect of the

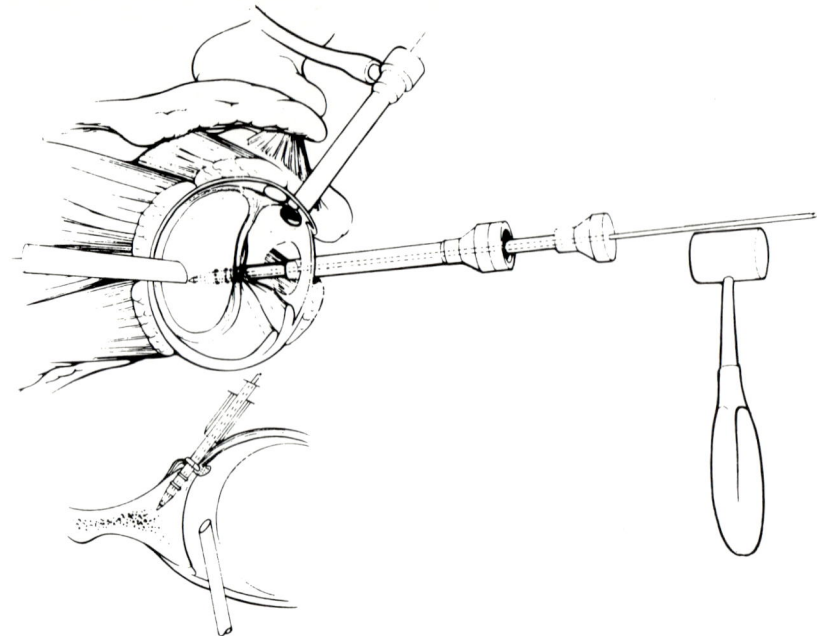

Figure 7   A biodegradable tac is then placed over the guide wire and impacted into place with a cannulated pusher.

labrum which begins posteriorly and extends anteriorly . . . including the 'anchor' of the biceps tendon to the glenoid." The arthroscopist must be careful not to mistake the normal mobility of the superior portion of the labrum or the labral sulcus for the SLAP lesion. In some cases, a meniscal-like labrum is present in which the supraglenoid insertion is recessed medial to the glenoid articular surface. In other cases, the superior labrum inserts directly on the edge of the articular margin. Snyder et al classified the SLAP lesion into four types based on arthroscopic findings:

Type I: Fraying of the superior labrum, but firm attachment of the labrum to the glenoid.
Type II: Stripping of the superior labrum and biceps tendon off the underlying glenoid, resulting in instability of the labral-biceps anchor.
Type III: Bucket-handle tear of the labrum with an intact biceps insertion.
Type IV: Bucket-handle tear of the labrum that extends into the biceps tendon.

In our experience, superior labral lesions are often associated with subtle forms of instability in which the affected patient may have a sense of "looseness" in the shoulder. Increased biceps activity has been noted in throwers with anterior instability, and the biceps may act as a secondary stabilizer of the shoulder. The forces incurred by this mechanism may help to explain the pathogenesis of the SLAP lesion in throwers and some patients with anterior instability.

While debridement of a Type III lesion may be of value if no instability is noted, simple debridement of the unstable superior labral lesions has not been highly successful in our experience. We have noted a resolution of the sensation of "looseness" after fixation of hypermobile (Types II and IV) superior labral lesions with an absorbable tac.

Nineteen patients were followed an average of 20 months (range, 9 to 41 months) after arthroscopic fixation of a superior labral lesion using the Suretac. The dominant arm was involved in 17 of the patients. The mechanism of injury was related to overhead sports in 10 patients, contact injury in five patients, and a traction injury in one patient. The remaining patients could not recall an inciting event. Symptoms included pain with overhead activity (all patients), painful clicking (six patients), and a sense of looseness (10 patients) in the shoulder. Eleven patients were noted to have subtle increases in glenohumeral translation, which resolved after fixation of the superior labrum. In each case, the hypermobile superior labrum was returned to its normal anatomic position, where it was fixed with one or two tacs. Two patients had overt anterior instability that necessitated concomitant stabilization.

Seventeen of the 19 patients (89%) were satisfied with the procedure. Nine of 10 overhead athletes (including four of four professional athletes) and two of three contact athletes returned to premorbid function. One patient required manipulation of the shoulder for postoperative restriction of motion. Two other patients lacked 15 to 20 degrees of rotation. Only one patient complained of significant pain. No patients complained of instability.

DISCUSSION

The biodegradable tac provides an alternative method of arthroscopic stabilization in patients with discrete lesions of the capsule or labrum. This method appears to be highly successful in the treatment of patients at high risk for recurrence after an acute episode of instability.

The tac is effective in restoring displaced Bankart lesions to their anatomical positions and in inducing these lesions to heal. If present, capsular laxity must be addressed concomitantly. Mild capsular laxity may be difficult to recognize, even with careful preoperative examination. Unrecognized capsular laxity appears to be highly associated with recurrent postoperative instability. Contact and overhead athletes have been reported to have poorer results after a variety of stabilization procedures, including open capsular repairs. Our patient base is skewed towards this active population, and our results may be less satisfactory as a result. While the results of arthroscopic stabilization procedures in such patients may be less encouraging than those in a more sedentary population, it is unclear if a matched population would fare better with an open procedure.

The tac appears to provide a satisfactory method for the arthroscopic treatment of unstable superior labral lesions. Secure fixation of the biceps anchor seems to be the key to successful treatment.

SUGGESTED READING

Altchek DW, Skyhar MJ, Warren RF. Shoulder arthroscopy for shoulder instability. In: Barr J, ed. American Academy of Orthopaedic Surgeons instructional course lectures. Park Ridge, Ill: AAOS, 1989:187.

Altchek DW, Warren RF, Wickiewicz TL, Ortiz G. Arthroscopic labral debridement: A three year follow-up study. Am J Sports Med 1992; 20:702–706.

Arciero RA, Wheeler III JH, Ryan JB, McBride Jr, JT. Arthroscopic Bankart repair for acute, initial anterior shoulder dislocations. Paper presented at annual meeting of the American Academy of Orthopaedic Surgeons, San Francisco, 1993.

Arciero RA. Arthroscopic Bankart repair of acute, initial anterior shoulder dislocations. Paper presented at Shoulder Arthroscopy Course, San Diego, 1993.

Bankart ASB. The pathology and surgical treatment of recurrent dislocation of the shoulder. Br J Surg 1938; 26:23–29.

Bowen MK, Warren RF. Ligamentous control of shoulder stability based on selective cutting and static translation. Clin Sports Med 1991; 10:757–784.

Hawkins RB. Arthroscopic stapling repair for shoulder instability: A retrospective study of 50 cases. Arthroscopy 1989; 5:122–128.

Morgan CD. Arthroscopic transglenoid Bankart suture repair. Oper Tech Ortho 1991; 1:171–179.

Pagnani MJ, Speer KP, Altchek DW, et al. Arthroscopic fixation of superior labral lesions. Paper presented at annual closed meeting of American Shoulder and Elbow Surgeons, 1993.

Perthes G. Uber operationen der habituellen schulterluxation. Deutsche Ztschr f Chir 1906; 85:199.

Rowe CR, Patel D, Southmayd WW. The Bankart procedure: A long-term end-result study. J Bone Joint Surg 1978; 60A:1–16.

Snyder SJ, Karzel RP, Del Pizzo W, et al. S.L.A.P. lesions of the shoulder (Lesions of the Superior Labrum Both Anterior and Posterior). Orthop Trans 1990; 14:257–258.

Snyder SJ, Karzel RP, Del Pizzo W. SLAP lesions of the shoulder. Arthroscopy 1990; 6:274–279.

Turkel SJ, Panio MW, Marshall JW, Girgis FG. Stabilizing mechanisms preventing anterior dislocation of the shoulder. J Bone Joint Surg 1981; 63A:1208–1217.

ARTHROSCOPIC CAPSULOLABRAL RECONSTRUCTION USING SUTURE ANCHORS

EUGENE M. WOLF, M.D.

The first known treatment of the unstable shoulder was that of Hippocrates. He was the first to observe that it was in the position of abduction and external rotation of the shoulder that recurrent dislocations took place. His infamous treatment consisted of placing a red hot poker in the axilla of the affected shoulder. The goal was to produce a severe burn that would lead to contractures of the axillary skin folds, thereby limiting elevation and rotation of the shoulder. Although modern operative treatment has become considerably more humane, the basic principle of limitation of motion has been the intentional or inadvertent hallmark of the surgical procedures of the twentieth century. This chapter limits the discussion to anterior traumatic instability, as opposed to the relatively rare, multidirectional atraumatic instability.

PREVENTION OF RECURRENT SHOULDER INSTABILITY

Are there any preventative measures that can be employed to keep this type of pathology from impacting the lives of millions of individuals? Anterior shoulder instability is, by definition, traumatic in nature. Recurrent anterior shoulder instability follows an initial event that produces a dislocation or subluxation. Thus the more precise questions are: Can we prevent the initial dislocation from occurring in the first place? After an initial dislocation, can we prevent recurrent episodes of instability? Unfortunately the evolutionary process of the shoulder has traded stability for mobility. The shoulder is the most mobile, as well as the most frequently dislocated, joint in the body. The first line of defense should be the prevention of the initial traumatic dislocation, but this poses a particularly difficult challenge in this era of increasing athletic activity levels for all ages of our population, not to mention vehicular and workplace trauma.

There are few predictive factors other than: (1) individuals who have had unilateral dislocations have a 25% chance of developing a bilateral problem, and (2) certain families exhibit a history of shoulder dislocations. These predictive factors would not justify the use of cumbersome protective harnesses that are available, but are extremely limiting and preclude any overhead activities. The best training and conditioning does not seem to have any impact in prevention, since the trauma involved in producing the initial dislocation is often significant and totally unexpected. Shoulder instability is as common in the highly trained athlete as it is in the ill conditioned individual.

Since we can do little to predict or prevent the initial dislocation, can we prevent the dislocations from recurring? The present "standard of care" in the treatment of an initial acute dislocation after reduction is 3 weeks of immobilization followed by a rehabilitation program. Unfortunately this "conservative" treatment program leads to a recurrence rate of over 90% in individuals less than 30 years of age, with a decreasing frequency of recurrence with increasing age.

The unstable shoulder joint is at risk for developing degenerative arthritis. The trauma of recurrent episodes of dislocations or subluxation damages the cartilaginous articular surfaces, erodes the labrum and glenoid rim, deepens the Hill-Sachs compression lesion, stretches the remaining capsular ligaments, and produces muscle atrophy of the shoulder girdle. Each recurrence facilitates and engenders more recurrences. The treatment of acute dislocations will remain an area of controversy for some years to come, but recent studies by Baker, Uribe, Ryan, and Arciero, have shown that early arthroscopic stabilization can reduce the recurrence rate to 10% without adding any significant morbidity. Early open operative stabilization has been shunned to this point because of the morbidity of standard open operative procedures. I believe that the first-time dislocator under the age of 30 should be given the option of immediate arthroscopic stabilization. This is the only treatment that permits restoration of the ligament-labral anatomy, and has the best chance of avoiding the risks of the arthritis of recurrent dislocation.

DIAGNOSIS

The clinical examination of the unstable shoulder can provide important information, but the diagnosis is made primarily by history. The history is as important to the shoulder as the examination is to the knee. ("The clinician has to examine knees, but listen to shoulders.") The mechanism of injury most commonly reported is one of sudden or forced external rotation and abduction. Occasionally an acute dislocation is produced in snow skiing accidents by external rotation and hyperextension. Recurrences can occur with little or no trauma. The position of the arm and the activity that produces the

recurrences are critical in determining the likely direction of the instability:

- External rotation and abduction = anterior instability
- Forward flexion = posterior instability
- Abduction = inferior instability

The most valuable clinical test for anterior instability is the "apprehension test." This is the patient's perception that the shoulder might "go out" when the involved extremity is externally rotated and abducted. Over time, this apprehension effectively reduces the range of motion in these planes. This measurable loss of motion is a natural protective mechanism. There may be tenderness noted on palpation of the anterior aspect of the shoulder especially if there has been a recent episode. *Although it is important to note all physical findings, it is possible that the examination of the unstable shoulder may be entirely normal.*

An examiner may be fortunate to have a patient relaxed enough to allow the instability to be appreciated in the office setting, and unfortunate enough to be unable to reduce a dislocation produced in the office. It is only under general anesthesia, that the type and degree of instability can be consistently and accurately assessed.

Classification of Anterior Instability

Three basic types of pathoanatomy of the glenohumeral ligament labral complex (GLLC) produce anterior shoulder instability.

Type 1: Glenoid avulsion of the GLLC (Bankart)

This lesion occurs at junction of the fibrocollagenous labrum with the cartilaginous glenoid surface and bony glenoid rim, and may extend to the periosteum of the scapular neck. A fracture of the glenoid rim may occur by avulsion at the time of the initial dislocation, or may occur via compression during recurrent dislocations. The Type 1 lesion is the most commonly found lesion.

Beware of "secondary" Type 1 labral lesions. These lesions may explain variation in the reported occurrence of Type 1 lesions, as well as some of the failures of repairs. These secondary labral lesions are due to the compression of the labrum as it rides out over the glenoid rim, but the primary pathology may be intraligamentous or at the humeral side.

Type 2: Insubstance tears, or diffuse laxity of glenohumeral ligaments

Bigliani has shown in fresh cadaver specimens, that the inferior glenohumeral ligament labral complex (IGLLC) stretches from 15% to 62% before failing. The ligament eventually failed at the glenoid insertion in 40% of the specimens, the substance of the ligaments in 35%, and at the humeral insertion in 25%. It is likely that there is some degree of strain (change in length) of the glenohumeral ligaments that occurs in the course of every dislocation, regardless of the type of lesion produced. Even a small amount of plastic deformation (stretching without gross tearing) of the IGL, without glenoid or humeral avulsions, may be enough to explain some cases of recurrent anterior instability. When there is gross insubstance tearing of glenohumeral ligaments, the healing response will make them extremely difficult to recognize "retroscopically". Subtle *intrasubstance* ligamentous lesions may also occur with plastic deformation, and are not grossly visible.

This type of instability is usually a diagnosis by exclusion. There are no accurate, objective methods (open or arthroscopic) of measuring "ligament or capsular laxity." This diagnosis is made in those cases where anterior instability has been documented radiologically, clinically, or by examination under anesthesia, but there are no significant intra-articular lesions of the IGLLC.

Type 3: Humeral avulsion of glenohumeral ligaments (HAGL)

This type of lesion was first recognized by Nicola. He actually performed "exploratory" procedures in 22 chronic, and five acute anterior dislocators, and found that 5 patients (19%) had avulsed the capsular ligaments from the humerus. In 1988 Bach and Warren reported on two cases of "lateral capsular ruptures" with bony avulsions from the humerus. All shoulders with anterior instability should be carefully explored at both the humeral and glenoid insertions of the glenohumeral ligaments.

Prospective Study

In a 2 year prospective study we found the following types of pathology in 64 patients with documented anterior instability: *Type 1*—Glenoid/Bankart (47 cases/73.4%), *Type 2*—Insubstance (11 cases/17.2%), and *Type 3*—Humeral/HAGL (6 cases/9.4%). There are any number of potential variations of each of these lesions, but this classification is based on the three possible areas of localization of the lesions.

In the diagnostic arthroscopy of chronic dislocation, the pathology is months or years old. A traumatic ligament avulsion from the glenoid, like any ligament injury, produces a healing response that might make the pathology difficult to recognize. The GLLC may be avulsed with or without a bony rim fragment, and may heal in a medialized and inferiorly rotated position. The attached ligaments become essentially nonfunctional. The "healed" Type 1 lesion (glenoid avulsion) may be difficult to recognize.

The repair process of the well-vascularized "insubstance" area is even more effective, and is even more difficult to recognize.

The body's attempt to heal the HAGL lesions poses similar diagnostic problems. Vascularity and fibrous responses vary enormously between individuals and injuries. *Only the experienced arthroscopic shoulder sur-geon, with a complete understanding of normal anatomy, and the knowledge of all the aspects of the potential intra-articular pathology of instability, will approach an acceptable success rate in the arthroscopic management of the unstable shoulder.*

Arthroscopic capsulolabral reconstruction (ACLR), using suture anchors, is a surgical approach that enables the surgeon to remedy those cases of instability due to Type 1 lesions at the glenoid rim. This same technique also permits a *concomitant capsular plication that is performed in all cases.* It is best to err on the side of plication, since it is impossible to calibrate the percentage of elongation of capsular ligaments that may have occurred during initial or repeated dislocations.

Those cases of anterior instability that are due to Type 2 intraligamentous lesions or to the Type 3 HAGL lesion are repaired with arthroscopic suturing/plication techniques, but without using suture anchors.

EXAMINATION UNDER ANESTHESIA

The examination of the glenohumeral joint under anesthesia (EUA) is performed systematically, and must include the following italicized elements:

The EUA must be performed in a *lateral decubitus position.* There are several reasons that make this position optimal, one of which is the need to apply the correct *axial compression* on the glenoid via the humerus and the humeral head. The weight of the arm provides just the right amount of pressure.

Matsen and Habermayer have both reported the suction cup effect of the intact labrum. When the labrum is disrupted, the suction effect is disrupted, and the humeral head can be more easily pulled from the glenoid. The sensory perception of this by the surgeon is critical to the diagnosis and can only be appreciated if the scapula, i.e., the glenoid, is stabilized. *Scapular stabilization* is thus another essential part of the EUA, and is best accomplished in the lateral decubitus position. Scapular stabilization in this examination is analogous to the necessary stabilization of the femur during Lachman's test in the knee. The degree of anterior translation of the humerus with respect to the glenoid cannot be appreciated without scapular stabilization. This is accomplished with the surgeon's stabilizing hand medial to the joint line. The thumb of this hand is in the infraspinatus fossa, and the fingers are over the anterior edge of the clavicle, medial to the coracoid. The surgeon's examining hand and arm is then used to balance the humeral head on the stabilized glenoid. With the humerus in the same plane as the scapula, the humeral head can then be "rocked out" and over the anterior rim. It reduces with a distinct "clunk".

From Turkel's work it is known that the IGL is the primary structure responsible for anterior stability of the glenohumeral joint. The role of the IGL increases with abduction and is maximal at 90 degrees. Thus, this examination needs to be performed in *90 degrees of abduction.* "Drawer tests" with the arm in an adducted position are of little value.

If there is any doubt about the degree or type of instability, the patient is examined *bilaterally*.

SURGICAL TECHNIQUE

The patient is placed in the lateral decubitus position, rotated back 20 degrees. A twin traction set-up is used, in which an axillary sling internally rotates the arm, relaxes the anterior capsule, and centralizes the humeral head on the glenoid. After induction of anesthesia, the table is rotated 120 degrees. The anesthesiologist stands at the umbilicus (180 degrees of access to the shoulder is necessary).

Materials used include a twin monitor arthroscopy set-up, an arthroscopic suture anchor kit, a threaded cannula, suture hooks, #1 PDS II suture (36 inch), a knot pusher, an arthroscopic periosteal elevator, and a 3M pump, with 1 mg of epinephrine per 3 liter bottle.

The pathology of anterior instability is best visualized from the anterior superior portal (ASP), but the procedure begins with the introduction of the of the arthroscope in the posterior superior portal (PSP), which is located at the posterior bony margin of the acromion. The PSP is made 1 cm medial to the posterolateral corner of the acromion. The portal incision is made at the *posterior bony margin*. The scope sheath with its blunt obturator are inserted through the deltoid and infraspinatus muscles. Palpate the posterior capsule and glenoid rim, and use the tip of the blunt obturator to dissect along the joint line. Direct the sheath and obturator at the tip of the coracoid and pop through the capsule into the joint.

The initial traction configuration is standard with 10 to 15 pounds applied distally, with the arm in approximately 45 degrees of abduction. The twin traction configuration is set up after all portals are made.

The anterior inferior portal (AIP) is then created. The sheath and blunt obturator are pushed across the joint, and the coracoid is palpated in the rotator cuff interval. The sheath and obturator are pushed through the cuff interval, lateral to the coracoid and proximal to the subscapularis tendon. This step can be achieved by palpation without visualization, or the scope can be inserted into the joint to visualize the superior border of the subscapularis where this portal is to be made. The sheath and obturator are pushed anteriorly through the rotator cuff interval, the deltoid, to the skin where an incision is made. The combination transduction cannula is then retrograded into the joint by maintaining contact with the sheath and obturator as its tip is backed into the joint.

The ASP is then created with an outside-in technique using a spinal needle to best localize the portal just anterior to the supraspinatus tendon, and at the level of the biceps. A cannula with a sharp obturator is used to enter the joint. This will be primarily a viewing portal. It is essential that the two anterior portals be made as far away from each other as possible to allow for comfortable triangulation.

Once the portals are made, switching sticks are used to move the scope to the ASP, the combination/outflow to the PSP, and an 8.5 mm cannula into the AIP. Now the entire IGLLC can be directly viewed, probed, and evaluated. The AIP is the "working portal," where a whisker and burr are used to prepare the lesion. The 8.5 mm Cannuloc threaded cannula is directed into the joint by the switching stick that fits into its cannulated obturator. The threaded cannula is literally screwed into the portal until it is seen entering the joint. The threads prevent the cannula from backing out and allows adjustment of the cannula during the case. This helps prevent the inadvertent loss of portals during the case, and the resulting extravasation that can make this difficult procedure impossible.

An arthroscopic pump and adrenaline (1 mg/3 liter bag) are indispensable for this complicated procedure.

A whisker blade is inserted in the AIP and a *synovial abrasion* of the anterior half of the joint is carried out. This relatively nonaggressive blade traumatizes the

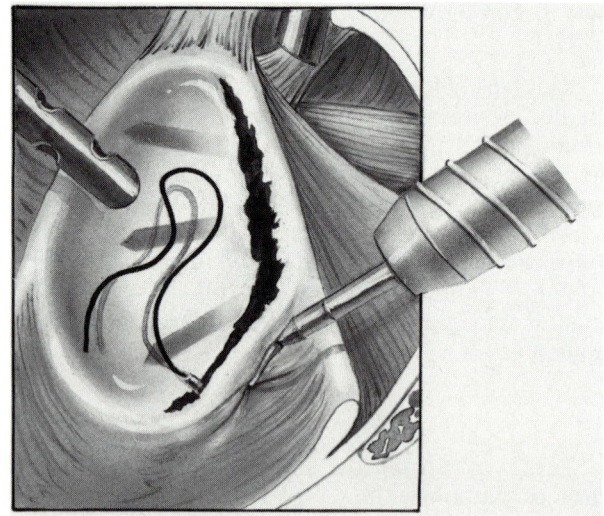

Figure 1 Suture placement.

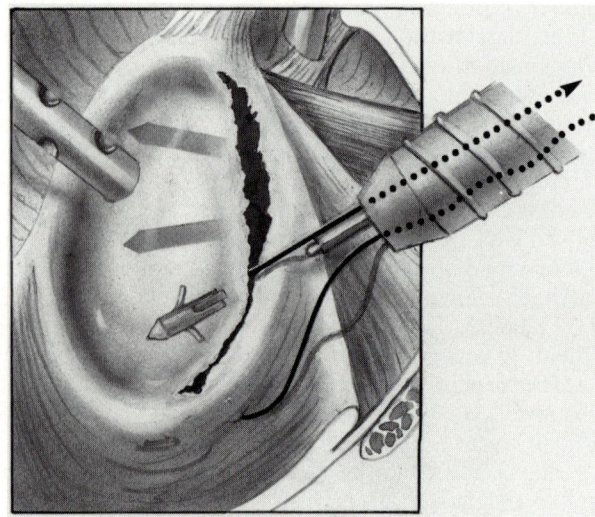

Figure 2 Anchor placement.

synovium and synoviocytes, without damaging capsular ligaments. This reduces the synovial environment and promotes a postoperative fibroblastic response from the synoviocytes.

The scapular neck is *aggressively burred* to produce a vigorous fibroblastic response. The burr is used to pock-mark the scapular neck so that the cancellous bone is seen. Care is taken to preserve the glenoid rim that may already be deficient.

Once the lesion is prepared, three drill holes are made in the anterior edge of the glenoid. The drill guide has a fish mouthed end that fits over the edge of the glenoid. The drill guide must be angled 20 degrees to the surface of the glenoid to ensure that the drill bit does not skive onto the cartilaginous surface, and that the anchors are located well below the subchondral bone. The hole made by these bits are deep enough to accommodate a second anchor in case of suture breakage.

A suture hook is used to pass a #1 PDS suture

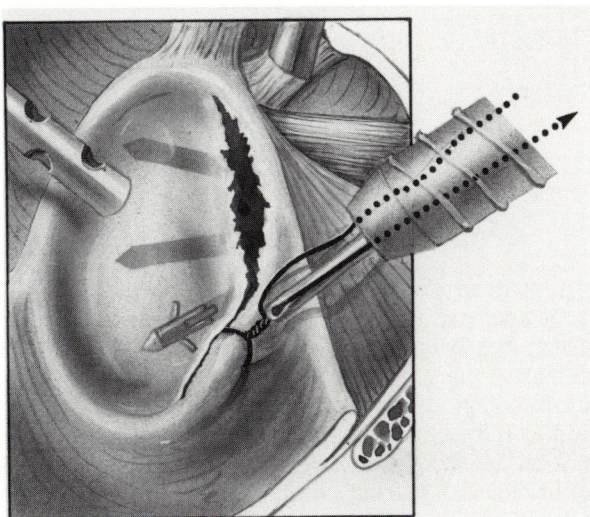

Figure 3 Knot tying.

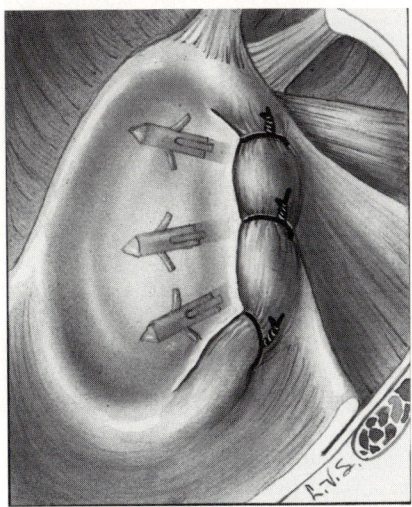

Figure 4 Closure of lesion.

through the substance of the IGL in the axillary pouch at the inferior pole of the glenoid, approximately 1 cm from the detached labral edge. The greater this distance, the greater the degree of capsular plication and reduction of capsular volume (Fig. 1). A more significant plication, and even a "global capsular plication" is necessary in younger, hyperlax individuals. In the all inside suturing approach, *only one suture can be placed and tied at a time.*

The first anchor, secured to it's inserter, is slid down the inside limb of the suture and inserted into the most inferior drill hole (Fig. 2). A common fishing knot is tied and slid down the cannula, thus reapproximating the GLLC to the glenoid (Fig. 3). This process is repeated two more times so as to completely close the lesion (Fig. 4).

POSTOPERATIVE CARE

ACLR is an out-patient procedure. The patient is discharged 2 to 3 hours after the operation. The involved extremity is immobilized for 3 to 4 weeks. We hold the younger (<30 years) males and more competitive athletic individuals for the full 4 weeks.

All patients are started on a home therapy program and given a home therapy kit. They receive an average of two 30 minute training sessions to ensure proper use of the kit.

Most patients return to noncontact sports at 3 months. The return to higher-risk athletic activities is at 6 months.

RESULTS

Sixty-four patients have been followed for 24 to 48 months. There have been no significant intraoperative or postoperative complications. Six patients (9.3%) experienced recurrence of instability. Three of these patients returned to contact sports before the recommended 6 month delay. Two patients were felt to have had a component of multidirectional instability. The other 58 patients (90.7%) returned to their prior activity levels without symptoms. Although the follow-up is still relatively short, and further study will likely reveal more recurrences, the success of this procedure is encouraging. The technique has evolved considerably since the prototypic days, and the ability to recognize the different types of pathology has improved dramatically. This should lead to improved results in subsequent series.

SUGGESTED READING

Bankart ASB. The pathology and treatment of recurrent dislocation of the shoulder joint. Br J Surg 1939; 26:23-29.

DePalma AF, Cooke AJ, Prabhakar M. The role of the subscapularis in recurrent anterior dislocations of the shoulder. CORR 1967; 54:35-49.

Gross RM. Arthroscopic shoulder capsulorrhaphy: Does it work? Am J Sports Med 1989; 17:495-500.

Hawkins RB. Arthroscopic stapling repair for shoulder instability: A retrospective study of 50 cases. Arthroscopy 1989; 5:122-128.

Hawkins RJ, Angelo RL. Glenohumeral osteoarthrosis. J Bone Joint Surg 1990; 72A:1193-1197.

Hovelius L, Akermark C, Albrektsson B, et al. Bristo-Latarjet procedure for recurrent anterior dislocation of the shoulder. Acta Orthop Scand 1983; 54:284-290.

Hovelius L, Thorling J, Fredin H. Recurrent anterior dislocation of the shoulder: Results after the Bankart and Putti-Platt operations. J Bone Joint Surg 1979; 61A:566-569.

Magnuson PB, Stack JK. Recurrent dislocation of the shoulder. JAMA 1943; 123:889-892.

May VR. A modified Bristow operation for anterior recurrent dislocation of the shoulder. J Bone Joint Surg 1970; 52A:1010-1016.

Morgan CD, Bodenstab AB. Arthroscopic Bankart suture repair: Technique and early results. Arthroscopy 1987; 3:111-122.

Moseley HF, Overgaard B. The anterior capsular mechanism in recurrent anterior dislocation of the shoulder: Morphological and clinical studies with special reference to the glenoid labrum and the glenohumeral ligaments. J Bone Joint Surg 1962; 44B:913-927.

O'Brien SJ, Neves MC, Arnoczky SP, et al. The anatomy and histology of the inferior glenohumeral ligament complex of the shoulder. Am J Sports Med 1990; 18:449-456.

Rowe CR, Patel D, Southmayd WW. The Bankart procedure: A long term end-result study. J Bone Joint Surg 1978; 60A:1-16.

Symeonides PP. The significance of the subscapularis muscle in the pathogenesis of recurrent anterior dislocation of the shoulder. J Bone Joint Surg 1972; 54B:476-483.

Torg JS, Balduini FC, Bonci C, et al. A modified Bristow-Helfet-May procedure for recurrent dislocations and subluxations of the shoulder: Report of 212 cases. J Bone Joint Surg 1987; 69A:904-913.

Turkel SJ, Panie MW, Marshall JL, Girgis RJ. Stabilizing mechanisms preventing anterior dislocation of the glenohumeral joint. J Bone Joint Surg 1981; 63A:1208-1217.

Wolf EM. Anterior portals in shoulder arthroscopy. Arthroscopy 1989; 5:201-208.

Wolf EM. Arthroscopic anterior shoulder capsulorrhaphy. Technique Orthop 1988; 3:67-73.

Wiley AM. Arthroscopy for shoulder instability and a technique for arthroscopic repair. Arthroscopy 1988; 4:25-30.

Zuckerman JD, Matsen FA. Complications about the glenohumeral joint related to the use of screws and staples. J Bone Joint Surg 1984; 66A:175-180.

SHOULDER REHABILITATION

MARTIN J. KELLEY, M.S., P.T.

Rehabilitation of the athlete's shoulder following injury or surgery creates a formidable challenge for the clinician. This is particularly true of the overhead athlete who places intense demands on the shoulder's osseous and soft tissue structures. Both contact and noncontact injuries often result in joint instability, myotendinous failure, fracture, neural trauma, and contusion. The most commonly treated pathologies encountered in the overhead athlete are glenohumeral joint instability, both traumatic and atruamatic, and rotator cuff tendonopathy, which can be primary or secondary in nature. Effective and safe shoulder rehabilitation requires an understanding of the unique anatomic and biomechanical characteristics of the shoulder complex, particularly related to sport-specific activity. When working with a postoperative athlete the clinician must have knowledge of the operative procedure, potential and associated surgical complications, and tissue healing parameters. As with all treatment, a comprehensive evaluation incorporating static, dynamic, and functional testing is essential to isolate and determine the extent of tissue involvement. Based on the evaluative findings, a rehabilitation course is established and progressed according to the involved structure's "reaction" to treatment. The ultimate goal for the treating clinician is to return the athlete to competition without reoccurrence of injury.

OVERHEAD SPORT DEMANDS

Overhead activity of the shoulder(s), either unilateral or bilateral, is required in throwing, racquet sports, spiking, and swimming. These activities involve repetitive high velocity, high torque end-range forces that test the physiologic limits of the capsuloligamentous-labral complex (CLLC) and rotator cuff. Velocities approaching 7500 degrees/sec are experienced during the acceleration phase of pitching while thousands of strokes are endured during each swimming sessions. The cocking position (abduction/external rotation) is extremely stressful to the athlete's shoulder, as is initial acceleration. During the initial acceleration phase the CLLC is completely tautened, creating, yet resisting, significant articular compressive and shear forces, respectively. The rotator cuff muscles are paramount to glenohumeral joint stability in mid-range where the capsule and ligaments are found "loose." Subsequently, as motion continues, and inconjunction with the static restraints, the rotator cuff assists in joint stabilization while experiencing violent torsional stresses at end-range. The deceleration phase of the overhead activity (throwing, tennis serve, spike) further challenges the structural integrity of the static restraints by distracting the joint surfaces. The rotator cuff is most vulnerable during arm deceleration since it must eccentrically contract at a high velocity. Eccentric activity is a causative factor in myotendinous strain.

The importance of the scapulothoracic muscle function is often overlooked, particularly if glenohumeral instability and/or rotator cuff pathology exist, thus rehabilitation can be incomplete. Not only do the scapulothoracic muscles provide a fixed proximal platform for the scapulohumeral and axiohumeral muscles to create force and distal movement of the humerus but they position the glenoid to maximize glenohumeral articular congruity, minimize CLLC tension, and reduce rotator cuff impingement. For example, during the swimming free-style stroke the scapular adductors are important in the recovery phase, directing the glenoid laterally, which results in reduced CLLC tension as the humerus elevates, horizontally abducts, and externally rotates. The serratus anterior is also important in scapular positioning in all overhead sports and is significantly and constantly active throughout all phases of the free-style stroke.

Regardless of the overhead sport, clearly the demands placed on the shoulder structures necessitate optimal flexibility, strength, and endurance.

PATHOLOGY

The following discussion is limited to glenohumeral instability and rotator cuff tendonopathy since these are the most commonly treated pathologies in the overhead athlete.

Glenohumeral Instability

Typically two groups of glenohumeral instability patients are described and designated by the acronyms TUBS and AMBRI (Table 1). The traumatic group typically experience glenohumeral joint dislocation due to an uncontrolled end-range force resulting in a breach in the stabilizing "envelope." The atraumatic group are characterized by subluxation/dislocation episodes without trauma resulting from a patcholous capsuloligamentous "envelope" that lacks end-range stabilizing ability and cannot provide the rotator cuff (which inserts into one-half the surface) with enough "grip" to translate force and develop dynamic stabilization. A third group of instability patients develops instability by repetitive end-range microtraumatic stretching of the CLLC, which eventually results in laxity of the capsule and ligaments as well as labral deterioration. Commonly, this group develops secondary rotator cuff impingement.

Table 1 Glenohumeral Instability Classification

Traumatic	Atraumatic
Unilateral	Multidirectional
Bankart lesion	Bilateral
Surgery required	Rehabilitation effective
	Inferior capsular shift required

Table 2 Rotator Cuff Pathology Classification

Primary compressive
Secondary compressive
Primary tensile
Secondary tensile
Macrotraumatic failure

Rotator Cuff Tendonopathy

The natural history of rotator cuff lesions is classically described as a progressive degenerative process ultimately resulting in tissue failure. Recently a new classification scheme of rotator cuff pathology has been applied to the athlete (Table 2). The cuff lesions are defined as primary or secondary (due to instability), tensile or compressive, and macrotraumatic. A tensile lesion is essentially cuff disruption due to overload, most times associated with eccentric activity as found during the deceleration phase of throwing. A compressive lesion exists when the rotator cuff is "truly" impinged by the overlying coracoacromial arch. The previously described lesions are microtraumatic and accumulative in nature compared to macrotraumatic tendon failure, which results from a single incident or, in the young athlete, is the end result of repetitive microtrauma displayed by a single event. The recent literature stresses that the intimate relationship between the CLLC and rotator cuff is not only anatomic, but functional. Balance is necessary for symptom-free overhead use; therefore, compromise to either the static or dynamic components will negatively impact the other.

REHABILITATION PRINCIPLES

Regardless of whether the athlete is postinjury or postsurgical, certain principles are closely followed. First, pain is always respected and rarely encouraged. The onset of pain following the introduction of a new exercise or a technique probably indicates the need for re-evaluation of the recent intervention. Modalities or exercises are therefore introduced one or two at a time. This also assists in identifying effective treatment interventions when the patient shows progress. Reactivity is a subjective means of qualifying the irritability of the involved structures and is based on both subjective and objective testing, i.e., pain with resistance, impingement sign. The patient's reactivity becomes the guide for program progression. Sometimes the patient will reach an "iatrogenic plateau" which essentially means further recovery is hampered by the very same factor that allowed some degree of recovery; the rehabilitation process. The plateau is characterized by stagnating mild tissue reactivity. By allowing the athlete a short but full rest from exercise, the tissue recovers as does the athlete's progress. A second principle followed is that current anatomic and biomechanical concepts are ingrained into the rehabilitation program. Thirdly, the progression of shoulder position or motion plane, during exercise, is from the nonprovocative to provocative. These positions and planes vary based on pathology or surgery but most commonly the least provocative position is somewhere between 20 and 55 degrees of scapular plane abduction. The plane of the scapula (POS) is advantageous in exercise performance for several reasons (Table 3). Utilization of the POS reduces tensile and torsional stresses to the rotator cuff and CLLC. Additionally, the POS is an inherently stable position for the glenohumeral joint if working with an athlete with

Table 3 Plane of the Scapula Rehabilitation Characteristics

Improved joint surface congruity
Reduced rotational stress to the CLLC and rotator cuff
The supraspinatus and deltoid are optimally aligned for elevation
Correlates with most functional activities

Table 4 Phases of Shoulder Rehabilitation

Phase I
  Rest from painful activity
  Anti-inflammatory therapy
  PROM and AAROM
  Joint mobilization
  Strengthening (submaximal → maximal)
    Isometrics
  Scapulothoracic strengthening
  Aerobic conditioning
Phase II
  Progress ROM
  Strengthening (sub-maximal → maximal)
    Manual and isotonic
      Multiangle isometrics
      Short-arc excursion
  Aggressive scapulothoracic strengthening
  Aerobic conditioning
Phase III
  Prophylactic stretching
  Strengthening/endurance (to full range and emphasize eccentrics then progress to sport specific positions)
    Variable and/or free-weight resistance
    Isokinetics
    Body blade
    Plyometrics
Phase IV
  Return to sport

instability. Provocative positions are typically at end range, particularly 90 degrees of coronal plane (or posterior) abduction and full external rotation. This position not only stresses the CLLC and twists the rotator cuff but can cause supraspinatus impingement against the posterior glenoid rim. Lastly, the patient's rehabilitation program is individualized based on reactivity, hyperelasticity/hypoelasticity, personality, goals, and surgical concerns/complications.

PHASES OF REHABILITATION

Obviously, whether the athlete is postinjury or postoperative will dictate how quickly they progress since the latter requires adequate time for the sites of tissue fixation to heal. However, if we approach the treatment as phases of progression, based on reactivity and signs and symptoms, then a single scheme of progression can be followed (Table 4). Determination of reactivity and not necessarily the severity of the involved tissue is essential in developing and advancing the rehabilitation program. For example, a patient with a significantly reactive supraspinatus tendinitis is initially treated more conservatively than a patient with a mildly reactive, small, full-thickness supraspinatus tear, even though the latter patient has greater structural damage.

Phase I

Regardless of whether rotator cuff inflammation is primary or secondary, due to instability resulting in impingement, appropriate rest from irritating activities is required. This includes terminating all painful exercises that were previously prescribed for the patient, i.e., the empty can. Countless times the patient will enter therapy and is already doing the empty can exercise (abduction in the POS while in full internal rotation). In most cases the patient admits that it is painful to perform even when elevating below 80 degrees. Although this exercise may be beneficial at some stage of rehabilitation, performing it can result in further irritation of the rotator cuff due to increased shear forces and direct cuff compression. Anti-inflammatory modalities may be utilized and include: phonophresis with either dexamethasone or hydrocortisone, iontophoresis using dexamethasone, ice massage, or ice. A short application of heat for 5 minutes with the anti-inflammatory medicine topically applied may assist in porous penetration. Positioning to optimize exposure of the targeted tissue is necessary. Oral NSAIDs may also be helpful. Transverse friction massage may be employed to an inflamed tendon in

efforts to promote scar tissue pliability and local blood flow.

Passive or active assisted range-of-motion exercises are initiated in pain-free ranges. Commonly, rotational exercises are performed at 45 degrees of POS abduction (Fig. 1). Glenohumeral joint mobilization, which is the performance of specific directional gliding of the humeral head relative to the glenoid, may assist in pain reduction and regain lost motion. If appropriate, pain-free submaximal resistance isometric exercises may be started either at the shoulder and/or elbow. Strengthening of the scapulothoracic muscles can be initiated without glenohumeral joint motion either by active contraction or manual resistance. Whenever possible the athlete should continue with aerobic conditioning on the bike, stairmaster, or equivalent device.

Phase II

As inflammation resolves modalities are discontinued and the intensity of stretching increased to approach the end range. If pain persists in certain (provocative) positions they are avoided. The strengthening program is also progressed, usually by manual resistance. The advantages of applying manual resistance to the athlete are real time feedback regarding pain, weakness, and apprehension. The clinician gains insight about provocative positions, planes, and ranges, in addition to resistance effort. Treatment may consist of multi-angle isometrics utilizing rhythmic stabilization at each angle chosen. For example, the arm may be moved from 30 to 90 degrees of POS abduction at 30 degree intervals (30,60,90). At each position the athlete is required to maintain a set position as the clinician varies the direction of force (rhythmic stabilization) (Fig. 2). This

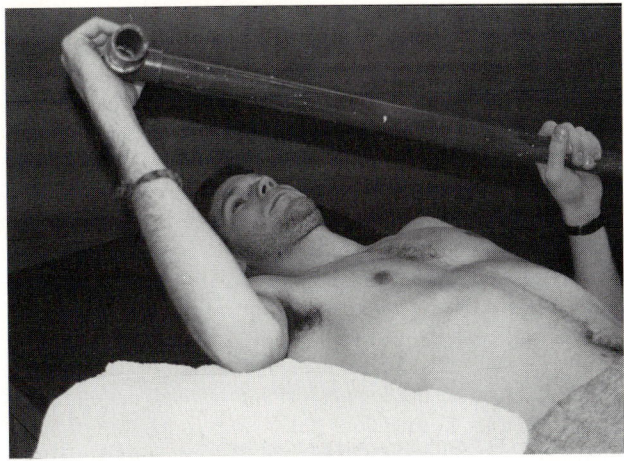

Figure 1 External rotation in 45 degrees of POS abduction.

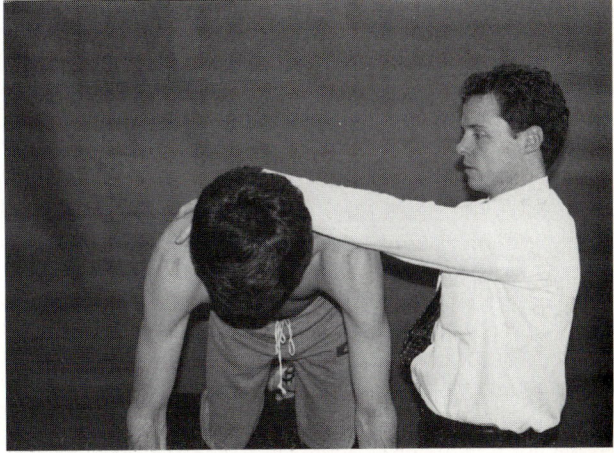

Figure 3 Quadruped (closed chain) position for serratus strengthening.

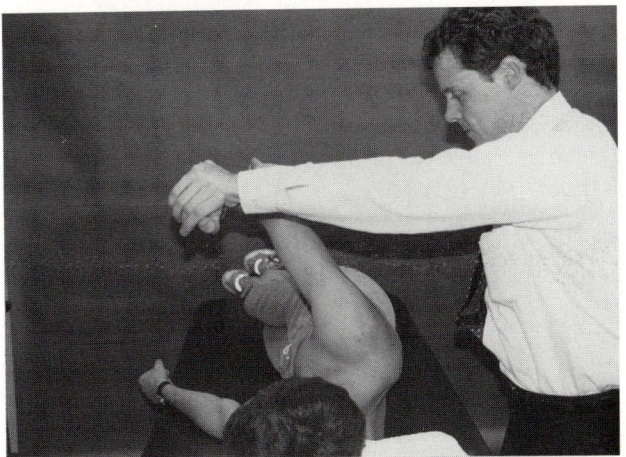

Figure 2 Rhythmic stabilization in POS.

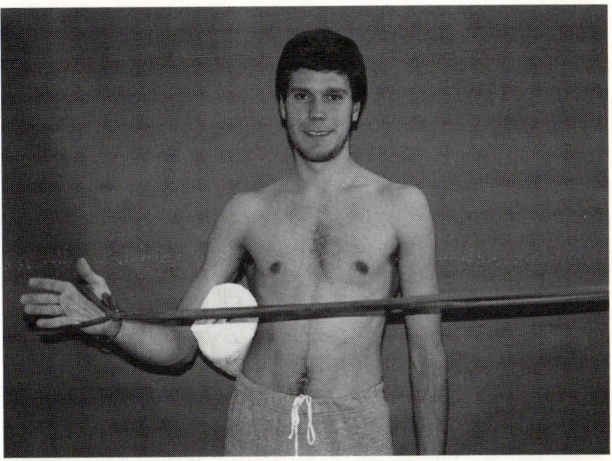

Figure 4 External rotation strengthening with bolster.

is an exceptional technique for regaining dynamic stabilization at different positions of elevation. Once painlessly tolerated, progression of movement toward provocative positions is begun and submaximal resistance through a short-arc of motion is attempted. Short-arc exercises may be achieved by performing rotation in 45 degrees of POS abduction or simple POS abduction. Scapular strengthening is further intensified with emphasis placed on the trapezius and serratus anterior since these muscles are critical to glenohumeral joint function (Fig. 3).

Based on the feedback from manual resistance, appropriate resistance equipment, i.e., elastic bands or light free weight, can be chosen. Adequate strength of the rotator cuff and deltoid can be achieved using light resistance; in fact, the ideal is to increase the repetition to improve muscular endurance. Exercises for the rotator cuff and deltoid are done by rotation, abduction, extension, and flexion then are progressed to combination motions. The scapulothoracic and elbow muscles are also strengthened in combination with the cuff and

deltoid. All too often the elastic band and free-weight exercises are performed incorrectly and/or painfully. Before any motion occurs at the glenohumeral joint the athlete is asked to "set" (slightly retract) the scapula into good anatomic position as opposed to the commonly seen position of protraction. The use of a small bolster, placing the arm in slight abduction, is usually beneficial when performing the rotational exercises; again, this is dependent on pathology and reactivity (Fig. 4). In the presence of a supraspinatus tendon lesion, placement of the arm in slight abduction slackens the tendon, thereby reducing passive irritating tendon tension. Additionally, restricting external rotation to 30 degrees further minimizes passive supraspinatus tension created by the coracohumeral ligament through its intimate relationship with the supraspinatus.

Phase III

At this phase the athlete should have relatively pain-free end range of motion and is performing a prophylactic stretching program. Manual resistance strengthening is progressed to full range and maximal resistance. Diagonal patterns and specific techniques of applying and sequencing isometrics, concentric and eccentric muscle activity are performed, which is called proprioceptive neuromuscular facilitation (PNF) (Fig. 5). PNF is extremely useful in regaining strength throughout the range but also in assisting in redeveloping glenohumeral joint proprioception, which is compromised following CLLC disruption. Eccentric activity is emphasized, particularly of the posterior cuff muscles since these muscles are subjected to damaging forces in the deceleration phase.

Manual resistive exercises are now applied in sport-specific activities. The pitcher is placed kneeling on his nonlead leg. The clinician can apply resistance at the hand while palpating and encouraging appropriate scapulothoracic motion. As before, treatment using manual resistance allows continued assessment of function. The swimmer is placed prone and dry land strokes are performed. Again, resistance can be applied to desired areas. Modifying shoulder position to replicate functional activities is useful when using the elastic bands and free weights.

Weight training using variable resistive devices or barbells are started with the same nonprovocative to provocative philosophy. Usually if the athlete has rotator cuff or CLLC pathology, loading the shoulder in the abducted/externally rotated position is avoided, particularly military press and behind-the-neck lat pull downs. These exercises may be modified to the POS.

Further endurance training is encouraged on the Upper Body Ergometer (UBE) or rowing ergometer. The UBE is commonly misused at the patient's expense because clinicians blindly follow the manufacturer's suggestions. Placing the athlete in a sitting position so that the machine's rotation axis is level with the glenohumeral joint requires the athlete to repetitively cycle against resistance in the impingement zone. The prudent clinician initially has the athlete perform the exercise in standing position (Fig. 6) to avoid the potential rotator cuff trauma; eventually the sitting position is used. Both the forward and backward direction are performed.

Another device found useful in strengthening, optimizing dynamic control, and endurance training is the Bodyblade® (Hymanson Inc., Playa Del Ray, Calif.) (Fig. 7). Small to large oscillations of a fiberglass rod are performed in multiple positions and various time intervals. Oscillating the blade requires short excursion, high-speed cocontraction muscle activity, particularly of the rotator cuff. Therefore, dynamic stabilizing training is achieved uniquely from other forms of exercise.

Isokinetic activity may be initiated for the glenohumeral rotators, both the short rotator cuff muscles and also the larger muscles, i.e., pectoralis major and latissimus. Because isokinetic dynamometers provide a

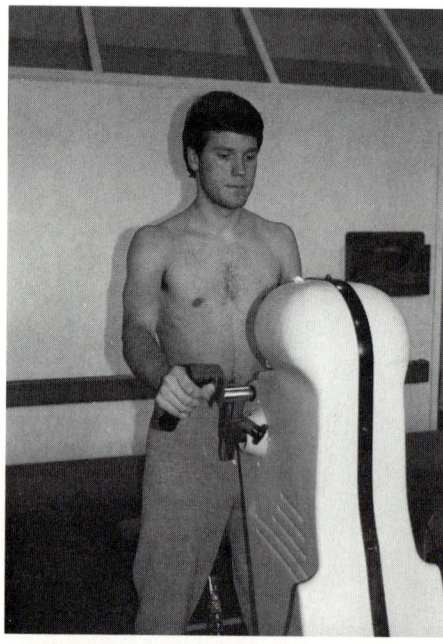

Figure 6 UBE in standing.

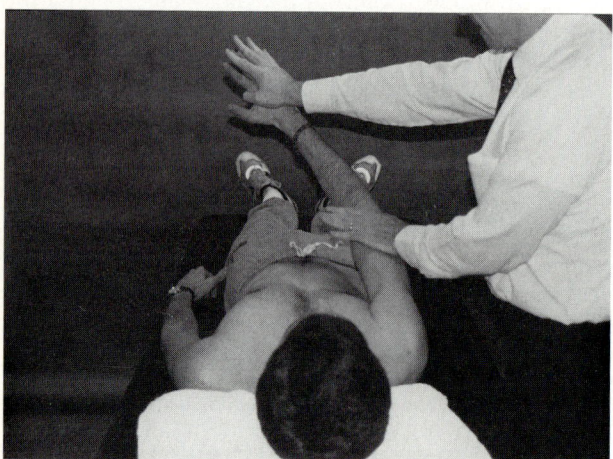

Figure 5 Eccentric strengthening of external rotators in a diagonal pattern similair to deceleration phase of throwing.

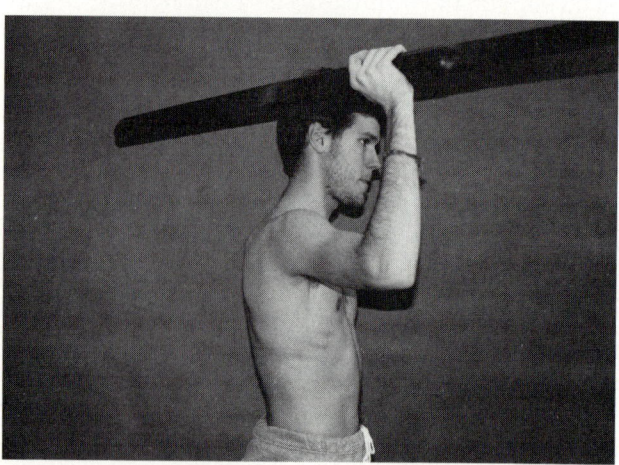

Figure 7 Strengthening with Bodyblade® in sport-specific position.

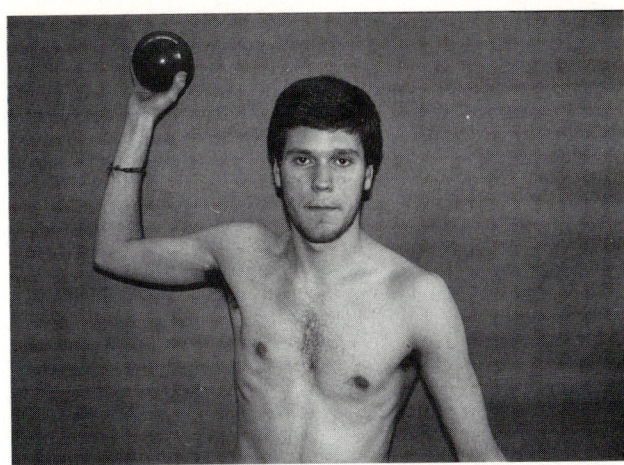

Figure 8 Plyometric training.

constant speed, maximal resistance can be achieved throughout the exercised range. Adequate dynamic stabilization and negligible myotendinous reactivity are a prerequisite to this mode of muscle strengthening. Usually speeds of 120 to 240 degrees/sec are used. Lower speeds result in increased concentric torque, however, an inverse effect occurs during eccentric activity, i.e., higher speeds-higher torque. Because of the potentially high torque produced the athlete is initially placed in the POS and progressed to the provocative cocking position.

Plyometric training using weighted balls has gained favor in shoulder rehabilitation since the physiologic stretch-shortening cycle of muscle can be replicated in sport-specific shoulder positions (Fig. 8). By catching and/or throwing a weighted ball (2 to 10 lbs) the adductors/internal rotators are eccentrically loaded, thus stretched, followed by a concentric shortening phase. These exercises appear to enhance muscle performance by neuromuscular control.

Phase IV

This is the phase when the athlete actually returns to his or her sport in a gradual manner. Regardless of the sport the athlete is allowed an accommodating entrance into the competitive sport. The pitcher performs an interval throwing program, the tennis player begins with forehands to backhands, while the swimmer performs low intensity interval training.

SUGGESTED READING

Clark JC, Harryman DT. Tendons, ligaments, and capsule of the rotator cuff. J Bone Joint Surg 1992; 74A:713.

Clark JC, Sidles JR, Matzen FA, III. The relationship of the glenohumeral joint capsule to the rotator cuff. Clin Orthop 1990; 254:29.

Ellman H, Hanker G, Bayer M. Repair of the rotator cuff: end-result study of factors influencing reconstruction. J Bone Joint Surg 1986; 68A:1136-1144.

Fleisig GS, Dillman CL, Andrews JR. A biomechanical description of the shoulder joint during pitching. Sports Med (Update) Fall/Winter 1991.

Johnston TB. The movements of the shoulder joint. A plea for the use of the "Plane of the Scapula" as the plane of reference in movements occurring at the humero-scapular joint. Br J Surg 1937; 25:252.

Kuhlman JR, Iannotti JP, Kelley MJ, et al. Isokinetic and isometric measurement of strength of external rotation and abduction of the shoulder. J Bone Joint Surg 1992; 74A:1320.

Matzen FA, Thomas SC, Rockwood CA. Anterior glenohumeral instability: the shoulder. In: Rockwood CA, Matzen FA, eds: Philadelphia: WB Saunders, 1990.

Meister K, Andrews. Classification and treatment of rotator cuff injuries in the overhead athlete. J Orthop Sports Phys Ther 1993; 18:413-421.

Neer CS II. Impingement lesions. Clin Orthop 1973; 173:70-77.

Nuber GW, Jobe FW, Perry JP, et al. Fine wire EMG analysis of the shoulder during swimming. Am J Sport Med 1986; 14:7.

O'Brien SJ, Neves MC, Arnoczky SP, et al. The anatomy and histology of the inferior glenohumeral ligament complex of the shoulder. Am J Sports Med 1990; 18:449-456.

Pappas AM, Zawacki RM, Sullivan TJ. Biomechanics of baseball pitching. Am J Sports Med 1985; 13:216-222.

Perry J. Anatomy and biomechanics of the shoulder in throwing, swimming, gymnastics and tennis. Clin Sports Med 1983; 2:247-270.

Sillman JF, Hawkins RJ. Current concepts and recent advances in the athlete's shoulder. Clin Sports Med 1991; 10:693-706.

Walch G, Boileau P, Noel E, Donell T. Impingement of the deep surface of the supraspinatus tendon on the posterior glenoid rim: An arthroscopic study. J Should Elbow Surg 1992; 1:239.

ANKLE SPRAIN: NONOPERATIVE MANAGEMENT

JOSEPH J. VEGSO, M.S., A.T.C.

It is a well-accepted fact that the ankle is the most frequently injured joint in athletes, representing 10% to 30% of all injuries. Although the incidence of injury to the ankle is high, relatively few patients come to surgery. This chapter presents an approach to nonoperative management of ankle injuries.

An accurate diagnosis is the obvious first step in the management of any ankle sprain. The standard grading system of I, II, and III is appropriate in defining the extent of ligamentous instability. In addition, a functional clinical grading system (Table 1) to supplement the instability classification has proved extremely helpful in instituting an appropriate course of treatment.

Grade III injuries in most situations are considered surgical problems, so this chapter focuses on grades I and II.

The ankle is an inherently stable joint: non-weight-bearing treatment is rarely appropriate and in fact may be detrimental. The common emergency room plan of crutches, Ace wrap, and advice to "stay off it for a while" may prolong the symptoms. The foot is held in the plantar flexed-inverted position, which places the injured ligaments under tension in an elongated position, and the foot is in a dependent position without the benefit of muscle action to increase venous and lymphatic return. Heat is also routinely prescribed after 24 hours, which by increasing the amount of swelling delays healing. One must be primarily concerned with the prevention of swelling in soft tissue injuries because increased swelling is directly related to loss of range of motion and an increase in recovery time. Therefore, heat should never be used in the acute or subacute phases of recovery. Individuals charged with the care of ankle injuries should not only encourage the use of ice but also strongly discourage the use of heat.

The appropriate initial treatment regimen consists of ice, compression, and elevation; this is easily recalled by the mnemonic "ICE" as mentioned by Brown. The use of cold in the acute and subacute stages of healing

Table 1 Functional Clinical Grading System for Ankle Sprains

Grade I	Minimal pain and swelling
	Stable joint
	Full range of motion
	Pain-free weight bearing
	Heel and toe walking
Grade II	Moderate pain and swelling
	Subtle joint or minimal anterior drawer
	Decreased range of motion
	Difficulty in weightbearing and ambulation
Grade III	Severe pain and swelling
	Unstable joint
	Minimal range of motion or inability to flex dorsally
	Inability to bear weight

in athletic injuries is well documented by Kalenak and colleagues and McMaster.

Physiologically, cold causes vasoconstriction, thereby decreasing blood flow and hemorrhage, with a resulting decrease of edema. Additionally, cold acts as a local anesthetic, which aids in the control of pain and secondarily to relieve muscle spasm. Ice is contraindicated for individuals with rheumatic conditions, decreased sensation, or vascular problems.

Frequently, grade II and even grade I sprains develop effusions that require aspiration, often of up to 5 ml of synovial fluid or blood. In addition to the aspiration, a single injection of a corticosteroid such as Kenalog-10 (triamcinolone acetonide) into the joint has been found to be extremely effective in controlling the inflammatory response.

IMMOBILIZATION

The need for support or immobilization is dependent on the individual's ability to bear weight. In cases of mild disability the individual is best supported by an adhesive strapping, an open Gibney in the acute stage followed by a closed Gibney boot.

The open Gibney is used to support the lateral and medial structures of the joint. However, it also allows freedom of movement in plantar flexion and dorsiflexion. It is left open along the dorsal aspect of the foot and ankle to allow normal circulation. The closed Gibney provides the same lateral and medial support, but is used in the subacute stage once edema and hemorrhage have begun to subside.

In individuals who require slightly more rigid support, an Unna boot made of Dome-Paste bandage is utilized. The Dome-Paste bandage is made of 3- or 4-inch wide gauze impregnated with a mixture of of zinc oxide and calamine. It is applied like an elastic bandage directly to the skin, with an elastic wrap over it. The bandage becomes semirigid within 24 hours and may be left on for 7 to 10 days. Weightbearing is permissible. This method of support is an ideal compromise between an adhesive strapping and a rigid cast. Crutches may be used to allow partial weight bearing with either method of support.

Rigid casting is reserved for individuals who are unable to bear weight following a grade II injury. Typically, a short-leg weight-bearing cast is applied for 1 to 3 weeks. When a rigid cast is used the foot must be placed as much in dorsiflexion and eversion as possible. During cast immobilization, strength in the upper leg and hip of the injured limb will decrease. Therefore, an exercise program designed to maintain strength must be instituted.

It is important to remember that cold therapy can and should be continued while the ankle is immobilized. Cold will penetrate tape, Dome-Paste, and plaster or fiberglass casts.

REHABILITATION

Ankle injuries are too often inadequately rehabilitated. Allman states that "the susceptibility of the ankle to ligamentous injury in athletics necessitates complete rehabilitation following surgery . . . and inadequately treated or poorly rehabilitated ankle injuries often result in instability." "On the other hand," says Klafs and Arnheim, "many sports physicians and trainers maintain that the best method is the moderately active approach, in which the athlete returns to competition much sooner than with the conservative treatment and completes his therapy through activity." Such is the dilemma facing the physician called upon to treat an athlete with an ankle injury.

Adequate healing must be guaranteed before the athlete may return to activity, and such activity must be without limitation in order that the individual may function safely and effectively. Therefore, a program with time constraints that meet these two objectives is warranted.

An accurate diagnosis followed by appropriate first aid are significant steps in the rehabilitation process. Standard first aid after ankle sprains includes ice, compression, and elevation simultaneously for 20 to 30 minutes. This procedure should be repeated four to six times daily for 48 to 72 hours. It is the author's opinion that heat should never be used as an independent modality in the treatment of ankle sprains.

Overnight treatment should consist of repeated cold therapy, in conjunction with an open Gibney strapping,

a soft foam horseshoe, and a loosely applied elastic bandage. The athlete should also be placed on crutches with instructions to bear as much weight as pain and range of motion permit. It is better to have athletes ambulate in a normal gait pattern with crutches than to allow them to limp. A ¼- to ⅜-inch heel lift often permits athletes to ambulate more comfortably in the acute stage. The open Gibney strapping procedure should be continued as long as the possibility of further swelling exists, usually for 48 to 72 hours. Crutch-assisted ambulation should continue until pain-free, normal ambulation is possible. Treatment protocols for ankle sprains by grade are outlined in Table 2.

Range-of-motion exercises for dorsiflexion may be initiated within 24 hours, depending on the severity of the injury. This should be done actively or in an active-assisted manner by having partial body weight provide the assistance, as shown in Figure 1A. A wedge board may also be used to perform this exercise (Fig. 1B). Calf stretching is also permitted as tolerated. Plantar flexion, inversion, and eversion should be avoided in the early treatment phase in order to permit healing.

It is important that non-weight-bearing activities designed to maintain strength and cardiorespiratory conditioning be implemented during the early phases of rehabilitation. Suggested activities include strength training on equipment such as Nautilus or Universal Gym, any other strength training equipment that does not require weight bearing, and swimming or arm cycling on a stationary bicycle.

Once swelling is controlled or begins to subside and the athlete is able to ambulate pain free, the second phase of the rehabilitation program may be initiated. This may begin as early as 24 to 48 hours after injury. Again, the time frame is dependent on the severity of the

Table 2 Treatment Protocol of Ankle Sprains by Grade

Grade I
 Accurate diagnosis
 ICE* (4 to 6 times daily)
 Aspiration and/or injection
 Taping or Unna boot for support or immobilization
  (3 to 5 days)
 Cardiorespiratory conditioning and total body strengthening
 Agility and functional activities

Grade II
 Accurate diagnosis
 ICE* (4 to 6 times daily)
 Aspiration and/or injection
 Unna boot or cast (1 to 3 weeks)
 Cardiorespiratory conditioning and total body strengthening
 Range of motion and strengthening exercises
 Agility and functional activities

Grade III
 Accurate diagnosis
 Surgical repair
 Cardiorespiratory conditioning and total body strengthening
 Range of motion and strength
 Agility and functional exercises

*Ice, compression, elevation.

injury. Ice treatments should continue as described previously. Support of the injured ankle for all nonathletic activities should be continued if necessary during this phase. This is best accomplished through the use of a loosely applied, closed Gibney strapping, which should be worn during all waking hours. If it is possible to have the ankle restrapped every day, the strapping should be removed and replaced by a loose-fitting elastic wrap overnight. If this is not possible, the strapping should remain on the ankle 24 hours a day for up to 3 days. However, the athlete must be cautioned with regard to possible tingling, numbness, blue toes, or constant, severe itching. Any of these signs warrant immediate removal of the tape.

Exercises in phase 2 are utilized to increase uniplane range of motion at the ankle joint and muscle strength in the lower leg. Exercises to increase plantar flexion are added to those performed in phase 1. Activities that would cause excessive inversion and eversion must still be avoided.

Toe raises are performed to increase strength in the posterior muscle group. They should be done on a wedge board, stool, or step so that the muscles work through a full range of motion. Heel and toe walking are also performed to improve muscular strength and endurance and neuromuscular function. The position of the feet should be changed so that they are inverted and everted while the heel and toe walking are performed. Dorsiflexion, inversion, and eversion strength can be increased through the use of surgical tubing, manual resistance, or isometric exercises at various angles.

A variety of other methods are employed to increase range of motion, strength, and muscular endurance of the ankle. The Elgin Ankle Exerciser and the Cybex II have proved extremely effective in rehabilitating injured ankles.

REINJURY

The most common reason for chronic pain and reinjury following an ankle sprain, in my experience, is decreased dorsiflexion. A simple method for determining whether an athlete has decreased motion is as follows: First, have the athlete place both feet (without shoes) on the floor, hip width apart and parallel. Next, instruct the athlete to bend both knees and both ankles while keeping the feet flat on the floor. Then, observe for a difference in motion. This test is an excellent indicator of the need for continuing or reinstituting a rehabilitation program.

Fiore and Leard, Freeman and colleagues, and others emphasize the importance of proprioceptive and neuromuscular function of the ankle joint. This aspect of rehabilitation is left to chance when the athlete is permitted to return to participation before functional, multiplane, and high-speed activities are incorporated into the rehabilitation program. Allowing this important aspect of rehabilitation to take place in the uncontrolled environment of practice or competition needlessly subjects the athlete to reinjury. It is therefore recommended

Table 3 Agility and Proprioceptive Activities

Heel and toe walking
Wobble board
Rope skipping
Straight ahead jogging
Straight ahead running
Backward running
Running circles: clockwise, counterclockwise, backward, and
    forward (5-yard diameter)
90-degree cuts while running
Running figure eights
Other sports-specific agility and skill activities

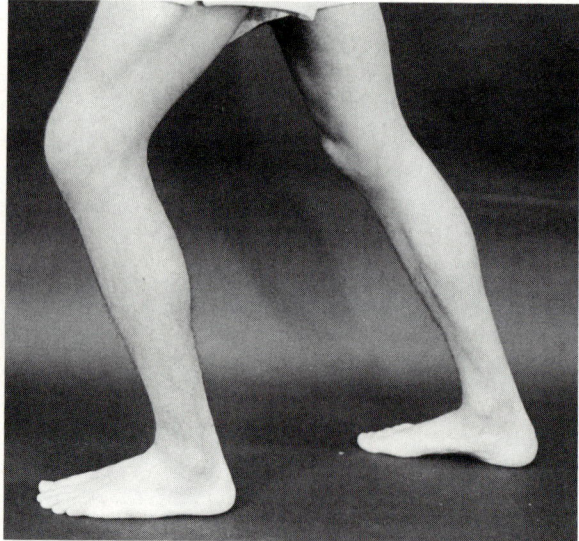
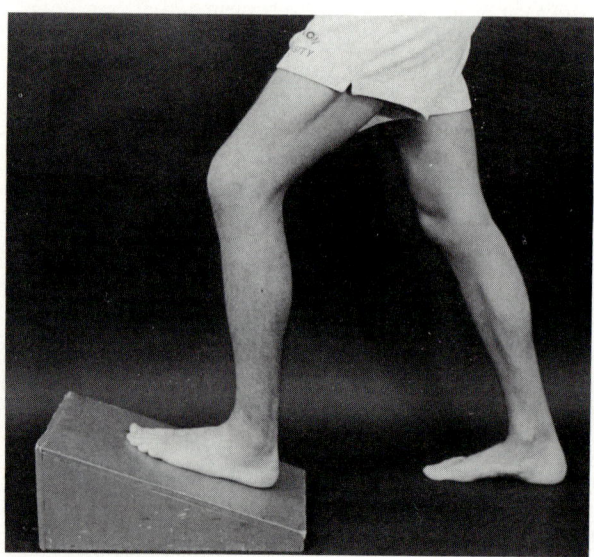

Figure 1 *A,* Ankle range of motion (dorsiflexion) is shown. The left ankle and the knee are flexed, and the foot is flat on the floor. *B,* Ankle range of motion on a wedge board (dorsiflexion) is shown. The left ankle and knee are flexed.

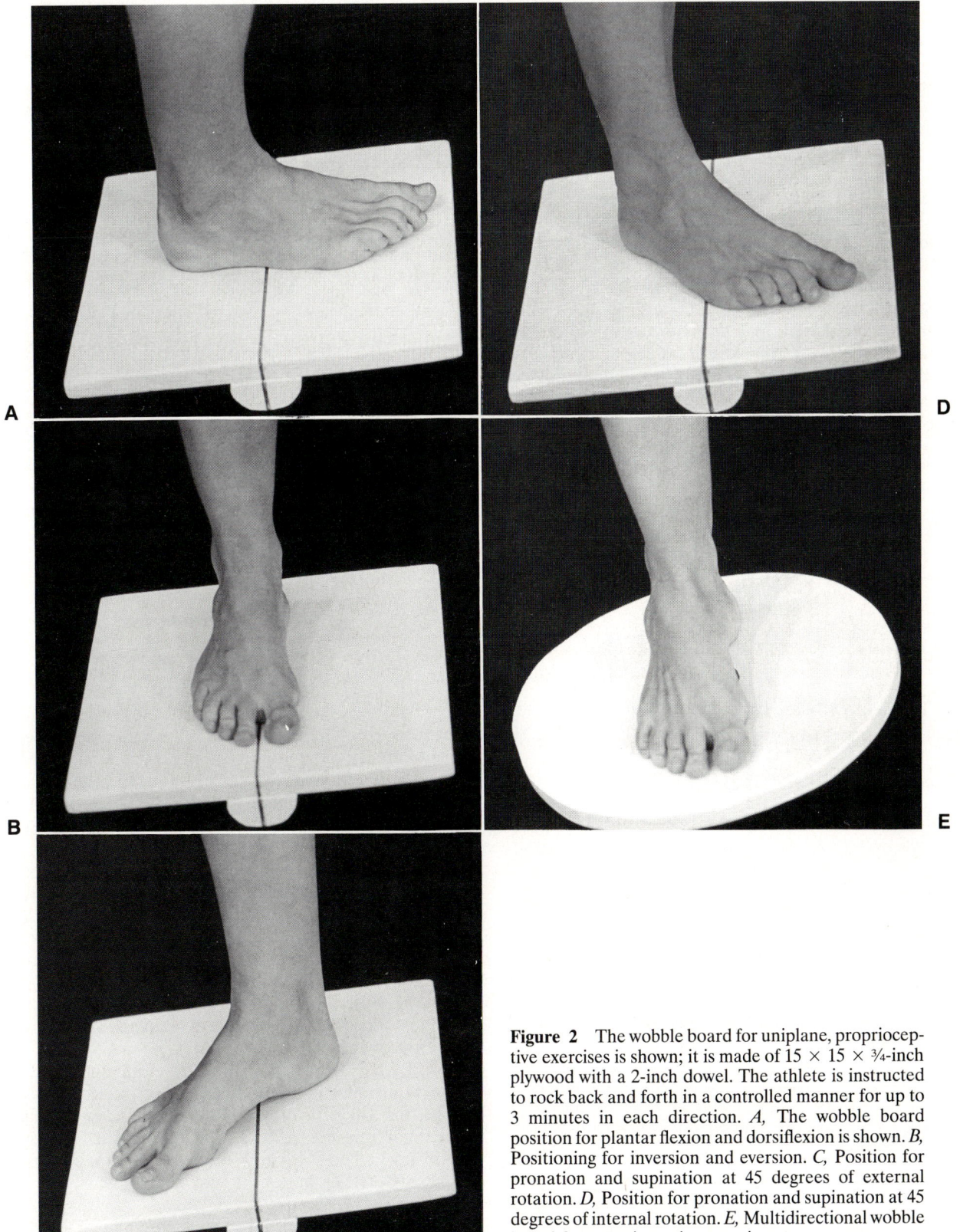

Figure 2 The wobble board for uniplane, proprioceptive exercises is shown; it is made of 15 × 15 × ¾-inch plywood with a 2-inch dowel. The athlete is instructed to rock back and forth in a controlled manner for up to 3 minutes in each direction. *A,* The wobble board position for plantar flexion and dorsiflexion is shown. *B,* Positioning for inversion and eversion. *C,* Position for pronation and supination at 45 degrees of external rotation. *D,* Position for pronation and supination at 45 degrees of internal rotation. *E,* Multidirectional wobble board for proprioceptive exercises.

that activities such as those listed in Table 3 should be used to redevelop proprioceptive and neuromuscular functions and to determine the athlete's ability to perform at a level necessary to return to activity safely (Fig. 2). The ankle should be supported with an adhesive strapping for these activities.

Once athletes are capable of performing all their sports-specific activities to the physician's, athletic trainer's, and coach's satisfaction, they are permitted to return to participation. An adhesive strapping should be used for participation following injury and should be continued throughout the season.

It is difficult and unwise to put time constraints on the rate of recovery or specific aspects of recovery. One may find that an athlete who suffers a grade I inversion sprain progresses through the entire rehabilitation program in 3 days; conversely, a nonsurgical grade II or greater inversion sprain may take up to 8 weeks before complete recovery is achieved. It seems, therefore, that a combination of the approaches recommended by Allman and by Klafs and Arnheim is appropriate. Emphasis should be placed on early and continued use of ice, the return to full range of motion, and the inclusion of activities designed to reintegrate neuromuscular function.

SUGGESTED READING

Allman FL. Rehabilitation following athletic injuries. In: O'Donoghue D, ed. Treatment of injuries to athletes. 4th ed. Philadelphia: WB Saunders, 1984.

Arnheim DD, Prentice WE. Principles of athletic training. 8th ed. St. Louis: Mosby-Year Book, 1993.

Blyth CS, Mueller, FO. An epidemiologic study of high school football injuries in North Carolina 1968-1972. Final report. Washington, DC: Consumer Products Safety Commission.

Brown A. Physical medicine in rehabilitation. Md State Med J 1970; 19:61.

Fiore RD, Leard JS. A functional approach in the rehabilitation of the ankle and rear foot. Athl Train 1980; 231-235.

Freeman MA, et al. The etiology and prevention of functional instability of the foot. J Bone Joint Surg 1965; 47B:678.

Garrick JG. The frequency of injury, mechanism of injury and epidemiology of ankle sprains. Am J Sports Med 1977; 5:241.

Jackson DW, Ashley RL, Powell, JW. Ankle sprains in young athletes—relation of severity and disability. Clin Orthop 1974; 101:201.

Kalenak A, et al. Athletic injuries: heat vs. cold. Am Fam Physician 1975; 12:131.

Mack RP. Ankle injuries in athletics. Athl Train 1975; 10:94.

McMaster WC. A literary review of ice therapy on injuries. Am J Sports Med 1977; 5:124.

Stanford Research Institute: National Football League 1974 Injury Study. Menlo Park, CA, June 1975.

LATERAL ANKLE RECONSTRUCTION FOR CHRONIC INSTABILITY

GEORGE A. SNOOK, M.D.

Chronic lateral ligament instability of the ankle is a condition resulting from inadequate healing of tears of the lateral ligaments of the ankle, specifically the anterior talofibular ligament (ATFL) and the calcaneofibular ligament (CFL). The situation arises because of the anatomic characteristics of the ankle and a casual attitude toward treatment of the original sprain.

ANATOMY—MECHANISM OF INJURY

The ankle is an inherently stable joint with support provided by the bony buttresses of the medial and lateral malleoli and the medial and lateral collateral ligaments. The support, however, is unequal, since the medial malleolus is short and does not completely embrace the talus, while the longer lateral malleolus extends to the subtalar joint. The opposite is true of the ligaments, since the medial collateral ligament is the wide, strong deltoid ligament, while the lateral collateral ligament consists of three thin, well-spaced bands: the ATFL, the CFL, and the posterior talofibular ligament (PTFL). The PTFL provides little or no support for varus instability of the ankle.

A varus force applied to the ankle, therefore, is resisted by the short medial malleolus and the relatively weak lateral ligaments. If the force is severe enough, the foot rolls over the medial malleolus and the ligaments rupture. A valgus force, on the other hand, is resisted by the larger lateral malleolus and the stronger deltoid ligament. If the force is too great in this direction a more serious fracture of the lateral malleolus occurs with rupture of the deltoid ligament.

The basic problem in the development of chronic lateral instability of the ankle is that, unlike the knee joint, the ankle is an inherently stable joint because of the bony supports. After a severe sprain the foot returns to its normal position and some healing of the ligaments takes place. The patient is soon able to walk, but if the joint is not protected the ligaments are subjected to constant motion and stretching, and they either heal elongated or are replaced with a mass of scar tissue. With the loss of integrity of the ligament supports, the ankle becomes unstable and subject to recurrent sprains.

DIAGNOSIS

The history usually is relatively simple. The patient complains of repeated sprains of the ankle, usually initiated by a major sprain on the first occasion. There is apprehension when walking on an uneven surface, and there are occasional sprains even on level terrain or when stepping off a curb.

The physical examination findings may be innocuous depending on the duration of time since the last injury. There may be tenderness over the ATFL. The most constant sign is a positive anterior drawer sign tested when the patient has no pain or tenderness. It is performed with the patient seated on an examining table and the knee flexed at 90 degrees. The lower leg is stabilized with one hand while the other hand grasps the foot at the heel and midfoot. With the foot at a right angle, it is drawn forward. A greater excursion in the injured ankle than in the normal ankle represents a positive anterior drawer test.

Roentgenograms should be taken, especially to determine the presence or absence of osteoarthritis or loose bodies.

Stress roentgenograms may be helpful when compared with similar films of the uninjured side. These must be considered only as an aid, because the results are variable and much depends on the position of the ligaments. The ATFL and the CFL form an arc. This arc makes the CFL the primary restraint when the ankle is at a right angle, while the ATFL is the primary restraint with the foot in plantar flexion. The ATFL is always torn in these injuries, while the CFL is torn in 20% to 90% of injuries depending on the investigator. Thus, stress roentgenograms may show normal results with the foot at a right angle, while the anterior drawer sign should always be positive.

The differential diagnosis should include neuromuscular weakness, osteoarthritis, loose bodies, and the impingement syndrome. This syndrome results from recurrent trauma to the joint capsule, synovial membrane, and articular cartilage. It can give the same clinical picture as recurrent ligament sprains, except that the anterior drawer sign is negative. Magnetic resonance imaging of the ankle may be of great assistance in making this diagnosis.

NONSURGICAL TREATMENT

Nonsurgical treatment of this condition consists of support, muscle strengthening, and development of position sense. Strengthening of the peroneal muscles is essential to this treatment regimen. This can be performed by resistance exercise of the ankle against rubber bands in abduction and plantar flexion. Development of position sense and protective reflexes can be done on a roller board or tilt table. The simplest form of support is a ¼-inch outer heel wedge in the shoe, which can be quite valuable on even surfaces although useless on uneven ground.

Although taping or ankle wraps can be used for athletic contests, they are not practical for everyday wear. Various types of laced or Velcro-fastened supports are available commercially.

SURGICAL TREATMENT

Surgical treatment is directed toward restoring stability to the lateral ankle while retaining a full range of motion to the joint.

Two types of procedures are currently in use: a direct repair of the ATFL as advocated by Brostrom and a replacement of the lateral ligaments by a tendinous substitute. The latter procedure can be further divided into those procedures that replace only the ATFL and those that replace both the ATFL and the CFL.

The repair procedure is the simplest of these operations: it does not sacrifice tendons and uses a smaller incision. When successful, it restores the normal anatomy. The author finds, however, that separating the ligament from the mass of scar tissue is not easy, and in very old cases the ligament is too short to repair and the surgeon is repairing only scar tissue. A second objection is that it does not solve the problem of the CFL. This operation is preferable for patients whose injury is no more than 6 months old.

There are a variety of reconstruction operations in current use. All of them use a portion or the whole of a tendon to replace the function of the injured ligaments. The peroneus brevis is the one most commonly used. Most of these operations replace the ATFL, and a few replace both ligaments.

I prefer the Chrisman-Snook procedure, which utilizes one-half of the peroneus brevis tendon and effectively replaces both the ATFL and the CFL.

Procedure

With the patient in the lateral position and the affected ankle uppermost, an incision is made starting at the base of the fifth metatarsal and extending proximally in a curved manner behind the lateral malleolus and up the leg for a distance of about 15 cm. The subcutaneous tissue is divided, hemostasis obtained, and a careful search made for the sural nerve. In most cases it is found alongside the proximal limb of the incision. It is carefully mobilized and retracted. A skin flap retaining the subcutaneous tissue is then mobilized anteriorly to expose the lateral malleolus. The sheaths of the peroneal tendons are opened throughout their length and the tendons mobilized. The peroneus brevis tendon is split longitudinally from its insertion at the fifth metatarsal to the musculotendinous junction. It is best to continue this split up along the tendon fascia that embraces the muscle, to ensure adequate length. One-half of the tendon is then detached proximally but left attached at the insertion. The graft is wrapped in a saline sponge and preserved. A drill hole is placed in the lateral malleolus from front to back at its widest part, starting with a small hole that is gradually enlarged until it is easy to pass the graft through it. Using the same drill bit that was

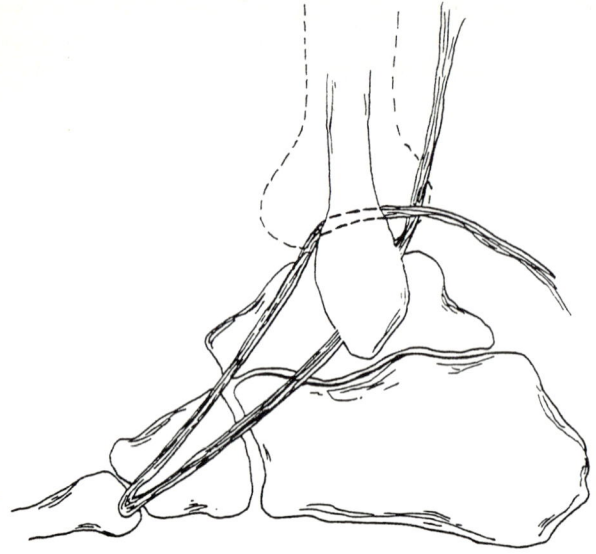

Figure 1 The free end of the divided peroneus brevis is passed through a drill hole in the distal fibula.

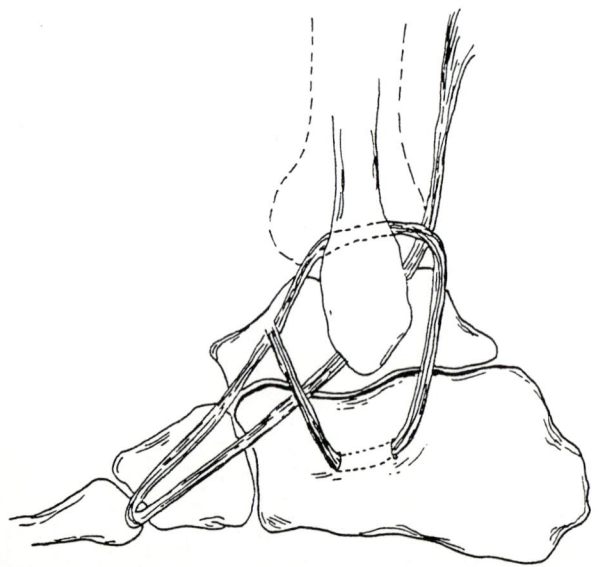

Figure 2 The free end of the tendon of the peroneus brevis is passed through a drill hole in the lateral wall of the os calcis and sewn back to itself to complete the ligament repair.

employed in the lateral malleolus, a tunnel is created on the lateral side of the os calcis just below the peroneal trochlea. This is done by making two holes in a "V" direction about 1 cm apart and then enlarging the holes with a curet.

The graft is next passed through the malleolar hole from front to back (Fig. 1). The foot is held in a neutral position while a tacking stitch is placed through the graft and periosteum to maintain the foot in this position against gravity. The peroneal tendons are replaced in their grooves, and the graft is brought inferiorly and through the os calcis tunnel and then proximally to be sutured to itself just in front of the lateral malleolus (Fig.

2). The ankle should be held in maximal dorsiflexion when anchoring the graft to itself.

The peroneal sheath is next closed behind the lateral malleolus to guard against subsequent subluxation of the peroneal tendons. The sural nerve is replaced and the wound closed.

POSTOPERATIVE CARE

A short-leg walking cast is applied in the operating room and ambulation is allowed on the cast as the patient may tolerate. At the end of 3 weeks, the cast is changed, the sutures removed, and a second walking cast is applied for 3 more weeks. This cast is then removed and the patient is started on an active exercise program.

Crutches are used for external support for as long as needed, usually 2 days to 1 week.

Range of motion in plantar flexion and eversion return rapidly. Dorsiflexion will return soon afterwards, but it may take several months before the final limit of inversion is reached. There may be slight loss of full inversion, but seldom more than 10 degrees. Physical therapy with whirlpool and joint mobilization can be helpful in regaining motion.

COMPLICATIONS

Aside from the complications common to any lower extremity operation (infection, thrombophlebitis), the patient should be warned about the risk of sural nerve neuritis and possible division of the nerve producing diminished or absent sensation along the lateral border of the foot. Neuritis is usually transient, and except for the rare tender neuroma the loss of sensation has not been troublesome to those few patients who have experienced it.

The incision just behind and below the lateral malleolus is apt to heal slower than the rest of the incision, and therefore the skin sutures should remain in place for 3 weeks.

One must be careful not to evert the ankle forcefully when performing the reconstruction, otherwise the patient may have trouble regaining inversion. Some athletes have experienced difficulty with a loss of dorsiflexion caused by making the second and third limbs of the reconstruction too tight. This can be prevented by placing the foot in maximal dorsiflexion and neutral rotation when suturing the third limb to the first at the last stage of the operation. This complication can be corrected by a Z-plasty lengthening of the second and third limbs of the graft.

RESULTS

In a long-term follow-up (4 to 24 years) of 48 operations, all but three patients had good or excellent results. The two patients with fair and the one with poor results experienced severe reinjury of the ankle with presumed damage to the reconstruction.

SUGGESTED READING

Brostrom L. Sprained ankles. III. Clinical observations in recent ligament injuries. Acta Chir Scand 1965; 130:560–569.

Cox JS, Hewes TF. "Normal" talar tilt angle. Clin Orthop 1979; 140:37–41.

Evans DL. Recurrent dislocation of the ankle. A method of surgical treatment. Proc R Soc Med 1953; 46:343–348.

Mandelbaum BR, Bartolozzi AR, Finerman GA, et al. The anterior capsular impingement syndrome in the ankle of the athlete: methods of diagnosis and treatment. Paper presented at the 13th Annual Meeting of the American Orthopedic Society for Sports Medicine, Orlando, FL, June 29, 1987.

Rubin G, Witten M. The talar tilt angle and the fibular collateral ligaments. J Bone Joint Surg 1960; 42A:311–326.

Ruth CJ. The surgical treatment of injuries of the fibular collateral ligaments of the ankle. J Bone Joint Surg 1961; 43A:229–239.

St Pierre R, Allman F Jr, Bassett FH III, et al. A review of lateral ankle ligamentous reconstructions. Foot Ankle 1982; 3:114–123.

Snook GA, Chrisman OD, Wilson TC. Long-term results of the Chrisman-Snook operation for reconstruction of the lateral ligaments of the ankle. J Bone Joint Surg 1985; 67A:1–7.

Stormont DM, Morrey BF, Kai-Nan A, Cass JR. Stability of the loaded ankle. Relationship between articular restraint and primary and secondary static restraints. Am J Sports Med 1984; 13:295–300.

SYNDESMOTIC ANKLE SPRAIN

DAVID A. FISCHER, M.D.

Ankle sprains are common in sports. Sprains are always painful and often disabling for the athlete. For the athletic trainer, they represent a large part of their effort on the field, especially during competitions. For the sports medicine practitioner they can be problematic if the sprain is severe, does not respond to typical treatments, or involves complications. Fortunately, most ankle sprains are of the lateral ligaments of the ankle and are relatively benign with little loss of playing time. However, sprains of the tibiofibular syndesmosis and associated connective tissues, although not common, are more serious and frequently prevent the athlete from competing for weeks or longer. It is important for medical personnel to be able to recognize syndesmotic sprains and understand their implications.

My experience with a professional football club indicates that about 60% of all significant ankle sprains involve the lateral ligaments, and the remaining 40% are of the syndesmosis. This proportion of syndesmotic sprains is probably higher than would occur in other sports and in other levels of competition. All of the syndesmotic sprains incurred by the professional football team occurred during games and none in practices, suggesting that the injury requires high energy circumstances not typically associated with a practice situation.

This notion is supported by the observation that syndesmotic sprains occur infrequently in sports with less contact, such as basketball and baseball, and are quite rare among strictly recreational athletes.

The mechanism of injury is not always clearly recalled by the player, and sometimes even game films are inconclusive. However, two mechanisms predominate, both involving forceful external rotation of the ankle. The first occurs when a player is lying on the field with the ankle externally rotated, and another player

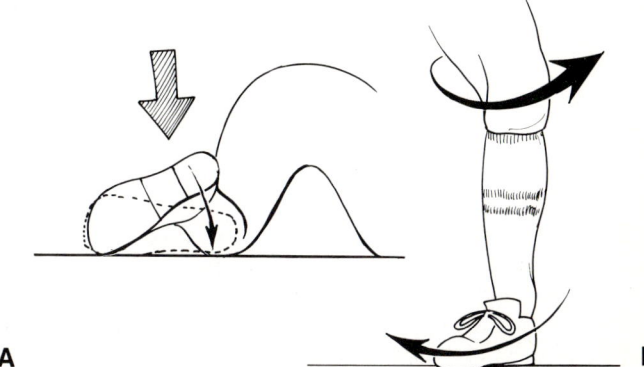

Figure 1 Mechanisms of external rotation sustained during football. *A,* Direct blow to the leg of a downed player whose foot was held in external rotation. *B,* Force applied to the lateral aspect of the knee while the player's foot was planted in external rotation. (From Boytim MJ, Fischer DA, Neumann L. Syndesmotic ankle sprains. Am J Sports Med 1991; 19:294; with permission.)

falls on the back of the leg and heel of the foot, applying a sudden further external rotation without the player's ability to compensate by externally rotating the entire leg at the hip (Fig. 1, *A*). The second mechanism involves a lateral blow to the knee or leg with the foot planted such that further external rotation occurs (Fig. 1, *B*). I believe these mechanisms are similar to those resulting in a Maisonneuve fracture. The first two stages of this soft tissue and fracture complex, as described by Pankovich, result in rupture of the anterior tibiofibular ligament, the interosseous membrane, and either a rupture of the posterior tibiofibular ligament or a fracture of the posterior tibial tubercle. To this extent the injury is a syndesmotic sprain; however, should the external rotation force and displacement continue, a typical Maisonneuve fracture of the proximal fibula can result.

Unfortunately, little can be done to prevent syndesmotic sprains. The nature of a running and cutting sport demands that the ankles not be restrictively braced, thus they must be left somewhat vulnerable to blows such as

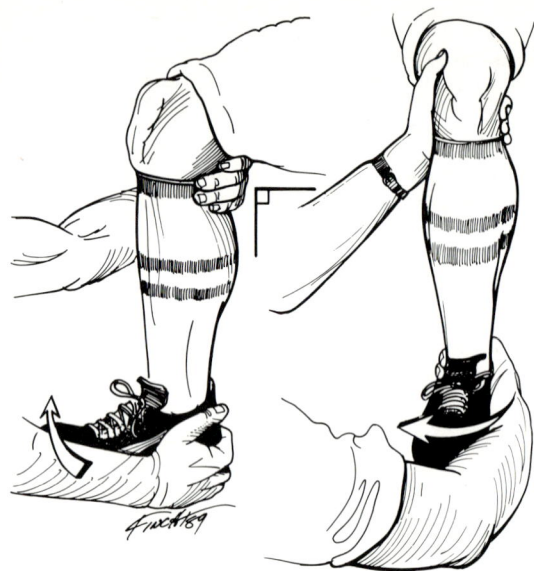

Figure 2 External rotation stress test is applied to the ankle in a neutral position with the knee flexed 90 degrees. (From Boytim MJ, Fischer DA, Neumann L. Syndesmotic ankle sprains. Am J Sports Med 1991; 19:294; with permission.)

those depicted in Figure 1. Also, in the example of football, the mechanisms of injury are inherent to the contact aspect of the sport. Artificial or natural turf has no bearing on the incidence of syndesmotic sprains in football players, nor does the type of shoe that is worn. Additionally, the player's team position does not seem to be a factor.

Since one cannot rely on the athlete to accurately describe the mechanism of the sprain, a diagnostic test that differentiates between lateral ligament ankle sprains and syndesmotic ankle sprains is practical and important. The key in the diagnosis of the syndesmotic sprain is to test for sensitivity to passive external rotation (Fig. 2). Passive external rotation of the foot and ankle will elicit significant pain in a syndesmotic sprain or lateral malleolar fracture. This test does not cause significant pain in even the most severe inversion sprain. A positive test will elicit pain in the anterolateral ankle, extending proximally in the leg for a variable distance. It is not uncommon for the athlete to complain of pain along the anterolateral leg extending 8 to 10 cm proximal to the ankle joint.

In my experience it has been virtually impossible for an athlete to continue competition with a syndesmotic ankle sprain and he or she is removed from play for ice, rest, and further evaluation including roentgenograms. These injuries frequently require 4 to 8 weeks of recovery and sometimes longer. Initial roentgenograms are generally normal with the exception of the avulsion of the posterior tibial tubercle visible on the lateral view.

The ankle joint mortise is generally anatomic and if a widening of the mortise is noted one must be certain that a Maisonneuve fracture of the proximal fibula is not present. Plastic deformation of the fibula without fracture resulting in a widened mortise is rare but does occur. Follow-up roentgenograms typically reveal calcification along the interosseous membrane and in the region of the posterior tibiofibular ligament.

I have found the management of this injury to be exceptionally frustrating. I have been unable to conclusively demonstrate any efficacy in the use of various orthoses, physical therapy modalities, cortisone injections, or braces. Pain associated with the calcification process in the interosseous membrane has been improved by the use of indomethacin, but I am unconvinced that it has, in fact, shortened the athlete's recovery time.

Typically an athlete recovering from this injury reaches a stage where there is little or no significant swelling and the gait is absolutely normal. Despite the normal appearance of the ankle to physical examination and normal function with light physical exercise, the athlete complains of persistent ankle pain with push-off and cutting maneuvers. It is at this point that either the courage of the athlete or the adequacy of the medical care, or both, can be questioned. This is most likely to happen when the diagnosis of a syndesmotic ankle sprain has not been made early, giving opportunity for the medical staff to inform the athlete and appropriate coaching personnel of the seriousness of the injury and the likelihood of a prolonged recovery. It is incumbent upon the sports medicine physician and athletic trainer to be familiar with this injury and its diagnosis.

SUGGESTED READING

Boytim MJ, Fischer DA, Neumann L. Syndesmotic ankle sprains. Am J Sports Med 1991; 19:294.

Edwards GS, DeLee JC. Ankle diastasis without fracture. Foot Ankle 1984; 4:305.

Fritschy D. An unusual ankle injury in top skiers. Am J Sports Med 1989; 17:282.

Guise ER. Rotational ligamentous injuries to the ankle in football. Am J Sports Med 1976; 4:1.

Hopkinson WJ, St Pierre P, Ryan JB, Wheeler JH. Syndesmosis sprains of the ankle. Foot Ankle 1990; 10:325.

Jackson R, Wills RE, Jackson R. Rupture of deltoid ligament without involvement of the lateral ligament. Am J Sports Med 1988; 16:541.

Katznelson AL, Lin E, Militano J. Ruptures of the ligaments about the tibiofibular syndesmosis. Injury 1978; 15:170.

Pankovich AM. Fractures of the fibula proximal to the distal tibiofibular syndesmosis. J Bone Joint Surg 1978; 60A:221.

Pankovich AM. Maisonneuve fracture of the fibula. J Bone Joint Surg 1976; 58A:337.

Taylor DC, Englehardt DL, Bassett FH. Syndesmosis sprains of the ankle. The influence of heterotopic ossification. Am J Sports Med 1992; 20:146.

ANKLE SPRAIN: OPERATIVE MANAGEMENT

CHAMP L. BAKER, M.D.
ANDREW A. BROOKS, M.D.

Ankle sprains are the most common injury in sports. The diagnosis and treatment of these injuries may be undertaken by a variety of health care professionals, such as family practitioners, emergency room physicians, pediatricians, orthopedic surgeons, physical therapists, athletic trainers, and chiropractors. However, despite the frequent occurrence of sprains, potentially serious injuries are frequently misdiagnosed and poorly managed. For some patients, an ankle sprain can lead to significant functional disability manifested by persistent instability and recurrent sprains.

Proper diagnosis and treatment of acute ankle sprains is dependent on the examiner's clear understanding of the ligamentous and muscular anatomy about the ankle.

ANKLE ANATOMY

The lateral side of the ankle has both static and dynamic structures that contribute to its stability. The static stabilizers are the joint capsule and four ligaments.

The capsule is attached to the articular margins of the tibia, fibula, and talus—except at the anterior aspect of the talus, where it is attached in front of the joint margin to the neck of the bone. Posteriorly, the capsule is also attached to the posterior talofibular ligament.

The anterior talofibular ligament is intracapsular and runs forward and almost horizontally between the anterior border of the distal fibula and the lateral neck of the talus. The calcaneofibular ligament is a cord-like extracapsular structure that runs from the inferior aspect of the lateral malleolar fossa and posteriorly to the lateral tubercle of the posterior aspect of the talus. Finally, the lateral talocalcaneal ligament, which crosses the subtalar joint, lies between the anterior talofibular and the calcaneofibular ligaments and blends with both.

The dynamic stabilizers of the lateral side of the ankle consist of the peroneus longus, brevis, and tertius muscles.

The medial ligaments of the ankle are less complex than those of the lateral side. The deltoid ligament is a thick, strong, fan-shaped ligament with a superficial and deep portion. The superficial fibers fan down from the medial malleolus to attach as a continuous sheath to the tarsal bones. The deep portion of the ligament attaches to the undersurface of the medial malleolus near its tip and runs more horizontally than the superficial fibers to attach to the medial surface of the talus.

MECHANISM OF INJURY

Acute lateral ligamentous injuries of the ankle are caused by rotational mechanisms, particularly plantar flexion and inversion. The ankle must be plantar flexed for ligamentous rupture to occur. In this position, the anterior capsule and anterior talofibular ligament are taut. With application of increasing inversion and internal rotation stress, a tear begins anteriorly at the capsule and anterior talofibular ligament and progresses posteriorly with complete or partial rupture of the calcaneofibular ligament. The posterior talofibular ligament is ruptured less often.

DIAGNOSIS

Patients who have lateral ankle sprains sometimes describe a popping or tearing sensation in the ankle at the time of injury. Depending on the severity of the tear, the patient may or may not be able to bear weight on the ankle. Typically patients with two torn ligaments will have difficulty walking.

The main purpose of the physical examination is to determine whether a ligamentous disruption severe enough to cause significant instability has occurred. Although the acutely injured ankle can be extremely difficult to examine, simple inspection can provide a great deal of information about severity of injury. The degree of swelling is usually dictated by the severity of the injury combined with timing of examination. With incomplete tears or minor injuries, symmetrical swelling confined to the ankle joint can be seen. Complete ligamentous disruptions tend to cause more diffuse swelling because the joint capsule is also torn, and the effusion is not well contained. Ecchymosis is usually not present initially. After 24 to 48 hours, the anterior and lateral portions of the ankle may become discolored, appearing blue and yellow secondary to hematoma organization and resorption. This discoloration may extend to the subcutaneous plane to involve the entire lateral side of the foot.

One of the key factors in assessing acute ankle sprains is the site of local tenderness. For example, tenderness under the lateral malleolus usually suggests avulsion of the anterior talofibular ligament from its fibular insertion—an injury of great significance. Local tenderness over the medial aspect of the ankle joint suggests the presence of an osteochondral fracture or a deltoid ligament tear. With a complete ligament tear, there may be a palpable defect along the course of the anterior talofibular ligament or calcaneofibular ligament.

The most important step in the physical examination is the test for instability of the ankle. Both lateral and anterior laxity should be measured. The anterior drawer test and talar tilt test, the two most commonly used to measure ligamentous laxity, should be performed on both ankles for comparison of the normal with the injured ankle.

The anterior drawer test evaluates the competency

of the anterior talofibular ligament. Disruption of this ligament causes abnormal anterior translation of the talus in relation to the tibia and, often, an increased anterior rotational laxity. This anterolateral rotatory instability of the ankle has been said to be analogous to that caused by ligamentous injuries of the knee. The test is usually done with the patient supine, the knee flexed 90 degrees, and the ankle secure on the examining table in 10 to 15 degrees of plantar flexion. This position maintains a lax posterior capsule and allows more specific testing of the anterior stabilizing structures. With one hand the examiner stabilizes the foot, while pushing the distal tibia posteriorly, thus allowing the foot to come forward in relation to the tibia (Fig. 1). Performed in this manner, the test causes minimal discomfort to the patient and is easily reproducible. An alternate method of performing the anterior drawer test is to have the patient sitting with the knee flexed 90 degrees and the ankle in the examiner's lap. The heel is grasped firmly with one hand, and the foot is pulled forward while stabilizing the tibia with the opposite hand. Another way is to stabilize the foot on the examiner's thigh and to push back on the tibia in relation to the fixed foot. This gives a reproducible test that causes minimal discomfort to the patient, particularly in a patient who has an acute injury. A positive anterior drawer test gives a sensation of subluxation of the talus and is indicative of anterior talofibular ligament injury. Occasionally a sulcus, or "suction sign," can be appreciated at the joint line.

The test for lateral instability is the talar tilt, or inversion stress, test. This test assesses damage to the calcaneofibular ligament and secondarily measures the competency of the anterior talofibular ligament. With the patient's leg hanging over the end of the examining table, the test is first done with the ankle at 10 to 15 degrees of plantar flexion and is repeated with the ankle in the neutral position. The patient's heel is cupped with one hand, the tibia is stabilized with the opposite hand, and an attempt is made to invert the talus and calcaneus on the fixed distal tibia (Fig. 2). If increased laxity is detected with the foot and ankle plantar flexed, the ankle must be retested in the neutral position. Laxity in the neutral position is more indicative of a tear of the calcaneofibular ligament. Increased inversion, in comparison with the uninjured ankle, is considered a positive test.

IMAGING STUDIES

Plain radiographs consisting of anteroposterior (AP), lateral, and mortise views are obtained of all acutely injured ankles. It is important to critically evaluate the routine films for avulsion fractures, syndesmotic injuries, and osteochondral injuries, as well as for occult fractures.

If the history and clinical examination demonstrate marked instability, stress radiographs of both ankles may be needed to document that laxity. A lateral anterior drawer stress radiograph is used to detect disruption of the anterior talofibular ligament. The radiograph is made while a posteriorly directed force is applied to the distal tibia either manually or with a commercial

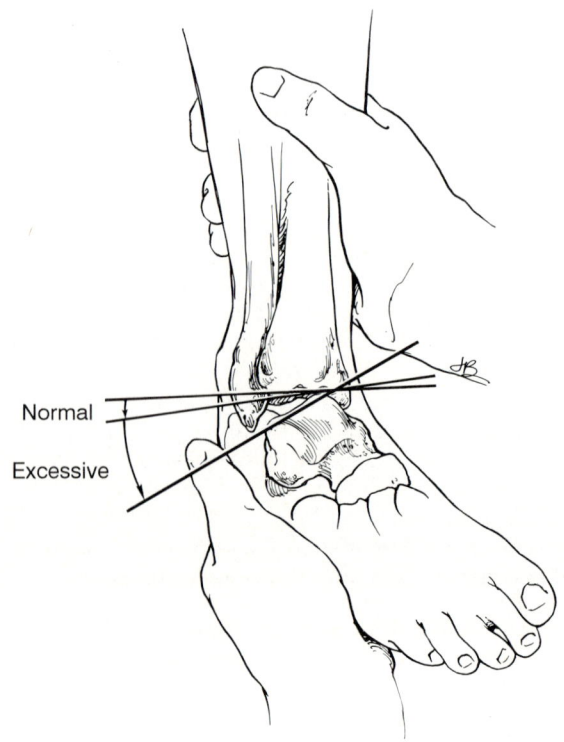

Normal

Excessive

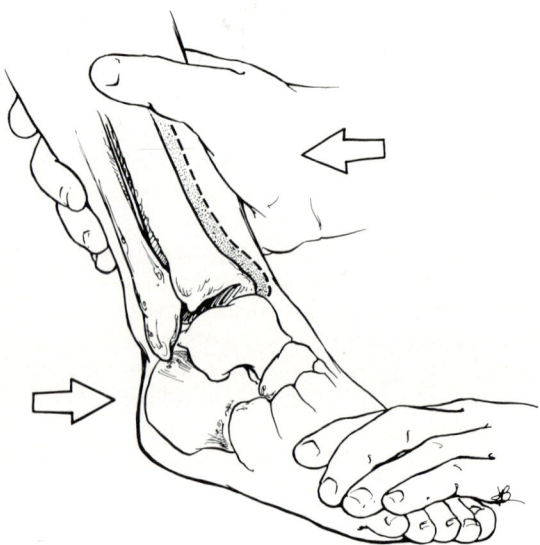

Figure 1 The anterior drawer test is done to detect abnormal anterior translation. With the foot stabilized in one of the examiner's hands, the distal tibia is pushed posteriorly with the other hand.

Figure 2 The talar tilt test is done to detect lateral instability. With one hand cupping the heel and one hand stabilizing the tibia, the examiner tries to invert the talus and calcaneus on the fixed distal tibia to detect excessive motion.

apparatus. A 3 mm side-to-side difference is considered abnormal. AP inversion stress radiographs are obtained to assess talar tilt. Again the stress is usually applied manually, but a commercial apparatus is available. An increase in talar tilt of 10 degrees or greater in the injured ankle over that of the uninjured ankle is considered abnormal and indicative of anterior talofibular ligament and calcaneofibular ligament rupture.

Additional radiologic studies, such as arthrograms, computed tomography (CT) scan, and magnetic resonance imaging (MRI), can be obtained to assess the extent of ligamentous rupture. However, in my experience, a physical examination and stress radiographs are adequate for the evaluation of most ankle sprains. Occasionally, MRI or CT may be warranted if there is a question of injury to surrounding tendons or bone. Ligamentous ruptures can be seen on MRI, but evaluation of the image requires an experienced radiologist or orthopedic surgeon.

CLASSIFICATION OF ANKLE SPRAINS

Ankle injuries are classified as grade I, II, or III. Grade 1 sprains usually involve stretching of the ligament without tearing and exhibit minimal tenderness and no measurable instability. Grade II sprains consist of partial macroscopic tears and are marked by tenderness over the involved structures and some instability. Grade III injuries consist of a complete tear of the lateral ligaments with marked tenderness and swelling (Fig. 3). Moderate laxity is present. More important than classifying ankle injuries by grade is determining whether the ankle is stable or unstable. Ankles that are stable or in which only one ligament is involved are classified as grade I or II and can be treated in a functional manner. Ankles with grade III injuries are unstable and have positive anterior drawer and inversion stress tests. This anterolateral rotatory instability is disabling and surgical repair may be indicated.

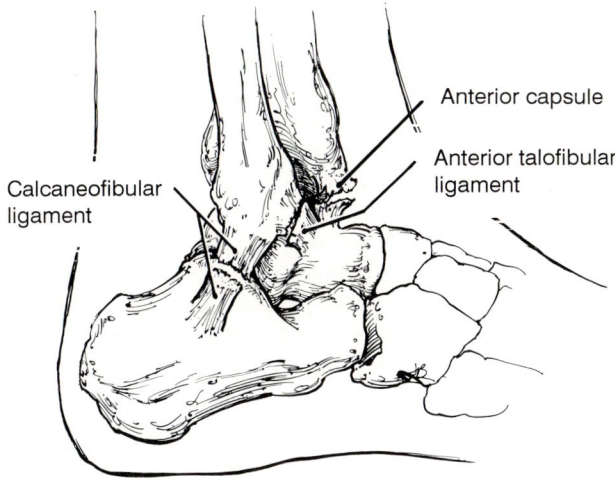

Calcaneofibular ligament

Anterior capsule

Anterior talofibular ligament

Figure 3 A grade III injury involves complete tearing of the lateral ligaments.

TREATMENT

Most physicians agree that grade I and II sprains can be successfully managed nonoperatively. The prognosis for these injuries is uniformly excellent or good. We use a functional treatment program initially consisting of ice, compression, elevation, and rest (RICE). The ankle is immobilized and protected with an off-the-shelf ankle stirrup device. Active range of motion exercises are started early and are followed by weight bearing as tolerated, proprioceptive retraining with a tilt board, and peroneal strengthening exercises.

Operative repair of unstable grade III ankle sprains is recommended in certain well-defined situations. Broström felt "primary surgical repairs should be considered, however, in young patients with a history of ipsilateral sprains and whose activities necessitate perfect ankle function." I believe surgical repair should be considered in athletes with unstable ankles that have tears of the anterior talofibular and calcaneofibular ligaments. These ankles usually have a talar tilt angle of greater than 20 degrees on the stress radiograph. A history of functional instability due to previous sprains is a secondary indication for surgical repair. Other conditions requiring surgery are an acute injury with a bony avulsion, a fractured lateral malleolus, or an associated osteochondral fracture of the talus in an unstable ankle.

Most patients in whom surgical repair is indicated are young high-performance athletes. Repair of grade III injuries provides a highly predictable and satisfactory outcome in these patients. A stable ankle is essential for an elite athlete to return to his or her previous level of performance.

TECHNIQUE OF REPAIR

Surgery is usually performed under general anesthesia and under tourniquet control. The patient is placed in the supine position with a bolster under the hip to allow easy access to the lateral aspect of the ankle. An oblique incision is centered over the anterolateral joint line (Fig. 4). Care is taken to locate and protect the intermediate dorsal cutaneous nerve anteriorly and the lateral dorsal cutaneous nerve distally. In an acute injury, a hematoma can usually be seen within the wound as the surgeon inspects the ankle joint. After the joint is irrigated, severe ligamentous and capsular disruption is readily visible. The joint is inspected through the tear in the capsule for osteochondral or chondral lesions. The peroneal sheath is identified distally and opened, and the tendons are dislocated laterally and retracted to allow visualization of the calcaneofibular ligament. A manual anterior drawer test at this time may demonstrate marked anterior instability and allow identification of the posterior talofibular ligament and its attachments on the inner fibular tip and the posterior aspect of the talus.

The calcaneofibular ligament, the anterior talofibular ligament, and the anterior capsule are repaired with nonabsorbable sutures (Fig. 5). If the calcaneofibular

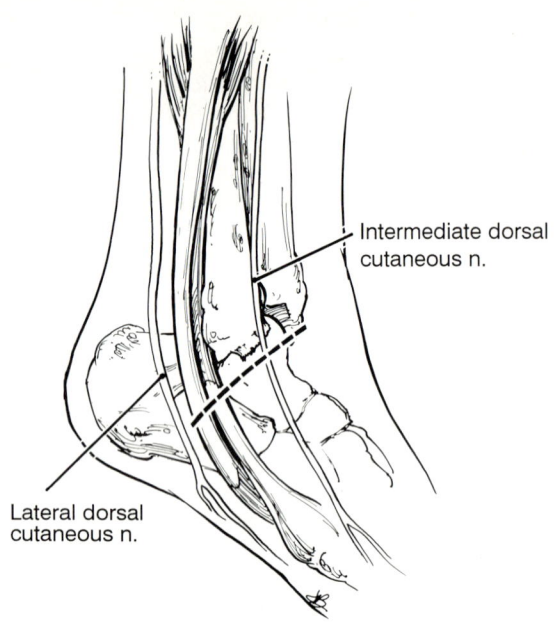

Intermediate dorsal
cutaneous n.

Lateral dorsal
cutaneous n.

Figure 4 Surgical approach to the joint is through an oblique incision that extends distally and ends at the tip of the fibula.

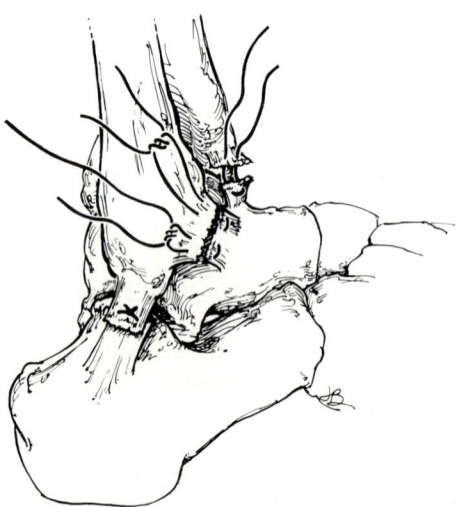

Figure 5 Nonabsorbable sutures are used to repair ligaments at the anatomical site of the tear.

ligament has been avulsed from the calcaneus or torn in midsubstance, the site of injury is identified and stitches are placed in the torn ligament. Mattress sutures are passed through adjacent soft tissue and left to be tied later.

The anterior talofibular ligament can usually be easily identified, and it is most often avulsed from either the fibula or talus, or it can be torn in midsubstance. Repair of the ligament depends on its site of rupture. When it is torn from the bony insertion, Mitek suture anchors (Mitek Surgical Products, Inc., Dedham, Mass.) are extremely helpful in reapproximating the ligament to

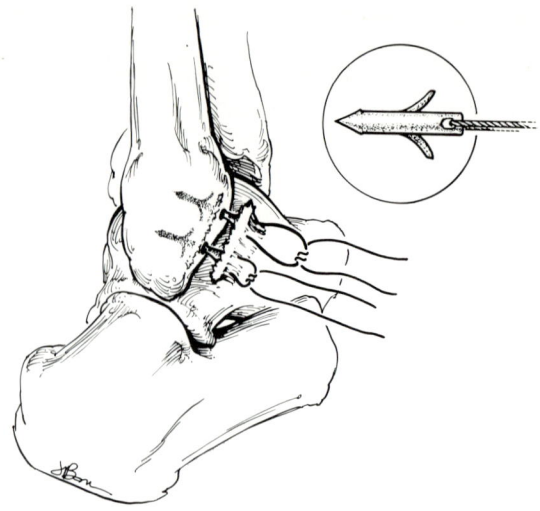

Figure 6 The avulsed anterior talofibular ligament is reapproximated to the fibula with Mitek GII suture anchors.

bone (Fig. 6). Next, sutures are placed in the rent in the anterior capsule to be tied later.

The ankle is placed in a dorsiflexed and everted position while the sutures in the anterior talofibular ligament are tied. Repairs are made in a pants-over-vest manner, which gives a double layer of repair. After sutures in the calcaneofibular ligament are tied, the anterior capsule can be repaired. The foot is held in the everted, dorsiflexed position throughout the remainder of the operation. Often, the dorsal retinaculum is used to reinforce the repair.

After the sutures are tied, the tourniquet is deflated and the ankle is retested for stability by anterior and varus stress testing. The skin is closed using subcuticular sutures. A local anesthetic administered after the procedure is completed will lessen postoperative pain. The operation can often be performed as same-day surgery.

POSTOPERATIVE CARE AND REHABILITATION

After surgery, the patient is placed in a U-shaped splint and a foot plate with the ankle in neutral dorsiflexion and slight eversion. When the patient is awake, alert, and comfortable, he or she can be discharged. The patient is instructed to remain non-weightbearing and to elevate the extremity with an ice pack over the operative site for the first 24 hours. Patients return in 7 to 10 days for removal of the sutures. At this time, the ankle is placed in a removable walking boot, and the patient begins gradual weightbearing.

At 3 weeks, the boot is removed, and the patient is fitted with a functional stirrup-type brace, or aircast. Active dorsiflexion, plantar flexion, and peroneal strengthening exercises are then begun. At 6 weeks after surgery, Achilles tendon stretching, proprioceptive retraining with a balance board, and resistive exercises are started. A patient can often return to agility sports at 8

significant laxity that is symptomatic in spite of adequate rehabilitation, surgical reconstruction is appropriate.

The history should include the exact time of the injury and what the athlete has done with the ankle since the injury. The degree of swelling, ecchymosis, and tenderness is related to the time between injury and presentation. It also reflects whether the athlete was wise enough to use crutches, ice, elevation, and some form of self-immobilization. The ability to prognosticate is significantly decreased without that knowledge. The mechanism is also a standard part of the history, although in many cases the athlete is really unable to accurately describe it. A general health history and specific musculoskeletal history is necessary as part of the initial evaluation. Athletes should be questioned about their normal level of activity and desires for future activity.

PHYSICAL EXAMINATION

Examination of the ankle is neither unique nor difficult. Observe for deformity, degree of edema, and amount of ecchymosis to help determine the degree of severity and rule out dislocation. Evaluate the neurovascular status with particular attention to function of the common peroneal nerve. On occasion, an inversion sprain can be severe enough to directly result in a traction neurapraxia of the common peroneal nerve that obviously alters the treatment time and the required protection. If the peroneal nerve is not functioning clinically, EMG Nerve Conduction Studies should be done at 3 weeks to determine the level and extent of the problem.

Palpate for focal areas of tenderness, paying particular attention to lateral and medial malleoli. Palpation of ligaments is next. Leave the ligaments most likely to be tender, based on history and observation, until last. Usually I examine the deltoid ligament first, then the posterior talofibular, the fibulocalcaneal, and the anterior talofibular. Finally, I palpate the anterior and posterior tibiofibular ligament area. The vast majority of patients with ankle sprains will present primarily with anterior talofibular tenderness and then secondarily with fibulocalcaneal tenderness. The one time I will consider stress roentgenograms for an acute case is when the anterior tibiofibular ligament is extremely tender to palpation, and the patient has pain with the so-called "squeeze test" or external rotation test. In that case, I do think it is worthwhile to get a syndesmotic stress view with the basic films.

RADIOGRAPHIC EVALUATION

Once the initial history and examination are completed, I normally order the standard three radiographic views of the ankle (AP, lateral, and mortise views). When the syndesmotic stress test is necessary, it is best if either I or one of the house staff perform this test personally rather than leaving it to the radiology technicians. The ankle is placed in position for a mortise view at 90 degrees dorsiflexion, the leg is stabilized, and the foot is externally rotated. If there is significant disruption of the syndesmosis, there will be visible widening. At that point it is the physician's personal decision whether to treat conservatively or resort to surgical intervention with a transfixion screw. In my practice, I do not surgically intervene unless the mortise is widened at rest without the stress being applied. As long as the mortise is in its normal dimension at rest, I go ahead with the treatment plan as outlined for severe sprain with the one exception that I delay weightbearing for 4 weeks. I would emphasize again that I do not do anterior stress or inversion stress views for acute ankle sprains. Those studies do not alter the treatment I recommend, and they are not adequate for future reference if the patient develops a chronic problem that requires further intervention. The use of MRI and CT arthrogram is equally inappropriate in my mind at this acute stage. I reserve both studies for patients with chronic problems or recurrent sprains.

TREATMENT

Phase I: Severe Edema

The athlete often comes in with severe edema about the ankle, occasionally so severe that the malleoli are not easily visualized. When I find marked edema in association with clinical findings of lateral ankle sprain and normal neurovascular status, I initiate phase I. Phase I is really directed toward controlling the initial inflammatory response and getting the patient ready for definitive treatment. I place the patient in a posterior splint with a compression dressing that is thin enough to allow some penetration of cold from cryotherapy. When possible, I use a compressive icing system, such as the "Cryo/Cuff Autochill by Aircast." I ask the patient to go home, elevate the ankle for 48 to 72 hours, and use crutches, nonweightbearing when standing. It is important to clarify to the patient what is meant by elevation. People often have the impression that sitting on a couch with their foot on a footstool is elevation, but it only represents less severe dependency. They need to understand that elevation means having the ankle above the level of the heart and that the higher it is above the heart the more effective the elevation will be.

If the athlete comes to my office within a few hours of the injury or has done a good job of rest, ice, and elevation prior to coming in, I bypass this phase and go directly to phase II.

Phase II: Initial Sprain Treatment

Phase II is started on those individuals who come in with minimal edema and ecchymosis and those who successfully complete phase I. When a phase-I patient returns after that first 48 to 72 hours of rest, ice, compression, and elevation, I re-examine the ankle. If the patient has been successful, he or she may progress to phase II; if not, I ask the patient to go home and more faithfully repeat phase I.

Patients are placed in a type of bivalve functional support. I personally use the "Air Stirrup by AirCast." I explain the concept of preventing inversion and eversion while allowing dorsiflexion and plantar flexion, and we discuss advantages of having a protected range of motion (ROM) that does not cause further damage. I ask patients to continue with icing a minimum of 3 hours a day, and I send them to physical therapy for instruction on a basic ROM program. They remove the AirCast twice a day to start alphabet writing and other forms of gentle, active ROM. They are advised to elevate the ankle as necessary to control edema, and they are encouraged to begin progressive weightbearing and to ambulate in the AirCast as tolerated. I explain that they need to wear a lace-up shoe over the AirCast and that the device is most effective when they are bearing full weight on the extremity. Most people achieve full weightbearing status within 48 hours of initiating this phase of the program. Phase II is expected to require 1 to 7 days, so I schedule the patient to return to see me in 1 week.

Phase III: Subacute Progression

At the time of the return visit 1 week into the functional protective bracing, I re-evaluate the ankle. Those patients that still have significant focal tenderness and are very apprehensive about going through an active ROM continue one more week at the phase II level. In most patients, the tenderness and the edema is dramatically decreased by the time of this visit, and they are able to go through a very comfortable, active ROM. I ask them to continue full weightbearing in the AirCast, continue working ROM, and see physical therapy for additional rehabilitation instruction. At this time, they start a progressive resistance exercise program. I prefer an elastic band program either with a commercially prepared figure-of-eight loop system or with Theraband. They also start working a balance-board routine with both feet on the board, as soon as they feel comfortable putting weight on the ankle without the AirCast. They are also encouraged to begin progressive activity in the AirCast with emphasis initially on the use of an exercise bike or one of the stair-step type machines; then progress to light jogging. Part of the treatment in this phase is psychological. Patients need to be reassured repeatedly that the bivalve functional protection device will protect them from further injury while they progress their recovery.

Phase IV: Return to Activity

When the patient has minimal tenderness, full ROM, and normal strength to clinical examination, they are allowed to progress to full activities. Patients are expected to continue the full rehabilitation program, including ROM work, progressive-resistance exercises, and the balance board. They resume activities wearing the AirCast and try taping under it to see whether that feels even better. Taping is not a requirement, but patients may prefer the additional support under the AirCast while playing. They are asked to wear the AirCast whenever they leave home or participate in sports. This progression to full activity normally occurs at 2 to 3 weeks but may take as long as 6 weeks in very severe sprains.

Phase V: Maintenance

From the time the patient resumes full activity as described under phase IV until 3 months after the injury, I require continued protection. Once they are totally asymptomatic, they are allowed to go either to an ankle lace-up or ankle tape for sports activities. My personal preference is the use of a lace-up, when it is used correctly, but the choice is left to the athlete and trainer. I ask patients to continue with the full rehabilitation program at least three times per week, and we progress with the understanding that they will resume the use of the AirCast if they develop any symptoms whatsoever during this time. I also emphasize that they have had a significant ankle sprain and that they need to accept maintenance-level rehabilitation as a way of life for the balance of their desired athletic career.

Phase VI: Long-term Maintenance

After 3 months, I ask them to do the maintenance rehabilitation program twice-a-week. I review the importance of choice of footwear, as well as condition of their shoes. If they have any residual clinical instability on examination or any sense of residual instability, I ask them to continue to wear a lace-up support, at least for sports activities.

DELTOID SPRAIN

Severe sprains of the medial or deltoid ligament are extremely uncommon. The vast majority of significant sprains of the deltoid that I have seen are related to lateral malleolar fractures and are part of a complex fracture-dislocation picture. In the case of focal tenderness over the deltoid without any associated lateral injury, I initiate treatment that would be phase III in the previously outlined lateral ligament sprain and progress activities as rapidly as tolerated. In the case of a true deltoid rupture associated with lateral instability, I fully agree with surgical intervention. In my experience, it is no longer necessary to open the medial side of the ankle in these patients. I have been very happy with arthroscopy to reduce any entrapped deltoid ligament or tendon on the medial side, and then fixation of the lateral side with plates or other device as necessary. That combination has not resulted in any clinical residual deltoid instability, and the patients have done uniformly well.

SYNDESMOSIS SEPARATION

As noted earlier, I do feel it is important to look for significant separation of the syndesmosis. If the separation is not apparent on resting films, and the patient's neurovascular status is intact, I attempt conservative treatment. The treatment plan is very similar to the one I use for the lateral ligaments, except that I do not allow weightbearing until 4 weeks after the injury. The entire treatment process is delayed 4 weeks, so every general guideline listed under lateral ligaments is 4 weeks longer with the syndesmosis. At the first indication of any widening of the syndesmosis at rest, I think surgical intervention is the preferred treatment; at this point there is no place for continued conservative treatment.

SUGGESTED READING

Barrett JR, Tanji JL, Drake C, et al: High- versus low-top shoes for the prevention of ankle sprains in basketball players: a prospective randomized study. Am J Sports Med 1993; 21:582–585.

Curtis MJ, Myerson M, Szure B: Tarsometatarsal joint injuries in the athlete. Am J Sports Med 1993; 21:497–502.

Edelman B: Get lateral stress x-ray for ruptured ankle ligaments. Orthopaedics Today 1993; 32–33.

Ferkel RD, Karzel RP, Del Pizzo W, et al: Arthroscopic treatment of anterolateral impingement of the ankle. Am J Sports Med 1991; 19:440–446.

Finsen V, Benum P: Osteopenia after ankle fractures. Clin Orthop 1989; 245:261–268.

Hensley JP, Saltrick K, Le T: Anterior ankle arthroplasty: a retrospective study. J Foot Surg 1990; 29:169–172.

Konradsen L, Holmer P, Sondergaard L: Early mobilizing treatment for grade III ankle ligament injuries. Am Orthopaedic Foot and Ankle 1991; 12:69–73.

Lassiter TE, Malone TR, Garrett WE: Injury to the lateral ligaments of the ankle. Orthop Clin North Am 1989; 20:629–640.

Meisterling RC: Recurrent lateral ankle sprains. The Physician and Sportsmedicine 1993; 21:123–132.

Rijke AM, Goitz HT, McCue III FC, Dee PM: Magnetic resonance imaging of injury to the lateral ankle ligaments. Am J Sports Med 1993; 21:528–534.

Stuart PR, Brumby C, Smith SR: Comparative study of functional bracing and plaster cast treatment of stable lateral molleolar fractures. Injury 1989; 20:323–326.

Wilkerson LA: Ankle injuries in athletes. Sports Med 1992; 19: 377–392.

SURGICAL ARTHROSCOPY OF THE ANKLE

J. SERGE PARISIEN, M.D.

Arthroscopic surgery is an accepted procedure for the management of various sports-related ankle disorders. Advances in instrumentation, refinement in techniques, and proper patient selection have resulted in the successful outcome widely reported to date.

INDICATIONS

From a review of the literature and from my own experience, the indications for ankle arthroscopic surgery can fall into the following categories: synovial impingement, transchondral fractures of the talus or osteochondritis dissecans, impingement exostoses, loose bodies, and post-traumatic disorders.

TECHNIQUES

General Principles

The procedure can be performed, on an out-patient basis, under general or regional anesthesia. The patient is placed in semisupine position with a bolster underneath the buttock and a tourniquet placed over the thigh area. A leg holder facilitates control of the lower extremity and a folded sheet underneath the heel maximizes plantar flexion and manual distraction (Fig. 1).

Various other positions of the patient have been advocated and have been used with success by some pioneers in the field. Johnson places the patient supine with the leg extended and stabilized in a leg holder. Andrews advocates flexion of the knee with the foot of the table bent at 90 degrees. Ferkel and Guhl, among others, place the patient supine with a sterile support for the foot and with the hip and the knee flexed over a nonsterile holder. Standard 4 mm 30 and 70 degree arthroscopes, or a short 2.7 mm 30 degree scope, small hand instrument sets, and small motorized instrumentation are very helpful. After joint distension with 20 or 30 mm of normal saline solution is obtained, two portals, the anterolateral, lateral to the common extensor tendons and peroneus tertius, and the anteromedial, medial to the tibialis anterior tendon, are mostly used in conjunction at times with the posterolateral portal. This latter point of entrance is posterior to the peronei tendons, close to the Achilles tendon, in order to avoid injury to the sural nerve.

In very tight ankles, mechanical distraction can be used. Although Guhl has for many years popularized the use of the invasive distraction device, at this time he, as well as Ewing, is advocating the use of a nondistraction method that offers less morbidity to the patient.

Specific Lesions

Synovial Impingement

Some patients with a history of multiple inversion injuries complain of pain and giving way aggravated by activities and disclose physical findings such as tenderness and swelling at the anterior or anterolateral aspect of the ankle without any evidence of objective signs of

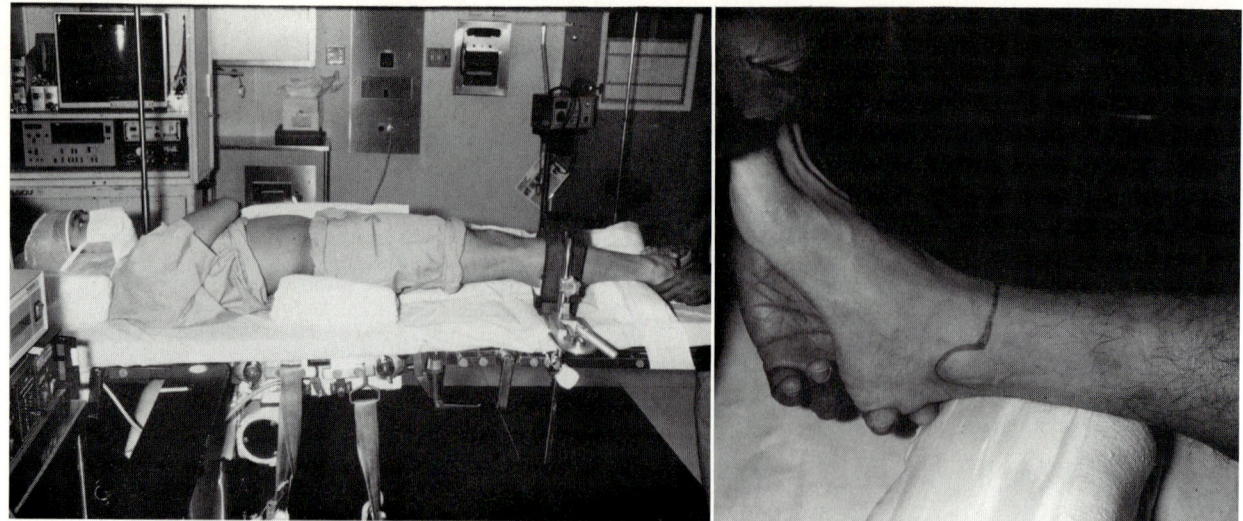

Figure 1 *A,* Patient in semisupine position with bolster underneath buttock. Internal rotation of hip improves access to posterolateral aspect of the ankle. *B,* Bolster underneath heel to maximize plantar flexion of ankle.

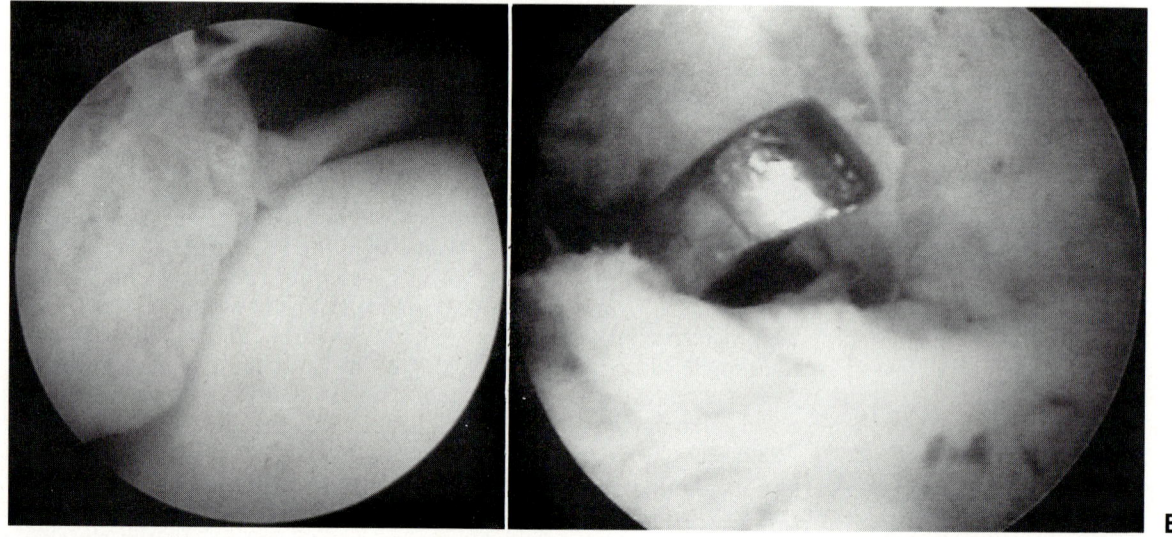

Figure 2 *A,* Synovial impingement anterolateral aspect, right ankle. *B,* Arthroscopic visualization of excision of adhesions, anterior aspect ankle.

instability. When conservative treatment for a period of at least 3 months consisting of the use of anti-inflammatory medication, physical therapy modalities, or the use of orthotics, is unsuccessful, arthroscopic surgery is indicated. A motorized shaver is used with the two standard anterior portals without joint distraction. It allows a careful, meticulous debridement of the hypertrophic synovitis and fibrous material at the anterolateral corner and the lateral talomalleolar space of the ankle (Fig. 2).

A thickening of the distal fascicle of the anteroinferior tibiofibular syndesmotic ligament, associated with chondromalacia of the corresponding surface of the talus, may also be found as described by Bassett. If it is responsible for the impingement, this offending struc-

ture should be excised with a combination of basket scissors and a motorized cutter.

A compression dressing is applied at the end of the procedure and the lower extremity is kept elevated for 1 or 2 days. Partial weight bearing progressing to full weight bearing after 1 or 2 days is advisable. Full range of motion (ROM) by the patient is encouraged. Return to sport activities is allowed as soon as the patient is asymptomatic.

Transchondral Fractures of the Talus

According to Berndt and Harty, these osteochondral lesions of the talar dome are usually secondary to an injury. Two types of lesions are generally described:

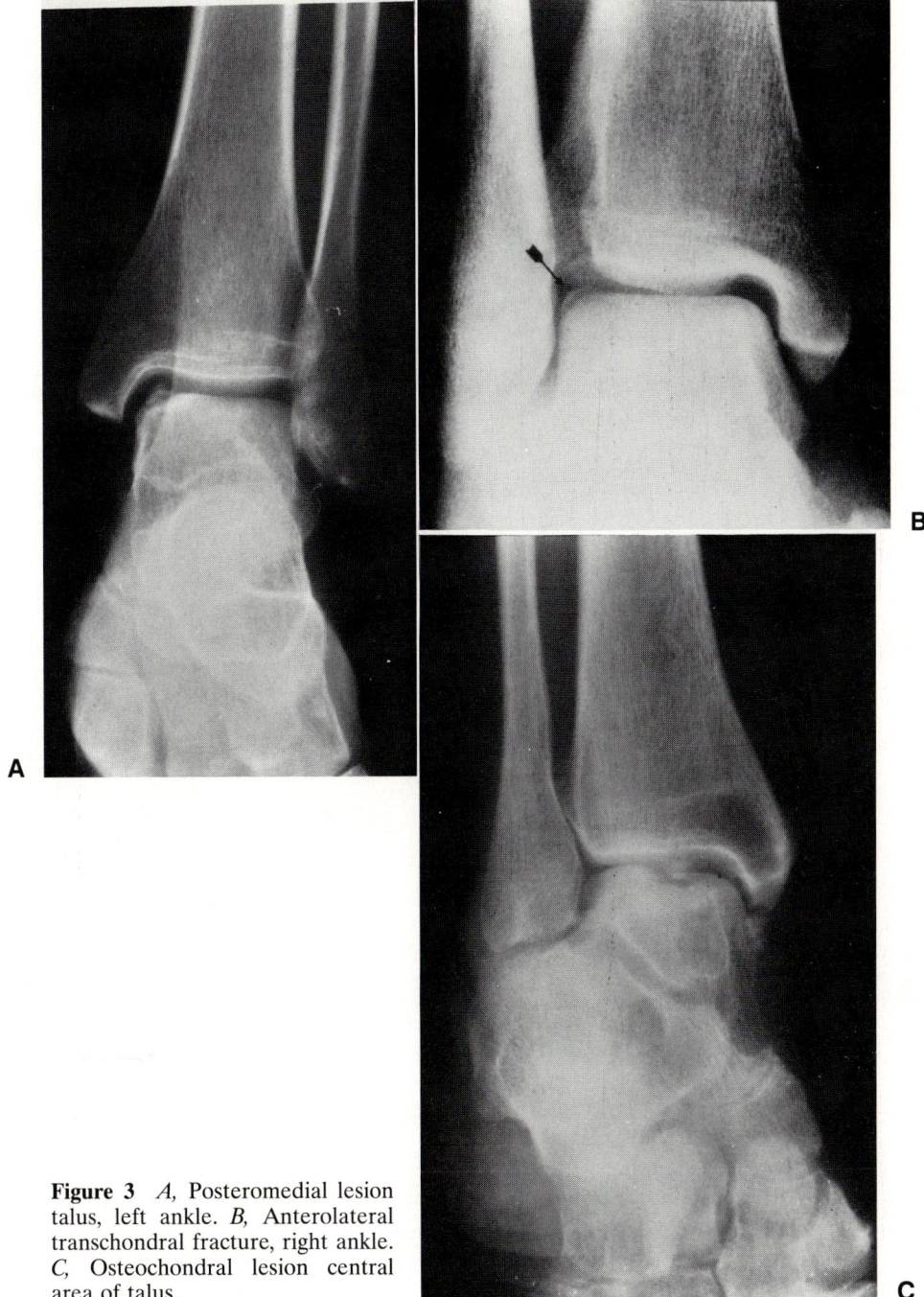

Figure 3 *A,* Posteromedial lesion talus, left ankle. *B,* Anterolateral transchondral fracture, right ankle. *C,* Osteochondral lesion central area of talus.

posteromedial and anterolateral (Fig. 3). The posteromedial talar lesion is caused by inversion, plantar flexion, and external rotation of the tibia on the talus. The anterolateral lesion is secondary to inversion and dorsiflexion injuries of the ankle. Some other locations (central or posterolateral) are less common. The lateral lesions are smaller and wafer shaped, while the posteromedial lesions are cup shaped.

The clinical presentation is often identical to a sprain, and without a strong awareness of this condition, the diagnosis is seldom made acutely. A history of inversion injury is usually present. Flick and Gould, in a review of more than 500 reported cases in the literature, have found the incidence of injury to be 98% for the lateral lesions and 70% for the medial lesions. Because some of the medial lesions appear to be atraumatic, some investigators feel that they represent true osteochondritis dissecans.

In an acute situation, the diagnosis is suggested by the presence of pain, swelling, and limitation of motion. In chronic cases, joint stiffness with a deep aching sensation and grinding can be found. Confirmation is obtained by x-ray examination (A-P, lateral, and internal oblique views), tomography or arthrotomography, CT

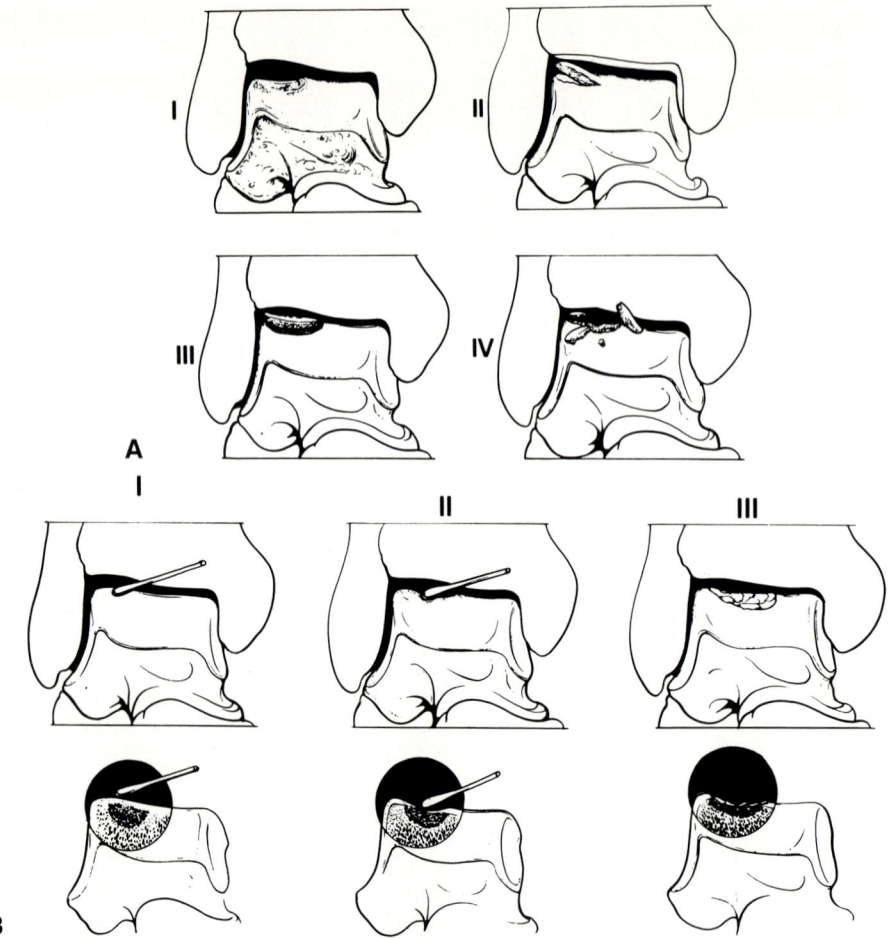

Figure 4 *A,* Radiographic staging of transchondral fracture. *B,* Arthroscopic grading. (From Parisien JS. Arthroscopic surgery in osteocartilaginous lesions of the ankle. In: McGinty JB, ed. Operative arthroscopy. New York: Raven Press, 1991; with permission.)

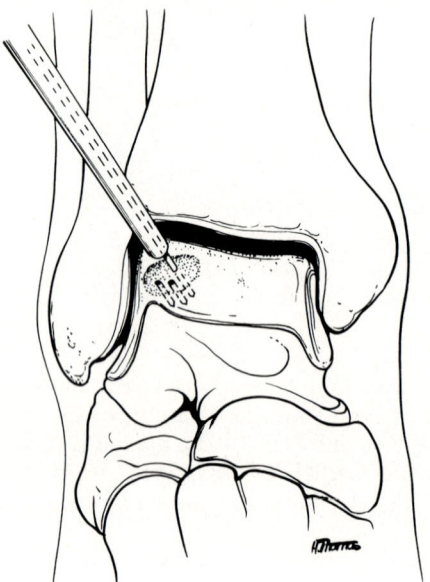

Figure 5 Drilling of anterolateral lesion. (From Parisien JS. Arthroscopic surgery in osteocartilaginous lesions of the ankle. In: McGinty JB, ed. Operative arthroscopy. New York: Raven Press, 1991; with permission.)

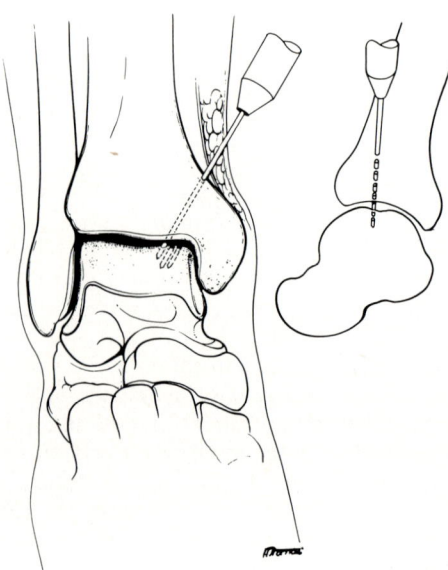

Figure 6 Drilling using the transmalleolar approach. (From Parisien JS. Arthroscopic surgery in osteocartilaginous lesions of the ankle. In: McGinty JB, ed. Operative arthroscopy. New York: Raven Press, 1991; with permission.)

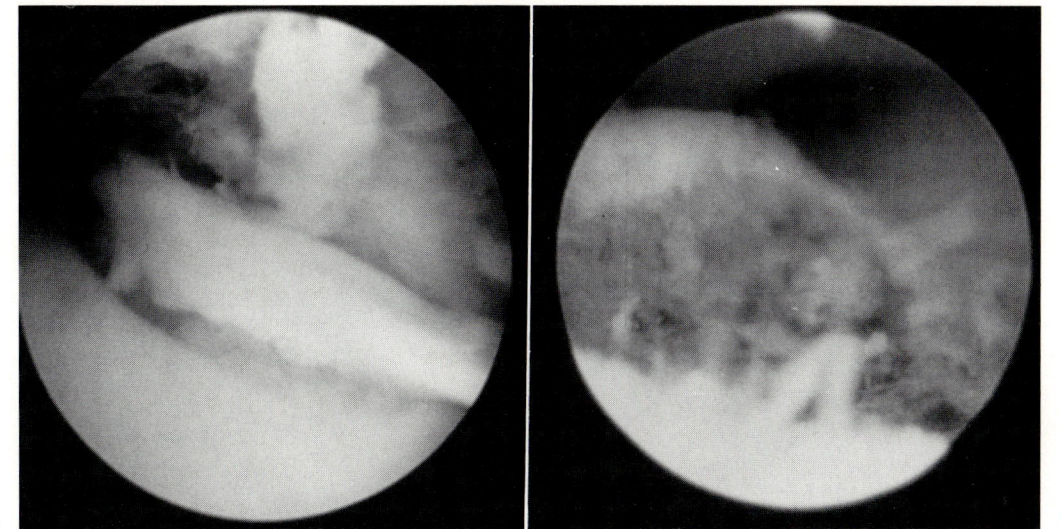

Figure 7 *A,* Transchondral fracture talus. *B,* Arthroscopic visualization of osteochondral bed after excision of transchondral fracture.

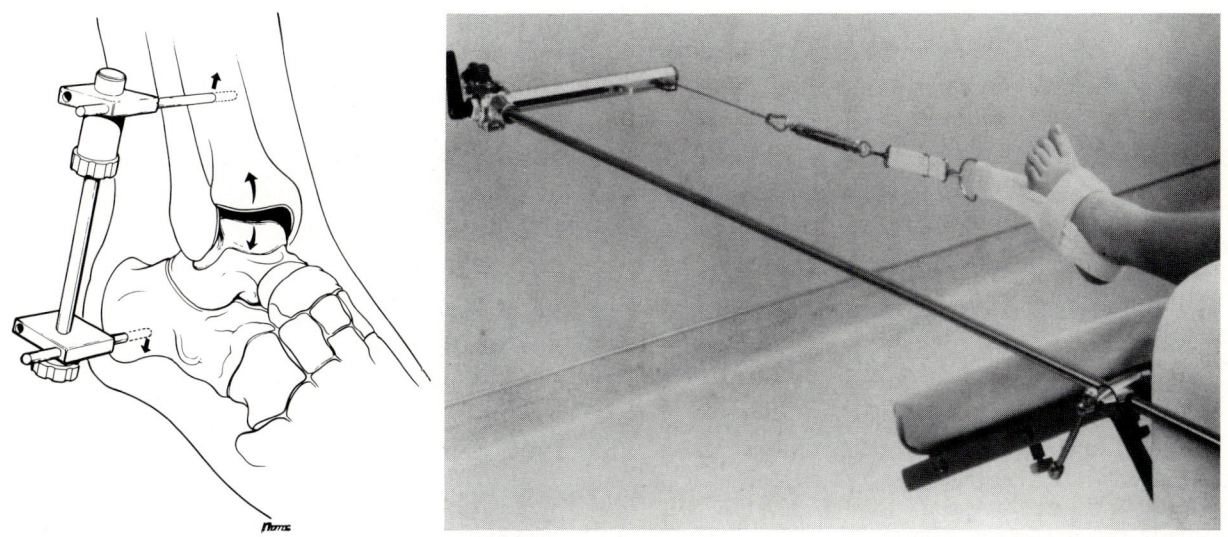

Figure 8 *A,* Mechanical distractor. (From Parisien JS. Arthroscopic surgery in osteocartilaginous lesions of the ankle. In: McGinty JB, ed. Operative arthroscopy. New York: Raven Press, 1991; with permission.) *B,* Noninvasive distraction. (Zimmer, Inc., Warsaw, Indiana) The apparatus is attached to the side of the operating table with the lower end flexed 70 degrees. Traction is applied through a sterile, disposable strap placed over the ankle.

(axial or coronal, with or without contrast material), or MRI. Although Berndt and Harty have classified transchondral fractures into four stages, according to the various degrees of stability of the lesion, the arthroscopic appearance seems to be more important in planning proper treatment when surgery is contemplated (Fig. 4). If the articular cartilage is degenerated, the fragment should be excised whether it is stable or not. When the articular cartilage is viable, the osteochondral lesion can be drilled or pinned according to the stability obtained after palpation. The technique varies according to the location of the pathology.

The anterolateral lesions are more accessible and require the use of the two standard anterior portals,

without joint distraction. Although there is no evidence in the literature yet of the benefits of simple drilling, the procedure can be easily performed with the scope placed anteromedially and the surgical instrument through the anterolateral portal (Fig. 5). An unstable osteochondral fragment with normal articular cartilage lining, without necrosis of the subchondral bone, can also be replaced and fixed by means of biodegradable pins or small screws. Excision of an unstable, nonviable osteochondral fragment is followed by debridement or drilling of the crater.

The posteromedial lesions, because of their location, may be a challenge even to the experienced arthroscopic surgeon. Drilling may be difficult using the

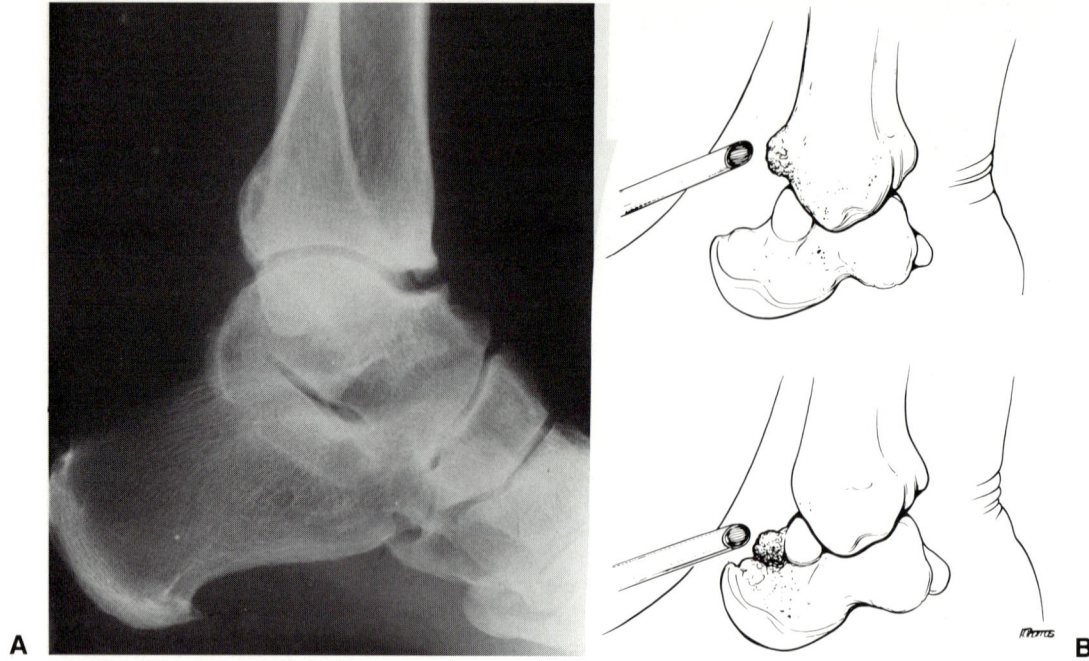

Figure 9 *A,* Radiograph of impingement exostoses. *B,* Excision of exostosis with motorized abrader. (From Parisien JS. Arthroscopic surgery in osteocartilaginous lesions of the ankle. In: McGinty JB, ed. Operative arthroscopy. New York: Raven Press, 1991; with permission.)

anterior portals. It may be necessary to resort to the use of the medial transmalleolar portal as advocated by Guhl (Fig. 6). After placing one wire in the desired location through the distal tibia, by dorsiflexing and plantar flexing the ankle, multiple drill holes can be placed into the talar lesion. The use of a cannulated reamer, while facilitating the placement of pins for fixation of a viable osteochondral fragment, carries the risk of potential fracture of the medial malleolus. Arthroscopic excision of a necrotic fragment followed by curettage and abrading the osteochondral defect can be performed without mechanical distraction (Fig. 7). The use of a 70 degree scope to improve the visualization of this posteriorly located lesion, coupled with a small instrumentation set, is mandatory for a successful outcome. In a very tight joint, mechanical distraction by invasive or preferably noninvasive means should be used (Fig. 8).

The postoperative management includes a period of non–weight-bearing, following drilling or fixation of the fragment. As far as excision is concerned, non–weight-bearing ambulation does not seem to be necessary, at least for a lesion of 1.5 cm diameter or less. Return to sports activities may take many months. Second-look arthroscopy has demonstrated the formation of fibrocartilage within the defect. However, the maturation of the tissue may take several months.

Exostoses

Direct trauma during forced dorsiflexion of the ankle can give rise to spur formation. These impingement exostoses can be found at the anterior lip of the

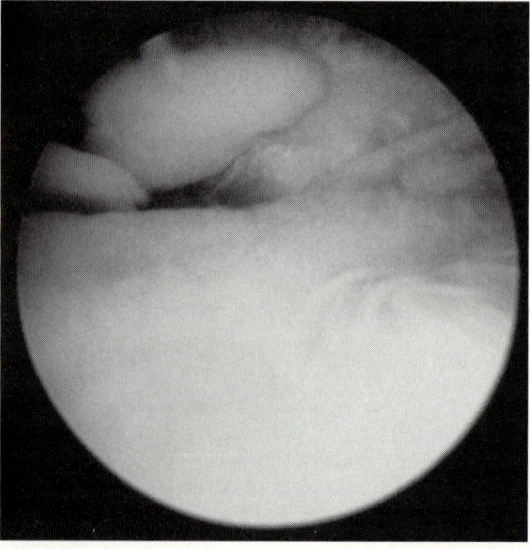

Figure 10 Arthroscopic visualization of multiple loose osteochondral fragments.

tibial plafond and/or at the opposing surface of the talus. They may be found in front of the medial malleolus, as well. O'Donoghue postulated that in football players, trauma due to forced dorsiflexion was responsible for spur formation in the anterior aspect of the ankle. He described a 45% incidence in this athletic population. Pain is caused by impingement of the bony spurs, as well as trapping of the chronically hypertrophied synovial tissue. Technetium bone scans, if obtained, will show an increased uptake in the area of the spur. However, plain

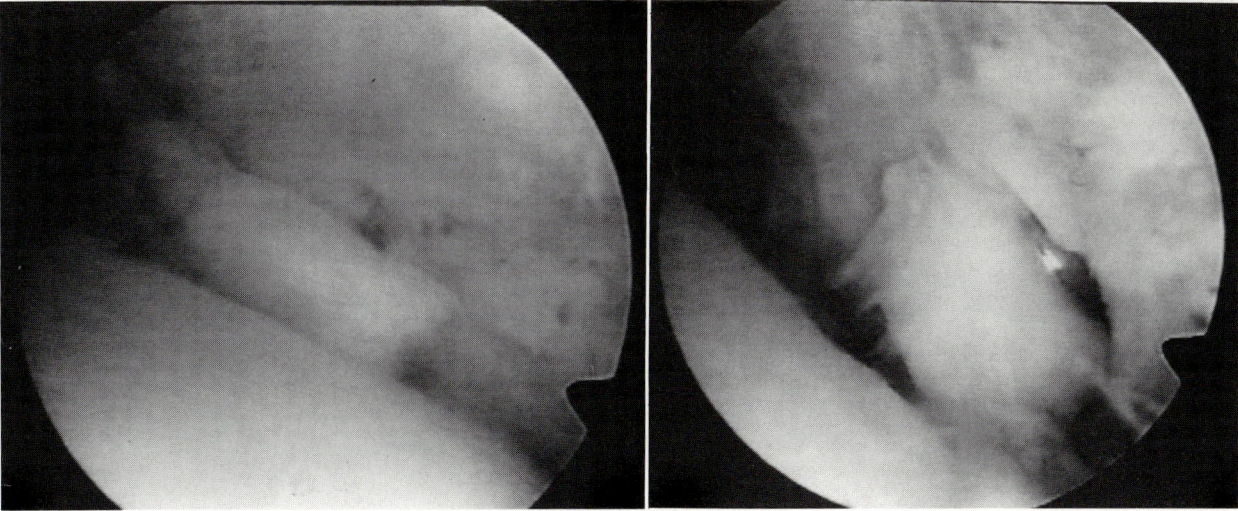

Figure 11 *A,* Arthroscopic visualization of loose osteochondral body, right ankle. *B,* Loose fragment being extracted from joint with grasping forceps.

lateral radiographs can also confirm the diagnosis. If conservative treatment consisting of the use of a heel-lift, associated with anti-inflammatory medication, fails to give symptomatic relief, arthroscopic resection of the painful spurs is advocated. This can be achieved with small osteotomes and small abraders, using the two anterior portals (Fig. 9). Active ROM exercises is begun immediately and full weight-bearing status is achieved gradually over a period of a few days.

To confirm adequacy of the excision, before completion of the procedure, it is advisable to switch the portals, in order to visualize the resected area from two different angles. Distraction is not necessary. The results are satisfactory if the spurs are not associated with joint degeneration.

Loose Bodies

Loose bodies, cartilaginous or osteochondral, can be the end stage of transchondral fracture or osteochondritis dissecans, part of a degenerative process of the joint, or less commonly due to synovial disease (synovial osteochondromatosis). They are usually diagnosed by basic x-ray examination or, in some situations, by computed axial tomography enhanced by air or CO_2. They can be located in the anterior or posterior pouch, or uncommonly in the medial or lateral gutter (Figs. 10 and 11).

Their arthroscopic excision, when they are not found posteriorly, is not difficult. When the loose fragment is anterior, with the scope placed through one anterior portal, a grasping forceps will ensure removal of the fragment through the opposite portal. For loose bodies found in the gutters, the use of a 70 degree scope will improve their visualization and facilitate their excision. The same approach is advocated for the removal of painful ossicles at the tip of the malleoli.

Posteriorly located loose bodies may require the use of a mechanical distraction (noninvasive or invasive)

coupled with the development of a posterolateral portal.

In the unusual situation of multiple loose bodies secondary to synovial osteochondromatosis, when dealing with a stage-three disease without synovial activity, no synovectomy is indicated. Complete removal of the loose fragments will be facilitated by the three portals technique associated with distraction. Full weightbearing, with active ROM, is advocated as soon as possible.

Post-Traumatic Disorders

Repeated traumatic episodes to the ankle of a very competitive athlete can cause generalized synovial hypertrophy, associated with chondromalacic areas, and loose chondral fragments. Chronic discomfort, intermittent swelling, and effusion are usually the sequelae of these intra-articular changes. Adequate joint debridement may give some lasting relief. Distraction combined with the three portals technique is advisable. However, with more advanced degenerative changes, the relief may only be temporary and usually will require a modification of life-style. Postoperatively, full weightbearing should be progressive with the use of nonsteroidal anti-inflammatory medication.

COMMENTS

Surgical arthroscopy of the ankle is a viable alternative to open arthrotomy in the management of many ankle disorders. Concerning the management of transchondral fractures or osteochondritis dissecans, despite the feasibility of drilling or fragment fixation, most published reports seem to support surgical removal of the lesion with curettage of the crater as the treatment of choice. Moreover, many physicians in the sports medicine community advocate early surgery for active individuals with persistent clinical symptoms. Operative arthroscopy of the ankle is not without complications, even in the hands of the experienced arthroscopic surgeon. The morbidity can be minimized by a good knowledge of the regional anatomy, familiarity with the instrumentation and surgical portals, and proper selection of patients.

SUGGESTED READING

Andrews JR, Previte WJ, Carson WG. Arthroscopy of the ankle: technique and normal anatomy. Foot Ankle 1985; 6:29–33.

Baker CL, Andrews JR, Ryan JB. Arthroscopic treatment of transchondral talar dome fractures. Arthroscopy 1986; 2:82–87.

Barber FA, Click J, Britt BT. Complications of ankle arthroscopy. Foot Ankle 1990; 10:263–266.

Basset FH III, Gates HS III, Billys JB, et al. Talar impingement by anteroinferior tibiofibular ligament. A cause of chronic pain in the ankle after inversion sprain. J Bone Joint Surg 1990; 72:55–59.

Berndt AL, Harty M. Transchondral fractures (osteochondritis dissecans) of the talus. J Bone Joint Surg 1959; 41:988–1020.

Campbell CJ, Ranawat CS. Osteochondritis dissecans: the question of etiology. J Trauma 1966; 6:201–221.

Ewing JW. Arthroscopic management of transchondral talar-dome fractures (osteochondritis dissecans) and anterior impingement lesions of the ankle joint. Clin Sports Med 1991; 10:677–687.

Ferkel RD. Soft tissue pathology of the ankle. In: McGinty JB, ed. Operative arthroscopy New York: Raven Press, 1991:713–725.

Ferkel RD, Fischer SP. Progress in ankle arthroscopy. Clin Orthop 1989; 240:210–220.

Ferkel RD, Guhl J, Van Buecken K, et al. Complications in ankle arthroscopy: analysis of the first 518 cases. Orthop Trans 1992–1993; 16:726–727.

Ferkel RD, Karzel RP, Del Pizzo W, et al. Arthroscopic treatment of anterolateral impingement of the ankle. Am J Sports Med 1991; 19:440–446.

Flick AB, Gould N. Osteochondritis dissecans of the talus (transchondral fractures of the talus): review of the literature and new surgical approach for medial dome lesions. Foot Ankle 1985; 5:165–185.

Guhl JF. New concepts (distraction) in ankle arthroscopy. Arthroscopy 1988; 4:160–167.

Hawkins RB. Arthroscopic treatment of sports-related anterior osteophytes in the ankle. Foot Ankle 1988; 9:87–90.

Martin DF, Curl WW, Baker CL. Arthroscopic treatment of chronic synovitis of the ankle. Arthroscopy 1989; 5:110–114.

Meislin RJ, Rose DJ, Parisien JS, Springer S. Arthroscopic treatment of synovial impingement of the ankle. Am J Sports Med 1993; 21:186–189.

O'Donoghue DH. Impingement exostoses of the talus and tibia. J Bone Joint Surg 1957; 39:835–852.

Parisien JS. Arthroscopic treatment of osteochondral lesions of the talus. Am J Sports Med 1986; 14:211–217.

Parisien JS, Shereff MJ. The role of arthroscopy in the diagnosis and treatment of disorders of the ankle. Foot Ankle 1981; 2:144–149.

Parisien JS, Vangsness T. Operative arthroscopy of the ankle. Three years' experience. Clin Orthop 1985; 199:46–53.

Parisien JS. Arthroscopic surgery in osteocartilaginous lesions of the ankle. In: McGinty JB, ed. Operative arthroscopy. New York: Raven Press, 1991:727–745.

Scranton PE Jr, McDermott JE. Anterior tibiotalar spurs: a comparison of open versus arthroscopic debridement. Foot Ankle 1992; 13:125–129.

Stone JW, Guhl JF. Ankle arthroscopy in the management of osteochondral lesions. In: Parisien JS, ed. Current techniques in arthroscopy. Philadelphia: Current Medicine, 1994:225–237.

Thein R, Eichenblat M. Arthroscopic treatment of sports-related synovitis of the ankle. Am J Sports Med 1992; 20:496–498.

SELECTED LESIONS AROUND THE TALUS

DAVID COLLINSON REID, M.D., F.R.C.S.(C), M.Ch. (Orth)

This chapter deals with a group of entrapment and impingement syndromes around the talus that may have the common features of a history of trauma, aggravated by activity and relieved by rest. Most of these are uncommon and some are rare; all have a high incidence of delayed diagnosis. Awareness of these potentially disabling conditions may lead to prompt, effective treatment. The most common of these is the osteochondral lesion of the talar dome. As with the other conditions, the presence of the lesion does not always mean that this is the cause of the symptoms. Caution must be observed at the outset concerning early aggressive surgical treatment, unless other causes of the symptoms have been ruled out. The very existence of some of these syndromes has been questioned, but in highly active individuals these otherwise quiescent lesions can prejudice the chances of successful performance. The meniscal lesion at the ankle, the anterior impingement syndrome, and the anterolateral corner compression syndrome all give intra-articular signs. The posterior talar compression syndrome is often peculiar to the ballet dancer or soccer player. The tarsal tunnel syndrome is a neural entrapment phenomenon, but its proximity makes a discussion under the single heading of "selected lesions around the talus" reasonable.

TRANSCHONDRAL FRACTURES OF THE TALUS (OSTEOCHONDRITIS DISSECANS)

Osteochondral lesions of the talar dome are uncommon, accounting for only 4% of all osteochondritic lesions and 0.9% of all fractures. The true incidence is unknown since frequently only symptomatic lesions are detected, and surprisingly even these are not always made obvious by standard diagnostic techniques.

Etiology

In 1959 Berndt and Harty suggested that trauma was the only significant factor in the development of these lesions, and the term "transchondral fracture" has been adopted. In cadaver studies, these authors reproduced lateral lesions with inversion and dorsiflexion and medial lesions with inversion, plantar flexion, and lateral rotation of the tibia on the talus (Fig. 1). Most authors

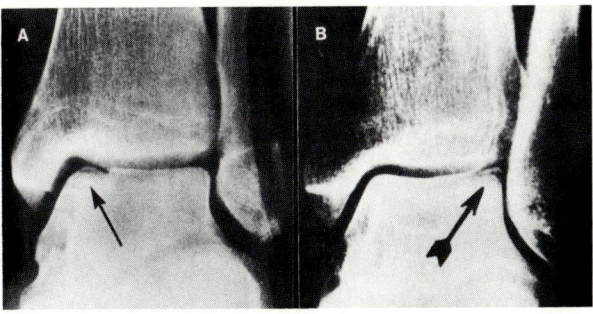

Figure 1 The most frequent sites of transchondral fractures are *A* posteromedial and *B* anterolateral. (From Pavlov H, Torg JS. The running athlete. Chicago: Year Book Medical Publishers, 1987; with permission.)

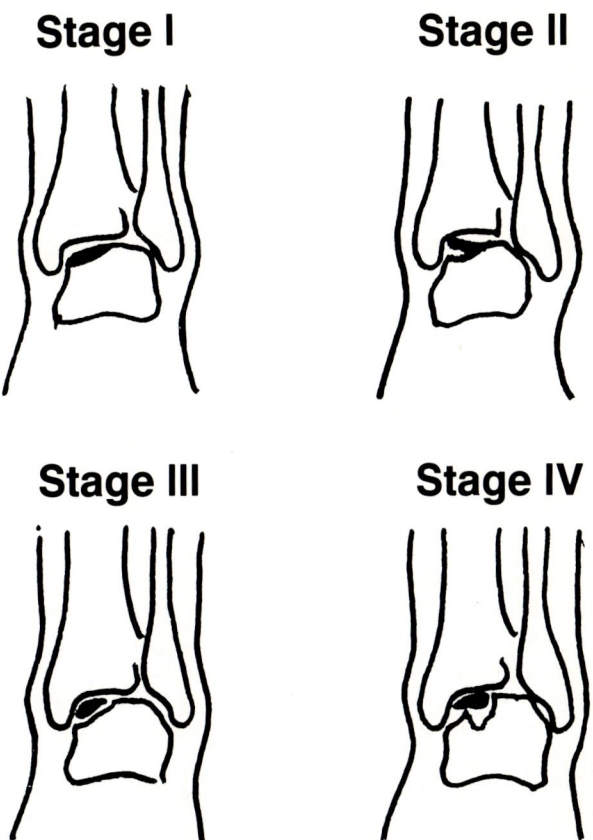

Figure 2 The four stages of osteochondral lesions according to Berndt and Harty. Stage I, a small area of compression. Stage II, a partially detached osteochondral fragment. Stage III, a completely detached fragment but remaining in situ. Stage IV, a detached, displaced fragment.

accepted their thesis. Nevertheless, some authors still support the idea of a separate clinical entity of osteochondritis dissecans evolving on an avascular basis. Many lesions are not visible on initial post-trauma films even in review. There is probably a spectrum of pathophysiology with acute shear fractures occurring at one extreme, as well as traumatic injury leading to injury to the subchondral vessels, resulting in delayed avascular collapse or separation. Perhaps at the other end of the scale are cases of idiopathic avascular necrosis due to systemic and local causes. Inasmuch as careful scrutiny has not shown that these lesions heal differently from others, further speculation as to cause is not warranted, and the lesion must be dealt with de novo, according to the symptoms. The undoubted association with trauma, in many cases, means that a high index of suspicion is important in considering this entity in the differential diagnosis of chronic ankle pain after injury. This may help reduce the unacceptable delay in diagnosis of from 3 months to 16 years, frequently discussed in the literature.

Signs and Symptoms

The major symptoms include a deep aching or pain aggravated by exercise. Ankle swelling, and occasionally crepitus, clicking, true locking, or a catching sensation, may also be present. The clinical signs include synovial thickening, effusion, and sometimes joint line tenderness and stiffness manifested as loss of range in one or both directions. In all cases, symptoms seem to be magnified by activity. In most people, there is a history of an inversion sprain or ankle fracture; occasionally, the lesion is associated with true or functional ankle instability.

Radiologic Examination

Radiographically the lesions typically can be seen to be located anterolateral or posteromedial on the dome of the talus (see Fig. 1). They may be classified according to the degree of separation (Fig. 2). Normally these lesions can be visualized in the routine ankle views, particularly in the internal oblique projection. However, an overpenetrated view of the plantar flexed ankle (x-ray

at 1 m with 70 kV) sometimes facilitates vision of the early posteromedial lesion. Tomography, computed tomography, or magnetic resonance imaging (MRI) allows accurate surgical planning if insufficient data are obtained from the plain films. Dipaola et al have recently correlated MRI changes with arthroscopic changes, allowing a comparison with previous plain radiographic staging (Table 1).

Treatment

The silent nature of many of these lesions means that all definitive surgical treatment must be preceded by a reasonable attempt at nonoperative therapy. The grades I and II lesions may do well with some protected weight bearing and nonsteroidal anti-inflammatory drugs (NSAIDs). In the series of Hagmeyer and van der Wurff, the stage I lesions treated nonoperatively were graded good, whereas the stage II lesions were mostly assessed fair to poor; the good results in stage II were from surgery. Symptomatic lesions of grade III are less likely to settle, but a trial of NSAIDs plus activity modification is worthwhile. If this is unsuccessful, surgery should be recommended. These findings have been endorsed recently by Pritch. If the patient is reluctant to undergo surgery, a patella-bearing, weight-

Table 1 Comparative Staging of Osteochondral Lesions

Stage	Radiographic*	MRI†	Arthroscopic
I	Compression lesion. No visible loose fragment.	Thickening of articular cartilage and low signal changes.	Irregular, softening or raised area of articular cartilage. No definable fragment.
II	Fragment visible but attached.	Articular cartilage breached. Low signal rim behind fragment indicating fibrous attachment.	Articular cartilage breached. Definable fragment, not displaceable.
III	Nondisplaced fragment without attachment.	Articular cartilage breached. High signal changes behind fragment indicating synovial fluid between fragment and underlying bone.	Articular cartilage breached. Definable fragment. Displaceable but still attached by some articular cartilage.
IV	Displaced fragment.	Loose fragment.	Loose fragment within defect or joint.

*Data from Berndt & Harty, 1959.
†Data from Dipaola, Nelson & Colville, 1991.

relieving ankle brace, worn for 6 weeks to 6 months, usually allows the symptoms to resolve. Alternatively a below-knee, non-weightbearing cast may be used, but this obviously has the disadvantage of more muscle wasting and joint stiffness for the competitive athlete. If a cast is worn, the period of immobilization should not exceed 6 to 8 weeks. The symptoms may return, however, with increased activity, and this approach is not really recommended. Canele and Belding felt that medial stage III lesions were more likely to settle with nonoperative treatment than the lateral stage III lesions. The displaced type IV lesion should be operated on promptly if symptomatic, particularly if it is causing joint locking, since it may damage the joint surface and predispose to osteoarthritis.

When explaining the surgical options to patients with grades I to II lesions, it is important to bear in mind the work of McCullough and Venngopal, who reported surprisingly few complications and very little evidence of joint degeneration in a 10 year follow-up; however, this series, like most in the literature, was small. Nevertheless, modification of activity may be a viable, preferable, and acceptable option for some young individuals. The degree of symptoms, level of competition, and ultimate athletic goals obviously all govern the decision whether and when to operate.

Surgical treatment may be directed at removing an undisplaced loose fragment, drilling an in situ fragment, or removing a displaced fragment and performing debridement. Depending on the size and position of the lesion, and the amount of normal laxity of the ankle, arthroscopic treatment is possible. The anterolateral lesion is the more amenable and it may even be possible to drill the bed. It should be stressed, however, that a well-performed arthrotomy procedure is preferable to a poorly executed arthroscopy.

Surgical Approaches

The position of the fragment determines whether the joint should be approached via an anterolateral, an anteromedial, or a posteromedial exposure.

Anterolateral Lesion. With the patient in the supine position, a large sandbag or wedge under the

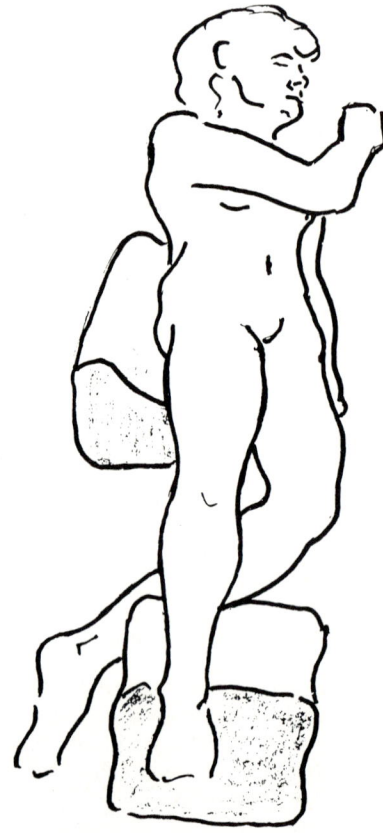

Figure 3 Patient positioned in the lateral decubitus position with the body tilted onto a support, giving access to both sides of the ankle by rotating the hip (after Parisien JS).

ipsilateral hip, and the leg supported on a well-padded box, the anterolateral ankle is easily exposed (Fig. 3). This is an excellent position for exposure of both medial and lateral ankle and can be used for most ankle surgery, including arthroscopy. Therefore the approach is described here in detail. An incision is made starting 5 cm proximal to the ankle joint, just medial to the crest of the fibula, curved down to approximately the level of the sinus tarsi. It is unfortunate that such a large exposure is usually necessary to perform this procedure well. The subcutaneous dissection is kept medial to the peroneus tertius, which is retracted laterally. Care must be taken to avoid damage to the cutaneous branch of the superficial peroneal nerve, which is retracted medially, along with the extensor digitorum tendons. The capsule is opened longitudinally, and since the malleolar and lateral tarsal arteries are usually divided, it is important to cauterize them before capsulotomy, in order to minimize postoperative hemorrhage. Blunt dissection and periosteal elevation of the capsule usually allow good visualization of the anterolateral lesion, which is facilitated by inversion and plantar flexion of the ankle. The lesion can be drilled or removed, and the edges trimmed. Attempts to secure the lesion with a bone peg or screw usually are not successful, and offer little in the way of improved functional outcome over removing the loose fragment and drilling the base.

Anteromedial Lesion. Thompson and Loomer advocate a medial incision that permits both an anteromedial and a posteromedial deep exposure, avoiding the need for osteotomy of the medial malleolus. An approach using a malleolar osteotomy provides an excellent view and is safe, but a longer recovery period is needed and therefore a soft tissue exposure is probably preferable in competitive athletes. It also eliminates the need for subsequent screw removal.

With the patient in the lying position, a 10 cm incision is curved posteriorly just posterior to the medial malleolus (Fig. 4). The anteromedial capsule and medial ligament are exposed. A 2 cm incision opens the capsule just anterior to the medial ligament. By maximal plantar flexion, the superomedial rim of the talus can be seen. If the medial talar lesion is too far posterior to be visualized, a second incision is made by retracting the tibialis posterior tendon anteriorly. The deep surface of the flexor retinaculum can be divided and the remaining

contents of the proximal tarsal tunnel carefully retracted posteriorly. It is not necessary to expose these structures separately to do this. At this point, maximal dorsiflexion usually allows access to the posteromedial half of the talus.

Arthroscopy. The supine position with a large wedge under the hip and the leg in a well-padded box, as previously described, usually permits access to the anterior, posterior, and lateral aspects of the ankle by rotation of the hip. The joint is distended with 10 to 15 ml of Ringer's lactate before the blunt probe is inserted. There are three anterior and one posterolateral portals, through which most lesions can be visualized. The anteromedial portal is medial to the tendon of the tibialis anterior, just lateral to the junction of the medial malleolus with the anterior joint space.

The anterocentral portal is lateral to the extensor hallucis longus, and care is needed to avoid the anterior tibial artery and deep peroneal nerve. The anterolateral portal is lateral to the peroneus tertius and the extensor digitorum longus tendons. Care is needed to avoid damage to the two terminal branches of the superficial peroneal nerve. The posterolateral portal is lateral to the Achilles tendon and approximately 2 cm above the tip of the lateral malleolus. The sural nerve and the short saphenous vein are vulnerable. It is rarely necessary to use the more dangerous posteromedial portal behind the flexor hallucis longus, and in very close proximity to the posterior tibial artery and nerve.

Once the scope is in the joint, a partial synovectomy may be necessary to visualize the more anteriorly placed fragment. The loose fragment is often best gripped with a small curved hemostat, the edges curetted and abraded with hand instruments. It may also be possible to drill the bed of an anterolateral lesion, but this is not a simple procedure.

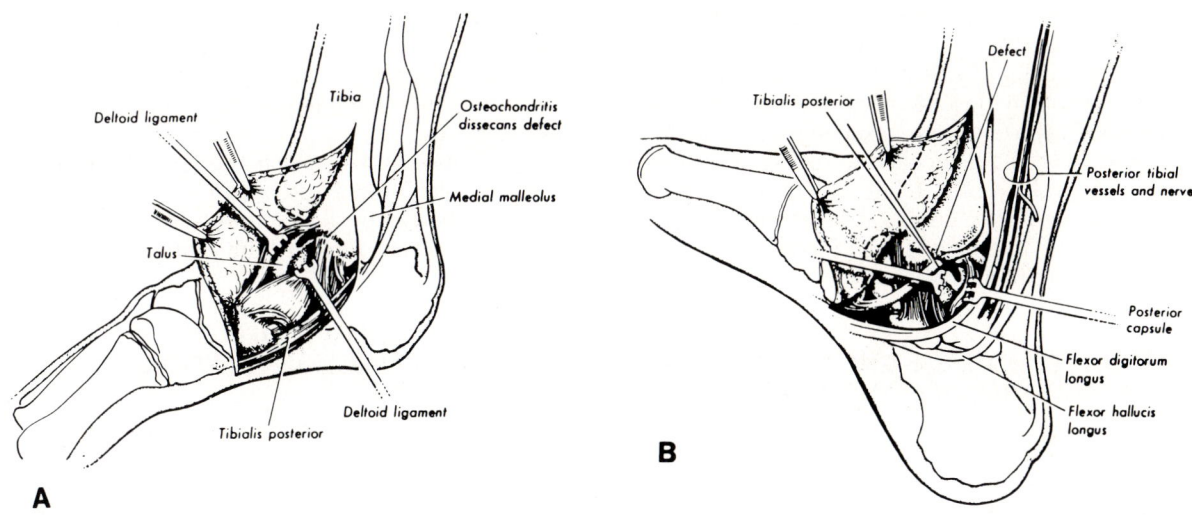

Figure 4 *A,* The anteromedial talus exposed in maximal plantar flexion. *B,* The posteromedial talus exposed via the same skin incision. (From Thompson JP, Loomer RL. Osteochondral lesions of the talus in a sports medicine clinic—a new radiographic technique and surgical approach. Am J Sports Med 1984; 12:460-463; with permission.)

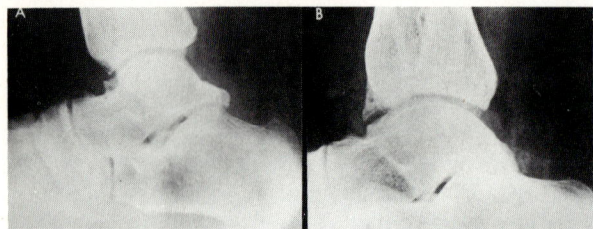

Figure 5 *A,* Hypertrophic spurs on the dorsal talus at the capsular insertion with normal joint space. *B,* Anterior tibial spur also associated with a painful limitation of dorsiflexion. (From Pavlov H, Torg JS. The running athlete. Chicago: Year Book Medical Publishers, 1987; with permission.)

TALAR ANTERIOR IMPINGEMENT SYNDROME

The talar anterior impingement syndrome is related to osteophytes on the neck of the talus or, more frequently, the anterior tibia. Dorsiflexion results in impingement of the bony spurs along with trapping and pinching of hypertrophied and chronically swollen synovium (Fig. 5).

These lesions occasionally are seen after repeated ankle inversion injuries and also are particularly associated with football linemen, in whom chronic repeated impingement stresses of the bony surfaces in dorsiflexion play a role in the etiology. Alternatively, the osteophytes may correlate with the tibial and talar attachments of the anterior capsule, and may relate to chronic traction stresses seen in runners and soccer players (see Fig. 5).

The athlete may simply complain of ankle pain and swelling proportional to the amount of activity. In mild cases this happens only with activities requiring sudden starts and stops or changes in direction, but in severe cases the symptoms occur with simple running or jogging. The feeling of pinching can be reproduced by forced dorsiflexion, and pain is experienced with palpation along the anterior talocrural joint line. Dorsiflexion is eventually limited by bony impingement as well as pain. Plain lateral radiographs help confirm the diagnosis. Support for the theory of chronic traction or compression stresses is lent by the usual absence of degenerative changes within the joint. For this reason, removal of the anterior synovium and resection of the osteophytes is usually all that is needed to relieve symptoms, and most athletes can return to full activity. With a small spur, it may be possible to do this arthroscopically, but it is usually necessary to open the joint for successful excision of adequate amounts of bone.

MENISCOID LESIONS OF THE TALOFIBULAR COMPONENT OF THE ANKLE

Wohlin and colleagues in 1950 described a series of patients who experienced chronic pain and swelling over the anterior and anterolateral ankle with activity. Often this is accompanied by a subjective feeling of instability and occasionally actual giving way. There is always a history of a moderately severe ankle injury.

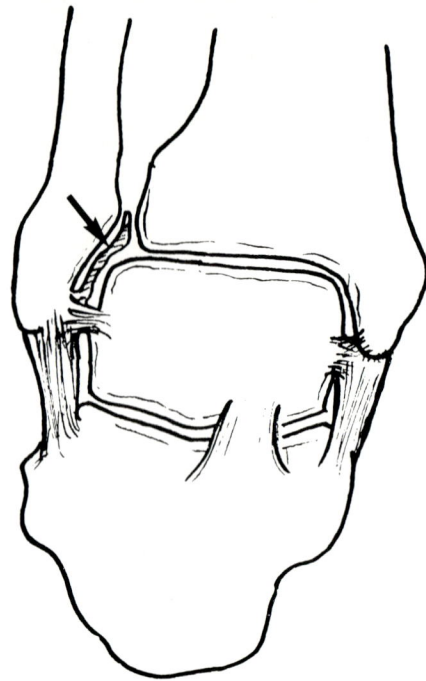

Figure 6 Schematic cross section of the talocrural joint showing a meniscoid lesion that may be related to the lateral ligament (after McCarrol JR).

There are two possible causes. This lesion may be secondary to traumatic synovial thickening, with incomplete resorption of the associated exudate. A small portion of inflammatory infiltrate persists between the fibula and the talus and eventually becomes hyalinized secondary to pressure, giving rise to these symptoms (Fig. 6). Other authors have suggested that these meniscoid lesions are tears of the anterior tibiofibular ligament in which the torn fragment becomes interposed between the talus and the lateral malleolus.

These lesions are rare, but it is important to consider the possibility of their presence in athletes who have persistent pain and swelling after inversion sprains, and in whom all roentgenographic and other diagnostic tests are negative.

Arthroscopy will reveal the lesion and the hyalinized, meniscoid-like band, and any redundant synovium may then be removed. Excision should cure the symptoms and prevent further joint irritation.

ANTEROMEDIAL DELTOID LIGAMENT IMPINGEMENT SYNDROME

A similar lesion is seen after disruption of the inferior tibiofibular articulation (with or without fracture of the fibula) with diastasis and rupture of the medial (deltoid) ligament of the ankle. Unrecognized incarceration of some of the ligament within the joint leads to chronic anteromedial ankle joint pain, sometimes with chronic swelling and disability with activity. Excision is often necessary, but the results are not always good because of the altered mechanics of the joint.

ANTEROLATERAL CORNER COMPRESSION SYNDROME OF THE ANKLE

Waller reported a syndrome that may be included in the spectrum of the previously described meniscoid lesion of the ankle. The athlete complains of pain located over the anteroinferior aspect of the fibula and the associated anterolateral talus, and the joint line. There is usually a history of inversion injury. The suspected etiology is a post-traumatic chondromalacia of the lateral wall of the talus, with associated synovial reaction.

It is suggested that pain and compression at foot strike makes the athlete, usually a runner, tighten the tibialis posterior and anterior tendons, and inhibits the peroneal tendons. This makes the runner susceptible to multiple inversion strains. The addition of a medial heel and inner sole wedge to the shoe may relieve impingement sufficiently to allow restoration of balanced inversion and eversion muscle action, and relieve symptoms. Walter claims that the symptoms are relieved in a matter of days in most cases. If the condition does not settle with modified activity, an orthosis, and a course of NSAIDs, arthroscopy should be considered to rule out other causes of the pain.

POSTERIOR TALAR COMPRESSION SYNDROME

Pain in the posterior ankle region may be incapacitating in ballet dancers and soccer players when due to impingement of an os trigonum or Stieda's process. This may be a diagnosis of exclusion in many instances, after Achilles tendinitis, peroneal tendinitis, and flexor hallucis longus tendinitis have been ruled out.

First described in 1804 by Rosenmuller, the os trigonum is present in at least 5% of feet, and as many as 38% of the adult population have an enlarged lateral process in the posterior surface of the talus (Fig. 7). It therefore is frequently present as an asymptomatic structure. Caution is warranted in oversubscribing symptoms to this normal anatomic variant. McDougall proposed three mechanisms for development of the os trigonum: (1) failure of fusion of the secondary ossification center, (2) repeated minor trauma with impingement against the posterior margin of the tibia, and (3) an acute fracture due to forced plantar flexion, occasionally in association with avulsion of the posterior band of the lateral ligament.

In the posterior talar compression syndrome, there usually is tenderness over the posterolateral aspect of the talus between the Achilles tendon and the peroneal tendons. The pain generally is reproduced by forced plantar flexion. The lack of tenderness over the peroneal tendons should help exclude the diagnosis of peroneal tendinitis.

A bone scan may be positive, but this is not

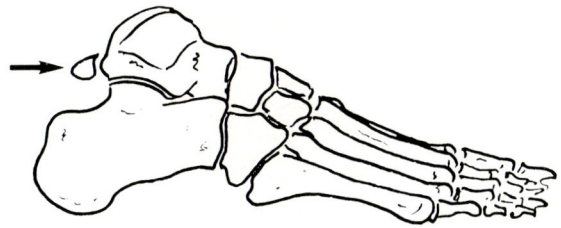

Os Trigonum

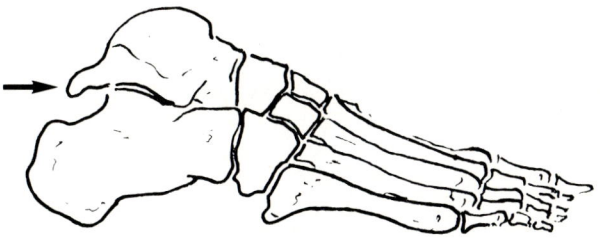

Stieda's Process

Figure 7 Lateral view of the foot showing an os trigonum and a Stieda's process.

mandatory to confirm the diagnosis. Forced plantar flexion radiography confirms the painful impingement, and temporary relief may be provided by infiltration of the area with 1% lidocaine (Xylocaine).

If modified activity and NSAIDs fail to relieve symptoms, excision of the os trigonum or Stieda's process, with adjacent release of the tendon sheath of the flexor hallucis longus, usually allows resumption of activities in about 1 month.

MEDIAL TARSAL TUNNEL SYNDROME

The medial tarsal tunnel syndrome represents a compression neuropathy of the tibial nerve or its terminal branches, the medial and lateral plantar nerves. The impingement frequently occurs in the distal two-thirds of the fibro-osseous canal, which has ill-defined limits. It begins a few centimeters proximal to the tip of the medial malleolus where the crural fascia starts to condense, forming a relatively unyielding roof, the flexor retinaculum. It ends where the medial and lateral plantar nerves enter or pass deep to the abductor hallucis. The anatomy is highly variable with regard to (1) the site at which the tibial nerve divides into the medial calcaneal, the medial plantar, and the lateral plantar nerves; (2) its terminal branches; and (3) the method by which it exits from the canal. The medial and lateral plantar nerves leave through separate fibrous openings or, on occasion, contiguously in one canal, sometimes piercing the abductor muscle (Fig. 8).

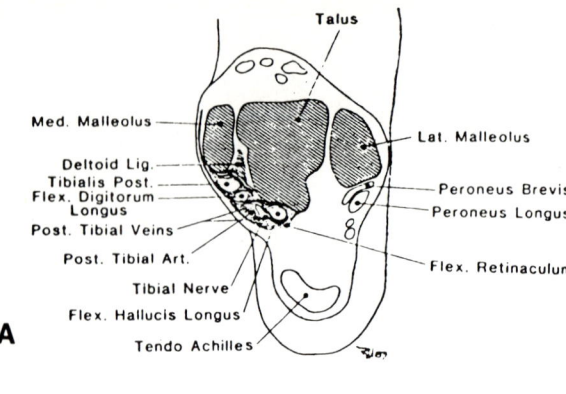

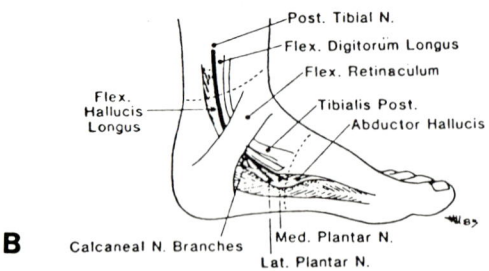

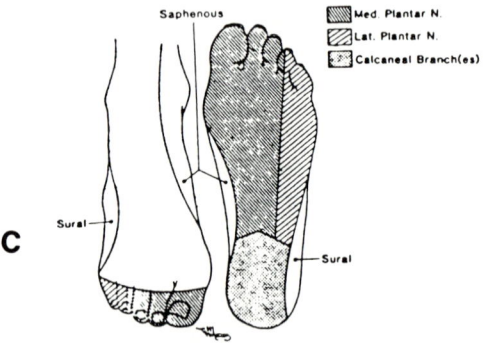

Figure 8 The relationship of the tendons and nerves of the tarsal tunnel *(A)* in cross section and *(B)* from the medial side. *(C)* The sensory areas supplied by the posterior tibial nerve terminal branches (after Kushner and Reid.)

Etiology

A variety of factors may lead to compromise of the nerve, and these may present in slightly different ways, contributing to a delay in diagnosis (Table 2).

Anatomic Factors. These include variations in the fibrous septa, areolar tissue, and retinaculum, which may be fibrous, may scar, or may swell with edema, limiting the space available for the contents of the tarsal tunnel. These may be secondary to trauma, aging, or repeated stresses. The nerve also may be compressed by dilated and engorged veins, and occasionally an arterial arch may cause symptoms. Variations in the anatomy of the abductor hallucis, including anomalous or accessory muscle, may involve the nerve distally. In athletes the repetitive stresses of running

Table 2 Etiology of Tarsal Tunnel Syndrome

Anatomic	*Tumor*
Septa	Neuroma
Areolar tissue	Lipoma
Retinacular	Synovial cyst
Vascular anomalies	Tendon tumors
Muscular variations	Neurolemmoma
Valgus alignment	
Trauma	*Inflammatory*
Fractures	Rheumatoid arthritis
Contusions	Ankylosing spondylitis
Postsurgical adhesions	Tenosynovitis
Sprains	Thrombophlebitis
Laceration	
Post-traumatic edema	
Post-traumatic adhesions	
	Miscellaneous
	Footwear
	Overuse syndrome
	Aging
	Fluid retention

may unmask these variations, particularly in the presence of a valgus heel and associated pronated forefoot, which may tighten the flexor retinaculum, the arch of the abductor hallucis, and the calcaneonavicular ligament.

Trauma. The tarsal tunnel syndrome can occur as a complication of ankle, calcaneal, or metatarsal fractures. In a review of 500 os calcis fractures, 10% developed tarsal tunnel syndrome and over one-fourth of these required surgical decompression. The syndrome also occurs with ankle sprains, tight casts, or hamstring injuries or postoperatively after osteotomies of the first ray or release of the Achilles tendon. All these causative conditions may have edema and secondary fibrosis as a common factor.

Tumor. In athletes, ganglion and post-traumatic synovial cysts constitute the most common neoplasms causing pressure in the canal. The symptoms may be intermittent, since such tumors swell with activity.

Miscellaneous. Chronic synovitis, ill-fitting footwear, inappropriate training surfaces, poorly graduated and planned training, fluid retention, pregnancy, and weight gain may all play a role. In addition, neuropathic conditions from a variety of systemic causes may precipitate the symptoms.

Clinical Picture

There appears to be no sex predilection and the onset is usually insidious. The most common complaint is of burning pain and paresthesia in the plantar aspect of the foot. Pain is exacerbated by activity and diminished by rest. The usual site is the great toe, followed in descending order of frequency by the remaining toes and the distal sole of the foot (Table 3). Symptoms occasionally occur in the medial plantar surface of the heel. Athletes may also report a "swollen or tight" sensation, as if there is an impending cramp in the arch of the foot.

Table 3 Clinical Data on Eight Patients with Medial Tarsal Tunnel Syndrome

Age	Sex	Sport	Occupation	Side	Duration (Mo)	Foot Alignment	Symptoms	Sensory	Motor EMG	Conservative Treatment	Findings at Surgery	Results
25	F	Runner, 40 mi/wk	Student	L	17	Normal	Pain into great toe after running	Hyperesthesia of great toe and medial foot Tinel +	None +	US Injection	Constriction by fibrous band in superior tunnel	Relief by 24 hr
35	M	Runner, 60 mi/wk Chronic tenosynovitis of tibialis posterior over 3-yr period	Teacher	L	38	Valgus heel Pronated forefoot	Numbness and paresthesia Nocturnal pain	Impaired pinprick Tinel −	None +	US TNS Injection	Thickening of nerve and fibrosis	Relief by 3 mo
22	F	Runner, 45 mi/wk	Student	R	15	Valgus heel Pronated forefoot	Burning sensation in great toe	Hyperesthesia Tinel +	None +	US Orthototic	Fibrosis of nerve	Relief in 1 mo
43	M	Runner, 65 mi/wk	Lawyer	R	5	Valgus heel Pronated forefoot	Burning sensation	Impaired pinprick Tinel −	None +	Orthotic	Fusiform thickening of nerve	Relief by 36 hr
19	F	Skater (skate pressure?)	Student	L	16	Prominent calcaneus	Burning sensation	Impaired pinprick Tinel −	None +	Modification of skates	Normal appearance	Relief in 24 hr
22	M	Soccer (post-contusion)	Phys. ed. teacher	L	8	Normal	Intense burning Nocturnal pain	Decreased pinprick over entire medial plantar nerve distrib. Tinel −	None +	US SWD Injection Mobilization	Dense scarring	Relief at 1 mo
33	M	Ice hockey (postfractured calcaneus)	Construction worker	R	14	Broadened heel	Intense burning Nocturnal pain	Paresthesia in foot and toes Tinel +	None +	Wax baths US Injection Mobilization	Dense scarring Neuroma	Relief at 6 wk
29	F	Runner, 80 mi/wk	Student	L	7	Valgus heel Pronated forefoot	Intense burning after running	Decreased tactile sensation Tinel −	None +	Orthosis US	Scarring near abductor hallucis muscle	Relief at 24 hr

EMG = electromyogram; US = ultrasound; TNS = transcutaneous nerve stimulation; SWD = shortwave diathermy.

For some individuals the pain may be worse at night, and they report that pain is relieved by hanging the foot out of bed, moving it, rubbing it, or getting out of bed and walking around.

Sensory signs include hypoesthesia to pinprick, diminished two-point discrimination, and a positive Tinel's sign (see Fig. 8). Sustained direct pressure reproduces or exacerbates the symptoms. It is difficult to detect associated weakness.

The definitive test is the nerve conduction study, of both the abductor digiti minimi and the abductor hallucis. Latencies of more than one standard deviation above the normal for the particular laboratory carrying out the test are considered positive, although evaluation of evoked sensory and motor potentials may be a more sensitive indication of a pathologic condition (see Table 3).

Treatment

Nonoperative

Modification of Activity. Advice should be offered with regard to the intensity of training, the building up of mileage, the impact of the terrain, the distance covered, and the spacing of training sessions.

Modalities. Most physiotherapeutic modalities should be aimed at reduction of edema and scarring. These may include the use of ice after activity, ultrasound, interferential therapy, lasers, and short wave diathermy. These may be successful when symptoms are recently acquired, but they rarely are of use for an established neuropathic condition.

Footwear and Orthoses. In view of the highly associated valgus heel and pronated forefoot, a trial of a medial arch support or medial heel wedge may be considered. Extremely tight lacing of shoes or skates may exacerbate the condition, as will shoes worn down at the lateral heel. Occasionally, when edema features highly in the etiology, support hose may be helpful.

Medication. Orally administered NSAIDs are most successful in acute-onset situations associated with tenosynovitis. Occasionally a trial of local injectable steroid is successful, but care should be taken to avoid direct injection into the vessel and nerve. Furthermore, skin atrophy can be troublesome in this situation; this can be minimized by a deep injection of steroid with only about 1 ml of accompanying lidocaine.

Operative

Surgical release may provide rapid relief from the symptoms of the compression neuropathy, although with denervation in established cases some signs may persist. Since it is difficult to localize the exact site of compression, the entire canal is released. The flexor retinaculum is completely divided and the posterior tibial nerve freed from encompassing fibrous tissue. The branches are explored where possible to mobilize them as far distal as the abductor hallucis muscle. Each hiatus for the medial and lateral plantar nerves is checked and released; if there is an accessory abductor hallucis, it is excised. Care is taken not to disrupt the fine calcaneal branches, since damage to these creates heel numbness. If there are tortuous veins present, they should be ligated proximally and distally and then excised. Even with careful dissection, it is impossible to identify unequivocal pathologic condition in about 25% of the cases; however, if previous neurophysiologic testing has confirmed the site of compression, relief can be obtained.

Partial weight bearing or limited walking with full weight bearing for 2 weeks is advised. By 3 weeks, more aggressive activity may be undertaken, including balance board work and running. It usually takes 4 to 6 weeks before a full return to sporting activities is possible. Recurrence of symptoms in a well-decompressed nerve is rare, and the only significant, but rare, long-term complication is subluxation of the tibialis posterior tendon.

This syndrome is not usually recognized early, which is unfortunate, since it often resolves promptly with nonoperative treatment in the early stages. For this reason, the variation in presentation and the multitude of etiologic factors have been stressed in this chapter in the hope that this syndrome will be included more often in the differential diagnosis of sources of medial talar, calcaneal, and medial foot pain.

SUGGESTED READING

Alexander AH, Lichtman DM. Surgical treatment of transchondral talar dome fractures. J Bone Joint Surg 1980; 62A:646–652.

Andrews JR, Drez DJ, McGinty JB. Symposium: Arthroscopy of joints other than the knee. Contemp Orthop 1984; 9:71–100.

Berndt AL, Harty M. Transchondral fractures (osteochondritis dissecans) of the talus. J Bone Joint Surg 1959; 41A:988–1020.

Brodsky AE, Khalil MA. Talar compression syndrome. Am J Sports Med 1986; 14:472–476.

Campbell CJ, Rangwat CS. Osteochondritis dissecans: The question of etiology. J Trauma 1986; 6:201–221.

Canele ST, Belding RH. Osteochondral lesions of the talus. J Bone Joint Surg 1980; 62A:97–102.

Cedell CA. Rupture of the posterior talotibial ligament with avulsion of a bone fragment from the talus. Acta Orthop Scand 1974; 45:454–461.

Dipaola JD, Nelson DW, Colville M. Characterizing osteochondral lesions by magnetic resonance imaging. J Arthros Rel Surg 1991; 7(1):101–104.

Distefano V, Sack JT, Whittaker R, Nixon JE. Tarsal tunnel syndrome. Clin Orthop 1972; 88:76–79.

Drez DM, Suhl JF, Gollehan DL. Ankle arthroscopy—technique and indications. Foot Ankle 1985; 2:138–143.

Flick AB, Gould N. Osteochondritis dissecans of the talus (transchondral fractures of the talus)—review of literature and new surgical approach for medial dome lesions. Foot Ankle 1985; 5:165–185.

Fu R, Delisa JA, Kraft GH. Motor nerve latencies through the tarsal tunnel in normal adult subjects: Standard determinations for corrected temperatures and distance. Arch Phys Med Rehabil 1980; 61:243–248.

Hagmeyer RH, van der Wurff M. Transchondral fractures of the talus on an inversion injury of the ankle: A frequently overlooked diagnosis. J Orthop Sports Phys Ther 1987; 8:362–367.

Hontas MJ, Haddard RJ, Schlesinger LC. Conditions of the talus in the runner. Am J Sports Med 1986; 14:486–490.

Kaplan PE, Kernahan WT. Tarsal tunnel syndrome. J Bone Joint Surg 1981; 63A:96–99.

Keck C. The tarsal tunnel syndrome. J Bone Joint Surg 1962; 44A:180–182.

Kushner S, Reid DC. Medial tarsal tunnel syndrome: a review. J Orthop Sports Phys Ther 1984; 6:39–45.

Langan P, Weiss CA. Subluxation of the tibialis posterior tendon: A complication of tarsal tunnel decompression. Clin Orthop 1980; 146:226–227.

Lindholm TS, Osterman K, Vankka E. Osteochondritis dissecans of elbow, ankle and hip: A comparison survey. Clin Orthop 1980; 148:245–250.

McCarroll JR, Schrader JW, Shelbourne KD, Rettig AC, Bisesi MA. Meniscoid lesions of the ankle in soccer players. Am J Sports Med 1987; 15:255–257.

McCullough CJ, Venngopal V. Osteochondritis dissecans of the talus: The natural history. Clin Orthop 1979; 144:264–268.

McDougall A. The os trigonum. J Bone Joint Surg 1955; 37B:257–265.

O'Farrell TA, Costello BG. Osteochondritis dissecans of the talus: the late results of surgical treatment. J Bone Joint Surg 1982; 64B:494–497.

Parisien JS. Arthroscopic treatment of osteochondral lesions of the talus. Am J Sports Med 1986; 14:211–217.

Parks JC, Hamilton WG, Patterson AH, et al. The anterior impingement syndrome of the ankle. J Trauma 1980; 20:895–898.

Pritch M. Arthroscopic treatment of osteochondral lesions of the talus. J Bone Joint Surg 1986; 68A:862–865.

Roden S, Tillegard P, Unander-Scharin L. Osteochondritis dissecans and similar lesions of the talus. Acta Orthop Scand 1953; 23:51–66.

Thompson JP, Loomer RL. Osteochondral lesions of the talus in a sports medicine clinic—a new radiographic technique and surgical approach. Am J Sports Med 1984; 12:460–463.

Waller JF Jr. Hindfoot and midfoot problems of the runner—symposium on the foot and leg in running sports. St Louis: CV Mosby, 1982:64.

Wohlin I, Glassman F, Sideman S. Internal derangement of the talofibular component of the ankle. Surg Gynecol Obstet 1950; 91:193–200.

PERONEAL TENDON DISLOCATION

IRA ZALTZ, M.D.
LYLE J. MICHELI, M.D.

Acute dislocation of the peroneal tendons is an uncommon injury. Consequently, its diagnosis is often overlooked until the patient presents with symptoms of chronic peroneal tendon subluxation. The acute injury is thought to occur while the ankle is dorsiflexed, the foot is everted, and there is an accompanying reflex contraction of the peroneal muscles. The injury has classically occurred in the downhill foot of the forward-falling skier. However, it has also been reported in football, rugby, gymnastics, tennis, water-skiing, and dancing.

PRESENTATION AND DIAGNOSIS

Acutely, the patient presents complaining of pain located over the distal aspect of the lateral malleolus and retromalleolar sulcus. A painful snap experienced at the time of injury should alert the physician to this particular injury. Physical examination reveals swelling and ecchymosis over the distal lateral malleolus and retromalleolar sulcus. Depending on the stability of the peroneal tendons, they may remain dislocated anterior to the peroneal groove or may have spontaneously reduced. Nevertheless, the stability of the tendons should be evaluated by stressing them with the ankle dorsiflexed and the foot everted.

Tenderness over the peroneal groove, often extending proximally up the tendon for several inches, and increased pain with provocative testing provide presumptive evidence of peroneal subluxation with retinacular tear.

Peroneal tendon subluxation must be differentiated from a sprain of the anterior talofibular ligament, as this is a frequent injury about the lateral aspect of the ankle and commonly diagnosed despite a history suggestive of peroneal tendon injury. In children, a Salter I injury to the fibular physeal plate must also be excluded.

Patients who fail conservative treatment for acute peroneal tendon dislocation or who are not diagnosed at the time of injury may present with chronically unstable peroneal tendons. They generally complain of activity-related pain and painful snapping over the distal lateral malleolus and retromalleolar sulcus. A history of ankle instability should be sought. Examination may reveal swelling over the course of the peroneal tendons and associated crepitus. Stressing the peroneal tendons often reproduces the painful snap and unstable feeling. Stability of the ankle joint should be thoroughly assessed in order to exclude chronic lateral ankle ligament insufficiency. Intra-articular causes of ankle "giving way" should be eliminated.

IMAGING

Patients presenting with either acute or chronic peroneal tendon subluxation should undergo routine anteroposterior, lateral, and mortise views of the ankle. A thin cortical fracture approximately 1 cm long seen on the mortise view is considered pathognomonic of peroneal subluxation and is present in approximately 15% of cases. Some authors have suggested obtaining computed tomography (CT) scans of acute cases in order to formulate a treatment plan based on the anatomy of the involved peroneal groove. Magnetic resonance imaging (MRI) shows signal changes in the soft tissues surrounding the ankle and may show attenuation of the peroneus brevis tendon, which has important implications in certain reconstructive procedures.

ANATOMY AND PATHOANATOMY

The peroneus longus and brevis muscles arise in the lateral compartment of the leg from adjacent surfaces of the fibula and interosseous membrane. Their tendons course distally in the peroneal groove on the posterior surface of the fibula. The peroneus brevis tendon, located lateral to the peroneus longus, turns around the lateral malleolus in a plantar and anterior direction to insert on the base of the fifth metatarsal. The peroneus longus turns in a plantar and medial direction coursing beneath the calcaneus to insert on the lateral aspect of the base of the first metatarsal. The middle portion of the lateral collateral ligaments of the ankle, the fibulo-calcaneal, lies deep to the tendons as they traverse the fibular groove.

The anatomy of the posterior fibula varies widely. In his dissections, Edwards noted that 82% of fibulae had definite grooves while 11% were flat and 7% were actually convex. Eckert and Davis reported a previously unrecognized dense collagenous structure located on the posterolateral rim of the fibula, which is distinct from the periosteum and peroneal retinaculum. They believe that this collagenous lip is a restraint for the peroneal tendons, and observed its involvement with various types of peroneal dislocations. In addition, Eckert and Davis observe that the superior peroneal retinaculum, a fascial band that blends with the fibular periosteum and is thought to assist in restraint of the tendons, is an inconstant structure of varying integrity.

In acutely dislocated tendons being treated by operative repair, Eckert and Davis classified all injuries into three groups. Grade I injuries, comprising 37 of 73 cases, occur when the superior retinaculum is separated from the collagenous lip and lateral malleolus. Grade II injuries, comprising 24 of 73 cases, occurs when the distal centimeter of collagenous lip as well as the superior peroneal retinaculum is elevated from the malleolus. Grade III injuries, comprising 12 of 73 cases, occurs when the collagenous lip is elevated from the fibula along with a thin shell of cortical bone.

A variety of findings have been reported in surgically treated cases of chronic peroneal subluxation. Das De and Balasubramanian, making comparison to the Bankart lesion, noted attenuation of the peroneal sheath, and elevation of the superior peroneal retinaculum and periosteum from the fibula in the majority of their cases. Pöll and Duijfjes reported rupture of the superior retinaculum in nine of 10 cases as well as stretching of the peroneal sheath. Multiple authors have described fraying of the peroneus brevis tendon in chronic lesions, and one group has reported on the association between peroneal subluxation and attenuation of lateral ankle ligaments.

TREATMENT

Treatment of acute peroneal tendon subluxation is the subject of some debate. While excellent results have been reported for the surgical treatment of acutely dislocated tendons, not all patients with subluxed tendons are symptomatic or disabled. Consequently, the precise surgical indications for repair of acutely dislocated peroneal tendons are not defined.

The goal of nonoperative treatment is to hold the peroneal tendons in their reduced position while their retinaculum heals or scars in place. This may be accomplished by means of casting, taping, or strapping with or without the use of pads. Escalas and co-workers reported that 28 out of 38 patients treated with "compressive bandages for several weeks" redislocated and required surgery. McLennan reported that patients with acute peroneal tendon subluxation can be treated conservatively with minimal morbidity and good functional results. Despite recurrent subluxation in some patients, results are still good or excellent. Stover and Bryan believe that treating patients with either acute peroneal dislocation or subluxation for 6 weeks in a non-weight-bearing short leg cast with the ankle positioned in slight plantarflexion will achieve excellent results even when there is an associated rim fracture. Eckert and Davis reported the largest series of operatively treated acute injuries. Seventy of 73 patients treated by either retinacular repair and fascial plication, with fracture reduction when necessary, achieved good results.

In contrast to acute treatment, there is no debate regarding the treatment of symptomatic chronically subluxed or dislocated peroneal tendons. The best results are achieved by operatively stabilizing the peroneal tendons in their anatomic position. The many procedures that have been designed to stabilize the peroneal tendons generally fall into four categories: periosteal reattachment, groove deepening, tenoplasty, and bone block. Generally, satisfactory results, in terms of tendon stability, residual discomfort, and functional recovery, have been reported for the many techniques.

Das De and Balasubramanian use sutures to reattach the periosteum to the fibular cortex and to imbricate the superior peroneal retinaculum in order to achieve reduction of the peroneal tendons. Zoellner and Clancy deepen the peroneal groove by creating a posterior osteoperiosteal flap, removing cancellous bone, and then impacting the flap deep within the fibula. Once the peroneal tendons are located within the deepened groove the repair is reinforced with a periosteal flap. Tenoplasty procedures include the classic described by Jones, which uses a strip of Achilles tendon anchored to the lateral malleolus to restrain the peroneal tendons. Rerouting the peroneal tendons beneath the calcaneofibular ligament by either dividing the tendons or temporarily elevating the ligament has also been reported. The original bone block procedure described by Kelly and later modified by DuVries enlarged the lip by sliding a sagittally cut piece of fibula posteriorly.

PREFERRED TREATMENT

Since 1977 we have used a modification of Kelly's procedure to repair chronically dislocated peroneal tendons. By sliding a slotted fibular graft distally instead of posteriorly, this procedure combines the advantage of a bone block procedure with that of a groove deepening procedure while preserving the fibro-osseous tunnel for the tendons to glide. At a mean 28.2 month follow-up we reported 91% excellent results judged by complete return to activities.

Technically, the procedure is accomplished with the patient in the supine position with a sand bag beneath the ipsilateral greater trochanter. A gently curved incision is made over the lateral malleolus in order to expose the distal 8 cm of fibula (Fig. 1). With the fibula exposed extraperiostally (Fig. 2), the osteotomy cuts are marked 6 to 7 cm proximally from the distal tip and 8 to 10 mm anteriorly from the lateral ridge. A mini-sagittal saw is used to make the proximal, anterior, and posterior cuts (Fig. 3). The distal periosteum and soft tissues must be left intact. The graft is then elevated from its bed using a curette, and can be mobilized distally by gently elevating the soft tissues from the undersurface of the remaining malleolus. Cancellous bone is then removed

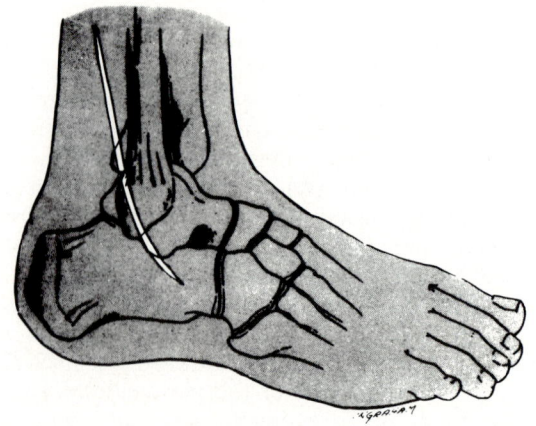

Figure 1 A gently curved incision is made over the lateral malleolus in order to expose the distal 8 cm of fibula. (From Micheli LJ, Waters PM, Sanders DP. Sliding fibular graft repair for chronic dislocation of the peroneal tendons. Am J Sports Med 1990; 17:68–71; with permission.)

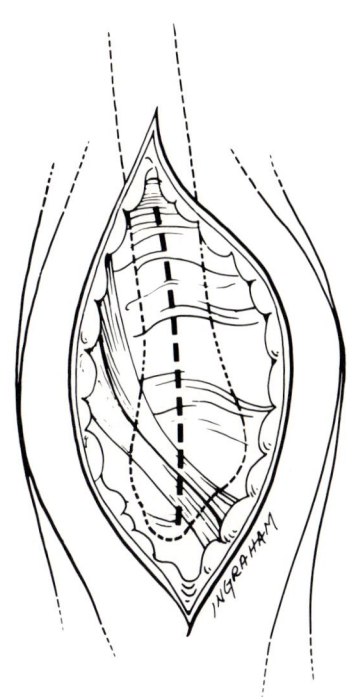

Figure 2 With the fibula exposed extraperiostally, the osteotomy cuts are marked 6 to 7 cm proximally from the distal tip and 8 to 10 mm anteriorly from the lateral ridge. (From Micheli LJ, Waters PM, Sanders DP. Sliding fibular graft repair for chronic dislocation of the peroneal tendons. Am J Sports Med 1990; 17:68–71; with permission.)

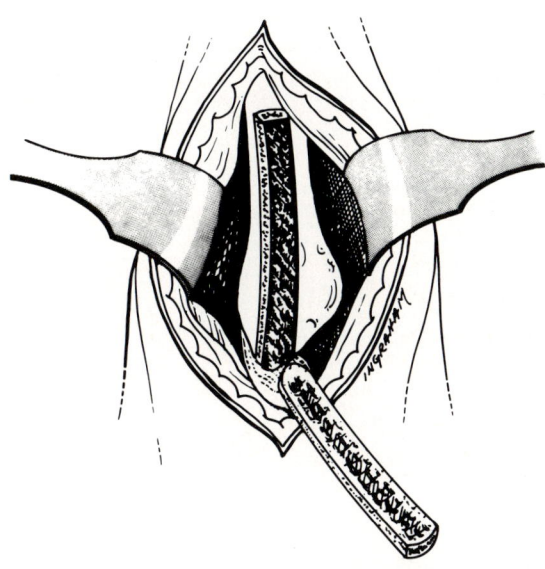

Figure 3 A mini-sagittal saw is used to make the proximal, anterior, and posterior cuts. (From Micheli LJ, Waters PM, Sanders DP. Sliding fibular graft repair for chronic dislocation of the peroneal tendons. Am J Sports Med 1990; 17:68–71; with permission.)

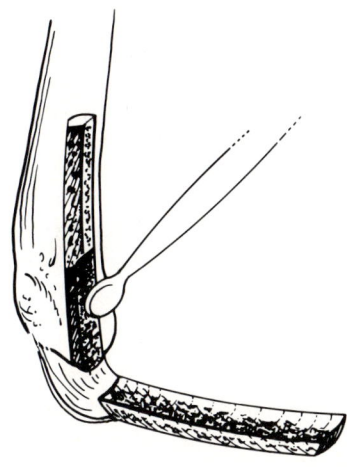

Figure 4 Cancellous bone is removed from the distal osteotomy bed in order to be able to deeply set the graft into the malleolus. (From Micheli LJ, Waters PM, Sanders DP. Sliding fibular graft repair for chronic dislocation of the peroneal tendons. Am J Sports Med 1990; 17:68–71; with permission.)

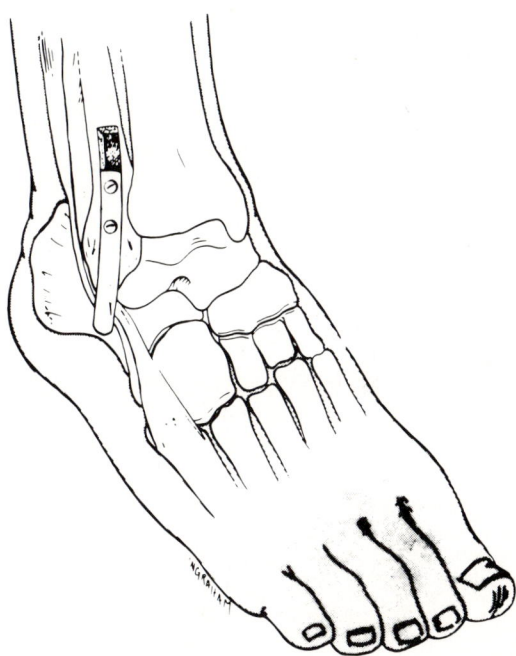

Figure 5 The reconstruction is fixed in place with two 3.5 mm AO cortical screws. (From Micheli LJ, Waters PM, Sanders DP. Sliding fibular graft repair for chronic dislocation of the peroneal tendons. Am J Sports Med 1990; 17:68–71; with permission.)

from the distal osteotomy bed in order to be able to deeply set the graft into the malleolus (Fig. 4). The graft is then slid distally between 1 and 1.5 cm and provisionally held by a Kirschner wire. The reconstruction is then tested, and, if successful, is fixed in place with two 3.5 mm AO cortical screws (Fig. 5). Intraoperative roentgenograms may be taken to check screw placement.

Postoperatively, the patient is immobilized in a

non-weight-bearing short leg cast for 4 weeks, and then a full weight-bearing cast for another 4 weeks. The patient is allowed to return to full activity once full ankle motion and strength are regained, which is approximately 6 weeks after cast removal.

One patient fractured her graft in a fall while figure skating. This healed uneventfully in a short leg cast, and the patient returned to her regular activities. Another patient was re-explored for pain. She was noted to have an exostosis at her osteotomy site and associated peroneal tenosynovitis. After resection of the exostosis, she now has an excellent result. There have been neither problems with shoe wear, loss of ankle motion, nor loss of eversion in any patient. Screws are removed only if the patient is symptomatic.

SUGGESTED READING

Arrowsmith SR, Fleming LL, Allman FL. Traumatic dislocations of the peroneal tendons. Am J Sports Med 1983; 11:142–146.

Brage ME, Hansen ST. Traumatic subluxation/dislocation of the peroneal tendons. Foot and Ankle 1992; 13:423–432.

Church CC. Radiographic diagnosis of acute peroneal tendon dislocation. Am J Roentgenol 1977; 129:1065–1068.

Das De S, Balasubramanian P. A repair operation for recurrent dislocation of peroneal tendons. J Bone Joint Surg 1985; 67B: 585–587.

Eckert WR, Davis EA Jr. Acute rupture of the peroneal retinaculum. J Bone Joint Surg 1976; 58A:670–673.

Edwards ME. The relation of the peroneal tendons to the fibula, calcaneus and cuboideum. Am J Anat 1928; 42:213–253.

Escalas F, Figueras JM, Merino JA. Dislocation of the peroneal tendons: Long-term results of surgical treatment. J Bone Joint Surg 1980; 62A:451–453.

Jones E. Operative treatment of chronic dislocation of the peroneal tendons. J Bone Joint Surg 1932; 14:574–576.

Martens MA, Noyez JF, Mulier JC. Recurrent dislocation of the peroneal tendons: Results of rerouting the tendons under the calcaneofibular ligament. Am J Sports Med 1986; 14:148–150.

Martin DF, Baker CL, Curl WW, et al. Operative ankle arthroscopy. Long-term follow-up. Am J Sports Med 1989; 17:16–23.

McLennan JG. Treatment of acute and chronic luxations of the peroneal tendons. Am J Sports Med 1980; 8:432–436.

Micheli LJ, Waters PW, Sanders DP. Sliding fibular graft repair for chronic dislocation of the peroneal tendons. Am J Sports Med 1989; 17:68–71.

Murr S. Dislocation of the peroneal tendons with marginal fracture of the lateral malleolus. J Bone Joint Surg 1961; 43B:563–565.

Pöll RG. The treatment of recurrent dislocation of the peroneal tendons. J Bone Joint Surg 1984; 66B:98–100.

Sarmiento A, Wolf M. Subluxation of peroneal tendons: Case treated by rerouting tendons under calcaneofibular ligament. J Bone Joint Surg 1975; 57A:115–116.

Sobel M, Warren RF, Brourman S. Lateral ankle instability associated with dislocation of the peroneal tendons treated by the Chrisman-Snook procedure: A case report and literature review. Am J Sports Med 1990; 18:539–543.

Stein RE. Reconstruction of the superior peroneal retinaculum using a portion of the peroneus brevis tendon: A case report. J Bone Joint Surg 1987; 69A:298–299.

Stover CN, Bryan DR. Traumatic dislocation of the peroneal tendons. Am J Surg 1962; 103:180–186.

Szczukowski M, St. Peirre RK, Fleming LL, Somogyi J. Computerized tomography in the evaluation of peroneal tendon dislocation: A report of two cases. Am J Sports Med 1983; 11:444–447.

Zoellner G, Clancy W Jr. Recurrent dislocation of the peroneal tendon. J Bone Joint Surg 1979; 61A:292–294.

I KNEE

PERIARTICULAR OVERUSE SYNDROMES

R. PETER WELSH, M.B., Ch.B., F.R.C.S.(C), F.A.C.S.
CHRISTINE HUTTON, M.B., Ch.B.

Periarticular knee pain can be troublesome to the athlete, diminishing performance and blunting the training effort. With athletic effort, overload or overuse syndromes are common. Symptoms may arise from the patellar mechanism, from the quadriceps tendon or the ligamentum patella at its origin and insertion, from the stabilizing retinacula, from the fat pads deep to the supra- and infrapatellar tendons, or from the synovial lining where it forms plicae or folds that run medially beneath the extensor mechanism and distally along the medial border of the patella to the distal fat pad. In addition, bursae may be aggravated not only in the prepatellar area but also deep to the infrapatellar tendon, as well as beneath the pes anserinus tendons on the medial side and the iliotibial tract on the lateral side. Any of these structures may be involved in the genesis of periarticular overuse syndromes around the knee.

EXTENSOR MECHANISM DYSFUNCTION

The most common presenting symptom is that of pain in or around the knee associated with running, jumping, or kicking activities, or with kneeling or crouching. Discomfort is commonly aggravated on ascending and descending stairs; a sensation of instability or crepitus may also be noted. On examination the only positive findings may be tenderness to palpation around or over the patella and its tendons, or to compression of the patella against the femoral condyles. It should be noted that there are no signs of internal derangement and there is no effusion, no loss of range of motion, and no ligamentous instability. There may be some mild quadriceps wasting and occasionally some retropatellar crepitus, but most commonly the examiner is unable to demonstrate major abnormality. This can lead him to discount the significance of the patient's complaints or to erroneously label the condition "chondromalacia." Both these approaches do the patient a gross disservice. A specific diagnosis should be made in every instance.

PATELLAR TENDINITIS (JUMPER'S KNEE)

Inflammation of the distal tendon of the quadriceps muscle (suprapatellar tendinitis), of the origin of the infrapatellar tendon (infrapatellar tendinitis), and of the insertion of the infrapatellar tendon (Osgood-Schlatter disease) are all overuse syndromes associated with running and jumping activities. Pain and tenderness are usually localized to the inflamed area. The discomfort tends to develop during the course of the activity and often persists afterward.

Initial treatment consists of physiotherapy with local ice frictions and ultrsonography, and strengthening and, more particularly, stretching of the quadriceps muscle in conjunction with oral nonsteroidal anti-inflammatory medication for 10 to 15 days. As with all tendinitis, aggressive treatment in the early stages is more successful than later treatment in the chronic established condition. The athlete is reassured that no harm is being done to the knee joint and is permitted to continue with sporting activities, but in modified form. If the provocative exercise involves springing and bounding, these must be discontinued and running or cycling exercises substituted. In all cases the intention should be to maintain the athlete's basic fitness while the condition is allowed to recover without continuing provocative stimuli.

In cases refractory to this regimen, local injection of steroid around the tendon and into the underlying bursa may be indicated. The injection of steroid can have a direct, deleterious effect on the collagenous structures. Injection, particularly of the infrapatellar tendon, should be limited to a maximum of two injections spaced at least 6 months apart lest the weakening of the tendon predispose to its rupture.

Surgical Treatment

On occasion the patellar tendinitis may become so pernicious that the athlete is forced to give up the chosen activity. Under such circumstances, when all conservative treatments have been exhausted, localized tenolysis has been most successful in reestablishing athletic capability.

In this minor procedure through a transverse skin incision, the ligamentum patella is split longitudinally along the direction of its fibers right at the lower pole of the patella. With a sharp dissection the ligamentum is reflected off the lower pole of the patella over an area of about 2 cm, retaining adequate supporting tissue on both the medial and lateral sides. The tendon may be degenerate, with granulation in the substance of the tendon; this degenerate tendon segment, which is usually quite small, is excised and sent for histologic examination. The exposed portion of the lower pole of the patella is then decorticated with an osteotome and the bed drilled with a fine drill point. Access to the infrapatellar fat pad is also gained; if this is hypertrophied, the redundant tissue is excised. A simple oversewing of the tendon is carried out with resorbable sutures, and the limb is protected in a soft dressing. Splint protection is afforded for 2 weeks; after suture removal, a light exercise program including hydrotherapy and bicycle exercises is begun. Isometric quadriceps and hip flexor-abductor exercises are maintained; return to running activity is allowed at 6 weeks.

The condition is not a common indication for surgery, but this simple procedure has been effective in athletes who have proved refractory to all other measures.

OSGOOD-SCHLATTER DISEASE

Osgood-Schlatter disease is a tendinitis in adolescents in which the tibial apophysis is involved. Pressures on the sensitive growth area evoke a local discomfort that can become very disabling. The conventional treatment of this condition has included complete immobilization in a cylinder cast in full extension for 6 weeks. However, in most instances one need not resort to such treatment; the use of an infrapatellar strap worn across the tendon during activity may decrease the pull on the tendon or the tubercle, as happens when a forearm band is used for tennis elbow. The mainstay of management of this condition involves restriction of jumping or bounding activities while the athlete is acutely tender, the use of local ice friction treatments, and diligent application to quadriceps stretching routines. By decreasing the pull on the quadriceps mechanism and making the quadriceps muscle more flexible, the load on the infrapatellar tendon and thus the impact on the tibial tubercle can be greatly reduced. Most athletes can continue their sports activity, but Osgood-Schlatter disease tends to be episodic, and there may be occasions for weeks at a time when restriction of activity becomes necessary. Most adolescents grow through this condition in the course of 2 to 3 years. However, the condition may continue into late adolescence or adulthood, with continuing problems around the tibial tubercle insertion. Local steroid injections may settle symptoms, but there are other instances when surgical treatment becomes necessary.

Surgical Treatment

X-ray review of patients with persistent symptoms around the tibial tubercle often reveals an ossific loose body in the tendon substance where the tibial tubercle apophysis has fragmented and one of the islands of bone has not united with the parent tibia. This local irritation is remedied by the excision of the loose fragment. A transverse incision at the tibial tubercle insertion followed by a longitudinal split in the tendon identifies the loose body; all fragments and any bursal reactive tissue are excised. The tendon is then oversewn and the leg protected in a soft dressing. Return to activity is allowed as symptoms dictate, but it usually takes 6 to 8 weeks before jumping and bounding activities can be recommended.

BURSITIS

Prepatellar Bursitis

Prepatellar bursitis (housemaid's knee) presents with pain and swelling in the bursal tissue over the anterior surface of the patella resulting from either direct trauma or repetitive irritation. A fluctuant swelling can be aspirated, local steroid injected, and a compression dressing applied. Follow-up care with anti-inflammatory medication and a therapy program with ultrasonography settles most cases. In long-standing cases, it may be necessary to consider surgical excision of the bursa.

Surgical Treatment

A transverse incision enables the prepatellar bursa to be completely shelled out and peeled off the surface of the patella. The tissues often are very extensively scarred and thickened; removal leaves a large space for potential hematoma formation. To control this, the prepatellar subcutaneous tissues should be sewn down to the fascia over the patella to close this space. A suction drain should be left in situ for 24 hours and a compression bandage applied for 2 weeks.

Infrapatellar Bursitis

Infrapatellar bursitis is a common accompaniment of infrapatellar tendinitis, associated also with the infrapatellar fat pad syndrome. Local steroid injection into the bursa through the ligamentum patella usually settles an infrapatellar tendon bursitis satisfactorily. At the time of surgery for infrapatellar tendinitis, this area should be thoroughly inspected for its possible involvement in the pathology.

Iliotibial Band Bursitis

Iliotibial band bursitis is a troublesome inflammation of the bursa underlying the distal portion of the iliotibial tract on the lateral aspect of the knee. It results from the friction forces associated with repetitive knee flexion and extension associated with impact loading of the knee, as in jogging. This is a perplexing condition that presents in an athlete with no previous indication of harm or injury. It may suddenly smite the athlete even in the course of a race event with a sharp pain over the lateral femoral condyle, and become so painful within a space of 100 yards that the athlete is forced to discontinue the activity completely. On walking the knee seems to improve spontaneously, but as soon as attempts are made to run again the sharp pain returns. On endeavoring subsequently to run, athletes find that they can often run for a short distance only to find the pain appear as suddenly as it had initially. This condition is often confused with internal derangements. Runners must recognize that with this condition they cannot persist in running farther than the threshold of discomfort allows. Maintaining a steady activity level over a reduced distance (even at an increased pace) often sees the condition disappear as mysteriously as it occurred. Ice friction treatments, ultrasonography, stretching and strengthening exercises, and oral anti-inflammatory medication are all adjunctive therapies often necessary to help alleviate this troublesome condition. On occasion, local steroid injection into the bursa may be indicated and surgical treatment may become necessary.

Surgical Treatment

There are class athletes whose condition fails to respond to local measures, modification of activity, and attention to the footwear and gait pattern. Their condition may warrant surgical release of the iliotibial tract and excision of the bursa.

A longitudinal incision is made over the lateral femoral condyle parallel to the upper border of the iliotibial tract. The fascia is incised longitudinally in the direction of its fibers, marking the upper margin of the iliotibial tract and releasing distally to the point of the femoral condyle and proximally for 2 inches. On flexion and extension of the knee, the fascial band is seen to have been freed and the bursa clearly revealed on flexion. Redundant bursal tissue can then be excised. Sutures are required only in the subcutaneous tissues and skin; a soft dressing is then applied. Light activity can commence when the sutures have been removed, with a return to running activity as symptoms allow.

Pes Anserinus Bursitis

Pes anserinus bursitis is an inflammation of the bursa underlying the sartorius, gracilis, and semitendinosus tendon complex on the medial aspect of the knee. This troublesome condition, which affects cyclists, runners, and swimmers, is treated locally with ultrasonography and ice frictions, these being the mainstays of therapy. Oral anti-inflammatory medication and local steroids may be necessary. Attention to footwear may be required, with particular concern for overpronation in runners. In swimmers, this bursitis can be very troublesome and associated with a medial ligament tendinitis; unless there is modification of the kick technique, this condition may prove refractory and jeopardize the athlete's ability to continue successfully in competitive swimming.

RETINACULITIS

Inflammation of the medial and lateral supporting structures presents with pain and tenderness over the retinacula where they play over the underlying femoral condyles, pinching the synovium and evoking pain from this source as a consequence of repetitive loading of the knee. It is important to distinguish this state from a true chondromalacia, for the prognosis is much different. Urgent attention to flexibility exercises, particularly stretching out the quadriceps, is essential to relieve pressures over the femoral condylar margins.

In the genesis of a tighter retinaculum and extensor mechanism, one must comment on the overzealous closure of the knee after arthrotomy. If the capsule is tightened unduly following a surgical arthrotomy of the knee, there can be a marked increase in the pressures over the condylar margins, increasing pressures on the patella as well. Postsurgical knee pain often stems from this tightening of the capsule, and postoperative stretching exercises for the quadriceps mechanism are therefore a very important adjunct to any surgical intervention in the knee.

FAT PAD IMPINGEMENT SYNDROMES

Impingement of the patellar fat pads or the synovium can be either acute or chronic in nature. Acute impingement can occur with sudden forced extension of the knee where the structures are caught between the patella or its tendons and the underlying femoral condyle. The mechanism of injury is elicited from the history, with pain and tenderness noted clinically medial and lateral to the patellar tendons or within the joint. The natural course of the injury is full recovery without intervention.

Chronic impingement syndromes often develop without specific history of trauma. With repetitive activity, the fat pad and synovium hypertrophy and become pinched between the patella and femur, where they are subject to repetitive low-grade trauma and become persistently symptomatic. This condition is often confused with chondromalacia patella because of the associated crepitus that is sometimes present. Careful examination differentiates the area of involvement from the patella, which remains completely smooth and uninvolved. Hoffa's syndrome can become troublesome to the athlete and may even require surgical excision of the hypertrophied tissue for satisfactory resolution.

At the outset, it is important to reduce patella loads with a program of flexibility exercises for the quadriceps muscle group. Avoidance of provocative overloading is most important, and discontinuation of springing activity may be necessary. The athlete with a fat pad syndrome is often found to be engaging only in intermittent activity. It is vital to even out the athletic effort and continue a program of regular, daily activity at a reduced but consistent level of performance. Local ultrasonography and ice frictions are sometimes of help; a steroid injection may be tried but is usually ineffective. On occasion, surgical treatment may become necessary.

Surgical Treatment

Arthroscopy of the knee should be performed to rule out completely any associated internal derangement or involvement of the articular surface of the patella. It is possible by arthroscopic technique to trim the infrapatellar fat pad to reduce the impingement between the lower pole of the patella and the femoral condyle. At the same time, a lateral retinacular release should be carried out and is best made through a separate 2 cm incision, exposing the retinaculum on the lateral side. A compression dressing is applied for 5 days before a light exercise routine is begun. Before the advent of arthro-

scopic surgical technique, an open fat pad excision was carried out, making a small arthrotomy and completely excising the infrapatellar fat pad. Should arthroscopic excision of the fat pad be inadequate, this treatment is still recommended. It should be emphasized that it is only in very rare instances that the fat pad need be excised; however, on occasion the symptoms can be extreme, as in the case of a pianist who had to give up her chosen profession because of fat pad sensitivity while operating the foot pedals. After excision of the fat pad, she returned to her "sport" without further problems.

SUGGESTED READING

Crenshaw AH, ed. Campbell's operative orthopaedics. 8th ed. St. Louis: Mosby-Year Book, 1992.
Kujala UM, Kuist M, Heinonen O. Osgood-Schlatter's disease in adolescent athletes. Am J Sports Med 1985; 13:236–241.
Terry GC, Hughston JC, Norwood LA. The anatomy of the iliopatellar band and iliotibial tract. Am J Sports Med 1986; 14:39–45.

PATELLAR PAIN SYNDROME: INSTABILITY AND LATERAL RETINACULAR RELEASE

S. C. CHEN, F.R.C.S.

Patellar pain in the young patient is usually due to chondromalacia patellae. This condition can arise as a result of:

1. Direct trauma causing a contusion of the articular cartilage.
2. Increased stress on the patellofemoral compartment in strenuous sporting activities.
3. Patellar malalignment, due to an increased Q angle, patella alta or baja, or an abnormal femoral condylar ridge.
4. Patellar instability such as recurrent subluxation or dislocation. Patellar malalignment or instability can cause chondromalacic changes due to abnormal pressure.

The earliest change in chondromalacia is edema of the articular cartilage that progresses to softening, fibrillation, and fissuring. The area affected may extend from a small isolated area to the whole of the articular surface. The areas most affected are the contact areas of the patella, usually the lateral facet, and less often the medial facet. The depth of cartilage affected can vary from the surface layer to the basal layer. Chondromalacia patellae does not necessarily progress to osteoarthritis unless the articular cartilage is eroded down to bone.

There are two types of patellar instability. In one there is an underlying pathologic condition such as an abnormal patella, a high or low patella, a deficient lateral femoral condyle, a lateral attachment of the ligamentum patellae, genu valgum, genu recurvatum, or contracture of the lateral patellar retinaculum and capsule. The other is a normal knee that has suffered an acute dislocation of the patella. The medial patellar retinaculum and capsule heal with undue laxity, so that the patella subsequently can dislocate or subluxate easily.

It is very common for patellar instability and chondromalacia to coexist. Insall maintains that patellar malalignment is primarily responsible for patellar pain and that the chondromalacic changes are a consequence of this.

CLINICAL FEATURES

A careful history taking will reveal any direct blows on the patella in sporting activities, such as kicks or falls on the knee. A feeling of giving way may be due to pain that results in sudden quadriceps inhibition or patellar instability. There may be a history of momentary locking due to maltracking of the patella. The knee may become swollen owing to associated synovial congestion and effusion. There may be a history of acute dislocation, recurrent dislocation, or subluxation of the patella.

Clinical examination reveals wasting of the vastus medialis. Tightness of the lateral and medial retinaculum is assessed by side-to-side movement of the patella. The patella may be tilted slightly laterally and during knee movement this lateral maltracking may be more obvious, especially during the last stages of extension. There may be patellofemoral tenderness during passive knee movement. It may also be present during quadriceps contraction while the patella is pressed against the lower femoral condyle. The undersurface can be palpated by pushing the patella to one side and then to the other; this may elicit tenderness. The apprehension test may be positive, indicating patellar instability.

The Q angle is measured, and if it is more than 20 degrees (normal = 14 degrees), there is lateral placement of the patella.

The height of the patella and the length of the ligamentum patellae are measured. Normally they should be the same. In patella alta, the ligament is longer than the height of the patella; in patella baja, the reverse is the case.

RADIOGRAPHY

Plain anteroposterior, lateral, and skyline views of the patella are taken. The anteroposterior view is taken with the knee extended. The lateral views are taken with the knee extended and flexed to 90 degrees. Measurements of the height of the patella and the ligamentum patellae are made in the knee-extended view. In the 90-degree flexed view, a line drawn across the front of the femoral shaft should skim over the top of the patella. If the patella is above this line, patella alta exists. Skyline views of the patella are taken at 30, 45, and 90 degrees of flexion. These will show lateral maltracking during flexion, if present (Fig. 1).

TREATMENT

Conservative treatment consists of (1) rest from sporting activities for at least 6 weeks and (2) physiotherapy, which should include shortwave diathermy or laser therapy and static quadriceps exercises with the knee in extension, so that the vastus medialis is strengthened and the patella is not subjected to increased pressure. It is important to note that the vastus medialis comes into play only in the last few degrees of knee extension.

Anti-inflammatory drugs, particularly aspirin-based agents, are given during this period. Compression bandages on the knee are discouraged because they increase pressure in the patellofemoral compartment. Intra-articular steroid injections are inadvisable since they can lead to increased degradation of articular cartilage.

In about 75% of patients with chondromalacia patellae, symptoms resolve after conservative treatment. If conservative measures fail and symptoms persist after 3 months, surgical treatment is undertaken.

RATIONALE OF SURGICAL TREATMENT—LATERAL RELEASE OF PATELLA

The object of surgical treatment is to decrease the pressure on the patellar surface and to correct any

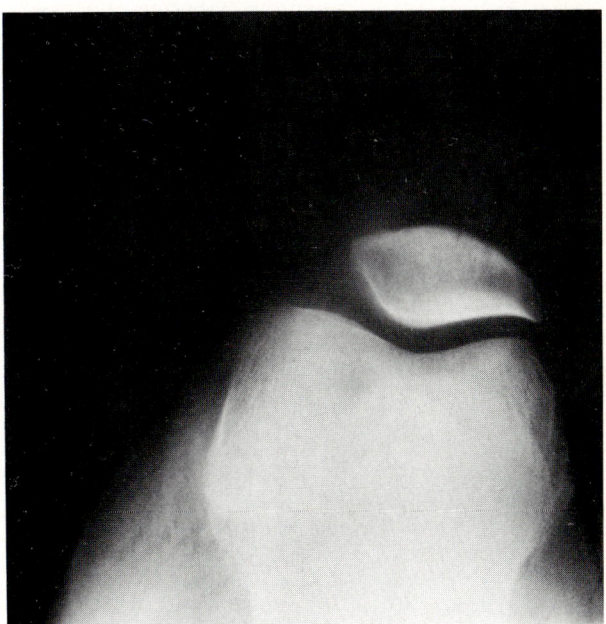

Figure 1 Skyline view of the patella with the knee flexed to 45 degrees to show a slight lateral malalignment.

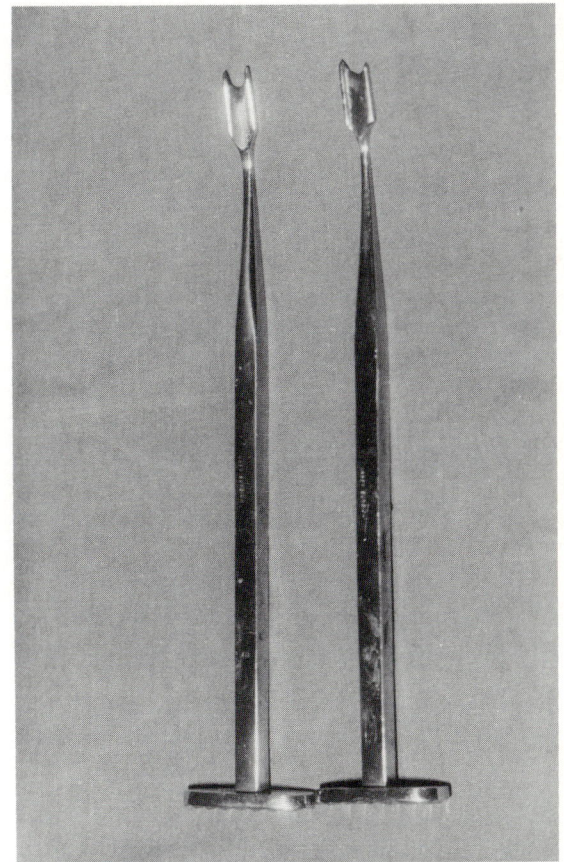

Figure 2 A pair of Smillie knives to show the curve of the blade and the two prongs of differing lengths.

malalignment. Lateral release of the patella achieves both objectives, by releasing the tethering effect of the patellar retinaculum and lateral capsule. It also interrupts the nerve supply to the patella from the lateral side, as neuromatous degeneration can cause symptoms. It is a simple procedure with a low morbidity rate, first described as an open procedure by Evans.

Procedure

A preliminary arthroscopic examination is carried out to confirm the diagnosis and to exclude any other pathologic condition. The arthroscope is introduced via an anterolateral portal. The same stab incision in the skin is employed in carrying out the lateral retinacular release with a Smillie knife. This knife comes in pairs, mirror images of each other, and both are necessary (Fig. 2).

The knee is kept fully extended during the closed

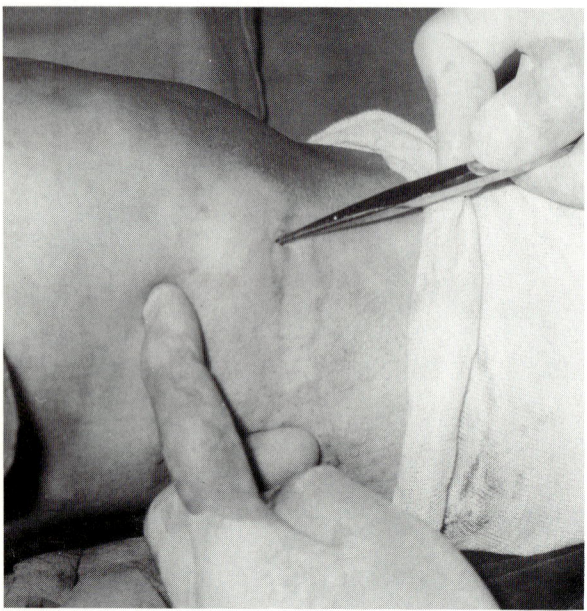

Figure 3 The Smillie knife is astride the lateral retinaculum. Note the finger palpating the knife through the skin, ascertaining its position as it is pushed along.

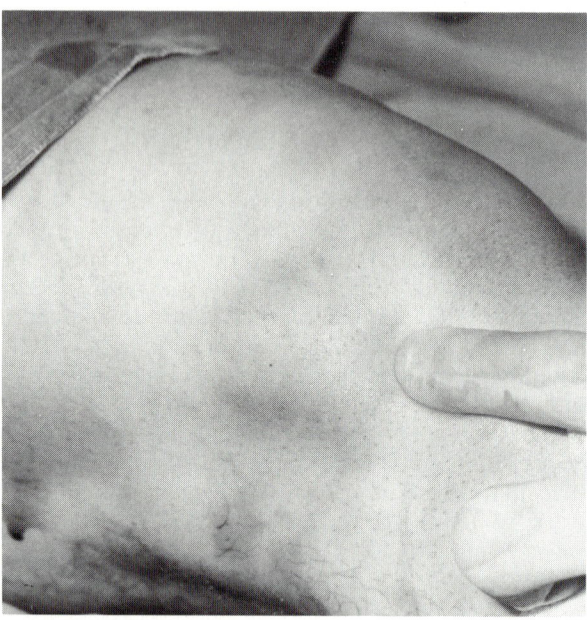

Figure 5 Sausage-shaped bulge on the lateral side of the patella following an adequate retinacular release.

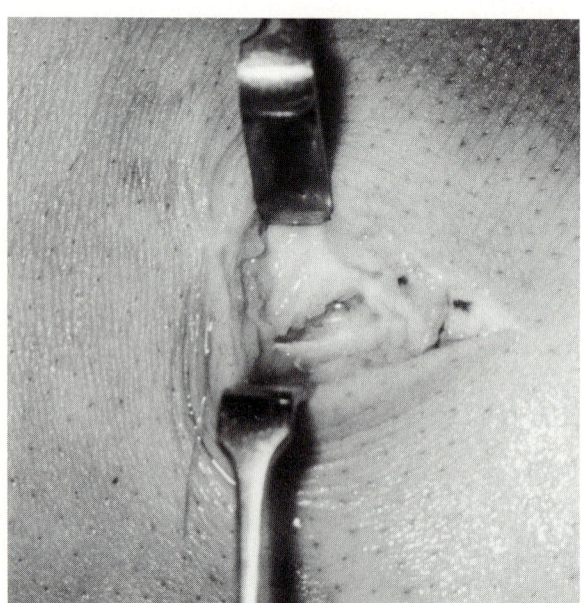

Figure 4 The lateral retinaculum has been exposed after a closed lateral release to show the incision made by the Smillie knife.

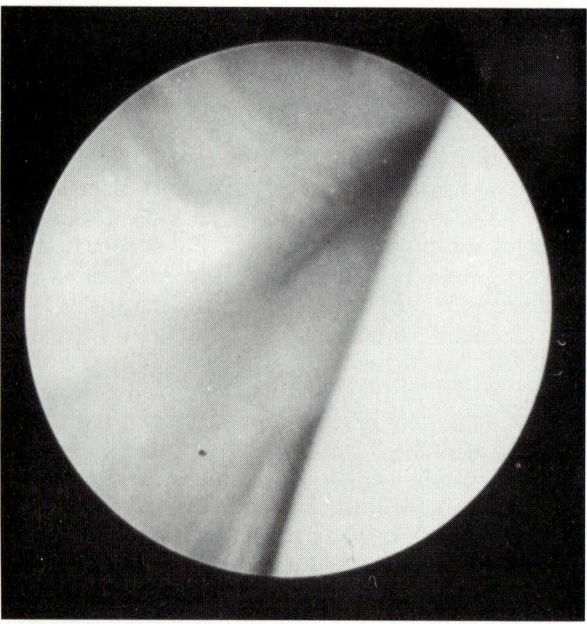

Figure 6 Arthroscopic view of the Smillie knife superficial to the synovial membrane.

lateral release to avoid damage to the intra-articular structures. The tibial tubercle, lateral border of the patella, and lateral joint line are identified by palpation. With the knee still distended with the Ringer's fluid after the arthroscopic examination (which helps in tensing the lateral retinaculum and lifting it from the lateral femoral condyle), the Smillie knife, with its tip curved outward, pointing upward, and the longer prong nearer the skin, is introduced through the stab incision (Fig. 3). The longer of the two prongs of the knife is inserted deep to the puncture wound in the retinaculum that was made during arthroscopy. The correct Smillie knife is used, to avoid cutting the retinaculum too medically and damaging the quadriceps muscle. A firm resistance is felt if the Smillie knife is astride the retinaculum. The knife tip is palpated through the skin and is guided upward and outward when pushed. By deviating laterally, the vastus lateralis muscle and lateral genicular vessels are avoided.

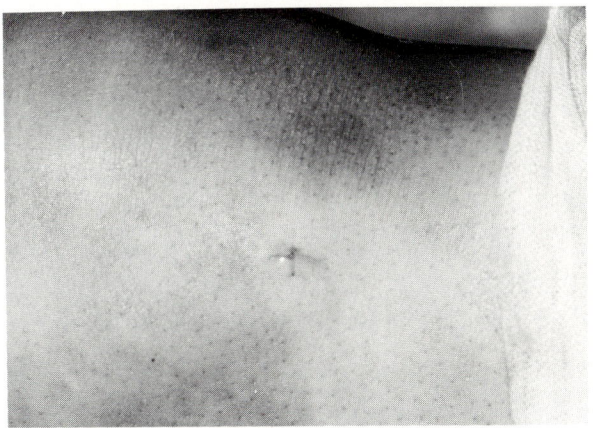

Figure 7 One absorbable stitch for the skin wound.

The retinaculum is divided for a distance equal to twice the height of the patella. Since the knee is fully extended during the procedure, the joint is closed anteriorly and therefore cannot be damaged (Fig. 4). The knife is removed. The other Smillie knife is then introduced with its tip curved outward, pointing downward, the longer prong nearer the skin. With the cutting edge astride the retinaculum, it is pushed down lateral to the ligamentum patellae. The patella is displaced medially to check that it is adequately released. The knee is also flexed and extended to ensure that the patella is tracking correctly. When the lateral retinaculum is divided adequately, a sausage-shaped bulge is seen along the lateral side of the patella, caused by the fluid distending the subcutaneous tissues and skin (Fig. 5). This usually disappears in about 3 months. The synovial membrane is not incised, and therefore the lateral femoral condyle cannot be damaged by the Smillie knife (Fig. 6). One absorbable stitch is used for the skin wound (Fig. 7).

Patients are allowed out of bed the day after surgery, and full weight bearing is permitted. During the first week they walk with the operated knee extended to prevent any effusion developing. They are discharged 2 days after surgery with instructions to carry out static quadriceps exercises and gentle mobilizing exercises for up to 30 degrees of flexion during the first week, and intensive quadriceps strengthening and knee mobilizing exercises are then instituted. By the end of the second week patients can return to work.

RESULTS

Ninety-three percent of patients with chondromalacia patellae responded well to a lateral release (Table 1). In patellar instability the incidence of excellent or good results was 81.5% in recurrent dislocations, 90% in recurrent subluxations, and 87% in acute dislocations (Table 2). There have been no complications in either series.

A simple closed lateral release procedure is carried out even if there is an underlying cause for the condition, such as an increased Q angle or a deficient lateral femoral condyle, since a large proportion of patients may have no further symptoms. A small proportion may require an additional operation such as a medial tibial tubercle transfer through a small transverse skin incision, or a patellectomy if the patellar surface is grossly

Table 1 Lateral Retinacular Release in Chondromalacia Patellae*

	No. of Patients	Relief from Symptoms	Failures
Male	24	23	1
Female	20	18	2
Total	44	41	3

*Average age, 23 years (range 9 to 57 years)

Table 2 Lateral Retinacular Release in Patellar Instability*

Grade	Recurrent Dislocation (n = 16)		Recurrent Subluxation (n = 10)		Acute Dislocation (n = 15)	
	Knees	Percent	Knees	Percent	Knees	Percent
Excellent or good	13	81.5	9	90	13	87
Fair or poor	2	12.5	1	10	2	13
Worse	1	6	0	0	0	0

*Average age, 20 years (range 13 to 35 years)

affected with severe chondromalacia. If the procedure is staged, many patients may be spared unnecessary surgery, prolonged immobilization, and possible complications. Furthermore, an unsightly scar is avoided.

Other forms of surgical treatment include proximal realignment, such as advancement of the vastus medialis if the Q angle is less than 14 degrees. The classic Hauser operation, which consists of lateral retinacular release, medial capsular reefing, and medial transfer of the tibial tubercle, is a major procedure involving at least 4 to 6 weeks in a plaster cast; the complete form may not be necessary. Furthermore the procedure can increase the pressure on the patellofemoral compartment and cause an unsightly large scar.

Chondroplasty, or shaving of the affected articular cartilage, is useful for severe forms of chondromalacia. It can be performed arthroscopically with a chondrotome. Multiple drilling of the shaved areas helps the regeneration of fibrocartilage. This can be combined with lateral release of the patella.

Elevation of the tibial tubercle can decrease pressure on the patellofemoral compartment, but can lead to greater instability if congenital abnormalities, such as patella alta or baja or a deficient femoral condyle, are present. It is a major procedure that may produce complications such as wound breakdown and a prominent anterior bone swelling below the knee.

PATELLOFEMORAL DYSFUNCTION

FRANK NOFTALL, M.D., F.R.C.S.(C)

Patellofemoral derangements are among the most common and most frustrating problems seen by orthopedic surgeons. Activities of daily living (e.g., going up and down stairs) place great demands on the patellar mechanism, let alone athletic activities. Although symptoms are often severe, overt pathology often is not evident.

Essential to an understanding of the patellofemoral arthralgias are the basic biomechanics of the patellofemoral joint, including patellar pressures and patellar excursion.

The patella increases the efficiency of the extensor mechanism by as much as 50%. The compressive force or joint reactive force of the patellofemoral joint is the resultant vector of the pull of the quadriceps mechanism and the resistance of the patellar tendon. The compressive force across the joint may be three to four times the body weight when a person goes up and down stairs, and is increased as flexion of the knee increases.

Another function of the patella is to translate the divergent forces of the quadriceps mechanism and transmit these to the patella tendon. Patellar excursion is determined by the resultant of these force vectors. Any anatomic, physiologic, or pathologic factor that alters this patellar function will affect the excursion of the patella and may lead to pain syndromes. Patellar excursion is affected by many factors. One of the most important is the so-called Q angle, which is formed by the line of pull of the quadriceps muscle and the line of the patellar tendon. This is normally a valgus angulation. The natural tendency is for the patella to displace laterally. This is resisted by the prominent lateral femoral condyle and trochlear groove, the fibers of the

vastus medialis distally, and the medial retinaculum. Any tightening laterally, laxity medially, or deficiency of the bone structures laterally increases the tendency of the patella to displace laterally.

Any factor that increases the Q angle also increases the tendency for the patella to displace laterally. Genu valgum, excessive external tibial torsion, and pes planus effectively increase the Q angle.

PATELLOFEMORAL ARTHRALGIA

Clinical Features

Patients with patellofemoral disorders generally have complaints when the patella is in a position of maximal compressive forces (again, during stair climbing and descending). They also complain of sensations of giving way, a feeling of instability or insecurity, and "locking" or catching sensations.

On examination there often is quadriceps atrophy. Effusions are not common but occasionally are seen. Stability test results are all normal in the patient with isolated patellar pain. Retro- or parapatellar pain sites can be elicited in most cases. Crepitus is often palpable but this may also be found in patients without any pain syndromes. The patellar excursion should be visualized throughout the range of extension to full flexion and back to extension, to observe any tendency toward lateral displacement or variation from the normal sinusoidal motion. Overall limb alignment, the Q angle, and finally the heel and foot position should be documented.

Radiologic Investigation

The radiologic investigation of patients with patellofemoral pain consists of plain film radiography including anteroposterior, lateral, intercondylar, and most important tangential (axial) views of the patella. Various techniques have been described for taking the axial view, and each has its own advantages and disadvantages. I believe that the techniques with the knee in 20 to 60 degrees of flexion probably are the most useful. The most important factors are consistency and reproducibility.

In recent years, computed tomographic (CT) scanning and MRI scanning have been used increasingly. These modalities will undoubtedly increase in usefulness, especially in refractory cases.

Radionuclide scanning is also being used but is mostly in the investigational stages.

Source of Pain and Management

Over the years, various theories have been put forward regarding the source of pain in patients with patellofemoral arthralgias; many of these are difficult to prove or disprove. Stimulation of nerve endings in subchondral bone, neuromatous degeneration in retinacular nerves, stretching and straining of the retinaculum and capsule, and impingement of the fat pad and/or synovium are among a few of the suggested sources of patellofemoral pain. The source of the pain in fact is actually not too important in this entity; it seems that regardless of the source, most cases of patellofemoral pain respond to conservative management, and only a few require surgical intervention.

The first step in management consists of modification of the provocative activity. The duration or intensity of the activity may have to be diminished. Sometimes a change of activity is necessary. The important point is that fitness must be maintained during the treatment process.

Physiotherapy is the mainstay of treatment of patellofemoral disorders, regardless of their cause. Strengthening exercises have to be explained appropriately, because certain exercises may actually aggravate the pain. Isometric quadriceps setting and straight leg raising, followed by progressive resisted exercises over the final 10 degrees of knee extension, are emphasized. Resisted exercises over the full range of motion are discouraged because of the excessive compressive forces generated and the tendency to intensify symptoms. Stretching of the quadriceps and hamstring groups is as important as strengthening. Shortwave diathermy and ultrasound techniques may be beneficial, especially in times of acute inflammation, but should not take the place of strengthening and stretching exercises. Faradic stimulation may also be helpful in selected patients. Orthotics aimed at correction of foot problems such as pes planus and heel valgus may be helpful when these conditions are contributing to abnormal patellar mechanics.

Anti-inflammatory medications have a limited role in the treatment of patellofemoral pain. They may provide some relief for patients experiencing acute exacerbations of pain or in whom there is evidence of inflammation or recent injury. They should be used over short periods in relatively high doses for maximal effect.

Two important points about patellofemoral pain need stressing. First, despite the presence at times of very significant symptoms, the majority of patients cause themselves no special harm or damage if they "play through" their pain. Second, before conservative management is to be considered a failure, it is necessary to be sure that patients have complied with the recommended therapy.

Surgical Treatment

Conservative management should be continued for at least 6 months. The patient should be disabled to the point of nonparticipation in work or sport.

Arthroscopy should be performed in all patients with patellofemoral pain who have reached the point of surgical intervention. The entire knee joint can be assessed and most of the pathology identified and initially dealt with.

The initial success of and enthusiasm for lateral retinacular release has not been sustained. The use of this relatively minor procedure should be reserved for patients having tight or contracted lateral structures, excessive lateral pressure, or radiographic evidence of lateral displacement or tilting of the patella. Avoidance of hematoma is mandatory, and patients should begin active rehabilitation early in the postoperative period. Again, as in conservative management, excessive loading of the patellofemoral joint must be avoided.

Fat pad hypertrophy and fibrosis may be one of the causes of patellofemoral pain identified at arthroscopy. The fat pad becomes impinged between the patella and the femur. Hoffa's syndrome is a definite entity, and arthroscopic excision is a very good form of initial surgical management. The fat pad is a substantial structure, and frequently a small medial arthrotomy is required to debride the structure adequately. Again, hemostasis is mandatory because of the very vascular nature of the fat pad.

Synovial hypertrophy and impingement may occur in the suprapatellar region. Arthroscopic excision in this region tends to be more satisfactory than with fat pad excision owing to greater accessibility and (usually) the smaller volume of tissue involved.

The medial plica syndrome can also be addressed arthroscopically. It is important not only to disrupt the continuity of the plica but to excise a segment, since it has been documented that the plica may heal and become symptomatic once again.

CHONDROMALACIA PATELLAE

One of the reasons for confusion with patellofemoral pain syndromes is that many similarly symptomatic disorders have been labeled as chondromalacia patellae. This led to much unnecessary surgery for minor conditions that did not warrant such aggressive therapy. True chondromalacia is a relatively rare entity and, comparing the number of patients with patellofemoral pain with those who actually undergo changes in the articular surface, the latter are in the minority.

The pathology of articular cartilage changes is well described. There are four stages: in stage I there is swelling and softening of the cartilage, in stage II fissuring, in stage III surface breakdown known as fasiculation, and in stage IV osteoarthritis.

As with any other condition affecting the patellofemoral joint, the first step in treating patients with chondromalacic changes is conservative. Physiotherapy aimed at quadriceps strengthening must be tempered with caution, for overloading the quadriceps may well aggravate the condition. It is important, however, to keep the quadriceps in good condition. All resisted exercises, deep knee bends, and crouches are to be avoided, as is any exercise involving knee flexion.

Obviously, any jumping, running, or squatting during sports activities may aggravate the condition; this is unavoidable. Maintenance of physical fitness may have to be supplemented by swimming or by cycling with the seat elevated. An athlete's training may have to be modified to avoid the intensification of symptoms. Anti-inflammatory agents may be helpful in acute exacerbations or if synovitis is present. Steroid injection is controversial and should probably be avoided in younger patients.

After an adequate trial of conservative management (at least 6 months), any patient who still has incapacitating symptoms may be considered for operative intervention. The first step is arthroscopic examination of the joint. This procedure allows the condition to be diagnosed and rules out other intraarticular pathology. Debridement of the joint can be accomplished, albeit sometimes with difficulty, using manual or mechanical devices. However, this does not address the underlying disorder causing the chondromalacia patellae. At the same time, if there is any evidence of excessive tightening of the lateral structures, a lateral retinacular release can be performed; if there is no such evidence, this will probably be unsuccessful.

The definitive procedure for the treatment of chondromalacia patellae unresponsive to less aggressive measures is elevation of the tibial tubercle. The true Maquet procedure is rarely performed today, because the original operation carried an unacceptably high degree of major complications, mainly skin breakdown and infections. This was attributed to the 2 cm of elevation initially described along with poor skin coverage. A number of modifications of the Maquet procedure have been reported. Most recommend 1 to 1.5 cm of elevation and no distal transfer of the tubercle. If any maltracking laterally or dislocation is present, this elevation can be combined with a medial transfer. Through elevation of the tibial tubercle, the patella gains mechanical advantage and becomes more efficient. This decreases patellofemoral pressure and reduces the joint reactive forces. A 1 cm elevation can produce approximately a 33% increase in efficiency, which is thought by most authors to be sufficient. The incidence of wound breakdown is markedly diminished but not completely eliminated.

Tibial tubercle elevation is usually combined with lateral retinacular release and frequently with open debridement. Degenerated cartilage should be excised, and any subchondral bone exposed should be drilled. If possible, early motion should be instituted. Undoubtedly, continuous passive motion will be used more frequently in the future in cases involving subchondral drilling. The patella should not be actively loaded during the postoperative period for at least 4 weeks. Depending on the technique, internal fixation can be avoided and early motion instituted if the bone graft is secure.

PATELLAR INSTABILITY

Patellar Subluxation

In the past, patellar maltracking and subluxation was too readily ascribed to patients with patellar symptomatology. It is undoubtedly the cause of patellar problems in many cases, but it has been overdiagnosed. This leads to the indiscriminate use of lateral retinacular release, and predictably poor results. Patellar maltracking is often difficult to diagnose except in the most obvious cases. Subluxation is often diagnosed on the basis of static x-ray films when it is a dynamic process. The biomechanics leading to maltracking and lateral subluxation have been described earlier.

Conservative treatment consists of anatomic and dynamic considerations. Foot alignment must be addressed, as pronated feet may cause an increased Q angle and lead to lateral subluxation of the patella. An orthotic to place the heel and foot in a more neutral or slight supinated position may be all that is necessary.

Patella-stabilizing braces have been used with reasonable success. The major problem with braces as well as orthotics is patient compliance. Orthotics generally are custom made, while patella-stabilizing braces are usually off the shelf and mass produced. There are a number on the market, most having a patellar groove that helps stabilize the patella from displacement while not putting any pressure directly on the patella. These tend to be useful only in very severe cases.

Physiotherapy concentrates on strengthening the vastus medialis portion of the quadriceps while increasing the flexibility of the quadriceps group; the latter is probably the more important. By a diligent stretching program, pressure on the patella is reduced and the muscle acts as a better shock absorber. With reduced tensions in this muscle group, there is less tendency for the patella to subluxate laterally.

Operative treatment is reserved for patients who have exhausted a comprehensive conservative program. Arthroscopy is performed to rule out other unsuspected intra-articular pathology. If this is discovered, it is dealt with first and the patient is observed to see if any improvement occurs. Patients should be markedly impaired in their activities to warrant surgical intervention.

Soft tissue procedures should suffice in most cases of true lateral subluxation. Since arthroscopy has been performed, a formal arthrotomy is unnecessary, and this decreases postoperative morbidity. A lateral retinacular release is performed either through a small incision in a semiopen fashion or through a formal incision. This may or may not be combined with a medial capsular plication and vastus medialis advancement. In most cases there is no need to transpose the tibial tubercle medially.

PATELLAR DISLOCATIONS

Acute Patellar Dislocation

When this occurs in the athlete it is a painful, worrisome, and potentially career-ending injury. As with any other dislocation, early reduction is of the utmost importance. Usually, simple extension of the extremity effects reduction and the injured person feels immediate relief. Most often the joint is reduced before the individual is examined. The history can be confused with that of an acute anterior cruciate injury. The physical examination usually gives the experienced examiner enough information to differentiate between the two conditions. Both, however, may show a painful hemarthrosis, but patients with an acute patellar dislocation have exquisite tenderness along the medial aspect of the patella, which intensifies on flexion of the knee. The anterior cruciate ligament stability tests should be normal.

X-ray films should be carefully examined to rule out osteochondral fractures; the lateral and skyline views are the most useful. If there is any doubt, arthroscopy should be performed. Small fragments should be removed, but repair of large osteochondral fragments with large areas of articular cartilage should be attempted; this is often difficult.

Simple cast immobilization in a stovepipe cast with the knee in full extension and molding to displace the patella medially is prescribed for from 4 to 6 weeks. During this time, quadriceps setting exercises are performed in conjunction with faradic stimulation if available. After cast removal, a patella-stabilizing brace can be used. Mobilization of the knee is begun. Return to sports activities is allowed only when full range of motion and full quadriceps rehabilitation, particularly flexibility, have been restored.

Recurrent Patellar Dislocation

With recurrent dislocations, soft tissue procedures are generally insufficient. However, before skeletal maturity there is no choice, as any operation that damages the proximal tibial growth plate could prove disastrous. Conservative treatment would consist of physiotherapy concentrating on medial quadriceps and a patella stabilizing brace. If conservative treatment fails, soft tissue plication medially with a lateral retinacular release and medial displacement of the tibial tubercle should be considered. Tibial tubercle displacement should only be done in the skeletally mature individual. This can be a very troublesome procedure, since internal fixation is required to hold the tubercle medially displaced, and if the soft tissue medial reconstruction is too tight it can lead to patellar problems postoperatively.

The medial displacement of the tibial tubercle can be combined with an elevation of the tubercle if chondromalacia patellae is present. This can be difficult to manage postoperatively: with chondromalacia it is important to institute motion as soon as possible, but because of the sometimes tenuous fixation of the tubercle it is often necessary to hold patients back from early motion until bone healing is secure.

SUGGESTED READING

Carson WC, et al. Patellofemoral disorder: parts I and II. Clin Orthop 185:165–186.
Insall J. Patellar pain. J Bone Joint Surg 65A:147–152.
Kettelkamp DB. Management of patellar malalignment. J Bone Joint Surg 63A:1344–1348.
Scuderi GR. The patellofemoral joint. Orthop Clin North Am, Oct. 1992.

PATELLAR DISLOCATION, SUBLUXATION, AND THE ELMSLIE-TRILLAT PROCEDURE

DAVID E. BROWN, M.D.

Patellar subluxations and dislocations occur frequently in athletes. The wide range of normal alignment patterns, the subtle misalignments that lead to symptoms, and the many causes of malalignment make the evaluation and management of these injuries difficult. Therefore, the clinician must first understand the etiology before an individualized treatment plan can be formulated.

Patellar malalignment may be caused by abnormalities occurring anywhere in the lower extremity. Excessive femoral anteversion, deficient or weak vastus medialis obliquus (VMO), tight vastus lateralis, abnormal insertion of the vastus lateralis, excessive genu valgum, shallow femoral trochlea, external tibial torsion with lateral insertion of the ligamentum patellae, and pes planus with hindfoot valgus are the most frequent factors leading to malalignment. Generalized joint laxity or trauma may exacerbate any of these factors.

EVALUATION

Complete patellar dislocations are easy to diagnose when the patient recalls the frightening sensation of displacement of the patella. It is more difficult to determine whether the patient is actually experiencing subluxations of the patella. However, episodes of buckling, momentary giving way, and "catching" are often symptoms of patellar instability. These may be associated with pain, swelling, and grinding.

The physical examination should include evaluation of rotational deformities of the hip and tibia and standing alignment of the hindfoot. Excessive femoral anteversion, external tibial torsion, and hindfoot valgus result in elevation of the quadriceps (Q) angle. Flexibility of the thigh musculature, particularly the vastus lateralis and iliotibial band, should be determined.

Knee examination should isolate the deficient VMO or tight lateral retinaculum, determine abnormal patellar mobility or tilting, and make a gross assessment of patellar tracking. The patellar apprehension test, if positive, is extremely helpful in isolating the cause of the patellar instability. I believe it essential to measure the quadriceps angle, in full knee extension. Normal values are generally considered to be 10 degrees for males and 15 degrees for females. When the Q angle is elevated, the patella tends to displace more laterally with active quadriceps contraction. Alternatively, the tubercle-sulcus angle may be used. This should be 0 degrees.

Other causes of knee pain and instability must be diligently sought, as they may coexist with patellar instability.

Radiographic evaluation should include one of the axial patellar views described by Merchant and Laurin and their colleagues. Nonstandardized axial views, especially if obtained in more than 30 degrees of knee flexion, rarely demonstrate patellar malalignment. The lateral view is evaluated for patella alta by the method of Insall and Salvati. Fulkerson described a computed tomographic (CT) method that allows evaluation of patellar position from full extension to 30 degrees of knee flexion, a range that may be more sensitive than that in the axial radiographs, since it correlates with the range of patellar instability. The CT scan is also the method of choice for quantifying femoral anteversion.

NONSURGICAL TREATMENT

Nonsurgical treatment should be given for 3 to 6 months unless evidence of an intra-articular loose body is seen. The vast majority of subluxators respond to an appropriate regimen aimed at alleviating or compensating for the cause of malalignment.

Rehabilitation of the deficient vastus medialis is nearly always required. Isometric quadriceps setting, straight leg-raising exercises, and progressive resistive exercises near terminal extension are emphasized. Bicycling (with the seat elevated) and swimming with a kick board are useful in developing quadriceps strength without irritating the patellofemoral articular surface.

Stretching of the quadriceps and hamstring muscles and mobilization of the patella to relieve a tight lateral retinaculum may reduce contact pressures in the patellofemoral joint. All these modalities are initially supervised by a physical therapist, but the patient must be willing to continue a maintenance program two to three times a week once the symptoms are alleviated.

A patella-stabilizing brace or McConnell taping helps to control mild lateral tracking or hypermobility. The brace additionally functions to keep the knee warmer during activity, often reducing the sensation of stiffness that most patients experience. When hindfoot valgus is present, a medial heel wedge and a shoe with a firm heel counter reduce overpronation and the resultant internal torsion of the knee. If relief of symptoms is obtained, a custom orthotic can be ordered.

SURGICAL TREATMENT

Surgical treatment should always include arthroscopy to complete the evaluation of patellar tracking, perform superficial chondroplasty, and evaluate the remainder of the knee for any pathologic condition. If possible, arthroscopy is performed under local anesthesia, without a tourniquet, to evaluate patellofemoral alignment under dynamic conditions and without the potential errors induced by tourniquet compression of the quadriceps muscles. An inferolateral portal immediately adjacent to the patella tendon and the superolateral portal are used to demonstrate lateral patellar subluxation or tilt.

Once this evaluation is complete, surgical realignment can be tailored to the needs of the patient. Surgical options include proximal soft tissue reconstruction (medial capsule imbrication and/or lateral retinaculum release), distal realignment (tibial tubercle or patella tendon transfer), and anterior displacement of the tibial tubercle. On rare occasions, femoral and tibial derotation osteotomies are required to correct severe rotational deformities.

Acute Patellar Dislocation

After the patella is reduced, the joint is aspirated, examination is carried out, and a complete set of radiographs are obtained. Any suspicion of an intra-articular loose body warrants arthroscopic examination. If excessive lateral subluxation is present, lateral release is performed. When the vastus medialis is avulsed from the superiomedial pole of the patella, an open repair is indicated. Postoperatively or after the injury, the knee is immobilized in extension, and weight bearing is allowed as tolerated. Within the first week, the patient is expected to perform active and passive motion in the first 30 to 40 degrees of flexion while wearing a patella-stabilizing brace.

This limited range-of-motion and quadriceps rehabilitation is prescribed to be carried out four times a day; extension immobilization is continued throughout the rest of the day for 4 weeks. The stabilizing brace is then worn for another 4 weeks while range-of-motion and more aggressive quadricep exercises are instituted.

Acute Patellar Subluxation

Short-term immobilization is occasionally necessary, but motion, rehabilitation, and resumption of activity are instituted as soon as possible. A careful search is performed for correctable causes of malalignment. High-intensity activities are delayed until complete quadriceps function returns and the patellar apprehension sign is negative.

Chronic Patellar Instability

Surgical reconstruction is indicated if there is failure to improve after 3 to 6 months of conservative therapy. Before surgical intervention, the surgeon must be able to confirm the clinical impression of subluxation or dislocation by radiography, arthrometry, or arthroscopy, much the same as for tibiofemoral or lateral ankle ligamentous reconstructions. Table 1 describes a treatment regimen based on the clinical diagnosis, objective findings, and radiographic findings.

Elmslie-Trillat Procedure

Diagnostic and therapeutic arthroscopy are completed, if not previously performed. A long, lateral parapatellar incision is made and a medially based skin flap is developed, exposing the medial retinaculum, tibial tubercle, and quadriceps tendon. Lateral release is accomplished from the insertion of the vastus lateralis to the tibial tubercle. The vastus medialis insertion is released and imbricated in a vest over pants fashion using multiple, absorbable mattress sutures. Distal advancement of the VMO may be required if the original insertion was too proximal.

An incision is then made on both sides of the tibial tubercle and the periosteum is elevated. The lateral side must be developed well, exposing at least 1 cm of the steep lateral tibial metaphysis. The interval between the patella tendon and fat pad is developed and a wide, curved osteotome inserted at a 45-degree angle to the horizontal, inclining to the medial side. The initial depth is 6 to 8 mm, gradually diminishing as the osteotome is driven distally 5 to 10 cm, leaving only a distal periosteal hinge. The tubercle is transferred medially 6 to 10 mm until the intraoperative Q angle is 10 degrees. This will result in 4 to 5 mm of anterior displacement. If additional anteriorization is desired, a local bone graft can be obtained from the lateral side of the tibial tubercle. A 10-cm osteotomy is necessary to improve the cosmetic appearance of the anteriorized tubercle. The tubercle is then held in its transferred position with a 3.2-mm drill bit, and the patellofemoral alignment is observed throughout the range of motion.

Frequently adjustments are made to the imbrication of the VMO, ensuring that the patella is centralized and

Table 1 Treatment Regimen for Chronic Patellar Instability

Diagnosis	Arthroscopic Findings, Radiographic Findings, Q Angle	Treatment Protocol
Subluxation	Patella tilt alone	Lateral release
Subluxation	Subluxation + tilt Q angle < 15 degrees	Proximal realignment
or	or Open physes	Medial capsule reefing Lateral release
Dislocation	Q angle ≥ 15 degrees	Elmslie-Trillat
	Grade II-III chondromalacia	Elmslie-Trillat + Further anteriorization with local bone graft

does not tilt. Once the alignment is deemed satisfactory, the drill bit is replaced with a 40-mm soft tissue screw. The tourniquet is released, alignment is re-examined, and meticulous hemostasis is obtained. The lateral side is left open and routine closure is accomplished over closed suction drainage. The knee is immobilized in a hinged knee brace in 0 degrees of flexion, and weight bearing is allowed as tolerated. Flexion to 40 degrees is begun at 2 weeks and increased to 90 degrees at 4 weeks. The brace is discontinued at 6 weeks. Quadriceps rehabilitation is begun immediately after the operation.

SUGGESTED READING

Brown DE, Alexander AH, Lichtman DM. The Elmslie-Trillat procedure: evaluation in patellar dislocation and subluxation. Am J Sports Med 1984; 12:104–109.

Cox JS. Evaluation of the Roux-Elmslie-Trillat procedure for knee extensor realignment. Am J Sports Med 1982; 10:303–310.

Ferguson RB, Brown TD, Fu FH, et al. Relief of patello-femoral contact stress by anterior displacement of the tibial tubercle. J Bone Joint Surg 1979; 61A:159–166.

Fulkerson JP. Anteromedialization of the tibial tubercle for patellofemoral malalignment. Clin Orthop 1983; 177:176–181.

Fulkerson JP, Schutzer SF, Ramsey GR, Bernstein RA. Computed tomography of the patellofemoral joint before and after lateral release or realignment. Arthroscopy 1987; 3(1):19-24.

Insall J, Salvati E. Patella position in the normal knee joint. Radiology 1971; 101:101–104.

Laurin CA, Dussault R, Levesque HP. The tangential x-ray investigation of the patellofemoral joint. Clin Orthop 1979; 144:16–26.

Merchant AC, Mercer RS, Jacobsen RH, et al. Roentgenographic analysis of patello-femoral congruence. J Bone Joint Surg 1974; 56A:1391–1396.

Schutzer SF, Ramsby GR, Fulkerson JP. Computed tomographic classification of patellofemoral pain patients. Orthop Clin North Am 1986; 17:235–248.

Shelbourne KD, Porter DA, Rozzi W. Use of a modified Elmslie-Trillat procedure to improve abnormal patellar congruence angle. Am J Sports Med 1994; 22:318-323.

ARTHROSCOPIC SURGERY OF THE KNEE UNDER LOCAL ANESTHESIA

JOSEPH S. TORG, M.D.

This chapter presents the technique for performing surgical arthroscopy of the knee under local anesthesia with intravenous (IV) sedation.

Augustin et al in 1955 described the use of local anesthesia in knee joint surgery in a review of 125 arthrotomies performed using lidocaine/epinephrine infiltration of the soft tissues. They described the method as "effective and uncomplicated; and easily accomplished and well accepted by the patient."

In the late 1970s, articles began to appear discussing the usefulness of local anesthesia in performing *diagnostic* arthroscopy of the knee—citing the reduced risk and morbidity to the patient as compared to general anesthesia. Only in the past 4 years have several articles appeared discussing local anesthesia for *surgical* arthroscopy of the knee.

SURGICAL PROCEDURE

Surgical arthroscopy of the knee can be performed under local anesthesia using the following method. An IV infusion is established, and an IV sedating agent is administered to the patient. The leg is prepared and draped. A tourniquet is not used. The patient is warned prior to each needle stick to help allay anxiety. Following the aspiration of effusion from the joint, 40 ml of a mixture of 1% lidocaine with 1:200,000 epinephrine is instilled into the knee. Five minutes is allowed for the agents to take effect, then 40 ml of saline is added to further distend the joint. Five milliliters of 1% lidocaine with 1:200,000 epinephrine is injected into the skin and subcutaneous tissues of each arthroscopic portal site. Generous portals are made, particularly in the capsular layer, to avoid tissue stretching and patient discomfort. One milligram of epinephrine is mixed with each 3,000 ml of saline irrigation.

The arthroscope is inserted into the knee, and inflow through the sheath is established. A separate egress cannula is used if needed. The arthroscopic examination and surgery are carried out with constant verbal communication between surgeon and patient. This facilitates manipulation of the leg and thorough examination of the entire joint by keeping patient anxiety and muscle tension to a minimum. The patient is encouraged to view the intra-articular problem and its treatment on the video monitor. When finished, the instruments are removed and the portals are closed with a 4-0 absorbable stitch in the subcutaneous layer and steri-strips. A compression dressing is applied to the knee for 3 days.

DISCUSSION

Surgical arthroscopy of the knee under general anesthesia is a well-established procedure that is effective in correcting many intra-articular problems. Intraoperative and postoperative morbidity of general anesthesia for this procedure, including cardiac arrhythmia, pneumonia, aspiration pneumonitis, nausea and emesis, and malaise and prolonged recovery time, have been noted by several authors. These problems are avoided with local anesthesia, and several large series have reported on its use in diagnostic arthroscopy of the knee. Within the last 3 or 4 years, there have been reports on the use of local anesthesia for surgical arthroscopy of the knee. However, because of reported difficulty with adequate visualization of the posterior regions of the joint, technical difficulty secondary to muscle spasm, as well as increased anxiety of both patient and surgeon, the widespread use of local anesthesia and surgical arthroscopy has been curtailed. I believe that the results of our combined retrospective and prospective studies clearly indicate that with meticulous attention to technical details and surgical techniques combined with the use of minimal therapeutic doses of appropriate IV sedative supplements all surgical arthroscopic procedures can be performed with local anesthesia.

I emphasize, on the basis of this extensive clinical experience, that the patient should not be overly sedated. Specifically, the patient should be relaxed but alert, conversant, and responsive to the inquiries and instructions of the surgeon. Again, based on clinical impression, the tendency to oversedate patients results in less rather than more relaxation as well as nonvolitional muscle spasm. Only if meticulous attention is paid to the technical details and a minimal dose of the appropriate IV sedative supplement used will there be a consistently successful outcome.

From our retrospective and prospective studies, we conclude:

1. All arthroscopic procedures of the knee performed under general anesthesia can be successfully performed with lidocaine and IV sedation.
2. Meticulous attention to technical details by the surgeon as well as patient relaxation and cooperation are needed to optimize surgical conditions.
3. Some form of IV sedation, preferably fentanyl, in minimal therapeutic dosage is recommended for optimal surgical conditions.
4. The use of minimal therapeutic doses of fentanyl does not significantly prolong the patient's recovery room stay nor does it result in postoperative nausea.
5. Fentanyl alone provides consistent patient comfort.
6. Arthroscopic surgery, with or without IV sedation, allows patients to be discharged from the ambulatory surgery facility earlier than those who received general anesthesia.

SUGGESTED READING

Augustin RW, MacAusland WR, Greenwald WF. Local infiltration anesthesia for knee surgery. J Bone Joint Surg 1955; 34:855–858.

Besser MIB, Stahl S. Arthroscopic surgery performed under local anesthesia as an outpatient procedure. Arch Orthop Trauma Surg 1986; 105:296–297.

Eriksson E, Haggmark T, Saartok T, et al. Knee arthroscopy with local anesthesia in ambulatory patients. Orthopedics 1986; 9:186–188.

Halperin N, Axer A, Hirshberg E, Agasi M. Arthroscopy of the knee under local anesthesia and controlled pressure irrigation. Clin Orthop 1978; 134:176–179.

Kitz DS, Robinson DM, Schiavone RA, et al. Discharging out-patients.

Factors nurses consider to determine readiness. AORN J 1988; 48:87–91.

Klein W, Schulitz KP. Outpatient arthroscopy under local anesthesia. Arch Orthop Trauma Surg 1980; 96:131–134.

McGinty JB, Matza RA. Arthroscopy of the knee. J Bone Joint Surgery 1978; 787–789.

McGuire DA, Frost JA, Floerchinger SL. Local anesthesia and arthroscopic surgery of the knee. Alaska Med 1986; 28(2):20–24.

Ngo I, Hamilton WG, Wichern WA, Andrea RA. Local anesthesia with sedation for arthroscopic surgery of the knee: a report of 100 consecutive cases. Arthroscopy 1985; 1:237–241.

Pevey JK. Outpatient arthroscopy of the knee under local anesthesia. Am J Sports Med 1978; 6:122–127.

MENISCAL REPAIR

JEFFREY R. KUHLMAN, M.D.

A better understanding of the biomechanics of the knee menisci during tibiofemoral load transmission and their importance in maintaining normal joint function has led to increasing efforts to preserve the meniscal cartilages whenever possible. Both animal models and clinical studies have documented acceleration in degenerative changes and deterioration in functional results with time after surgical removal of the menisci.

The load transmission and shock absorption characteristics of the menisci are dependent on normal anatomic and histologic structure. The wedge-shaped cross-section of each meniscus allows for congruency at the tibiofemoral articulation, thereby increasing articular contact area and reducing peak contact stresses. The menisci facilitate transmission of 40% to 50% of the load in the medial compartment and 65% to 75% of the load in the lateral compartment. At the microstructural level, the menisci are composed primarily of circumferential collagen fibers with strong bony attachments at the anterior and posterior horns. With axial compression of the knee joint, "hoop stresses" are developed within these circumferential fibers, which serve to further dissipate the load across the joint. Any attempts to repair the menisci must recreate this normal anatomy to be of functional significance.

Without the protective effects of the meniscus, articular cartilage wear is accelerated as demonstrated by the finding of a 40% incidence of marked degenerative joint disease at long-term (average 17 years) follow-up of knees having undergone total medial meniscectomy. Even more rapid degenerative changes can be expected after lateral meniscectomy due to the greater percentage of load transmission through the meniscus in the lateral compartment. Not only total meniscectomy but also partial meniscectomy is detrimental to the articular surfaces. As demonstrated in the dog model, the degree of degenerative changes occurring after partial meniscectomy is proportional to the extent of tissue resected. While arthroscopic partial meniscectomy presents distinct advantages over total meniscectomy, removal of even 16% to 34% of the meniscus can increase joint contact forces by 350%.

In order to preserve a torn meniscus, healing must be possible at the tear site. Meniscus cartilage demonstrates both extrinsic and intrinsic pathways of healing. The extrinsic pathway is dependent on vascularity, relying on the influx of undifferentiated mesenchymal cells for production of fibrovascular scar tissue. Vascularity has been demonstrated in the outer 25% to 33% of the menisci, with slightly greater vascularity at the anterior and posterior horns. The lateral meniscus in the area of the popliteus hiatus is relatively avascular. In contrast to the extrinsic pathway, the intrinsic pathway relies on the inherent capability of meniscal chondrocytes to proliferate and synthesize matrix if given the proper environment and is not dependent on blood-borne mesenchymal cells. Recent research with growth factors found in the fibrin clot has focused on ways to turn on this intrinsic pathway of healing.

INDICATIONS FOR REPAIR

Certain meniscal tears do not require surgical treatment and can be expected to heal clinically without excision or stabilization. Generally, vertical longitudinal tears less than 1 cm in length or involving less than 50% of the vertical width of the meniscus are considered stable, and a probe is unable to evert or subluxate the free edge into the joint. Similarly, small (< 3 mm) radial tears may be left alone.

For those unstable tears that require treatment, two considerations are important when contemplating repair. First, the meniscus must be capable of generating a healing response sufficient for a satisfactory rate of clinical healing. Second, the repaired meniscus must retain its mechanical properties for participation in load transmission. Only vertical longitudinal (bucket handle) tears located in the vascular periphery of the menisci satisfy both of these conditions. While radial and complex tears can be stimulated to heal, animal studies have demonstrated that the wide fibrovascular scar that results does not allow normal function to be maintained.

The meniscal tear most amenable to repair is therefore a vertical longitudinal (bucket handle) tear greater than 1 cm in length, involving greater than 50% of the width of the meniscus, and within 4 to 5 mm of the meniscosynovial junction. Approximately half of such tears occur in either acute or chronic anterior cruciate ligament (ACL) deficient knees. A simple classification system of vertical longitudinal tears pertinent to prognosis is based on the vascularity present on either side of the tear. *Red-red* tears are peripheral meniscal separations, with good vascularity both on the synovial and meniscal sides of the tear. *Red-white* tears occur within the vascular peripheral third (4 to 5 mm) of the meniscus; the peripheral rim retains a blood supply whereas the inner fragment is devoid of vascularity. *White-white* tears are those within the avascular inner two-thirds of the meniscus and have no vascularity on either side of the tear. Both red-red and red-white tears are capable of fibrovascular healing through the extrinsic pathway.

Meniscal repair should not be attempted when there is significant damage to the body of the meniscus and the tear site does not coapt nicely. A retear of a previously repaired meniscus is not a contraindication to a repeat attempt at repair, provided the tear site can be coapted. Multiple longitudinal tears, i.e., double bucket handle tears, are best treated by resection of the inner fragment and repair of the more peripheral tear. Meniscal repair in the ACL deficient knee should generally be performed in conjunction with a reconstructive stabilization procedure, as the results of the meniscal repair will be dependent on the grade of functional instability of the knee.

TECHNIQUES OF REPAIR

Meniscal repair may be performed through an open incision, through the arthroscope, or by employing a combination of arthroscopic and open methods. While certain locations of tears are more amenable to one technique than another, several considerations are common to all repair techniques.

Sutures of size 0 to 2-0 provide adequate strength for repair, and either absorbable or nonabsorbable suture material may be used. Vicryl and Dexon retain minimum strength at 3 weeks in an inflammatory synovial fluid environment and are not recommended for routine use. PDS retains 40% of its strength after 6 weeks in the joint and loses all of its strength by 9 weeks. However, this seems to be adequate for meniscal repair as no significant difference in healing rates between PDS and nonabsorbable suture have been demonstrated. While nonabsorbable suture (i.e., braided polyester) raises a theoretical concern of possible articular cartilage scuffing by the exposed material, this complication has not been seen during repeat arthroscopy.

Correct suture technique is critical for adequate coaptation of the tear and strength of the repair. Vertical mattress sutures provide greater pull out strength than horizontal mattress sutures, which in turn are stronger than the "end knot" technique (multiple overlapped knots placed at the end of a single strand of suture, which is then pulled up against the meniscal surface). Sutures should be placed no more than 5 mm apart from each other. Especially in larger tears, it is important that the sutures be placed variously on the superior and inferior surfaces of the meniscus to prevent puckering and maintain coaptation at the tear site. If a concomitant ACL reconstruction is performed, the sutures should be placed before but tied after the ligamentous surgery.

Stimulation of the healing response by preparation of the tear site has been demonstrated to increase healing rates, especially in chronic tears. Abrasion of both sides of the tear as well as the perimeniscal synovium with either a rasp or a motorized shaver creates fresh surfaces for healing and stimulates increased blood flow for influx of mesenchymal cells. Implantation of an exogenous fibrin clot, formed by agitating 30 cc of venous blood obtained from the patient, has been advocated as a method to turn on the intrinsic pathway of healing and thus obtain repairs in white-white tears. In a dog model, the fibrin clot acted as a chemotactic and mitogenic stimulus, causing a proliferation of fibrous connective tissue in the meniscus defect that eventually modulated into fibrocartilaginous tissue. However, this repair tissue always remained grossly and histologically different from normal meniscal tissue. Similar results have been demonstrated with application of a fibrin sealant containing endothelial cell growth factor (ECGF). In clinical practice, use of an exogenous fibrin clot may provide further stimulus to healing of isolated meniscal tears in the vascular periphery when the generalized hemarthrosis from an ACL reconstruction will not be present, but can not be relied upon to induce healing of avascular white-white tears. Other possible methods for stimulating healing of white-white tears, such as the creation of vascular access channels or excision of the peripheral meniscal rim, are to be condemned on the basis that they disrupt normal meniscal anatomy and function.

The four methods of suture placement techniques currently available include: (1) open repair, (2) "inside-out" arthroscopic repair, (3) "outside-in" arthroscopic repair, and (4) "all-inside" arthroscopic repair.

Open Repair

Open meniscal repair, first reported by Annandale in 1885, is best suited for posterior peripheral detachments of the menisci, and for technical reasons is limited to tears within 2 mm of the meniscosynovial junction. Exposure of the tear site is through a standard posteromedial or posterolateral approach.

On the medial side, a 4 cm vertical skin incision is made at the posteromedial corner just behind the palpable posterior edge of the superficial medial collateral ligament with the knee flexed. Dissection is continued down to the deep fascia, which is divided along the anterior border of the sartorius. The sartorius, medial hamstrings, and sartorial branch of the saphenous nerve are retracted posteriorly with the knee flexed. Blunt dissection with a finger, or a Cobb elevator if needed, is next required to separate the semimembranosus and medial head of the gastrocnemius from the underlying posterior capsule. An oblique capsular incision along the posterior edge of the posterior oblique ligament provides entrance into the joint and exposure of the tear.

On the lateral side, a 4 cm vertical incision is made at the posterolateral corner just behind the fibular collateral ligament with the knee flexed. The iliotibial band is identified and split in line with its fibers just anterior to the biceps femoris. The biceps femoris is gently retracted posteriorly, protecting the underlying common peroneal nerve. Blunt dissection carefully develops the interval between the lateral head of the gastrocnemius and the underlying posterior capsule, further protecting the peroneal nerve and popliteal neurovascular structures. An oblique capsular incision along the posterior border of the popliteus tendon provides entrance into the joint and exposure of the tear.

Visualization of the superior meniscosynovial junction and peripheral 2 to 3 mm of the posterior meniscal horns is possible through these approaches. Tears located more centrally are obscured by the femoral condyles. Once the tear has been identified and abraded, vertical mattress sutures are placed with a small curved needle to reapproximate the meniscus rim and capsular bed. Sutures may be tied either inside or outside the capsule. Absorbable suture is then used to repair the capsular incision.

Advantages of open meniscal repair include direct visualization of extremely peripheral tears and detachments, ease of tear site preparation, and the ability to precisely place vertical mattress sutures for greatest stability of repair. Additionally, if all sutures are tied inside the capsule, there is no concern of posterior capsular entrapment or tethering, which could result in flexion contracture postoperatively. Disadvantages include the inability to visualize and suture tears greater than 2 mm from the meniscal periphery. Also, placement of sutures for some tears may be more difficult than with arthroscopic approaches, especially on the lateral side in the area of the popliteus tendon.

Inside-Out Repair

Arthroscopic techniques for meniscus repair achieved popularity in the early 1980s. The inside-out arthroscopic meniscus repair, pioneered by Henning, was the first such technique developed. Straight or curved cannulas are introduced into the knee through the anterior arthroscopic portals in order to deliver the long tapered needles of a double-armed suture into the substance of the meniscus and across the tear site. Recovery of the needles outside the joint thus allows a mattress type suture to be placed across the meniscus tear. Either horizontal or vertical mattress sutures may be placed depending on the orientation of the cannulas within the joint.

As most tears suitable for repair are located in the posterior horns, blind recovery of the needles places the popliteal neurovascular structures at extreme risk. A small posteromedial or posterolateral approach, as previously described, is necessary for exposure of the posterior capsule and placement of a popliteal retractor (Fig. 1). Commercially available retractors (Stryker) are specially designed to fit in the space between the head of the gastrocnemius and posterior capsule and deflect the needles away from midline as they exit through the posterior capsule. A sterile teaspoon serves this purpose equally well. Once all needles are recovered, tension is placed on the sutures as the meniscus is viewed arthroscopically and the quality of the repair observed. The knots of the mattress sutures are tied snugly over the posterior capsule.

Advantages of the inside-out arthroscopic suturing technique include the precise placement of mattress sutures under direct arthroscopic visualization and the ability to suture tears located up to 5 mm from the meniscal periphery. Proper preparation of a peripheral tear is more difficult than with open techniques and may require a posteromedial portal. Although passage of the needles from inside the joint places the posterior neurovascular structures at risk for inadvertent laceration, this risk is minimized by proper technique including a posterior incision with correct placement of a popliteal retractor.

Outside-In Repair

Reports of catastrophic neurovascular complications after early attempts at inside-out arthroscopic meniscus repair (*without* use of a posterior incision) prompted the development of outside-in arthroscopic repair techniques. Safe passage of suture needles from outside the joint is based on identifiable anatomic landmarks. On the lateral side, needles are passed from the posterolateral corner with the knee near 90 degrees of flexion. The safe zone for passage lies anterior to the biceps femoris, thereby avoiding the common peroneal nerve. On the medial side, the saphenous nerve must be avoided as it traverses near the posteromedial corner of the joint. With the knee flexed, the safe zone lies anterior to the pes tendons at the joint line. Alternatively, as suggested by Morgan, the suture needles may be passed with the knee near full extension just posterior to the palpable pes tendons, 2 cm behind the posteromedial corner.

A straight or curved 18 gauge needle with trochar is directed into the joint and through the peripheral meniscal rim at the site of the tear. At this point, firm counter pressure with a probe is required to continue passage of the needle through the inner segment of the torn meniscus. The needle is generally directed through the concave superior surface of the meniscus. Once passed, the trocar of the needle is removed and a suture threaded into the joint (Fig. 2, *A*).

Two options are available for tying the suture. A second cannulated needle may be passed from outside-in and a suture snare used to pull the free end of the suture

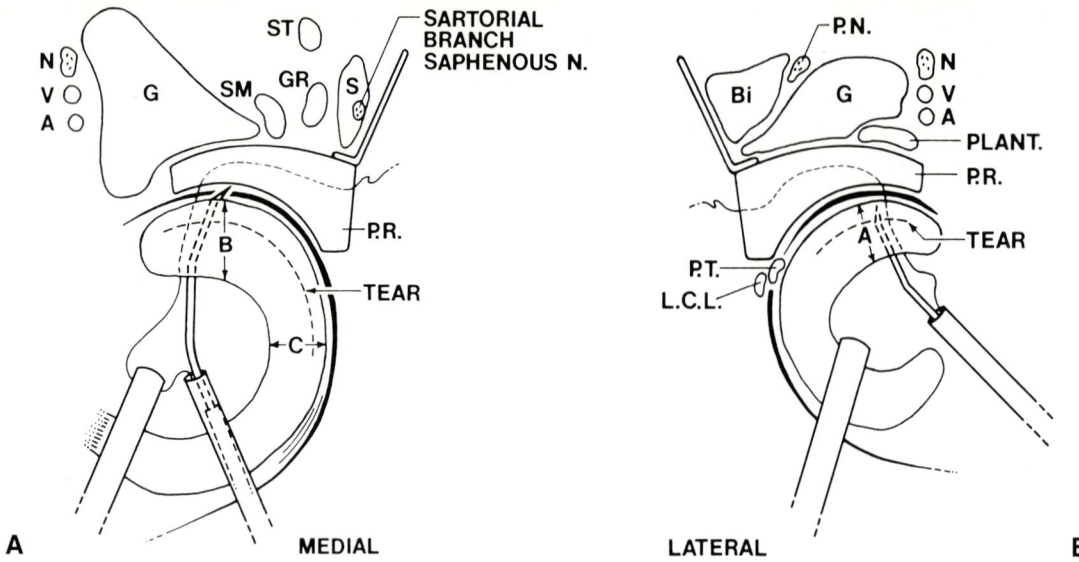

Figure 1 Inside-out arthroscopic meniscus repair. *A,* On the medial side, the popliteal retractor is positioned behind the posterior capsule and in front of the hamstring tendons and medial head of the gastrocnemius muscle. The repair needle may be placed through either the anteromedial or anterolateral portal and should be directed into the popliteal retractor, thereby protecting the neurovascular structures. *B,* On the lateral side, the popliteal retractor is positioned behind the posterior capsule and in front of the biceps tendon and lateral head of the gastrocnemius muscle. This protects the common peroneal nerve and the popliteal neurovascular structures. Identical approaches are used for open meniscal repairs of posterior peripheral tears. PR = popliteal retractor, S = sartorius, GR = gracilis, ST = semitendinosus, SM = semimembranosus, G = gastrocnemius, N = tibial nerve, A = popliteal artery, V = popliteal vein, PN = common peroneal nerve, Bi = biceps femoris, PLANT = plantaris, PT = popliteus tendon, LCL = lateral collateral ligament. (From Henning CE, Lynch MA, Yearout KM, et al. Arthroscopic meniscal repair using an exogenous fibrin clot. Clin Orthop 1990; 252:64-72; with permission.)

back through the meniscus and outside the joint, thus creating a horizontal mattress suture. Alternatively, the free end of the suture may be brought out of the joint through an anterior portal and overlapping end knots (mulberry knot) tied. As tension is placed on the back end of the suture, the end knot is pulled back into the joint and snugged up against the meniscal surface, thus coapting the tear (Fig. 2, *B*). Although this leaves a large knot of suture material in the joint, no deleterious effects of the suture on either the meniscus or the articular cartilage have been documented at second look arthroscopy. Whichever technique is used, a small skin incision is needed posteriorly to retrieve the multiple suture tails in the subcutaneous tissue so that they can be tied over the deep fascia.

While the outside-in technique offers the advantage of control over where the needles pass in relation to the neurovascular structures, some control is lost over where the needles (and suture) pass through the meniscus. Also, the end knot technique provides the least secure fixation of the meniscus in terms of pull out strength. Nevertheless, with a sufficient number of sutures passing close to the free edge of the meniscus, adequate stability of the repair can be obtained.

All-Inside Repair

The all-inside repair was developed by Morgan as an arthroscopic technique designed to eliminate the risk of neurovascular complications from needle passage. It is best for tears in the most posterocentral portions of the posterior horns, as the instruments may have difficulty reaching other tears. Tears up to 3 to 4 mm from the meniscosynovial junction are amenable to repair by the all-inside technique.

Visualization of the tear is with a 70 degree arthroscope passed through the intercondylar notch and into the posteromedial or posterolateral compartment. A posteromedial or posterolateral portal is required for the suturing instrumentation. A specially designed suture hook is used to place vertically orientated sutures through the tear; these sutures are similar to those sutures that would be placed with an open repair technique (Fig. 3, *A*). The knots are tied intra-articularly with an arthroscopic knot pusher through the posterior portal (Fig. 3, *B*).

The all-inside repair technique offers the advantages of vertically orientated sutures, no needle passage out of the joint, and no posterior capsular entrapment or tethering as all sutures are tied within the joint. However, this is a technically demanding technique requiring special instruments, and addresses those tears that are more easily treated with suturing through an open repair technique.

POSTOPERATIVE CARE AND REHABILITATION

Specific rehabilitation protocols following meniscus repair are controversial and continue to evolve. A

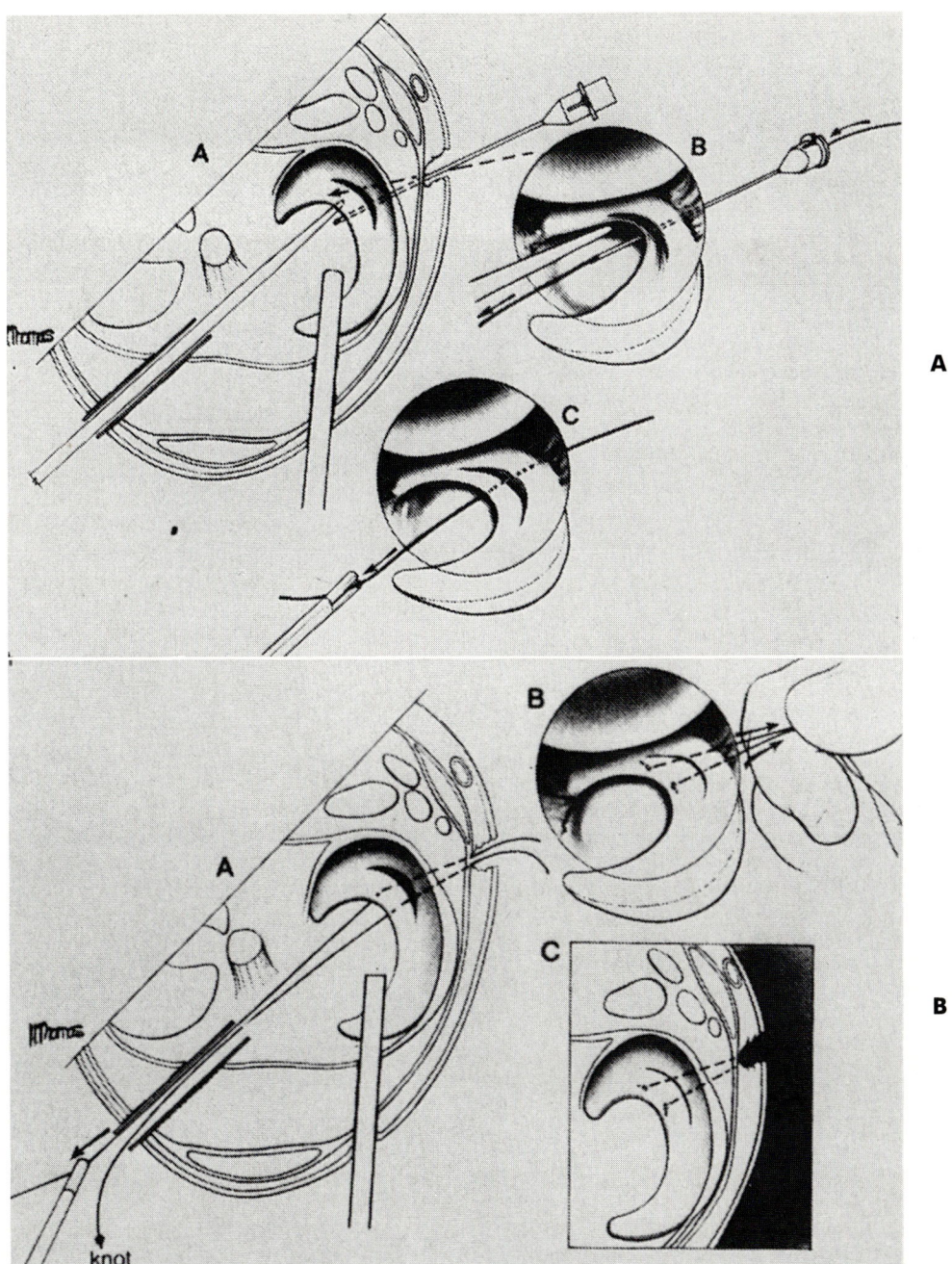

Figure 2 Outside-in arthroscopic meniscus repair. *A,* The meniscus tear is reduced with a probe as a spinal needle is passed percutaneously from the posteromedial corner and across the tear. Suture is then threaded through the needle and brought out of the knee through an anterior portal. *B,* The procedure is repeated until a sufficient number of sutures have been placed across the tear. End-knots are tied and then pulled back into the joint against the meniscal surface, thus securing the tear. The multiple suture tails are tied to each other over the deep fascia. (From Warren RF, Hanley S, Bach BR. In Parisien JS, ed. Arthroscopic surgery. New York: McGraw-Hill, 1988:130; with permission.)

general consensus is that isolated meniscal repairs (no ligamentous surgery) should be protected for 4 to 6 weeks with limited weight bearing. Some authors allow full weight bearing in extension. Strict immobilization has been associated with loss of motion after meniscus repair and is not recommended. A canine model has demonstrated good healing rates with adequate suture fixation without the need for immobilization or restricted weight bearing.

When a meniscus repair is performed in conjunction with a ligament reconstruction, early motion is mandatory to prevent arthrofibrosis. In general, a therapy protocol similar to that used for ligament reconstruction alone is followed.

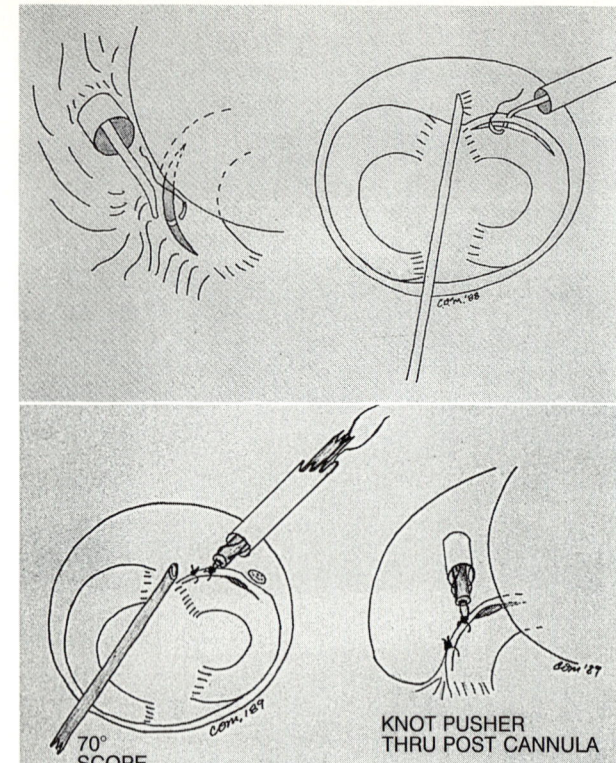

Figure 3 All-inside arthroscopic meniscus repair. *A,* A specially designed suture hook is placed through a posterolateral portal while the tear is visualized with a 70 degree arthroscope positioned through the intercondylar notch from an anteromedial portal. A vertically orientated suture is placed and threaded through the suture hook. *B,* The sutures are tied with an arthroscopic knot pusher through the posterolateral portal. All sutures are completely intra-articular. (From Morgan CD. The "all-inside" meniscus repair. Arthroscopy 1991; 7:120-125; with permission.)

The amount of time needed for maturation of the repair tissue at the tear site is not known. In the dog model, the tear is filled by fibrovascular scar within 6 weeks. By 6 months, mature fibrocartilage is present but this tissue is still grossly and histologically different from normal meniscus. In humans, 3 to 4 months are required to see arthroscopic evidence of healing, and abnormal MRI signal persists in arthroscopically documented healed tears at time points greater than 1 year. Current recommendations are that return to pivoting athletics not be allowed for 4 to 6 months after meniscal repair.

RESULTS OF MENISCAL REPAIR

Results of both open and arthroscopic meniscal repair in appropriately selected tears have been very favorable. Clinical healing rates (no mechanical symptoms suggestive of meniscal pathology) are reported to be approximately 90% in most series. As determined by second look arthroscopy or postoperative arthrograms, meniscal healing may involve greater than 90% of the height of the tear (fully healed), between 50% and 90% of the height of the tear (partially healed), or less than 50% of the tear height (not healed). Both fully healed and partially healed menisci render a clinically successful result. Using this system, reports have documented 75% to 80% of repaired menisci as completely healed, 15% as partially healed, and 5% to 10% as failures.

In the stable knee, results of meniscal repair do not decrease appreciably with time. Long-term follow-up at 5 to 10 years demonstrates low retear rates in the range of a few percent. While no series has follow-up of sufficient duration to document prevention of development of degenerative changes after successful meniscal repair, early reports have shown a difference in Fairbanks changes between knees undergoing meniscal repair versus meniscectomy.

In the unstable ACL deficient knee, the prognosis for a sutured tear is dependent on the degree of functional instability of that knee. While some studies have reported retear rates only slightly greater than those in stable knees, others have documented retear rates approaching 10% per year in the unstable knee. Laboratory studies have also documented increased loading of the medial meniscus in the ACL deficient knee. When a repairable meniscus is encountered in an ACL deficient knee, stabilization through a ligamentous reconstruction procedure is strongly recommended. Meniscal repair without ligament reconstruction is acceptable only in those individuals willing to greatly modify activities, and a higher retear rate must be acknowledged.

Certain factors have been looked at as determinants of the probability that a given repairable tear will heal. The width of the peripheral rim of meniscus at the tear strongly correlates with rates of healing. Tears with rim widths of 0 to 2 mm show higher rates of healing than those with rim widths of 3 to 5 mm. Length of the tear does not strongly influence the rate of healing as long as proper suture stabilization is accomplished. The age of the tear does not affect the chance of healing if proper tear site preparation (rasping, shaver debridement) is performed and there has been no damage to the body of the torn meniscus over time. Also, the age of the patient does not affect healing as long as there are no degenerative cleavage components to the tear. Medial and lateral meniscal tears heal equally well, and no difference is seen in healing rates between open and arthroscopic suturing techniques. Significantly increased healing rates are observed when meniscus repair is performed in conjunction with intra-articular ACL reconstruction, most likely secondary to the hemarthrosis and resulting generalized inflammatory response. As mentioned previously, the use of an exogenous fibrin clot implanted at the tear site may increase the chances of healing for isolated meniscal tears through a similar mechanism.

SUGGESTED READING

Arnoczky SP, Warren RF. The microvasculature of the meniscus and its response to injury: An experimental study in the dog. Am J Sports Med 1983; 11:131-141.

Cooper DE, Arnoczky SP, Warren RF. Meniscal repair. Clin Sports Med 1991; 10:529-548.

DeHaven KE, Black KP, Griffiths HJ. Open meniscus repair: Technique and two to nine year results. Am J Sports Med 1989; 17:788-795.

Hanks GA, Gause TM, Handal JA, et al. Meniscus repair in the anterior cruciate deficient knee. Am J Sports Med 1990; 18:606-613.

Henning CE, Lynch MA, Yearout KM, et al. Arthroscopic meniscal repair using an exogenous fibrin clot. Clin Orthop 1990; 252:64-72.

Morgan CD, Wojtys EM, Casscells CD, et al. Arthroscopic meniscal repair evaluated by second-look arthroscopy. Am J Sports Med 1991; 19:632-637.

Newman AP, Anderson DR, Daniels AU, et al. Mechanics of the healed meniscus in a canine model. Am J Sports Med 1989; 17:164-175.

Newman AP, Daniels AU, Burks RT. Principles and decision making in meniscal surgery. Arthroscopy 1993; 9:33-51.

O'Meara PM: The basic science of meniscsus repair. Orthop Rev 1993; 22:681-686.

Scott GA, Jolly BL, Henning CE. Combined posterior incision and arthroscopic intra-articular repair of the meniscus: An examination of factors affecting healing. J Bone Joint Surg 1986; 68A:847-861.

ARTHROSCOPIC REPAIR OF MENISCAL TEARS

ROLAND P. JAKOB, M.D.
JOHN C. EDWARDS, M.D.

A relatively common injury of the knee in athletes is a traumatic tear of one of the menisci. These tears may be either an isolated injury or may be associated with an injury to one of the stabilizing ligaments of the knee, usually the anterior cruciate ligament (ACL). The advent of arthroscopy has led to an evolution in the treatment of these injuries. Once treated by open total meniscectomy, the goal now is to preserve as much meniscal tissue as possible. The reasons for this change in attitude, and a technique that has been employed since 1982 by the senior author (RPJ), are presented in this chapter.

BACKGROUND

The menisci perform a vital role in protecting the articular cartilage of the knee joint. The medial meniscus transmits approximately 50% of the contact forces in the medial compartment with the lateral meniscus transmitting an even higher percentage in the lateral compartment. Seedholm and Hargreaves showed that removal of 16% to 34% of meniscal tissue would increase the contact forces between the articular surface of the femur and tibia by approximately 35%. Clinical proof of these increased forces that are borne across the knee joint was offered by Fairbanks in 1948 when he first described the degenerative changes seen on radiographs in previously meniscectomized knees. Several other authors have confirmed these results. The study of Johnson et al was particularly dramatic, showing osteoarthritic changes in 40% of previously meniscectomized knees at 17 years while only 6% of the contralateral knees in this group showed the same degenerative changes.

The introduction of the arthroscope into the armamentarium of the orthopedic surgeon allowed for more conservative meniscal surgery. Treatment could be directed to resection of only that part of the meniscus that was damaged in an attempt to preserve as much of the remaining nondamaged tissue as possible. Confirmation of this approach was suggested by Cox and Cordell when they showed in an animal model that the amount of degeneration seen in the knee joint was directly related to the amount of tissue excised. This has been further validated by several clinical trials to date.

The next logical step in the treatment of these injuries would be to attempt to repair the torn portion of the meniscus, and in that way conserve even more of its protective function. Actually, attempts to repair meniscal tissue date back to the late 1800s, when the first account of meniscal reattachment was published by Annandale. In 1936, King successfully reattached a meniscus in a canine model and observed that repairs were possible in the vascular periphery, but not towards the avascular center. Arnoczky and Warren showed that the peripheral one-fourth to one-third of the human meniscus was vascular and could therefore mount a healing response. This vascular portion appears to be age related in that the fetal meniscus has a rich vascular supply that extends into the central third of the meniscus. By age 11 most of the vessels are gone from this region. This theoretical healing capability has been proven by the numerous reports in the literature, employing many different arthroscopic and open techniques, which have shown that clinical healing occurs in approximately 80% to 90% of meniscal repairs.

INDICATIONS

The clinical studies mentioned in the previous section have led to an increased understanding of the variables that effect healing in meniscal repairs, and have therefore led to an evolution in our indications for this procedure. Although each case is evaluated individually, our current indications for meniscal repair are:

1. Longitudinal tears that are at least 15 mm long and located in the vascular zone or in the junction of the vascular and nonvascular zone.
2. Longitudinal tears that are diagnosed at the time of ACL reconstruction.

3. Isolated tears that meet the criterion of indication 1 above in a ligamentously stable knee.

Our contraindications include:

1. Degenerative type meniscal tears in patients older than 40.
2. Flap or radial type tears.
3. Meniscal tears in an ACL insufficient knee when the patient is unwilling to undergo reconstruction of the ACL.
4. Tears in vigourly athletic patients who are unwilling to undergo the extended rehabilitation that accompanies meniscal repair.
5. "Leave alone" tears.
6. Tears found at the time of diagnostic arthroscopy that do not fit with the clinical symptoms.
7. Incomplete tears on either the superior or inferior surface of the meniscus.
8. Cleavage-type tears in the older patient with osteoarthritic changes without typical meniscal symptoms.
9. Lateral meniscal tears found at the time of ACL reconstruction that are short (<15 mm), in the periphery, and that cannot be displaced into the joint with an arthroscopic probe.

TECHNIQUE

In order for a technique to be successful it needs to be relatively simple, reproducable, and safe. The senior author (RPJ) has employed an arthroscopic "inside out" technique over the last 10 years that allows accurate placement of the stiches in the torn meniscal fragment. This is accomplished by the use of a series of needles of three different curvatures that fit into three canulas of corresponding curvatures (Fig. 1). The needles are thin (1.2 mm) and resemble a sewing machine needle with a hole that is situated 15 mm from the end of the needle. The tip of the needle itself looks like that of a Keith needle. The different curvatures allow precise placement of the sutures to different parts of the meniscus, depending upon where the tear is located. The technique will be described in detail using the example of a relatively common "bucket-handle" tear of the medial meniscus.

Diagnostic Arthroscopy

A diagnostic arthroscopy is performed through routine medial and lateral parapatellar portals located at the respective border of the patellar ligament. The 30-degree arthroscope is introduced into the knee joint through the lateral portal, and an arthroscopic probe is placed through the medial portal.

The tear is evaluated and determinations are made as to its location, extent, shape, thickness, and stability. This allows the tear to be classified, and a decision is made as to whether the dislocated bucket is in good enough shape to warrant refixation. If meniscal repair is decided upon, the next step is the debridement of both

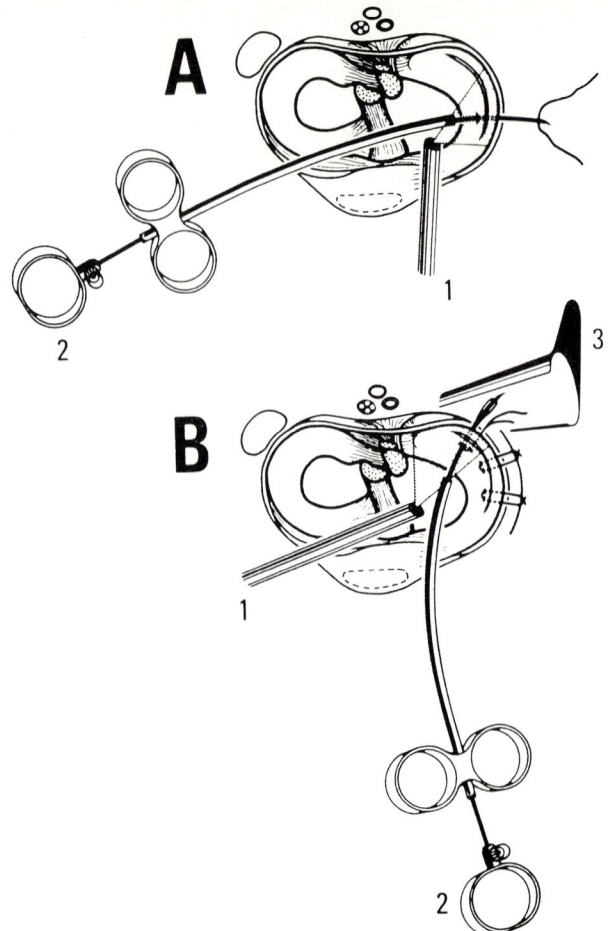

Figure 1 *A*, For the middle one-third of the meniscus the needle with least curvature is inserted from the opposite compartment. *B*, For the posterior horn the most curved needle is inserted from the ipsilateral compartment. A Henning retractor secures safe posterior perforation.

fragments with the aid of arthroscopic rasps and shavers. A small shaver with a curved tip has been found to be particularly useful in this circumstance, because it allows the lesion to be reached at a mechanically advantageous angle. The remaining meniscus is closely examined for any secondary tears, and any unstable portions of the rim are removed at this time.

Reduction of Bucket-Handle Tear

The bucket-handle tear is now reduced with the aid of the blunt trocar that is used to introduce the arthroscope into the knee joint. The addition of a valgus stress on the knee may facilitate the reduction of the meniscus in the event that difficulty with this maneuver is encountered. (A varus stress is used for a tear of the lateral meniscus.) With the meniscus reduced, any radial tears of the bucket-handle itself can now be debrided.

Approach to Posterior Corner

With a medial meniscus tear, an approach to the posteromedial structures is undertaken. Great care is taken to protect the saphenous nerve and its branches in this region. Late discomfort and decreased skin sensation in the distribution of this nerve is one of the most common complications following meniscal repair on the medial side. A small portion of the medial gastrocnemius is detached so that a retractor can be inserted posteriorly that will protect the posterior structures when the needles are passed from inside the knee out through the posterior capsule.

On the lateral side the most important structure encountered is the common peroneal nerve. It is protected by directly exposing it, and then inserting a retractor posterior to the fibular head. The retractor then acts as a barrier between the nerve and the penetrating needles. With these posterior incisions, and utilizing a curved needle inserted from the contralateral portal, sutures can be placed within 1 cm of the posterior attachment without risking any of the neurovascular structures.

Placement of AO Distractor

At this stage the AO distractor is routinely placed in case of tight ligaments (Fig. 2). One short Schanz screw is inserted in the adductor tubercle and the other is inserted 3 cm distal to the joint line for the medial meniscus. (Corresponding sites are selected for the lateral meniscus.) The screws are inserted to a depth of 40 mm, which avoids their catching the opposite cortex. We have observed in cadaver knees that a unicortical screw will loosen before the distraction necessary to injure the ipsilateral collateral ligament can be applied. However, this is not the case when both cortices are engaged, because in this situation the distractor becomes far more efficient at generating increased tension. Although some may argue that the use of the distractor as described by Henning unnecessarily complicates the procedure, we have found it allows improved visualization of the posterior horn of the meniscus, permits more precise suturing of the meniscus, and helps avoid scoring of the articular cartilage with the arthroscopic instruments. It also avoids having to have an assistant hold the compartment open during the procedure.

Placement of Sutures

The sutures are now placed in the meniscus with the different needles and corresponding canulas depending on the location of the tear. Posterior sutures are placed using the most curved needle that is passed through the ipsilateral portal. More anterior sutures are placed with less curved needles passed through the contralateral portal. In order to accomplish this the arthroscope needs to be changed from one portal to the other. The last 1 to 2 cm of the posterior horn can be sutured with "an outside-in" technique to avoid damage to the neurovascular structures in the posterior aspect of the knee. (See section on the outside-in technique for more details.)

Four to five sutures are placed on the upper surface and three to four are placed on the undersurface with a distance of 6 to 7 mm between sutures. Although technically more demanding, placement of sutures in the undersurface of the meniscus are mechanically superior

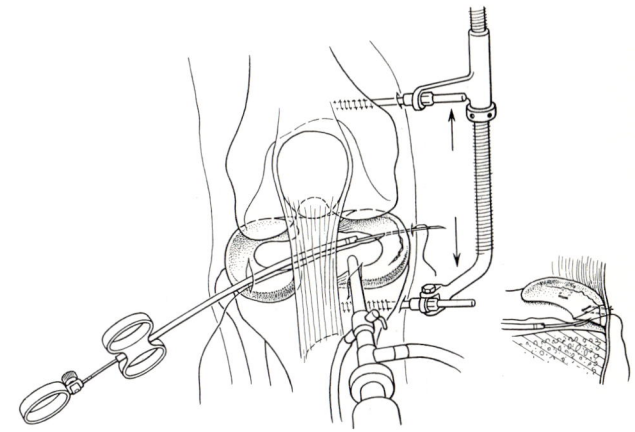

Figure 2 Use of the AO femoral distractor.

and are more apt to reduce the meniscus anatomically. The suture materials are an absorbable and nonabsorbable "O" monofilament suture. The nonabsorbable sutures are used for the more peripheral parts of the meniscus while the absorbable sutures are placed in the more central parts.

Closure

The AO distractor is removed, and the efficacy of the repair is checked with gentle probing of the tear. The sutures are then tied with moderate tension over the capsule, making sure that a branch of the saphenous nerve has not been caught in the knots. The subcutaneous tissue and skin are then closed in a routine fashion.

Outside-In Technique

As stated previously, the outside-in technique is used for tears that are 1 to 2 cm from the attachment of the posterior horn or for rare tears of the anterior horn of either meniscus. Popularized by Warren, the technique consists of placing two spinal needles either through a capsular exposing incision or percutaneously from outside the joint into the meniscus. The needles pierce the meniscus approximately 6 mm from each other. Monofilament sutures are passed through both needles and brought out through the arthroscopic portal with the aid of an arthroscopic grasper, and the spinal needles are removed. A double "dilating" knot is tied approximately 8 to 10 cm from the end of one of the sutures, and then the two ends are tied together with a single square knot. The opposite end of the suture that has the dilating knot (the end that is outside the capsule at the entry point of the spinal needle) is then pulled until the dilating knot and the square knot are delivered out through the capsule. This suture is then cut, and the two ends of the other suture are tied over the posterior capsule (Fig. 3). An alternative approach to this same technique is to pass a loop of suture through the second spinal needle and then arthroscopically place the first suture through this loop. As the loop is pulled back out

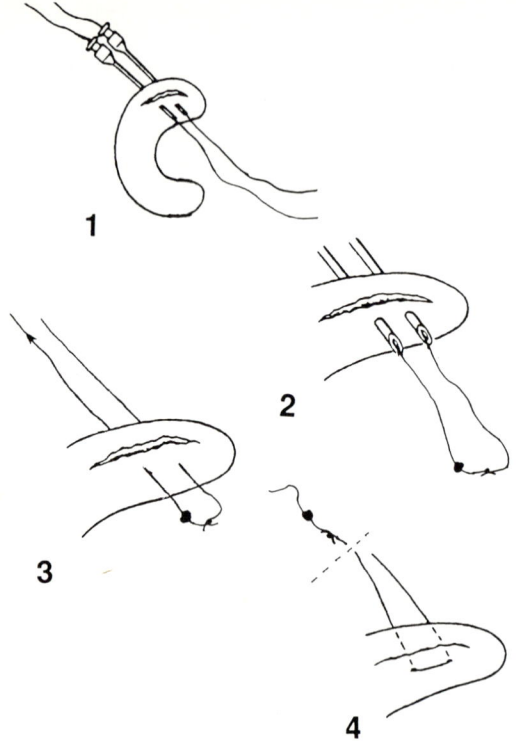

Figure 3 Outside-in technique of Warren (see text for details).

through the spinal needle, the end of the first suture is then delivered out through the posterior capsule. Both techniques arrive at the same point, with the ends of the first suture being tied over the posterior capsule.

Another outside-in technique described by Tiling and Röddecker also starts with spinal needles being placed into the meniscal tissue. Their sutures are once again delivered out through one of the arthroscopic portals with the aid of an arthroscopic grasper. However, in their technique each suture is then threaded with several small absorbable buttons to form a cone-shaped disc. Both sutures are then pulled back into the joint, and as the discs make contact with the meniscus they hold it in place. These two sutures are then tied over the capsule. This technique is particularly elegant when dealing with tears of the anterior horn.

POSTOPERATIVE PROTOCOL

Postoperatively, the knee is allowed a range of motion between 20 and 90 degrees of flexion for 6 weeks. In this way the increased anteroposterior motion of the meniscus that accompanies extreme ranges of motion of the knee are limited during its healing phase. Return to active competition is restricted for 4 months.

COMPLICATIONS

Most of the early complications of arthroscopic meniscal repair dealt with injury to the neurovascular structures. With the use of posterior counter incisions, and with the placement of a finger or retractor to protect these structures when suturing the posterior horn, these complications have been greatly decreased. However, care still needs to be taken to avoid injury to the saphenous nerve and vein on the medial side, and the peroneal nerve on the lateral side. The peroneal nerve is particularly vulnerable if the needle is allowed to exit posterior to the fibular head.

RESULTS

Of the 54 ruptured menisci, 42 (78%) healed without further injury. Reruptures occurred in 12 patients (22%). In 6 patients this occurred with minimal trauma after 2½ to 24 months, and 6 patients sustained another significant injury while participating in athletic activity 1 to 2 years after the repair. Ten of the twelve reruptures were treated by arthroscopic partial meniscectomy. A successful secondary refixation was performed in an 18-year-old female who had shown partial healing on the arthrogram at 4 months and who complained of some discomfort, and in a 35-year-old male whose cleavage plane was very peripheral with an otherwise intact anteriorly subluxated meniscal body. Four of the twelve patients had a partial anterior cruciate tear as a possible cause of the recurrence.

Of the 12 reruptures, 4 were longitudinal tears and 8 were bucket-handle tears. The type of retear resembled the initial lesion (e.g., the cleavage plane was the same).

The number of retears was compared with the duration of symptoms prior to refixation. The average duration of symptoms prior to the arthroscopic refixation in those 12 patients with retears was 21 days; thus, we were dealing with a group of relatively fresh meniscal tears.

Control arthrograms as suggested by Scott et al were performed at about 4 months after refixation in 29 of 54 patients, indicating meniscal defects in 7 cases (24%). Four of these seven patients had some subjective complaints, and in six of the seven patients we found objective signs such as a moderately positive McMurray sign.

In a long-term follow-up study, 32 of the initial 54 patients that were reported on in 1988 were available for follow-up. Of these 32 patients 28% ultimately went on to rerupture their meniscus, with 60% occurring in the first 6 months; there were no reruptures between 44 and 82 months. Twenty-five of the patients consented to MRI examination, and 96% of them had grade 3 to 4 changes in the repaired menisci. In that most of these patients were symptom free, the conclusion was reached that MRI is an invalid diagnostic tool for menisci that have been previously repaired.

DISCUSSION

Although meniscal repair has been shown to be very successful, particularly when associated with a reconstruction of the ACL, there are several issues that need to be considered when dealing with athletes. One of these issues is the rehabilitation time. The 4 months of healing that we require before allowing an athlete to return to his sport usually results in the loss of a season. This is of particular interest in isolated tears of the meniscus because the results are less predictable than when associated with a reconstruction of the ACL, and because a simple arthroscopic meniscectomy will allow a much quicker return to participation. For this reason, many athletes will opt for the latter even though they may pay for it down the road with earlier degenerative changes in their knee joint. (Those meniscal tears that are associated with an ACL reconstruction are less of a problem in that the time required for rehabilitation of the ligament reconstruction allows plenty of time for the meniscus to heal.)

Due to the inherently better healing potential of the lateral meniscus, one author (Beaufils) questions the necessity of suturing acute lateral meniscal tears, and proposes leaving them alone.

The question routinely arises as to whether or not some preventive measures could be taken to protect the structures of the knee joint. Bracing the knee in high-risk sports such as football has been advocated at times as a means of protecting the structures of the knee, but two studies found that incidence of injury actually increased in the braced population. One of the studies also found that there was increased risk of injury to the ipsilateral foot and ankle. Currently about the best protective measure for the menisci is a good general conditioning program that includes all the muscles that cross the knee joint. These muscles act as the main shock absorbers to the forces that cross the knee during ambulation, and when they are weak or unconditioned the increased forces are borne directly by the articular cartilage and menisci.

SUGGESTED READING

Ahmed AM, Burke DL. In vitro measurement of static pressure distribution in synovial joints. Part 1: Tibial surface of the knee. J Biomech Eng 1983; 105:216–225.

Arnoczky SP, Warren RF. Microvasculature of the human meniscus. Am J Sports Med 1982; 10:90–95.

Barber FA, Stone RG. Meniscal repair, an arthroscopic technique. J Bone Joint Surg (Br) 1985; 67:39–44.

Beaufils P, Bastos R, Wakim E, et al. The meniscus lesion on the reconstruction of anterior cruciate ligament. Mensicus repair or abstension. Rev de Chirurg Orthop 1992; 285–291.

Benedetto JP, Glotzer W, Kunzel KH. The vascularization of the menisci. Morphological basis for the repair. Acta Anat (Basel) 1985; 124: 88–92.

Buckwalter JA, Rosenberg LC, Hunziker EB. Articular cartilage: composition, structure, response to injury, and methods of facilitating repair. In Ewing JW, ed. Articular cartilage and knee joint function: Basic science and arthroscopy. New York: Raven Press, 1990.

Clancy WG, Graf BK. Arthroscopic meniscus repair. Orthopaedics 1983, 6:1125–1129.

Clark CR, Ogden JA. Development of the menisci of the human knee joint: morphological changes and their potential role in childhood meniscal injury. J Bone Joint Surg (Am) 1983; 65:538–547.

Cox JS, Cordell LD. The degenerative effects of medial meniscus tears in dogs' knees. Clin Orthop 1977; 125:236–242.

De Haven KE. Commentary. Repair of peripheral meniscus tears, a preliminary report. Am J Sports Med 1981; 9:213–214.

De Haven KE. Meniscus repair—open versus arthroscopic. Arthroscopy 1985; 1:173–174.

De Haven KE. Meniscus repair in the athlete. Clin Orthop 1985; 198:31–35.

Fairbanks TJ. Knee joint changes after meniscectomy. J Bone Joint Surg (Br) 1948; 30:664–670.

Grace TG, Skipper BJ, Newberry JC, et al. Prophylactic knee braces and injury to the lower extremity. J Bone Joint Surg (Am) 1988; 70:422–427.

Heatly FW. The meniscus—can it be repaired? An experimental investigation in rabbit. J Bone Joint Surg (Br) 1980; 62:397–402.

Hendler TL. Athroscopic meniscal repair, surgical technique. Clin Orthop 1984; 190:163–169.

Henning CE. Arthroscopic repair of meniscus tears. Orthopaedics 1985; 6:1130–1132.

Jakob RP, Ballmer PM, Zuber K, Stäubli HU. Meniscus repair with special reference to arthroscopic technique. In Jakob RP, Stäubli H-U, eds. The knee and the cruciate ligaments. Berlin, Heidelberg: Springer-Verlag, 1990.

Jakob RP, Stäubli H-U, Zuber K, et al. The arthroscopic meniscal repair. Techniques and clinical experience. Am J Sports Med 1988; 16:137–142.

Johnson RJ, Kettlekamp DB, Clark W, et al. Factors affecting late results after meniscectomy. J Bone Joint Surg (Am) 1974; 56: 719–729.

Morgan CD, Casscells SW. Arthroscopic surgery: repair of peripheral detachment of the meniscus. Contemp Orthop 1986; 2:3–12.

Newman AP, Daniels AU, Burks RT. Principles and decision making in meniscal surgery. Arthroscopy 1993; 9:33–51.

Northmore-Ball MD, Dandy DJ. Long-term results of arthroscopic partial meniscectomy. Clin Orthop 1982; 167:34–42.

Roeddecker K, Giebel GD, Lohscheidt C, Nagelschmidt M. Arthroscopic repair of traumatic longitudinal meniscal tears. A 3- to 5-year follow-up. Surg Endosc 1993; 7:46–51.

Ronrich P, Schworm B. Experience with open meniscus refixation. Results of follow-up in 17 cases. Beitr Orthop Traumatol 1990; 37:547–551.

Rosenberg TD, Paulos LE, Wnorowski DC, et al. Arthroscopic surgery: meniscus refixation and meniscus healing. Orthopaedics 1990; 19:82–89.

Rosenberg TD, Scott S, Paulos LE. Arthroscopic surgery: repair of peripheral detachment of the meniscus. Contemp Orthop 1985; 10:43–50.

Scott GA, Jolly BL, Henning CE. Combined posterior incision and intraarticular repair of the meniscus. An examination of the factors affecting healing. J Bone Joint Surg (Am) 1986; 68:847–861.

Seedholm BB, Hargreaves DJ. Transmission on the load in the knee with special reference to the role of the menisci. Part I: Anatomy, analysis and apparatus. N Engl J Med 1979; 8:207–219.

Seedholm BB, Hargreaves DJ. Transmission of the load in the knee joint with special reference to the role of the meniscus. Part II: Experimental results discussion and conclusions. N Engl J Med 1979; 8:220–228.

Teitz CC, Hermanson BK, Kronmal RA, Diehr PH. Evaluation of the use of braces to prevent injury to the knee in collegiate football players. J Bone Joint Surg (Am.) 1987; 69:2–9.

Warren RF. Meniscectomy and repair in the anterior cruciate ligament-deficient patient. Clin Orthop 1990; 252:55–63.

Wirth CR. Meniscus repair. Clin Orthop 1981; 157:153–160.

PROXIMAL REALIGNMENT AND LATERAL RETINACULAR RELEASE FOR PATELLAR SUBLUXATION AND DISLOCATION

GILES R. SCUDERI, M.D.
W. NORMAN SCOTT, M.D.

Anterior knee pain is a common complaint that brings a patient for evaluation. Through a careful history, physical examination, and radiographic evaluation the problem can be diagnosed.

HISTORY AND PHYSICAL EXAMINATION

Patients with patellar subluxation or dislocation clearly describe a giving way, especially while walking straight ahead, and in the case of patellar dislocation, the complete lateral displacement of the patella and resultant locking of the knee in flexion. Patients who clearly describe recurrent lateral patellar dislocations are candidates for proximal patellar realignment and lateral retinacular release.

Those patients who are subluxors are sometimes more difficult to diagnose and special attention needs to be given to evaluating laxity of the medial supporting structures and tightness of the lateral retinaculum. The Sage test has been helpful in assessing a tight lateral retinaculum. While the patient is supine, the relaxed knee is flexed 20 degrees, and the examiner attempts to displace the patella medially. Medial excursion of the patella less than one-quarter its greatest width is considered positive for a tight lateral retinaculum. Quantitatively, 10 mm of medial displacement is considered normal, whereas 5 mm or less indicates a tight lateral retinaculum.

The patellar glide test is also useful in assessing patellar mobility. Again, the relaxed knee is flexed 20 to 30 degrees and the examiner displaces the patella medially and laterally. Prior to displacement the examiner divides the patellar into quadrants. Usually the normal patella glides two quadrants in both the medial and lateral direction. A medial glide of one quadrant is consistent with a tight lateral retinaculum, similar to a positive Sage sign. A lateral patellar glide of three or more quadrants is indicative of lax medial restraints. When the patella displaces medially three or more quadrants, the patella is considered hypermobile.

The quadriceps (Q) angle is helpful in determining the alignment of the extensor mechanism. The Q angle is measured by drawing an imaginary line from the anterior-superior iliac spine to the center of the patella. A second line is drawn for the center of the patella to the tibial tubercle. The intersection of these two lines forms the Q angle. In males, the Q angle is normally 8 to 10 degrees while in females the normal value is from 10 to 20 degrees. Insall considers a Q angle greater than 20 degrees as abnormal, whereas Hughston believes that a Q angle greater than 10 degrees is abnormal and should be corrected.

The tubercle sulcus (TS) angle allows measurement of the patella position at 90 degrees of flexion. The benefit of this measurement is that the patella is engaged in the sulcus and any rotational anomalies can be observed. The TS angle is determined by a line from the center of the patella to the tibial tubercle and the angle formed with a line perpendicular to the transepicondylar axis passing through the center of the patella. Normally the TS angle is 0 degrees while an angle greater than 10 degrees is considered abnormal.

RADIOGRAPHIC EVALUATION

The radiographic evaluation provides further information in confirming the diagnosis. Several methods of measuring the patellar height from lateral radiographs have been reported. The Insall-Salvati ratio, which describes the patellar height as a ratio between the length of the patellar tendon and the longest vertical length of the patella, has been popular. The average patellar height based on this ratio was 1.02. Blackburne and Peel have reported their assessment of patellar height as the ratio between the perpendicular distance from the tibial articular surface and the inferior margin of the patellar articular surface and the length of the patellar articular surface. They found this ratio to be 0.8 in normal subjects. Caton and Linclau offer another measurement of patellar heights, which has been described as the vertical patellar height. This method relies on establishing another ratio. The distance from the inferior most point of the patellar articular surface to the anterior edge of the tibial articular surface and the length of the patellar articular surface. Scuderi recently demonstrated the vertical patellar height to be 0.97 in males and 0.96 in females with a standard deviation of 0.14.

Axial radiographs provide essential information concerning the patellofemoral articulation. Our preference is the Merchant view, which is a tangential radiograph of the patellofemoral joint with the knee flexed 45 degrees. This view allows measurement of the sulcus angle and the congruence angle. The sulcus angle measures the depth of the femoral sulcus while the congruence angle measures the degree of patellar subluxation. The congruence angle is measured by bisecting the sulcus angle in order to establish a reference line. A second line is then drawn from the apex of the sulcus angle to the lowest point of the patellar crest. The angle between these two lines is the congruence angle. By convention, the line bisecting the sulcus angle is considered 0 degrees. If the angle falls lateral to this line, it is given a positive value, while those medial to it are given a negative value. Merchant reported the congruence angle should be less than +16 degrees to be considered normal. Aglietti et al subsequently noted that the upper limit of a normal congruence angle be considered +4 degrees. Our feeling is similar to that of Aglietti, that a congruence angle greater than +4 degrees is indicative of patellar subluxation.

TREATMENT

Although the arthroscopic lateral retinacular release is an appealing procedure for dividing tight lateral structures, it does not restore normal orientation to a malaligned extensor mechanism. This failure of the lateral release to centralize the patella is supported by the patients who continue to experience patellar subluxation and dislocation. Although distal realignment procedures have been used commonly to treat this group of patients, we prefer to address this problem proximally. A proximal patellar realignment and lateral retinacular release is intended to release the tight lateral structures and reinforce the supporting medial structures. This includes advancing the vastus medialis obliquus, altering the dynamic pull of the quadriceps musculature and restoring patellofemoral congruence.

Madigan et al in 1975 originally described a method of quadricepsplasty for recurrent patellar subluxation. Technical problems with reorientation of the pull of the vastus medialis obliquus compromised the results. This led other surgeons to develop other techniques to realign the extensor mechanism proximally. Insall et al in 1979 described the proximal "tube" realignment as a quadricepsplasty that was later modified to the proximal patellar realignment with advancement of the vastus medialis and imbrication of the medial capsule. An important component of this procedure was an extensive lateral retinacular release that was extended into the vastus lateralis. Proximal realignment improves the dynamics of the vastus medialis, while the lateral retinacular release extending into the distal fibers of the vastus lateralis improves patellar tracking.

Surgical Technique

Before the open realignment procedure, an arthroscopic evaluation of the knee is performed. This allows treatment of associated lesions, such as meniscal tears, which may not be fully appreciated at the time of arthrotomy.

The knee is approached through a straight midline skin incision followed by a medial parapatellar arthrotomy. This arthrotomy extends in a straight line through the quadriceps tendon from the upper edge of the vastus medialis, over the patella and down the medial edge of the patellar tendon to the tibial tubercle (Fig. 1, *A*). A lateral retinacular release extending through the synovial membrane and into the lower fibers of the vastus lateralis is performed prior to medial advancement. The lateral superior geniculate artery is usually cut at the time of the lateral release, so it is important to identify this vessel and cauterize

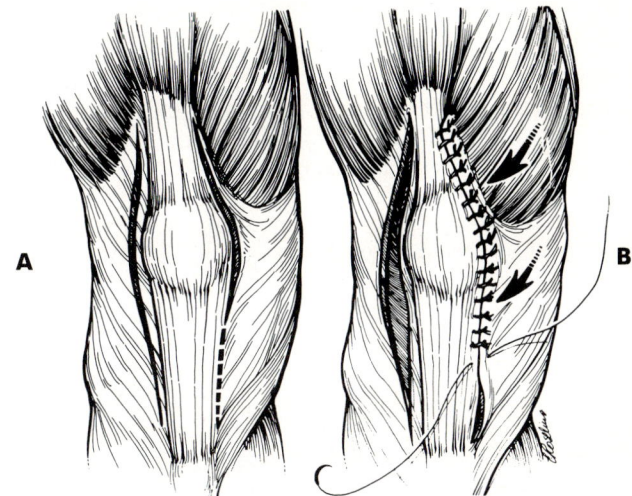

Figure 1 *A,* The medial parapatellar arthrotomy extends from the quadriceps tendon to the tibial tubercle and the lateral retinacular release includes the lower fibers of the vastus lateralis. *B,* The medial flap including the vastus medialis obliquus is advanced laterally and distally. From Scuderi GR: Extensor mechanism injuries: Treatment in ligament and extensor mechanism injuries of the knee. Scott WN, ed. St. Louis: Mosby-Year Book, 1991; with permission.)

Table 1 Surgical Results

Clinical Grade	Characteristics
Excellent	No pain and full participation in all sports
Good	Mild pain and participation in all sports
Fair	Moderate pain, mild limitation of function, and partial improvement compared with the preoperative condition
Poor	Moderate or severe pain, instability, limited function, and no improvement compared with the preoperative condition

it in order to avoid hemarthrosis. Medial capsular tightening and advancement of the vastus medialis is accomplished by overlapping the medial flap on the quadriceps tendon and patella by approximately 1 cm. This closure is held with several provisional sutures and should move the insertion of the vastus medialis to a more lateral and distal position (Fig. 1, *B*). At this point, the pneumatic tourniquet is released so that there is no pressure on the quadriceps muscle during the intraoperative assessment of patellar position. The patella is determined to be centralized if it tracks entirely within the intercondylar sulcus with no medial or lateral tilt through a full arc of motion. Care should be taken not to overtighten the medial capsule or rotate the patella at the time of closure. Following this evaluation, the arthrotomy is closed with multiple horizontal mattress stitches utilizing No. 0 absorbable sutures. Distally along the patellar tendon, there is little advancement and the closure tends to be side-to-side. The subcutaneous tissue and skin incision are closed in a routine fashion and a soft bulky dressing is applied.

Postoperative Care

Postoperatively, continuous passive motion and cryotherapy are begun with the patient allowed full weightbearing with crutches as soon as pain permits. A structured rehabilitation program is initiated and when the patient can actively flex to 120 degrees and perform straight leg-raising exercises, progressive resistance exercises are begun. The patient is allowed to resume recreational activities when the quadriceps strength as tested by a Cybex dynamometer is 90% of the contralateral side.

RESULTS

A previous review of 52 patients (60 knees) with a diagnosis of either patellar subluxation or dislocation who underwent a proximal realignment and lateral release was conducted. There were 25 females and 29 males with an average age of 22 years (range, 11 to 37 years). The average duration of radiographic and clinical follow-up was 3.5 years (range, 2 to 9 years). These patients were divided into two groups. Group 1 included 21 patients (26 knees) who had recurrent patellar dislocations. Group 2 included 31 patients (34 knees) who were diagnosed as recurrent patellar subluxation.

Intraoperatively, the severity of chondromalacia of the patella was graded according to the classification of Outerbridge. The operative procedure was similar for all patients and no other operative procedure including shaving of the articular cartilage was performed on the patella.

At final follow-up patients were graded on a clinical scale as seen in Table 1. Eighteen (30%) of the 60 knees were graded as excellent; 31 (51.7%) as good; 6 (10%) as fair; and 5 (8.3%) as poor. The degree of chondromalacia present at the index operation was not a prognostic factor since 81.6% of the knees had a good or excellent result, regardless of the extent of chondromalacia patella. The presence of grade IV changes did not

PATELLA SCORE POST-OP

Last Name ______ First Name ______ Med. Rec. No. ______

Date of Surgery ______ Date of Exam ______

Side ○ Left ○ Right ○ both Sex ○ Male ○ Female

	None									Severe
Pain at Rest	○ 10	○ 9	○ 8	○ 7	○ 6	○ 5	○ 4	○ 3	○ 2	○ 1
Walking	○ 10	○ 9	○ 8	○ 7	○ 6	○ 5	○ 4	○ 3	○ 2	○ 1
Stairs	○ 10	○ 9	○ 8	○ 7	○ 6	○ 5	○ 4	○ 3	○ 2	○ 1

	None									Constant
Giving Way	○ 10	○ 9	○ 8	○ 7	○ 6	○ 5	○ 4	○ 3	○ 2	○ 1
Limp	○ 10	○ 9	○ 8	○ 7	○ 6	○ 5	○ 4	○ 3	○ 2	○ 1
Swelling	○ 10	○ 9	○ 8	○ 7	○ 6	○ 5	○ 4	○ 3	○ 2	○ 1

	No Difficulty									Unable
Running	○ 10	○ 9	○ 8	○ 7	○ 6	○ 5	○ 4	○ 3	○ 2	○ 1
Jumping	○ 10	○ 9	○ 8	○ 7	○ 6	○ 5	○ 4	○ 3	○ 2	○ 1
Squatting	○ 10	○ 9	○ 8	○ 7	○ 6	○ 5	○ 4	○ 3	○ 2	○ 1
Sitting	○ 10	○ 9	○ 8	○ 7	○ 6	○ 5	○ 4	○ 3	○ 2	○ 1

Would you have surg. again? ○ yes ○ no

Are you satisfied with results of operation? ○ yes ○ no

Has knee ever dislocated following surg? ○ yes ○ no

Figure 2 Patellar Visual Analog Score (PVAS) and outcome evaluation.

result in clinical failure, however, a poor outcome was always associated with progression to patellofemoral arthritis.

With our early experience there was an equal number of male and female patients, and we noted that gender was a significant prognostic factor, regardless of diagnosis. The female patients did not do as well and we speculate that factors such as a broader pelvis, increased femoral anteversion, and genu valgum result in residual forces that continue to direct the patella laterally. Age at the time of the index procedure also influenced the clinical result. All patients in the second decade of life at the time of surgery had an excellent or good result, while no one in the fourth decade or older had better than a good result.

Objectively the clinical results correlated with improvement of the congruence angle as radiographically measured on the Merchant view. Patients who were graded good or excellent tended to have a greater improvement in their postoperative congruence angle. This observation was noted in both group 1 and group 2 and implies that centralization of the patella in the femoral sulcus influences the final outcome.

There was no instance of medial dislocation in our series and the lateral redislocation rate was 1.2%. This is superior to the redislocation rate, ranging from 5% to 25% in other studies.

Recently, 10 patients from our original cohort were re-evaluated and rated according to a visual analog patellar scoring system, as well as the Tegner and Lysolm activity score. The patellar visual analog score (PVAS) is a subjective evaluation and has a maximum score of 100 (Fig. 2). Scores of 85 to 100 are rated as excellent, 70 to 84 as good, 55 to 69 as fair, and those less than 54 as poor. The Tegner and Lysolm activity score is graded from 0 to 10 and includes activities of daily living, recreational and professional sports.

This group of 10 patients included one bilateral case for a total of 11 knees. There were eight females and two males, with an average length of follow-up of 13.8 years (range, 10 to 15 years). At the latest follow-up, the PVAS revealed 73% excellent or good results, 18% fair, and 9% poor. The average postoperative activity score was 5.2. This distribution of satisfactory results is only slightly less than our original report and was not influenced by the original degree of chondromalacia. In the original report the rate of redislocation was 1.2%. This later review revealed no further increase in this incidence of redislocation.

In our outcome study the results were evaluated according to the patient's expectations. All patients indicated they would have the surgery again, yet one patient was not satisfied with the results of surgery. Surprisingly, this patient's original diagnosis was recurrent subluxation and she had no chondromalacia at the time of the index procedure at the age of 14. Now, 14 years postsurgery, she has a PVAS of 63 and an activity score of 3. She did indicate, however, that she would have the same procedure again.

Radiographically, this group also demonstrated that the congruence angle, as measured on the Merchant view, maintained its corrected position in follow-up as long as 15 years. There was no evidence of degenerative changes in the medial patellofemoral joint or medial subluxation.

SUGGESTED READING

Aglietti P, Insall JN, Cerulli G. Patellar pain and incongruence: I. Measurements of incongruence. Clin Orthop 1983; 176:217–224.

Hughston JC. Subluxation of the patella. J Bone Joint Surg 1968; 50:1003–1028.

Insall JN, Aglietti P, Tria AJ. Patellar pain and incongruence: II. Clinical application. Clin Orthop 1983; 176:225–232.

Insall JN, Bullough PG, Burstein AH. Proximal "tube" realignment of chondromalacia patellae. Clin Orthop 1979; 144:63–69.

Madigan R, Wissinger HA, Donaldson WF. Preliminary experience with a method of quadricepsplasty in recurrent subluxation of the patella. J Bone Joint Surg 1975; 57A:600–607.

Scuderi GR. Surgical treatment for patellar instability. Orthop Clin North Am 1992; 23(4):619–630.

Scuderi G, Cuomo F, Scott WN. Lateral release and proximal realignment for patellar subluxation and dislocation. J Bone Joint Surg 1988; 70A:856–861.

ANTEROMEDIALIZATION OF THE TIBIAL TUBERCLE

JOHN P. FULKERSON, M.D.
DAVID A. BUUCK, M.D.

Anterior knee pain has been a continuing source of consternation to the orthopedist, primary care physician, and physical therapist. This chapter discusses the indications and use of the anteromedialization of the tibial tubercle (AMZ) for chronic malalignment of the knee extensor mechanism and associated lateral and distal medial facet articular lesions of the patella. The indications for this procedure are quite specific and most causes of anterior knee pain, including mild malalignment, may still be treated conservatively.

A thorough history and physical, appropriate radiographic evaluation, and intensive physical therapy should distill these patients down to a select few that meet the indications for this procedure. Patient expectations need to be realistic. Return to pain-free activities of daily living (ADL) are the goal. Return to competitive sports is possible, but less likely. The surgery has been quite successful with regards to relieving pain and instability while the complication rate remains low.

AMZ is a highly effective technique for transferring the tibial tuberosity when anteriorization is desired in addition to medial shift of the patellar tendon insertion. Prompt primary bone healing can be achieved, allowing rapid rehabilitation with substantially improved patellofemoral mechanics. No bone grafting is necessary to achieve anteriorization. Realignment of the patellofemoral mechanism and relief of patellofemoral contact stresses may be achieved. This procedure was first described in 1983 and we now have over 130 cases in our series.

HISTORY

The office evaluation of the patient with anterior knee pain should include a complete review of the factors leading to the visit. One should determine if there is a specific injury leading to the pain, particularly blunt trauma or a dislocation of the patella, suggesting a frank articular lesion. If the pain has come on insidiously, one must suspect an underlying problem with extensor mechanism malalignment and resulting maldistribution of contact stresses on the patella and trochlea.

In the patient with blunt trauma and chondral injury, physical therapy may be counter productive in the immediate postinjury period. These people benefit from rest, gentle range of motion (ROM) exercise, and cryotherapy. It is inappropriate to place these patients in a program of vigorous early exercise against resistance.

In those with no history of trauma, nonsteroidal anti-inflammatory drugs (NSAIDs), icing, physical therapy, and taping techniques are the mainstays of nonoperative therapy.

Ask the patient about inability to sit for long periods, pain on climbing stairs, swelling, grating under the kneecap, history of patellar dislocation, episodes of giving way, sensation of weakness, pending litigation, Workman's Compensation, and pain at night.

The evaluation of the patient with anterior knee pain requires one to keep an open mind and to seek a more definitive diagnosis. There are many causes of anterior knee pain, including extensor mechanism malalignment, articular lesions, loose bodies, retinacular tightness, patellar and quadricep tendonitis, apophysitis, Hoffa's disease, tight iliotibial band, neuroma, scar formation from old arthroscopy portals, tumor, fracture, bursitis, bone bruise, plica, and painful osteophytes.

PHYSICAL EXAMINATION

Physical examination of the patellofemoral joint is done in a careful, systematic manner. The active and passive ROM of the knee are recorded, taking care to note any extensor lag or contractures. The soft tissues about the patella are carefully palpated for tightness and painful areas, specifically noting tenderness in the patellar and quadriceps tendons as well as the medial and lateral retinaculum. Feel for increased warmth in the affected knee. Run the back of your thumbnail over

any former arthroscopy portals to try and elicit any scar or neuroma pain (Thumbnail test). With the knee extended and muscles relaxed, use both thumbs to check the lateral retinaculum for tightness by trying to elevate the patella to neutral. Evaluate carefully for any effusion. It is rare for patients with isolated patellofemoral pain and chondromalacia of less than Outerbridge grade 2 to have a true effusion.

Place the knee through full ROM while applying moderate pressure to the patella with the palm of one hand. Note at what degrees of flexion you feel crepitus or elicit pain. This helps in determining the proximal–distal location of an articular lesion if present. If you feel the crepitus and elicit pain with the knee towards full extension, the lesion is most likely more distal. If the symptoms are elicited in more flexion, the lesion is more likely proximal.

While seated in front of the patient, have him/her slowly flex and extend the knee. Note any abrupt lateral motion of the patella as the knee moves into extension. Normally the patella moves very gently from lateral to medial as the knee is flexed and engages the trochlea at about 15 to 20 degrees of flexion. Palpate the medial and lateral facets for pain as well as the medial and lateral walls of the trochlea, which occasionally have painful osteophyes. Note any snapping bands of tissue as the patient flexes and extends the knees.

Check the patient for excessive tightness of the hamstrings and quadriceps. With the patient supine, flex the hip to 90 degrees and then try and straighten the knee. With the patient prone and your fist on their buttock, you should easily be able to get the foot to touch your fist. If they have difficulty with either of these manuevers, a stretching program may be of benefit. Measure the quadriceps circumference and compare both sides. Look at the VMO and note its development.

Check the patient standing for excessive femoral anteversion, planovalgus feet, tight iliotibial band, excessive pronation when walking, and knee valgus that suggest lateralization of the extensor mechanism and/or tilting of the patella. We do not routinely record the "Q" angle, as the measurements are quite subjective and have not been helpful in our evaluation. We believe it is more helpful to describe the pattern of patella tracking.

Finally, though the presenting complaint may be anterior knee pain, the menisci and ligaments are evaluated.

RADIOGRAPHIC EVALUATION

At the initial evaluation, plain roentgenograms are obtained. Anteroposterior (AP) and lateral roentgenograms are done of the affected knee. We also get a Merchant view, a tangential view of the patellofemoral joint with the knee flexed at 45 degrees and the beam angled 30 degrees from the horizontal. This view gives us a rough idea of the tilt and/or subluxation of the patella. The mildly maltracking patella will sometimes appear to track normally at higher degrees of flexion as the contact forces increase, making this view advantageous to pick up more subtle tracking problems. Disadvantages of this view are image overlap and the inability to image the patellofemoral joint in early flexion. The surgeon is responsible for making sure this view is taken properly for reproducible results. Too often, the x-ray film is taken in too much flexion and it is hard to draw any conclusions from the view as the mildly maltracking patella normalizes with increase flexion.

If the patient has failed conservative therapy and a surgical procedure such as an arthroscopy, lateral release, or AMZ is being considered, a computed tomographic (CT) scan showing mid-patella transverse images of the patellofemoral joint may be of benefit. These are routinely taken at 0, 15, 30, and 45 degrees of knee flexion. They are also taken with and without active quadriceps tension. This allows the surgeon to measure tilt and subluxation accurately on the CT scan. This becomes extremely important in the surgical algorithm.

We are beginning to order bone scans on a small subset of patients. These include people who have suffered blunt trauma with pain that is difficult to localize, patients who have failed previous surgery, and patients with suspected reflex sympathetic dystrophy. Bone scans help in localizing areas of irritation on the patella and trochlea that are not seen on plain roentgenograms.

NONOPERATIVE MANAGEMENT

In the patient diagnosed with tilt or subluxation of the patella, the mainstays of therapy are NSAIDs, physical therapy consisting of stretching and strengthening the quadriceps and hamstrings, patellar mobilization techniques, and McConnell taping techniques. We limit the use of modalities to icing the knee frequently, especially after therapy for periods of 15 minutes. We have not found other modalities such as ultrasound, electrical stimulation, or friction massage to be of much benefit for this subset of patients.

SURGICAL INDICATIONS

While conservative management remains the cornerstone of treatment for patients with anterior knee pain, some patients are still unable to do ADLs pain free. The indications for an AMZ are specific and are described using the classification described by Fulkerson and Schutzer (Tables 1 and 2).

Type I. Patients with subluxation only and no tilt of the patella on CT or roentgenogram are good candidates for the AMZ. These patients need to have the entire extensor mechanism realigned. If the patient has subluxation only and his/her articular cartilage is normal or just softened, a flatter osteotomy is desired. This allows for more medialization of the tubercle. If the patient has more significant articular lesions or milder subluxation,

Table 1 Fulkerson-Schutzer Classification of Patients with Patellofemoral Pain

Type I	A)	Patellar subluxation, with no articular lesion
	B)	Patellar subluxation with grade 1–2 chondromalacia
	C)	Patellar subluxation with grade 3–4 arthrosis
	D)	Patellar subluxation with a history of dislocation and minimal or no chondromalacia
	E)	Patellar subluxation with a history of dislocation, with grade 3–4 arthrosis
Type II	A)	Patellar tilt and subluxation with no articular lesion
	B)	Patellar tilt and subluxation with grade 1–2 chondromalacia
	C)	Patellar tilt and subluxation with grade 3–4 arthrosis
Type III	A)	Patellar tilt with no articular lesion
	B)	Patellar tilt with grade 1–2 chondromalacia
	C)	Patellar tilt with grade 3–4 arthrosis
Type IV	A)	No malalignment and no articular lesion
	B)	No malalignment and grade 1–2 chondromalacia
	C)	No malalignment and grade 3–4 arthrosis

From Fulkerson JP, Hungerford D. Disorders of the patellofemoral joint. Baltimore: Williams & Wilkins, 1990; with permission.

Table 2 Treatment Recommendations (Failed Conservative Treatment and Intolerable Patellofemoral Pain or Instability *Not* Complicated by Reflex Sympathetic Dystrophy)

Type I	A and B)	Lateral retinacular release (VMO advancement if necessary), if mild, AMZ otherwise
	C)	Lateral retinacular release and AMZ
	D)	Acute dislocation—selective arthroscopy and reconstruction of osteochondral damage; consider lateral retinacular release; delay reconstruction. Recurrent dislocation—lateral retinacular release (VMO advancement or realignment if necessary)
	E)	Lateral retinacular release and AMZ
Type II	A and B)	Lateral retinacular release (VMO advancement if necessary) if mild, AMZ otherwise
	C)	Lateral retinacular release, careful debridement, and AMZ
Type III	A and B)	Lateral retinacular release
	C)	Lateral retinacular release, careful debridement, and AMZ
Type IV	A)	Continue nonoperative treatment; look for another pain source
	B)	Consider arthroscopic debridement in selected patients Arthroscopic debridement and possible tibial tubercle anteriorization—15 to 20 mm in severe cases, using AMZ with offset bone graft

a steeper cut will give you more anteriorization, giving less contact forces and changing the location of the stresses to a more proximal position. It also prevents you from doing much medialization. All AMZs require a complete lateral release so that there are no structures keeping the patella from being transferred to its new position. Vastus medialis obliquus (VMO) advancement is used uncommonly.

Type II. Patients with subluxation and tilt of the patella are treated with an AMZ along with a lateral release. As above, the steepness of the cut is decided by evaluating the severity of the subluxation, which determines how much medialization you want. The articular surface is also visualized by arthroscopy and direct vision to determine how much you need to anteriorize the patella to change the contact forces. These patients will have inconsistent results with lateral release alone as nothing has been done about subluxation.

Type III. Patients with pure tilt are usually treated with an isolated lateral release if articular cartilage is 0 to 2 in the Outerbridge classification. Patients with articular lesions that are more severe did not have as reproducible a result and are best treated with a lateral release and a steep AMZ to significantly anteriorize the patella and correct the tilt. There is no need to medialize these patients because subluxation is not the problem.

On rare occasions, we have had to go back and perform a steep AMZ on patients who had isolated tilt and normal or grade 1 cartilage that did not improve after a lateral release.

Type IV. Patients with no malalignment of the patella and more advanced degrees of articular degeneration are occasionally candidates for an AMZ. Lesions occurring from blunt trauma may fall in this category. People with lesions on the lateral facet or distal-medial facet will tend to do better than those with proximal-medial lesions. These patients require a steep AMZ along with the lateral release to alter the contact forces. An offset bone graft may be necessary to give proper patella tracking. In addition, the articular cartilage is debrided to remove any loose fragments that may continue to cause irritation. Do not take any more than is necessary and do not bevel.

We have never done an AMZ for the purpose of placing the tubercle more proximal to correct a patella baja and do not advocate this. If the subluxation is felt to be due in part to a patella alta, the osteotomy should be shorter rather than longer. With a shorter length of bone in the osteotomy, you have more distal transfer of the extensor mechanism when you rotate the pedicle.

Absolute contraindications to this surgery are skeletally immature patients, active infection, or evidence of reflex sympathetic dystrophy. A past history of infection that has resolved is not a contraindication, but the patient must be evaluated for any evidence of quiescent infection such as a sedimentation rate and a bone scan.

A relative contraindication to this procedure is the knee with articular lesions on the more proximal portion of the patella, especially medial. By anteriorizing the tubercle, you are shifting the forces to a more proximal location. When you medialize, you are displacing the forces more medially.

PATIENT EXPECTATIONS

Preoperative discussion with patients about their expectations of the surgery is imperative. The major goal of surgery is to achieve a stable, pain-free knee with ADLs. Return to activities such as swimming, biking, walking, and golf are reasonable expectations. Return to competitive sports such as basketball, tennis, and running is possible, but less likely. Competitive athletes who are about to undergo this procedure need to be counseled on the possibilities of not returning to their previous level of sport.

People with sedentary jobs can usually return to work within 3 to 6 weeks of surgery. People who have light duty return to work at 2 to 6 months depending on the demands of their job. Patients who work high-demand factory or construction jobs may return to work at 4 to 6 months, but this is quite variable and some are never able to return to their preinjury level of work. Each case must be evaluated individually.

Patients must be advised of the risks and complications of the surgery. They need to be aware that they will have a prominent "bump" on their knee after moving the tubercle and that kneeling may be difficult.

All patients need to be counseled that some of them will want to have their hardware removed at some point, usually at about 1 year. Because of the prominence of the tubercle, the screws are occasionally painful when a patient kneels.

SURGICAL TECHNIQUE

Under tourniquet control and using standard surgical preparation, an arthroscopy using a proximal superomedial portal as well as an anterolateral peripatellar portal is done to ensure that anteromedial transfer of the tubercle is warranted. No leg holder is used and the end of the table is left up. If there is lateral tilt and lateral patellar articular damage, a lateral release alone is done. If anteromedial tibial tubercle transfer is most appropriate, an incision is made beginning at the midpole of the patella and just lateral to the lateral facet. The incision is carried down 10 to 12 cm to a point on the anterior tibial crest. The patellar tendon is identified by sharp dissection and a complete lateral release is done, taking care to release the vastus lateralis obliquus tendon. The lateral release should stay within about 1 cm of the patella as this allows the tissues to separate once they are cut. Stay out of the vastus lateralis tendon itself. Any infrapatellar contracture is released because this may tether your transfer. The patella should be able to be turned 90 degrees and may be inspected by direct vision.

A Kelly clamp is now placed behind the patellar tendon to better define its edges. Incisions are made longitudinally into the periosteum parallel to the anterior crest of the tibia just medial to the crest and at the muscular origin of the anterior compartment on the lateral side, reflecting the periosteum and tibialis anterior muscle belly to expose the entire lateral tibia for 10 to 12 cm. The periosteum is elevated and Cobb elevators are placed carefully behind the posterolateral cortex of the tibia to protect the neurovascular structures.

A Hoffman drill guide is used to direct two ⁹⁄₆₄-inch drill bits (extra long) at an oblique angle, allowing a cut very close to the anterior tibial crest medially. The bits are placed from anteromedial to posterolateral. The first two bits are placed at opposite ends of the guide, taking great care to keep these parallel and fixing the guide in place throughout the osteotomy. The most proximal bit is drilled first. It is started just medial and proximal to the insertion of the patellar tendon on the tibia. The most proximal drill bit penetrates the lateral tibial cortex at or anterior to the posterolateral corner of the tibia, depending on how steep you want your osteotomy. We do not advocate having the drill bit exiting out behind the posterolateral cortex as the neurovascular structures (anterior tibial artery and deep peroneal nerve) are at risk. With the proximal bit in place, the guide is angled distally and anterior until the distal bit engages the most anterior portion of the crest. *By having your distal bit as anterior as possible, your distal pedicle hinge is small and makes moving the osteotomy easier when the time comes.* Take some time sliding the guide up and down on the two bits prior to drilling your distal bit. When the guide slides easily, you are assured that your bits are parallel. Make sure that your bit does not walk when you drill. Keeping the guide close to the tibia will help prevent this from occurring.

The guide is now firmly in place, anchored by the two bits at opposite ends. These are approximately 8 cm apart. Load another bit in the drill of the same size. Your guide should move smoothly up and down the bits. Take the guide off and make sure you are parallel. If not, redrill one or both of your holes. With your first two bits and guide in place, drill the remaining holes in the guide using the same bit, creating a parallel line of holes that are bicortical (Fig. 1). Move the Cobb elevators down the posterolateral cortex, taking care to protect the soft tissues. Prior to drilling each hole, move the guide smoothly up and down your first two bits and the bit you

are about to drill to ensure you are parallel. Make sure your bit does not walk as you drill. After all of your holes are drilled, remove the guide. Remember, this procedure gives the surgeon great variability in angle of the osteotomy (Fig. 2). A steeper cut requires that the guide be started more anterior on the medial side, while a flatter cut allows you to place the guide a little more posterior. The bits will exit more posterior on the lateral side with a steep cut than with a flatter cut, which will come out more anterior.

The osteotomy may be completed with osteotomes or an oscillating saw. We prefer an osteotome because this gives us better control. The osteotomy consists of three distinct cuts. The first one is accomplished with a 2 inch osteotome beginning on the lateral side. The osteotome is held at a 45 degree angle from the floor, aiming down at the tibia (Fig. 3). It is directed at an angle

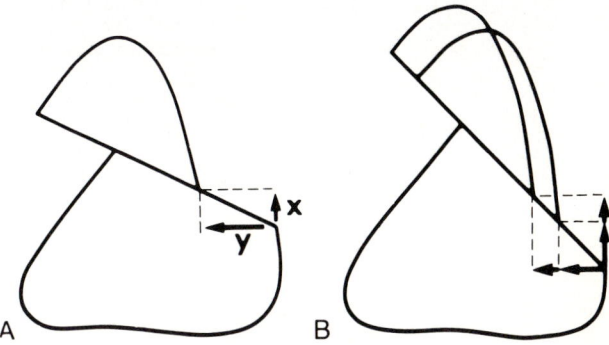

Figure 2 The osteotomy may be varied from a relatively flat cut (*A*) to a steeper cut (*B*). Although (*A*) will give you less anteriorization, you will get more medialization. (From Fulkerson JP, Hungerford D: Disorders of the patellofemoral joint. Baltimore: Williams & Wilkins, 1990; with permission.)

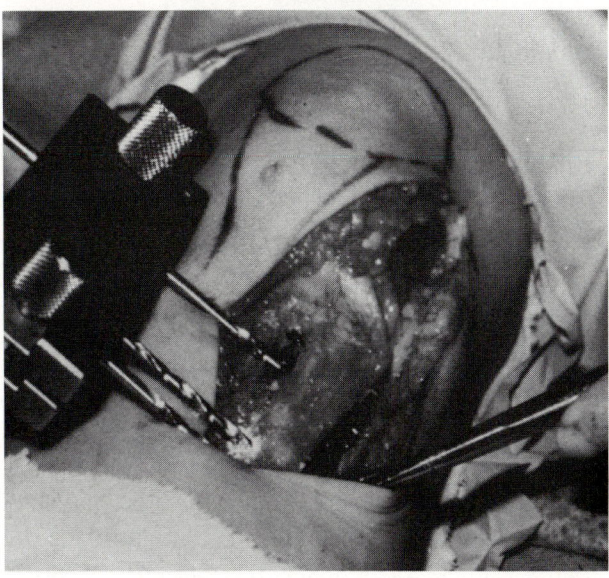

Figure 1 Parallel placement of your drill bits is imperative for a satisfactory osteotomy. (From Fulkerson JP, Hungerford D. Disorders of the patellofemoral joint. Baltimore: Williams & Wilkins, 1990; with permission.)

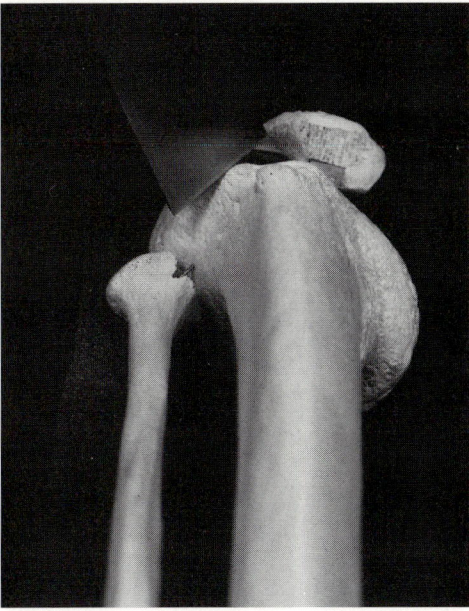

Figure 3 Placement of the osteotome for the proximal-lateral cut, looking distal–proximal.

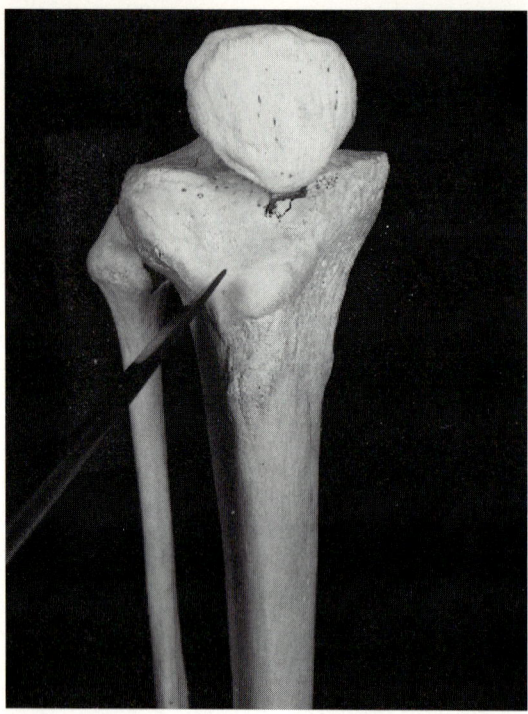

Figure 4 Angle of osteotome for proximal-lateral cut, looking anterior-posterior.

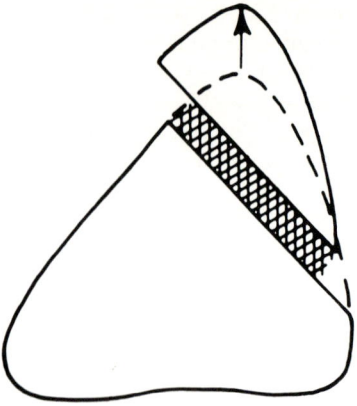

Figure 5 Adding local bone graft from proximal tibia increases ability to anteriorize. (From Fulkerson JP: Operative management of patellofemoral pain. Ann Chir Gynecol 1991; 80:224–229; with permission.)

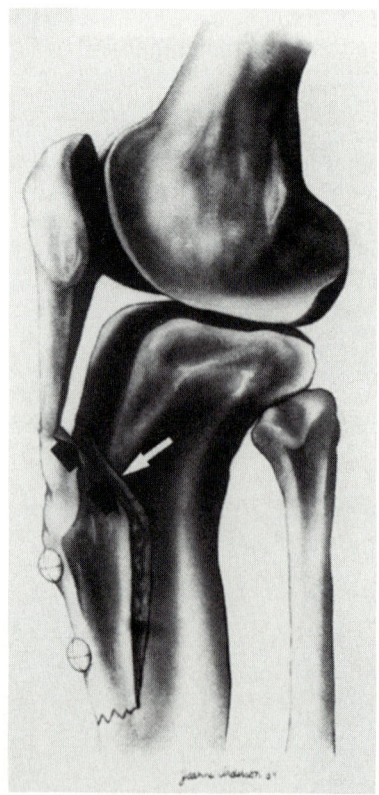

Figure 6 Screw placement in AMZ. (Adapted from Fulkerson JP: Anteromedialization of the tibial tuberosity for patellofemoral malalignment. Clin Orthop 1983; 177:176–181; with permission.)

that will connect the most proximal hole on the lateral side to an area a few millimeters proximal to the insertion of the tendon (Fig. 4). This is an oblique cut that avoids cutting into the broad metaphyseal region of the tibia. The cut is complete once the osteotome engages the most proximal hole. With a retractor holding the tendon out of the way, a one-half inch osteotome is then directed from the most proximal point of the previous cut across the tibia from lateral to medial at an angle that travels from distal–lateral to proximal–medial. This angle just needs to be off the horizontal to allow for the osteotomy to be moved. This cut ends at the medial edge of the tendon. With the 2 inch osteotome, the final cut is made. This final cut connects the drill holes on the medial side. The angle of the osteotome is matched to the angle of your two parallel bits. The holes are connected by the osteotome, taking great care to stay in the osteotomy plane. Once you have penetrated the lateral cortex with your osteotome, the drill bits may be removed and you can use your osteotomy plane as your guide to complete the cut.

You should be able to slide your bone pedicle anteriorly and medially now. The length of this bone pedicle is usually 5 to 8 cm long and allows good surface contact. With great care not to fracture the pedicle itself except at its most distal point, the bony fragment is carefully mobilized and displaced medially such that it will slide anteriorly and medially. If advancement of the tuberosity is desired, a segment of the distal pedicle may be removed and the remaining fragment advanced. This may be desirable if any laxity of the patellar tendon is

noted following anteromedialization or if there is patella alta.

Up to 17 mm of anteriorization may be obtained with the steepest AMZ, but occasionally more is desired or the patients' anatomy does not allow that much. It is then possible to take local bone graft, including cortex, from the proximal tibial metaphysis and place it between the tibia and bone pedicle (Fig. 5).

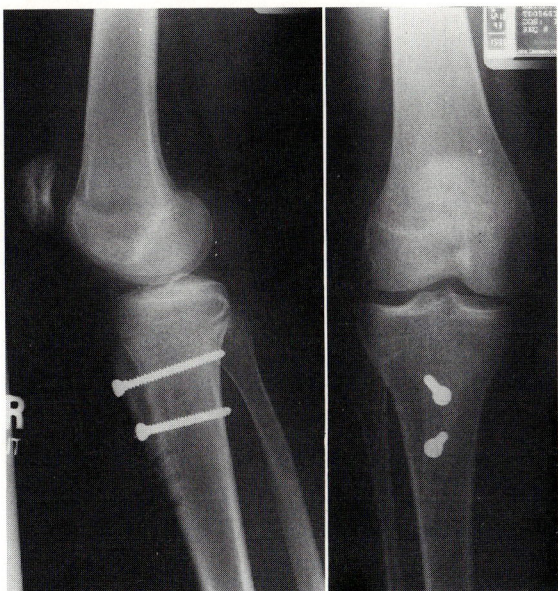

Figure 7 Postoperative x-rays of anteromedialization of the tibial tubercle.

We test the bone pedicle in several positions to determine how medial we want to place it. The pedicle is held down with pressure by the thumb and the knee is ranged. You can get a finger under the patella with your other hand as you go through a ROM and try to determine your best position. You want to medialize enough to stop the subluxation, but not so much that your patella subluxates medially. Only rarely do we add a medial imbrication to this procedure and the vast majority of patients do not need this. We feel that medial imbrication has a tendency to tip the patella posteriorly and increase the contact forces on the medial facet more than we would like. In the rare instance a medial imbrication is done, the VMO is advanced just to take up the slack, but not overtightened.

Once the best position is determined, a drill hole is made through the pedicle and into the cortex of the tibia distal to the tibial tuberosity. The anterior hole is made with a 4.5 mm drill bit. The hole is then countersunk. A guide is placed in this hole and a 3.2 mm bit is used to drill the posterior cortex. This is depth-gauged, tapped, and the 4.5 mm cortical screw is hand tightened until snug. Do not overtighten because you may fracture the bone pedicle or cause the osteotomy to slide posterior. A second screw is placed about 2 cm distal to the first one and at a slightly divergent angle (Fig. 6).

At this point, the tourniquet is released and hemostasis obtained. Care is taken to inspect the edges of the cut synovium and the fat pad; both have been problem areas for bleeding. The anterior compartment fascia is not closed. The wound is closed loosely in layers. Skin closure has not been a problem in over 130 cases to date. Sterile dressings are applied, and the knee is placed in an immobilizer. Bleeding has not been a problem because compression of most of the exposed bone is achieved, but Hemovac drainage and Cryocuff are advisable. Bone wax is not used as we do not want to introduce a foreign body into the operative field. If the patient is discharged on the same day, the hemovac is removed in the recovery room prior to discharge. An x-ray is taken in the recovery room to check for screw placement (Fig. 7).

REHABILITATION

Patients are discharged on crutches, partial weight bearing. They are instructed to take the brace off several times a day beginning Day 1 postoperatively to work on getting their ROM back. They are also instructed in straight leg raises and quad sets to get their strength back.

Sutures or staples are removed at 1 to 2 weeks. Their weight-bearing status is kept at toe touch until 6 weeks. The immobilizer comes off at 4 to 6 weeks, but crutches are used for protection up to 6 to 8 weeks postoperatively. A roentgenogram may be taken at 6 weeks, 3 months, 6 months, and 1 year to follow the healing. Because of the secure primary bone healing with compression across the osteotomy, prompt healing and early rehabilitation have been possible in most patients.

Formal physical therapy is instituted at 1 to 2 weeks if the patient is having difficulty getting the motion back, or if the patient is unable to perform the exercises as prescribed.

COMPLICATIONS

This surgical procedure is very forgiving. There have been very few significant complications over the years. Intraoperatively, care must be taken to preserve the neurovascular structures posteriorly. Hemostasis must be achieved. A long, tapered osteotomy gives more surface area for healing and reduces the chances for non-unions.

In our series of over 130 patients, there have been no skin sloughs and no compartment syndromes. There have been two tibial shaft fractures that occurred about 6 weeks postoperatively when the patient twisted his leg while arising from a chair. This was treated in a cast and healed uneventfully. There have been few deep vein thromboses, but these are rare since the protocol to get the knee moving right away was implemented. There have been two non-unions that healed with bone grafting.

RESULTS

The results have been quite gratifying over the past 10 years since this procedure was introduced. This procedure has an advantage over the Maquet and Elmslie-Trillat in that the surgeon has many options for the angle at which he chooses to make his osteotomy.

The senior author (JPF) has previously published the results of his first 30 AMZ patients with at least

2-year follow-up. Twelve of these patients had at least 5-year follow-up; 93% had good to excellent results reported subjectively and 89% had good to excellent results objectively. The results do not seem to deteriorate with time. Good results have been reported in 75% of patients with advanced articular lesions, although none reported an excellent outcome.

SUGGESTED READING

Fulkerson JP. Awareness of the retinaculum in evaluating patellofemoral pain. Am J Sports Med 1982; 10:147–149.

Fulkerson JP. Anteromedialization of the tibial tuberosity for patellofemoral malalignment. Clin Orthop 1983; 177:176–181.

Fulkerson JP, Becker GJ, Meaney JA, et al. Anteromedial tibial tubercle transfer without bone graft. Am J Sports Med 1990; 18:490–497.

Hauser EDW. Total tendon transplant for slipping patella. Surg Gynecol Obstet 1938; 66:199–214.

Maquet P. Advancement of the tibial tuberosity. Clin Orthop 1976; 115:225–230.

Merchant AC, Mercer RL, Jacobsen RH, Cool CR. Roentgenographic analysis of patellofemoral congruence. J Bone Joint Surg 1974; 56A:1391–1396.

McConnell J. The management of chondromalacia patellae: a long-term solution. Austral J Physiother 1986; 32:215–223.

Outerbridge RE. The etiology of chondromalacia patellae. J Bone Joint Surg 1961; 43B:752–757.

Post WR, Fulkerson JP. Distal realignment of the patellofemoral joint. Orthop Clin North Am 1992; 23:631–643.

Schutzer S, Ramsby G, Fulkerson J. Computed tomographic classification of patellofemoral pain patients. Orthop Clin North Am 1986; 17:735.

Schutzer SF, Ramsby GR, Fulkerson JP. The evaluation of patellofemoral pain using computerized tomography. A preliminary study. Clin Orthop 1986; 204:286–293.

Trillat A, DeJour H, Couette A. Diagnostic et traitement des subluxations recidiventes de la rotule. Rev Chir Orthop 1964; 50:813–824.

PREPATELLAR BURSITIS

JOHN ALBRIGHT, M.D.
DAN FOSTER, M.A., ATC

As the term for a "wine sac" in the Greek language, the word *bursa* provides both an excellent description of the gross structural form of this anatomic entity and a hint about its usual functional role as a fluid-filled cushion. First described by Alexander Monro in 1788, there are actually over 150 bursae throughout the body. They are located in places at which friction would otherwise develop between tissue layers. From the clinical perspective, some bursae are quite superficial and others are sufficiently deep that they are identifiable only when they are symptomatic. The *praepatellaris subcutanea* (prepatellar bursa) is an easily palpable and very vulnerable structure located between the hard surface of the patella and the skin. Usually only 1 to 2 cm in diameter, the prepatellar bursa of the knee is distinctive in the way it facilitates the excessive freedom of movement enjoyed by the skin over the bone surface. In their normal state, bursae are small sacs whose thin walls are lined with synovial cells, as well as many large and delicate blood vessels and filled with a few milliliters of viscous fluid that is sufficient to merely moisten the synovial surfaces and allow a friction free gliding of one structure over the other. In the pathologic state, prepatellar bursae often expand to the point that they obscure the entire anterior aspect of the knee.

CLASSIFICATION OF PATHOLOGIC STATES BY ETIOLOGY

There are three basic causes of inflammation of bursae: mechanical irritation, infection, and crystal deposition. By far, the most common in an athlete is a history of mechanically induced trauma imparted directly to the prepatellar surface. This presentation of symptoms will vary according to the severity and repetitiveness of the trauma and the history of previous bursitis episodes.

Acute Mechanical Bursitis

Most patients with mechanically induced prepatellar bursitis can remember the day, if not the time and place, of the initial traumatic episode that produced an unusually dramatic and painful swelling. The index episode is usually initiated with one or several repeated sharp blows directly to the anterior surface of the patella. In sports, the speculation that the hardness of the playing surface may be a primary factor is partially supported by the higher incidence of this type of pathology in football practices and games played on artificial turf rather than natural grass. Those sports that put an athlete at greatest risk of prepatellar bursitis appear to be wrestling and football. It is also obvious that those two sports present more inherent risk of a direct blow of the anterior aspect of the knee with the playing surface than others.

Chronic Mechanical Bursitis

Chronic bursitis can develop in individuals who have a recurrence of significant acute episodes. It can also develop in a much less dramatic, more insidious form in those individuals exposed to the cumulative effects of repeated minor trauma. The swelling and tenderness of chronic bursitis is much more difficult to resolve and often recurs with minimal trauma.

Septic Bursitis

Staphylococcus aureus is the cause of septic prepatellar bursitis in more than 95% of the reported cases, with beta-hemolytic *Streptococcus pneumoniae* and *Staphylococcus epidermidis* as the two next most common organisms. We have also cultured *Streptococcus bovis* (a nonenterococcal Group D streptococcus). Others have reported *Haemophilus influenzae* and *Pseudomonas* species in the general population. There are also rare reported cases of anaerobic streptococci as well as fungi and mycobacteria. The occurrence of the anaerobic group of organisms makes the obtaining of cultures in an anaerobic environment worthwhile.

Septic bursitis can develop with or without an antecedent history of traumatic bursitis. However, it is suggested by many authors that the fibrosis and decreased ability to clear foreign matter associated with chronic bursitis not only predisposes the development of septic bursitis but also makes nonoperative management much less effective. In the general public, most patients with septic bursitis do have a history of recent or frequent trauma to the bursa. Watkins reported that coal miners who knelt for long hours each day so commonly developed chronic and often septic prepatellar bursitis that they coined the term "beat knee."

In athletes also, most infections are felt to be a result of local trauma; such as the infection of an abrasion, or as a result of a direct penetration of the skin by a foreign body. Minor mat and turf abrasions are extremely common and, in those cases where superficial wounds are not found, they may have healed prior to the infection becoming clinically evident. The incubation time from initial seeding to full blown infection is often nearly a week. The fact that *Staphylococcus aureus* is the principal infector and also is a common inhabitant of skin supports the concept of a local infection rather than hematogenous spread.

Crystal Induced Bursitis

Crystal induced bursitis is by far the least common type of bursitis in the athletic population. The diagnosis is made by looking for crystals under the polarizing light microscope. Crystals from gout and rheumatoid arthritis have both been reported in bursae but are not likely in an athlete. However, when infection is persistent, keep in mind that crystal induced bursitis can coexist with infection.

DIAGNOSIS

Clinical Presentation

Given its superficial location, the diagnosis of prepatellar bursitis should be relatively simple to make.

Since bursae only are of clinical importance when they are inflamed, the diagnosis hinges on the detection of one or all of the cardinal signs of inflammation (e.g., rubor, calor, dolor, and tumor). The most important feature for making the diagnosis is the anatomic location of the swelling. In prepatellar bursitis, the swelling appears in the subcutaneous tissue, on the anterior aspect of the knee. In its milder forms, the edges of the inflamed bursa may be localized to the patellar borders. However, often the swelling can spread over the entire anterior, medial, and lateral aspects of the joint to give the appearance of joint effusion. Because this tissue plane has no natural barriers, in its most dramatic presentations the swelling may be expanded to below the tibial tubercle and half the way up the thigh. In any instance, the posterior aspect of the knee is not usually swollen, full extension is comfortable while flexion beyond 50 to 60 degrees produces pain anteriorly, and the patient recognizes that the swelling is not located inside the knee joint. Patellar ballottement is not present.

Acute Mechanical Bursitis

Usually the clinical picture develops over the course of several hours so that, with those practices and competitions held in the evenings, the athlete may even awaken the next morning with symptoms. Swelling, warmth, redness, and pain and tenderness, are essential for making the diagnosis of acute bursitis. As noted above, the extent of the swelling varies greatly but has been seen to cover three sides of the knee from just below the tibial tubercle to the mid-thigh region. Usually, the primary complaint of the patient is pain, which is associated with the expansion of the hematoma as it dissects along the subcutaneous tissue planes. These symptoms usually have reached a maximum within 12 to 24 hours after onset and will diminish progressively thereafter. However, left untreated, the uncomplicated blood filled bursa will remain enlarged for several weeks to several months. Often, in the more dramatic presentations of an initial episode of acute aseptic bursitis, clotting blood can be aspirated from the bursa. The use of a large bore needle should be considered particularly for use in the aspiration when clotted blood is likely to be present. If it is an acute recurrent bursitis, it is very likely that the fluid will be yellow and free of any gross blood.

Chronic Mechanical Bursitis

The diagnosis of chronic prepatellar bursitis includes a spectrum of clinical presentations that are most easily sorted out by obtaining a detailed history from the patient. The most common situation is the knee that is subjected to repeated trauma on a long term basis (e.g., an entire competitive season) without ever having sufficient time between traumatic episodes to recover from the inflammatory process. At the other extreme are those patients who have had one or two significant, previous acute episodes but develop recurrences more readily in the same knee with little provocation despite achieving a seemingly adequate period of quiescence between acute episodes.

In our experience, the high recurrence risk patients can be picked out by follow-up examination for residuals in patients recovered from acute prepatellar bursitis. It is not uncommon that a residual area of mild induration and local tenderness may remain for weeks or months. These patients remain at risk for recurrence of the acute process. Even after the tenderness is gone, in a significant group of patients, the prepatellar area is often left with a peculiar palpable ring of subcutaneous tissue that outlines the margins of the residual scar tissue. Depending on the magnitude of the acute process and the number of preceding incidents there have been, the amount of scar tissue can be barely palpable or grossly obvious. This scar tissue usually presents as a visible and palpable rim of tissue that encircles the patella but may be quite wide of it. Within the margins of this ring may be small somewhat mobile, nodular masses that resemble loose bodies. Instead, they are usually fibrotic bands bridging from one wall to another under no tension. In the extreme cases, small pockets or large masses of fluid may even remain within the fibrotic area even though there are no other signs of inflammation. It appears that the more dramatic the clinical findings in these "asymptomatic" patients, the greater the chances of the recurrence of either an aseptic or a septic episode.

Septic Bursitis

The symptoms of septic bursitis are often less severe than infections in other parts of the body. The presence of sepsis can be overlooked and treatment delayed several hours or longer because the symptoms are not initially that impressive. In our experience, proper treatment has been delayed in several cases even though we are keenly aware of the possibility. While obtaining an aspirate of the bursal fluid is a necessity, the Gram stains are usually negative and the cultures may take 48 to 72 hours to become positive, if they ever do.

The main distinguishing clinical feature is the downhill course of the clinical picture with time. In mechanical bursitis, the symptoms are at a maximum within 12 to 24 hours after the index trauma, with a plateau or even improvement seen thereafter. When infection is developing, the symptoms gradually, but steadily increase with time. According to North et al the average time from the onset of the first signs and symptoms and the diagnosis is 2 days in acute cases and as many as 12 days when there is a subacute development. Eventually, most all patients with septic bursitis develop swelling, pain, and tenderness. As many as two thirds have chills and fever as their presenting symptoms. By this point in the development, the involved area is very warm and erythematous. The area of erythema may also spread well beyond the margins of the bursal swelling. Regional inguinal lymph nodes are often also swollen and tender.

Crystal-Induced Bursitis

In order to rule out crystal induced inflammation, a polarized light microscopic examination should be requested for all aspirated fluids. However, in athletes, crystal analysis is only cost efficient if the patient has a history of gout or rheumatoid arthritis. Monosodium urate crystals will be noted in gouty bursitis and cholesterol crystals will be seen in rheumatoid arthritis.

Examination of Bursal Fluid

All inflamed prepatellar bursae should be aspirated in order to establish the precise diagnosis as well as to relieve the patients' acute discomfort. Sterile technique should be strictly adhered to. The area to be aspirated should be the most fluctuant. This spot is usually located in the original prepatellar confines of the bursa in its normal state. If, however, there are any areas of abrasion or laceration, an aspiration site should be chosen that keeps as far away from the lesion as possible. The target area should be cleansed thoroughly at least three times with povidone-iodine soap or an equivalent prep solution. After sterile draping, a 25 gauge needle is used to numb the skin with a subcuticular wheal of a local anesthetic. An 18 gauge needle is then used to aspirate the fluid. If nothing is aspirated through this size needle because of viscous fluid, fibrinous clot, or tissue fragments, then a 16 or even a 14 gauge needle should be used.

The most important place to send any fluid aspirated is to the bacteriology lab for Gram staining and cultures with sensitivity testing. If there is sufficient fluid, then also obtain a white cell count (WBC) and differential count. While there is some debate about the necessity of obtaining glucose levels from the aspirate, it is our opinion that, if there is sufficient fluid, this is one test that should be done if possible. We have experienced situations where the Gram stain smear and the cultures proved to be negative and the WBC count was not characteristically high until 24 hours later but the glucose in the initial bursal aspirate was 50% of that in the venous blood sample. This meant that antibiotic therapy was started much earlier because of this test result alone. Therefore, we conclude that, while the glucose value is not always low in septic cases, there is sufficient evidence to support it as a valuable adjunct to assist in making the diagnosis in the difficult cases. To date, lactic acid tests of the bursal fluid appear to be of little value in differentiating traumatic arthritis and bursitis.

DIFFERENTIAL DIAGNOSIS

Knee Joint Effusion

As noted above, the more dramatic cases of prepatellar bursitis can indeed look similar to knee effusions and if the inciting blow to the knee was sufficient, there may even be a concomitant intra-articular swelling. However, careful examination and inquiry should be sufficient to establish the extra-articular location of the pathology. Also noted previously, in cases where there is any doubt, the patient will tell the examiner (if asked) that the joint itself is not involved. If the patient is uncertain or for some other reason there remains a doubt about the location of the swelling, a simple examination of the location of the fluid in relation to the patella may be helpful. As opposed to joint swelling, in prepatellar bursitis the patella is readily palpable beneath the skin, but lies deep to the swelling. Attempts to palpate the patella produce pitting, with an imprint of the examiners finger sustained for some time after it is withdrawn. Furthermore, once the patella is reached by palpation, it is not buoyed up away from the femur by intra-articular fluid as it would be with a joint effusion, and therefore is not ballotable.

Quadriceps Rupture

The subcutaneous swelling that is associated with a quadriceps rupture can indeed be confused with prepatellar bursitis at first glance. However, distinguishing features of an extensor mechanism disruption include: inability to actively extend the knee against resistance; joint swelling; a palpable defect in the extensor mechanism immediately proximal to the superior pole of the patella; and an easily moveable patella despite contraction of the quadriceps muscle mass.

Patellar Tendonitis

In mild and acute cases, or when the residuals of acute prepatellar bursitis are present as a small fibrous mass or ring to indurated tissue, the inferior bursal edge may lie directly over the primary site of patellar tendonitis. Palpation of the rest of the rim of scar tissues makes the differentiation obvious. Furthermore, maximum contraction of the quadriceps against resistance in the fully extended knee does not produce pain in the case of the bursitis.

Thrombophlebitis

According to North et al, adenopathy and swelling of the entire involved extremity has been seen to the point that the clinical picture can mimic thrombophlebitis. While we have never seen this situation, swelling anterior to the knee is not expected to occur in thrombophlebitis.

RATIONALE FOR TREATMENT

As mentioned above, it is often nearly impossible to distinguish the cause or temporal classification of the full-blown clinical presentation of prepatellar bursitis. They are all usually grossly swollen, dramatically painful, hot to the feel, and exquisitely tender to the touch. Aspiration of the fluid for analysis is the cornerstone of the recommended management plan.

Acute Mechanical Bursitis

Initial Episode

The expected clinical picture of an initial episode of acute mechanical bursitis is as follows. The history is compatible with a first injury. The bursal aspirate is bloody, and it clots upon standing. The expected laboratory findings include: Gram stain and cultures negative; WBCs less than 5000 to 10,000; with mostly mononuclear cells; and the bursal glucose is greater than 70% of the venous blood value. The recommended treatment for the initial episode of prepatellar bursitis is aspiration, compressive wrap, nonsteroidal anti-inflammatory agents, and immobilization for approximately 1 week. Then, if all swelling and tenderness have cleared, the athlete is allowed to return to action with a knee pad for protection. It is important to note that in some sports like wrestling and football, a negative history (where the athlete does not recall preceding symptoms) may not be totally reliable. The impression of it being an initial acute episode is enhanced if the aspirate is bloody.

Particularly in wrestlers, noncompliance is a major issue that can affect the intended result of any treatment plan. Regardless of the sport, athletes are informed that they will indeed be helped to get back into competition as soon as possible without danger of recurrence. They are made aware that the appearance of a recurrence involves the frustration of doubling their time-loss from competition. Recurrence also means that the knee can become increasingly sensitive to even minor subsequent bumps stirring up the inflammation as well as making the bursa vulnerable to infection. They are told that recurrence, with or without infection, may mean that they will need to have surgery to correct the problem.

They are informed that because a main principle behind the treatment is to get one side of the expanded bursal wall to stick down to the other; they are not to remove the immobilizer or bend their knee until they are told it is safe to do so. Until proven otherwise, all competitive athletes should be suspected of being so intent on returning to competition that they will become noncompliant as soon as the intense initial pain has subsided. As a preventive measure, they are informed that in our experience with prepatellar bursitis in UI varsity wrestling team members, being noncompliant and attempting to rush back into action too soon has repeatedly resulted in a fourfold increase in both recovery time and recurrence rate. For maximum emphasis, they are also told the story about one exceptionally uncooperative college wrestling team member who kept ignoring the advice he had been given, and wound up needing surgical excision of the bursae. However, to set the record for exceptional noncompliance, he ran 3 miles in his cylinder cast a few days after surgery. He accounted for the longest "missed practice" time on record (69 days) because he developed a large draining hematoma in the wound site, which was delayed in its resorption because of continued banging on the front of the cast.

Recurrent Episodes

For the first recurrence, the clinical presentation is expected to be the same as the initial one except that the aspirate may be straw colored fluid rather than blood. For the first recurrence, the same management plan described above (e.g., aspiration, compressive wrap, immobilization, and nonsteroidal anti-inflammatory agents) is repeated with the possible addition of a more prolonged rest and immobilization period. While this conservative approach may seem futile to the patient when it did not work the first time, we have seen more than one individual experience a permanent remission after a second and even a third and a fourth recurrence. Given that observation as a basis for discussion, when the problem arises in the middle of a competitive season, the athlete should be informed that the recovery time of a few weeks is much less if the conservative regimen works than if we must resort to surgery. In our experience under ideal circumstances, a mean of 34 days out of practice or competition should be anticipated postoperatively. Therefore, in general, it may be best to inform patients to expect that it will take at least 6 weeks before the wound will be healed enough for the patients to be able to return to their sports without fear of complications or recurrence of the symptoms. They are presented this information in the form of a challenge as a target time to beat by being diligent in following the suggestions of their physician.

It should be understood by the sports medicine physician that surgery is rarely needed in the general population for this problem. Even in athletics, when the inciting factor can be avoided, conservative treatment should be given a longer trial. Only when the nature of the individual's sport renders them vulnerable to repeated traumatic episodes should surgical excision of the bursa be considered.

Chronic Mechanical Bursitis

Chronic prepatellar bursitis is an entity that is clinically and histologically distinct from acute bursitis. If the diagnosis of chronic bursitis is accompanied by chronic pain and inflammation or frequent superimposed acute recurrences, it is recommended that surgical excision be considered.

Septic Bursitis

It is important to begin antibiotic treatment with a bactericidal antibiotic as soon as possible after the onset of an infection. Given that *S. aureus* and other Gram positive organisms are responsible for an overwhelming majority of septic bursae, dicloxacillin or some equivalent penicillinase-resistant antibiotic should be initiated on an empiric basis. Ideally, the drug of choice will be suggested by the results of the Gram stained smear and confirmed by the antibiotic sensitivity tests done on the cultures. However, once an adequate aspirate has been obtained, therapy should begin. Whether an intravenous or oral administration is preferable depends on the circumstances. Indications for admission and intravenous administration include: pre-existing thick scar tissue from chronic bursitis, recurrence of infection, the presentation of a full-blown acute initial episode with systemic symptoms, or merely the anticipation of compliance problems in questionable cases. In these instances patients should be told to anticipate that they will need 10 to 14 days of intravenous management with bed rest, elevation, and hot compresses before it is safe to use oral medications.

On the other hand, it is important to note that oral administration of the proper medication can produce adequate antibiotic levels in the infected prepatellar bursa. It has been shown by Ho and Tice that by using oxacillin (500 mg qid) in patients with symptoms less than 1 week an average of 4 to 5 days was needed to reach sterility. Patients with an onset that is greater than 1 week can expect that more than 9 days of treatment will be required. Therefore, it is safe to establish a routine of a 10 to 14 day course of oral antibiotic therapy for an uncomplicated case of septic bursitis. In this instance, the patient should be followed closely (e.g., every 3 to 4 days) until the situation is totally under control. Repeat aspirations may be indicated; however, the effectiveness of this procedure must be questioned each time it is felt to be indicated. If the fluid accumulates too rapidly or the cultures continue to be positive with elevated white cell counts, then we suggest resorting to other measures. Establishment of better drainage can be accomplished with a stab wound, breaking up any loculations with a hemostat and then irrigating with sterile normal saline. A quarter-inch plain gauze wick that is advanced slowly over 24 to 48 hours may provide a better chance for controlling the symptoms in the more resistant cases. However, in these cases, operative management with an open bursectomy should always be considered as a definitive alternative once the systemic symptoms and the advancing local symptoms are brought under control. When dealing with an athlete who is concerned with minimizing the time they are out of action, the chances of later developing a sterile bursitis as a residual of the septic episode also becomes an important consideration.

The use of intrabursal steroid injections are mentioned only for the sake of completeness as we do not have extensive first hand experience with this method. No good studies have been done to assess the effectiveness of this form of treatment. On the other end, there are many documented complications from the use of these drugs including: infection, skin atrophy, delayed diagnosis, and impaired host defense against infection.

SURGICAL TECHNIQUE

A variety of incisions can be used successfully for excision of the prepatellar bursa. Given the usual grossly enlarged size of the bursa being removed, we have found that a transverse incision centered over the proximal one-half or even the superior pole of the patella is best for two reasons. First, the spread of the margins of the pathologic tissue usually is equal in all directions. This means that the scar tissue may be expected to have spread over the medial and lateral margins of the patella up to the posterolateral and posteromedial borders of the knee joint capsule. The transverse incision allows easy extension in this direction to provide adequate exposure of these recesses if needed. The second advantage of this incision is the observation that the athlete is more likely to be able to continue kneeling comfortably afterwards. For the sake of efficiency and to best ensure that all of the tissue involved is resected, it should be a goal to dissect the bursa and its surrounding scar tissue as one single mass.

The subcutaneous dissection should be carried at the margin of the pathologic tissue around the entire circumference of the lesion. Especially in long-standing cases, the identification of the bursal border is usually difficult. In these cases, it is usually easiest to identify the bursal border medially or laterally, and this is where dissection in the correct tissue plane should begin. The surgeon should work circumferentially around the entire bursa by stripping it cleanly away from the normal tissues with a dissection scissors for the most part and with blunt finger dissection where possible. Staying in the correct tissue plane is facilitated by maintaining tension on the bursal sac with Alice clamps. If there is sufficient fluid present inside the bursa at the time of resection, it is best to leave the structure completely intact. The intact fluid filled sac provides a much appreciated line of demarcation where the borders of the mass end and the adjacent soft tissue begins. However, if the walls are perforated and the fluid is allowed to run out, the use of tension through the Alice clamps still facilitates the identification of the correct tissue plane. Distally, the pathologic mass may be stuck down directly to the tibia or the patellar tendon. Proximally, it may be stuck down to the quadriceps mechanism. When the adhesions extend to the right or left of the midline, the fascial compartment of the quadriceps muscle may be easily entered by mistake. After excision of the bursa is accomplished, achievement of hemostasis should be achieved with the tourniquet down.

POSTOPERATIVE MANAGEMENT

If there is any question of a continued postoperative trickling of blood, a drain should be used with a bulky, compressive dressing and some form of knee immobilizer. These measures are all needed to prevent hematomas. If such hematomas do develop, they will be very slow to resorb and should be aspirated and rewrapped in a compressive dressing. After the immediate postoperative period, the knee should be protected with a cast or knee immobilizer for 6 to 8 weeks. Isometric quadriceps muscle strengthening can be initiated early in this period but flexion of the knee should be put off at least 2 to 3 weeks until the acute cellular inflammatory phase of the repair process has definitely subsided. Return to action should not be allowed until the entire repair process has been completed.

PREVENTION

Knee Pads

The simplest means of preventing future episodes of prepatellar bursitis is to discontinue that activity predis-

posing the individual to it. Unfortunately, this is not practical in the dedicated athlete. Therefore, while there are no studies that prove effectiveness, it is believed that in order to maximize the athlete's safety during competition some form of protective padding is indicated. A knee sleeve that uses viscoelastic material as padding and extends from below the tibial tubercle to above the superior pole of the patella appears to offer the best protection in wrestlers. We have also custom-made a pad that appears to be effective. It is constructed as follows:

1. Cut the packing bubbles into six rectangular sheets measuring about 5 inches by 8 inches. The size of the pad can be varied depending on individual needs, but this size is appropriate for most adult males.
2. Use a scalpel blade to cut a patellar relief hole out of the center of three of the bubble sheets. The holes should be about 3 inches in diameter or the size of the patient's patella.
3. Lay the six sheets of bubbles together in a stack. Place zonas tape along the sides of the bubble sheets so that half of the tape width is on the flat surface of the top sheet and the other half is folded over the edge toward the bottom. Turn the pad over and follow the same taping procedure in order to tightly close the cut edges of the bubble sheets.
4. Prewrap the knee over the area where the bubble pad will be placed.
5. Place the bubble pad so that the hole encircles the patella and the top surface is smooth. Prewrap the bubble pad to the knee. This protects the bubble pad so that it can be reused.
6. Secure the pad to the knee using 3 inch elastic tape. To prevent slippage, attempt to secure the corners of the pad by crossing the corners at angles with the elastic tape. Tape should be applied to the skin just above the pad and below in order to prevent slippage.

Cleansing Mats

There is no question that cleansing of the mats in wrestling is an essential part of a prevention program. In order to keep the mats free of bacteria and viruses, it is recommended that the following protocol be observed:

1. Clean the mats about 2 hours before each practice so that the cleaner has about 30 minutes to dry.
2. When cleaning the mats, wear clean socks; no shoes and no bare feet.
3. Sweep the mats free of dirt and debris with a clean, dry, dust mop. Use a systematic approach to sweep away from walls. Overlap each lane (width of the mop) until the total mat area is swept.
4. Prepare at least one pail of warm water (2 gallons). Mix Virex or other similar concentrate in the pail (1 oz Virex to 1 gallon water).

5. If room fans or heaters are available, turn them on to help dry the mats.
6. Soak the mop in the cleaning solution and strain about one-half of the solution from the mop.
7. Use a back-and-forth motion of the floor mop to cover about a 3 foot wide lane and one-half length of the mat for each fresh application.
8. Start in one corner and systematically overlap each lane until the mat area is covered.
9. Use a fresh mop every one-half length of the mat and change buckets after mopping one full mat. If the water gets dirty before finishing a mat, change to a fresh bucket.
10. Allow the solution to dry.
11. Dump the solution and thoroughly rinse the bucket until the bucket water is clean. Scrub the bucket at least once per week with Lysol or similar disinfectant cleaner. Strain the mops with fresh water until the strained solution is clear.
12. Wipe each bucket dry and strain each mop dry.
13. Store the bucket upside down and elevated off the floor. Store the mop with the mop head in the air not on the floor.

SUGGESTED READING

Caruso JJ, Sheckman PR. Septic subcutaneous bursitis: Report of sixteen cases. J Rheumatol 1979; 6:96–102.

Ho G, Su EY. Antibiotic therapy of septic bursitis. Arthritis Rheum 1981; 24:905–911.

Ho G, Tice AD, Kaplan SR. Septic bursitis in the prepatellar and olecranon bursae: An analysis of 25 cases. Ann Intern Med 1978; 89:21–27.

Ho G, Toder JS. Antibiotic therapy of septic arthritis and septic bursitis. Orthopaedics 1984; 7:1571–1576.

Larson RL, Osternig LR. Traumatic bursitis and artificial turf. J Sports Med 1974; 2:183–188.

Monro A. A description of all the bursae mucosae in the body. Edinburg: Elliot, 1788.

Mysnyk MC, Wroble RR, Foster DT, JP Albright. Prepatellar bursitis in wrestlers. Am J Sports Med 1986; 14:46–54.

North HH, Zimmerman B, Ho G. Septic bursitis: Confirming the diagnosis and treating appropriately. J Musculoskeletal Med 1992; 9:52–64.

Sharrard WJW. Aetiology and pathology of beat knee. Br J Industr Med 1963; 20:24–31.

Soderquist B, Hedstrom SA. Predisposing factors, bacteriology, and antibiotic therapy in 35 cases of septic bursitis. Scand J Infect Dis 1986; 18:305–311.

ILIOTIBIAL BAND FRICTION SYNDROME

MARC A. MARTENS, M.D.

An iliotibial band (ITB) friction syndrome may be considered as an overuse syndrome caused by friction between the ITB and the lateral femoral epicondyle.

In sports where repetitive knee flexion past 30 degrees is required, the ITB is especially susceptible to irritation. Therefore this syndrome is typically observed in runners and has been described as the "jogger's knee," but also football players and cyclists present this exertional pain syndrome. We have seen it in patients who participate in a large variety of sports. But most often the initiation of the pain syndrome was related to running or cycling as part of their training.

PATHOMECHANICS

ITB friction syndrome may be the result of a combination of extrinsic and intrinsic factors. Extrinsic factors are improper training conditions including: (1) running or cycling on an oblique surface causing a pelvic tilt; (2) a sudden increase in running or cycling distance; and (3) an improper cycle sit with f.i. cleats too far

internally rotated or a saddle that is not well positioned. *Intrinsic factors* are anatomic factors including: (1) a varus knee deformity that predisposes for this friction syndrome between the lateral femoral epicondyle and the over-riding iliotibial band; (2) leg length discrepancy; and (3) forefoot pronation.

Symptoms

Only a few patients present an acute onset of pain related to an unusually strenuous activity. All patients complain of pain at the lateral side of the knee, in some cases radiating proximally or descending. Pain recurs during the sports activity after a pain-free start. The length of the pain-free time is variable between individuals but tends to become progressively shorter when the patient tries to continue sports activities. When pain appears during the sports activity, it becomes progressively worse. Most patients complain only of pain during sports activity but in some instances pain persists a few days, especially on stairwalking.

Clinical Examination

Clinical examination reveals a localized tenderness on the lateral epicondyle and the typical pain can also be reproduced by an active flexion-extension of the knee while the examiner exerts with the thumb a pressure on the lateral femoral epicondyle. There is at this maneuver a painful arc with a maximum at 30 degrees of knee flexion.

Diagnosis

The diagnosis is based on clinical symptoms and signs. But because signs subside with rest, the clinical examination performed shortly after activity is more relevant. Roentgenographic examination remains negative. An echography may show an aberrant picture around the lateral femoral condyle with localized edema.

Differential Diagnosis

The differential diagnosis includes chondromalacia patellae, torn or discoid lateral meniscus, biceps or popliteus tendinitis, or a stress fracture.

The fact that many patients undergo a diagnostic arthroscopy for a suspicion of a torn lateral meniscus, illustrates that the syndrome may be overlooked and mistaken for other pathology.

TREATMENT

Conservative Treatment

Conservative treatment should not only imply measures to control the inflammation by anti-inflammatory drugs, icing and local steroid injections, since they will only give a temporary relief of symptoms. More important is to look for and to correct the predisposing extrinsic and intrinsic factors.

A period of rest is often indicated and stretching exercises of the ITB seems to be very effective to overcome the friction syndrome.

An early correct diagnosis and adequate conservative treatment are important in order to avoid long periods of sports inactivity and progressive worsening of the symptoms due to chronic and sometimes irreversible soft tissue changes due to chronic inflammatory reaction of the tissues between the bone and the ITB.

Surgical Treatment

Indication

When a sufficiently long period (minimum 3 months) of conservative treatment, including rest and stretching exercises, does not resolve the pain syndrome, surgical treatment may be considered for the group of patients who are motivated for surgery because of inability for further sports performances. Although 3 months should be the minimum period before surgery is considered, most of my patients suffered from this syndrome for a much longer period before surgery.

The mean of 9 months of preoperative complaints for a group of surgically treated patients in my group's report on surgical treatment for ITB friction syndrome illustrates that surgery is only indicated in selective cases.

Surgical Technique and Postoperative Care

Frequently macroscopically inflammatory tissue is observed over and around the lateral femoral epicondyle. One should take care not to touch or to excise this tissue since that could damage or perforate the underlying knee synovia, which could cause postoperative bleeding and synovial reaction with persistent filling of the subcutaneous space with synovial fluid arising from the intra-articular cavity that is leaking through the perforated synovial layers. Careful hemostasis is needed after release of the tourniquet and the leg is put in a splint for a few days. The patient may return to sports activity after 3 to 4 weeks.

Results

Patients are very satisfied with surgical results. All pursued their previous sports activity at preoperative levels.

Complications

In our practice we have encountered a few benign hematomas. From elsewhere we have seen a more serious complication, namely a perforation of the synovial layer of the knee with persistent effusion and filling of the subcutaneous space on the lateral side of the knee with synovial fluid. Repeated aspiration, rest, and immobilization did not successfully solve the problem and revision surgery with suturing of the synovial defect was necessary in order to solve this complication. One should be very careful not to dissect or resect the tissues underneath the ITB.

SUGGESTED READING

Evans P. Functional and clinical aspects of the iliotibial tract. J Bone Joint Surg 1981; 63B:633.

Firer P: Aetiology and results of treatment of iliotibial band friction syndrome. J Bone Joint Surg 1990; 72B:742.

Henderson I: Iliotibial band friction syndrome. J Bone Joint Surg 1989; 71B:879.

Martens M, Libbrecht P, Burssens A: Surgical treatment of the iliotibial band friction syndrome. Am J Sports Med 1989; 17: 651–654.

Noble CA: Iliotibial band friction in runners. Am J Sports Med 1980; 8:232–234.

Renne JW: The iliotibial band friction syndrome. J Bone Joint Surg 1975; 57A:1110–1111.

QUADRICEPS AND PATELLAR TENDON RUPTURES

CHRISTOPHER W. SIWEK, M.D.

Injuries to the extensor mechanism of the knee have been recognized and described since the times of Galen. Samuel of England is credited with the first published case of quadriceps tendon rupture in English literature, in 1838. Treatment of these injuries consisted of immobilization and limited weight bearing until Lister in 1878 first practiced suture of the knee extensor. Charles McBurney reported the first successful repair of the quadriceps tendon in North America in 1887. McMaster in 1933 published his experimental studies on ruptures of tendons and muscles in animals. He concluded that ruptures of the quadriceps and patellar tendons rarely occur through their substance, but rather are sustained at the musculotendinous junction or insertion of the tendon into the bone. During the last half-century, several different methods have been described, dealing with repairs and reconstruction of neglected, delayed ruptures of extensor mechanism of knee joint.

MECHANISM AND LEVEL OF RUPTURE

Continuity of the extensor mechanism of the knee is disrupted as a result of sudden, powerful contracture of quadriceps muscle against the weight of the body applied to the affected extremity. The actual moment of tearing occurs when the knee is in a mild flexion, the patella firmly held against the femoral condyles by the pull of quadriceps muscle and the force continuing.

The mechanism of rupture for quadriceps as well as patellar tendons is the same. The level of rupture is determined by predisposing factors.

It appears to me that the single most important factor is the individual's age. The natural physiologic aging process "favors" patellar tendon ruptures in individuals younger than 40 years of age and quadriceps tendon ruptures in those above that age. Males sustain injuries six times more often than females, according to my study. Other predisposing factors include diabetes, rheumatoid arthritis, gout, psoriatic arthritis, hyperparathyroidism, systemic lupus erythematosus, and nephritis. Ruptures of patellar tendons in athletes following multiple knee injections with steroids have also been documented.

EXAMINATION

Ruptures of the quadriceps and patellar tendons are uncommon considering all the trauma that occurs about the knee. The severe hematoma that often accompanies the acute rupture may conceal the important diagnostic signs. Much too frequently, these ruptures are misdiagnosed in the acute stage of knee injury. In my study, 39% of ruptures have been missed on the initial examination. Testing of the extensor mechanism should be an essential part of the total comprehensive knee evaluation. It is of utmost importance that an early diagnosis be established in order to ensure good final results. During examination, one must look for loss of active knee extension or inability to maintain a passively extended joint against gravity. If the rupture does not extend through medial and lateral retinacula, the patient may have limited, weak, active extension, but still is not able to maintain the completely extended knee joint against gravity. Lack of complete active extension, accompanied by local tenderness and hemarthrosis, strongly suggests at least a partial tear. Complete ruptures are always associated with a palpable soft tissue defect. The rent is easily identifiable in quadriceps tendon, owing to a larger mass of the tissue. However, it may be difficult to palpate a rent in the patellar tendon at the time of swelling and hemarthrosis. In this situation, one should examine the joint while the patient is sitting on a table with his or her legs hanging down. Examination is done by comparing both patellar tendons. The examiner sits in front of the patient, identifies both patellar tendons by placing his thumbs on them, and asks the patient to slowly extend both knees. The examiner should immediately feel "sudden tension" under the thumb that is over the normal patellar tendon, but this tension is absent on the affected side. Proximally (patellar tendon rupture) or distally (quadriceps tendon rupture), a displaced patella may also be observed clinically or radiographically. Old untreated ruptures with partial return of function may be a diagnostic problem. Although partial return of quadriceps function in these cases may occur several weeks after the injury, the disability remains.

QUADRICEPS TENDON RUPTURES

Occurrence

As noted previously, this lesion usually occurs in individuals who are past the fifth decade in age. I have reviewed 117 cases, published from 1880 to 1978, in which the age of the patient was given. There were 69 quadriceps tendon ruptures, and all but four occurred in patients 40 years of age or older. In my own study, 78% of quadriceps tendon ruptures occurred in the fifth decade of life or later.

The tears are transverse in nature and begin in the central portion of the rectus femoris, traversing its entire thickness. Only on rare occasions is the tear limited to the rectus femoris; usually it extends laterally and medially, implicating the fibrous expansions of the vastus lateralis and medialis for varying distances. Most of the injuries are observed at the level of the quadriceps tendon attachment to the patella. The margins of the tear are ragged, and tissues are infiltrated with blood. Intratendinous tears do not occur so frequently, and once such a tear is found a "pathologic tear" should be suspected. Systemic diseases, as previously mentioned, or prior steroid infiltrations should be included in the differential diagnosis.

Microscopic examination of tissue from the rupture site shows local degenerative changes, including a decreased level of collagen in fibers of the tendon, fibrotic degeneration, and infiltration.

Diagnosis

The diagnosis is made readily, provided that correct interpretation is given to the clinical features. Frequently the true nature of the lesion is overlooked because the examiner does not suspect the possibility of a rupture of the quadriceps tendon and depends too heavily on roentgenographic findings, which are not always helpful. The clinical findings are directly related to the extent of the tear and the degree of separation of fragments. The cardinal clinical features are a history of stumbling, with severe pain above the knee and subsequent inability to extend the joint.

In complete tears, including synovial membrane, a large hemarthrosis is present. Upon flexion of the knee, the bloody content of the joint is displaced into the suprapatellar pouch and is easily observed as an "abnormal" bulge at the level of rupture. One can palpate a soft tissue defect above the patella. The patella itself may be displaced distally, and it has increased side-to-side motion when compared with the unaffected leg. Roentgenograms may reveal a distally displaced patella, and soft tissue technique may demonstrate the rent itself. If the tear occurs at the tendo-osseous junction, small fragments of avulsed superior pole of the patella appear to be displaced proximally, being retracted with the rectus femoris.

Small tears within the rectus femoris alone may be difficult to diagnose. This may be especially true in obese individuals. These patients still have active extension against gravity, but never complete extension. The examiner may reverse the test: rather than asking the patient to extend the joint, he should bring the knee to complete extension and ask the patient to maintain it. In cases of tear, one always notices a "drop" of the leg of varying degrees. During the examination, the patient complains of increased pain in the suprapatellar region owing to quadriceps tension. In some of these diagnostically difficult cases, a computed tomographic (CT) scan has been helpful in identifying the rupture, its extent, and its location.

Proper diagnosis of small tears can be easily missed. I have observed that this incorrect diagnosis is most often made in the emergency room. Usually the history and physical examination fit into a pattern of "sprained knee," and the patient is given some kind of knee splint. Because the knee support allows some mobility, reasonable comfort, and noticeable steady improvement, the patient may continue this incorrect therapy for several weeks. Disappointment comes when the patient cannot regain full quadriceps strength and is unable to climb stairs or walk on an inclined plane without risk of falling. Return to even mild recreational sport activity is impossible.

Treatment

Repair of the defect should be achieved by surgical intervention in all cases of tear of the extensor mechanism. Adequate assessment of the tear should be made in order to achieve proper and lasting repair. Treatment is generally divided into early and late repair. Distinction between these two phases is made more by the amount of retraction of quadriceps, by difficulty of end-to-end approximation, and by the amount of scar tissue formation than by the actual time from rupture to repair. These findings vary from case to case. In the past I have used 2 weeks as a cut-off time between early and late repairs, but in many instances I was able to make primary repairs with end-to-end suture in tears as old as 3 weeks, and in small tears even older. I would suggest that we use the term "late repair" when, because of time loss, surgical treatment is more extensive and requires additional reinforcement of suture, other than just end-to-end repair. In my experience, no additional reinforcement has been necessary in early repairs or in cases in which end-to-end approximation is achieved without significant strain and tension.

Preferred Methods for Early Repairs

Techniques of repair may vary according to the level of rupture. If the tear is intratendinous and an adequate amount of tissue is available for approximation, an end-to-end suture repair is sufficient. In cases in which the quadriceps tendon is avulsed from patellar attachment, longitudinal holes have to be drilled in the patella for placement of sutures to secure the repair.

Surgical Technique (End-to-End Repair)

A midline anterior longitudinal skin incision is begun about 10 cm proximal to the superior pole of the patella. In tears involving large portions of medial and lateral retinaculum, the incision may have to be extended proximally for an additional 5 to 7 cm. Distally, the incision ends at the joint level. After subcutaneous and fatty tissues are dissected, the rupture is exposed with its hematoma and ragged edges. All clots are removed and the cavity is well irrigated. The entire quadriceps tendon and the suprapatellar pouch area are examined and damage is assessed. The edges of the tendon are trimmed of all devitalized and frayed strands of tissue. If the synovial membrane of the suprapatellar pouch is torn, it should be repaired first. If there is difficulty in approximation, a towel clip should be placed in the rectus femoris tendon at the proximal side of the wound and traction applied distally. A rent in the quadriceps tendon should be closed with heavy, absorbable horizontal mattress sutures. Deep layers are closed first; suturing is continued outward through the middle layers of the vastus medialis and lateralis to the most anterior tendon of the rectus femoris. The suture line is tested under direct vision. The knee is passively flexed to 90 degrees and the repair carefully examined. Subcutaneous and skin closure is done with the knee in 45 degrees of flexion to avoid tight suturing and future tissue contractures, which may delay recovery of range of motion. The entire procedure is done without tourniquet control. The tourniquet is applied, but used only if necessary; an inflated tourniquet causes additional retraction of the proximal fragment and distorts the anatomy of the thigh muscles. Meticulous hemostasis is done to avoid hematoma formation.

Surgical Technique (Tendon-to-Bone Repair)

The technique differs slightly in cases of avulsion of the tendon from the superior pole of the patella. An avulsed rectus is less frayed than with an intratendinous rupture. There is always a good thick stump of tendon to work with. Attention should be directed toward debridement and preparation of the patella for acceptance of the tendon, and proper placement of holes drilled through the body of the patella. By means of a small curette, the edge of the superior pole is "cleaned" from remaining fragments of tendon and sclerotic bone; damage to articulating surface is avoided. With a drill sized 3/32, three holes are made in the following fashion. A sponge is placed onto the floor of the defect to prevent bone fragments from falling into the knee joint. The first hole is drilled centrally, starting at the proximal pole of the patella just superior to the articulating surface. The drill should exit at the lower portion of the body of the patella, making the hole at least 2 cm long; otherwise, fracture may occur. A small guide wire may be placed into the hole to ensure parallel placement of two additional holes. The lateral holes should be at least 1 cm away from the central one, but well within the body of the patella. Two separate heavy sutures are placed through the holes and the rectus femoris (Fig. 1). Additional reinforcing sutures are placed through the superior layer of the rectus femoris. The remaining portion of tear within both vastus muscles are closed as described previously. The use of more than three holes in the patella is unnecessary and may weaken the bone. Occasionally, I use Bunnell's pull-out wire to secure the repair for the period of healing.

Late Repair

Neglected cases exhibit marked disability because of lack of stability in the affected extremity.

Many of these patients must depend on a cane or a brace in order to walk. The quadriceps muscle becomes contracted and extensive adhesions develop. The edges of ruptured tendon become thickened and sclerotic.

Debridement and excision of devitalized tissue should be the first step in surgical repair. All necrotic tissues at the rupture site must be evacuated in order to have vital substances for approximation. Failure to achieve this may result in poor delayed healing and possible re-rupture. Release of adhesions, mainly between the quadriceps and the femur, may allow for

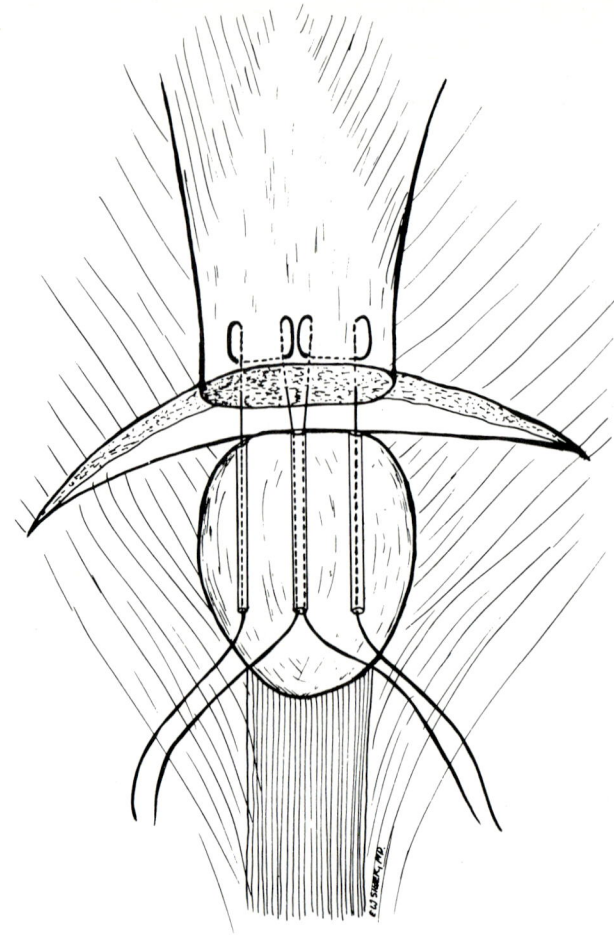

Figure 1 Tendon-to-bone repair of quadriceps tendon rupture. Two separate heavy sutures are placed through the holes in the patella and the rectus femoris.

additional distal displacement of the stump. Meticulous hemostasis must be achieved. If good approximation is possible, I prefer to repair by means of the tendon-to-bone technique already described. Sutures passed through drilled holes make the repair more secure. At this point, after the rent itself is closed, routine testing of suture line by knee flexion is done, and about 90 degrees of flexion should be possible. The surgeon has to bear in mind that excessive tension of the extensor mechanism will cause limited range of motion and may produce painful patellar symptoms, particularly in active sports-oriented individuals.

The next step in late repairs of the quadriceps tendon is reinforcement of the rupture. The least traumatic and most adequate repair is achieved by means of the Scuderi-type inverted V-flap, taken from the rectus femoris and crossed over the suture line. The triangular flap is based 2 cm above the side of the rupture, and it covers the entire width of the rectus. A height of 6 to 8 cm is sufficient for the triangle. An even thickness of 3 to 4 mm (about one-third the full thickness of the tendon) is stripped, starting from the apex of the triangle and ending 2 cm above the rupture level. The flap is inverted and tacked down to the distal portion of the extensor mechanism covering the rent. Depending on the quality of the repair, an additional pull-out wire can be used for protection and may remain in place throughout the healing process. In late repairs, I prefer to anchor the pull-out wire to the transverse tibial pin rather than place the pin through the patella. In the latter case, demineralization of the patella occurs owing to prolonged disuse, and additional transverse holes may dangerously weaken the patella, subjecting it to fractures.

One further step is taken in the repair of a neglected quadriceps tendon rupture when, despite releases, approximation of the edges of the rent is not possible. A lengthening of the quadriceps tendon by the "sliding" method of Codivilla is used. Occasionally, I have reinforced the suture line with a wide strip of fascia lata obtained from the same side. This is used instead of the Scuderi inverted V-flap in cases in which the area is already weakened by a quadriceps-lengthening procedure. The reinforcing strip is sutured to the vastus muscles above, and to the patella and its medial and lateral retinacula below.

Postoperative Management

After the operation the knee is maintained in complete extension. Compression dressings and a conventional knee splint are applied. In less reliable patients, a long leg cast is preferred. Routine wound care is given to the operated site. The patient uses crutches and is allowed "toe touch" for balance only. Quadriceps setting and leg raising with assistance are initiated as soon as postsurgical pain and soreness permit. Two weeks after surgery, sutures are removed. The leg is placed in a brace with adjustable hinges at the knee level. Passive range of motion starts 3 weeks after repair and does not exceed 60 degrees until the fifth postoperative week. The patient is allowed partial to full weight bearing as tolerated, beginning the third postsurgical week. Quadriceps stimulation is used if necessary. The brace is discontinued between the fifth and the seventh week. Judgment regarding the optimal time to discontinue the immobilization is based on the size of the tear and the "soundness" of the repair. Range of motion is continued since full recovery seldom is obtained at this point. Strengthening exercises should include a comprehensive program to regain complete balance of all muscle groups in the leg.

Mild, recreational, noncontact sports activity may be initiated 3 to 4 months after surgery, depending on the severity of the tear. Competitive sports should not be allowed until the full strength of the quadriceps muscle is achieved.

Results

Early repair of the quadriceps tendon, with adequate postoperative physical therapy, gives excellent results. Thirty patients whom I studied regained quadriceps strength comparable with that of the opposite leg, and range of motion measured 120 degrees (in older patients) or more.

Late repair greatly diminishes the chance of regaining satisfactory function postoperatively. In my study, the main obstacle to better results was limited range of motion. Of six patients who underwent delayed repair, only one regained more than 90 degrees of knee flexion. Five of them had persistent quadriceps atrophy.

Since quadriceps tendon ruptures occur in the older population, the timing of physical therapy after repair is very important. In patients with adequate secure repairs, strengthening exercises and range of motion should begin soon after surgery. In motivated patients, complete recovery can be expected.

PATELLAR TENDON RUPTURES

Occurrence

Rupture of the patellar tendon is very rare and occurs mostly in individuals below the age of 40. In a group of 33 patients whom I studied, only one sustained injury after the age of 40 (the patient was 47); the remaining 32 were under 40. The incidence of patellar tendon rupture is about equal to that of quadriceps tendon rupture, and the mechanism is the same.

Most commonly, the lesion comprises complete avulsion of the tendon from the inferior pole of the patella, and the tear extends into both medial and lateral retinacula. Occasionally, small fragments of bone are avulsed from the patella. A healthy patellar tendon does not rupture through its substance, and if such a lesion is found one should suspect underlying causes other than the injury. Effects of injudicious steroid injections in young athletic individuals have to be included in the differential diagnosis. Bilateral simultaneous ruptures also are suspect for systemic diseases. There is no mention of such a case in the literature, all reported simultaneous, bilateral ruptures being associated with a variety of "predisposing factors."

I have seen cases in which some longitudinal fibers of the patellar tendon have been detached from the patella and others from the tibial tubercle (Fig. 2), causing severe shredding of the tissue. This "spaghetti-like" effect makes direct suturing impossible, and fascia lata graft is necessary to restore continuity.

Injuries to the distal portion of the patellar tendon are usually associated with avulsion fractures of the tibial tubercle, often preceded by Osgood-Schlatter disease.

Diagnosis

A detailed history helps to recreate the actual moment of injury, which should strongly suggest rupture of the extensor mechanism. The cardinal sign—lack of active extension—is always present. Proximal migration of the patella is easily noted clinically and radiographically. In more difficult cases, one can make comparisons

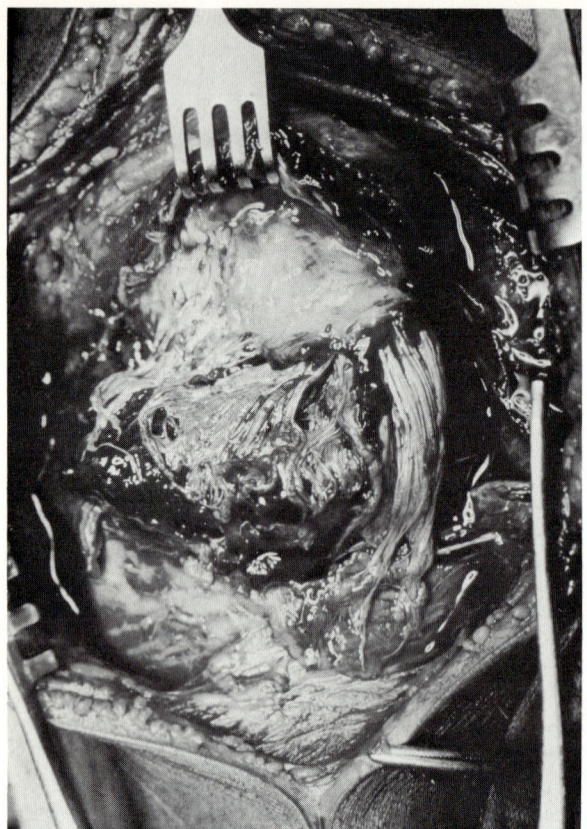

Figure 2 Patellar tendon rupture. Some longitudinal fibers have been detached from the patellar tendon and others from the tibial tubercle, causing severe shredding of the tissue.

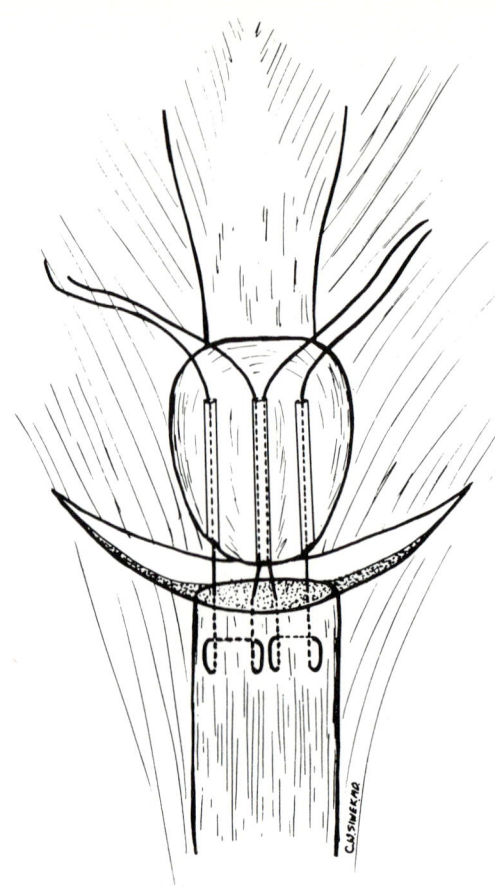

Figure 3 Bone-to-tendon repair of patellar tendon rupture. The main supporting sutures are opposed (see text).

with the opposite knee. If swelling obscures the pathology, a test of "sudden tension," as described previously, may be of value.

Treatment

Ruptures should be repaired at the earliest opportunity. In early repairs, surgical technique differs according to the level of injury. Delayed suturing may require additional preoperative or intraoperative procedures. Regardless of the type of injury and the surgical technique used, gentle handling of the tissues is important. The fat pad should remain undisturbed and its normal contact with the patellar tendon preserved, since it serves as a very important blood supply to the tendon. Any debridement at the rupture site must be adequate, but careless excision of tissue should be avoided. Functionally disabling patella baja may result if an excess of tendon is removed.

Actual repair of the patellar tendon, as opposed to quadriceps tendon repair, does not give a sense of "soundness" and security. The patellar tendon is susceptible to longitudinal separations of its fibers, and placement of sutures under excessive traction may cause additional shredding of the tendon. Sutures have to be passed through "tight" healthy portions of tendon in a manner that will not cause strangulation of tissue. I

routinely use pull-out wires to avoid tension on the suture line and weakening of the repair.

Preferred Methods
Bone-to-Tendon Technique

This repair is a mirror image of the technique described for quadriceps tendon avulsion from the superior pole of the patella.

The skin incision extends from 5 cm above the superior pole of the patella to the tibial tubercle in straight anterior fashion. The entire patellar tendon is exposed and the quality of tissue noted. The avulsed end of the tendon is debrided by sharp transverse dissection, removing enough frayed fragments to leave a thick wide stump for repair. The main supporting sutures are opposed (Fig. 3). The same technique may be used in cases of fracture of the inferior pole of the patella when comminuted fragments are excised.

Tendon-to-Tendon Technique

As already mentioned, one should suspect "pathologic" rupture when a tear has occurred transversely through the substance of the tendon. In these patients direct mattress suturing is not strong enough to maintain continuity of the tendon, even with the leg immobilized in full extension. Quadriceps contractures may cut the sutures through fragile tendon, causing separation of fragments. On the other hand, more vigorous and more bulky suturing may strangulate the tissue.

I reinforce the suture line with a strip of fascia lata obtained from the same side. The strip has to be three times the length of the ruptured tendon and 1.5 cm wide in order to be sufficient for repair. Two tunnels are made, one at 1.5 cm to 2 cm above the inferior pole of the patella and the second 1 cm below the attachment of the patellar tendon to the tibial tubercle. A high-speed air drill with a 3 mm burr is excellent for shaping the edges of the tunnels. When this instrument is used, chipping of bone and fractures is easily avoided. One has to ensure that edges of both tunnels are smooth and round to prevent them from cutting into a fascia lata graft. Before final repair is made, a pull-out wire is passed through the superior pole of the patella, and sufficient distal traction is applied. Wires are anchored to the transverse tibial pin. Excessive traction on the patella is avoided since it may result in a patella baja. The graft is rolled into a cord and passed through both tunnels (Fig. 4). The entire graft is tucked down to both sides of the patellar tendon. The wound is closed in the usual manner.

Delayed Repairs

Despite delay, primary approximation of fragments is possible in many cases. These ruptures can be treated by one of the techniques described above. In severely neglected cases, preoperative skeletal traction may be necessary to overcome contractures and adhesions of the quadriceps mechanism. The following are indications for preoperative traction: (1) marked clinical and radiographic proximal displacement of the patella, (2) an inability to move the patella manually to its anatomic position, and (3) a loss of free passive side-to-side motion of the patella (indicative of severe adhesions).

Traction is applied through a 9⁄64-inch Steinmann pin placed transversely into the patella. The size of the pin largely depends on the size of the patella. To avoid skin tension, the skin is displaced proximally before pin insertion, and a maximum of 2 kg of weight is applied. It may take a few days to 2 weeks before adequate displacement is obtained. Progress of the traction is checked clinically or radiographically. During the period of traction, the knee is engaged in passive range of motion. This is done most comfortably with the patient lying on the unaffected side.

When satisfactory distal displacement of the patella is achieved, surgical repair follows. After routine exposure of the lesion, a second Steinmann pin is inserted into the proximal tibia. The patella is brought to its anatomic position and maintained there by wiring both Steinmann pins together. Actual repair of the patellar tendon is made by means of the tendon-to-tendon technique already described.

A patellar tendon that is not performing its function because of rupture quickly undergoes disuse, degeneration, and disintegration. In these severe cases, one may

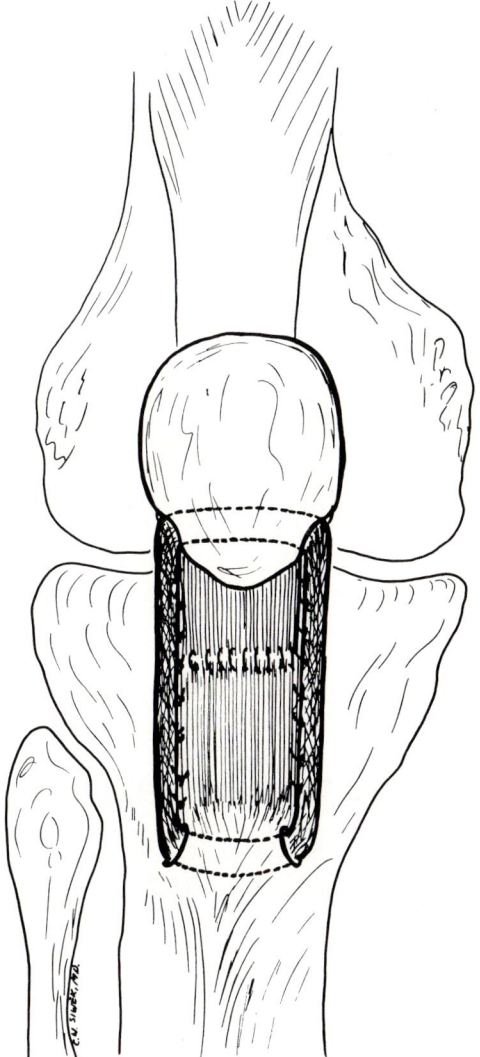

Figure 4 Tendon-to-tendon repair of patellar tendon rupture. The graft is rolled into a cord and passed through both tunnels (see text).

have to reconstruct the entire patellar tendon, and I prefer to use the distal tendinous portion of the semitendinosus muscle as a substitute for the patellar tendon. The tendon is looped through transverse tunnels in the patella and proximal tibia and then sewn onto itself. After wound closure, a long leg cast is applied, incorporating both pins.

Postoperative Care

For early repairs with good strong approximation, postoperative management is the same as for early repairs of quadriceps tendon ruptures.

In delayed repairs of the patellar tendon, judgment of postoperative management is based on the extent of rupture, the quality and availability of tissues for approximation, and the actual strength of the suture line at the conclusion of surgery. If pins and wires have been used, they should be maintained for 4 to 5 weeks. Cast immobilization with the knee in full extension is continued for 7 to 8 weeks postoperatively.

In early repairs, mild, recreational, noncontact sports activity may be initiated 3 to 4 months after surgery. Prolonged recovery in delayed repairs may extend this time to 6 months.

Results

In my study, 25 patients underwent early repairs of patellar tendons. Twenty of them obtained excellent results with full range of motion and strength of quadriceps muscle equal to that of the opposite leg. Four patients were unable to obtain full active extension, even though passive extension was possible. One patient re-ruptured his patellar tendon 8 weeks after the original repair, while attempting to play football on a recreational level.

Results of seven late repairs in my study were directly related to but he had other medical problems that did not allow him to receive a proper course of therapy. In the remaining five ruptures, motion ranged from full extension to 130 degrees of flexion. Good quadriceps strength was regained despite persistent atrophy of thigh muscles.

SUGGESTED READING

Feagin J, Jackson D. Quadriceps contusion in young athletes. J Bone Joint Surg 1973; 55A:95–105.

Grenier RE, Guimont A. Simultaneous bilateral rupture of the quadriceps tendon and leg fractures in a weight lifter: a case report. Am J Sports Med 1983; 11:145.

Kamali M. Bilateral traumatic rupture of the infrapatellar tendon. Clin Orthop 1979; 142:131.

McCouister Evarts C. Surgery of the musculo skeletal system. New York: Churchill Livingstone, 1983:195.

Rao J, Siwek C. Bilateral spontaneous rupture of the patellar tendons. Orthopaedic Rev 1978; 7:5.

Siwek C, Rao J. Rupture of the extensor mechanism of the knee joint. J Bone Joint Surg 1981; 63A:932–937.

ISOLATED MEDIAL COLLATERAL LIGAMENT TEAR: NONOPERATIVE MANAGEMENT

PETER A. INDELICATO, M.D.

Over the past 10 years, the approach to the management of major ligament tears of the knee has changed significantly. Whereas the pendulum has swung in favor of a more aggressive surgical approach to tears of the anterior cruciate ligament (ACL) and, to a lesser degree, the posterior cruciate ligament (PCL), it has generally swung in the opposite, more conservative, direction regarding tears of the medial collateral ligament (MCL). This chapter outlines an approach to the nonoperative management of complete tears of the MCL and describes the current philosophy when this occurs as an isolated lesion and also in combination with tears to other major ligaments of the knee.

FUNCTIONAL ANATOMY

The MCL that is referred to here, has been labeled, in the past, "the superficial medial collateral ligament" or "tibial collateral ligament." It has a proximal attachment site at the medial femoral condyle and a distal attachment site at the metaphyseal flair of the tibia, 4 to 5 cm below the medial joint line deep to the pes anserinus insertion. Deep to these parallel superficial fibers is the medial capsule to which is firmly attached the periphery of the medial meniscus. The posterior oblique ligament is a discrete thickening of the posteromedial capsule of the knee and is frequently injured simultaneously along with the MCL. The primary function of the MCL is to resist medial joint opening when a valgus load is applied to the knee joint.

PHYSICAL EXAMINATION

The key to an accurate diagnosis is a careful history and physical examination. Frequently some valgus force is applied to the involved knee, resulting in disruption of some portion of the ligament. If the force is large enough, a complete rupture occurs and the physical examination reflects the degree of damage in most cases. It is critical to follow some basic principles when performing the examination; namely, the patient must be relaxed and the opposite knee must be used as a control to determine the presence and degree of asymmetrical medial joint opening. This medial joint opening, coupled with the quality of the "end-point," should be accurately assessed. The focus of the examination should be to determine the degree of abnormal medial opening to valgus stress with the knee in full extension and 30 degrees of flexion.

Abnormal (asymmetrical) medial laxity detected with the knee in full extension and 30 degrees of flexion is suggestive of significant structural damage to not only the MCL and posterior oblique ligament but also the ACL and/or PCL. Abnormal medial laxity detected with the knee in 30 degrees of flexion and none in full extension is indicative of damage to only the MCL and possible underlying capsule. A negative Lachman test with a firm "end-point" is usually sufficient evidence to rule out significant damage to the ACL. The key to a successful treatment plan for the nonoperative management of complete tears of the MCL is to rule out significant structural damage to the ACL and/or PCL. This can usually be accomplished by physical examination alone. It is sometimes necessary to reexamine the patient in order to rule out coexisting ACL/PCL damage.

The need to rule out other damage, particularly to the meniscus, may occasionally necessitate diagnostic studies such as an MRI or arthroscopy.

TREATMENT OF COMPLETE "ISOLATED" TEARS OF THE MCL

When a complete tear of the MCL is established on physical examination, and no other pathology is detected, a protocol aimed at establishing motion in the knee followed by recovery of strength in the thigh usually allows a safe and early return to sports. The protocol described below is one that has evolved with time and has become more aggressive as experience is gained. It is divided into three phases.

Phase 1

Initial pain and swelling dictate the early course of management. Usually the initial discomfort requires immobilization and protected crutch walking ambulation. It is important to immobilize the knee in full extension during this initial phase in order to minimize the risk of a flexion contracture and also to facilitate isometric quadriceps exercises. In addition, it allows the patient easier gait ambulation with the knee straight. Early weight bearing is encouraged and the patient is instructed to place as much weight on their involved foot as is comfortable. This initial phase usually takes 10 to 14 days. During this time the patient is instructed to remove the light weight immobilizer and move their knee through a comfortable range of motion for 10 minutes at least four or five times a day. In addition, the patient should sleep with the immobilizer in place, again to minimize the development of a flexion contracture. The patient is allowed to progress to Phase 2 when they can ambulate without a noticeable limp.

Phase 2

Once the patient can walk without a noticeable limp, resistive strengthening exercises to the quadriceps and hamstring muscles are begun. "Open" and "closed" chain kinetic exercises, along with isometric and isokinetic exercises, are all utilized. The goal is to recover the strength, power, and endurance in the involved thigh and calf as quickly as possible. At the beginning of Phase 2, the patient is given a functional hinged brace that allows full motion of the knee and is instructed to wear this all the time except when exercising, showering, or sleeping. The exercise protocol is usually supervised by a trained physical therapist or trainer experienced with knee injuries. When possible, the patient should perform these strengthening exercises three or four times a week. After 2 or 3 weeks, a "baseline" strength test is performed to establish the remaining deficiency that exists between the quadriceps and hamstrings muscle groups in both thighs. The goal is to achieve at least an 80% recovery of strength, power, and endurance before the formal program is considered complete. Aerobic exercises such as swimming, riding a stationary bicycle, and jogging in chest-deep water are encouraged as soon as the patient finds these activities comfortable.

The spontaneous occurrence of an effusion is very unusual once the initial swelling subsides after the injury. If it occurs, a repeat history and physical examination should be performed in order to discover the cause. The most likely causes are a subclinical "bone bruise" or an occult cruciate and/or meniscal tear. Infrequently, patients experience posteromedial discomfort during strengthening exercises to the hamstring muscles and this most likely is a result of the anatomic connections between the semimembranosus and the posterior oblique ligament. If discomfort occurs, this particular exercise is temporarily discontinued until the pain experienced when doing it has disappeared. If anterior knee pain develops in the retropatellar area during quadriceps strengthening exercises, the exercise program is modified to accommodate this patellofemoral pain. Limiting the strengthening exercise to the final 30 degrees of extension is usually sufficient to solve the problem.

Phase 3

Once the patient has achieved 80% recovery of strength, the final stage of rehabilitation is begun; that being a supervised program of agility drills under the watchful eye of an experienced physical therapist or trainer. During these workout sessions, the patient is made to wear the functional brace, otherwise they may discontinue its use for normal activities of daily living. The program begins with the patient performing slow, "lazy" figure-of-eight drills making, at first, large circles and then progressing to "tighter" circles over the course of time. Simultaneously, straight ahead sprinting and sudden stopping is begun. Within a few days, if there are no complaints, the patient is allowed to begin backpedaling and carioca drills that should progress with intensity over time.

TREATMENT OF COMPLETE TEARS OF THE MCL AND ACL/PCL

There is some controversy regarding the management of complete tears of the MCL when it coexists with a complete tear of the ACL and/or the PCL. Shelbourne et al have recently advocated a nonoperative approach for the MCL and a primary reconstruction either the ACL or PCL.

My approach is more dependent on the physical

examination. If the knee is unstable to valgus stress in 30 degrees of flexion, but stable in full extension, I first perform a primary reconstruction of the ACL and then re-evaluate the medial laxity while the patient is still under anesthesia. If the laxity examination shows that the medial laxity decreases from 3 + to 1 + or 2 +, I feel that a primary repair is not required. If, however, there is no decrease in the abnormal laxity following the cruciate reconstruction, I then perform a primary repair of the damaged medial structures.

If the knee has evidence of ACL and/or PCL damage and is unstable to valgus stress testing in full extension, I routinely perform a primary repair of the medial structures. Surgical exposure usually reveals significant structural damage to the posterior capsule, which is also meticulously repaired. Careful attention is paid to not "overtighten" the posteromedial capsule and iatrogenically create a flexion contracture.

The postoperative management is modified to include the immediate use of a CPM device to minimize the risk of arthrofibrosis. When the patient can easily maintain a range of motion from 0 degrees extension to over 90 degrees of flexion out of the CPM device, the device is discontinued. The protocol from this point on is similar to our routine for ACL reconstructions.

SUGGESTED READING

Bergfeld J. Functional rehabilitation of isolated medial collateral ligament sprains. First, second and third-degree sprains. Am J Sports Med 1979; 7:207–209.

Bosch U, Kasperczyk WJ. Healing of the patellar tendon autograft after posterior cruciate ligament reconstruction — a process of ligamentization. Am J Sports Med 1992; 20:558–566.
Derscheid GL, Garrick JG. Medial collateral ligament injuries in football: non-operative management of grade I and grade II sprains. Am J Sports Med 1981; 9:365–368.
Ellasser JC, Reynolds FC, Omohundro JR. The non-operative treatment of collateral ligament injuries of the knee in professional football players: An analysis of seventy-four injuries treated non-operatively and twenty-four injuries treated surgically. J Bone Joint Surg 1974; 56:1185–1190.
Hastings DE. The non-operative management of collateral ligament injuries of the knee joint. Clin Orthop 1980; 147:22–28.
Indelicato PA. Non-operative treatment of complete tears of the medial collateral ligament of the knee. J Bone Joint Surg 1983; 65:323–329.
Indelicato PA, Hermansdorfer J, Huegel M. The non-operative management of complete tears of the medial collateral ligament of the knee in intercollegiate football players. Clin Orthop 1990; 256:174–177.
Jones RE, Henley MB, Francis P. Non-operative management of isolated grade III collateral ligament injuries in high school football players. Clin Orthop 1986; 213:137–140.
Shelbourne KD, Porter DA. Anterior cruciate ligament medial collateral ligament injury: non-operative management of medial collateral ligament tears with anterior cruciate ligament reconstruction. A preliminary report. Am J Sports Med 1992; 20:283–286.
Warren LF, Marshall JL. The supporting structures and layers on the medial side of the knee: an anatomical analysis. J Bone Joint Surg 1979; 61:56–62.

ARTHROSCOPICALLY ASSISTED RECONSTRUCTION OF THE ANTERIOR CRUCIATE LIGAMENT

ALEXANDER A. SAPEGA, M.D.

Any individual with chronic, symptomatic anterior cruciate ligament (ACL) deficiency unresponsive to knee rehabilitation and bracing, or any active athlete with acute disruption of the ACL, is a potential candidate for ligamentous reconstruction. One surgical option for these patients that is rapidly becoming the treatment standard in the field of athletic trauma surgery is arthroscopically assisted ACL reconstruction. Simply stated, this represents intra-articular ACL reconstruction without an open arthrotomy. It is properly referred to as "arthroscopically assisted" because extra-articular incisions, although limited, are still needed for graft harvesting and/or bone tunnel drilling. It therefore is not strictly an arthroscopic procedure. The basic surgical method can be applied to the placement of any ACL graft or substitute that can be placed through tibial and femoral bone tunnels, with only slight modification for prosthetic ligaments that require femoral "over-the-top" placement.

There are some obvious clinical advantages to this surgical method, such as lower perioperative morbidity, easier institution of voluntary joint motion, less intra-articular scar formation, and improved cosmetic results. Technical advantages include better visualization of the landmarks within the intercondylar notch before graft placement and the ability to evaluate the ACL substitute critically once it is in place to check for osseous contact-abrasion or impingement with knee motion. Controlled distention of the joint and lavage with the arthroscopic irrigant solution often allow the arthroscopic portions of the procedure to be performed with the limb tourniquet deflated, thus cutting ischemia time by 75% or more. Perhaps the only disadvantages relative to traditional open surgery are the greater dependence on surgical instrumentation and the fact that a good deal of patience and technical skill with the arthroscope are necessary.

ANATOMIC CONSIDERATIONS

The ACL is a broad, ovoid-sectioned ligament that, when viewed in extension, is composed of a continuum of parallel fibers (Fig. 1), with no detectable physical boundaries between different fiber "bundles." Different portions of the ligament's macrostructure are therefore best referred to as "fiber regions," which are arbitrarily distinguished by their geographic area of insertion on the tibia. Because of its noncylindric shape and its broad osseous insertional areas (maximal diameter, 17 to 30 mm), it is not yet technically feasible to reconstruct surgically the entire macrostructure of the normal ACL. A reasonable surgical alternative is to reconstruct the most functionally significant portion of the ACL in as anatomic a manner as possible. Given the limited diameter (6 to 12 mm) of the tibial and femoral bone tunnels generally employed for graft placement during ACL reconstruction, the surgeon can only direct the ACL substitute through approximately one-half of each anatomic insertional area. In choosing which half of the ACL fibers to reconstruct (anterior, central, or posterior), biomechanical factors come into play.

BIOMECHANICAL CONSIDERATIONS

Arms and colleagues consider that the anterior or, more specifically, the anteromedial fiber region should be the choice for selective reconstruction. Graf stated that the anteromedial fibers are the most isometric of any in the ACL. My own laboratory studies have confirmed Graf's conclusion, and also demonstrate that

the anterior fibers of the ACL act as the principal restraint to anterior tibial translation at both 15 and 90 degrees of flexion (Figs. 2 and 3). This is consistent with the original observations of Rosenberg and Rasmussen and the data of Hollis and associates. Based on the weight of available experimental evidence as well as clinical experience, I actively attempt to reconstruct the anteromedial fiber region as anatomically as possible during surgery rather than the central fiber core of the ACL. This involves the use of intra-articular landmarks as well as intraoperative "isometry" testing, as described later.

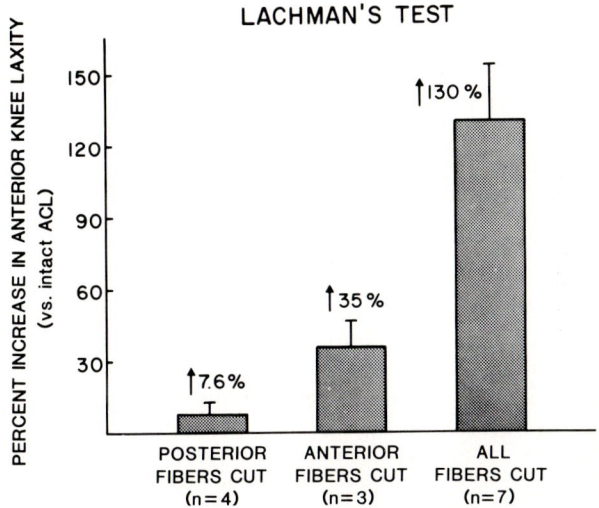

Figure 2 The results of standard manual Lachman's testing before and after selectively cutting the anterior and posterior 50 percent of the ACL fibers in seven fresh knee preparations, instrumented as described by Sapega and colleagues (error bars = SEM).

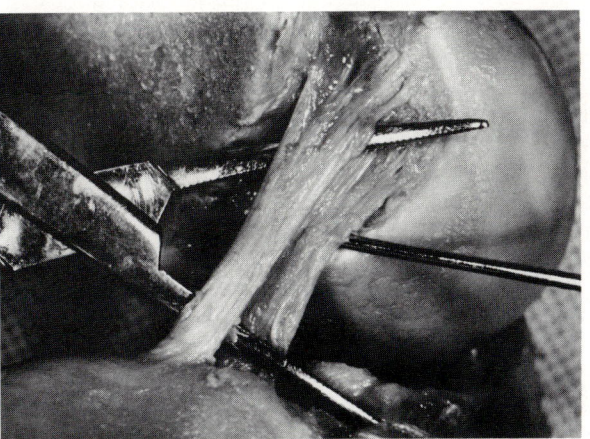

Figure 1 Fiber-splitting dissection shows that, aside from a limited degree of proximal and distal fiber fanning, the parallel arrangement of fibers seen on the medial surface of the ACL (knee in extension) is maintained throughout the ligament's substance. No anatomically separate fiber "bundles" are visible.

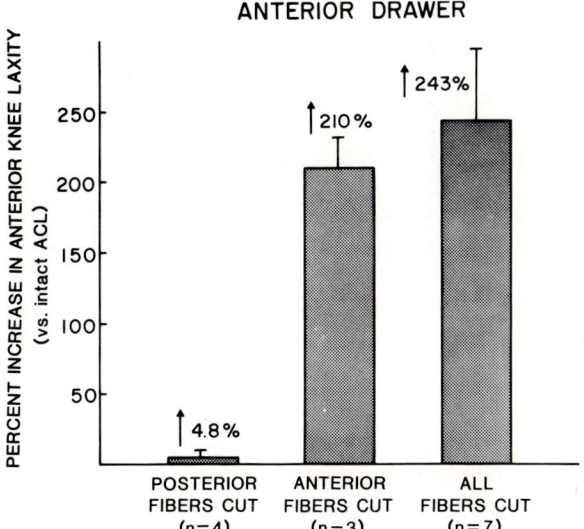

Figure 3 The results of standard manual anterior drawer testing before and after selectively cutting the anterior and posterior 50% of the ACL fibers (same knee preparations as in Figure 2).

My current personal preference for the ACL substitute is a combined semitendinosus and gracilis autograft. According to the data of Noyes and colleagues, the combined strength of these two tendons (approximately 120% of normal ACL strength) compares favorably with the calculated strength of a 9.5 mm (10 mm bone tunnel) patellar tendon graft (100% of normal ACL strength). The tensile strength of the semitendinosus and gracilis tendon tissue, in terms of load capacity *per unit cross-sectional area,* is almost twice that of patellar tendon tissue; thus, considerable overall tensile strength can be packed into an osseous tunnel of limited diameter (6.5 to 7.5 mm). This permits precise, selective fiber region reconstruction and theoretically minimizes inhomogeneous loading within the graft caused by differential fiber length behavior within the graft as the knee moves through its range of motion. Harvesting the semitendinosus and gracilis tendons involves a minimum of operative morbidity, leaves the extensor mechanism undisturbed, and produces no detectable loss of leg strength in either knee flexion or internal tibial rotation. Leaving the natural distal osseous attachments of these tendons intact provides satisfactory tibial fixation and avoids troublesome hardware irritation under the distal incision. My use of a double fold-over stapling technique (three staples, incorporating two 180 degree folds of the graft within a rectangular cancellous bed) on the femoral side has allowed immediate postoperative weight bearing as tolerated, without any detectable loss of stability. Clinically, the long-term biologic fixation of this soft tissue graft has not been observably different from that of bone-block grafts.

Regardless of the type of ACL autograft or allograft employed, there is a theoretical place for the use of a ligament augmentation device (LAD) to reinforce the waning tensile strength of the graft at or later than 4 weeks after surgery, when the patient is beginning to resume normal daily activities with only a brace for support. Owing to United States governmental restrictions regarding the use of the current, commercially available polypropylene LAD, since 1986 I have empirically employed six heavy strands of nonabsorbable suture (three woven into each tendon) for graft augmentation. No known complications have resulted. From a biologic standpoint, this technique should be no different than open primary repairs of the ACL with nonabsorbable suture material. The mechanical efficacy of this particular technique, however, has not been evaluated in any controlled studies.

SURGICAL TECHNIQUE

The technique described here represents my currently preferred method of arthroscopically assisted ACL reconstruction. Although the choice of available drill guide instruments and the means of performing intraoperative "isometry" testing (if this is desired) necessarily create variations in technique, the basic steps are generally similar for all methods employing tibial and femoral bone tunnels. The addition of a supplemental

lateral extra-articular procedure is considered optional, in accordance with the preference of the surgeon. I generally do not employ lateral, extra-articular "back-up" procedures for simple anterolateral rotatory instability, but will perform a supplemental posteromedial capsular reefing and gastrocnemius-semimembranous tenodesis for patients exhibiting significant chronic anteromedial rotatory instability.

To obtain a consistently high degree of surgical precision and accuracy in the intra-articular placement of the tendon grafts, intraoperative "isometry" testing is quite helpful. I employ a drill guide system that combines the technical capabilities of drill guide instruments with those of an isometer gauge system, to allow the performance of intraoperative isometry testing without the need to drill pilot holes in the tibia or femur. This permits the testing of as many prospective bone tunnel sites as needed to achieve ideal graft placement, with little time expenditure, before any guide pin placement or tunnel drilling. See the chapter *Intraoperative Isometry Testing* for more information.

All required arthroscopic meniscus-articular surface work is generally completed before the intraarticular reconstruction is begun. Tourniquet use is minimized. With adequate joint distention, tourniquet inflation can generally be avoided whenever the arthroscope is in use. Only two portals are required for the procedure, a low anteromedial (inferomedial) portal and an anterolateral portal. The use of a suprapatellar medial or lateral portal for placement of an inflow cannula is helpful, but optional.

Intercondylar notch preparation begins with clearance of soft tissue scar and obstructive anterior cruciate remnants, followed by intercondylar notch widening ("notchplasty") with a high-speed motorized burr or resector (Fig. 4). The degree of widening needed depends on the degree of intercondylar notch stenosis secondary to the cruciate insufficiency, if chronic. Good visualization and clearance for ACL substitute placement must be obtained, from the anterior inlet of the intercondylar notch to its posterior outlet, directly adjacent to the "over-the-top" position.

A 1½ inch extra-articular incision is made over the tibial insertion of the semitendinosus and gracilis tendons. These are identified and detached proximally at their musculotendinous junction in a closed fashion with a tendon stripper. The distal tibial insertions are left intact. A 2 to 2½ inch lateral extra-articular incision is made to expose the metaphyseal flare of the femur. Both incisions serve as drill guide access points and external bone tunnel exit sites.

The drill guide-isometer gauge system is set up as shown in Figure 5. Maintaining the arthroscope in the lateral portal, the tips of the drill guides' aimer arms are initially positioned by visual judgment into what appear to be the areas of greatest isometry, corresponding to the anatomic attachment areas of ACL's anteromedial fibers. The femoral guide employs a posterior, "over-the-top" approach for the introduction of its aimer arm. The tibial guide has a cannulated aimer arm, through which passes a heavy monofilament suture that spans the

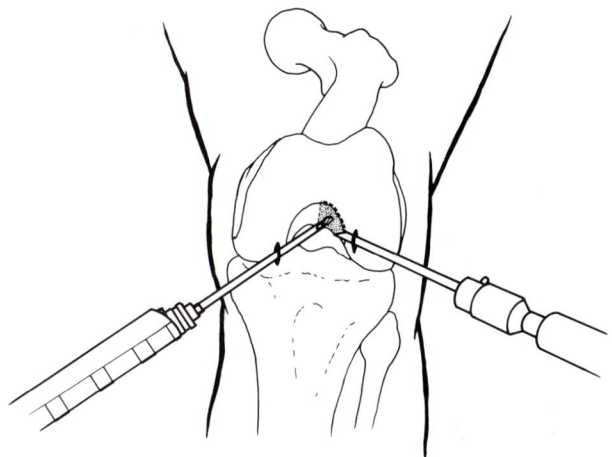

Figure 4 Using anterolateral and inferomedial portals, clearance of obstructive ACL remnants followed by widening of the intercondylar notch ("notchplasty") is performed with a high-speed resector and/or burr. (Reproduced with permission from ACL Drill Guide Instructional Manual. Andover, MA: Dyonics, Inc.)

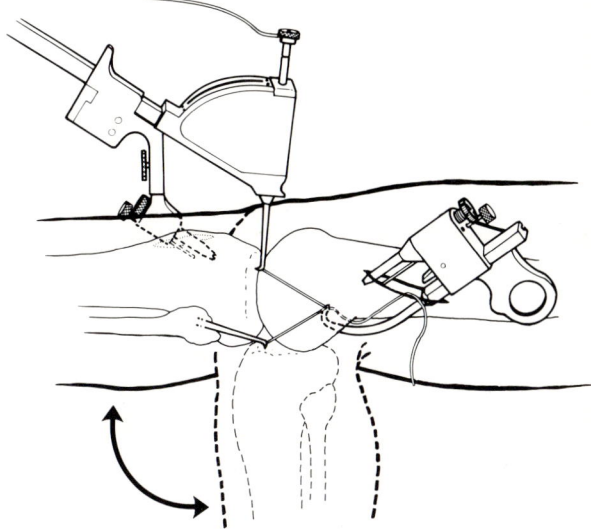

Figure 5 The drill guide-isometer instrument system used by the author. Operative isometry testing is performed with both guides in place, without the use of any pilot bone tunnels. The isometer gauge is located within the body of the tibial drill guide; it measures the changes in length of the segment of suture in between the two guide arm tips as the knee is passively brought through a range of motion. (Reproduced with permission from ACL Drill Guide Instructional Manual. Andover, MA: Dyonics, Inc.)

intra-articular distance between both aimer arm tips. It is tied to the femoral aimer tip and slides freely in and out of the tibial aimer arm tip as the distance between these two tips changes with knee motion. Within the body of the tibial guide, the suture is fixed to a spring-loaded "isometer" (suture excursion) gauge, which registers the changes in intra-articular suture length on an external read-out scale.

The knee is then passively flexed to at least 100 degrees and brought back out to full extension (see Fig. 5). The changes in read-out scale position followed by the suture excursion marker indicate, in millimeters, the changes in linear distance between the tips of the tibial and femoral aimer arms (prospective bone tunnel sites) as the knee is brought through its range of motion. If the initially selected sites on the tibia and femur yield what is thought to be an optimal separation distance profile through the range of motion, the intra-articular tips of the guide's aimer arms are left in place and 3/32 inch guide pins are drilled (from outside to inside) through the guide pin sleeves clamped to the tibia and femur.

If the excursion profile yielded by the gauge indicates that a nonoptimal or unacceptable graft length change profile would be provided by the tibiofemoral points selected, either the femoral or tibial guides may be unclamped and their aimer arm tips maneuvered to a different site on the femur or tibia. The testing process is then repeated as described above. This is continued until the optimal tibial and femoral points are found. When the tibial aimer arm is properly positioned at the anteromedial fiber insertion area, an isometer gauge reading that indicates only aimer arm tip *separation* as the knee is flexed generally indicates that the femoral aimer arm has been positioned "anterior" (arthroscopist's perspective) to the normal attachment site of the anteromedial fibers. A gauge reading that demonstrates *only* aimer tip *approximation* with knee flexion, with *no*

reseparation back toward the starting distance by 100 degrees of flexion, generally indicates that the femoral aimer arm has been positioned "posterior" (arthroscopist's perspective) to the anatomic anteromedial fiber insertion area.

Under simulated intraoperative isometry testing conditions, cadaver studies have shown that the anatomic centers of the anteromedial fiber region's osseous insertion areas naturally exhibit a small (1.5 to 3 mm) deviation from true isometry, demonstrating a characteristic pattern of decreasing tibiofemoral distance from 0 to 30 degrees of flexion, followed by reseparation with further flexion through 120 degrees. The anatomic central and posterior fiber attachment sites demonstrate somewhat similar patterns but with a greater deviation from isometry. Although the ideal suture excursion gauge measurement to search for intraoperatively has not yet been definitively established, I believe that deviations from true isometry greater than 1.5 mm should be evaluated in terms of their *pattern* (i.e., directions) of change in tibiofemoral distance over the range of motion. If sites demonstrating absolute changes of 1.5 mm or less cannot be found, deviations from isometry up to 3 mm should prove acceptable as long as the directional profile of the deviation follows a relatively anatomic (or what might be termed a "physiometric") pattern. Once the final tibiofemoral tunnel sites are selected and the guide pins drilled, the latter will be seen to exit the tibia and femur at intra-articular locations that either match, or are slightly offset from, the points occupied by the tips of the tibial and femoral aimer arms. This will depend on whether or not the drill guides were preset to provide an intentional guide pin offset (see below). The drill guides are removed and the guide pins are then overreamed with an appropriately sized cannulated bone drill. The internal entrances of the bone tunnels are meticulously radiused with an internal radiusing tool or arthroscopic bone tunnel rasps.

The tendon grafts are drawn up the tibial bone tunnel, across the joint, and out of the femoral tunnel. With tension placed on the grafts external to the femoral tunnel, the knee is brought through a range of motion while the degree and pattern of tendon excursion in and out of the femoral tunnel are observed externally. This should match the isometer gauge reading obtained just before the guide pins were drilled.

The intra-articular span of the graft is observed arthroscopically while the knee is brought through a full range of motion. It must be seen that no impingement of the graft by the roof of the intercondylar notch occurs in knee extension, and that no significant lateral (notch) wall contact abrasion occurs during knee motion. If either of these phenomena is observed, supplementary notch clearance is performed.

With firm manual tension on the grafts, they are fixed to the femur by the previously described stapling technique. The knee joint angle selected for graft tensioning and fixation depends on the graft excursion profile observed, as described above. With a perfectly isometric graft, the joint angle does not matter. With a "physiometric" graft length profile, i.e., one that matches the normal, slight deviation from isometry exhibited by the anteromedial fibers, a joint angle of 80 to 90 degrees of flexion is generally selected. This allows full knee extension without excessive graft tension.

Standard wound closure procedures are followed. Drains usually are not needed. A sterile electrical muscle stimulation electrode is placed over the distal vastus medialis, followed by application of a compression dressing. A long-leg rehabilitation brace is applied, its hinges generally set to allow joint motion from 20 to 90 degrees of flexion.

ECCENTRIC (OFFSET) GUIDE PIN PLACEMENT

As originally observed by Clancy and colleagues, ACL substitutes tend to lean toward the leading edges of their intra-articular bone tunnel entrances, producing an undesired shift in the effective fixation points of the graft. This effect is magnified when a radius is put on the tunnel entrance to minimize graft abrasion (Fig. 6). Tests in my laboratory using simulated bone tunnels and a variety of actual fresh tendon preparations have indicated that the degree of this graft shift error depends on the relative match between graft and tunnel diameters; well-fitted cylindric grafts shift the least and loosely fitted and/or flat (e.g., patellar tendon) grafts shift the most (Fig. 7). Special corrective graft positioning within the bone tunnel is often possible with bone-block grafts, but otherwise one or both of the bone tunnels must be drilled in a slightly offset or eccentric

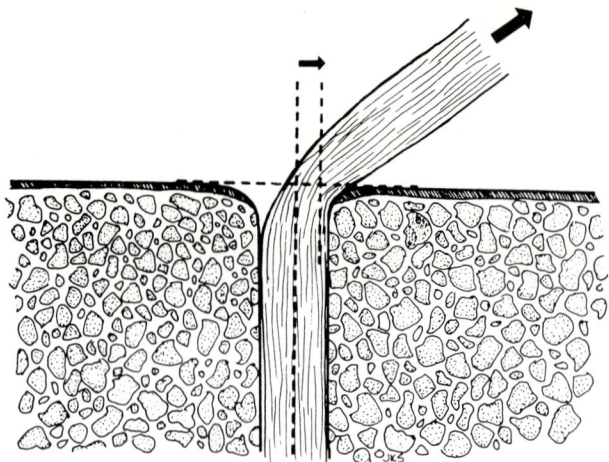

Figure 6 Schematic illustration of how the central fiber of a tendon graft shifts off center at an intra-articular bone tunnel entrance. (Reproduced with permission from ACL Drill Guide Instructional Manual. Andover, MA: Dyonics, Inc.)

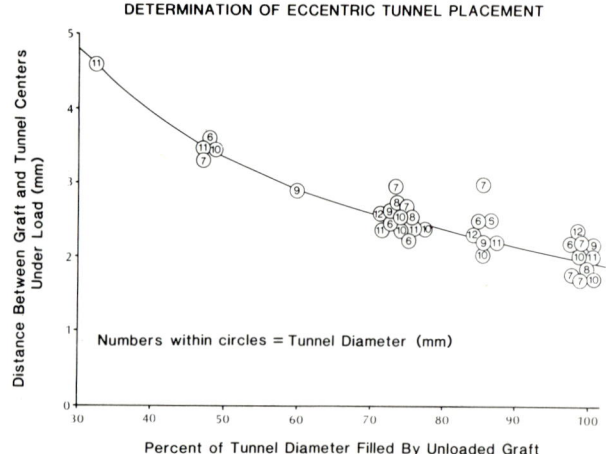

Figure 7 Graph of measured off-center tendon shift versus the relative size match between the graft and its tunnel. The more snugly a tendon graft is fitted in its tunnel, the less is the eccentric shift. The absolute tunnel diameter does not matter nearly as much as the relative fit of the graft within it.

location to the desired graft center points, to compensate for this error.

The drill guide system that I employ provides for a variable degree of eccentric guide pin (tunnel center) placement. A 3 mm offset is selected for the semitendinosus-gracilis graft. The orientation of the tibial guide's aimer arm, when positioned properly in the knee through the inferomedial portal, provides that its offset is in the desired anteromedial direction. When the femoral guide is properly placed in the knee, its orientation provides that its offset is in the "posterior" (arthroscopist's perspective) direction. No superior offset (toward the middle of the roof of the notch) is provided because this only applies to the *flexed* knee position, and tends to reverse itself in extension. In contrast, the posterior offset is applicable through the greater part of the functional range of knee motion.

POSTOPERATIVE REGIMEN

Electrical muscle stimulation (2 hours per day) and active range-of-motion exercise is begun within 72 hours. If no chondroplastic or meniscal repair work has been performed, weight bearing and careful ambulation are allowed as tolerated. Transfer from the long-leg rehabilitation brace to a functional ACL brace, stationary bike exercise, and isokinetic quadriceps work (limit, 30 degrees from full extension and using an "antishear" device) are generally instituted by the end of the third postoperative week. The rehabilitation regimen becomes progressively more active over time, straight running being allowed at 6 months and return to sport at 10 months.

SUGGESTED READING

Arms SW, Pope MH, Johnson RJ, et al. The biomechanics of anterior cruciate ligament rehabilitation and reconstruction. Am J Sports Med 1984; 12:8–18.

Clancy WG, Nelson DA, Reider B, et al. Anterior cruciate ligament reconstruction using one-third of the patellar ligament. J Bone Joint Surg 1982; 64A:352–359.

Girgis FG, Marshall JL, Al-Monagem ARS. The cruciate ligaments of the knee joint. Clin Orthop 1975; 106:216–231.

Graf B. Biomechanics of the anterior cruciate ligament. In: Jackson DW, Drez D, eds. The anterior cruciate deficient knee. St. Louis: CV Mosby, 1987:55.

Graf B. Isometric placement of substitutes for the anterior cruciate ligament. In: Jackson DW, Drez D, eds. The anterior cruciate deficient knee. St. Louis: CV Mosby, 1987:102.

Hollis JM, Marcin JP, Horibe S, et al. Load determination in ACL fiber bundles under knee loading. Trans Orthop Res Soc 1988; 13:58.

Lipscomb AB, Johnston RK, Snyder RB, et al. Evaluations of hamstring strength following use of semitendinosus and gracilis tendons to reconstruct the anterior cruciate ligament. Am J Sports Med 1982; 10:340–342.

Noyes FR, Butler DL, Grood ES, et al. Biomechanical analysis of human ligament grafts used in knee-ligament repairs and reconstructions. J Bone Joint Surg 1984; 66A:344–352.

Odensten M, Gillquist J. Functional anatomy of the anterior cruciate ligament and a rationale for reconstruction. J Bone Joint Surg 1985; 67A:257–261.

Rosenberg TD, Rasmussen GL. The function of the anterior cruciate ligament during anterior drawer and Lachman's testing. Am J Sports Med 1984; 12:318–322.

Roth JH, Kennedy JC, Lockstadt H, et al. Polypropylene braid augmented and nonaugmented intra-articular anterior cruciate ligament reconstruction. Am J Sports Med 1985; 13:321–336.

Sapega AA, Moyer RA, Schneck C, et al. Intraoperative "isometry" testing during anterior cruciate ligament reconstruction: anatomical and biomechanical considerations. Submitted for publication.

Sapega AA, Moyer RA, Schneck C, et al. The biomechanics of intra-operative "isometry" testing during anterior cruciate reconstruction. Trans Orthop Res Soc 1988; 13:130.

ARTHROSCOPICALLY ASSISTED RECONSTRUCTION OF THE ANTERIOR CRUCIATE LIGAMENT USING PATELLAR TENDON AUTOGRAFT

ROBERT D. BRONSTEIN, M.D.
KENNETH E. DeHAVEN, M.D.

The indications, technique, and postoperative care of anterior cruciate ligament (ACL) reconstruction have evolved considerably over the past 15 years and are continuing to evolve. Although much is now known regarding the anatomy of the ACL and of graft behavior, the techniques of reconstruction that have been developed result in at best an imperfect substitute for the normal ligament. Although our technique will continue to change as well, we present our currently preferred surgical treatment for the athlete with ACL deficiency.

This regimen has reliably provided good results and can be learned by most surgeons with advanced arthroscopic skills.

INDICATIONS FOR AND TIMING OF ACL RECONSTRUCTION

Although most individuals with ACL deficiency will experience functional instability and reinjuries if they continue to pursue activities that place high demands on their knees, we have had patients who function quite well even at the highest levels of demand. We therefore present operative and nonoperative options to all patients with an acute ACL injury and actively involve them and their families in the decision for initial surgical or nonsurgical treatment.

In the absence of multiple ligamentous disruption, ACL reconstruction is not recommended until the post-traumatic synovitis has resolved and the athlete has regained essentially full range of motion (ROM) of the knee. Although there is no absolute timetable, acute reconstruction is associated with a higher incidence of arthrofibrosis. We have found that most (but certainly not all) patients regain their motion sufficiently to lower their arthrofibrosis risk by 3 weeks from injury. As our therapy regimen is the same during this time frame for individuals undergoing operative or nonoperative treatment, it gives anyone who is uncertain about their choice the time to learn about the injury and make an informed decision regarding treatment.

PATIENT POSITIONING

Currently, most of our ACL reconstructions are performed under continuous epidural anesthesia, which is also utilized for early postoperative analgesia. A careful examination is performed under anesthesia to document the complete laxity profile and patients with a Grade III (grossly positive) pivot shift examination are treated with an iliotibial band tenodesis in addition to the intra-articular reconstruction.

The patient is positioned with a blanket roll under the thighs and both knees flexed 90 degrees over the end of the operating table (Fig. 1). An above knee (thigh high) compressive stocking is placed on the contralateral lower extremity and that foot is rested on a padded stool. A well-padded tourniquet is placed high on the operative thigh and a removable lateral post is positioned at the level of the distal femur. This set up allows access to the entire knee and distal thigh and allows for knee motion from full extension to 90 degrees of flexion. After the extremity is prepped and draped, the knee joint and portal sites are infiltrated with a total of 40 ml of 0.5% bupivacaine with epinephrine 1:200,000 equally mixed with 1% lidocaine to decrease intraoperative bleeding prior to tourniquet inflation.

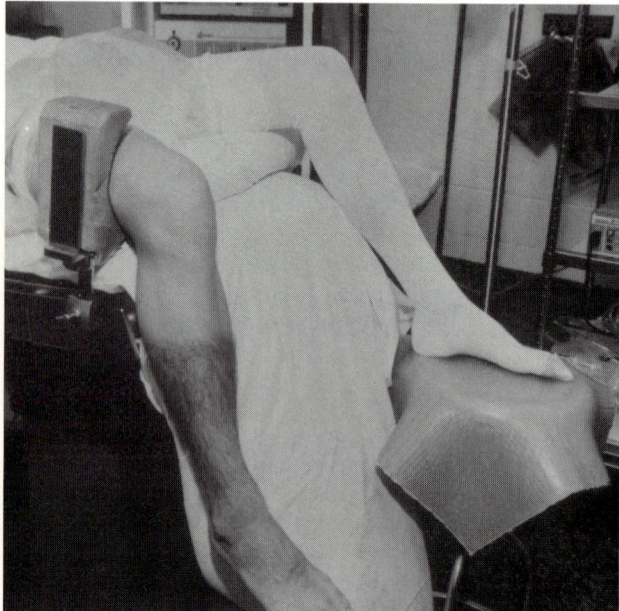

Figure 1 Patient positioning for a right ACL reconstruction. The operative extremity is positioned to allow full extension and flexion to at least 90 degrees. The nonoperative extremity is supported on a padded sitting stool.

OPERATIVE PROCEDURE

Our procedure for arthroscopically assisted reconstruction of the ACL is a two-incision technique using a central third patellar tendon autograft. We prefer this graft because of its strength and the advantages of the bone blocks for fixation. In addition, harvesting the graft is usually a surprisingly low morbidity procedure. While the concern is frequently raised about extensor mechanism problems associated with patellar tendon graft harvest, only one study to date has documented this to be the case and several other studies have reported no increase in the incidence of patellofemoral pain or quadriceps weakness.

The surgical procedure begins with a standard arthroscopic examination of the knee. We use an arthroscopic pump with the inflow through the arthroscope and outflow through a superior medial portal. Any meniscal pathology is addressed at this time. If a meniscus repair is indicated, the repair sutures are placed but are not tied until the completion of the ligament reconstruction unless open meniscus repair is carried out, when the repair is performed after the ACL reconstruction has been completed. The tibial stump and any remaining femoral fibers of the ACL are resected with a synovial resector and hand bitters. We routinely expose the lateral border of the posterior cruciate ligament (PCL) so it can be protected throughout the remainder of the procedure. Anterior synovium is also resected as required to provide visualization of the anterior horns of both menisci. The arthroscopic cautery is helpful for hemostasis during soft tissue debridement and is used to further resect the tibial stump of the ACL to the bone to aid in making the tibial tunnel.

Notchplasty

After the soft tissue has been cleared, we assess the need for a notchplasty. The purpose of the notchplasty is to allow adequate space for a 10 mm graft to lie between the lateral wall of the notch and PCL as well as to fully visualize the posterior outlet of the intercondylar notch (Fig. 2). A ridge of bone is usually present along the lateral wall of the notch anterior to the over-the-top position ("residents ridge"), and it is important not to mistake this ridge for the true posterior outlet. It is also important not to perform too extensive of a notchplasty, especially posteriorly, which will have the effect of lateralizing the femoral attachment of the graft. The notchplasty, when necessary, is performed with a 4.0 mm motorized burr and smoothed with a rasp.

Following adequate notchplasty we mark the point of the proposed femoral tunnel with the burr. This dimple indentation is centered approximately 7 mm anterior to the over-the-top position at the junction of the roof and sidewall of the notch, as the femoral tunnel is usually 10 or 11 mm in diameter. Ideally, there should be a thin posterior wall of bone after the femoral tunnel is drilled.

The arthroscopic pump and the cautery in conjunction with our preoperative injection of bupivacaine with

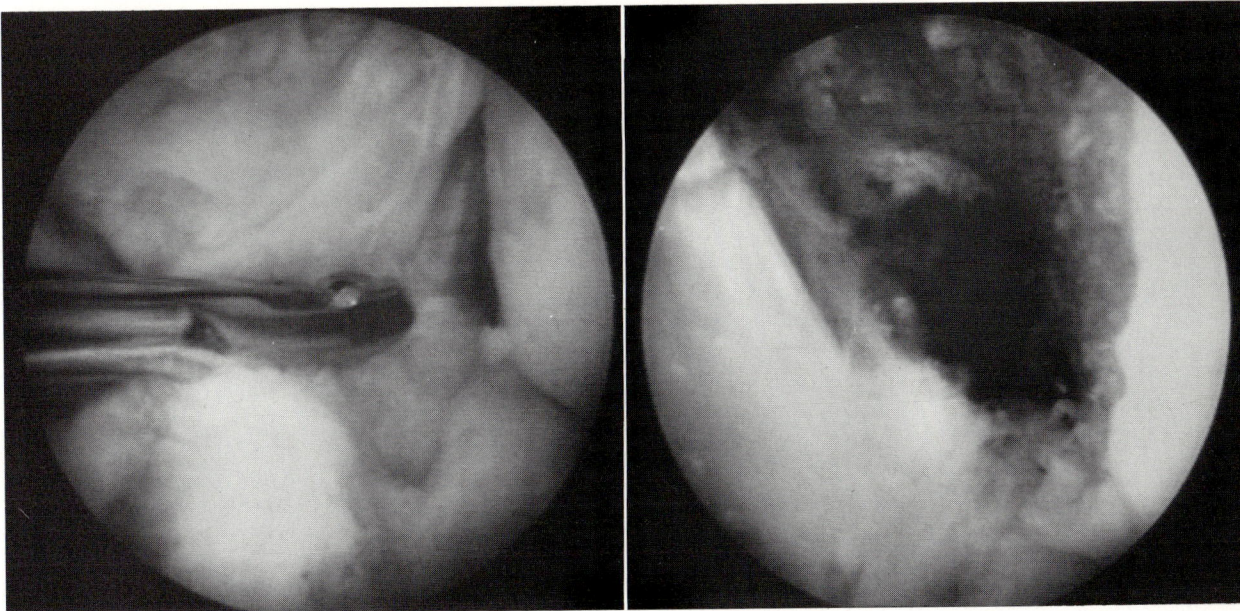

Figure 2 A probe on the posterior cruciate ligament demonstrates a stenotic notch (*A*), which is widened (*B*) to allow visualization of the notch outlet and provide space for a 10 mm graft.

epinephrine usually allows us to complete the notch-plasty without inflation of the tourniquet. Following the notchplasty, the extremity is exsanguinated with an esmarch bandage and the tourniquet is inflated. In an average sized patient we inflate the tourniquet to 150 mm Hg above the patient's systolic blood pressure. For larger thighs a higher pressure may be required.

Graft Harvest

Attention is then given to harvesting the graft. A mid-line anterior skin incision is made from the inferior pole of the patella to the tibial tubercle. Mobility of the patella usually allows the graft to be taken without extending the incision further proximally. The incision is deepened to the level of the paratenon of the patellar tendon. After nicking the paratenon with the scalpel, the paratenon is opened proximally and distally with the Metzenbaum scissors. The paratenon is then reflected medially and laterally to fully expose the patellar tendon.

The width of the patellar tendon is measured at it's mid point, and a central one-third graft is harvested. We use a fresh #10 scalpel blade keeping the knee flexed to provide tension on the tendon and using a forceps to hold the split open behind the blade. With this method we are able to visualize tendon fibers and keep our incision from cutting across the fibers. For this reason we do not use double blade knives.

When the split has been completed to the inferior pole of the patella and to the tibial tubercle the knee is extended and the foot placed on a padded Mayo stand. The tendon incisions are then extended over the tibial tubercle for a distance of 2.5 cm, taking care to protect the lateral and medial tendon insertions. The medial and lateral incisions are then connected with a transverse incision.

An oscillating saw is then utilized to make the initial bone cuts in the tibial tubercle. Taking note of the width of the saw blade and accounting for the path of the blade oscillations, 10 mm deep cuts are made. The transverse cut is made with a ¼ inch straight osteotome, which is also utilized to complete the cuts and remove the bone block. We make the block as rectangular in shape as possible so that it can be fashioned and shaped to best fit the round bone tunnels.

To make the patellar cuts, tension is applied from the tibial bone block through the graft while the assistant applies thumb pressure to the superior pole of the patella (Fig. 3). This delivers the patella into the wound, thereby avoiding a larger incision. The patellar cuts are made similar to the tibial cuts except the transverse cut is made with the saw to minimize potential damage to the patellofemoral joint from hitting on the osteotome. A patient with a small patella may require taking a shorter bone block to avoid injury to the quadriceps tendon.

The bone plugs are then fashioned with a rongeur and sized using cylinders that will match a round hole. The graft should easily pass through the hole in the sizer but should fill the hole as completely as possible. The bone that is removed from the bone blocks is saved. Two holes are made in each block from the cancellous surface with a short-chucked guide wire and a #5 Ethibond suture is passed through each hole. The graft is kept moist in a kidney basin, which is placed inside an instrument basket to prevent it from being accidentally discarded or knocked off the scrub table.

Tunnel Placement

A 5 cm lateral incision is then made extending proximally from the lateral epicondyle in line with the iliotibial band (ITB). The adipose tissue is reflected from

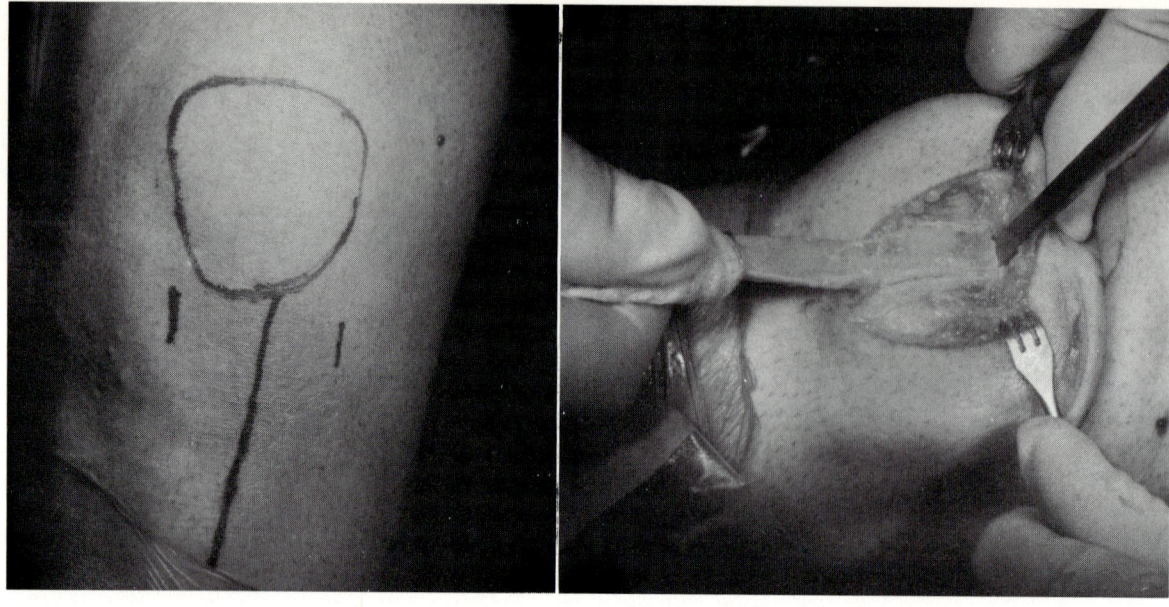

A   B

Figure 3 An incision is made from the inferior pole of the patella to the tibial tubercle (*A*). By applying traction to the graft and with thumb pressure on the superior pole, the patella can be delivered into the incision without extending the incision (*B*).

the ITB with a dry sponge and the ITB is incised in line with its fibers 2.5 cm anterior to its posterior border. The vastus lateralis muscle is elevated from the ITB and the lateral intramuscular septum to expose the lateral femur. Distally, perforating branches of the lateral superior geniculate artery will be encountered and should be cauterized.

The arthroscope is then reinserted and any clotted blood is removed with the synovial resector. The Acufex Protract tibial drill guide (Acufex Micosurgical, Mansfield, Mass.) is set at 50 degrees with the tip placed directly anterior to the PCL off the edge of the medial tibial spine ("J" ridge) and the external barrel set medial to the tibial tubercle and above the superior border of the pes anserinus. The guide wire is drilled into place. This position within the posterior portion of the ACL tibial insertion should prevent the graft from impinging on the roof of the notch when the knee is in full extension. Although the normal ACL has a broad tibial insertion that extends anterior to this point, the anterior insertion of the normal ligament is flattened, and this anatomy cannot be reproduced with a graft.

After its position is verified, the guide wire is overdrilled to the appropriate diameter, taking care to avoid diverging from and cutting the guide wire. We "catch" the drill in a curette inside the joint to protect the PCL and femoral articular cartilage.

An Acufex femoral gaff that has been modified with reduced radius of curvature is then passed (under direct arthroscopic visualization) from the anteromedial portal past the over-the-top position and out the lateral wound. Care is taken to keep the gaff in contact with the posterior condyle during passage. A #2 nylon suture (Excursion Filament, Dyonics, Inc., Andover, Mass.) is tied to the gaff prior to passage for use with isometry.

The suture is then removed from the gaff and passed through the hole in a modified rear entry femoral drill guide (Acufex Microsurgical, Mansfield, Mass.) (Fig. 4). The rear entry guide is brought back into the knee with the gaff and gaff is disengaged. The guide is seated into the previously made dimple and the suture is pulled through the tibial tunnel with the nerve hook. Isometry can then be performed from the proposed femoral tunnel through the tibial tunnel (Fig. 5). We aim for 2 mm or less excursion as the knee is brought from full flexion to full extension with the tightening occurring in extension. If our proposed position yields unsatisfactory excursion, the location of the femoral guide can be adjusted anteriorly or posteriorly until the excursion is acceptable before the guide pin is inserted.

The femoral tunnel guide wire is then drilled from the lateral femur at the flare of metaphysis. Care is taken to assure a sufficiently anterior entry point on the lateral surface of the femur so that a 10 to 11 mm drill hole will not break out the posterior cortex. If the K-wire is correctly positioned it is overdrilled under arthroscopic control, using a curette through the anteromedial portal to protect the PCL from the drill bit. The resulting tunnel should have a thin shell of bone posteriorly.

Tunnel preparation is completed with the Gore Smoother TM (W.L. Gore & Associates, Inc., Flagstaff, Az.) that is passed from proximal to distal. While applying a posterior force on the smoother to prevent anterior tunnel drift, the tunnels are rasped and champhored as the knee is brought through a ROM from 90 degrees to full extension. The Smoother should move easily in all knee positions, especially in complete extension, thus assuring the absence of notch impingement (Fig. 6).

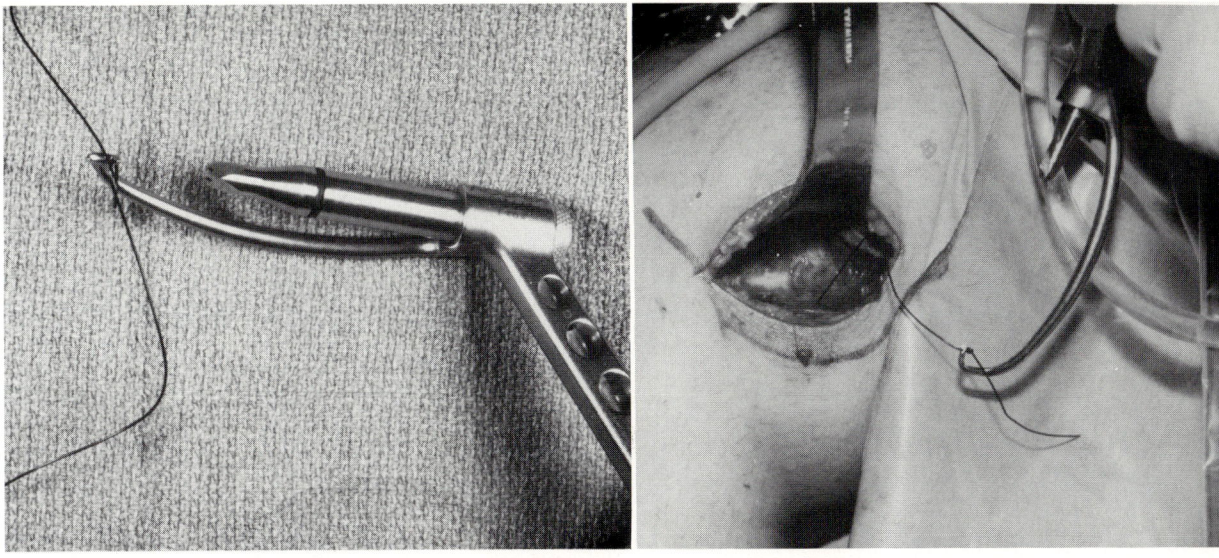

Figure 4 *A,* Acufex femoral drill guide modified with a drill hole to allow placement of a #2 suture. *B,* The guide with the attached suture may be placed at the proposed femoral site for isometric testing prior to drilling the femoral tunnel.

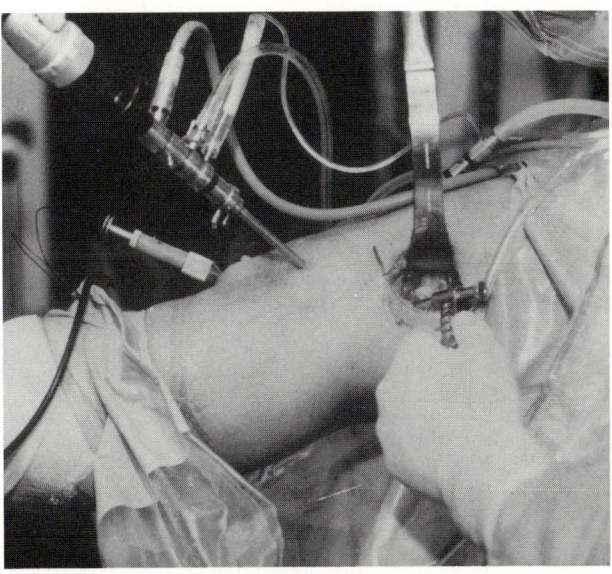

Figure 5 Isometry is tested as the knee is brought from full extension to 90 degrees of flexion. No more than 2 mm of excursion should be accepted.

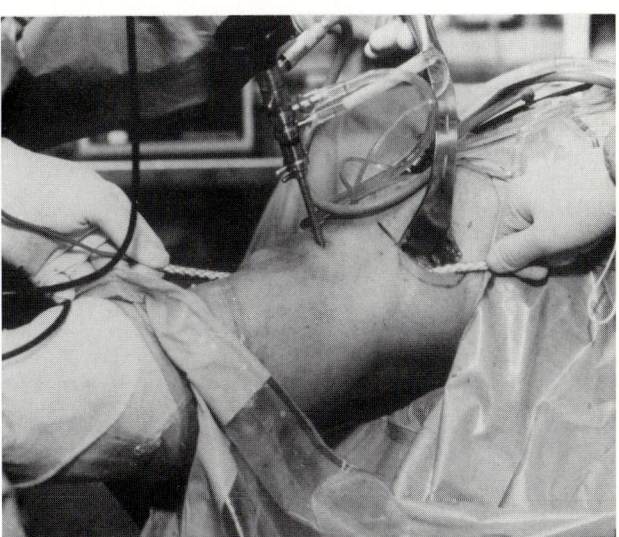

Figure 6 Easy movement of the Gore Smoother as the knee is brought to full extension from 90 degrees of flexion assures the absence of notch impingement. Posterior pressure is applied as the Smoother is used to prevent anterior tunnel drift.

Graft Insertion and Fixation

The patellar tendon graft sutures are then pulled through the joint from proximal to distal using the Smoother as it is removed from the joint. The graft is then pulled through the joint with the knee slightly flexed. It is important that both tunnel entrances are clear of soft tissue to allow smooth graft passage.

We pass the graft with the cancellous surface directed anteriorly and the femoral block all the way to the bottom of the femoral tunnel, which puts the tendon as posterior as possible in the femoral tunnel. With the tibial bone block entirely within its tunnel, we secure the bone block with a cannulated interference screw. The screw is positioned inferiorly in the tunnel to place as much bone as possible between the screw and the tibial plateau.

Proximal fixation is achieved with an obliquely directed bicortical 4.5 mm malleolar screw and washer (Synthes, Paoli, Pa.). The screw is placed 1.5 cm proximal to the lateral entrance to the femoral tunnel and is obliquely directed from distal to proximal (Fig. 7). The sutures through the femoral bone block are then securely tied over the screw and washer with the knee near full extension. By using a screw 5 to 10 mm longer

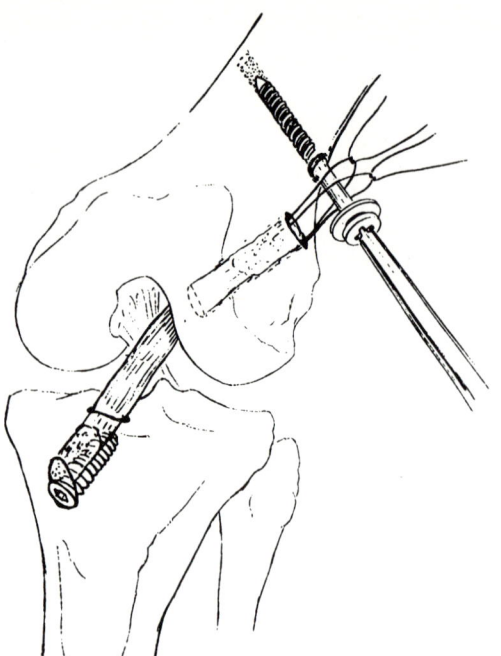

Figure 7 Femoral fixation is performed by tensioning over an obliquely placed Synthes 4.5 mm malleolar screw and washer with the knee in full extension. Tension can later be adjusted by advancing or reversing the screw. (From Diment MT, Sebastianelli WJ, DeHaven KE. Arthroscopically assisted anterior cruciate ligament reconstruction using a central-third patellar tendon autograft and two incisions. Op Tech Sports Med 1993; 1:45–49; with permission.)

than the measured length, the graft can be tensioned after fixation by advancing the screw.

The knee is then placed through a ROM and stabilities rechecked. The graft is visualized and probed to recheck graft tension. If necessary, we can increase the tension of the graft by advancing the obliquely directed femoral fixation screw.

If preoperative examination revealed a Grade III (grossly positive) pivot shift, an ITB tenodesis is then performed. The posterior portion of the split ITB is held firmly to a spot 1 cm proximal and posterior to the lateral epicondyle (Krackow's point) as the knee is brought through a full ROM. If the ITB is easily held in its position without undue tension throughout a ROM it is fixed to this spot (after denuding and "fish-scaling" the cortex) with a low profile screw with soft tissue washer (Concept Linvatec, Largo, Fla.).

At the completion of the cruciate reconstruction, any meniscal repair sutures are tied, the tourniquet is deflated, and hemostasis is obtained. The ITB is reapproximated with interrupted absorbable sutures. The bone saved from trimming the bone blocks and from drilling the tunnels is firmly tamped into the patellar defect and also the tibial tubercle defect if there is sufficient bone. The paratenon is closed over the tendon defect, leaving the tendon itself alone. The remainder of closure is in a standard fashion. Suction drains are utilized.

POSTOPERATIVE CARE AND FOLLOW-UP

Postoperatively, the patient is placed in a long leg hinged knee splint locked at full extension. Passive ROM and quadriceps and hamstring isometric exercises are begun on the first postoperative day. Prophylactic antibiotics are continued for 24 hours postoperatively. Touchdown weight bearing begins on the second day and the patient is discharged on the second or third postoperative day.

At 10 to 14 days the patient is seen in the office and the brace is unlocked during the day. We continue locking the brace in extension at night until 6 weeks after surgery. While early weight bearing is routinely progressed as tolerated (with the brace locked in extension), whenever meniscus repair has also been performed progression to full weight bearing is delayed until after 6 weeks after surgery. Progressive resistance exercises for the quadriceps are limited from 90 to 60 degrees to prevent undue graft forces until 5 months postoperatively. Return to full sports is allowed when full criteria are met after 7 months (average 9 months). We recommend using an ACL brace for high-risk activities (in the hope of helping prevent reinjuries) for at least the initial year after returning to sports.

SUGGESTED READING

Acker JH, Drez D. Angulation of fixation screw in knee ligament procedure. Orthopaedics 1989; 12:823–826.

Cosgarea AJ, Sebastianelli WJ, DeHaven KE. Prevention of arthrofibrois following ACL reconstruction using one third patellar tendon autograft. Am J Sports Med (in press).

Furia JP, Zambetti GJ. An injection technique to create a bloodless field in arthroscopically assisted anterior cruciate ligament reconstruction. Am J Sports Med 1992; 20:406–409.

Graf B, Uhr F. Complications of intra-articular anterior cruciate ligament reconstruction. Clin Sports Med 1980; 7:835–848.

Howell SM, Taylor MA. Failure of reconstruction of the anterior cruciate ligament due to impingement by the intercondylar roof. J Bone Joint Surg 1993; 75A:1044–1055.

Lephart SM, Fu FH, Harner CD. Effects of two selected anterior cruciate ligament reconstructions on the quadriceps mechanism and functional status of athletes. Presented at AAOSM Annual Meeting, Orlando, Fla., 1991.

Lephart SM, Kocher MS, Harner CD, Fu FH. Quadriceps, strength and functional capacity after anterior cruciate ligament reconstruction: Patellar tendon autograft versus allograft. Am J Sports Med 1993; 21:738–743.

Levitt R, Uribe J, Michalow A. The effect of removal of mid third patellar tendon on return of quadriceps strength in ACL reconstruction. Presented at AOSSM Annual Meeting, Orlando, Fla., 1991.

Noyes FR, Butler D, Paulos LE. Intra-articular cruciate reconstruction. I: Perspectives on graft strengths, vascularization, and immediate motion after replacement. Clin Orthop 1983; 172:71–77.

Re LP, Weiss RA, Rintz KG, et al. Anterior knee pain in the anterior cruciate ligament reconstructed knee. Presented at American Academy of Orthoapedic Surgeons 12th Annual Meeting, AOSSM Specialty Day, San Francisco, 1993.

Strum GM, Friedman MJ, Fox JM. Acute anterior cruciate ligament reconstruction. Clin Orthop 1990; 253:184–189.

Warren R, Sgaglione NA, Wickiewicz T, et al. Primary repair with semitendinosis tendon augmentation of acute anterior cruciate ligament injuries. Am J Sports Med 1990; 18(1):64–73.

ARTHROSCOPICALLY ASSISTED ANTERIOR CRUCIATE LIGAMENT RECONSTRUCTION USING PATELLAR TENDON GRAFT AND ENDOSCOPIC TECHNIQUE

ANDREW M. WONG, M.D.
PETER A. INDELICATO, M.D.

Since the first published reports of anterior cruciate ligament (ACL) replacement, the surgical techniques have undergone a multitude of changes and refinements. With the development of the arthroscope, a new generation in ACL surgery was introduced as better visualization of the knee with less surgical trauma became possible. The surgical options have been expanded even further as a variety of natural tissues and synthetic materials have been used as ligament substitutes with varying degrees of success. The use of autogenous tissue, however, remains the "gold standard" and is the preferred source of graft among our patients. We currently only use bone-patellar tendon-bone constructs and our surgical technique has evolved from a two-incision technique to a one-incision arthroscopically assisted procedure. This chapter shares our method of endoscopic reconstruction and discusses the goals and potential pitfalls to successful surgery.

RATIONALE

Most surgeons currently use either hamstring tendon or patellar tendon as the primary sources of autograft tissues. Patellar tendon grafts with accompanying patellar tibial bone have the distinct advantage of long-term bone-to-bone healing and the bony surfaces allow utilization of interference screws for internal fixation that can be placed arthroscopically. By performing the operation predominantly through the arthroscope, we avoid extensive dissection of the knee joint and exposure of the interior to the ambient environment with desiccation of the articular cartilage. Avoiding an arthrotomy leads to less disruption of the normal anatomy with less pain, edema, and hemarthrosis in the immediate postoperative period. The decrease in discomfort may allow for faster mobilization and prevent painful inhibition of quadriceps activity. The arthroscope gives excellent visualization of the ACL attachment sites for thorough debridement without damaging adjacent structures such as the posterior cruciate ligament and menisci. It also promotes precise graft placement, particularly on the femoral side where the intercondylar ridge (residents' ridge) and soft tissue can obscure visualization of the "over-the-top" position. The replacement graft can be examined dynamically through the arthroscope for evidence of impingement or laxity at various joint positions.

We offer all our patients the option of using allograft bone-tendon-bone tissue, but only approximately 30% choose to use this tissue source. The primary reason for refusal of donor patellar tendon and bone is the potential risk of disease transmission. Although estimates in the orthopedic literature place the risk of contracting the human immunodeficiency virus (HIV) at approximately one in a million, the magnitude of this risk and the chance of hepatitis transmission are interpreted differently by each patient. Since we cannot guarantee the safety of each piece of donor tissue, we make no personal recommendations regarding tissue choice and leave the final decision to each individual. The only instance in which we do not offer the use of allograft tissue is in the patient with multiple failed allograft ACL reconstructions. In this limited group, we prefer autograft patellar tendon if available with the hope that the patient's own tissue will lead to better graft incorporation and lower chance of failure.

SURGICAL TECHNIQUE

Arthroscopy and Graft Harvesting

ACL reconstruction through our endoscopic technique begins with a thorough examination of the involved limb under anesthesia followed by an arthroscopic evaluation. A tourniquet is placed around the upper thigh, but is generally not used during the diagnostic arthroscopy in order to maximize tourniquet time during the reconstructive portion of the operation. A standard diagnostic arthroscopy is performed by placing our inflow cannula in the superolateral portal and the arthroscope through an anterolateral portal. The anteromedial portal is larger and placed more anterior than the usual "soft spot" portal to provide better access to the femoral tunnel and subsequent interference screw placement (Fig. 1). During the arthroscopy, any associated meniscal injuries are addressed and the integrity of the articular cartilage is noted and recorded via intraoperative photographs or videotape.

For those patients who are particularly concerned about cosmesis, harvesting of the patellar tendon graft can be performed as the first step. Following removal of the graft, the medial and lateral skin edges can be retracted away from the midline and the anterolateral and anteromedial arthroscopy portals can be established directly through the joint capsule without penetrating the skin and creating additional scars.

We harvest the central one-third or 10 mm of the patellar tendon through a longitudinal incision that is placed slightly medial to the midline. By placing the incision closer to the medial edge of the patellar tendon, a second incision over the tibia is not necessary during the creation of the tibial tunnel. The harvesting incision can simply be retracted distally to obtain access to the anteromedial surface of the tibia at the level of the tibial

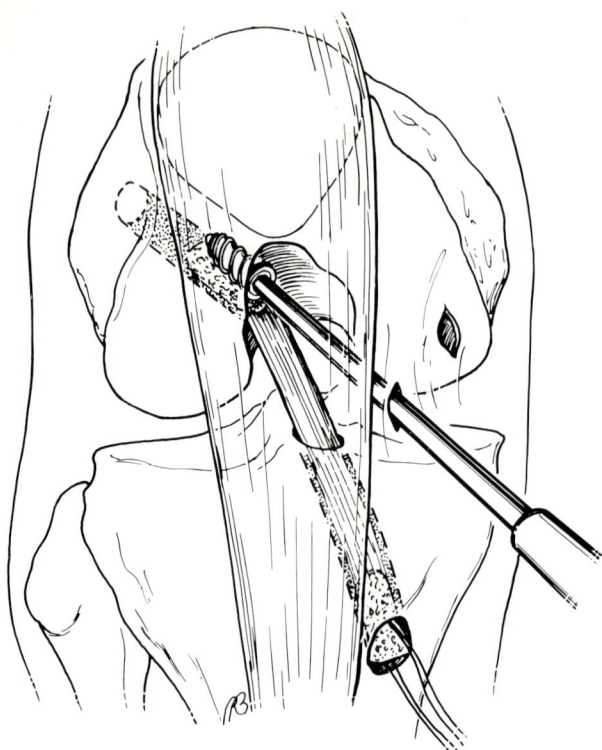

Figure 1 The anteromedial portal should be placed just medial to the edge of the patellar tendon and just above the joint line for subsequent femoral interference screw placement. A standard soft-spot portal will make this screw placement difficult because the medial femoral condyle will obstruct placement. (From Christian/Indelicato: Allograft anterior cruciate ligament reconstruction with patellar tendon: An endoscopic technique. Op Tech Sports Med 1993; 1(1); with permission.)

tubercle. The skin incision is begun at the inferior pole of the patellar and ends at the proximal portion of the tibial tubercle. There is a fair amount of skin mobility in the superior-inferior direction and this should be assessed prior to incision so that the shortest possible skin incision is made. The incision is taken down through the subcutaneous tissues and onto the patellar tendon sheath. A small cut is made in the sheath and it is then divided longitudinally with Metzenbaum scissors. Distally the sheath blends in intimately with the tendon and can be difficult to identify. A graft 10 mm wide is measured in the center of the tendon and parallel longitudinal incisions are made through the tendon along its entire length. Counter pressure applied to the tendon as it is divided makes it easier to follow the orientation of the fibers and maintain a constant graft width. Avoid penetrating the patellar fat pad during harvesting as disruption will lead to fluid extravasation and some loss of visibility and distention during the procedure.

Several cutting guides and jigs are available to assist in the patellar and tibial osteotomies but we find these unnecessary and perform the bone cuts free-hand. The bone plugs should also be 10 mm wide and approxi-

mately 20 mm long. The periosteum overlying the bone is incised and then a small oscillating saw is used to first make the longitudinal cuts in the bone. The blade is held perpendicular to the bony surface of the patella and angles inward on the tibia to create a triangular-shaped bone plug. The longitudinal cuts are connected by a transverse cut with extreme care to connect the corners of the osteotomies to prevent fracture or splintering of the bone as it is removed. A one-quarter inch osteotome is placed into the patellar saw cuts first and the bone block is elevated out of its bed. This block and the patellar tendon are then lifted distally as the soft tissue connected to the underside of the tendon is sharply divided. For the tibial bone plug, a second horizontal osteotomy is made with the osteotome just proximal to the site of bony attachment of the patellar tendon. This will allow the bone block to be taken out of the tibia without involving the anterior articular surface of the proximal tibia.

Once the graft is taken out of the knee, it is placed on the back table where the tibial bone plug is further contoured to a triangular shape, which facilitates passage into the femoral tunnel and provides a large, bony surface for internal fixation. The patellar bone plug is modified to a trapezoidal shape with the free edge wider for press fitting into the tibial tunnel (Fig. 2). The patellar bone plug and its corresponding tibial tunnel are at least as large as the tibial bone plug and its femoral tunnel, but we often make them 1 mm larger to make graft passage easier through the tibia en route to the femur. Two 1.5 mm drill holes are made through each bone plug and a no. 5 nonabsorbable Tevdek or TiCron suture is passed. The holes must be placed away from the edge of the plug to prevent fracture when tension is applied to the sutures. These sutures will act as "handles" for graft passage and can also be tied over a screw for fixation if interference screws cannot be utilized.

The patellar tendon defect is closed with interrupted 2-0 absorbable suture. We prefer to repair the tendon with figure-of-eight sutures placed in the deep posterior substance of the tissue. This avoids strangulation of the full thickness of the tendon and permits the anterior half of the tendon to heal without tension. The patellar tendon sheath is closed as a separate layer to prevent scarring of the tendon to the sheath and interference with normal gliding and nutrition.

The arthroscope is returned to the knee through the previously established portals and the ACL graft site is prepared.

Tunnel Preparation

The old ACL is debrided using a 4 or 5 mm aggressive meniscal shaver or full radius resector. An understanding of the anatomic shape of the tibial ACL attachment is essential to allow for adequate debridement without inadvertently resecting the intermeniscal ligament or damaging the tibial attachment of the menisci. An appreciation of the fan-shaped ACL footprint also aids in placement of the new graft at the

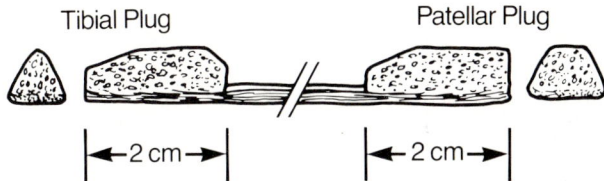

Figure 2 Specially contoured bone plugs at either end of the preparation facilitate graft passage, screw placement and interference or press fit (see text). (From Christian/Indelicato: Allograft anterior cruciate ligament reconstruction with patellar tendon: An endoscopic technique. Op Tech Sports Med 1993; 1(1); with permission.)

proper site (Fig. 3). For stenotic intercondylar notches, a notchplasty is performed by removing bone from the medial wall of the lateral femoral condyle at the entrance of the notch. The amount of bone to be removed depends on the degree of stenosis and often up to 5 mm of bone will be taken away to provide adequate exposure. This is done best with a one-quarter inch osteotome or 6 mm round or egg-shaped burr. Any remaining soft tissue attached to the lateral wall of the notch is removed at this time with particular attention paid to any tissue blocking the "over-the-top" position. The anterior intercondylar ridge (residents' ridge) can be mistaken for the true over-the-top position and this area must be debrided smooth to avoid this error and to provide visualization of the correct position. Bone is not resected routinely from the anterior aspect of the roof of the intercondylar notch unless impingement of the graft in extension is noted after placement.

After the notchplasty and debridement of the lateral wall of the intercondylar notch is completed, a pilot hole for the femoral tunnel is selected. A point 5 to 6 mm anterior to the over-the-top position and the junction of the roof and the wall is identified and marked with a small angled curette. The distance from the over-the-top position to this point should be equal to one-half the diameter of the bone plug to be used on the femoral side. If the roof of the intercondylar notch represents 12 o'clock on the clock face, this point is placed at the 1 o'clock position for a left knee and at the 11 o'clock position for a right knee. This results in an appropriate sized femoral tunnel with an intact back wall of bone approximately 1 to 2 mm thick. A tunnel placed too far posteriorly can result in a deficient back wall as a result of fracturing through the back of the tunnel at the time of reaming, which preludes the use of interference fixation. The pilot hole can then be widened with either a curette or burr. It is important to make the pilot hole large enough to identify during the "dry" phase of the arthroscopy when bleeding can often obscure the surface of the bone.

A variety of tibial drill guides are available for ACL reconstruction, but they are all based on essentially the same principles. In the system we use, the tibial drill guide is designed such that the tip of the guide is placed in the center of the old ACL footprint just lateral to the medial intercondylar eminence. Depending on the type of system used, the tip of the guide will be anywhere from

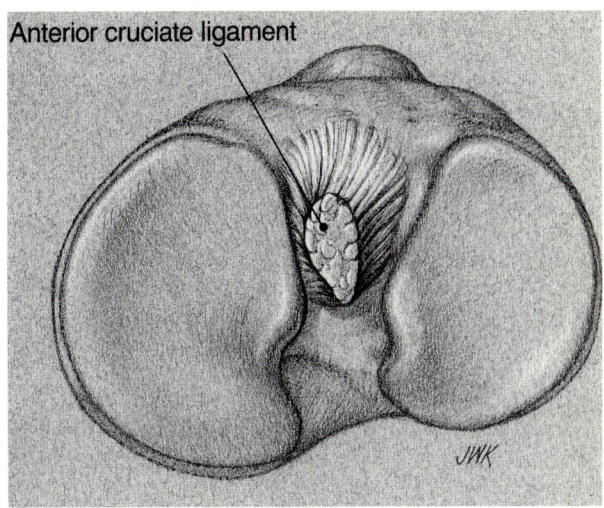

Figure 3 Note the fan-shaped tibial attachment site. (From Brown/Indelicato: Complications of anterior cruciate ligament reconstruction. Op Tech Orthop 1992; 2(2):125–135; with permission.)

5 to 7 mm anterior to the posterior cruciate ligament (PCL). The main goal is for the tibial tunnel to be centrally placed in the site of the old ACL attachment to prevent impingement, divergent tunnel angles, or mechanical insufficiency in resisting tibial translation (Fig. 4). With the tip of the guide placed through the anteromedial portal and into the ACL footprint, the tibial drill sleeve is placed against the medial aspect of the proximal tibia. A point 5 to 6 cm below the joint line and just medial to the tibial tubercle should be selected. The length of the tibial tunnel must be sufficient to keep the patellar plug contained within the bony tunnel for potential interference fit fixation and this can be ensured by drilling a tunnel that subtends an angle of 50 to 60 degrees with the horizontal (Fig. 5). A tunnel that is more proximal and horizontally oriented will be too short and have an increased risk of fracturing through the thinned anterior cortex of the tibia. A longer, more vertically oriented tunnel will be too long and may make access to the femoral pilot hole through the tibial tunnel impossible.

The location of the drill sleeve is then marked on the tibia, a periosteal flap is raised, and a 1 by 1 cm area of tibial bone is exposed. Extend the previously made skin incision 1 to 2 cm if it does not have enough mobility to expose the necessary tibial surface. With the knee in 75 to 90 degrees of flexion the drill sleeve is placed against the bone and a 2.4 mm guide pin is drilled from the anteromedial face of the tibia into the center of the ACL footprint. The guide pin is advanced far enough to demonstrate that it will remain just lateral to the PCL and not impinge on its fibers. The aiming device is removed and a cannulated reamer is placed over the guide pin. The size of the reamer should correlate with the size of the patellar bone plug determined at the start of the case. The reamer is advanced over the guide pin until it can be seen within the joint with care taken to

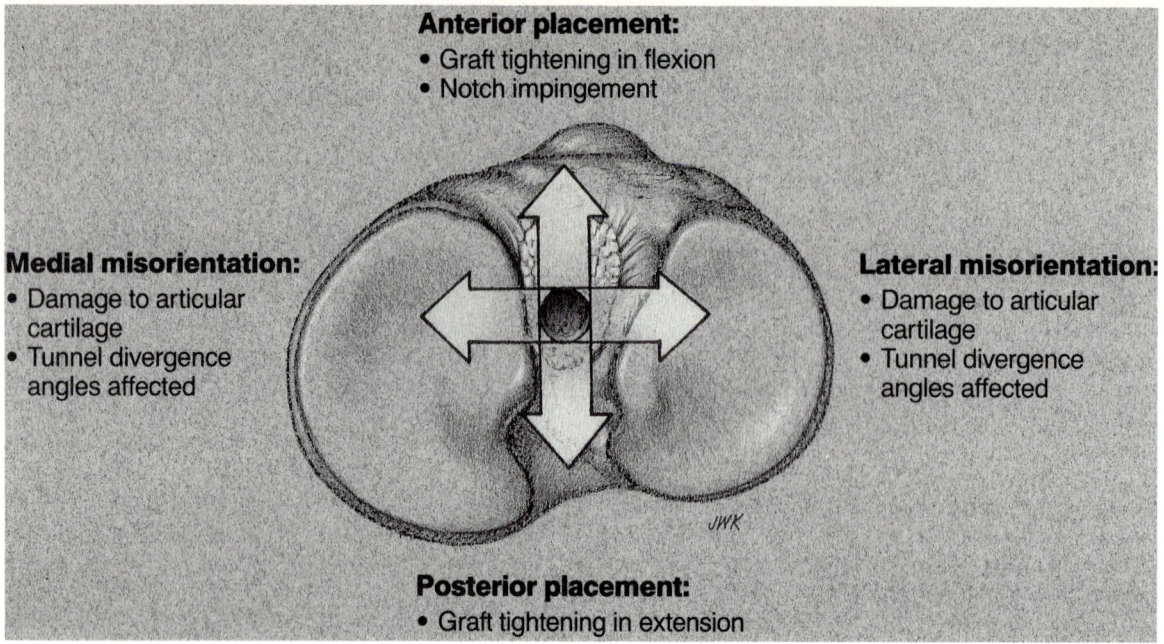

Anterior placement:
• Graft tightening in flexion
• Notch impingement

Medial misorientation:
• Damage to articular cartilage
• Tunnel divergence angles affected

Lateral misorientation:
• Damage to articular cartilage
• Tunnel divergence angles affected

Posterior placement:
• Graft tightening in extension

Figure 4 Improper placement of tibial drill hole could lead to an increased incidence of postoperative failure. (From Brown/Indelicato: Complications of anterior cruciate ligament reconstruction. Op Tech Orthop 1992; 2(2):125–135; with permission.)

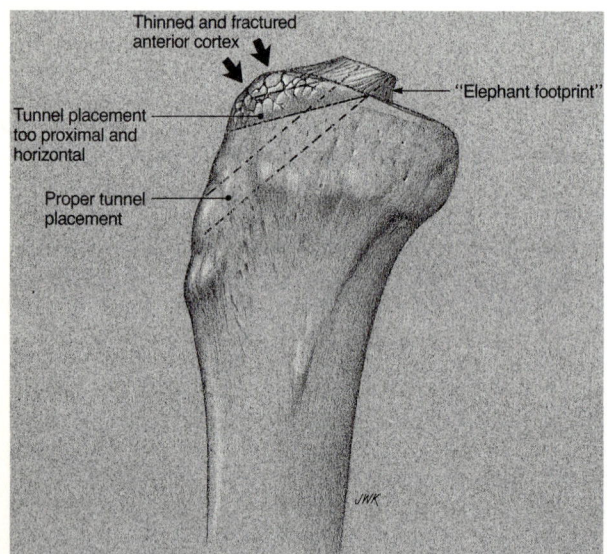

Thinned and fractured anterior cortex

Tunnel placement too proximal and horizontal

"Elephant footprint"

Proper tunnel placement

Figure 5 Appropriate placement of the tibial drill hole is located on the posterior "footprint" of the tibial attachment site. (From Brown/Indelicato: Complications of anterior cruciate ligament reconstruction. Op Tech Orthop 1992; 2(2): 125–135; with permission.)

prevent injury to the PCL. The bone shavings from the reaming are saved for later use as bone graft. The knee is then irrigated and a plug is placed in the entrance of the tibial tunnel to allow the knee to be reinflated with saline. A combination of curette, arthroscopic shaver, and burr is used to chamfer the back wall and lip of the newly created tunnel to prevent graft impingement or wear against sharp bony edges. This will also assist in the removal of any remaining ACL stump, which is often found around the edges of the tunnel. The knee is then drained of all fluid and the femoral tunnel is prepared.

The knee is flexed to 90 degrees and the leg is placed over the edge of the table. A second 2.4 mm guide pin is passed through the tibial tunnel and its tip is placed in the previously selected pilot hole. If the hole is obscured by blood, the inflow may be turned on to flush the joint. Otherwise, the inflow should remain off to decrease fluid loss through the tibial tunnel. Since this guide pin crosses the knee joint, extreme care should be taken to prevent any flexion or extension of the limb. If motion of the knee occurs, the guide pin will bend and reaming will become difficult and lead to possible pin breakage. The guide pin is advanced until it engages or exits through the lateral cortex of the femur. The pin must be securely in bone to allow for over-reaming and accurate tunnel alignment. A reamer that corresponds to the size of the tibial tubercle bone plug is then placed over the guide wire. To avoid damage to the PCL, this reamer is passed manually through the tibial tunnel and tapped gently with a mallet. Once it has safely passed the PCL and is against the bone of the lateral wall of the intercondylar notch, it is tightened onto a drill and the guide pin is over-reamed until it exits the lateral femoral cortex. The reamer is backed out of the femoral tunnel and once the tip can be seen within the knee, it is pulled out manually to again avoid damage to the PCL. The guide pin may remain within the reamer and be removed at the same time or it may stay engaged in the bone. If the pin comes out with the reamer, the tip should be inspected to confirm that the pin did not break from binding against the reamer and that it was removed in its entirety.

The entrance of the femoral tunnel must be chamfered smooth to prevent impingement or damage to the allograft. In a fashion similar to chamfering the tibial tunnel, a curette is passed through the anteromedial portal and the anterior edge of the tunnel is gently smoothed and all bone reamings are removed. At this time, the tunnel is inspected and the back wall is measured and checked for evidence of fracture or "blow out." As mentioned previously, a competent back wall should be approximately 1 to 2 mm thick. It can be probed with a nerve hook anteriorly through the entrance and posteriorly from the over-the-top position. If the back wall of the femoral tunnel is blown out, then interference fixation is not possible and screw and washer fixation is necessary.

Once the femoral tunnel has been reamed and chamfered, a large Beath pin is passed through the tibial tunnel and guided into the femoral tunnel under arthroscopic visualization. This is best done with the knee held in 90 degrees of flexion over the edge of the table. The Beath pin we use has an eye at its base similar to a large sewing needle and a slotted groove down its entire length (Fig. 6). This groove accommodates a smaller guide pin that can be used for the cannulated interference screw. The Beath pin is firmly advanced until its tip exits out the lateral thigh. The sutures attached to the tibial bone plug (femoral side) are threaded through the eye of the pin and are brought out to the skin surface as the pin is pulled all the way through and out the thigh (Fig. 7). A clamp is placed on the ends of the sutures and used to pull the tibial bone plug through the tibial tunnel and into the femoral tunnel under direct arthroscopic guidance. Just before the tibial bone plug enters the femoral tunnel, the patellar bone plug will usually wedge itself against the entrance of the tibial tunnel. This bone plug can be gently advanced by tapping its base with a bone tamp as constant tension is applied to the sutures exiting the anterolateral thigh. Arthroscopically, the tibial bone block and patellar tendon should be seen to advance as a unit. Before it is firmly engaged in the femoral tunnel, the position of the graft must be checked to ensure that it is oriented in the optimum position.

The tendon side of the graft should be placed posteriorly to reproduce more closely the normal orientation of the anteromedial portion of the ACL on the femur. The patellar bone plug is rotated 90 degrees to place its cortical side on the medial wall of the tibial tunnel. This effectively rotates the graft and places the tendon "on edge" to decrease the likelihood of impingement on the lateral wall of the notch and increase its resistance to failure.

With the graft in its appropriate orientation, it should be further advanced with gentle tapping until the tibial bone plug is well seated in the femoral tunnel and the bone-tendon interface can be seen. The tension of the graft is manually checked by tugging on the tendon with a nerve hook. If the tension is satisfactory, a 7 by 25 mm cannulated interference type screw is placed to secure the tibial bone plug within the tunnel. The screw should be placed anteriorly, opposite the side of the

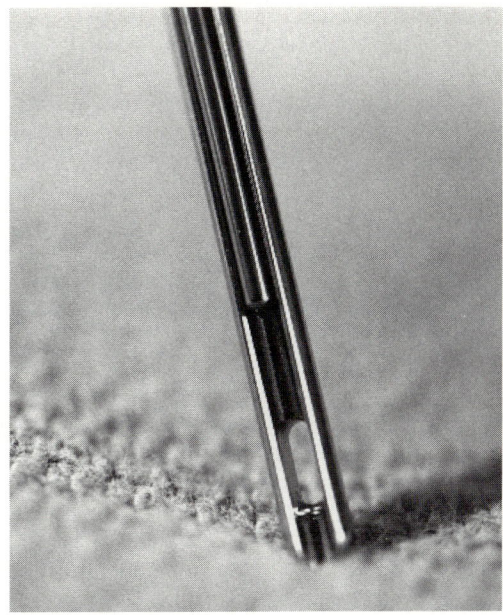

Figure 6 Close-up photograph of slotted groove in the Beath pin.

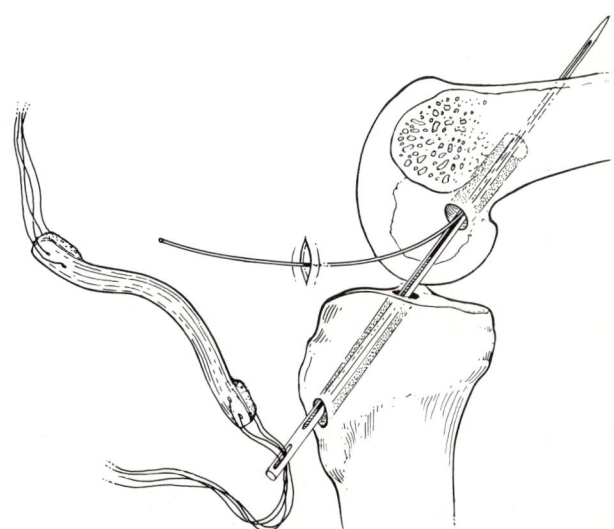

Figure 7 Beath pin with sutures through eye traversing joint and exiting anterolateral thigh. The cannulated interference screw guide wire enters through the arthroscopy portal and exits with the Beath pin.

bone-tendon attachment, and directed parallel to the bone plug to prevent screw divergence that can lead to fixation failure. If a blow-out of the posterior wall of the tunnel is present, then interference screw fixation should not be attempted. A second incision should be made over the lateral aspect of the thigh and brought through the iliotibial band and onto bone. A 6.5 mm screw and washer can be placed through this incision and firmly fixed in the femur, directed away from the tunnel opening. This screw acts as a post and the sutures of the tibial bone block can be tied under tension beneath the screw head and washer. Once it is securely tied, the screw can be further advanced to ensure increased tension.

The knee is then extended into 30 degrees of flexion and manual tension is applied to the sutures on the patellar bone plug. If tunnel length and orientation are correct, the patellar bone block should be counter-sunk completely in the tibial tunnel. A second 7 by 25 mm interference screw is tightened into place away from the site of the tendon-bone attachment on the graft. It is often helpful to use the cannulated screw system and place the guide wire between tunnel and bone block interface to help direct the screw to its proper location. If the bone plug is not completely within the tunnel, then a trough must be created in the tibia just distal to the tunnel opening. The trough should be large enough for the bone block to rest flush with the surface of the tibia after it is secured in place by one or two medium bone staples. This fixation can be augmented by tying the sutures of the patellar bone plug around a 6.5 mm screw and washer placed in the tibia to act as a post.

The knee is then re-examined and tested for Lachman, pivot shift, and anterior drawer signs. Under arthroscopic visualization, the knee is brought through a full range of motion (ROM) to check for impingement, particularly in full extension. If bony impingement on the graft is seen, the anterior roof of the notch is burred down as an extension of the notchplasty. We like to obtain at least 2 mm of clearance between the notch and the graft. Once the examination and ROM is considered satisfactory, the tourniquet is released, hemostasis is obtained, and a small suction drain is placed in the anteromedial incision and brought out through a separate stab wound distally. If interference type screw fixation has been used for the patellar bone block, we pack the opening of the tibial tunnel with any bone graft saved from the reaming of the tunnels. The surgical wounds are closed with absorbable sutures and the knee is immobilized in full extension. We stress the need for full extension postoperatively. Additionally, a cold device that has an inflatable bladder filled with ice water to decrease postoperative swelling and pain is applied immediately.

POSTOPERATIVE COURSE

For the past 1.5 years we have been performing this procedure on an out-patient basis with the assistance of a visiting home health nurse who administers pain medications and intravenous antibiotics for the first 24 hours. Our patients have all expressed a great deal of satisfaction with this method and prefer the out-patient setting over standard hospital overnight stays. Patients are kept in the knee immobilizer for the first 4 days, during which they perform isometric quadriceps setting exercises and straight leg raises. They are also instructed preoperatively on prone leg stretching, which is begun the evening following surgery. They are permitted to be weight-bearing as tolerated with crutches. Following the fourth postoperative day, patients are allowed to be out

of their immobilizer to perform passive ROM exercises several times per day. Again, this is taught preoperatively but we instruct them again in clinic to ensure that the exercises are done passively without subjecting the graft to shear stress from active flexion and extension. At 3 weeks, we fit them with a de-rotation brace and begin closed chain exercises and strengthening. Tests of quadriceps strength dictate the rate of advancement to straight line running and eventual "cutting" type drills with most patients returning to sports participation by 6 months.

DISCUSSION

Many surgeons advocate the use of anterior "outside-in" and rear entry "over-the-top" type of drill guides for drilling of the femoral tunnel. Both require exposure of the lateral femur through the iliotibial band and the vastus lateralis. Our method of single incision arthroscopically assisted ACL reconstruction avoids the routine use of the second lateral incision and its potential complications. The approach to the femur often necessitates ligation of the lateral-superior geniculate artery and vein to reduce postoperative bleeding. The rear entry guide uses a passer that must pierce or elevate the posterior capsule in order to properly position the guide. This places the posterior neurovascular structures at risk for accidental penetration or injury. The anterior guide has its tip in the anatomic ACL position within the femoral notch and permits drilling of a guide pin from the lateral supracondylar region towards the notch. This is a safer method of pin placement and may have the advantage of accurate interference screw placement down the tunnel under direct visualization through the lateral opening. The use of a cannulated screw system reduces the chance of screw divergence under the arthroscopic method and eliminates the need for a lateral incision without sacrificing accuracy. As mentioned previously, if interference screw fixation is not possible, a lateral incision is necessary in order to tie the graft to a screw and washer. Finally, with the single incision technique, there is no chance of muscle herniation through the iliotibial band defect if the soft tissue repair fails and cosmetically there is no skin scarring on the lateral thigh.

COMMENTS

As our understanding of disease transmission and testing methods improve, we may be able one day to offer patients risk-free surgery with allograft tissues. Until this occurs and the long-term success of allografts is know, we fortunately have many autogenous tissues at our disposal for use as graft material in those patients who are unwilling to use donor sources. We cannot overemphasize the technical demands of this reconstruction technique and the potential errors that can be made from a lack of understanding of ACL anatomy and inadequate surgical exposure. A mastery of good arthroscopy skills is of paramount importance. Although a number of devices are available for measuring graft position and assisting with tunnel placement, a reliance on these instruments does not allow for individual differences in anatomy. Malalignment of the tibial or femoral tunnels can lead to graft impingement and failure, or alterations in knee biomechanics with loss of motion or recurrence of instability.

Overall we have found autograft ACL reconstruction with endoscopic assistance to be an excellent procedure with high patient and surgeon satisfaction. Patients have also been very pleased with the cosmesis of the operation and those who have chosen to return to athletics have done so without the use of external bracing or with any modifications in their activity levels.

SUGGESTED READING

Arnoczky S. Anatomy of the anterior cruciate ligament. Clin Orthop 1983; 172:19–25.

Barrack RL, Bruckner J, Kneisel J, et al. The outcome of non-operatively treated complete tears of the ACL in active young adults. Clin Orthop 1990; 259:192–199.

Buseck M, Noyes FR. Arthroscopic evaluation of meniscal repairs after ACL reconstruction and immediate motion. Am J Sports Med 1991; 19:489–494.

Clancy WG Jr, Nelson DA, Reider B, Narechania RG. Anterior cruciate ligament reconstruction using one-third of the patellar ligament, augmented by extra-articular tendon transfers. J Bone Joint Surg 1982; 64A:352–359.

Clancy WG, Ray J, Zoltan D. Acute tears of the anterior cruciate ligament: Surgical versus conservative treatment. J Bone Joint Surg 1988; 70A:1483–1488.

Donaldson W, Warren R, Wickiewicz T. A comparison of acute ACL examinations: Initial versus examination under anesthesia. Am J Sports Med 1985; 13:5–10.

Engebretsen L, Benum P, Fasting O, et al. A prospective randomized study of three surgical techniques for treatment of acute ruptures of the anterior cruciate ligament. Am J Sports Med 1990; 18:585–590.

Feagin JA, Curl W. Isolated tear of the anterior cruciate ligament: A five-year follow up study. Am J Sports Med 1976; 4:95–100.

Indelicato P, Bittar E. A perspective of lesions associated with ACL insufficiency of the knee: A review of 100 cases. Clin Orthop 1985; 198:77–80.

Johnson RJ, Beynnon BD, Nichols CE, et al. Current concepts review: The treatment of injuries of the anterior cruciate ligament. J Bone Joint Surg 1992; 74A:140–151.

Kurosaka M, Yoshiya S, Andrew J, Drish J. A biomechanical comparison of different surgical techniques of graft fixation in an anterior cruciate ligament reconstruction. Am J Sports Med 1987; 15:225–229.

Marder RA, Raskind JR, Carroll M. Prospective evaluation of arthroscopically assisted anterior cruciate ligament reconstruction: Patellar tendon versus semitendinosus and gracilis tendons. Am J Sports Med 1991; 19:478–484.

Noyes F, Butler D, Grood E, et al. Biomechanical analysis of human ligament grafts used in knee ligament repairs and reconstructions. J Bone Joint Surg 1984; 66A:344–352.

Noyes FR, Mangine RE, Barber S. Early knee motion after open and arthroscopic ACL reconstruction. Am J Sports Med 1987; 15:149–160.

Sachs R, Reznik A, Daniel D, Stone M. Complications of knee ligament surgery. In: Daniel D, ed. Knee ligaments: Structure, function, injury, and repair. New York: Raven Press, 1990: 505.

Shelbourne KD, et al. Arthrofibrosis in acute ACL reconstruction: The effect of timing and rehabilitation. Am J Sports Med, 1991; 19:332–336.

Shelbourne D, Nitz P. Accelerated rehabilitation after anterior cruciate ligament reconstruction. Am J Sports Med 1990; 18:292.

Sherman M, Lieber L, Bonamo J, et al. The long term follow-up of primary ACL repair: Defining a rationale for augmentation. Am J Sports Med 1991; 19:243–255.

INTRAOPERATIVE ISOMETRY TESTING DURING RECONSTRUCTION OF THE ANTERIOR CRUCIATE LIGAMENT

ALEXANDER A. SAPEGA, M.D.

Isometry testing as a guide to anterior cruciate ligament (ACL) graft placement was originally introduced as a possible means of preventing knee joint contractures and/or graft failures caused by the excessive and unnatural stresses encountered by a misplaced graft during postoperative knee motion. It has now evolved beyond that point, to where its intention is to ensure precise anatomic reconstruction of select, "priority" fiber-regions of the ACL, with graft length-changes that duplicate the natural mechanical behavior of those fibers.

The most functionally important region of the wide (10 to 12 mm midsection; 20 to 30 mm insertional zone), rather flat ACL is the frontal, more isometric section (Fig. 1), at least in terms of restraint to anterior tibial excursion in the Lachman's and anterior drawer test positions. Precise anatomic reconstruction of these priority fibers entails the selection of graft attachment sites that will cause the majority of graft fibers to behave in a near-isometric fashion, with their limited deviation from isometry following a *normal physiologic pattern* (slight tightening between mid-flexion and full extension). Such physiologic graft fiber-length behavior has aptly been termed "physiometric." "Near-isometric" behavior is a less specific term, since it implies only a less precise, "absolute value" criterion when assessing deviations from isometry (i.e., it specifies only the *degree* of deviation, rather than both the *degree* and *direction/pattern* of deviation).

Whether testing for isometry or physiometry, knowledge of the practical considerations for performing such testing in the operating room is equally important to understanding the theory behind it.

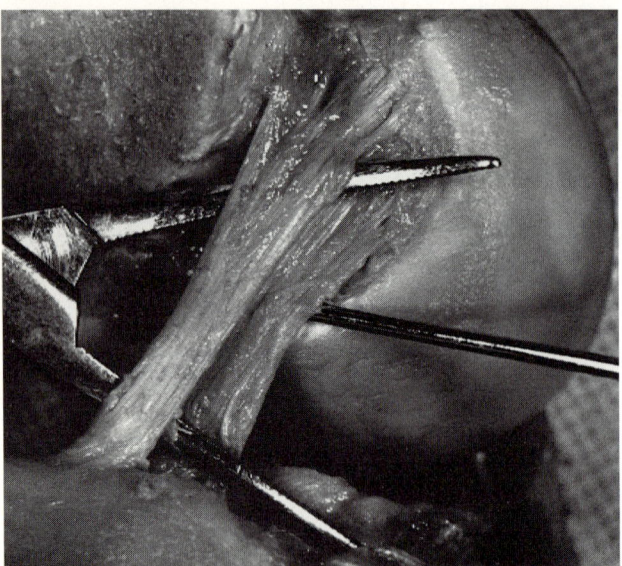

Figure 1 Anatomic dissection demonstrating the more isometric and so-called "priority" fibers for anterior cruciate ligament (ACL) reconstruction. The normal ACL is so broad in dimension that even a 10 mm wide graft cannot effectively reconstruct its entire macrostructure. Therefore, even if graft placement is *within* the normal anatomic fiber attachment zones on the tibia and femur, some choice regarding specific fiber-region reconstruction still remains for the surgeon. The fibers demonstrated above are the most isometric and most functionally important of the ACL. They also typically appear as the most dense and well-organized (low signal) fibers on magnetic resonance imaging.

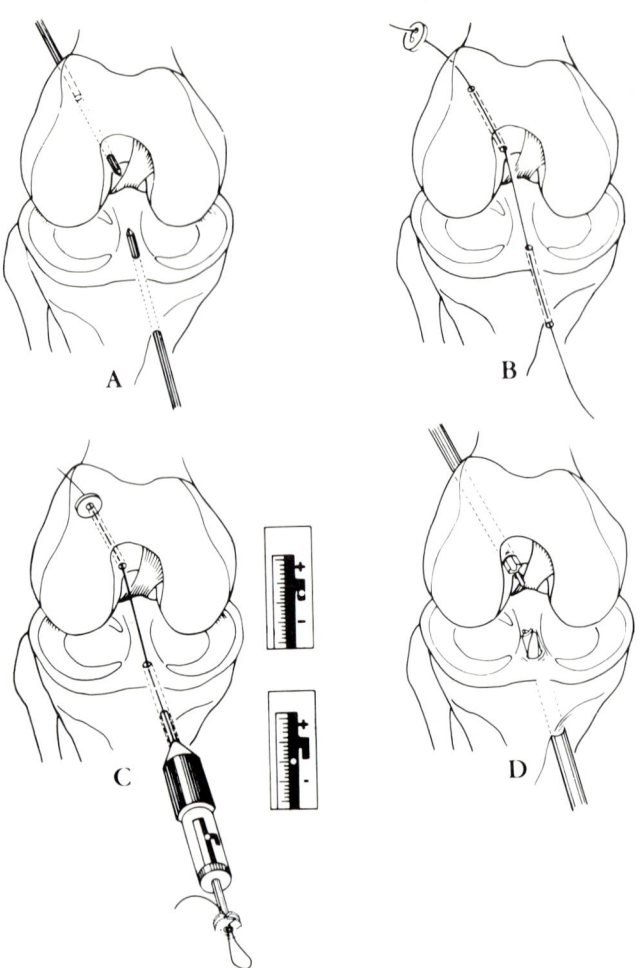

Figure 2 Original technique for intraoperative isometry testing during ACL reconstruction as introduced by Graf. (From: Graf B. Isometric placement of substitutes for the ACL. In: Jackson DW, Drez D, eds. The ACL deficient knee. St. Louis: CV Mosby, 1987; with permission.)

WHY IS NEAR-ISOMETRIC OR PHYSIOMETRIC GRAFT PLACEMENT IMPORTANT?

In addition to providing precise anatomic reconstruction of the more functionally important anterior or anterocentral ACL fibers, grafts with the appropriate minimal deviations from isometry have been shown to restore normal knee kinematics more successfully than frankly nonisometric grafts, even if the latter were still within the anatomic osseous attachment zones of the ACL. Near-isometric or physiometric anteromedial fiber grafts are less likely to loosen or stretch out during postoperative continuous passive motion and are more mechanically efficient at resisting anterior tibial translation forces than less isometric, more vertically oriented grafts. Another point to consider is that a previous review of 37 failed ACL reconstructions revealed femoral tunnel misplacement (too far anterior, yielding excessive graft tightening in flexion, or too far posterior, yielding excessive graft tightening in extension) in 51%.

EVOLUTION OF ISOMETRY TESTING TECHNIQUE

Intraoperative isometry testing during ACL reconstruction has evolved through three phases of develop-

ment since the basic technique was introduced by Graf in 1987 (Fig. 2). In that early, first phase of implementation, perfect graft isometry was considered the ideal, ultimate objective. The surgeon was simply instructed to find sites on the tibia and femur that demonstrated the least possible deviation from isometry during joint motion. A 1.5 or 2 mm maximum change in tibiofemoral separation distance was generally considered acceptable, but no stipulation was made with regard to the *direction* or *pattern* of that tibiofemoral distance change. In addition, early isometry testing was often only performed through a limited range of motion (0 to 90 degrees), which was not a very strict criterion when compared with full-range (0 to 120+ degrees) testing. In essence, this phase of the technique employed a nonspecific, absolute value criterion for determining acceptable isometric graft placement, demonstrated only through a limited range of joint motion. The principal drawback of this initial approach was that a graft demonstrating 2 mm of *lengthening* between extension and flexion was considered equally desirable to a graft that demonstrated 2 mm of *slackening* from extension to flexion (as we know now, the latter is far more representative of actual ACL fiber behavior). No distinction was made between these divergent graft behaviors under the original absolute value concept of isometry. Today, prospective graft fixation sites that would produce 2 mm of graft tightening (length increase) between 0 and 90 degrees of flexion would generally be rejected out of hand, as this is really 3 to 4 mm away from ideal behavior, and possibly moreso with greater knee flexion. The other limitation of early phase isometry testing was that no particular attention was given to the joint motion and loading conditions in effect during intraoperative testing. No instructions or guidelines were available regarding the manner in which passive knee joint motion was to be accomplished, much less the appropriate way to deal with gravitational joint distraction effects or the absence of functioning secondary ligament stabilizers such as the collateral or posterior cruciate ligaments. At times, this resulted in skewed and inconsistent isometer readings.

The second phase in the evolution of intraoperative isometry testing took place about 1989, when it was proven in the laboratory that the joint motion and loading conditions employed while testing for isometry (e.g., gravitational effects, superimposed anterior versus posterior tibial translation force, the presence or absence of congruent joint surface contact during joint motion) had a significant effect on the readings registered by isometer test gauges. Many surgeons had also empirically observed by that time that errant readings were easily obtained if normal tibiofemoral tracking kinematics during passive motion were disturbed by inadvertently applied tibial rotation forces, passive anterior tibial subluxation allowed by the absence of ACL restraint, or tibiofemoral subluxations in other directions allowed by lax collateral or posterior cruciate ligaments. Also, it was becoming apparent that the ACL is not a genuinely isometric structure. When it became obvious that perfect isometric graft placement was rarely if ever achieved, attention turned toward an analysis of the characteristics of the residual deviations from isometry that could never quite be eliminated, particularly when a 0 to 120 degree range of test motion was employed. This led to the bypassing of the absolute value concept of isometry testing, in favor of the third and current phase of this intraoperative testing technique.

Currently, it is recommended that surgeons seek out tibiofemoral graft attachment sites (bone tunnel sites) that will lead to minimal changes in graft length during knee motion, in a pattern that *mimics* the *normal* length change behavior of the most nearly isometric, anterior fibers of the ACL. Seeking a specific physiologic pattern of site-to-site distance change (i.e., physiometric behavior: slight tibiofemoral approximation of 1.5 to 2 mm as the knee is brought from extension to 30 degrees of flexion, a mid-range neutral or inflection zone, and then partial reseparation as the knee advances past 90 degrees and reaches 120 degrees

of flexion) has now generally replaced perfect isometry as the criterion for ideal graft placement. In addition, the specific joint motion and loading conditions employed while ranging the knee are recognized as being of critical importance.

I still use an isometer device routinely during ACL reconstruction, seeking graft attachment sites that demonstrate a tibiofemoral separation distance change profile matching the physiometric length change profile of the anteromedial fibers of the ACL. Isometer readings are recorded while: (1) taking care to avoid application of unwanted axial tibial rotation or valgus-varus forces during joint motion, (2) maintaining congruent tibiofemoral joint surface contact, and (3) preventing anterior tibial subluxation by maintaining a mild posterior drawer force at all times. If significant posterior cruciate ligament laxity is present, no attempt is even made to obtain isometer readings. Under these circumstances ACL graft placement must be based strictly on anatomic landmarks because normal tibiofemoral kinematic tracking is nearly impossible to reproduce. In cases of medial collateral ligament deficiency, extra care is taken to avoid valgus tibial rotation during motion as isometer readings are being recorded.

HOW IMPORTANT IS IT TO PERFORM INTRAOPERATIVE ISOMETRY TESTING?

The importance of intraoperative isometry testing varies greatly with the experience of the surgeon. While gross errors in graft placement by the inexperienced surgeon can be avoided through properly performed isometry or physiometry testing, I would agree that experienced surgeons need not feel compelled to perform intraoperative isometry testing on a routine basis, unless they consistently wish to strive for theoretical perfection by "fine tuning" their graft placements. It has been my experience that anatomic variations from individual to individual prevent perfect physiometric graft placement via the use of anatomic landmarks alone. No amount of surgical experience allows one to account for such individual anatomic variation in condylar cam mechanics. Paulos et al recently commented on the utility of intraoperative isometry testing in the following fashion: "We believe this is an essential part of the ACL reconstruction. We have been surprised to find that nearly 25 percent of the initial femoral anatomic attachment sites selected at surgery are subsequently changed because of the use of the isometer." While I would not disagree, it is important to state that meticulous care must be taken to observe and control the joint motion and loading conditions under which isometer readings are taken, when using these devices to fine tune graft placement. In addition, various other technical considerations must be kept in mind regarding the avoidance of measurement errors by the isometer itself and by the drilling of bone tunnels concentrically about the tibiofemoral points ultimately selected by the isometer.

INTERPRETATION OF ISOMETER GAUGE READINGS

A knowledge of the anatomic-mechanical relationships that govern the degree and pattern of isometer excursion gauge readings is essential to surgeons who utilize this technique as a guide in graft placement. Such testing was never meant to substitute completely for surgical judgement and familiarity with anatomic landmarks; thus the technique is greatly facilitated (much less trial and error work) if the surgeon takes the first step correctly by selecting sites for testing that are relatively anteromedial on the tibia and high and posterior (arthroscopist's perspective) in the intercondylar notch, as originally advocated by Clancy. Once the appropriate general region has been reached, fine tuning of graft placement can be accomplished. Tibial site selection *can* significantly affect isometry test readings, at least at this stage of final adjustment. It must be remembered, however, that intercondylar notch impingement of the graft in knee extension remains an over-riding anatomic consideration governing tibial placement unless the surgeon is prepared to deal with this by performing a notchplasty as needed.

In general, if an ideal *femoral* site has been selected, an isometer reading that demonstrates an excessive increase in tibiofemoral site separation distance between 90 degrees of flexion and full extension can be corrected by moving the tibial site more anterior, and vice versa. The corollary is that given an ideal *tibial* site, an isometer reading that demonstrates too much of an increase in tibiofemoral site separation distance between 90 degrees flexion and knee extension can be corrected by moving the femoral site toward the frontal inlet of the intercondylar notch, and vice versa.

In my opinion, prospective tunnel centers that demonstrate *any* degree of separation (future graft tightening) between full extension and 90 degrees of flexion are undesirable, even if only by 0.5 or 1 mm. Such sites are likely to move even further apart with flexion greater than 90 degrees, representing a clearly "unbalanced" situation (when flexing the knee, the amount of graft tightening between 90 degrees and 120 degrees should never exceed the degree of initial graft slackening observed between 0 and 30 degrees, which should rarely if ever be greater than 2 mm).

SUGGESTED READING

Acker JH, Drez D: Analysis of isometric placement of grafts in ACL reconstruction procedures. Am J Knee Surg 1989; 2:65–70.

Brand MG, Daniel DM: Considerations in the placement of an intra-articular anterior cruciate ligament graft. Operative Tech Orthop 1992; 2:55–62.

Buzzi R, Aglietti P, Pisaneschi A, et al: Intra-articular reconstruction of the anterior cruciate ligament (ACL): An experimental study of the isometric attachment points. Italian J Sports Traumatol 1987; 9:243–253.

Clancy WG, Nelson DA, Reider B, et al: Anterior cruciate ligament reconstruction using one-third of the patellar ligament. J Bone Joint Surg 1982; 64A:352–359.

Fleming B, Beynnon BD, Johnson RJ, et al: Isometric versus tension measurements: A comparison for the reconstruction of the anterior cruciate ligament. Am J Sports Med 1993; 21:82–88.

Friederich NF, et al: How important is isometric placement of cruciate ligament substitutes? 1989 A.A.O.S. Scientific Exhibit. Accepted for Publication, Acta Ortho Scandinavica, Supplementum.

Graf B: Isometric placement of substitutes for the anterior cruciate ligament. In: Jackson DW, Drez D, eds. The anterior cruciate deficient knee. St. Louis: CV Mosby, 1987: 102.

Hefzy MS, Grood ES, Noyes FR: Factors affecting the region of most isometric femoral attachments. Am J Sports Med 1989; 17:208–216.

Johnson R, Beynnon B, Nichols C, et al: Current concepts review – The treatment of injuries of the anterior cruciate ligament. J Bone Joint Surg 1992; 74:140–151.

O'Brien WR: Isometric placement of anterior cruciate ligament substitutes. Operative Tech Orthop 1992; 2:49–54.

O'Meara PM, O'Brien WR, Henning CE: Anterior cruciate ligament reconstruction stability with continuous passive motion. Clin Orthop 1992; 277:201–209.

Paulos LE, Cherf J, Rosenberg TD, et al: Anterior cruciate ligament reconstruction with autografts. Clin Sports Med 1991; 10:469–485.

Penner DA, Daniel DM, Wood P, et al: An in vitro study of anterior cruciate ligament graft placement and isometry. Am J Sports Med 1988; 16:238–243.

Sapega AA: Arthroscopically assisted reconstruction of the anterior cruciate ligament. In: Torg JS, Welsh P, Shephard RJ, eds. Current therapy in sports medicine, ed 2. Philadelphia: BC Decker, 1989: 292.

Sapega A, Moyer R, Schneck C, et al: Testing for isometry during reconstruction of the anterior cruciate ligament. J Bone Joint Surg 1990; 72:259–267.

Yaru NG, Daniel D, Penner D: The effect of tibial attachment site on graft impingement in an anterior cruciate ligament reconstruction. Am J Sports Med 1992; 20:217–220.

NONOPERATIVE MANAGEMENT OF MEDIAL COLLATERAL LIGAMENT TEARS WITH ANTERIOR CRUCIATE LIGAMENT RECONSTRUCTION

K. DONALD SHELBOURNE, M.D.
THOMAS E. KLOOTWYK, M.D.

In combined ligament injuries of the knee involving the medial collateral ligament (MCL) and the anterior cruciate ligament (ACL), the MCL injury should be treated nonoperatively while the ACL is reconstructed with an autogenous central one-third patellar tendon graft. This recommendation is based on our clinical observations and gradual changes in our treatment protocol of 142 patients with this injury pattern who were treated with reconstructive ACL surgery over the last 10 years.

Previous recommendations for treatment of this combined ACL/MCL injury were for repair and reconstruction of all damaged structures. Surgery was most often performed shortly after the injury. However, this treatment resulted in an unacceptably high rate of postoperative stiffness. Therefore, our approach to the patient with a combined ACL/MCL injury has progressively changed regarding our recommendation of surgical reconstruction of the ACL tear and the timing of the surgery.

DIAGNOSIS

The combined ACL/MCL ligament disruption occurs with both contact and noncontact knee injuries. The ACL injury can be predictably diagnosed in most cases by taking a careful history. Questions that should be asked of the patient are: (1) Did you feel or hear a "pop" in your knee?; (2) Did you feel you had significantly injured your knee?; (3) Did you feel as if your knee came apart?; (4) Were you able to continue playing?; and (5) Was there significant swelling within 1 to 2 hours? Positive responses to these questions are frequently heard from patients with an ACL tear. On examination, a positive Lachman test is diagnostic of the ACL disruption.

The MCL injury is diagnosed and graded by the physical examination. Palpation along the course of the MCL will localize the site of the tear and can have critical implications in the rehabilitation process. The MCL is the primary medial stabilizer to valgus stress of the knee in 30 degrees of knee flexion. With the knee in greater degrees of extension, the ACL and the posterior cruciate ligament assume greater responsibility in preventing medial opening. It is important to correlate the amount of valgus opening with the degree of knee flexion when testing for MCL injuries. When testing the integrity of the MCL alone, the knee should be in 30 degrees of flexion.

The amount of medial knee opening comparing the injured knee to the contralateral knee is a direct measure of damage to the medial capsuloligamentous complex. The MCL injury is graded on a scale of I to III based on tenderness, laxity, and the presence of a distinct endpoint with valgus stress testing. A grade I injury has tenderness, no laxity with valgus stress testing at 30 degrees of knee flexion, and a solid endpoint. A grade II injury is similar, but there is some degree of medial laxity with a firm endpoint still detectable. A grade III injury represents a complete disruption to the MCL with significant medial opening and no detectable endpoint with valgus stress testing.

TREATMENT

Associated Meniscal Pathology

In a review of ACL/MCL injured patients Shelbourne and Porter describe the associated meniscal injury patterns. There exists a predictable pattern of meniscal pathology. Contrary to previous thinking, tears to the body of the medial meniscus are not frequently associated with combined ACL/MCL injuries. Overall only 10% of these combined ligament injury patients had medial meniscal tears. In contrast, lateral meniscal tears were present in 71% of grade II MCL and 32% of grade III MCL injuries. At least 50% of these lateral meniscal tears were felt to be repairable. Lateral chondral injuries were present in 17% of grade II MCL injuries and in 8% of grade III MCL tears. Of significant note is that meniscal injury was absent in 60% of grade III MCL tears. The results of this study revealed that the more common injury associated with an ACL/MCL injury is a lateral meniscal tear.

Our current data reflect a similar meniscal tear pattern with ACL/MCL injuries. Of 142 patients with ACL/MCL injury and subsequent ACL reconstruction, 80 (56%) had lateral meniscus tears compared to 22 (15%) with medial meniscus tears. The associated lateral meniscal tears were usually radial and/or posterior peripheral and the less common medial tears were peripheral. All of these tears tended to be stable and either heal or remain asymptomatic. We continue to take an aggressive approach at meniscal preservation. Of the 80 lateral meniscus tears, 56 (70%) were repaired or left alone, and, of the 22 medial meniscus tears, 13 (59%) were repaired or left alone. To date, none of these patients have developed postoperative meniscal symptoms. Additionally, in treating over 40 patients with ACL/MCL injury nonoperatively, none have required further treatment for symptomatic meniscal tears. As our knowledge of the natural history of stable meniscal tears has increased, we continue with an aggressive approach of meniscal preservation.

With a consistent, predictable meniscal injury pattern and our present treatment approach, we have not found a need for a magnetic resonance imaging (MRI) evaluation in most of our patients. We have found that the ligament injuries can be diagnosed on physical examination alone and the meniscal pathology can be appropriately treated at the time of a delayed reconstruction.

Timing of ACL Surgery and Treatment of MCL

The two most significant advancements in the treatment of ACL/MCL injuries in the past 10 years have been in the nonoperative treatment of the MCL portion of the injury and in the delay of the surgical reconstruction.

The increased incidence of arthrofibrosis with acute ligament reconstructions has been well established. This potential complication is especially applicable to the ACL/MCL injured patient. We have noted that patients who sustain a MCL tear from the femoral origin have difficulty regaining their full range of motion (ROM). This results in minimal residual medial laxity before a reconstructive procedure. The avoidance of immediate surgery with emphasis on appropriate preoperative rehabilitation greatly decreases the incidence of arthrofibrosis after ACL reconstructive surgery.

Since we have found that acute surgery is not necessary to address the associated meniscal pathology, the initial focus of our treatment can be on the MCL. Shelbourne and Baele compared two groups of patients who had sustained ACL/MCL injuries. One group underwent repair of the MCL with an autogenous patellar tendon ACL reconstruction and a second group had an ACL reconstruction without repair of the medial side. No patient in either group had postoperative functional or objective instability. The group that underwent MCL repair had an increased incidence of residual stiffness. With these results noted, our approach to the ACL/MCL injured patient who desires surgical reconstruction is one of conservative treatment of the MCL injury with a delayed reconstruction of the ACL.

It is well accepted that all degrees of isolated MCL injuries can heal with stability and excellent functional results with nonoperative treatment. Similar excellent results in regard to medial stability can be obtained with a nonoperative treatment of the MCL injury associated with an acute ACL tear. There exists laboratory data utilizing animal models investigating MCL healing in the presence of an ACL deficient knee. This biomechanical animal study revealed healing of the injured MCL is adversely affected in the absence of an ACL. However, this study does not reflect our clinical experience. The nonoperative treatment of a MCL injury associated with an acute ACL tear has resulted in predictable stable MCL healing in clinical trials. Satisfactory healing of the MCL can occur as long as secondary giving-out episodes are not allowed to occur during the healing phase prior to the ACL surgery.

Rehabilitation of Acute Injury

We utilize a similar principle of treatment in dealing with the combined ACL/MCL injury as we do with an isolated ACL tear. As with treatment of an isolated ACL tear, the first step of treatment when dealing with a combined ACL/grade I or II MCL injury is rehabilitation. Early treatment emphasizes control of pain and swelling, restoration of knee ROM, and the use of crutches until gait is normalized. We have found the knee Cryo/Cuff of great value in treating acute knee injuries. The cold compression provided by this device assists in pain relief and helps control swelling. A knee immobilizer is used to provide support until the patient has regained good leg control and is comfortable during ambulation.

The initial treatment of a combined ACL/grade III MCL injury is different. Control of pain and swelling are still emphasized, but rehabilitation to restore ROM is altered depending on the location of the MCL injury. We have found that when the MCL tears from its femoral insertion site or in its midsubstance, the injured knee tends to become stiff. At times it can be difficult for the patient to regain all of the preinjury knee ROM. Therefore, rehabilitation aimed at ROM is stressed. As the rehabilitation progresses, the injured knee is easily protected by a hinged brace that provides collateral support and allows full extension and flexion.

In contrast to MCL injuries off the femur or midsubstance, the MCL tears from the tibia insertion site have a tendency to heal with residual valgus laxity. We have found that a brief period of immobilization with the knee in approximately 30 degrees of flexion assists the MCL healing and results in less residual medial laxity. After a 2 week delay, ROM rehabilitation is initiated.

An uncommon injury pattern can occur when the ACL/MCL and posteromedial structures are injured. This includes injury to the posterior oblique ligament. On examination these injuries exhibit laxity to valgus stress testing at zero degrees even though the posterior cruciate ligament is intact. In the early treatment of this injury, the knee is protected from early terminal extension, but otherwise the postinjury rehabilitation is the same with control of pain and swelling by using the Cryo/Cuff and a simple immobilizer to provide support until the gait pattern is normalized.

Planning for Treatment of ACL Deficiency

With the knowledge that the MCL injury will heal satisfactorily with appropriate nonoperative care, the decision of whether to treat the torn ACL with reconstruction must be made. Those patients who sustain a combined MCL injury off the femur will have some added knee stability due to medial scarring which can mask the underlying ACL instability at a later time. It is important when treating the younger athlete to be aware of this "relative" stability afforded by the MCL off the femur injury pattern and treat them according to the known ACL instability. We counsel our patients based on their activity desires as to whether they should undergo an ACL reconstruction. Those patients who wish to continue aggressive athletic activity, especially activity that involves cutting, twisting, or pivoting motions, are best treated with an ACL reconstruction. This group includes most young athletic individuals and high-demand patients.

We are often faced with lower-demand patients with a combined ACL/MCL injury with the MCL tear being proximal off the femur. These patients usually do well with conservative treatment of the MCL and develop enough stability to be functional with activities of daily living.

Those patients who elect nonoperative treatment are guided through the final phases of rehabilitation. This includes restoration of full ROM, closed chain functional activities, and a functional progression of lower-risk athletic activities such as biking, stairstep machines, and straight ahead running. Patients are counseled on the importance of avoiding risky activities. An ACL brace may be used for the patient who participates in an occasional higher-risk activity.

Patients who elect to proceed with ACL reconstruction are treated with an appropriately timed arthroscopy and autogenous patellar tendon ACL reconstruction. Shelbourne and Mohtadi in separate reports have noted an unacceptable high rate of arthrofibrosis with acute ACL reconstructions. Reconstructive surgery should be delayed until the patient has regained full knee ROM including full hyperextension, has no swelling, and has resumed a normal gait pattern. This usually translates into a 7 to 8 week delay between injury and reconstruction. If the patient does not have full ROM even after 2 months of delay, further preoperative rehabilitation is prescribed until the knee has regained full ROM. This can certainly be the situation when dealing with the combined ACL/MCL injury with the MCL injured off the femur. This delayed reconstruction approach allows for a much easier and more rapid postoperative rehabilitation. As previously noted, this delay does not jeopardize the eventual treatment of any associated meniscal pathology. This treatment approach has greatly decreased postoperative knee stiffness.

The additional advantage of a surgical delay is allowing the patient to mentally prepare for the reconstruction. School, work, and family schedules can be appropriately arranged. All reconstructed patients follow our accelerated rehabilitation program and the preoperative delay allows the patient to fully understand this rehabilitation program, which provides for a smoother postoperative course.

SUGGESTED READING

Fetto JF, Marshall JL. Medial collateral ligament injuries of the knee: A rationale for treatment. Clin Orthop 1978; 132:206–218.

Indelicato PA. Nonoperative management of complete tears of the medial collateral ligament. Orthop Rev 1989; 18:947–952.

Inoue M, McGurk-Burleson E, Hollis JM, et al. Treatment of the medial collateral ligament injury: The importance of anterior cruciate ligament on the varus-valgus knee laxity. Am J Sports Med 1987; 15:15–21.

Jokl P, Kaplan N, Stovel P, et al. Non-operative treatment of severe injuries to the medial and anterior cruciate ligament of the knee. J Bone Joint Surg 1984; 66A:741–744.

Kannus P. Long-term results of conservatively treatment medial collateral ligament injuries of the knee joint. Clin Orthop 1988; 226:103–111.

Mohtadi NG, Webster-Bogaert S, Fowler PJ. Limitation of motion following anterior cruciate ligament reconstruction: A case control study. Am J Sports Med 1991; 19:620–625.

Shelbourne KD, Baele JR. Treatment of combined anterior cruciate ligament, and medial collateral ligament injuries. Am J Knee Surg 1988; 1:56–58.

Shelbourne KD, Klootwyk TE, DeCarlo MS. Clinical development of preoperative and postoperative ACL rehabilitation. In: Feagin JA Jr ed. The crucial ligaments, ed 2. New York: Churchill Livingstone, 1994.

Shelbourne KD, Porter DA. Anterior cruciate ligament-medial collateral ligament injury: Nonoperative management of medial collateral ligament tears with anterior cruciate ligament reconstruction. Am J Sports Med 1992; 20:283–286.

Shelbourne KD, Wilckens JH, Mollabashy A. Arthrofibrosis in acute anterior cruciate ligament reconstruction: The effect of timing of reconstruction and rehabilitation. Am J Sports Med 1991; 19:332–336.

Wasilewski SA, Covall DJ, Cohen S. Effectg of surgical timing on recovery and associated injuries after anterior cruciate ligament reconstruction. Am J Sports Med 1993; 21:338–342.

ACCELERATED REHABILITATION AFTER ANTERIOR CRUCIATE LIGAMENT RECONSTRUCTION

K. DONALD SHELBOURNE, M.D.
ROCCI V. TRUMPER, M.D.

Reconstruction of the anterior cruciate ligament (ACL) has received considerable attention during the past 2 decades. Although treatment advances have changed the operative management of this injury, the primary goals of treatment remain constant. These include restoration of knee stability, limiting surgical morbidity, and a successful return to full activities.

The mid-third autogenous patellar tendon graft is the most common graft source used for ACL reconstructive surgery. However, a number of surgeons have chosen alternative grafts due to the potential morbidity associated with harvesting of this graft source. The most common of these complications include knee stiffness, anterior knee pain, and quadriceps weakness.

In lieu of searching for a graft source equal to the patellar tendon in restoring knee stability, we have focused on minimizing the postoperative morbidity associated with its use. The most significant contribution to this effort has been in the area of perioperative rehabilitation. This began in the 1980s when we observed that patients strictly following our rehabilitation protocol were progressing more slowly than those who were advancing their activities as tolerated contrary to our guidelines. These noncompliant patients had fewer complications without an increased incidence of instability. The key differences we observed between these two groups were: (1) patients who regained full hyperextension early did not exhibit increased instability but had fewer complaints of anterior knee pain and stiffness with return to full activities; (2) patients who developed good leg control and were able to ambulate with a normal gait pattern immediately after surgery had better patellar mobility, less patellofemoral pain, and regained their strength much faster; and (3) if a large hemarthrosis developed after reconstruction, this limited progression of rehabilitation with a trend toward recurrent effusions and prolonged strength loss. Since that time, we have continued to critically examine and modify the rehabilitation guidelines with a continued trend toward fewer limitations and an earlier return to full activities.

This approach has significantly limited the morbidity commonly associated with autogenous patellar tendon grafts. In addition, we have noted that by critically assessing graft placement and our ability to reproduce this position, we have continued to decrease our KT-1,000 and functional instability failures despite allowing a much faster return to full sporting activities. We feel we are now able to offer the patient the "gold standard" in ACL reconstruction without the increased morbidity commonly associated with its use.

BASIC REHABILITATION CONCEPTS

Achieving optimal results using the accelerated rehabilitation protocol requires an understanding of some key concepts. The most critical of these is full knee extension. It is important to note that most patients exhibit a small amount of hyperextension when the knee is fully extended. The term full knee extension actually refers to hyperextension equal to the contralateral knee. The importance of this can not be overemphasized. Achieving and maintaining full knee extension, simply stated, equates to prevention of surgical morbidity. A stiff knee lacking full extension rarely leads to complaints of instability, but often results in a dissatisfied patient with anterior knee pain, quadriceps weakness, and a poorly functioning knee. These complaints if allowed to develop can often be lessened by postoperative arthroscopic scar resection and restoration of full knee extension. However, it is best to prevent problems by obtaining full extension before and immediately after surgery, rather than treat them once they occur.

Patient education is a second major key to a successful postoperative course. With our rehabilitation program few patients require more than four or five physical therapy visits. These visits are aimed at patient education and rehabilitation guidance with emphasis on avoiding postoperative problems. It is vital for the patient to fully understand the rehabilitation goals and

Table 1 Phases of Rehabilitation Following ACL Surgery

Phase I (Preoperative rehabilitation of the injured knee):
 Regain full ROM
 Minimize swelling
 Review postoperative rehabilitation program
 Mental preparation for surgery
 Arrange school, work, family schedule for surgery
Phase II (0 to 2 weeks postoperatively):
 Obtain full knee extension (hyperextension)
 Allow wound healing
 Maintain active quadriceps leg control
 Minimize swelling
 Achieve 90 degrees of flexion
Phase III (3 to 5 weeks postoperatively):
 Resume a normal gait pattern
 Improve flexion to 135 degrees
 Begin closed chain quadriceps strengthening
Phase IV (From 5 weeks postoperatively):
 Isokinetic and KT-1000 stability testing
 If strength is adequate, start lateral shuffles, cariocas, jumping rope, light running program
 Start sport specific activities and return to competition as rehabilitation progress allows

how they can be achieved. A smooth postoperative course is characterized by a patient who takes responsibility for achieving the rehabilitation goals.

Finally, organization of the perioperative protocol is worthy of brief discussion. Our accelerated protocol can be separated into a four-phase program. These phases are helpful in guiding the patient and physician during the preoperative and postoperative course. However, it may be more appropriate to think of rehabilitation as a step-wise progression. For example, the patient must control swelling before realizing a full range of motion (ROM). We have found that motion, and full knee extension in particular, is a prerequisite to a rapid return of quadriceps strength. Quadriceps strength is a must for a successful return to full activities. Failure to proceed in a step-wise fashion results in a frustrating and prolonged postoperative course. This is well demonstrated by the patient who attempts to participate in functional activities before achieving a return of 70% quadriceps strength. The result is often a swollen knee that functions poorly.

An outline of the accelerated protocol is given in Table 1. These are merely guidelines and each patient's progress should be individualized. Although each phase has a general time period assigned to it, very few time constraints are placed on patient progress with the exception of the first 2 postoperative weeks where we focus on limiting swelling and maintaining full knee extension. When the goals of a specific rehabilitation phase are achieved, the patient is ready to proceed to the next phase.

REHABILITATION PROTOCOL

Phase I

Preoperative preparation of the patient is the foundation for a successful postoperative recovery.

Delaying surgery until the patient has a normal appearing knee with no swelling and normal ROM will limit surgical morbidity. Operating on an acutely injured knee without restoring full knee extension preoperatively is associated with an increased incidence of postoperative knee stiffness. Most patients require 3 to 6 weeks before their swelling is minimal and motion has returned to normal.

Two special circumstances deserve mention. The first involves the patient with a concomitant medial collateral ligament (MCL) injury. These individuals are particularly prone to have motion problems if reconstructed in the acute period. This is particularly true if the MCL injury is off the medial femoral condyle. In this setting, 6 to 10 weeks of preoperative rehabilitation are often required before the knee is ready for the reconstructive procedure.

The second circumstance involves the individual with a chronic ACL deficient knee who presents with a locked bucket handle meniscal tear and a flexion contracture greater than 10 degrees. Simultaneous management of the meniscal pathology and ligament instability can result in an increased incidence of postoperative stiffness. We have found that a two-staged approach can effectively eliminate this problem. Our preferred treatment includes initial care of the meniscal tear through outpatient arthroscopic repair followed by a delayed reconstructive procedure when knee motion has returned to normal. This not only serves to minimize the chances of having motion problems after the ACL reconstruction, but allows for an aggressive approach toward meniscal preservation. A second-look arthroscopy at the time of reconstruction will allow for evaluation of the meniscal repair and hopefully encourage us to repair more of these torn menisci.

Finally, the patient's psychological frame of mind is critically important. It is normal to feel depressed and/or angry for a short time after a major knee injury. This frame of mind is not conducive to a smooth postoperative recovery. Patients need to be well informed and mentally prepared for the procedure. This often involves scheduling around school vacations or work.

Delaying surgery until the patient and the knee is ready for ACL reconstruction will not compromise ultimate stability. However, it will serve to significantly limit the incidence of postoperative morbidity.

Phase II

Phase II consists of the initial 2 weeks after surgery. The goals of this phase include (1) minimizing swelling, (2) establishing and maintaining full knee extension, (3) obtaining knee flexion to 90 degrees, and (4) demonstrating good quadriceps leg control. This period is the most critical and emphasis must be placed on avoiding problems as opposed to solving them once they occur. For this reason, most patients remain in the hospital for approximately 2 days after surgery. During these first 2 days patients begin to understand the rehabilitation process and take responsibility for obtaining the goals outlined for them.

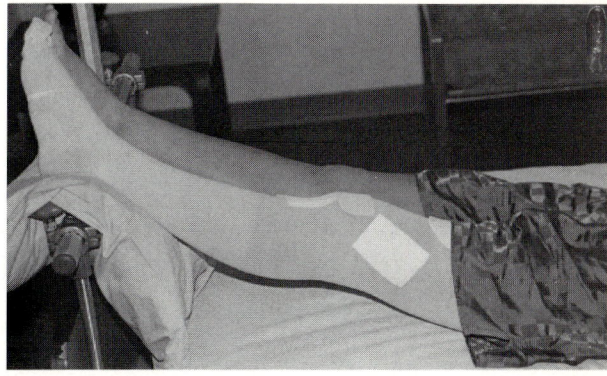

Figure 1 Full knee extension is achieved by placing the patient's heels on the bed frame and allowing the knee to relax into hyperextension. A 2.5-pound weight may be applied to the proximal tibia to aid in gaining full extension.

Following surgery a Cryo/Cuff and Tecnol immobilizer are applied to the operative leg. The splint is removed when the patient returns to the room and the leg is placed in a continuous passive motion (CPM) machine with a ROM from 0 to 30 degrees. The CPM machine serves to effectively elevate the knee and aid in keeping the patient comfortable. Extension exercises are started almost immediately by placing the patient's heels on the end of the bed frame and allowing the knee to relax into full extension as shown in Figure 1. A 2.5-pound ankle weight may be applied to the proximal tibia to aid in obtaining full knee extension. This is repeated every waking hour for approximately ten minutes.

The following day the patient continues the extension exercises during the waking hours. In addition, flexion exercises are initiated by allowing the knee to bend over the side of the bed three times a day during meals. Leg control is enhanced by performing short arc quadriceps contractions from 90 to 30 degrees. Prior to discharge a shower is allowed with a plastic bag covering the operative extremity. Full weight-bearing is encouraged and serves to facilitate patellar mobility and leg control.

We have found that this program for the first 2 days after surgery allows us to eliminate problems postoperatively and minimizes the need for physical therapy to undo problems that may develop.

After discharge the patient continues much of the same at home. The CPM machine is utilized for approximately 1 week and the Cryo/Cuff is used almost continuously except during extension exercises and meals. Full weight-bearing ambulation is allowed but should be kept to a minimum during this initial phase of rehabilitation as it may result in knee swelling, which will slow the rehabilitation.

An increase in activity is allowed during the second week. Many patients return to school or work on a part-time basis. Liberal use of the Cryo/Cuff and extension exercises must be continued. Knee swelling serves as the best guide in determining the amount of activity allowed.

The most urgent aspect of this phase is obtaining and maintaining full knee extension. Failure to achieve

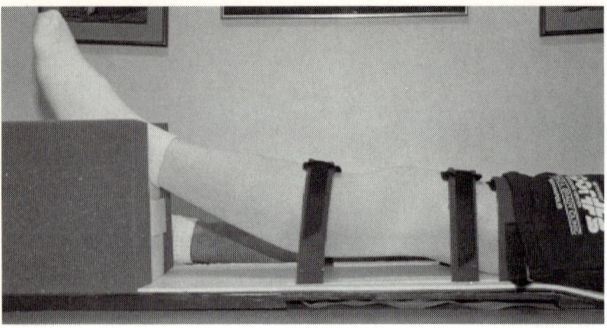

Figure 2 The extension board is useful for patients who have difficulty gaining full knee extension. The heel is elevated while straps above and below the knee joint serve to promote knee extension.

full extension early often leads to a permanent loss of knee motion and subjective symptoms upon return to activity. If the knee is allowed to remain in the flexed position the patellar tendon graft will not fit snugly in the intercondylar notch. As a result, scar tissue will fill the space and act as a "door stop," preventing terminal extension, which can cause anterior knee pain and crepitus. Flexion has a lower priority during the initial phase of rehabilitation although we obtain near 90 degrees of knee flexion prior to discharge to prevent patellar entrapment.

Occasionally patients have difficulty maintaining full knee extension. If this situation develops, it must be recognized and aggressively addressed at this phase of the rehabilitation to prevent it from becoming a more difficult problem later.

In most cases, management of this problem includes utilization of an extension board, as shown in Figure 2. The patient's heel is placed on an elevated pad at the end of the board while straps above and below the knee serve to extend the joint. Liberal use of the board is continued until the patient can easily achieve full knee extension.

The use of an extension cast also is occasionally required. In particular, a cast seems to be most useful in two circumstances. The first is the patient who returns at the 1 week postoperative visit with 5 degrees or more short of full extension. A full extension cast in this individual during sleep at night can eliminate the flexion contracture and also decrease knee swelling and allow a resumption of the program. The second involves the patient who reports a very stiff and bent knee each morning. This situation is best treated by applying an extension cast, bivalving it, and having the patient wear it while he or she sleeps at night.

Both the extension board and casting are well tolerated and effective methods of limiting knee extension problems. With an understanding of the importance of full knee extension, patients are eager to do whatever is necessary to achieve this goal.

Phase III

Phase III of therapy encompasses the general period from 2 to 5 weeks following reconstruction. Emphasis is placed on (1) achieving a normal gait pattern, (2) maintaining full knee extension, (3) increasing knee flexion, and (4) quadriceps strengthening.

By the third week patients should be ambulating without aids and without limping. Flexion exercises such as wall slides are continued, but the importance of maintaining full knee extension must be emphasized. Quadriceps strengthening is also an important part of preparing for a return to sport specific activities. The best tolerated strengthening programs usually include closed chain exercises such as a stair-step machine, stationary bicycle, and leg press exercises.

Phase IV

Very few time constraints are placed on a return to full activities. We have found that a 70% return of quadriceps strength seems to be the necessary level for successful participation in sports specific activities. Any attempt to return before this level of strength is obtained often results in a sore and swollen knee. Rehabilitation should therefore focus on strengthening until this 70% level is achieved. Thereafter, strength will continue to improve with less emphasis on strengthening by resumption of participation in functional activities. It is not uncommon for patients to start these activities as soon as 5 weeks after surgery. Early involvement in lateral shuffles, cariocas, jumping rope, or shooting baskets is progressed as the patient becomes more comfortable and confident on the reconstructed knee.

It is important to remember that most patients require 2 to 3 months of sport specific activities before returning to a competitive level. Realistically, this means that an athlete who plans on returning to competition 6 months after reconstruction needs to begin playing full-court basketball or equivalent at 3 to 4 months after surgery.

Although little scientific support exists for functional bracing, we have continued to encourage its use during the first competitive season. Most patients can anticipate bouts of patellar tendon soreness and occasional swelling during the preseason drills. Avoiding severe patellar soreness early in the season, and in particular during two-a-day practices, is important to a successful return as the season progresses. Judicious use of a day off and limiting practice to once a day will often serve to minimize these problems. Very few patients experience the same difficulties the following season.

DISCUSSION

It is believed that maturation of the reconstructed ligament is preceded by initial weakening as shown by previous animal studies. This graft weakening is accompanied by formation of a vascular sheath and revascularization by 6 to 8 weeks after the procedure. A more recent human study has demonstrated that the reconstruction graft is repopulated with new host fibroblast as early as 3 weeks after reconstructive surgery. Amiel et al have presented evidence that suggest the patellar tendon graft does respond to its environment. In addition, we now know that the healing ligament demonstrates both collagen synthesis and degradation, the balance of which is shifted toward synthesis during the inflammatory stage. Collagen synthesis and organization is also known to be influenced by applied stress in transplanted connective tissue. These observations would lead us to believe that the reconstructed patellar tendon graft is not a nonviable structure with little adaptive potential, but is actually a living construct with the ability to respond in a positive fashion to applied stress. This concept of "ligamentization" is central to the accelerated rehabilitation protocol.

To date we have been unable to identify any detrimental effects of the accelerated protocol. While using the same surgical technique before accelerated rehabilitation (before 1987) and after accelerated rehabilitation (after 1987) we have seen an improvement in KT-1,000 values. At a minimum follow-up of 2 years, the patients prior to 1987 had an average KT-1,000 manual maximum difference of 2.8 mm. Patients following the accelerated protocol have had an average KT-1,000 manual maximum difference of 2.1 mm. This improvement is most likely the result of our enhanced ability to reproduce the surgical technique with correct positioning and tensioning of the patellar tendon graft. Regardless of the reason, it appears that resumption of full weight-bearing and an early return to functional activities actually serves to strengthen the patellar tendon graft instead of "stretching" it out as previously hypothesized.

The major advantage of the accelerated protocol lies in its ability to limit the incidence of postoperative morbidity. Patients who obtain full knee extension before and immediately after surgery rarely exhibit the surgical complications commonly associated with this procedure. Knee stiffness, patellofemoral pain, and quadriceps weakness are rarely encountered. Less than 1% undergo subsequent procedures for flexion contractures. Also, we have discovered that most patients are able to return to full activities much sooner than previously thought with no detrimental effects.

SUGGESTED READING

Amiel D, Kleiner JB, Akeson WH. The natural history of the anterior cruciate ligament autograft of patellar tendon origin. Am J Sports Med 1986; 14:449–462.

Andriacci T, Sabiston P, DeHaven K, et al. Ligament: Injury and repair. In: Woo SL, Buckwalter JA, eds. Injury and repair of the musculoskeletal soft tissues. Park Ridge, Ill: American Academy of Orthopedic Surgeons, 1987:103.

Arnoczky SP, Tarvin GB, Marshall JL. Anterior cruciate ligament replacement using patellar tendon. J Bone Joint Surg 1982; 64A:217–224.

Clancy WG, Narechania RG, Rosenberg TD, et al. Anterior and posterior cruciate ligament reconstruction in rhesus monkeys. J Bone Joint Surg 1981; 63A:1270–1284.

Fullerton LR, Andrews JR. Mechanical block to extension following augmentation of the anterior cruciate ligament: A case report. Am J Sports Med 1984; 12:166–168.

Klein L, Lunseth PA, Aadalen RJ. Comparison of functional and non-functional tendon grafts. J Bone Joint Surg 1972; 54A: 1745–1753.

Krippaehne WW, Hunt TK, Jackson DS, Dunphy JE. Studies on the effect of stress on transplants of autologous and homologous connective tissue. Am J Surg 1962; 104:267–272.

Mohtadi NG, Webster-Bogaert S, Fowler PJ. Limitation of motion following anterior cruciate ligament reconstruction: A case control study. Am J Sports Med 1991; 19:620–625.

Paulos LE, Rosenberg TD, Drawbert J, et al. Infrapatellar contracture syndrome: An unrecognized cause of knee stiffness with patella entrapment and patella infera. Am J Sports Med 1987; 15:331–341.

Rougraff B, Shelbourne KD, Gerth PK, et al. Arthroscopic and histologic analysis of human patellar tendon autografts used for anterior cruciate ligament reconstruction. Am J Sports Med 1993; 21:277–284.

Sachs RA, Daniel DM, Stone ML, et al. Patellofemoral problems after anterior cruciate ligament reconstruction. Am J Sports Med 1989; 17:760–765.

Shelbourne KD, Johnson GE. Locked buckethandle meniscus tears in chronic ACL-deficient knees. Am J Sports Med (in press).

Shelbourne KD, Nitz P. Accelerated rehabilitation after anterior cruciate ligament reconstruction. Am J Sports Med 1990; 18: 292–299.

Shelbourne KD, Wilckens JH, Mollabashy A, et al. Arthrofibrosis in acute anterior cruciate ligament reconstruction: The effect of timing of reconstruction and rehabilitation. Am J Sports Med 1991; 19:332–336.

POSTEROLATERAL KNEE INJURIES

CHERIE A. HOLMES, M.D.
BERNARD R. BACH, Jr., M.D.

Injuries to the posterior cruciate ligament (PCL) and posterolateral structures of the knee are uncommon but highly debilitating. Although our understanding of injuries to the anterior cruciate ligament (ACL) is far superior, improvements have been made in the last decade to further our understanding of the pathomechanics, pathoanatomy, and surgical treatment of posterolateral knee rotatory instability. This pathology and its resultant disability must be understood completely by the practitioner before treatment since the physical examination often presents a confusing picture with subtle findings and complex instability patterns. Only through knowledge of the anatomy, biomechanics, mechanisms of injury, and natural history can a clear plan for diagnosis and treatment be formulated.

ANATOMY AND BIOMECHANICS

Seebacher et al have described the anatomy of the posterolateral knee (Fig. 1). They have classified it into three layers. Layer I is comprised of the iliotibial band anteriorly, the superficial biceps tendon posteriorly, and their individual expansions. The peroneal nerve lies deep to layer I and posterior to the biceps tendon. It is important to remember that its fascial attachments can tether the nerve, especially as it proceeds distally when performing the Clancy biceps tenodesis reconstructive procedure.

Layer II is formed by the quadriceps retinaculum anteriorly and two patellofemoral ligaments posteriorly. Of the posterior structures, the proximal ligament attaches to the lateral intermuscular septum while the distal ligament inserts into the fabella (if present) or into the lateral gastrocnemius muscle extension to the posterolateral capsule. Layer II also contains the patellomeniscal ligament.

Layer III consists of the lateral joint capsule with its direct tibial and femoral attachments and the lateral meniscus along a horizontal plane. The coronary ligament, which is the capsular attachment to the meniscus, contains a hiatus for passage of the popliteus tendon, which runs superolaterally. The lateral capsule forms two discrete laminae posterior to the iliotibial tract; the more superficial encompasses the LCL, with the LCL lying superficial to layer III. The superficial lamina ends posteriorly at the fabellofibular ligament. The coronary ligament is formed by the deeper lamina and passes posteriorly to the arcuate ligament. The "Y"-shaped arcuate ligament, along with the fabellofibular ligament reinforces the posterlateral capsule by spanning medial to and between the popliteus muscle and tendon from the styloid process of the fibular to the posterior femur. The posterior tibia is the point of origin of the popliteus muscle, which then passes superolaterally in a more

tendinous fashion lying between the coronary ligament and the synovial membrane.

Marshall noted that the long head of the biceps tendon becomes tendinous 7 to 10 cm proximal to the tendon. Prior to insertion, the long head splits into three layers: superficial, deep, and the layer that encompasses the LCL.

The clinical studies by DeLee and Baker and Hughston and the sequential and combined sectioning studies by Jakob, Gollehan et al, and Grood et al have contributed to our understanding of the primary and secondary restraints of the posterolateral corner and the pathoanatomy of posterolateral insufficiency. They have helped clarify the differentiation from PCL injuries. These studies demonstrated that posterior translation at all angles of flexion, but primarily at 90 degrees, is the result of sectioning of the PCL. Loss of the PCL, however, did not increase external rotation significantly. Isolated sectioning of the LCL and isolated sectioning of the arcuate ligament complex both produced significant increases in primary external rotation, the former mostly at 30 degrees of flexion, the latter at various degrees. Neither affected varus instability. When both ligaments underwent combined sectioning, both primary varus angulation and primary external rotation increased markedly at 30 degrees of flexion. This also resulted in a mild degree of posterior translation. When PCL sectioning was added to this instability pattern significant posterior translation from 30 degrees to 90 degrees was noted.

The clinical implication of these biomechanical studies is that minimal posterolateral rotation is found in an isolated PCL injury. When combined with a poster-

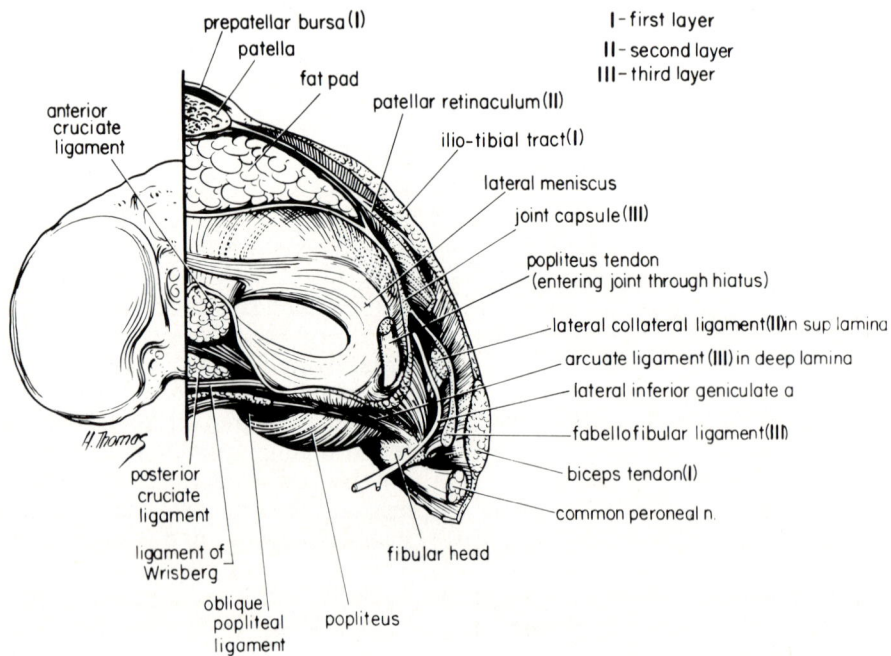

Figure 1 The three-layer concept of the posterolateral corner of a right knee is depicted. (From Seebacher JR, Inglis AE, Marshall JL, Warren RF. The structure of the posterolateral aspects of the knee. J Bone Joint Surg 1982; 64(A):536-541; with permission.)

olateral injury, posterolateral rotation will be more extensive and more easily viewed at 90 degrees of knee flexion. When occurring as an isolated entity, a posterolateral injury will have greater posterolateral rotation at 30 degrees as opposed to 90 degrees of knee flexion.

MECHANISM OF INJURY

Vehicular accidents and sports injuries are the most common causes of posterolateral ligamentous trauma. Disruption of the posterolateral complex occurs when a posterior force is directed against the medial aspect of the proximal tibia when the knee is extended. This produces a hyperextension force with a varus moment. However, isolated posterolateral injury is extremely uncommon. Most commonly it occurs in association with either PCL or other ligamentous injuries, as is seen in knee dislocations.

CLINICAL HISTORY AND PHYSICAL EXAMINATION

Careful examination of the knee is important since injuries to the posterolateral structures as well as the PCL are often missed. A history of the injury mechanism is foremost in determining the potential injury pattern. Evaluation of the anterior or anteromedial tibia for abrasions or lacerations should be performed. A tense effusion as seen with ACL injuries is uncommon. The posterolateral corner of the knee should be palpated for tenderness or swelling and inspected for ecchymosis. Open injuries mandate prompt irrigation and debridement in the operating room.

A thorough neurovascular examination is required since posterolateral injury is often associated with other ligamentous injuries, as can be seen in knee dislocations. If knee dislocation is suspected, an arteriogram is mandatory. If vascular compromise is grossly obvious, the arteriogram should be bypassed for immediate surgical exploration.

Gait abnormalities are not uncommon. Patients may be observed to ambulate with the foot externally rotated. Instability associated with stairs, particularly while descending, or while walking down ramps is frequently noted. One must attempt to differentiate these symptoms from a patellofemoral basis. If chronic posterolateral instability exists, a varus thrust at the knee may be evident. Noyes and co-workers have popularized the concept of increased tensile forces ("lateral lift off") accompanied by increased medial compartment compressive forces as an explanation for increased medial knee symptoms in many of these patients. Patients may complain of pain, fatigue, and giving way and rotational movements may be difficult.

Evaluation for posterolateral instability requires examination of both the PCL and posterolateral corner. The posterior drawer exam is performed at 90 degrees of flexion in neutral, internal, and external rotation to determine associated evidence of PCL injury. The

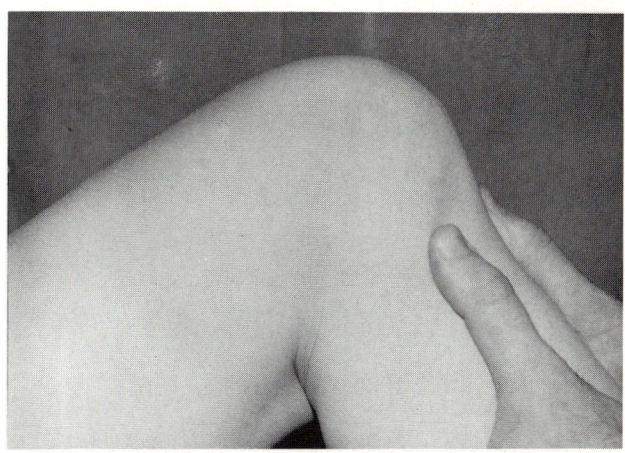

Figure 2 Physical examination of this right knee demonstrates a combination of posterior translation and posterolateral rotation consistent with a combined PCL posterolateral injury. (From Bach BR Jr, Jewell BF, Dworsky B. Posterolateral knee reconstruction using Clancy biceps tenodesis—surgical technique. Am J Knee Surg 1993; 6:97-103; with permission.)

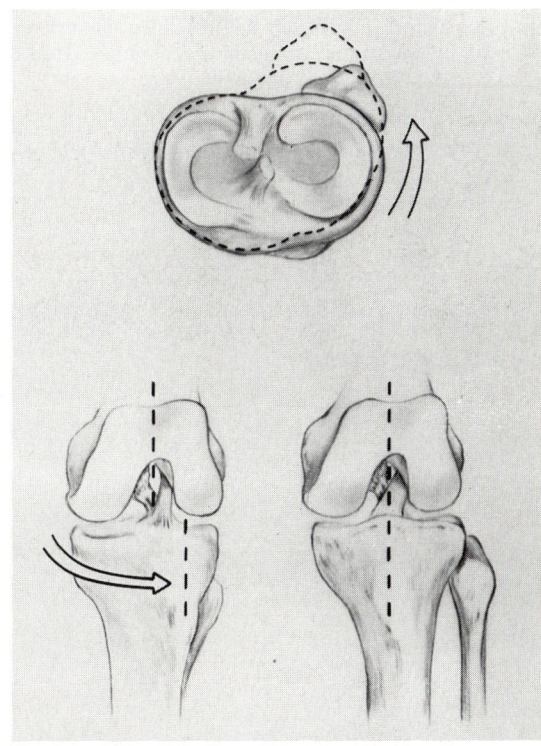

Figure 3 Posterolateral rotation. (From Bach BR Jr, Jewell BF, Dworsky B. Posterolateral knee reconstruction using Clancy biceps tenodesis—surgical technique. Am J Knee Surg 1993; 6:97-103; with permission.)

normal knee has an anterior tibial step-off of approximately 10 mm. A decrease in this step-off is suggestive of a PCL injury. This should be correlated with the degree of posterior displacement and the quality of the end-point. Varus and valgus laxity is evaluated at both 0 degrees and 30 degrees to assess the collateral ligaments.

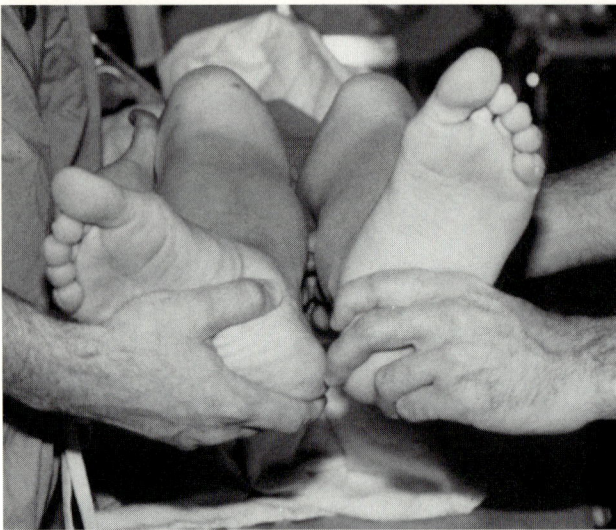

Figure 4 This injured right knee demonstrates an increased thigh-foot angle. Posterolateral rotation was observed more so at 30 degrees than at 90 degrees. The patient sustained a low velocity soccer related posterolateral knee dislocation. Physical examination revealed a grade 3 posterior drawer, grade 3 varus laxity and an obvious posterolateral laxity. (From Bach BR Jr, Jewell BF, Dworsky B. Posterolateral knee reconstruction using Clancy biceps tenodesis—surgical technique. Am J Knee Surg 1993; 6:97-103; with permission.)

Additionally, posterolateral injury can cause varus instability at full extension without injury to the PCL.

The posterolateral drawer and the external-rotation recurvatum test as described by Hughston is performed to assess posterolateral laxity. The former is executed with the knee at 80 to 90 degrees of flexion and 15 degrees of external rotation of the foot. Posterior movement of the lateral tibial plateau on the lateral femoral condyle is assessed. In contrast to the isolated PCL injury, where straight posterior translation is noted, the examiner will observe a combination of posterior translation accompanied by external tibial rotation. Posterolateral rotational assymetry must be compared to the contralateral knee (Figs. 2, 3, and 4). The external rotation recurvatum test is performed in the supine position with both knees in full extension while grasping the great toes. The amount of pathologic knee hyperextension and external rotation of the tibia is assessed.

Two other tests used to determine posterolateral laxity are the reverse pivot shift as reported by Jakob and the prone external rotation test described by Cooper. The reverse pivot shift can be elicited by taking the knee from a 90 degree flexed position, where the knee is subluxed, to a full extended position under valgus load and tibial external rotation, where the knee is in the relocated position. In contrast to the pivot shift phenomenon of ACL insufficiency, the knee is subluxed in

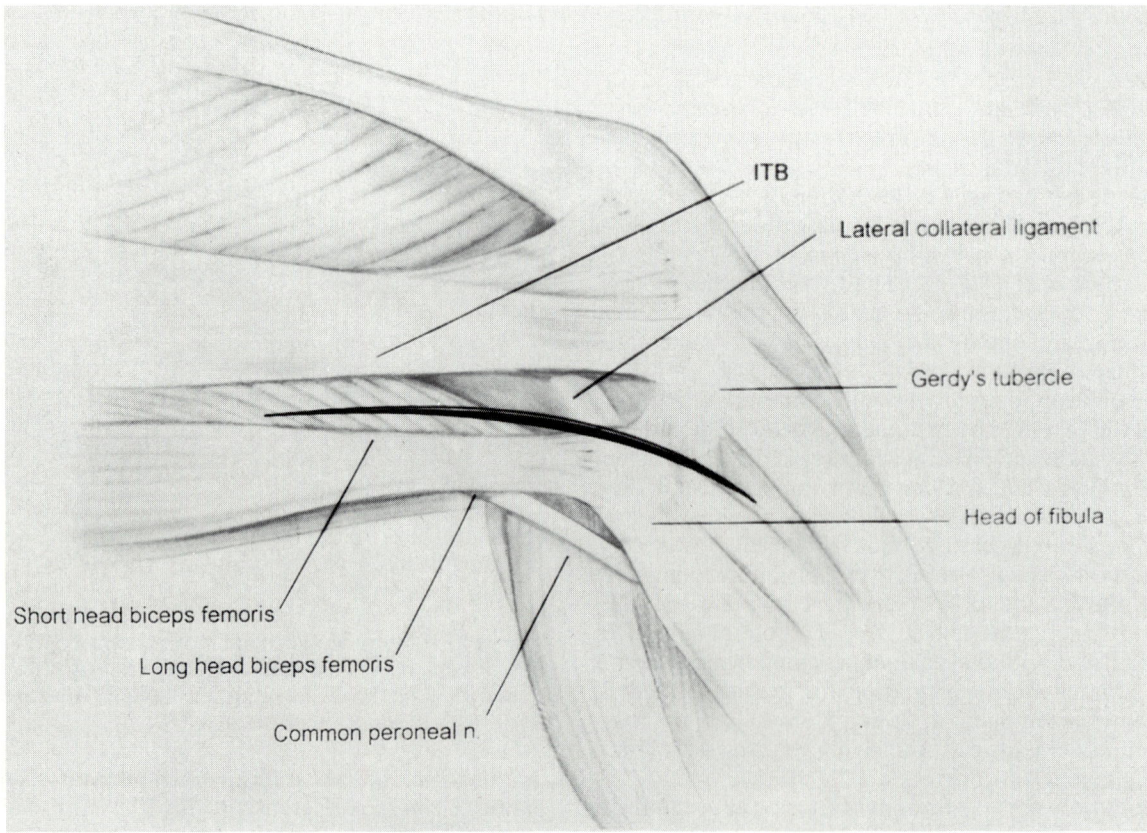

Figure 5 The skin incision is fashioned midway between Gerdy's tubercle and the fibular head and is approximately 6 inches in length. (From Bach BR Jr, Jewell BF, Dworsky B. Posterolateral knee reconstruction using Clancy biceps tenodesis—surgical technique. Am J Knee Surg 1993; 6:97-103; with permission.)

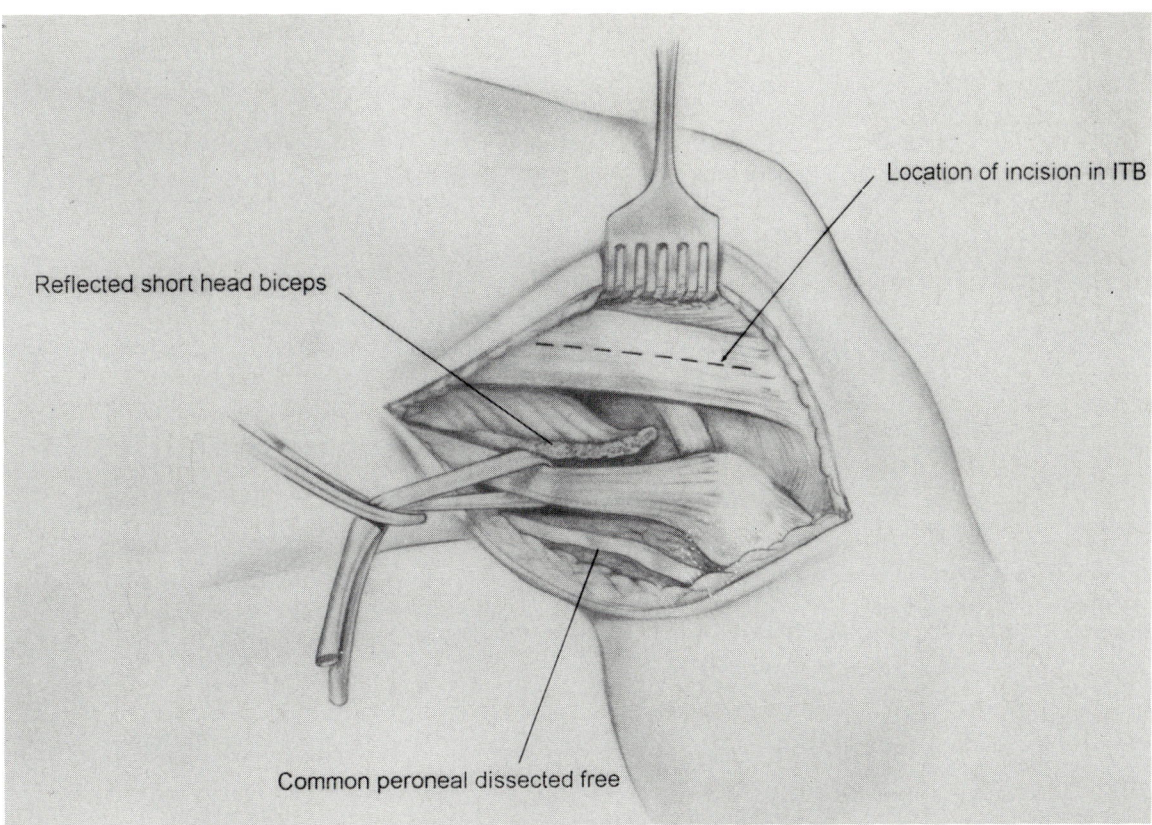

Reflected short head biceps

Location of incision in ITB

Common peroneal dissected free

Figure 6 This schematic illustration summarizes identification and dissection of the peroneal nerve, incision and isolation of the long head biceps tendon, and reflection of the short head bicep muscle fibers from the tendon. The dotted line indicates the subsequent incision that will be made into the midsubstance of the iliotibial band. (From Bach BR Jr, Jewell BF, Dworsky B. Posterolateral knee reconstruction using Clancy biceps tenodesis—surgical technique. Am J Knee Surg 1993; 6:97-103; with permission.)

flexion and reduces in extension. This test, however, lacks specificity since Cooper showed that 35% of normal patients examined under anesthesia demonstrated a reverse pivot shift finding. The prone external rotation test has provided greater specificity. The knee is stabilized in the prone position at 30 and 90 degrees. The foot is forcefully externally rotated while the medial border of the foot is measured relative to the axis of the femur. As with all the tests, significant variation exists in external rotation from patient to patient and the injured extremity must be compared with the contralateral side.

Instrumented testing for posterolateral laxity of the knee has not been shown to correlate with the clinical examination, as the KT-1000 measures anterior posterior translations rather than rotations. It is not routinely used as part of the physical examination, other than to assess the magnitude of translations associated with ACL or PCL injuries.

RADIOGRAPHIC EVALUATION

Plain radiographs can be helpful in determining ligamentous injuries. Avulsion of the fibular head or Gerdy's tubercle are highly suggestive of injury to the lateral or posterolateral structures. Posterior translation, posterior sag, or posterior tibial avulsion may also be evidence of an associated PCL injury. Chronic posterolateral insufficiency, especially if associated with PCL loss, may show increased evidence of tricompartmental degenerative changes, as evidenced by the marked elevation in contact pressures in all three compartments in the sectioning study by Skyhar et al.

Magnetic resonance imaging (MRI) can be helpful in diagnosing injury to the PCL, but it is usually inadequate in differentiating full from partial tears. It can be utilized to identify concomitant soft tissue injuries, especially those in the posterolateral corner. It should be emphasized that MRI is used as an adjunct to the clinical examination and not in place of a carefully performed physical examination.

As mentioned previously, chronic posterolateral instability may be associated with a varus, hyperextension stance clinically evidenced as a varus thrust during the gait cycle. Full-length, standing lower extremity radiographs help identify abnormal alignment while abnormal gait mechanics can best be determined by gait analysis in a gait lab. These are useful in assessing the need for tibial osteotomy before soft tissue procedures, as recommended by DeLee. Soft tissue procedures will

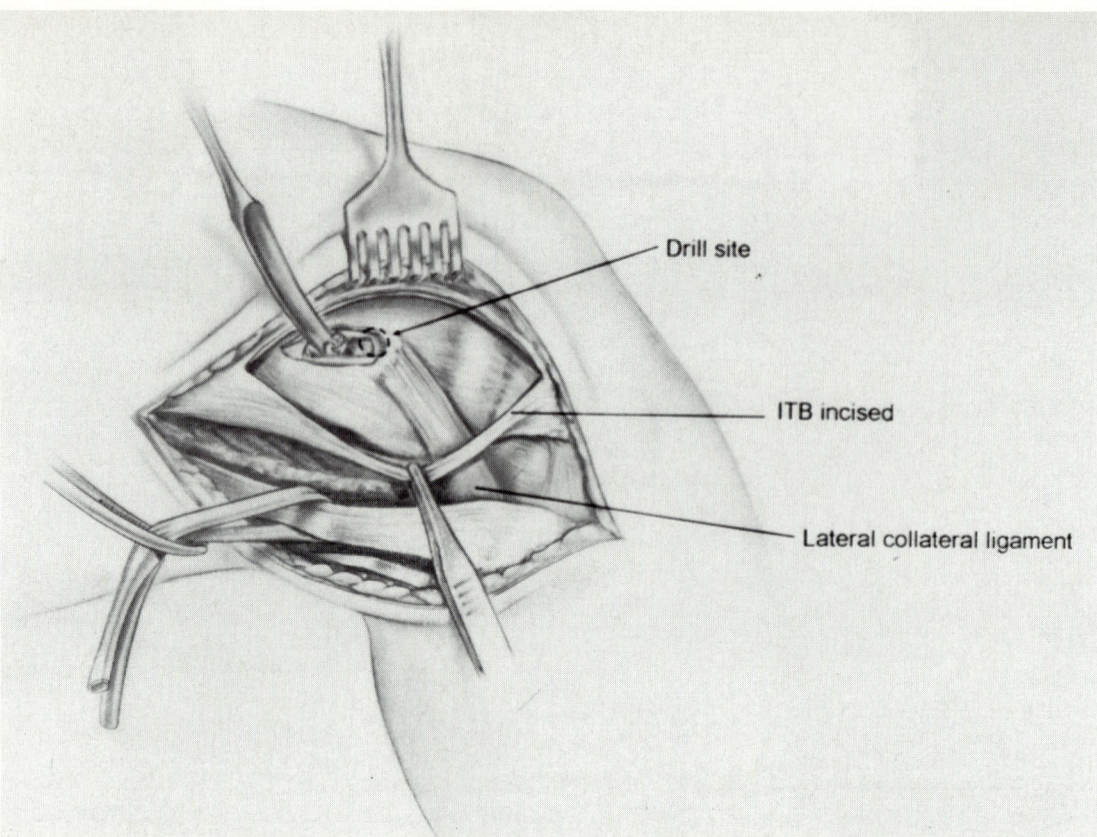

Figure 7   The iliotibial band incision has been performed and is retracted posteriorly. The lateral collateral ligament is identified and its origin at the lateral femoral epicondyle is confirmed. A Cobb gauge is used to create a trough for the transferred biceps tendon. (From Bach BR Jr, Jewell BF, Dworsky B. Posterolateral knee reconstruction using Clancy biceps tenodesis—surgical technique. Am J Knee Surg 1993; 6:97-103; with permission.)

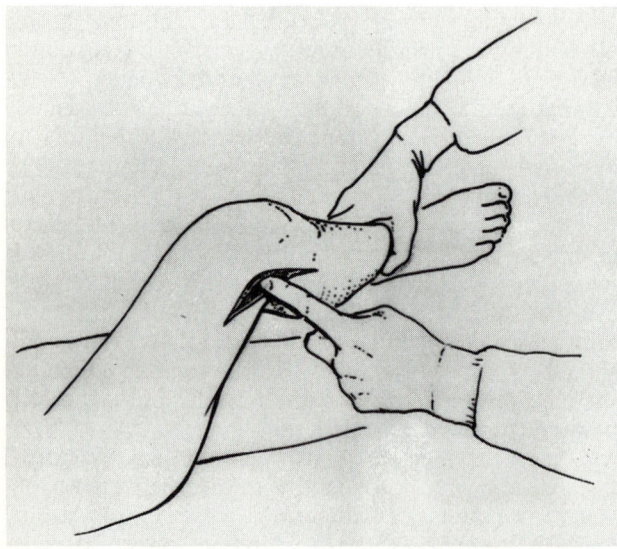

Figure 8   Confirmation of the lateral collateral ligament is performed by placing the knee in a "figure four" position. (From Bach BR Jr, Jewell BF, Dworsky B. Posterolateral knee reconstruction using Clancy biceps tenodesis—surgical technique. Am J Knee Surg 1993; 6:97-103; with permission.)

more than likely fail if the static or dynamic malalignment is left unaddressed.

TREATMENT

Vigorous quadriceps strengthening through closed chain exercises may be helpful in treating the patient with low grade isolated posterolateral instability. However, since most of these injuries are associated with other ligamentous injuries, nonoperative treatment is usually found to be insufficient to give stability to the knee. Either the posterolateral corner should be addressed independently and the patient re-examined, or the posterolateral laxity in conjunction with the other ligamentous injuries needs to be reconstructed.

No true consensus exists in the literature to clarify the surgical indications or surgical treatment for posterolateral instability. General agreement is that operative treatment of acute posterolateral instability has more success than chronic posterolateral instability. When found in conjunction with low grade PCL injuries, we have found that addressing the posterolateral instability alone provides adequate stability to the knee.

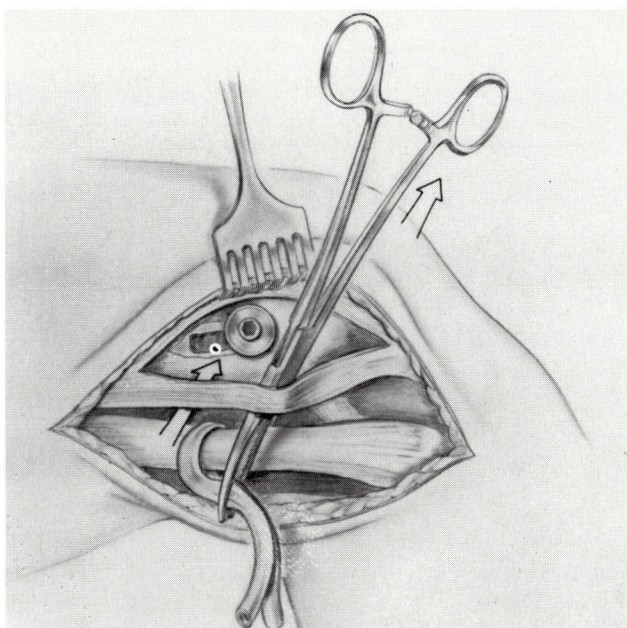

Figure 9 Transfer of the biceps tendon through the incision in the posterior intermuscular septum so that the tendon is placed medial to the iliotibial band. A screw and washer assembly has been secured at the origin on the lateral collateral ligament. (From Bach BR Jr, Jewell BF, Dworsky B. Posterolateral knee reconstruction using Clancy biceps tenodesis — surgical technique. Am J Knee Surg 1993; 6:97-103; with permission.)

Cooper maintained that a 10 degree difference in external rotation or assymetry of varus angulation both assessed at 30 degrees of flexion is significant enough instability to require reconstruction. High tibial osteotomy, as recommended by DeLee (personal communication) for those patients with varus malalignment, is a potential alternative to, or used as an adjunct prior to posterolateral reconstruction.

Various surgical procedures have been popularized including popliteus tendon recession, popliteus tendon bypass, reconstructions using allograft tissues, posterolateral corner advancements, iliotibial band rerouting procedures, and biceps tendon tenodesis procedures. Clancy is credited with the description and popularization of the biceps tenodesis. The biceps femoris muscle is a powerful knee flexor, external rotator, and posterolateral tibial subluxor. Tenodesis of the biceps will help negate its subluxing effects while simultaneously reinforcing and advancing the posterolateral structures.

SURGICAL TECHNIQUE

After performing a meticulous bilateral physical examination under anesthesia, the knee is prepped and draped, antibiotics administered preoperatively, and the tourniquet is left deflated. An attempt is made to perform as much of the procedure as possible without the use of the tourniquet. Routinely, tourniquet times

have been less than 40 minutes. Arthroscopy is performed if there is evidence of meniscal injury, or to assess injury to the cruciate structures or articular surfaces. The goal of this procedure is to transfer the biceps femoris tendon medial to the iliotibial band and secure at the origin of the LCL. The rationale for the procedure is to eliminate the deforming flexion and rotational forces of the biceps tendon, to augment and parallel the LCL tissue, and to tighten the posterolateral structures.

With the knee flexed to 30 degrees a 6 inch incision is made following the line of the iliotibial band, placed midway between the biceps and the iliotibial band and ending half way between the fibular head and Gerdy's tubercle (Fig. 5). Anterior and posterior skin flaps are created. The peroneal nerve is identified and dissected free of its surrounding fat and fascia from the biceps femoris muscle proximally to the fibular head distally (Fig. 6). We feel that release of the nerve helps prevent nerve entrapment after transfer and tenodesis of the biceps tendon. The fascia just anterior to the biceps tendon is identified next and a longitudinal incision is made in the line of the biceps tendon. The muscle fibers of the short head of the biceps are then elevated proximally for 6 to 8 cm off the medial surface of the tendon and the tendon is then retracted with a small penrose drain (Fig. 6). An incision is then placed in the thick mid-third of the iliotibial band (ITB), extending in the line of its fibers to Gerdy's tubercle (Fig. 7). With further knee flexion the posterior part of the ITB will relax, allowing greater exposure of the LCL. Better palpation of the LCL can be accomplished by placing the knee in a figure-of-four position (Fig. 8).

The bony dissection at this point parallels the original dissection. The lateral femoral epicondyle and supracondylar metaphyseal area are elevated free of periosteum and prepared with an osteotome or ¼ inch curved gauge see (Fig. 7). This helps promote in-growth and scarring at the tenodesis site, preventing future failure. The isometric point for the tenodesis as determined by Legyt et al is identified just slightly anterior and cephalad to the LCL. A 3.2 mm drill hole is placed in this spot and either a 6.5 mm AO screw and washer, or preferably a 20 mm Concept low profile screw with 2.5 mm offset washer are inserted, leaving 1.5 cm still protruding from the bone surface.

The biceps tendon is passed through an incision in the posterior intermuscular septum. It is transferred anteromedial to the iliotibial band (Fig. 9). Flexing the knee to 90 degrees and using a ¾ in. Cobb elevator, the tendon is levered over the screw and washer while slowly extending the knee to 0 degrees (Fig. 10). Care is taken to ensure that the entire tendon is transferred over the hardware. The screw is tightened flush with the femur while the knee is held in full extension and the foot in neutral rotation. Gentle range of motion of the knee makes certain that the tendon does not dislocate or sublux from its new position and that the iliotibial band does not snap over the screw and washer (Fig. 11)

The knee is re-examined at 30 and 90 degrees, checking for posterolateral spin and reduction of the thigh-foot angle. Since with this procedure we have

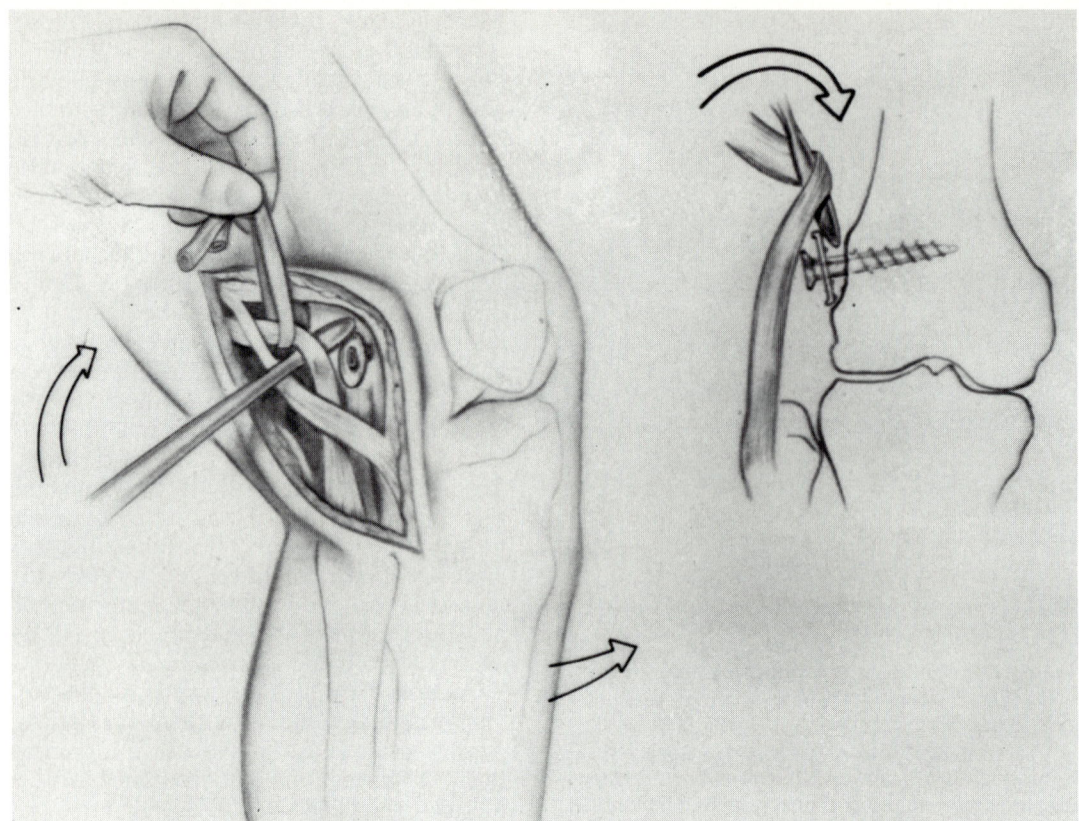

Figure 10 The tendon is transferred over the screw head by levering the tendon while the knee is slowly entended. Enough of the screw must be prominent to permit complete transfer of the tendon. (From Bach BR Jr, Jewell BF, Dworsky B. Posterolateral knee reconstruction using Clancy biceps tenodesis—surgical technique. Am J Knee Surg 1993; 6:97-103; with permission.)

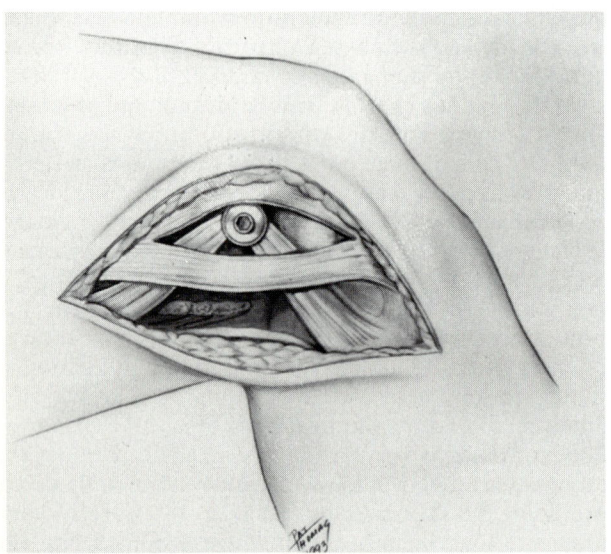

Figure 11 The tenodesis has been secured in extension and the foot in neutral rotation. This view in flexion depicts the new orientation of the tendon transfer. It is acting as a sling, effectively tightening the posterolateral corner. Also note that the distal portion of the transfer parallels the lateral collateral ligament. (From Bach BR Jr, Jewell BF, Dworsky B. Posterolateral knee reconstruction using Clancy biceps tenodesis—surgical technique. Am J Knee Surg 1993; 6:97-103; with permission.)

observed additionally a one grade decrease in the posterior drawer, the senior author prefers to address only posterolateral insufficiency in those patients with combined posterolateral injury and grade one to two PCL drawer.

Following re-examination, the tourniquet is released and the newly re-routed biceps tendon is sutured to the LCL complex. The peroneal nerve is checked again for any impingement by fascial bands before closing the middle third of the iliotibial band with interrupted Vicryl sutures. The subcutaneous tissue is approximated with Vicryl sutures over a Hemovac drain placed in the posterior flap region. The skin is closed with a running subcuticular pull-out suture. Placing the knee in a postoperative brace at 20 to 30 degrees of flexion in the first 24 hours helps relieve early hamstring spasm. The brace is subsequently locked in full extension and the patient is made touch-down weight bearing for the first 6 weeks.

RESULTS

While the literature does not clearly define long-term results of surgical reconstruction, we feel that guidelines can be formulated for addressing the conservative and operative treatment of posterolateral instability. In our patients with a valgus or neutral alignment, we have had favorable results with the Clancy biceps tenodesis procedure. However, these reconstructions represent less than 5% of our overall knee reconstruction procedures and the wide variety of associated pathology (i.e., combined ACL or PCL injuries) results in an extremely heterogeneous patient study group, making overall evaluation and conclusions difficult.

SUGGESTED READING

Bach BR Jr, Jewell BF, Dworsky B. Posterolateral knee reconstruction using Clancy biceps tenodesis-surgical technique. Am J Knee Surg 1993; 6(3): 97–103.

Clancy WG. Repair and reconstruction of the posterior cruciate ligament. In: Chapman MW, ed. Operative orthopaedics. Philadelphia: JB Lippincott, 1988:1651.

Cooper DE, Warren RF, Women JP. The posterior cruciate ligament and posterolateral structures of the knee: Anatomy, function and patterns of injury. Instr Course Lectures. 1991; 40:249–270.

Covey DC, Sapega AA. Current concepts review injuries of the posterior cruciate ligament. J Bone Joint Surg 1993; 75(A): 1376–1386.

Girgis FG, Marshall JL, Almonajem ARS. The crucial ligaments of the knee joint: Anatomical, functional and experimental analysis. Clin Orthop 1975; 106:216–231.

Gollehon DL, Torzilli PA, Warren RF. The role of posterolateral and cruciate ligaments in the stability of the knee. J Bone Joint Surg 1987; 69(A):233–242.

Grood ES, Stavers SF, Noyes FR. Limits of movements in the human knee. J Bone Joint Surg 1988; 70(A):88–97.

Hughston JC, Jacobson KE. Chronic posterolateral rotatory instability of the knee. J Bone Joint Surg 1985; 67-A:351–359.

Hughston JC, Norwood LA. The posterolateral drawer test and external rotational recurvatum test for posterolateral rotatory instability of the knee. Clin Orthop 1980; 147:82–87.

Jakob RP, Hassler H, Staeubli HU. Observations on rotatory instability of the lateral compartment of the knee. Acta Orthop Scand 1981; 191(suppl):1–31.

Noyes FR, Stowers SF, Grood ES, et al. Posterior subluxations of the medial and lateral tibiofemoral compartments: An in vitro ligament sectioning study in cadaveric knees. Am J Sports Med 1993; 21:407–414.

Seebacher JR, Inglis AE, Marshall JL, Warren RF. The structure of the posterolateral aspects of the knee. J Bone Joint Surg 1982; 64(A):536–541.

Shelbourne KD, Benedict F, McCarroll JR, Rettig AC. Dynamic posterior shift test: An adjunct in evaluation of posterior tibial subluxation. Am J Sports Med 1989; 17:275–277.

Shino K, Horibe S, Ono K. The voluntarily evoked posteriolateral drawer sign in the knee with posteriolateral instability. Clin Orthop 1987; 215:179–186.

Skyhar MJ, Warren RF, Ortiz GJ, et al. The effects of sectioning of the posterior cruciate ligament and posterolateral complex on the articular contact pressure within the knee. J Bone Joint Surg 1993; 694–699.

Wascher DC, Grauer JD, Markoff KL. Biceps tendon tenodesis for posterolateral instability of the knee. Am J Sports Med 1993; 21:400–406.

ARTHROSCOPICALLY ASSISTED RECONSTRUCTION OF THE POSTERIOR CRUCIATE LIGAMENT

D. C. COVEY, M.D.
COMMANDER, MEDICAL CORPS, U.S. NAVY

Except for avulsion fractures, treatment of injuries to the posterior cruciate ligament (PCL) has been controversial. Some authors have recommended operative treatment of both acute and chronic isolated PCL tears, while others have recommended surgery only when a PCL tear is combined with other ligamentous injury, causing multidirectional instability. If surgical treatment is selected, the surgeon is faced with choices regarding operative technique (open versus arthroscopically assisted), the type of graft most appropriate for the reconstruction (autogenous tissue or allograft, with or without synthetic augmentation), and whether to aim for an isometric as opposed to an anatomic reconstruction of the PCL; since both cannot be achieved with a single 10 to 12 mm wide graft.

Indications for PCL reconstruction include pain and functional limitations (that may include instability) caused by posterior tibial subluxation, and the presence of a 2+ to 3+ posterior drawer sign. Combined PCL and posterolateral injuries are usually treated operatively with PCL reconstruction, and a concomitant extra-articular posterolateral procedure.

This chapter describes my current method of arthroscopically assisted PCL reconstruction that incorporates graft placement guidelines based on recent anatomic and biomechanical studies of the PCL. The surgical goal is to approximate, as near as possible, the normal anatomy of the PCL, while minimizing the operative morbidity.

ANATOMIC AND BIOMECHANICAL CONSIDERATIONS

The name PCL is derived from the ligament's spatial orientation and its site of insertion on the posterior tibial shelf. The ligament is surrounded by a fold of synovium that is reflected from the posterior capsule, making the PCL extrasynovial yet intra-articular. The PCL has a large origin (12 by 32 mm) on the medial femoral condyle that resembles a horizontally oriented semicircle, with a convex inferior boundary that parallels the articular margin of the condyle. The smaller quadrilateral tibial insertion zone is located on an inclined, recessed shelf inferior to the articular surface of the plateau. As a reflection of the disparate sizes of the areas of the PCL's origin and insertion, the cross-sectional area of the ligament decreases from its proximal to distal bony attachments.

Traditionally, the macroscopic anatomy of the PCL has been considered to be composed of two bands or bundles, variously termed anterior or anterolateral, and posterior or posteromedial. The anterior fiber group, that comprises the bulk of the ligament, has been observed by most investigators to tighten with knee flexion and relax with extension. The relatively small cross-sectioned posterior fiber group has been described as being slack in flexion and tight in extension.

It may be overly simplistic to describe the functional morphology of the PCL in terms of just two reciprocally functioning bundles. Some authors have characterized the the PCL as having anterior, central, and posterior fibers, while a recent report viewed the PCL in terms of four consistent fiber-regions (Fig. 1) that are delineated by osseous attachment sites, fiber orientation, and

mechanical behavior during knee motion. Contemporary studies also indicate that the PCL is not composed of anatomically distinct bands or bundles, but is actually a continuum of fibers, different portions of which are taught or slack depending on the angle of knee flexion.

The PCL is the primary restraint to straight posterior translation of the tibia. Isolated PCL rupture has little effect on tibial rotational laxity or varus and valgus angulation unless there is associated injury of the extra-articular restraints. Rupture of the PCL combined with injury to the posterolateral (arcuate) complex results in a marked increase in both varus angulation and tibial external rotation when the knee is flexed 90 degrees, but only small increases in these motions occur at full extension.

PCL fiber strain (the percent change in fiber length) varies markedly in different regions of the ligament. Strain in the anterior-most fibers has been shown to

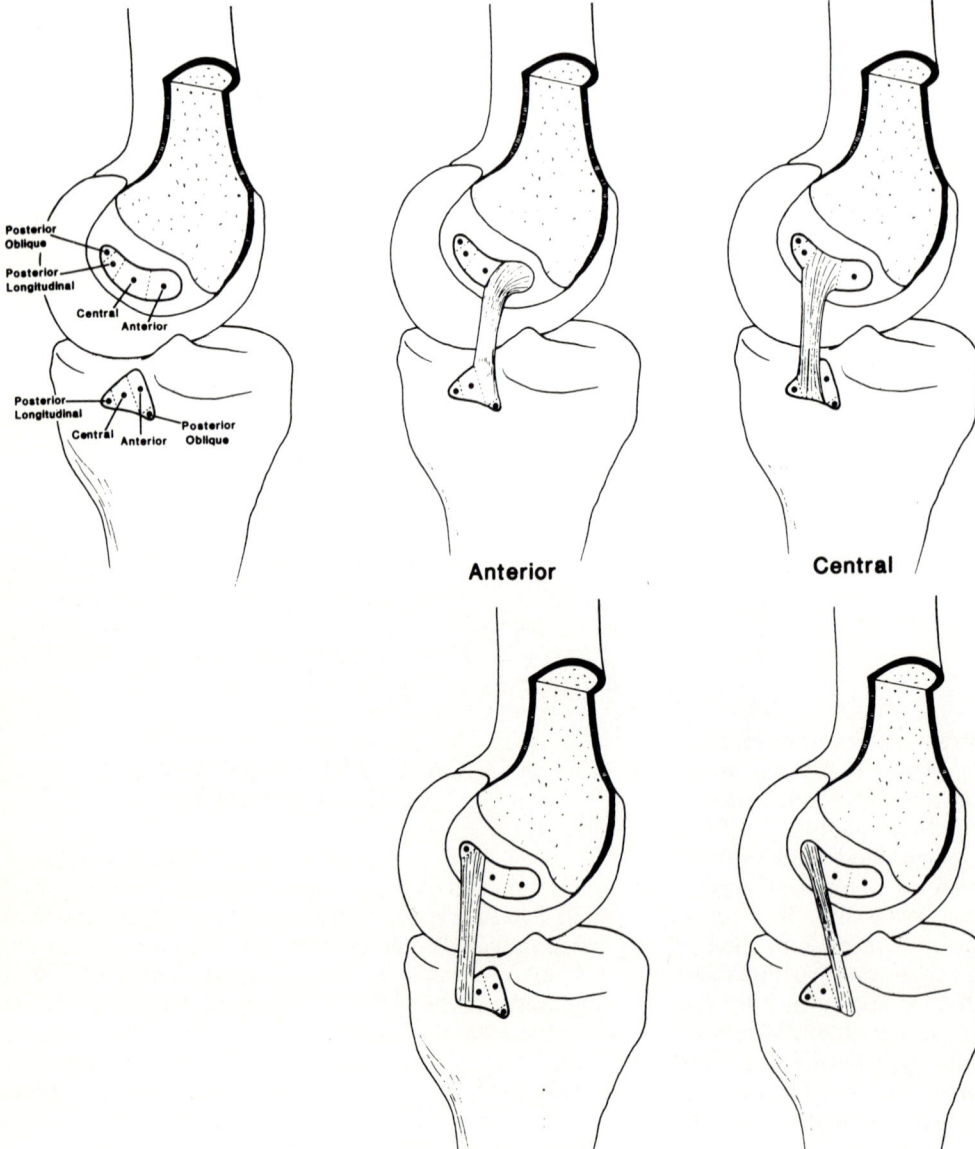

Anterior

Central

Posterior Longitudinal

Posterior Oblique

Figure 1 Anatomic schematic drawings showing the four fiber regions of the posterior cruciate ligament (PCL) and their osseous sites of attachment on the medial femoral condyle and posterior tibial shelf. (From Covey DC, Sapega AA. Current concepts review. Injuries of the posterior cruciate ligament. J Bone Joint Surg 1993; 75A:1376–1386; with permission.)

increase from 10 to 120 degrees of knee flexion, being markedly higher in magnitude than strain in the posterior-most fibers. Studies examining the end-to-end length behavior of different fiber regions within the PCL have shown that the magnitude and pattern of length change during knee motion are governed primarily by the site selected within the large area of the femoral origin, and are less dependent on the location within the tibial insertion zone.

My intraoperative experience has borne out the predictions of several recent laboratory investigations; that is, as graft placement becomes more anatomic, it becomes less isometric. An anatomically faithful reconstruction of the principal fiber bulk of the PCL requires femoral tunnel placement in the attachment zone of the anterior and central fibers. The 4 to 5 mm of end-to-end length increase that the anterior and central fiber regions normally exhibit with knee flexion in vivo requires that a graft substituting for these fibers (constituting the principal fiber bulk of the PCL) be tensioned and fixed near 90 degrees of flexion.

OPERATIVE TECHNIQUE

With the patient supine on the operating table, an examination under anesthesia is performed to corroborate the clinical impression of isolated or combined PCL injury. A tourniquet is placed on the upper thigh, and the operative limb placed in an arthroscopic leg holder, or alternatively, off the side of the operating table. An arthroscopic pump is used routinely, and may obviate the need to inflate the tourniquet. From an anterolateral portal, a 30 degree arthroscope is used to visualize the intercondylar notch region, verify injury to the PCL, and to perform a standard arthroscopic examination of the entire knee joint, noting any articular cartilage or meniscal injury. After appropriate treatment of any meniscal pathology, a 5.5 mm motorized shaver is placed through an anteromedial portal to remove scar tissue and remnants of the PCL. The soft tissue debridement begins at the anteromedial inlet of the intercondylar notch and extends posteriorly in a progressive fashion. The fibrous attachment of the PCL to the medial femoral condyle is excised nearly down to bone, leaving only a small footprint of fibers that will serve to delineate the ligament's zone of origin. Care should be taken to avoid damage to an intact anterior cruciate ligament (ACL).

The region of the distal tibial stump must be adequately visualized to facilitate its resection prior to drilling the tibial tunnel. The posterior tibial insertion area is viewed either with a 30 degree, or preferably a 70 degree arthroscope inserted via a frontal portal, or with a 30 degree arthroscope through a posteromedial portal, as needed (Figs. 2 and 3). Specially designed currettes and rasps introduced through the anteromedial portal may be used to assist removal of all soft tissue between the posterior border of the central tibial plateau and the most distal and posterior fiber attachment site of the PCL. The posterior joint capsule attaches to the posterior tibial shelf just distal to the PCL. It is usually

faster and more efficient to perform this step using a 5.5 mm motorized shaver inserted through a posteromedial portal while watching from the front with a 70 degree arthroscope angled downwards.

Several ligament substitutes have been used for arthroscopically assisted PCL reconstruction. Autogenous or allograft bone-patellar tendon-bone prepara-

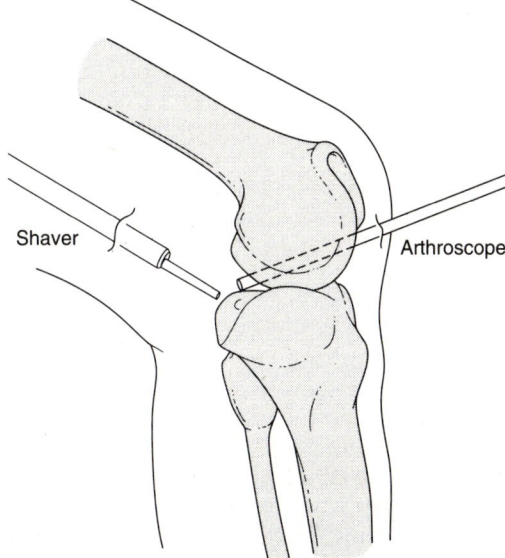

Figure 2 A posteromedial arthroscopic portal is helpful for viewing the tibial attachment of the PCL, resecting the tibial stump, and for visualization prior to drilling the tibial tunnel. (From Covey DC, et al. Arthroscopic-assisted allograft reconstruction of the posterior cruciate ligament. Technique and biomechanical considerations. J Orthop Tech 1993; 1:91–97; with permission.)

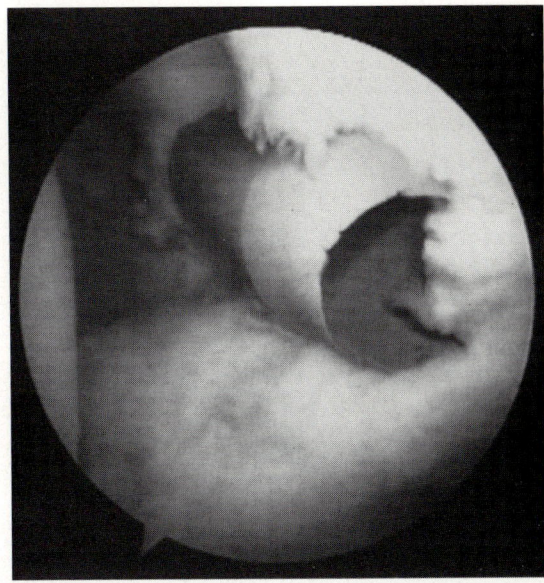

Figure 3 An instrument cannula placed through a posteromedial portal is viewed with the arthroscope in the anterolateral portal.

tions, or Achilles tendon allograft are reasonable choices for this procedure. My current preference is sterilely harvested, fresh-frozen, and irradiated Achilles tendon allograft. The tendon and attached portion of calcaneus is allowed to thaw in normal saline at room temperature for 30 to 60 minutes prior to use. Antibiotics may be added to the thawing solution according to the surgeon's preference. The calcaneal bone is fashioned into a rough cylinder that will pass through a 12 mm sizing tube without difficulty. The tendon is trimmed and then tubularized to the same diameter using two sutures of number 5 Ticron. Two additional sutures of number 5 Ticron are placed through drill holes in the calcaneal plug to act as a leader.

The PCL tibial drill guide is placed through the anteromedial portal and positioned at the approximate sagittal midpoint of the tibial attachment of the PCL, with the tip of the guide presumably hooked over the posterior tibial shelf (Fig. 4). A 3 cm incision is made over the anteromedial tibia to expose the bone just below the level of the tibial tubercle. A guide pin is advanced well into the tibia, and anteroposterior and lateral roentgenograms or fluoroscopy are used to verify satisfactory position of both the drill guide and guide pin in relation to the anatomic PCL tibial insertion zone (Fig. 5). Since the popliteal artery is immediately posterior to the confluent tibial attachment of the PCL and posterior capsule, arthroscopic visualization combined with a drill stop, fingertip, and/or a retractor, may be used to protect the neurovascular structures when over-reaming the pin and exiting the tibial cortex. A broad radius is placed on the proximal tunnel edge with a burr or bone rasps to provide a graduated, curved surface (instead of a sharp edge) for the graft to wrap around as it changes direction. This broad tunnel edge radius shifts the effective graft fixation point proximally somewhat, thus

it is important to achieve distal tibial tunnel placement initially.

Selection of the intra-articular site for the femoral bone tunnel involves identification of the anterior and central fiber attachment areas using femoral landmarks. With the knee in 90 degrees of flexion, a point at the 2 o'clock position of the intercondylar notch (right knee) approximately 6 mm posterior to the articular surface of the medial femoral condyle will place the center of the bone tunnel a few millimeters anterior to the junction of the anterior and central fibers. This will result in graft placement that reconstructs the so-called "antero-central bulk" of the anatomic PCL. A generous radius is then placed on the posterior tunnel margin to protect the graft from edge-carving, and to shift the effective femoral fixation point back to the junction of the anterior and central fiber regions. The femoral drill guide is passed through the anteromedial portal, and the tip of the aimer arm is placed at the position noted above (Fig. 6). A 3 cm oblique incision is positioned equidistant between the medial epicondyle and the medial patellofemoral joint to allow proper extra-articular seating of the drill sleeve. The femoral tunnel is drilled with a guide pin followed by an 11 or 12 mm cannulated reamer (Fig. 7).

Confirmation of proper femoral guide pin placement before over-reaming can be accomplished with an isometer gauge. Documenting the change in tibiofemoral separation distance as the knee is moved through the range of motion allows a prediction of graft length changes after placement and fixation. The isometer's

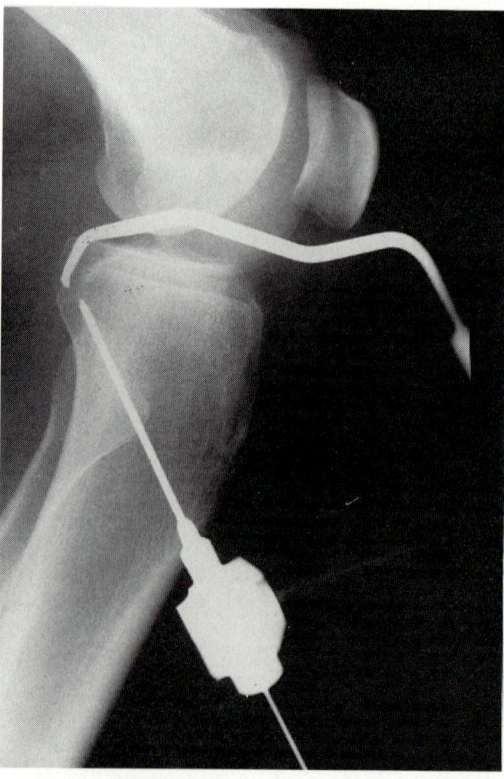

Figure 5 A lateral roentgenogram of the knee with the tibial guide in place confirms the guide tip's position in relation to the posterior tibial shelf.

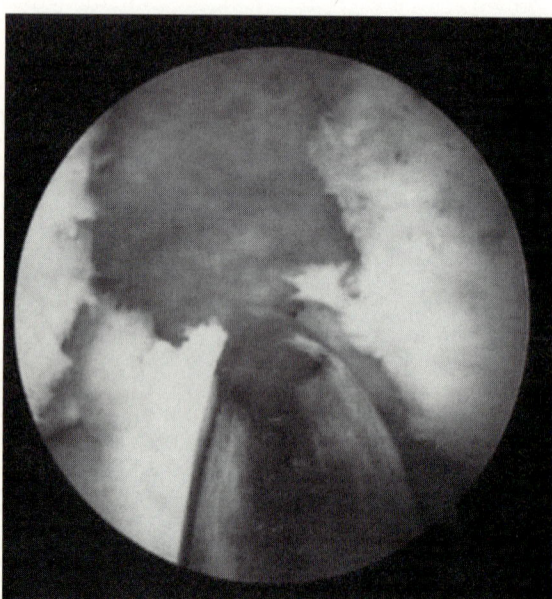

Figure 4 Arthroscopic view of the tibial guide hooked over the posterior tibial shelf (viewed from an anterolateral portal).

excursion suture can be centralized in the tibial tunnel using a reversed cannulated drill, with the suture excursion gauge fixed externally. The proximal end of the suture is threaded through the preliminary femoral guide pin hole and secured external to the femoral cortex

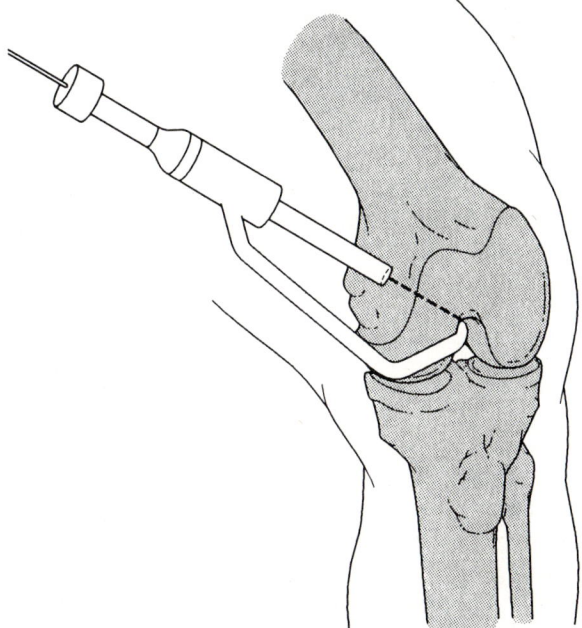

Figure 6 The tip of the femoral drill guide is placed through the anteromedial arthroscopic portal, and is positioned on the medial femoral condyle at approximately the 10 o'clock or 2 o'clock position (left or right knees, respectively), 6 mm posterior to the articular surface. (From Covey DC, et al. Arthroscopic-assisted allograft reconstruction of the posterior cruciate ligament. Technique and biomechanical considerations. J Orthop Tech 1993; 1:91–97; with permission.)

by a clamp or several overhand knots. While ranging the knee, it is important to apply a proximally-directed force to keep the tibiofemoral joint surfaces in full, congruent contact at all joint positions, and avoid tibial rotation forces. Care should be exercised to prevent posterior tibial subluxation while taking suture excursion readings. The so-called isometric point of the PCL's femoral attachment lies at the insertion of the far posterior oblique fibers, thus the suture excursion reading expected when reconstructing the main fiber bulk of the PCL is approximately 4 to 6 mm of increasing tibiofemoral distance (i.e., future graft tightening) with knee flexion from 0 to 90 degrees.

After the femoral bone tunnel preparation is completed, a curved, wire suture passer is placed through the tibial tunnel, across the joint, and out the femoral tunnel in order to pull-through a suture leader of number 5 Ticron. With the suture leader pulled through the joint, and the knee positioned at 90 degrees of flexion, the Achilles tendon allograft is directed into the tibial tunnel, through the joint, and out the femoral tunnel, leaving the calcaneal bone plug in the tibial tunnel (the reverse may also be performed as desired). The calcaneal bone plug is then secured with an interference screw. With the proximal graft end tensioned, but not yet secured, the allograft is viewed with the arthroscope as the knee is brought from a position of full extension to approximately 110 degrees of flexion. Manually detectable tightening of the graft should be noted at its free end (as it is pulled into the femoral tunnel) when the knee is flexed from 0 to 90 degrees, plateauing after that. Such a nonisometric graft will not undergo plastic deformation if it is tensioned and fixed at or near the joint position of maximum intra-articular graft length. With the knee flexed (generally 70 to 90 degrees) a firm anterior tibial drawer force is applied and the proximal allograft is tensioned and fixed to the femur in a

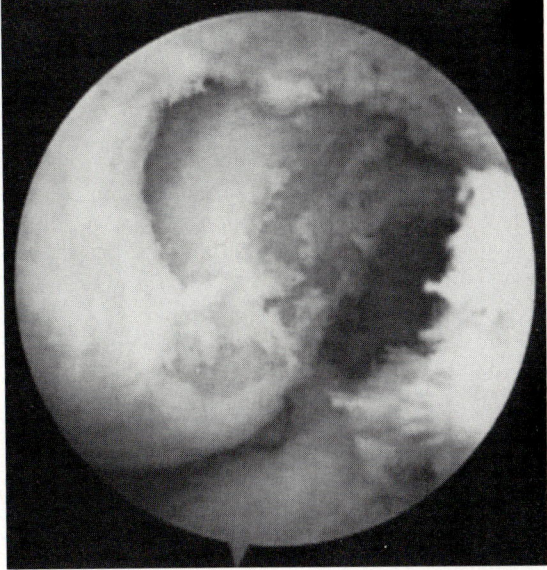

Figure 7 Arthroscopic view of a 12 mm femoral tunnel positioned so that the graft will approximate a reconstruction of the anterocentral fiber bulk of the PCL.

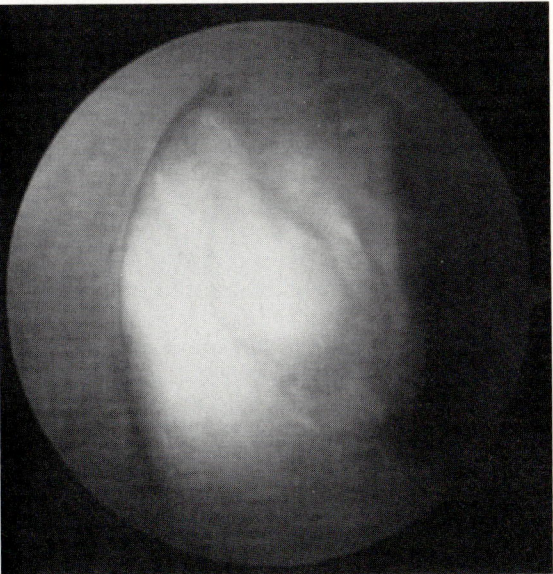

Figure 8 An Achilles tendon graft placed to reconstruct the anterocentral fiber bulk of the PCL.

prepared bed using a large spiked washer and screw developed by Concept. Fixation may be enhanced if the soft tissue end of the graft is split in a bifid fashion, wrapping each arm around the screw in opposite directions before tightening the washer. Proper graft placement allows full range of motion while eliminating preoperative posterior tibial sag in flexion (Fig. 8). After wound closure, the knee is placed in a postoperative hinged brace at full extension where the graft is somewhat slackened, and thus unloaded.

POSTOPERATIVE MANAGEMENT

The patient begins isometric quadriceps and hip abductor exercises in the hospital, and is discharged on the first or second postoperative day, weight-bearing as tolerated with the brace locked at full extension. These exercises are continued at home three times per day, and the patient uses crutches only as needed. At the first clinic follow-up, 7 to 10 days later, the patient is instructed to unlock the hinged brace three times per day to perform supine, gravity-induced knee flexion from 0 to 70 degrees under active quadriceps control. Only isometric hamstring exercises in full extension are permitted at this point. The patient is encouraged to bear full weight on the operated limb. Three weeks after surgery the patient is placed in a functional brace with full range of motion (ROM). The patient is instructed on standing one-quarter squats with full body weight while keeping the trunk erect. At 4 to 6 weeks postoperatively, bicycle exercises are added. The functional brace is worn full-time until the sixth postoperative week, when it can then be removed for sleep only. A progressive quadriceps strengthening program is emphasized, while hamstring strengthening advances at a slower pace emphasizing closed-kinetic-chain exercises. At 16 weeks postoperatively, the functional brace may be discontinued for nonstrenuous activities. Six months after surgery, open-kinetic-chain hamstring exercises may be instituted, and the patient is allowed to begin a supervised jogging program. Full return to athletic activity is anticipated 10 to 12 months postoperatively.

DISCUSSION

The results of PCL reconstructive surgery are not yet comparable to those achieved with anterior cruciate ligament reconstruction. Future technical refinements should further improve the surgical outcome. Variables such as chronicity of injury, associated ligament or cartilage damage, type of graft, graft augmentation, and the postoperative rehabilitation protocol, all play a part in determining the final clinical result after reconstruction.

PCL reconstruction with an allograft offers several advantages. Use of allograft obviates the need for autogenous tissue, thus sparing the ipsilateral patella and patellar tendon (the most commonly used autograft) from surgical trauma. In the PCL-deficient knee, the patella is already at risk for degenerative arthritis due to abnormal joint contact forces resulting from increased posterior tibial translation. Additionally, quicker patient rehabilitation may be expected due to decreased operative morbidiy. Technical benefits of using Achilles tendon allograft include sufficient graft length and initial strength, and one nonosseous end that facilitates making the 90 degree turn required to direct the graft from one bone tunnel into the other. This maneuver may be more difficult with a bone-patellar tendon-bone preparation.

Arthroscopically assisted PCL reconstructive surgery is technically challenging and not without risk for complications. There is a potential danger to the popliteal artery and other structures in the popliteal fossa during tibial guide pin placement, and during the over-reaming procedure. To ensure adequate visualization, the surgeon should debride the PCL tibial insertion area thoroughly. Use of intraoperative roentgenograms or fluroscopy, a fingertip and/or retractor, a drill stop, and arthroscopic visualization of the exiting pin or reamer while making the tibial tunnel will help reduce the risk of neurovascular injury. To minimize the risk of neurapraxia, tourniquet time should not exceed 2 hours. Potential late complications include loss of knee ROM, avascular necrosis of the medial femoral condyle, increased posterior laxity, and the possibility of adverse immune sequela from the use of allograft. Allograft ligament reconstruction also raises the concern of infectious disease transmission from the implanted tissue.

Clancy and co-workers have long recommended that the intra-articular position of the femoral drill hole should coincide with the principal anatomic center of the PCL attachment, similar to the technique I now employ. This differs from an isometric graft placement technique, which reconstructs the more posterior, vertical fibers of the PCL. Although nearly isometric, these fibers make up only a very small portion of the bulk of the PCL. A femoral drill hole centered on the osseous attachment zone of these fibers will result in a graft that is oversized for its location, precluding an anatomic approximation of the main fiber bulk of the PCL.

Biomechanical investigations now suggest that the optimal location for the femoral tunnel is slightly anterior to the center of the PCL attachment, resulting in a graft that unslackens and becomes tight between 0 and 90 degrees of knee flexion, simulating the in vivo behavior of the majority of PCL fibers. Reason indicates that the graft that best approximates and maintains normal PCL anatomy will have the greatest likelihood of restoring normal tibiofemoral kinematics.

SUGGESTED READING

Bomberg BC, Acker JH, Boyle J, Zarins B. The effect of posterior cruciate ligament loss and reconstruction on the knee. Am J Knee Surg 1990; 3:85–96.

Clancy WG, Shelbourne KD, Zoellner GB, et al. Treatment of knee joint instability secondary to rupture of the posterior cruciate ligament. J Bone Joint Surg 1983; 65A:310–322.

Clancy WG, Timmerman LA. Arthroscopically assisted posterior cruciate ligament reconstruction using autologous patellar tendon graft. Operative Tech Sports Med 1993; 1:129–135.

Covey DC, Sapega AA. Anatomy and function of the PCL. Clin Sports Med 1994 (in press).

Covey DC, Sapega AA. Current concepts review: Injuries of the posterior cruciate ligament. J Bone Joint Surg 1993; 75A:1376–1386.

Girgis FG, Marshall JL, Al Monajem ARS. The cruciate ligaments of the knee joint: Anatomical, functional and experimental analysis. Clin Orthop 1975; 106:216–231.

Gollehon DL, Torzilli PA, Warren RF. The role of the posterolateral and cruciate ligaments in the stability of the human knee. J Bone Joint Surg 1987; 69A:233–242.

Grood ES, Stowers SF, Noyes FR. Limits of movement in the human knee joint: Effect of sectioning the posterior cruciate ligament and posterolateral structures. J Bone Joint Surg 1988; 70A:88–97.

Jackson DW: Use of allografts for anterior cruciate ligament reconstructions. AAOS Bull 1992; 40:10–11.

Jackson DW, Proctor CS, Simon TM: Arthroscopic assisted PCL reconstruction: A technical note on potential neurovascular injury related to drill bit configuration. Arthroscopy 1993; 9:224–227.

Keller PM, Shelbourne KD, McCarroll JR, Rettig AC. Nonoperatively treated isolated posterior cruciate ligament injuries. Am J Sports Med 1993; 21:132–136.

PROPHYLACTIC KNEE BRACES

DAVID L. MONTGOMERY, Ph.D.

Knee orthoses have been in existence for many years as part of the treatment and protection of injured knees. The practice of wearing knee braces as a protective measure when participating in contact sports started proliferating in the early 1980s. North American football has been both the causative stimulus for the development of prophylactic knee braces and the predominant test mode for these devices.

The knee is frequently the site of sport injuries, especially in football. No other injury category compares to the knee in terms of numbers, rate of occurrence, participation time loss, or the necessity for surgical intervention. Using data from the Pennsylvania State University football team between 1972 and 1983, Whiteside et al calculated that players had an 18.1% chance of receiving a time-loss knee injury during the combined spring and fall seasons. Hewson et al estimated that players in high-risk positions (linemen, linebackers, tight ends) had a 23% chance of suffering a knee injury in a single season and a 64% chance of at least one knee injury during a 4-year collegiate career.

The high incidence of knee injuries to collegiate football players and the health costs associated with these injuries resulted in an available market for manufacturers of knee braces. Prophylactic bracing was advocated as one solution to this serious problem. Stimulated by testimonial evidence from athletes and trainers as well as a sales pitch by manufacturers attributing unrealistic benefits to bracing, there was a threefold increase in the use of preventive knee braces. In spite of a paucity of scientific documentation to support their efficacy, an unproven solution was promoted with little thought given to the consequences of implementation.

Initially, athletes, trainers, and coaches were hesitant about endorsing prophylactic braces with concerns that they were: expensive, hot, heavy, causing pistoning, slipping, restricting mobility, causing leg muscle cramps, weakening supporting muscles and ligaments, and perhaps increasing injuries because of new force vectors.

The scientific community has been cautious in its endorsement or rejection of knee braces. What began as an untested practice, now continues with evidence that is equivocal. In 1985, the Sports Medicine Committee of the American Academy of Orthopaedic Surgeons (AAOS) as well as the American Orthopaedic Society for Sports Medicine voiced reservations about knee braces.

CLASSIFICATION OF KNEE BRACES

The AAOS classified knee braces into three types—prophylactic, functional, and rehabilitative. Rehabilitative knee braces are designed to allow protected motion of injured knees that have been treated operatively or nonoperatively. Functional knee braces are designed to provide stability for unstable knees. Prophylactic knee braces were introduced to prevent or reduce the severity of damage to the knee joint caused by contact and noncontact injuries. Several of the modern braces cannot be distinctly categorized since they combine features from two classifications.

BRACE DESIGNS

To understand how braces function, it is necessary to examine the structure of the knee joint (Fig. 1). The lateral collateral ligament (LCL) and the medial collateral ligament (MCL) provide stability when the leg is extended. The MCL is the primary restraint against valgus loading. The menisci act as shock absorbers. When the knee is flexed, the cruciate ligaments assist to keep the bones in proper alignment. In contact sports, blows to the side of the knee are a common cause of injury. The lateral force may cause the inside of the knee to "open-up," resulting in a tear to the MCL. Similarly, a medial force may cause injury to the lateral collateral structures of the knee, although this type of injury is less frequently observed. The MCL and/or cruciate ligaments may also be injured during foot fixation with an

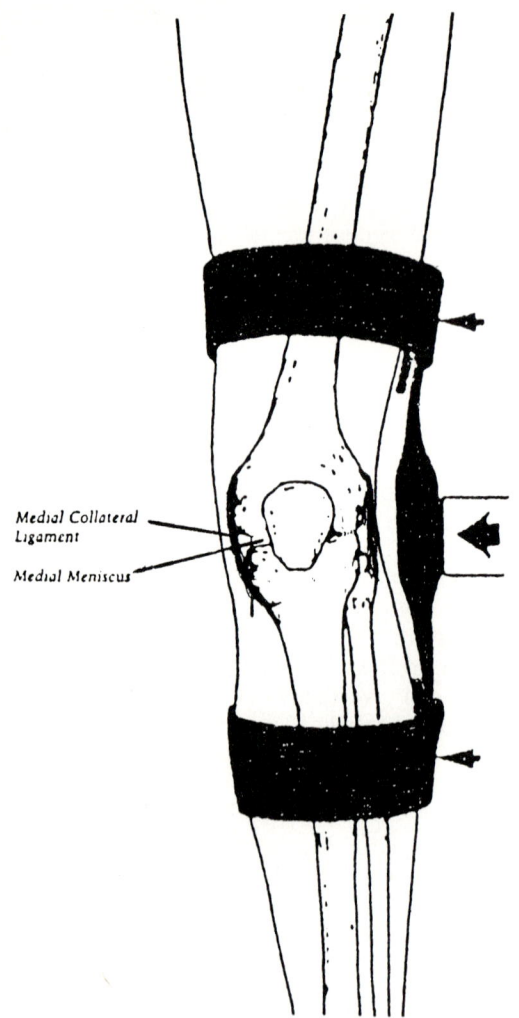

Medial Collateral Ligament

Medial Meniscus

Figure 1 Application of lateral force to a prophylactic knee brace. (From Montgomery D, Koziris P. Knee brace controversy. Sports Medicine. 1989; 8:262, with permission.)

abduction, external rotation load placed on the knee.

The ideal knee brace should permit normal anatomic knee movements. Motion about the knee joint includes six degrees of freedom—flexion, extension, varus, valgus, internal rotation, and external rotation—as well as three translational motions—distraction-compression, medial-lateral, and anterior-posterior. While several manufacturers of knee braces claim anatomic properties for their braces, none of the current devices available to sport participants can simulate all degrees of freedom of motion.

Prophylactic braces may be categorized by two design types. One type consists of bars and hinges. Theoretically, the lateral posts of the brace dissipate the energy from a lateral blow to the knee, thereby protecting the knee from injuries caused by "opening-up" the knee. The hinges may be placed on the lateral and/or the medial side of the knee. The hinges may also include "stops," which are designed to restrict the range of extension and flexion movement. The hinge may be

monocentric, biaxial, polycentric, or multiaxial cams. Designs claiming to be anatomic utilize a multiaxial cam action permitting anterior translation during flexion. The second category of braces is constructed with plastic cuffs that encircle the thigh and calf muscles. The braces are held in place by straps, elastic wraps, or taping over the thigh and lower leg.

Prophylactic knee braces claim to protect the knee from impact forces. The three principal factors that determine the impact response characteristics of a brace/knee composite are force distribution, energy absorption, and energy transmission. Baker et al applied lateral loads to cadaver knees in extension and at 20 degrees of flexion with and without braces. With the knee in full extension, prophylactic braces have a limited capacity to protect the MCL from direct lateral stress. In flexion or with a change in direction of the load, the protective effect was greatly reduced.

Using a surrogate knee model, Van Hoeck et al concluded that preventive braces absorb 15% to 30% of the energy of a direct blow. They caution that energy absorption would be significantly lower under athletic competition conditions with the addition of anterior-posterior and rotational forces. In an excellent study of 1,396 cadets at the U.S. Military Academy at West Point, Sitler et al examined the efficacy of bracing in an athletic environment in which the athletic shoe, playing surface, athlete exposure, knee injury history, and brace assignment were either statistically or experimentally controlled. Direct lateral knee contact resulted in fewer ($p = 0.08$) MCL injuries when prophylactic knee braces were used.

Using information from cadaver knees and a surrogate knee model, an impact safety factor of 1.50 has been recommended as a protection standard for prophylactic knee braces. This value corresponds to a load reduction of 30% in the MCL and an overall ligament protection of 50%. The clinical significance of brace-induced MCL preload has been examined by France and co-workers using impact loading of a surrogate knee model. Six commercially available brace types were studied. Over 500 impact tests were performed on the surrogate knee in unbraced versus braced conditions. Tests were conducted for three impactor masses (23, 75, and 127 kg), two flexion angles (0 and 30 degrees), and free or constrained limb positions. Impact safety factors were calculated for each test condition and brace type. Brace induced MCL preload in vivo was negated by joint compressive forces. Only one brace (Don Joy) exceeded the minimum impact safety factor. For the six types of braces, the average impact safety factor ranged from 1.18 to 1.51. The six braces performed differently depending on the mass and speed of impact and the degree of constraint of the limb. Braces that tested well under some conditions, tested poorly when subjected to other variables, suggesting that both material properties and mechanical design were important factors in brace function.

According to the AAOS Committee on Sports Medicine, the ideal prophylactic knee brace would have the following characteristics:

- adaptive to various anatomic shapes and sizes
- supplement the stiffness of the knee to injury-producing loads from contact and noncontact stresses
- cost effective and durable
- does not interfere with normal knee function
- does not harm other players
- does not increase injuries to the lower extremity
- documented efficacy in preventing injuries

ADVERSE EFFECTS OF BRACING

Four potentially adverse effects associated with lateral bracing have been described: MCL preloading, center axis shift, premature joint line contact, and brace slippage.

1. "MCL preloading" is an increased static MCL tension associated with brace application. The significance of this observation remains unclear.

2. "Center axis shift" is a shift of the axis of valgus rotation from the center of the knee laterally toward the brace.

3. Premature contact of the center of the brace with the lateral bony structures of the knee decreases brace efficiency by reducing the effective lever arm. Joint line contact may concentrate forces normally distributed along the lateral surface of an unbraced leg directly in the knee joint and possibly cause more damage to knee ligaments than that incurred in the unbraced condition. Premature joint line contact results from improper brace fit, material properties, structural properties, and fixation techniques.

4. Brace slippage relates to the fit and fixation of the brace on the knee. It is influenced by knee varus/valgus angulation, paddle contour, hinge design, and brace fixation technique. A poorly designed brace that does not adapt to changing limb contours or one that slips could be harmful to the patient by concentration of forces at the joint line with the potential for increased ligament or bone damage.

EPIDEMIOLOGICAL STUDIES OF PROPHYLACTIC BRACES

The most frequently posed question by practitioners is "Can lateral bracing reduce knee injuries?" As we approach the mid-1990s, a conclusive answer concerning the effectiveness of existing prophylactic braces cannot be made. The multitude of models currently on the market differ in design, materials, and construction. Other confounding factors must be considered, such as: the normal fluctuation in the incidence of injuries from year to year; alterations in footwear and playing surfaces; changes in rules, coaches, and coaching techniques; changes in medical staff; and changes in diagnostic and therapeutic approaches to injuries. Since these factors influence injury rates, they must be carefully evaluated before ascribing any change in injury patterns to the use of prophylactic bracing.

Ten clinical and epidemiological studies have not resolved the question. Five reports support prophylactic knee bracing, three show no significant change in knee injuries with bracing, and two show an increase in the incidence of injuries with knee bracing. Since some of the data show no protective effect, the trend in recent years has been a decrease in use of prophylactic knee braces. Sports medicine practitioners should examine these studies since a summary tally may present a biased perspective. A critical analysis offers more insight. The references are included in the suggested readings.

Epidemiologic data are limited in their ability to provide direct answers. The ten studies used a variety of methods, populations, and brace types. It is not surprising that the conclusions disagree about the effectiveness of prophylactic knee braces. The major methodologic difficulty in these studies has been an inadequate control group. The use of separate periods of time for bracing and nonbracing has the effect of confounding other changes that may have occurred over the same time period. Two studies that have come to different conclusions are presented in greater detail. These studies show the dilemma facing sports medicine practitioners who would like to make a recommendation on knee bracing.

Most studies on the effectiveness of knee bracing have been conducted with a limited sample size at a single institution. The retrospective investigation by Teitz et al attempted to control for many of the known biases and utilize a large sample. Injury data were collected on 6307 football players from 71 schools in 1984 and 5445 players from 61 schools in 1985. In 1984, 36% of the players wore knee braces and in 1985, 44% of the players wore braces. In both years, the players who wore the preventive braces had a significantly increased rate of injury to the knee when compared with the rate of injury in players who did not wear braces (for 1984, 11.0% compared with 6.0%; for 1985, 9.4% compared with 6.4%). It concluded that so-called preventive braces are not preventive and may in fact be harmful. Despite the purported value of the brace in the prevention of MCL injuries, there were significantly more injuries to the MCL among players who wore braces (for 1984, 7.6% compared with 3.5%; for 1985, 5.4% compared with 3.6%). The increased injuries among players who wore braces occurred during contact. For the ACL and the meniscus, there were no significant differences in the overall incidence of injury between braced and unbraced players.

Recent evidence suggests a possible role for prophylactic braces in specific populations based on level of play and the size of players. Sitler and associates examined the efficacy of bracing to reduce knee injuries in 1,396 cadets participating in intramural tackle football over two seasons. Injuries were defined as an acute knee trauma resulting in the absence from at least one day of practice following the injury. This prospective, randomized study accounted for such factors as shoes, playing surface, athlete-exposure, and knee injury history. Bracing significantly reduced the frequency of knee injuries. Defensive players who wore knee braces had fewer knee injuries than controls. This was not true of offensive players with no difference in injuries between the brace and control conditions.

Should prophylactic knee braces be recommended to patients or athletes? Based on current clinical studies, several organizations (the AAOS, The Medical Society of the State of New York, and the Journal of Bone and Joint Surgery) and sports medicine practitioners have stated that prophylactic braces do not reduce knee injuries and therefore should not be recommended for this purpose. France et al stated "no physician, coach, or athletic organization should recommend these braces as mandatory equipment or, on the other hand, prevent their use." Based on their biomechanical research, France and Paulos recommend that prophylactic braces not be abandoned but improved and further evaluated through well-controlled prospective clinical studies.

PRESCRIPTION OF BRACES

The most common prophylactic braces worn by U.S. college athletes are the Omni, McDavid Knee Guard, Don Joy, and Stromgren. If you are convinced that the evidence supports the efficacy of knee braces, several factors must be considered when the physician prescribes a knee brace.

1. Purpose—prophylactic versus rehabilitative or functional
2. Cost—custom design versus "off-the-shelf" model
3. Activity—recreational versus competitive, contact sport
4. Weight of the brace
5. Comfort to the skin
6. Ventilation of the limb
7. Varus and valgus alignment of the limb
8. Location of the hinge axis
9. Effect on athletic performance
10. Durability
11. Proper fit to avoid brace slippage
12. Educating the patient to the importance of proper application

The cost of mandated bracing is an issue that must be addressed. Based on statistics of the number and severity of MCL injuries, Garrick and Requa estimated the cost of surgical intervention versus the cost of mandatory bracing. The net costs of mandatory bracing exceeded the costs of no-bracing by $41 per player. Hewson found that the average cost to equip a single player with a brace (including cost of the brace, personnel time in assisting with the application of the brace, and wrapping supplies) was about $400 per season. For teams with limited budgets, the cost factor may determine brace usage.

SUGGESTED READING

American Academy of Orthopaedic Surgeons. Knee Braces Seminar Report. Chicago: 1985, p 1.

American Academy of Orthopaedic Surgeons. A position statement: The use of knee braces. Chicago: American Academy of Orthopaedic Surgeons, 1987.

Anderson G, Zeman SC, Rosenfeld RT. The Anderson knee stabler. The Physician and Sportsmedicine 1979; 7(6):125–127.

Baker BE. The effect of bracing on the collateral ligaments of the knee. Clin Sports Med 1990; 9:843–851.

Baker BE, VanHanswyk E, Bogosian SP, et al. The effect of knee braces on lateral impact loading of the knee. Am J Sports Med 1989; 17:182–186.

Coughlin L, Oliver J, Berretta G. Knee bracing and anterolateral rotatory instability. Am J Sports Med 1987; 15:161–163.

Cowell HR. College football: To brace or not to brace. J Bone Joint Surg 1987; 69(A):1.

France EP, Paulos LE. In vitro assessment of prophylactic knee brace function. Clin Sports Med 1990; 9:823–840.

France EP, Paulos LE, Jayaraman G, Rosenberg TD. The biomechanics of lateral knee bracing. Part II: Impact, response of the braced knee. Am J Sports Med 1987; 15:430–438.

Garrick JG, Requa RK. Prophylactic knee bracing. Am J Sports 1987; 15:471–476.

Grace TG, Skipper BJ, Newberry JC, et al. Prophylactic knee braces and injury to the lower extremity. J Bone Joint Surg 1988; 70(A):422–427.

Hansen BL, Ward JC, Diehl RC. The preventive use of the Anderson knee stabler in football. The Physician and Sportsmedicine 1985; 13(9):75–81.

Hewson GF, Mendini RA, Wang JB. Prophylactic knee bracing in college football. Am J Sports Med 1986; 14:262–266.

Hewson GF, Wang JB, Mendini RA. Prophylactic knee bracing in college football. Nashville, Tenn: American Orthopedic Society for Sports Medicine, 1985.

Johnston JM, Paulos LE. Prophylactic lateral knee braces. Med Sci Sports Exerc 1991; 23:783–787.

Legwold G. Are prophylactic knee braces prophylactic? The Physician and Sportsmedicine 1985; 13(9):27–28.

Montgomery DL, Koziris PL. The knee brace controversy. Sports Med 1989; 8:260–272.

Paulos LE, Drawbert JP, France P, Rosenberg TD. Lateral knee braces in football: Do they prevent injury? The Physician and Sportsmedicine 1986; 14(6):119–124.

Paulos LE, France EP, Rosenberg TD, et al. The biomechanics of lateral knee bracing. Part I: Response of the valgus restraints to loading. Am J Sports Med 1987; 15:419–429.

Potera C. Knee braces: Questions raised about performance. The Physician and Sportsmedicine 1985; 13(9):153–155.

Quillian WW, Simms RT, Cooper JS. Knee-bracing in preventing injuries in high school football. Int Pediatr 1987; 2:255–256.

Requa RK, Garrick JG. A review of the use of prophylactic knee braces in football. Pediatr Clin North Am 1990; 37:1165–1173.

Requa RK, Garrick JG. Clinical significance and evaluation of prophylactic knee brace in football. Clin Sports Med 1990; 9:853–869.

Rovere GD, Bowen GS. The effectiveness of knee bracing for the prevention of sport injuries. Sports Med 1986; 3:309–311.

Rovere GD, Haupt HA, Yates CS. Prophylactic knee bracing in college football. Am J Sports Med 1987; 15:111–116.

Ryan AJ, Grant TT, Rosenfeld RT, et al. Knee braces to prevent injuries in football. The Physician and Sportsmedicine 1986; 14(4):108–118.

Schriner JL. The effectiveness of knee bracing in preventing knee injuries in high school athletes. Med Sci Sports Exerc 1985; 17(2):254.

Sitler M, Ryan J, Hopkinson W, et al. The efficacy of a prophylactic knee brace to reduce knee injuries in football. Am J Sports Med 1990; 18:310–315.

Stuller J. Bracing the unstable knee. The Physician and Sportsmedicine 1985; 13(2):142–156.

Taft TN, Hunter S, Funderburk CH. Preventative lateral knee bracing in football. Nashville, Tenn: American Orthopedic Society for Sports Medicine, 1985.

Teitz CC, Hermanson BK, Kronmal RA, Diehr PH. Evaluation of the use of braces to prevent injury to the knee in collegiate football players. J Bone Joint Surg 1987; 69(A):2–9.

Van Hoeck JE, Brown TD, Brand RA. A surrogate knee model for dynamic loading studies of prophylactic braces. In: Rekow ED, Thacker JG, Erdman AG, eds. Biomechanics in sports: A 1987 update. New York: American Society of Mechanical Engineers, 1987, p 35.

Whiteside JA, Fleagle SB, Kalenak A, Weller H. Manpower loss in football: A 12-year study at the Pennsylvania State University. The Physician and Sportsmedicine 1985; 13(1):103–114.

Wirth MA, DeLee JC. The history and classification of knee braces. Clin Sports Med 1990; 9:731–741.

REFLEX SYMPATHETIC DYSTROPHY OF THE KNEE

BRETT C. HYNNINEN, M.D.
DAVID L. JACKSON, M.D.

Reflex sympathetic dystrophy (RSD) of the knee, while relatively uncommon, is a diagnosis that deserves consideration in the athlete with knee pain who does not respond to treatment. Although RSD of the knee has been described in the literature, it is often not included in the differential diagnosis of knee pain until late in the workup. The term *RSD of the knee* may be a slight misnomer, because the syndrome usually affects the entire extremity. Trauma to the knee most likely causes retrograde changes in the lumbar sympathetic chain, which subsequently causes abnormal sympathetic activity throughout the lower limb.

Reflex sympathetic dystrophy is a term used to describe a disorder consisting of neurovascular and dystrophic changes in the extremity characterized by severe pain, swelling, stiffness, and discoloration. During the Civil War, a persistent burning pain associated with trophic changes in soldiers with gunshot wounds of the peripheral nerves was noted and referred to as "causalgia." Since that time, numerous authors have noted similar syndromes and used a variety of terms to describe these conditions. The term *reflex sympathetic dystrophy* has been used to encompass all of the entities.

RSD is associated with a wide variety of inciting events such as trauma, surgery, stroke, myocardial infraction, and radiculopathy. It has been reported that RSD is present to some extent in one of every 2,000 accidents involving an extremity.

CLINICAL PICTURE

RSD has been described as an excessive or exaggerated response to an injury in an extremity with several characteristics including intense or unduly prolonged pain, vasomotor disturbances, delayed functional recovery, and various associated trophic changes. Patients often complain of a burning, stabbing, or crushing pain. Patients with RSD of the knee have similar complaints. Diffuse tenderness is often present with occasional point tenderness at the medial aspect of the knee. Pain may be constant or intermittent. Gait may or may not be affected. Patients complain of a burning or aching pain. Sensitivity to cold and night pain are common. Stiffness is also a common feature of RSD of the knee; some suggest that it is so prevalent that it may help distinguish RSD from patellofemoral syndrome. These patients, however, have been found to have a full range of motion under anesthesia unless intra-articular changes have occurred. Swelling is also a common complaint in patients with RSD of the knee. On examination, bogginess through the capsular area is sometimes noted; however, a significant effusion is seldom appreciated. As the syndrome progresses, the patient may complain of buckling or locking of the knee secondary to muscular weakness and capsular changes such as synovitis and fibrosis.

On physical examination, sudomotor changes such as hyperhidrosis early in the syndrome and dryness later on are noted. Prolonged capillary refill may be seen due to vasomotor instability. Patients complain of pain upon ranging the knee. Discoloration may be present. Cutaneous hypersensitivity (even to light touch) may be present. Patients are often on narcotics at time of presentation, as well as involved in litigation.

Pain associated with RSD can continue for a prolonged period, with the majority of patients complaining of pain for longer than 6 months.

While most patients with RSD of the knee appear to be psychologically stable, some authors have noted a syndrome of diathesis personality in which the patients have a low pain threshold, insecurity, constantly complain, blame others, avoid responsibility for their health, place the physician on the defensive, and enjoy a poor state of health for secondary gain. We have not found these attributes in most of the patients we have treated for RSD.

Involvement of the patellofemoral joint in RSD of the knee has been reported from 65% to 100%. The average time from onset of symptoms to diagnosis is 29 months with an average of 1.6 surgeries on the knee prior to diagnosis. Signs and symptoms of RSD of the knee should be sought before any surgery to the knee is considered.

Histologic changes have been noted in the vascular tissue, bone, and joints of patients with RSD of the knee. Initial vasoconstriction is seen followed later by vasodilatation with increased blood supply to the tissues around the joint. Increased blood flow is seen in the affected extremity. Synovitis has been noted in patients with RSD of the knee, increasing with the duration of the syndrome.

ETIOLOGY

It is generally accepted that autonomic dysfunction plays a major role in the pathophysiology of RSD, however, the exact mechanism is unclear. Numerous authors have proposed theories as to the possible origin of RSD, yet none have been confirmed. In 1943, Livingston proposed that reverberating circuits within the spinal cord cause the perception of chronic peripheral sensory nerve irritation. These circuits are felt to be triggered by intense painful stimuli. These reverberating circuits in turn increase sympathetic efferent activity. Melzak thought that prolonged pain could leave "memory traces," making an individual more susceptible to recurrent pain. Sunderland suggested that injury to sympathetic efferent fibers may cause retrograde changes in the sympathetic ganglia with transsynaptic degeneration in neurons form self-sustaining circuits. Doupe, Cullen, and Chance proposed that injury may allow ephaptic transmission between sensory afferents and sympathetic efferents. Roberts suggested that Wide Dynamic Range (WDR) neurons in the dorsal horn may respond to mechanoreceptor activity initiated by efferent sympathetic activity. These WDR neurons could become activated in the absence of cutaneous stimulation, producing sympathetically maintained pain.

Many precipitatory factors for RSD of the knee have been identified including diabetic amyotrophy, L3-4 spinal nerve irritation, femoral nerve palsy, hysterical personality disorder, patellar and femoral condyle fractures, osteoarthritis, meniscal tears, and sensory nerve injury. RSD of the knee has also been reported following arthroscopy for patellofemoral pain, total knee replacements, lateral release, patellectomy, high tibial osteotomy, and chondral shaving for chondromalacia. A small number of cases have been reported without any apparent etiology.

DIAGNOSIS

Diagnosis of RSD of the knee is primarily clinical. Pain, swelling, and stiffness are almost universal complaints. Osteopenia, discoloration, sudomotor changes, temperature changes, trophic changes, and vasomotor instability are usually present.

Roentgenographic studies have been used to aid in diagnosis. Transient patchy osteopenia is seen but the degree of decalcification may vary. Plain films are usually not adequate to make the diagnosis because it takes 30% to 50% of demineralization to occur before changes are seen on x-ray, which may take as long as 12 weeks to develop. The distribution of osteopenia is usually greatest in the patella followed by global osteopenia, osteopenia in the distal femur, and osteopenia of the patella with distal femur. The sunrise or merchant view is essential when looking at RSD of the knee because the patella is so often involved.

Three-phase bone scan is often used to confirm the diagnosis. Bone scan has been found to be positive in 60% of patients with RSD by showing either asymmetric blood flow or increased periarticular activity in multiple joints of the affected extremity. Bone scan may be positive in asymptomatic joints in the extremity, which return to normal after healing has occurred in the affected joint. Patients with RSD of the knee often have increased uptake in the hip and foot indicating that the pathologic process affects the entire extremity.

Thermography has also been used to aid in the diagnosis of RSD. Decreased heat emission involving several dermatomes throughout the affected extremity is seen. Initially, increased temperature may be seen on thermography with surface vasodilatation and warmth due to total ablation of sympathetic activity. This is followed later by cooling in the affected extremity, with decreased temperature becoming the predominant finding. Sensitivity of thermography has been reported between 89% and 100%. Thermography may be helpful in the future to monitor the efficacy of treatment for RSD of the knee.

A positive response to sympathetic blockade is felt by some to be essential in making the diagnosis of RSD. Sensitivity however has not been 100%. A false-positive response may be obtained if the patient reports numbness with relief secondary to the blocking of somatic sensory nerves.

TREATMENT

Treatment consists primarily of sympathetic interruption. Adjuvant therapy such as physical therapy, trigger point injections, psychological counseling, pneumatic compression, and transcutaneous electrical nerve stimulation (TENS) have also been utilized. No specific treatment protocol is consistently beneficial; however, sympathetic intervention appears to be the most essential component of any protocol.

The success rate of sympathetic blockade has been reported to be as high as 90% with RSD. Onset of relief can occur within minutes and last for weeks. In RSD of the knee, sympathetic interruption can be obtained with a lumbar sympathetic block. Early intervention appears to produce the best results. Response rate is partially dependent on the skill of the practitioner.

Sympathetic blockade can also be obtained via continuous epidural infusion. Cooper placed indwelling lumbar epidural catheters with bupivacaine (Marcaine) followed by narcotics in 14 patients with RSD of the knee. In 11 of 14 patients, the symptoms resolved. Two of 14 continued to complain of intermittent aching, while one patient had no relief.

Intravenous (IV) regional blocks using lidocaine (Xylocaine) and methylprednisolone (Medrol) have also been used to treat RSD. Hannington-Kiff used IV guanethidine (Esimil, Ismelin) and 80% of patients with causalgia reported pain relief at 15 week follow-up. Regional IV guanethidine may work by depleting norepinephrine from synaptic vesicles in sympathetic efferent fibers by either blocking its presynaptic reuptake and/or preventing the release of norepinephrine upon arrival of the action potential.

Surgical sympathectomy is sometimes used with response to surgery varying in the literature from 12% to 97%. Katz and Hungerford found a "good" response in 65% of patients with RSD of the knee while 35% had a "fair" response. Sympathectomy may be an option if the patient fails to have complete relief following a series of four blocks. Failure of sympathectomy has been reported and may be due to collateral reinnervation of postganglionic sympathetic efferent fibers. Postsympathectomy pain (sympathalgia) has been reported in 20% to 40% of patients and can be managed with anticonvulsants. Trigger points are often present in RSD and trigger point injections may be of some benefit.

Many medications have been used to treat RSD of the knee. Tietjen found that some patients benefited both psychologically and physiologically from short-term use of oral corticosteroids. Steroids may help decrease swelling and fibrosis. Tietjen suggested that aspirin or NSAIDs also may help decrease synovitis associated with RSD of the knee.

Oral sympatholytic medications such as phenoxybenzamine (Dibenzyline), guanethidine, prazosin (Minipress, Minizide) and propranolol (Inderal) have been used to treat RSD, as have calcium channel blockers. Prough found that 7 of 11 patients with RSD obtained some relief with nifedipine (Adalat, Procardig).

Physical therapy plays an essential role in the treatment of RSD. Its importance probably lies more in counteracting dystrophic changes in muscles and joints than in reversing the pathologic process. Caution must be exercised by the therapist as aggressive passive range of motion may increase pain. Deep friction massage, increased tactile stimulation, and TENS have proved somewhat beneficial. Both heat and cryotherapy may be helpful. Tietjen reported that an alternating hot and cold whirlpool may be effective. Reduction of edema is essential and best achieved with elevation and compression.

There are also psychologic complications associated with chronic pain. Increased sympathetic firing has been demonstrated with stress or arousal. Biofeedback, hypnosis, and other relaxation techniques may therefore be of some benefit.

SUGGESTED READING

Cooper D, DeLee J, Ramamurthy S. Reflex sympathetic dystrophy of the knee. J Bone Joint Surg 1989; 71:365–369.

Doupe J, Cullen C, Chance G. Post traumatic pain and causalgia syndrome. J Neurol Neurosurg Psychiatry 1944; 7:33–48.

Ficat R, Hungerford D. Disorders of the patellofemoral joint. Paris: Masson, 1977.

Hannington-Kiff J. Intravenous regional sympathetic block with guanethidine. Lancet 1974; I:1019–1120.

Hannington-Kiff J. Relief of causalgia in limbs by regional intravenous guanethidine. Br Med J 1979; 2:367–368.

Katz M, Hungerford D. Reflex sympathetic dystrophy affecting the knee. J Bone Joint Surg 1987; 69:797–803.

Kozin F, Soin J, Ryan L, et al. Bone scintigraphy in the reflex sympathetic dystrophy syndrome. Radiology 1981; 138:437–443.

Livingston W. Pain mechanisms. New York: Macmillan, 1943.

Lofstrom J, Cousins M. Sympathetic neural blockage of upper and lower extremities. In: Neural blockage in clinical anesthesia and management of pain. 2nd Ed. Philadelphia: JB Lippincott, 1988:461.

Melzack R. Phantom limb pain: Implications for treatment of pathologic pain. Anesthesiology 1971; 35:409–419.

Ogilvie-Harris D, Roscoe M. Reflex sympathetic dystrophy of the knee. J Bone Joint Surg 1987; 69:804–806.

Payne R. Neuropathic pain syndrome, with special reference to causalgia and reflex sympathetic dystrophy. Clin J Pain 1986; 2:59.

Prough D, McLeskey C, Boehlin C, et al. Efficacy of oral nifedipine in the treatment of reflex sympathetic dystrophy. Anesthesiology 1985; 62:796–799.

Raskin N, Levinson S, Hoffman P, et al. Postsympathectomy neuralgia amelioration with diphenylhydantoin and carbamazepine. Am J Surg 1974; 128:75–78.

Raven T. The radionuclide flow study and liquid crystal thermography in the early detection of reflex sympathetic dystrophy. 12th Annual meeting of American Academy of Thermology, Baltimore, 1983.

Roberts W. An hypothesis on the physiologic basis for causalgia and related pains. Pain 1986; 24:297.

Sunderland S. Pain mechanisms in causalgia. J Neurol Neurosurg Psychiatry 1976; 39:471–480.

Tietjen R. Reflex sympathetic dystrophy of the knee. Clin Orthop 1986; 209:234–243.

Tracy G, Crockett F. Pain in the lower limb after sympathectomy. Lancet 1957; I:12–14.

Uematsu S, Hendler N, Hungerford D, et al. Theromography and electromyography in the differential diagnosis of chronic pain syndrome and reflex sympathetic dystrophy. Electromyogr Clin Neurophysiol, 21.

KINETIC CHAIN EXERCISE IN KNEE REHABILITATION

RANDAL A. PALMITIER, M.D.

Kinetic chain exercises have become a key component in lower extremity rehabilitation. Recent research has shown that these exercises, when prescribed correctly, are capable of neutralizing knee shear forces and reducing patellofemoral compression while effectively exploiting the specificity of training principles that are so important in rehabilitating the injured athlete. It is imperative that rehabilitation professionals supervising such programs thoroughly understand the kinetic chain principles if they hope to take full advantage of all the benefits kinetic chain exercises have to offer. This requires some basic knowledge of the terminology and biomechanics. After acquiring this foundation, practical application of the principles is less confusing and more rewarding.

TERMINOLOGY

The open and closed kinetic chain terminology was derived by Steindler from the closed kinematic and link concepts used by mechanical engineers. The link concept deals with rigid overlapping segments connected in series by pin joints. The system is considered closed if the terminal ends are connected to a rigid framework, thus preventing translation of the first or last joint in the series. Kinematics have to do with joint motion. A closed kinematic chain movement at one joint leads to movement at all other joints in a predictable manner. If the system is open, i.e., one end is not fixed to the framework, joint motion is not predictable.

Steindler was interested in joint forces or kinetics and suggested that if each human extremity were considered a series of rigid segments, muscle recruitment and joint forces would differ under different limb loading conditions. He coined the terms *open* and *closed kinetic chain* to make this distinction. Specifically, an open kinetic chain exists when the peripheral joint of the extremity can move freely, as when waving the hand or moving the foot forward in the swing phase of gait. A closed kinetic chain exists whenever the foot or hand meet resistance, as in the push-up or when rising from a squat. Steindler hastened to point out that a true closed kinetic chain only exists during isometric exercise, when neither the proximal nor distal joint center moves.

In the 1980s these theoretical principles found practical application in knee rehabilitation. Researchers had shown that traditional seated knee extension exercises, which were universally used to strengthen the quadriceps, placed significant strain on the anterior cruciate ligament (ACL). The force of quadriceps contraction transferred by way of the patellar tendon to the tibial tubercle resulted in a tendency for anterior tibial translation that could only be checked by the ACL. These forces were considered high enough to endanger the healing graft in an ACL reconstructed knee or stretch the secondary restraints in the ACL deficient knee. In 1985 Henning et al published their landmark study, which suggested that strengthening the lower extremity in the weight bearing posture did not place excessive strain on the ACL. The closed kinetic chain terminology was used to describe this type of exercise and was quickly adopted by the rehabilitation community.

Closed kinetic chain exercises for the lower extremity include squats, leg presses, and stationary bike, while the traditional seated knee extension is considered an open kinetic chain exercise. Joint forces and specifically ACL shear forces are indeed different during the two types of exercise, but using the open and closed kinetic chain terminology to make the distinction is inaccurate and confusing. As Steindler pointed out, neither type of exercise is truly a closed system since either the proximal

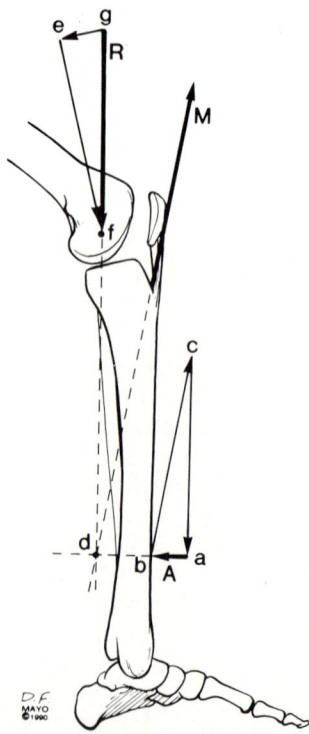

Figure 1 Force diagram. A = applied force; M = quadriceps muscle force; R = joint reaction force; f = knee instant center of rotation; a,b,c, = triangle formed by force vectors in equilibrium; used to determine length of unknown vector, R; d = common point of intersectin of three force system in equilibrium; e-g = shear component of R; e-f = normal component of R. (From Palmiter RA, An KN, Scott SG, et al. Kinetic chain exercise in knee rehabilitation. Sports Med 1991; 11(6):402-413; with permission.)

Adapted with permission from Palmiter RA, An KN, Scott SG, et al. Kinetic chain exercise in knee rehabilitation. Sports Med 1991; 11(6):402-413.

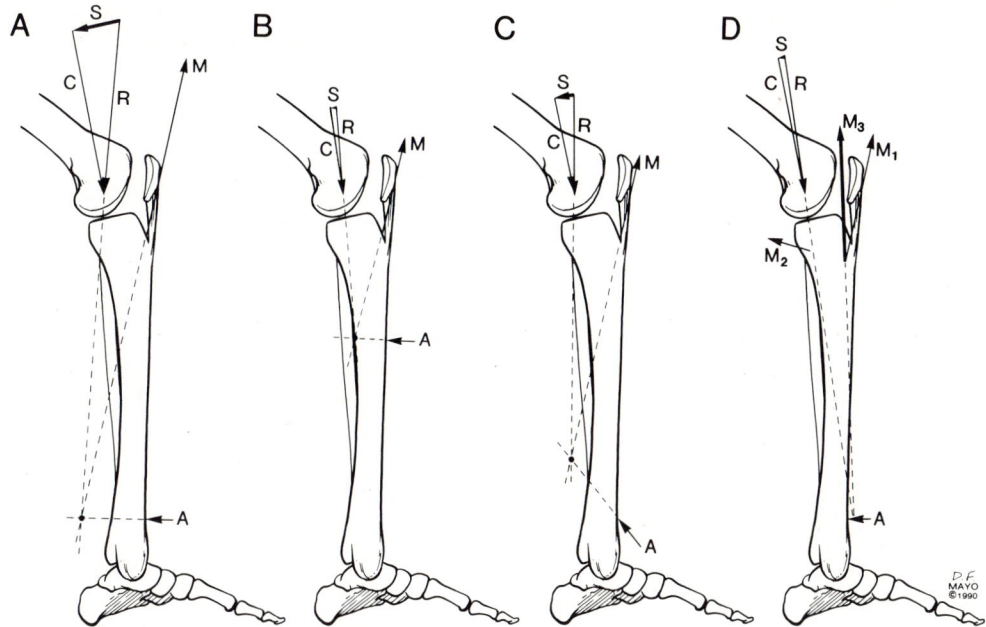

Figure 2 Force diagrams demonstrating altered joint reaction force. In each example, C represents the compression component of the joint reaction force and S represents the shear component of the joint reaction force. *A,* Knee extension exercise with force applied on distal tibia. *B,* Knee extension with force applied proximally. *C,* Axial orientation of applied load. *D,* Quadriceps and hamstring co-contraction. (From Palmiter RA, An KN, Scott SG, et al. Kinetic chain exercise in knee rehabilitation. Sports Med 1991; 11(6):402-413; with permission.)

or distal joint center moves. Conversely, one could consider both closed kinetic chain exercises since the limb meets resistance in each situation.

The hip, knee, and ankle comprise the lower extremity kinetic chain. Exercises like the squat recruit all three links in unison while seated knee extensions isolate only one link of the chain. As such, the seated knee extension is not a kinetic chain exercise at all and should be differentiated from exercises like the squat by calling it a joint isolation exercise. The squat should simply be called a kinetic chain exercise; further description with open or closed only confuses the issue.

BIOMECHANICS

Knee shear is reduced during kinetic chain exercise through hamstring co-contraction and the axial orientation of the applied force. This can be demonstrated with simple force diagrams. Figure 1 is a force diagram on the seated knee extension exercise. The system has been simplified such that only three fundamental forces are acting on the tibia: the applied force *(A)*, the quadriceps muscle force *(M)*, and the joint reaction force *(R)*. If the tibia is in equilibrium, the line of application of all three forces must pass through a common point *(d)*. Therefore, if the direction and point of application of *M* and *A* are known, the direction of *R* can be determined. Vector *R* can then be resolved into its components, ef (compression) and eg (shear). The shear force is directed posteriorly, indicating that if it were not for soft tissue constraint, the tibia would

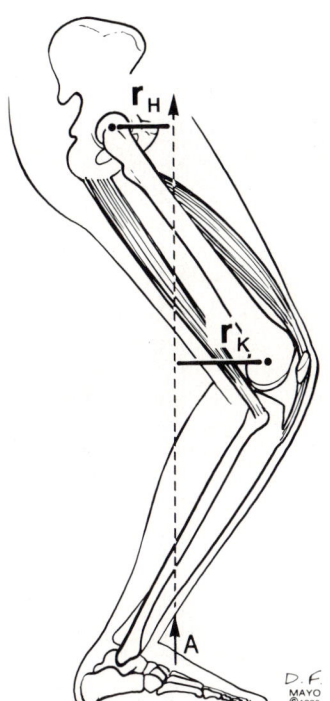

Figure 3 Diagrammatic representation of the induction of muscular co-contraction due to flexion moments caused by the applied force. A = applied force; rH = hip moment arm; rK = knee moment arm. (From Palmiter RA, An KN, Scott SG, et al. Kinetic chain exercise in knee rehabilitation. Sports Med 1991; 11(6):402-413; with permission.)

tend to translate anteriorly. Studies have shown that 86% of this soft tissue constraint is provided by the ACL.

Figures 2A, B, and C show how variation in the location and orientation of the applied force influences the knee shear force. When A is applied proximally on the tibia, as in 2B, knee shear is dramatically decreased. Figure 2C shows the effect of changing the orientation of the applied force. If the force is applied with a more axial orientation, the shear component of the joint reaction force is, once again, smaller.

Figure 2D shows the dramatic decrease in joint shear that occurs with hamstring co-contraction. In this situation, simultaneous contraction of the quadriceps, M1, and hamstrings, M2, produces a net force vector M3. As can be seen, the joint reaction force R, caused by this net force, has a much smaller shear component than that seen during isolated quadriceps contraction. Kinetic chain exercise induces hamstring co-contraction. The reason for this is illustrated in Figure 3. Consider a force A applied to the distal tibia. Since the hip and knee are unconstrained, the force creates a flexion moment at both joints. The hamstrings contract to stabilize the hip and the quadriceps contract to stabilize the knee. Activity in the biarticular hamstring muscle group, induced for hip stability, helps neutralize the tendency of the quadriceps to cause anterior tibial translation. A similar phenomenon oc-

curs at the ankle joint if the force A is applied to the bottom of the foot. Tension in soleus, which would be induced to stabilize the ankle flexion moment, will have an indirect effect on knee shear. During exercise, the lower extremity kinetic chain is recruited when the hip, knee, and ankle are unconstrained and the force is applied axially, causing triarticular flexion. Therefore, knee shear forces are reduced by the mechanisms illustrated in both 2C and 2D.

During seated leg extensions, the force is applied perpendicular to the tibia and causes a flexion moment at the knee only. Such joint isolation during exercise does not take advantage of the secondary stabilizing effect of other muscles in the lower extremity kinetic chain. In other words, the kinetic chain is not exploited, and the term kinetic chain should not be used in describing such exercises.

INEFFECTIVE EXERCISES

The preceding principles must be understood in order to prevent errors in exercise prescription. Moments at the hip and knee will vary depending on the type of exercise performed. Figure 4 illustrates two weight-bearing exercises that do not neutralize knee shear. In Figure 4A, the intersection of the force lines on bodyweight and the support force from the wall define

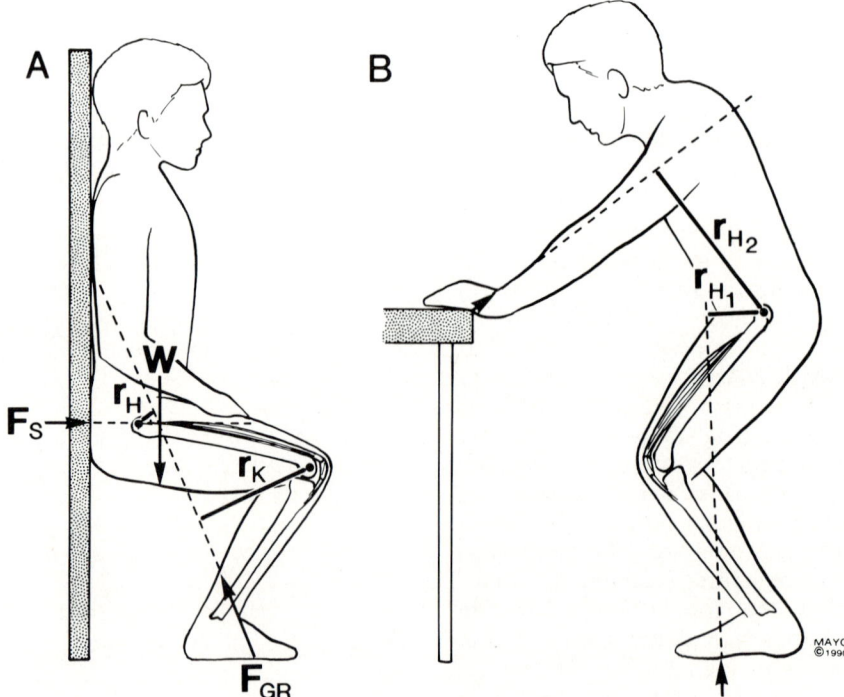

Figure 4 Hamstring co-contraction is minimal in these two exercise situations. *A,* The intersection of force line A (support force) and W (body weight) defines a point through which the force line of the ground reaction force must pass producing a large knee moment, rK, and a small hip moment, rH; *B,* Arm support can easily stabilize the hip flexion moment arm of the ground reaction force, rH1. (From Palmiter RA, An KN, Scott SG, et al. Kinetic chain exercise in knee rehabilitation. Sports Med 1991; 11(6):402-413; with permission.)

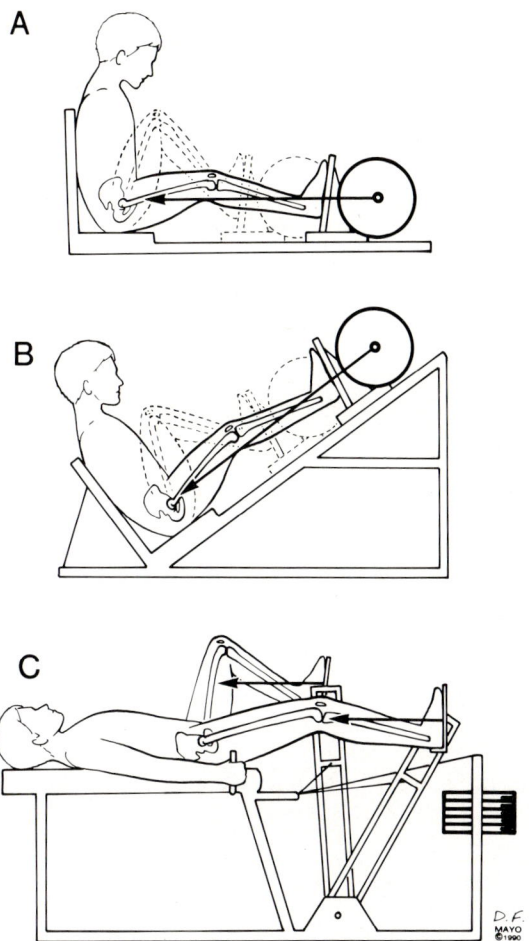

Figure 5 Illustration of the line of force application relative to the tibia, hip, and knee for various leg press exercise situations. (In *A,* the resistance is applied horizontally via a pulley system). (From Palmiter RA, An KN, Scott SG, et al. Kinetic chain exercise in knee rehabilitation. Sports Med 1991; 11(6):402-413; with permission.)

the point through which the ground reaction force line must pass. As can be seen, the knee moment created by this force is large while the hip moment is small. In Figure 4*B,* the large moment arm of the upper extremity support force allows the arm to easily overcome the hip flexion moment. Both of these exercises approach the joint isolation scenario, but are commonly used in rehabilitating patients who are too weak to do unsupported squats.

The leg press is another form of kinetic chain exercise for the weak postoperative or postinjury patient. It is a more stable exercise that allows the patient to exercise with less than body weight and allows exercise of one leg at a time. Unfortunately, none of the leg press machines presently available on the market take full advantage of the kinetic chain. As can be seen in Figures 5*A* and 5*B,* the line of force application produces little if any hip flexion moment. On the other hand, at the bottom of movement there is an extremely large knee

movement. A more biomechanically sound leg press is pictured in 5*C.* The foot plate moves in an arc, which results in an increase in both hip and knee flexion moments as the leg goes through the movement. It is my understanding that several companies are working on such a machine. Until adequate equipment is developed, kinetic chain exercises such as multiangled isometric leg press, power squats, stair climbing, and stationary biking should be emphasized to neutralize knee shear.

BENEFITS OF KINETIC CHAIN EXERCISE

Decreased shear at the knee is not the only advantage to the use of kinetic chain exercise in knee rehabilitation. Walking, running, jumping, climbing, and rising from a chair are all activities that exploit the kinetic chain. The lower extremity is usually used in this manner and should, therefore, be rehabilitated in this manner. Specificity of training is an accepted concept in rehabilitation and sports medicine. It involves improving strength and coordination of the injured athlete with exercises that are similar to the sporting activity itself. Central nervous system engram patterning results from precise repetition of movement. Repetitive deviation from the correct movement pattern can result in substitution patterning. A substitution pattern is an incorrect and inefficient muscular recruitment pattern that can hinder performance and lead to injury.

The importance of this concept in lower extremity rehabilitation becomes evident when the kinesiology of kinetic chain exercise is studied. Consider the simultaneous hip and knee extension that occurs when rising from a squat. The rectus femoris and the hamstrings are both active. As the hip extends, the rectus femoris lengthens while the hamstrings shorten, but as the knee extends the rectus femoris shortens as the hamstrings lengthen. The result at the muscular level might be called a pseudoisometric contraction, due to simultaneous concentric and eccentric contractions at opposite ends of each muscle. This so-called concurrent shift cannot be reproduced with isolation exercises.

Neural adaptation is another benefit of strength training that will be affected by the type of exercise chosen. The literature has repeatedly shown that strength gains seen during the first 4 weeks of training are primarily due to neural adaptation, not muscular hypertrophy. Since the neural adaptation that occurs in the lower extremity will differ dramatically as a function of whether the kinetic chain is recruited or the joint is isolated, lower extremity rehabilitation protocols must incorporate kinetic chain exercise early.

SUGGESTED READING

Grood ES, Suntay WJ, Noyes FR, et al. Biomechanics of knee extension exercise. J Bone Joint Surg 1984; 66A:725–734.
Henning CE, Lynch MA, Glick JR. An in vivo strain gauge study of

elongation of the anterior cruciate ligament. Am J Sports Med 1985; 13(1):22–26.

Lutz GE, Palmitier RA, An KN, et al. Comparison of tibiofemoral joint forces during open-kinetic-chain and closed-kinetic-chain exercises. J Bone Joint Surg 1993; 75A:732–739.

Lutz GE, Stuart MJ, Sim FH. Rehabilitation techniques for athletes after reconstruction of the anterior cruciate ligament. Mayo Clin Proc 1990; 65:1322–1329.

Palmitier RA, An KN, Scott SG, et al. Kinetic chain exercise in knee rehabilitation. Sports Med 1991; 11(6):402–413.

Paulos L, Noyes FR, Grood E, et al. Knee rehabilitation after anterior cruciate ligament reconstruction and repair. Am J Sports Med 1981; 9(3):140–149.

Steindler A. Kinesiology of the human body under normal and pathological conditions. Springfield Il: Charles C. Thomas, 1973.

I FOOT

METATARSALGIA AND OTHER COMMON PROBLEMS

R. PETER WELSH, M.B., Ch.B, F.R.C.S.(C), F.A.C.S.

"When the foot aches, the whole body aches!" To the athlete with pain in the forefoot, the whole athletic performance is indeed compromised, and there are few injuries more frustrating to cope with than these ill-defined and often unresponsive maladies.

CLINICAL ENTITIES

Common foot problems include:

Intermetatarsal ligament strains and intermetatarsal bursitis
Morton's metatarsalgia
Stress fractures
Freiberg's infraction
Metatarsal prolapse and plantar callosities
Sesamoiditis
Bunions and bunionettes
Hallux rigidus
Hammer and claw toes

Intermetatarsal Ligament Strains and Intermetatarsal Bursitis

The running sports impose tremendous loads on the forefoot with impact forces of up to three times body weight at foot-plant and push-off. The intermetatarsal ligament complex is subject to tremendous strain, particularly with the demands of hard surface running, and with aging there is also a gradual splaying of the forefoot, imposing undue stress on this structure. Furthermore, inflammation of the intermetatarsal bursae occurs in response to the jostling motion with running activity, and this results in an ill-defined forefoot pain in the region between adjacent metatarsal heads and necks. Tender to touch, sensitive to loads, this condition may completely preclude running activity.

Morton's Neuroma

Morton's neuroma is a more distinctive entity; symptoms are quite specific, often with a lancinating jab of pain on footfall and an associated neuritis in the form of parasthetic sensations spreading down the adjacent borders of the affected toes in the digital nerve distribution. This condition is defined pathologically as a neuroma, but in reality is due to the bursitic involvement of the neurovascular complex at its intermetatarsal digital bifurcation.

Stress Fractures

Repetitive cycling of any structural element may lead to the development of fatigue fractures. Bone shows such a breach in the rigid cortex of the metatarsal neck area and occasionally near the base of the metatarsal.

In runners and dancers, other sites of these fractures are of course the distal fibular 2 inches above the tip of the lateral malleolus, the tibia about the junction of the proximal and mid one-third, and occasionally the tibial plateau and the femoral condyle. Very rarely a stress fracture may be seen in the neck of the femur.

The breach in the cortex sets up an intense subperiosteal reaction, which is very painful and does not settle until there is new bone formation sufficient to consolidate the fracture focus. Radiographs may not be positive in the initial stages, and changes may not be observed until periosteal new bone is noted 3 to 4 weeks after injury. A technetium bone scan is often helpful in the early stages in differentiating a stress fracture from a simple intermetatarsal foot strain. The scan is positive only if there is actual bone involvement.

Freiberg's Infraction

A rare avascular necrosis of the metatarsal head, most commonly the second, is occasionally seen as a cause of metatarsalgia. The condition is known as one of the osteochondroses and is in fact akin to Perthes' disease of the hip. The metatarsal head is rendered dysvascular, and then, with regeneration, new bone is laid down on the old scaffold, but not before a fracture or partial collapse of the head distorts the shape of the metatarsal and deranges the metatarsal phalangeal articulation, leading in late stages to degenerative arthritis of the joint.

Metatarsal Prolapse and Plantar Callosities

Abnormal weight-bearing pressures beneath the metatarsal head result in the development of painful callosities. The collapse of the transverse arch of the foot sees the weight borne preferentially on the middle metatarsals instead of the first and fifth. Similarly, the development of an arthritic tendency at the base of the metatarsal may result in loss of flexibility in the foot and abnormal weight distribution across the forefoot without the normal resilience being shown at this level.

With prolapse of the metatarsal head, the prominence of the bone causes abnormal loading on the weight-bearing bursal pad with secondary thickening of the overlying skin, producing a hard callus.

Sesamoiditis

If the abnormal pressures are maldistributed beneath the first metatarsal head, it is often the metatarsal sesamoids that bear the brunt of the load. Associated sesamoiditis and bursal inflammation may result. Furthermore, the sesamoids, which are bones in the tendon of the short flexor of the great toe, are also subject to fracture and developmental abnormalities (they are often bipartite), and in the older individual they are subject to arthritic change in their articulation with the metatarsal head.

Bunions and Bunionettes

A bunion is a painful bursitis overlying the medial prominence of the first metatarsal head. A bunionette is a similar condition on the lateral aspect of the foot in relation to the fifth metatarsal head. In the great toe a bunion may be associated with hallux valgus or hallux rigidus, whereas a bunionette may also be associated with abnormal weight bearing on the plantar aspect of the foot.

Hallux Rigidus

A disabling arthritis of the first metatarsophalangeal (MTP) joint results in gross limitation of first metatarsal joint movement, particularly in extension. This markedly limits participation in any of the running or jumping sports, for without adequate dorsiflexion, push-off is severely inhibited. Often there is a strong familial tendency in the development of this condition, although it may also arise as a consequence of trauma involving the first MTP joint.

Hammer and Claw Toes

A flexion deformity of the interphalangeal joints of the toes may result in abnormal pressure areas with callus or corn formation overlying the prominence of the angulated joint. A hammer toe is associated with flexion at the distal interphalangeal (DIP) joint and extension at the MTP joint. A claw toe maintains a normal articulation at the MTP joint that involves a clawing or flexion deformity at either the proximal interphalangeal (PIP) or DIP joints.

CLINICAL ASSESSMENT

The clinical diagnosis of the above conditions is obvious in most instances. In others, such as hallux rigidus, review of radiographs is required to confirm the extent of the condition, and if doubt exists in defining whether or not a metatarsal neck pain is related to a stress fracture, a technetium bone scan may be required.

In completing the assessment, particular care should be taken on examining the hindfoot, noting the mobility of associated ankle subtalar and midtarsal joints as well as the characteristics of the foot and the heel plant, and whether there is a varus or valgus disposition of the heel that will misdirect the forefoot placement. In all instances the neurovascular status of the extremities should be carefully evaluated. The foot itself should never be examined in isolation from the rest of the patient. Particular importance is placed in the overall examination, noting the total limb alignment and whether there is a varus or valgus deformity or rotational anomaly of the limb more proximally. Any limb length inequalities should be noted and any rotational abnormality in the hip, femur, or tibia documented. The knee joint function, particularly patellar mechanics, is of vital concern with regard to the functioning of the foot. A tendency to genu valgum with a subluxating patella due to an increased "Q" angle leads invariably to a displacement of the forefoot with a valgus tendency of the heel at foot-plant, resulting in abnormal hyperpronation of the forefoot.

Finally, in the clinical assessment, any abnormalities of the spine and its development should be noted; for example, scoliosis may affect foot mechanics.

MANAGEMENT OF METATARSALGIA AND FOOT DISORDERS

Management of these conditions may require (1) modification of sports activity, (2) footwear adaptation, (3) use of orthotics and other podiatric appliances, (4) physical therapies, (5) medications, and (6) surgery.

Modification of Sports Activity

Participation in many of the running and jumping sports must be modified. Acute strains of the forefoot require rest from provocative loading; stress fractures cannot be subjected to more than normal daily walking and must heal completely before running can be resumed. Hallux rigidus may put an end completely to the career of a dancer or jumper because of the inability to dorsiflex the great toe joint.

Footwear Adaptation

Footwear must be both protective and supportive, comfortably conforming to the foot. An arch support system should be adequate, but not bulky; of particular importance is the adequacy of heel control, which directs forefoot plant and push-off. Pressure points should be eliminated by stretching at sites of local irritation, or areas of pressure should be bridged so that the sensitive area fits into a relative recess.

Different conditions dictate particular footwear requirements. With hallux rigidus, a stiff shank or even a rocker bottom sole may be of great assistance, whereas in many sports a stiff shank may result in excessive loading of the heel at the bone-tendon junction and a predisposition to Achilles tendinitis. Obviously, footwear requirements must be tailored to the needs and condition of the patient.

Use of Orthotics and Other Podiatric Appliances

Customized adaptation of footwear can play a major part in the management of foot disorders.

Orthotics should in most instances be regarded as a temporary aid, just as a back brace aids an acutely injured spine. Most foot disorders suffered acutely are self-limiting, and a soft orthotic may assist by allowing continuance of the sports activity while the healing process occurs. However, once the injury has healed, the device should be discarded. Therefore, it makes no sense for athletes who have run successfully for perhaps 5 or 10 years to feel that, because of a single foot injury, they must forever persist with an orthotic support in the shoe. Only if an injury proves recurrent and major structural abnormality is seen to benefit from the use of an orthotic should a more permanent device be prescribed.

It should be remembered that an orthotic device occupies space in a shoe and adds weight to the foot, and that by the employment of these aids, even a subtle alteration of foot-plant and push-off must call for compensatory adjustment in the gait pattern elsewhere, at the level of the knee, hip, or spine.

The type of orthotic employed varies according to the condition from which the patient suffers. Orthotics may be of great value in acute long arch strains, in which case an arch support and scaphoid cookie greatly reduce load on the arch structure. A more rigid device is required for the patient with hallux rigidus to restrict pressures on the great toe joint, but such rigidity may throw loads at the heel and cause Achilles tendinitis.

In managing metatarsal problems, there is no need for the major building-in of a long arch system into the orthotic; all that is required is a metatarsal pad support beneath the metatarsal neck to elevate and separate the metatarsal heads and reduce their compressive tendency on weight bearing. This device also may be very effective in the management of Morton's neuroma.

There has been a great tendency to overprescribe orthotics for what is termed the hyperpronated or flat foot. There is such a wide range of what may be considered the normal arch height that to offer orthotics arbitrarily to the flatter-appearing foot totally disregards how that individual may function with that particular foot form. The arbitrary prescription of orthotics in these instances can be more harmful than beneficial, but if injury does prove resistant to other forms of treatment, and proven benefit is obtained by a soft orthotic device, prescription of more permanent orthotics should be considered. Otherwise, most orthotics should be used on a temporary basis to assist the athlete through the

healing of an injury. It is probably better to further customize the footwear itself than to add redundancy in the form of orthotic devices to the athlete's shoes.

In most instances, soft, resilient orthotics are preferred to the more rigid materials often prescribed. Even though these more rigid materials may prove more durable in regard to the life of the device itself, it is better to have a system that conforms more to the texture of both the shoe and the foot structures than to have a rigid interface between the foot and the shoe.

Other appliances that may be useful are doughnut protective devices over pressure points to prevent friction between the foot and the shoe, e.g., over a bunion or hammer toe prominence. Care must be paid in general to the skin of the foot, with careful attention to any cracks or ulcer areas. A tendency to interdigital fungal infection usually can be handled adequately with topical antifungal agents.

Physical Therapies

As a species, man has lost much of his capacity to individual control of the intrinsic musculature of the foot. Physical therapy aimed at assisting intrinsic function can be of extreme benefit. In this regard, faradic foot baths may be employed to initiate intrinsic response, and teaching of intrinsic exercises may be of considerable benefit.

Passive stretching of deforming digits and stiffening toes is a worthwhile endeavor.

Local measures, such as icing and ultrasound, may have empiric value; if no benefit is obviously arising from their employment, treatment should be discontinued.

Medications

Systemic medication has little place in the management of most of these conditions, but local steroid injections between the metatarsal heads may settle acute bursitis and benefit a Morton's neuroma. Sesamoiditis may also respond to local infiltration. As a general rule in most treatments, if one injection does not help, there seems little justification for continuing treatments of that type, and if one injection works, there is no cause for further treatment.

Surgery

Foot problems of some athletes prove to be both refractory to treatment and sufficiently disabling to preclude any sports participation. These require definitive surgical treatment.

Morton's Neuroma. Local interdigital exploration allows the resection of the involved bursal scar tissue enveloping the bifurcation of the digital nerve and interdigital space. Tourniquet control of circulation greatly aids the dissection in these instances, and a web space incision is favored: this gives a clear view of the whole intermetatarsal space both dorsally and on the plantar aspect.

Freiberg's Infraction. Metatarsal neck osteotomy decompresses the involved metatarsophalangeal joint in addition to easing the weight-bearing load on the affected metatarsal head.

Metatarsal Prolapse and Plantar Callosities. Elevation of the affected metatarsal head by metatarsal neck osteotomy decompresses the lesser and overlying calloused skin. An oblique osteotomy just proximal to the head allows the head to slide up and shorten slightly. Weight bearing is allowed immediately, but the fracture requires 4 to 6 weeks to unite. The return to sport may be delayed 2 to 3 months by swelling and tenderness.

The patient should be closely observed postoperatively for transfer of weight from one metatarsal to the adjacent metatarsal head, which may necessitate another decompressive osteotomy.

Sesamoiditis. Excision of the sesamoids for nonunion, avascular necrosis, or osteoarthritis can be extremely rewarding. Care must be taken to avoid injury to the digital nerves or flexor tendon.

Bunions. If the bunion is associated with hallux valgus, the local excision of the bunion must always be carried out in conjunction with correction of the hallux valgus. In addition, any degree of metatarsus varus should be corrected by metatarsal osteotomy, preferably at the base of the first metatarsal.

Preservation of the intact joint should be practiced whenever possible, and procedures such as the McBride procedure are preferred to excisional remedies such as a Keller procedure.

Bunionettes. The fifth metatarsal head should never be excised in the athlete, or a tendency to rolling over and a sense of weakness will always prevail. Instead, in addition to a local bunionette excision, an oblique medializing osteotomy of the neck of the fifth metatarsal allows both correction of the lateral deviating metatarsal head and upward correction of any abnormal weight-bearing pressure point.

Hallux Rigidus. In the athlete, excisional arthroplasty may be necessary, with excision of the base of the proximal phalanx removing sufficient bone to permit adequate dorsiflexion of the joint. Careful capsular reconstruction is essential, but tension on the great toe joint must be minimal at the conclusion of the procedure. The use of interposition material, as with Silastic arthroplasty, has little place in the athlete; these materials cannot prove durable to the repetitive load demands of active athletic endeavor.

Metatarsophalangeal fusion has a definite place in certain individuals. It provides a totally pain-free, strong push-off, but limits the type of footwear that can be used, and its success relies on complete mobility of the associated joints at the DIP and the base of the first metatarsal.

Greater morbidity of this procedure, the risk of nonunion, and the necessity for careful technical considerations in obtaining the correct angle of the MTP joint make this a demanding technique. In general, the excisional procedure is favored in dancers and jumpers.

Hammer and Claw Toes. For hammer toes with PIP hyperextension, if the joint remains mobile and the MTP joint is not subluxated, a flexor to extensor tendon transfer is recommended.

If the PIP deformity is fixed, an interphalangeal fusion is preferred; if the MTP joint is concurrently subluxated, a partial excision of the base of the proximal phalanx is added.

For claw toes at the DIP joint, a Jones repair, excising a transverse dorsal elipse of skin, tendon, and a bone wedge at the DIP joint, provides a completely durable correction.

SUGGESTED READING

Bossley CJ, Cairney PC. The intermetatarsophalangeal bursa: Its significance in Morton's metatarsalgia. J Bone Joint Surg 1980; 62B:184.

Mann RA. DuVries's Surgery of the Foot. 4th ed. St. Louis: CV Mosby, 1978.

Mann RA, Clanton TO. Hallus rigidus: Treatment by cheilectomy. J Bone Joint Surg 1988; 70A:400.

Myerson MS, Shereff MJ. The pathological anatomy of claw and hammer toes. J Bone Joint Surg 1989; 71A:45.

Richardson E. The foot in adolescents and adults in Campbell's operative orthopaedics. 7th ed. St. Louis: CV Mosby, 1987:829.

SOFT TISSUE INJURIES

G. JAMES SAMMARCO, M.D., F.A.C.S.

Soft tissue in the foot serves to support, nourish, and provide sensation, in addition to controlling the position of the bone structures. At the same time, it acts as a shock-absorbing mechanism for high loads created during weight bearing.

The foot may be divided into the forefoot, midfoot, and hindfoot; special conditions occur in each of these areas. Two types of problems occur in soft tissue: the acute injury arising from a single traumatic event or several and the chronic tissue problems associated more commonly with overuse. Certain principles should be followed when treating injuries to soft tissue.

An acute injury is often the result of a single traumatic episode. This presents with swelling, tenderness, significant pain, and decreased joint motion, all of which interrupt sports activity. Restriction of motion and application of ice and a compression dressing while the leg is elevated above the level of the waist (acronym, RICE) are recommended as principles of acute care. Restriction of motion is achieved with a cast, splint, or brace. The principle of elevation is simply that "water flows downhill." Although it does not reduce edema, ice does provide a certain anesthetic effect to the skin, thereby reducing the pain. Restriction of motion relates to the particular part injured. The player is encouraged to move the remaining part of the foot: e.g., if the subtalar joint is injured and placed in a splint, the player is encouraged to elevate the leg and move the toes. This creates a "milking" action that helps reduce edema. The injury is reassessed in a few days and a rehabilitation program is started. This includes stretching, range-of-motion exercises, and power building to develop proprioception. The use of the foot and ankle exerciser board or "wobble board" is helpful (Fig. 1). If surgery is indicated, there should be a specific diagnosis; early return to the field should be expected if surgery is not required. During surgery a bloodless field is to be preferred in order to delineate tissue structures, avoid cutaneous nerves, and visualize vessels. For surgery on the toes and small joints, loupe magnification is helpful. When the athlete returns to sports activities, taping or bracing may be required with a modification of the shoe.

For chronic injuries due to overuse syndromes, a treatment regimen should include a warm-up program to deal specifically with the injured foot (Table 1). Warming up the foot before exercise is as important as stretching. Functional bracing and strapping, in addition to nonsteroidal anti-inflammatory drugs (NSAIDs) are important adjuncts to treatment.

NAIL INJURIES

Acute problems of the nails can occur from trauma such as a crush creating an acute *subungual hematoma*. Repeated minitrauma of the toe may produce a chronic subungual hematoma, "black toe," and is usually asymptomatic. The acute subungual hematoma is drained by means of a small drill held through the nail into the hematoma, allowing the blood under pressure to escape. A second, more traditional method is to heat the end of a paper clip under an alcohol lamp until red hot (Fig. 2). The hot tip is pressed directly over the nail, creating a hole into the hematoma and allowing the blood under pressure to escape. The nail is not removed but is taped in place to protect the nail bed; it may be lost at a later date, but meanwhile the nail bed begins to heal. Removal of the nail exposes the tender matrix to repeated painful trauma, and it may take 1 year for the hallux toenail to regrow.

Onycholysis, delaminating of the nail on its end, occurs as a result of weight bearing on the tip of the toe or repeatedly striking a hard object with the end of the nail. Partial avulsion can occur, but if the condition is chronic, as in toe dancers, no treatment is needed since the condition is asymptomatic. This should not be confused with paronychia, ingrown toenail, or onychomycosis.

SKIN INJURIES

The skin of the sole may be 7 mm thick. It is well fixed through fibrous septa to deep tissue and lacks sebaceous glands. Beneath lies a compartmentalized subcutaneous fat layer that acts as a shock-absorbing cushion. This is in contrast to the skin of the dorsum of the foot, which may be less than 1 mm thick and overlies several fascial layers that permit excellent mobility.

A *tear of the plantar skin* is caused by overstretching of the flexion creases of the proximal hallux or small toes. Tension on the foot is caused by running, stopping, or turning either barefoot or in a light shoe. This is treated by gentle cleansing and prophylactic antibiotic ointment until healing occurs. This condition does not prevent participation in sport.

Ill-fitting shoes force the toes into a hammer toe position, causing ulceration and *corns* on the dorsal aspect of proximal interphalangeal (PIP) joints and on the toe tufts and adjacent toes. The condition is corrected by changing shoes and padding the toes. In athletes with flexible hammer toe and chronic corns, a doughnut-shaped foam rubber pad is taped to the top of each corn. Such pads can also be placed between the toes

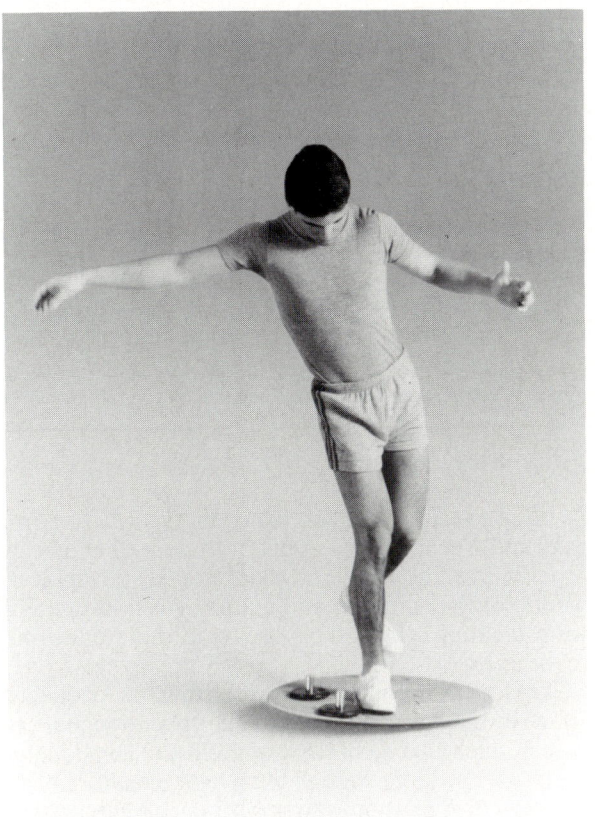

Figure 1 Athlete using the foot and ankle exercises board (BAPS BOARD). The foot is placed in the center and rotated. Proprioception, range of motion, and strength are developed after injury.

Table 1 Flexibility Program for the Foot and Ankle

Non-Weightbearing Exercises

Do each exercise 10 times a day. Increase repetitions of each exercise by 5 each day up to a total of 30 repetitions.
Do the program 3 times daily.
Exercise slowly and to the maximal stretch.

1. Sit on floor with legs straight in front. Place towel around ball of foot. Grasp both ends of towel with hands, and pull foot toward knee. Stretch to a count of 5. Release.
   Repeat the above, except pull more with right hand to bring foot to the right, then pull with left hand to bring foot to the left.
   Repeat with knee bent about 30 degrees.
2. Sit on floor with legs straight out. Flex foot upward toward face and curl toes under at the same time. Now point foot downward and bring toes up at the same time. The sequence is: Foot up, toes down, foot down, toes up.
   Sit on floor with legs straight out in front, putting foot flat against wall. With heel and ball of foot flat against wall, pull toes toward face. Hold to a count of 5. Relax.
   Do the same exercise with knee bent 30 degrees.
3. Sit in chair with knee bent and foot flat on floor under knee. Keep heel and ball of foot on floor, and raise toes. Keeping toes up, slide foot back a few inches, and relax toes. Raise toes again and slide foot back a few more inches. Keep raising toes and sliding foot back until you can no longer keep heel on floor while raising toes. Bring foot back out to starting position.
   Repeat from starting position. Raise heel, keeping toes flat on floor, then press down again. Lean upper body forward for increased stretch.
   Same position as above. Slide foot forward as far as you can, keeping both toes and heels in contact with floor. At this point, keep heel in place and knee straight. Flex foot up toward knee, then point foot and press toes onto floor. Keep stretching and pointing foot.
   Repeat from starting position, except keep toes curled as you stretch and point foot.
4. Sit with knees parallel, foot flat on floor. Pull inside edge of foot toward you (supinate), keeping outside edge on floor. Hold to a count of 5. Flatten foot, then bring outside edge of foot toward you (pronate), keeping inside edge on floor, including big toe. Hold to a count of 5. Don't let knee move during this exercise.
   Sit with feet flat on floor. Claw toes and inch foot forward as toes claw, then release. Separate toes between clawing. Inch out as far as possible, then slide back and start again.
5. Sit with feet flat on floor. Raise big toe, then second, progressing to little toe. Reverse and go from little toe to big toe.
   Sit with feet flat. Slightly lift heel, putting weight on lateral borders of feet. Roll from little toe to big toe, then back through heel without letting heel touch down. You are making a complete circle around ball of foot. Repeat and reverse.

Progressive Weightbearing Exercises

1. Between two chairs, using them for support: Stand with one foot 12 inches in front of the other, feet flat on floor. Rock forward onto front foot, so that weight is on this foot, leaving back foot in contact with floor, toes on floor, heel lifted. Rock all the way back so that front foot is on heel and toes are pulled back. Change position of feet and repeat.
   Between two chairs, stand on good leg. Swing affected leg all the way back, knee flexed, foot pointed, then swing leg forward to an extended leg, foot and toes pulled toward you (dorsiflexed). Keep repeating.
2. Stand with back to wall, feet directly under shoulders, weight evenly distributed. Slowly bend knees and do not raise heels. Go to point of maximal stretch and hold 5 counts, then rise up and repeat.
   Standing as above, at the bottom of knee bend, roll onto balls of the feet to maximal arch, then roll down, then straighten legs. Repeat.
3. Stand on a step with feet parallel, heels hanging off edge so that calves are maximally stretched. Pull all the way up onto toes, slowly, then lower all the way down to maximal stretch. Repeat up to 10 times. Repeat with feet turned out, then turned in. Progress to using 5 to 10 pound ankle weights.
4. Stand with all the weight on one leg. Keep knee straight and raise to a fully arched foot, slowly, then lower down. Repeat up to 20 times.
   Stand with all the weight on one leg. Bend knee and keep heel down, then straighten knee and pull up to a full arch. Slowly lower heel, keeping knee straight. Repeat.
5. Stand, rock back on heels, claw toes. Walk on heels and then walk with toes clawed around pencils.
   Walk on heels with 1 to 3 pound ankle weights wrapped around forefoot.
6. Standing, raise and lower inner sides of feet with toes clawed.
   Stand with feet parallel, on balls of feet, weight on outer borders of feet, knees about 4 inches apart. Roll the weight from fifth metatarsal to big toe in a circuiar motion. Heels stay off floor. Do this exercise with feet turned in, then with feet turned out.

to prevent soft corn formation. A neglected soft corn can become infected and develop a *web space abscess.* Diagnosis of an abscess is made by clinical examination that reveals tenderness and redness in the web space. A sinogram can help confirm the diagnosis if the clinical diagnosis is in doubt. Treatment consists of incision and drainage of the abscess with administration of appropriate antibiotics. The player may resume activities in 10 days when healing has occurred. Recurrent or persistent soft corn formation is treated by excision of the underlying cartilaginous osteophyte through a longitudinal incision above the flexion crease line on the side of the toe (Fig. 3). The edges of the corn are not excised, because they will resolve when the underlying protuberance is removed. Sports activity is restricted until the wound heals.

Blisters result from two concomitant forces, normal force and shear force, applied to feet that are not properly conditioned. The skin breaks down at the junction of the cornified and maturing cell layers. Fluid forms, creating a bleb. This occurs in the areas of high pressure.

Treatment is symptomatic, relieving the loadbearing surface by taping a closed cell foam rubber doughnut pad (¼-inch thick) to the bottom of the foot. The doughnut hole should be large enough to include the entire blister. An alternative method is to apply benzoin circumferentially about the blister, followed by a moleskin patch with a hole cut out for the blister. A small amount of Vaseline should be applied to the center area. To prevent recurrent blisters, recommended prophylaxis includes applying a single layer of Micropore paper tape over the

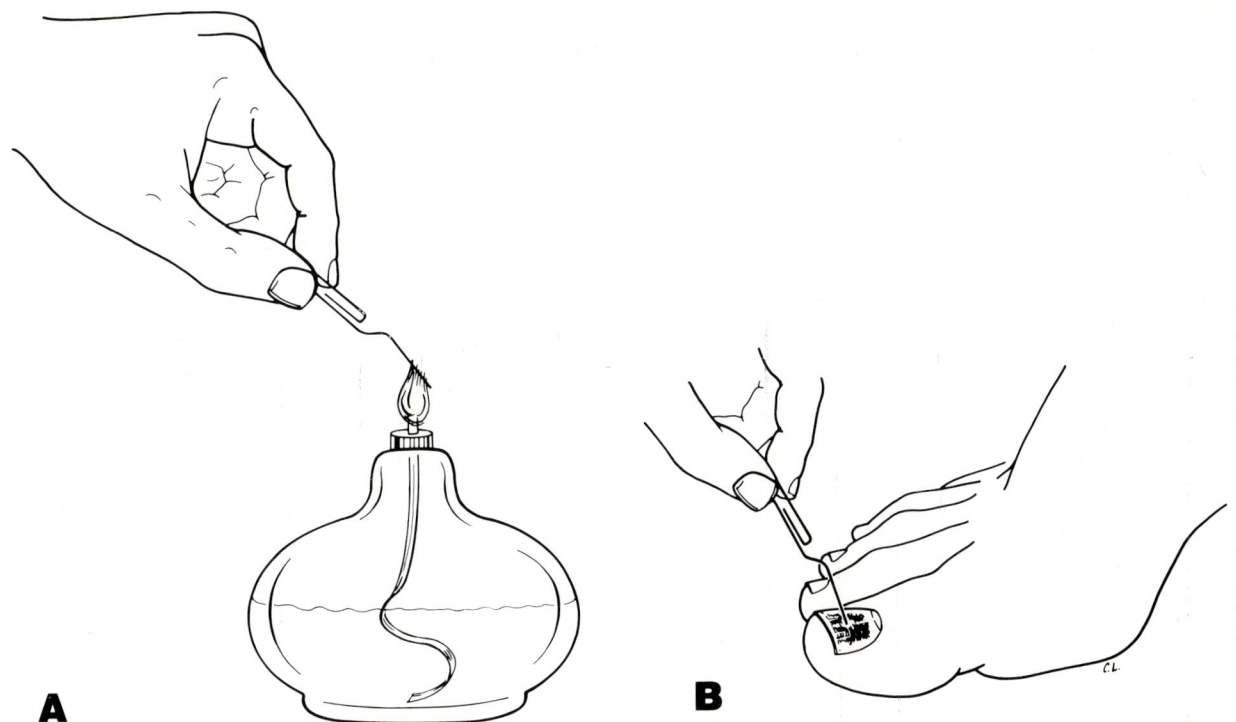

A

B

Figure 2 Acute hallux subungual hematoma causes pain from pressure beneath the nail. A paper clip is heated in the flame of an alcohol lamp *(A)* and pressed through the nail *(B),* creating a hole into the blood and relieving pressure.

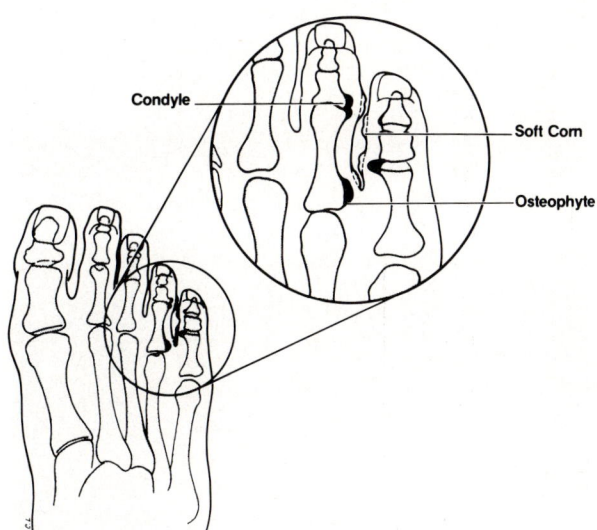

Condyle

Soft Corn

Osteophyte

Figure 3 Diagram of the region of soft corn formation between the toes. As the toes are pressed together in the shoe, pressure against a condyle or osteophyte and sweat cause skin maceration, and chronic pressure necrosis develops.

area at risk, and wearing double-thickness socks and properly fitted shoes. A graduated fitness program increases skin tolerance. A thick sock or a special double-layered sock also helps reduce normal and shear forces on the skin.

PUNCTURE WOUNDS

The puncture wound is the most underrated injury to soft tissues of the foot. Penetrating objects must pass through the shoe and sock before entering the skin, carrying both normal flora and pathogens. The most serious error is to underestimate the nature of the wound in light of a history of a penetrating injury and foot x-ray films revealing no evidence of radiopaque objects. In fact, most puncture wounds in which foreign bodies are found are caused by nonradiopaque objects such as ordinary glass, splinters, thorns, and plastic. Close follow-up is an important principle of treatment. Radiographic examination using soft tissue technique, with special views such as metatarsal head views or lateral and oblique views of the heel with thick emulsion film, may be necessary. The history is important, since the patient may relate that only part of the object was recovered. Gentle cleansing and prophylactic antibiotics are recommended. I prefer to use cephalexin (Keflex), 500 mg every 6 hours. The wound is examined after 48 hours for the presence of swelling, redness, increasing tenderness, and signs of early abscess formation. It may be necessary to perform incision and drainage. Magnetic resonance imaging (MRI) is helpful to determine whether a nonradiopaque foreign body is present. The incision should be positioned in the region of the puncture wound, avoiding a site directly beneath the metatarsal head or other bony weight-bearing prominence. Meticulous care is taken to explore the area of abscess

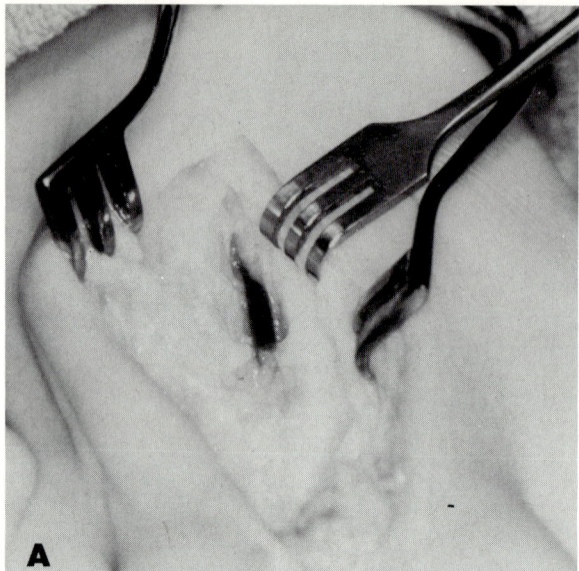
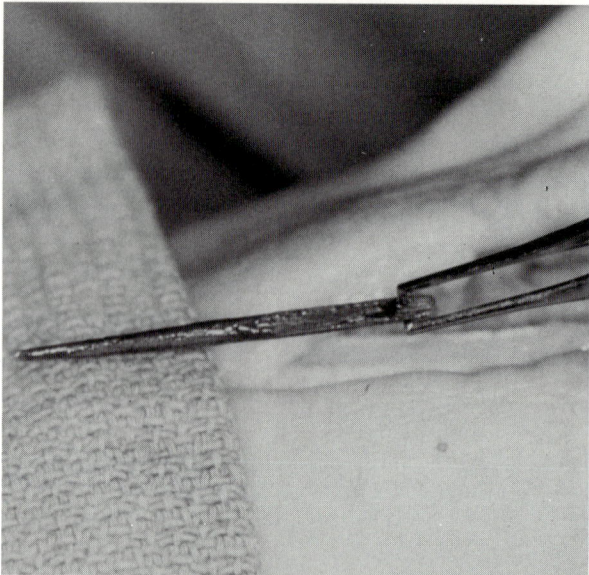

Figure 4 Operative photographs of a foot abscess with a toothpick 1 year after injury. The patient's report of recovering only a small amount of toothpick from the ball of the foot went unheeded. Two subsequent plantar incisions for the abscess failed to reveal the other half of the toothpick, which had migrated to the base of the metatarsal. A third dorsal incision revealed the source of the bimicrobial infection.

thoroughly without violating the unaffected, compartmentalized fat pad on the sole. At the time of surgery, both aerobic and nonaerobic cultures are obtained. Polybacterial infections are common (Fig. 4). Thorough examination of the wound is necessary to ensure that a foreign body is not present, since migration can occur quickly (Fig. 5). Postoperatively, a splint is applied. Cephalosporin antibiotic coverage is continued postoperatively until the operative culture and sensitivities are returned. The patient is then placed on appropriate specific antibiotics.

Rehabilitation is begun without weight bearing after 5 days. A weight-bearing program is added when the wound has healed.

LESSER TOE INJURIES

Soft tissue injuries of the lesser toes can have two causes: (1) external trauma related to jamming, crushing, and ill-fitting shoes; and (2) internal trauma due to lesser toe deformity or laxity of joint ligaments. Crushing injuries to the toes can occur either from player contact or from off-the-field injuries. Acute treatment includes elevation of and compression dressing to the forefoot. After edema begins to subside, active motion of the toes with elevation is started. If blebs have developed, the toe is protected with a soft dressing. The player is allowed to return to sports when symptoms permit. Uncommonly, dislocation of the PIP or distal interphalangeal (DIP) joint can occur, usually associated with fracture. After closed reduction, the toe is "buddy" taped to the adjacent toes for 3 weeks.

If flexible hammer toes are repeatedly traumatized

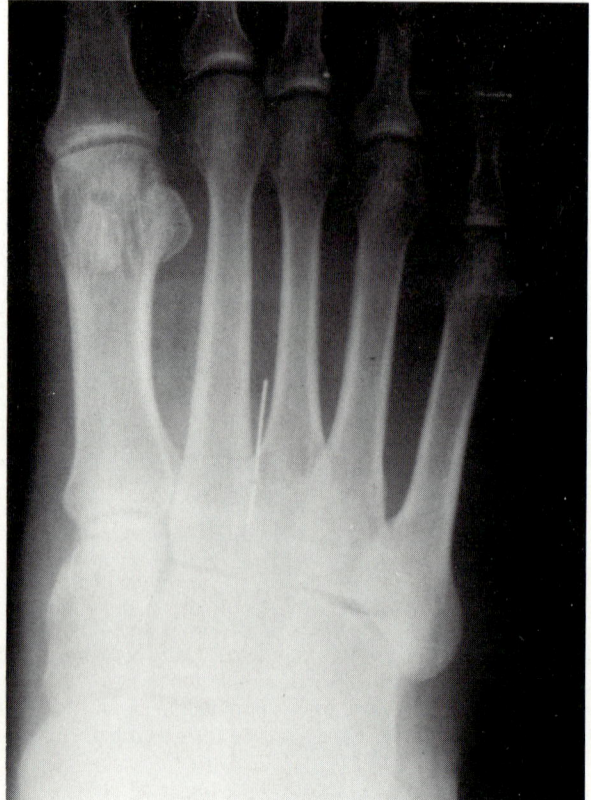

Figure 5 X-ray photograph of a foot 20 years after a puncture wound. No object was originally found at the entrance wound near the ball of the foot, no x-ray films were taken, and the pain and swelling eventually subsided. The needle has migrated to the midfoot.

and become symptomatic, a flexor-to-extensor tendon transfer of the modified Girdlestone type or one of its variants is recommended. Such surgery should be timed for the off-season, since 1 month is necessary for healing. For players with toes prone to repeated injury, a semirigid full-insole orthosis provides rigidity beneath the forefoot.

A player with cock-up fifth toe deformity is at risk for injury to the toe. Taping and padding between the fourth and fifth toes, as well as laterally, prevents corn and blister formation. Persistent symptoms warrant surgical correction and can be timed for a period of laying off. I recommend a partial proximal phalangectomy of the toe. Recovery takes 6 weeks.

HALLUX INJURIES

The great toe is subject to the most injuries. *Interphalangeal (IP) injuries* are usually caused by acute flexion either in a soft shoe or when barefoot. Repeated injury about the IP joint can cause arthritis and osteophyte formation, which predisposes the hallux to additional trauma. "Buddy" taping the hallux to the second toe helps prevent recurrence of the injury.

With the advent of artificial turf, the incidence of hyperextension injuries has increased. *Turf toe* is caused by jamming the forefoot, forcing the hallux into hyperextension at the metatarsophalangeal (MTP) joint causing strain and avulsion of the plantar plate. To this is added a valgus stress, and the medial collateral ligaments may be partially avulsed. Although most such injuries are initiated on artificial turf, recurrent injuries occur on both artificial and natural turf. Symptoms include severe pain beneath the first metatarsal head medially, with swelling of the hallux and decreased range of motion. An antalgic gait is noted. Radiographic examination may reveal avulsion fractures from the proximal phalanx or metatarsal head at the attachment of collateral ligaments. The sesamoids may be retracted, indicating avulsion of the plantar plate from the proximal phalanx. Rarely, a fractured sesamoid is noted, but even dislocation of the hallux has been reported. Treatment includes rest, ice application, elevation, and a compression dressing. The player is seen after 48 hours and, depending on the severity of the symptoms, a rehabilitation and stretching program is begun. Recurrence is prevented by restricting hyperextension of the hallux at the MTP joint. To achieve this, 1 inch tape is looped over the dorsum of the proximal phalanx, criss-crossing on the sole (Fig. 6A). Tight circumferential tape is not recommended, because it may cause circulatory compromise. Additional protection with a foot orthosis stiffened beneath the forefoot and hallux helps to prevent hyperextension. Sports shoes with a steel plate in the metatarsal region also help prevent hyperextension of the hallux. Counseling for acceptance of the orthosis may be required, since players often consider this to be a minor problem. Long-term sequelae of turf toe include hallux rigidus and hallux valgus. Surgical treatment of the acute injury is limited to the unreducible dislocation of the MTP joint.

Football players are also prone to hyperflexion injuries at the MTP joint, as are ballet dancers and runners. The mechanism in noncontact activities such as running or dancing is simply that of tripping. In contact sports, blocking or tackling from behind, and landing on the hallux with the added force of a tackler, contribute

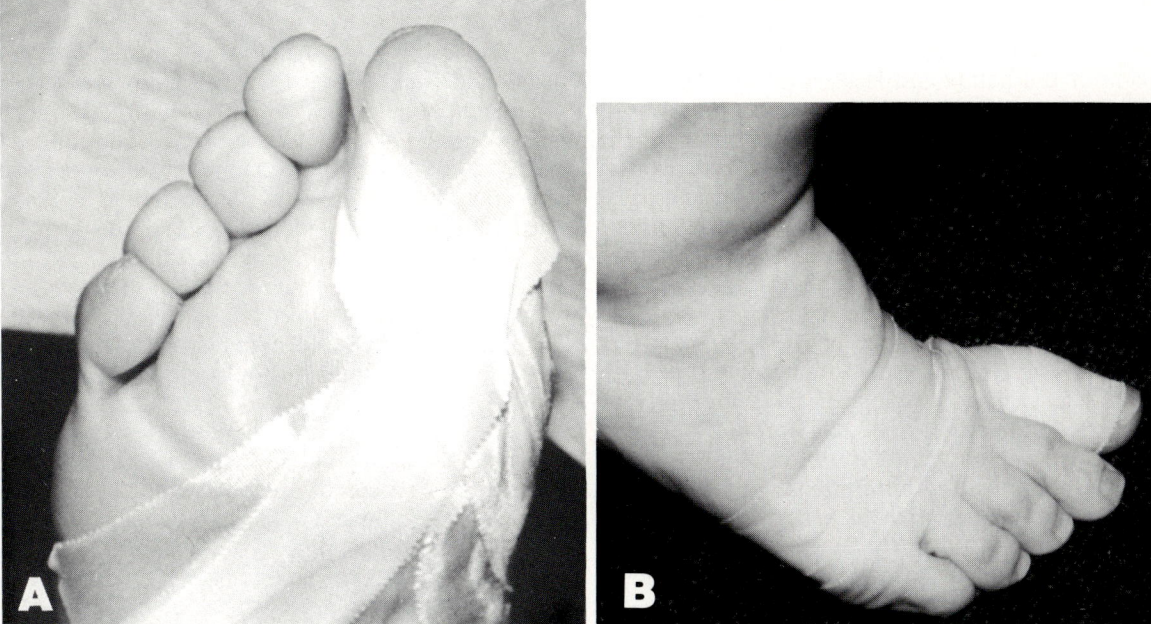

Figure 6 Recurrent turf toe prevention. *A,* The plantar aspect of the foot with dorsally looped 1 inch tape criss-crossed on the sole. *B,* Hyperextension of the hallux metatarsophalangeal joint is restricted. This may be combined with a stiff hallux extension in a foot orthosis to prevent reinjury.

to the force of the injury. Compression dressing, elevation, and ice are indicated, followed after 48 hours by a rehabilitation program as dictated by the subsidence of symptoms. A subsequent decrease in range of motion may occur. Long-term sequelae are similar to those for turf toe.

Acute bursitis of the MTP joint is caused by poorly fitted shoes or repeated medial trauma. Symptoms of pain and swelling may follow acute injuries, such as turf toe or tripping injuries, and may reflect an associated collateral ligament injury. The condition may also develop from chronic pressure and irritation at the medial metatarsal head. Treatment includes a doughnut-shaped closed foam pad taped over the medial first metatarsal head. The doughnut hole should be large enough to permit the tender area to settle within the opening. The pad should be thick enough (at least 5 mm) to prevent contact of the tender bursa with the shoe. NSAIDs are also prescribed.

PLANTAR FASCIITIS AND PLANTAR HEEL PAIN

Acute conditions of the plantar fascia include acute fasciitis in its proximal, middle, or distal parts. Complete rupture can occur near the calcaneal insertion. More commonly, *acute plantar fasciitis* occurs along the medial border of the middle part of the fascia anterior to its insertion. It is caused by strain with microrupture of the fascia following increased exercise after a period of laying off. The origin of the flexor digitorum brevis muscle is closely associated with the middle section of the plantar aponeurosis. The abductor hallucis and abductor digiti quinti muscles also take origin in part from the medial and lateral portions of the plantar aponeurosis, respectively. Acute fasciitis in this region may be associated with acute intrinsic muscle strain. Diagnosis is made by palpation in the tender region. Dorsiflexion of the hallux and lesser toes tightens the plantar fascia, permitting localization to a specific point. The principle of treatment is to maintain flexibility while decreasing inflammation and protecting the foot from additional injury. Active motion with elevation and ice packs accompanied by NSAIDs is prescribed. A foot and ankle flexibility program is started (see Table 1). Shoes should be changed if needed and double-thickness socks worn. Taping the arch is helpful during the acute stages, but if symptoms persist a semirigid foot orthosis is recommended. These should be custom molded to the foot to provide an even distribution of load. *Acute rupture of plantar fascia* in the posterior medial portion requires time away from play until symptoms subside (Fig. 7). The diagnosis may be difficult to differentiate from a stress fracture since the tender area is near the calcaneal tuberosity.

Heel pain (calcaneodynia) may be caused by avulsion of the fascia from its insertion on the calcaneus, entrapment of the nerve to the abductor digiti quinti, or stress fracture of the inferior calcaneal tuberosity. A thin or atrophic heel fat pad contributes to the symptoms. Diagnosis may be difficult since more than one condition

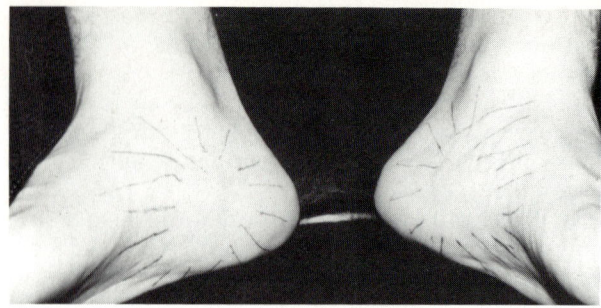

Figure 7 The foot of a 15-year-old male soccer player with acute bilateral plantar fascia rupture. The most symptomatic areas are plantar and plantar medial, as outlined on the skin. Conservative treatment failed, necessitating bilateral partial plantar fasciectomies. The player returned to practice 2 months postoperatively.

may exist at the same time. The athlete complains of heel pain of acute onset, but not generally associated with a traumatic episode. Tenderness is present directly beneath the calcaneal tuberosity or slightly distal to it. Symptoms are present in the morning upon rising; they tend to subside during the day, only to increase at the beginning of practice. During strenuous activity the pain may decrease again, but recur after a work-out. Runners find that they are unable to sustain their usual distance.

Radiography of the heel may reveal a localized area of osteoporosis or heel spur, which is found in 50% of patients with calcaneodynia. However, it is difficult to implicate such a common finding as the sole cause of the pain. Bone scans may indicate periostitis or stress fracture in the tuberosity. A computed tomographic (CT) scan may confirm a stress fracture, but nerve conduction velocities are ineffective in revealing a nerve entrapment.

Treatment of calcaneodynia includes a heel lift fashioned from ½ inch-thick Silastic pad or closed cell foam rubber pad with a central cut-out in the tender area. The diameter of the aperture should be 3 cm so that the entire tender area is relieved of pressure. The hole may be eccentrically placed if the tender region extends into the distal medial aspect of the heel. This can be taped to the heel or glued into the shoe. A foot and ankle flexibility program is prescribed. If shoes are worn or cleats protrude against the soft tissue, new, properly fitted shoes are ordered. When symptoms persist, a foot orthosis with a similar cut-out in the heel is prescribed. NSAIDs are helpful.

Chronic pain in the heel may be related to repeated tearing and healing of the plantar fascia. An olive-sized mass may be palpable distal to the fascial insertion. Occasionally, injection of 1 ml of beta-methasone (Celestone) mixed with 1 ml of 1% lidocaine (Xylocaine) is given. I do not recommend more than three injections at 1 month intervals. A 3 cm (1½ inch) 25 gauge needle is used and injection is made into the area of discrete tenderness. Relief of pain during injection indicates that corticosteroid has been placed in the symptomatic region. Severe and disabling symptoms that last longer

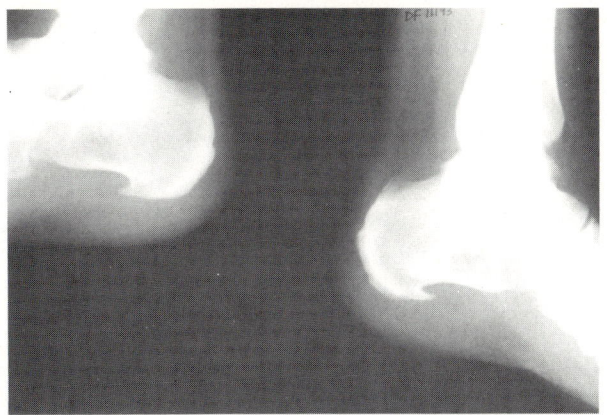

Figure 8 X-ray photograph of heels showing bilateral heel spurs. These lie beneath the plantar fascia and superficial to the nerve to the abductor digiti quinti. These may be removed during plantar fasciectomy to relieve pressure on the nerve if necessary.

than 6 months and significantly alter performance may require surgical intervention. However, these patients represent only a small percentage of symptomatic cases.

Surgical technique includes an oblique medial incision 4 cm in length above the heel pad, curving upward proximally at the heel and curving plantarward distally to the anteromedial border of the weight-bearing heel pad. Dissection is made with loupe magnification to avoid small branches of cutaneous nerves that are present. The medial calcaneal nerve is identified posteriorly, and the nerve to the abductor digiti quinti is located at the posterior margin of the wound passing beneath the origin of the abductor hallucis muscle. Constricting bands of fascia are divided. The plantar fascia is then located deep to the heel fat pad and cleaned on its superficial and deep surfaces. An area of scarred aponeurosis may be visible, usually the size of a small olive; it may be more than 1 cm in length. The median half of the central part of the aponeurosis is excised. The specimen measures 2 cm by 1 cm. Palpation laterally in the wound ensures that aponeurosis has not been completely divided. Care is taken to protect neurocirculatory structures passing between the plantar aponeurosis and the inferior calcaneus. If a heel spur is present and palpable from beneath the heel, it is excised (Fig. 8). A compression dressing is applied postoperatively, and restricted weightbearing with crutches is prescribed until the wound heals. A foot orthosis is recommended early in rehabilitation. Competitive play is permitted when symptoms subside.

DISORDERS OF POSTERIOR HEEL

The differential diagnosis of disorders of posterior heel pad includes insertional tendinitis of the Achilles tendon, retrocalcaneal bursitis, and heel pain secondary to symptomatic posterolateral calcaneal process, "pump bumps," or calcaneal apophysitis (Sever's disease).

Insertional tendinitis of the Achilles tendon occurs at its insertion onto the posterior calcaneus; it encompasses the lower two-thirds of the surface of the latter. Diagnosis is made simply by palpating the posterior calcaneus at the insertion of the tendon. Tenderness is noted medially, posteriorly, and laterally. Radiographs are not helpful, although fragmentation of the posterior calcaneal apophysitis (Sever's disease) may be seen in athletes who have not completed their growth. A ½ inch elevation of the heel and NSAIDs are recommended for both conditions. A combined heel cord stretching and foot and ankle flexibility program is begun. Padding the counter of the sport shoe to relieve direct pressure on the plantar insertion is also helpful. Symptoms may continue for 6 months.

Retrocalcaneal bursitis (Haglund's disease) is caused by inflammation of the bursa that lies between the superior calcaneus and the anterior border of the Achilles tendon. The cause of retrocalcaneal bursitis is pressure and irritation on the bursa between the posterior superior calcaneal tuberosity and the Achilles tendon. Pain is elicited by medial and lateral palpation of the bursa anteriorly just above the tendon insertion. Symptoms are increased by passive dorsiflexion of the ankle. This can be confirmed by injecting 1 ml of 1% lidocaine into the bursa through a 25 gauge needle, with consequent relief of pain. X-ray films may reveal a prominent posterior superior tuberosity. Treatment includes a ½ inch heel lift, NSAIDs for 3 weeks, and a flexibility program for the foot and ankle. If symptoms do not subside over several months, excision of the bursa is recommended. I prefer a medial longitudinal incision 3 cm long; the bursa is excised along with the portion of the posterior superior calcaneal tuberosity.

A tight shoe with a stiff counter can irritate the posterior lateral calcaneus and cause a painful callus and periostitis ("pump bump"). A prominent lateral heel border emerges as a response to irritation from the shoe counter. Treatment includes changing the shoe type so that a padded heel counter comes into contact with the tender region. The shoe may be modified by cutting the counter to accommodate the tender area. A horseshoe-shaped pad made of ⅜ inch felt or closed cell foam rubber may be used to pad around the tender area. The aperture within the U should be large enough so that all the tender area is included in the opening. When the pad is placed in the shoe or taped to the heel, the entire area should remain nontender when pressure is exerted against the posterior lateral heel.

If these forms of conservative management fail to relieve symptoms, excision of the tuberosity is recommended. I prefer a medial longitudinal incision 4 cm in length. The posterior superior tuberosity of the calcaneus is removed along with the prominent "pump bump" on the lateral border with a high-speed oscillating micro-saw. A medial incision avoids a hypertrophic tender scar laterally. Palpation over the lateral area of prominence ensures that no bone protrusion remains. The attachment of the calcaneus is long and broad, and a portion of the tendon insertion is elevated to ensure that enough bone has been removed. If more than 50% of the Achilles tendon is detached, sutures are placed through the calcaneus to reattach that portion back to the bone. The patient is placed in a short leg cast. Failure of this procedure usually results from too little bone being removed. A cast will considerably decrease the amount of immediate postoperative pain. After 2 weeks the cast is removed and a cast boot with a variable hinge is applied. Motion is increased gradually and the patient is permitted full weightbearing. The boot is discontinued 3 weeks later.

NERVE INJURIES

Traumatic neuritis can occur in any of the peripheral nerve branches to the foot. The *cutaneous branch of the superficial peroneal nerve* is irritated by pressure from a shoe at the tarsometatarsal or talonavicular joints more often than from a direct blow. Symptoms may be caused by osteophytes pressing upward from articular joint margins and entrapping the nerve against outer footwear. Symptoms are caused by stretching the irritated nerve. Irritation of the *intermediate cutaneous branch of the superficial peroneal nerve* causes pain on the dorsum of the foot. A positive Tinel's sign may be elicited not only on the dorsum of the foot but also at the exit of the nerve from the deep fascia of the leg in the anterior compartment, 15 cm above the ankle. A fasciotomy may be necessary to relieve symptoms caused by nerve entrapment at the fascial opening.

Trauma from both walking and running can cause irritation of the *interdigital nerve* between the third and fourth metatarsal head (Morton's neuroma). The nerve in this area often receives branches from both the medial and lateral plantar nerves. It is much less common for neuroma to occur in other interdigital nerves. Symptoms may be elicited by pressing the web space dorsally and plantarly between the finger and thumb while compressing the foot medially and laterally. The patient experiences paresthesia in the third and fourth toes. If symptoms are not relieved with a metatarsal pad or a foot orthosis including a metatarsal pad, along with antiinflammatory medication, surgical excision is indicated. A dorsal incision is recommended and loupe magnification is used to avoid injuring cutaneous nerves and the artery that accompanies the nerve proximal to the neuroma. A flexibility program is started as soon as the wound heals, and return to play is permitted as symptoms subside, usually within 1 month.

Injury to the *proper digital nerve* is uncommon. Symptoms include metatarsalgia associated with paresthesia along the medial hallux. A Tinel's sign is elicited medially and proximally to the tibial sesamoid as the nerve passes through dense connective tissue before passing medially to the tibial sesamoid. If NSAIDs and appropriate padding do not relieve persistent symptoms that significantly alter performance, excision of the neuroma is recommended. My experience indicates that neurolysis on the weight-bearing aspect of the forefoot carries a poor prognosis. Neurectomy is the treatment of choice. The patient should

be advised that the neuroma may recur proximally and require additional resection.

TARSAL TUNNEL SYNDROME

The tarsal tunnel syndrome is rarely caused by direct trauma to the tibial nerve at the posterior medial ankle. Post-traumatic causes are often associated with calcaneal or ankle fractures or dislocation at the subtalar or ankle joints. Unlike the carpal tunnel syndrome, the tarsal tunnel syndrome has many causes and occurs more often in middle-aged athletes. Symptoms begin insidiously, the only consistent symptoms being pain daily and occasionally at night, and burning on the sole with prolonged standing, walking, and running. Other symptoms are so variable and inconsistent that patients have often been diagnosed as having interdigital neuroma and undergo surgery, only for symptoms to persist postoperatively. Electromyography and nerve conduction velocity studies may give objective evidence of entrapment or injury to the posterior tibial nerve or its branches as it divides into the medial and plantar nerves.

Treatment of this condition is difficult. Antiinflammatory medication together with a foot orthosis helps. A flexibility program performed twice daily is prescribed. Surgery is reserved for patients with symptoms that are significantly disabling and have caused modification of life-style. Neurolysis of the posterior tibial nerve and its branches is performed with loupe magnification under tourniquet control.

I have found that the most common causes of the tarsal tunnel syndrome are scarring of the tibial nerve, a small vascular loop passing through or around the nerve at its terminus, giving a "vascular leash" effect, cysts, anomalous muscles, and varicosities surrounding the nerve. The most consistent operative finding is a thickened fibrotic region of the tibial nerve within 1 cm of its division. Other anatomic variants of the nerve have been found in addition to those described. The ankle is splinted for 2 weeks postoperatively, after which a supervised physical therapy program is begun. The athlete should be advised that recovery may take 6 months.

ACUTE LIGAMENT SPRAINS

The mechanism of foot strain occurs most commonly through plantar flexion and inversion. Less commonly, forced dorsiflexion may occur. Strain is common at the lateral tarsometatarsal joints, Chopart's joint, or the subtalar joint. In addition to symptoms of lateral ankle ligament injuries, such as pain with giving way, tarsometatarsal strain produces pain with weightbearing at the fourth and fifth tarsometatarsal joints. Radiographs are negative or may show only chip fractures dorsally. Treatment of the acute injury includes an Ace bandage, NSAIDs, and limited weight bearing with crutches. If symptoms are severe and pain persists, cast immobilization for 2 weeks may be necessary. A physical therapy program of whirlpool, power building, and use of a foot and ankle exerciser board follows (see Fig. 1). When the athlete returns to the field, an ankle support is prescribed to help prevent plantar inversion. If symptoms persist, bone scan and CT scan help rule out stress fracture and arthritis. Subtalar strain is characterized by tenderness in the region of the sinus tarsi. This is treated in a similar manner. If symptoms persist, however, MRI may reveal the formation of a cyst, a ligament tear, or outpouching of the posterior facet joint into the sinus tarsi. Symptoms may persist for several months. Surgical exploration is reserved for the most severe cases unrelieved by conservative measures.

TRAUMATIC CYSTS

Traumatic cysts are uncommon in the foot but do occur at the MTP joints. They develop over a short time, giving symptoms of an expanding soft tissue mass in the web space, most commonly at the second MTP joint (Fig. 9). The forefoot appears broadened and the involved toe may become angulated, giving the appearance of a cross-over toe. The use of thick emulsion x-ray film and soft tissue technique may reveal the presence of a mass. CT and MRI may confirm the presence of a mass, often shaped like a dumbbell, that is expanded superiorly and inferiorly. The cyst, filled with synovial fluid, is distinct from a ganglion cyst, which is chronic in nature and filled with gelatinous material. Treatment consists of aspiration or simple excision through a dorsal incision, and the athlete is permitted to return to sports when the wound is healed.

TENDINITIS

Inflammation of tendons in the foot occurs primarily in those of the extrinsic muscles. The intrinsic muscles have short tendons with short excursions pulling in a straight line. Although cramping can occur, this is usually of short duration in the plantar aspect of the foot. The most commonly affected tendon is the *tibialis posterior tendon*. Tendinitis is present from the tendon insertion at the navicular tuberosity, extending beneath the medial malleolus into the posterior calf. Redness and swelling may be present. Painful active inversion against resistance aids in the diagnosis. Treatment of the mild condition includes NSAIDs, strapping, or an ankle orthosis as well as a foot and ankle flexibility program.

Although uncommon, acute avulsion of the tendon from its insertion requires open repair. Through a 6 cm medial incision over the tendon, the ligamentous canal is opened and a tenosynovectomy performed if indicated. The avulsion may be transverse, in which case the tendon is advanced and attached through drill holes in the navicular tuberosity with 2-0 braided polyester sutures. A cast is applied for 6 weeks postoperatively. If a longitudinal disruption of the fibers is found, indicating a more chronic condition, it is repaired with 5-0 polyester sutures. The tendon sheath is not closed. (The treatment

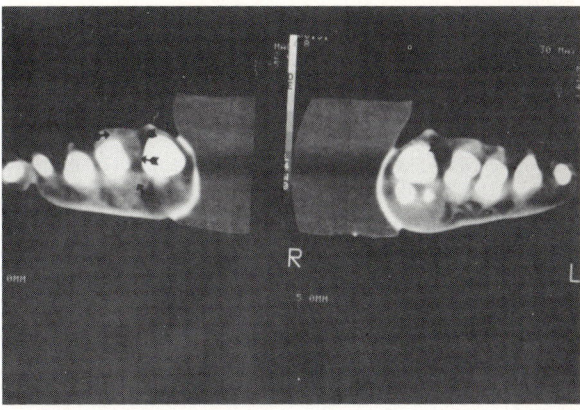

Figure 9 Axial CT scan of the right and left forefoot through the region of the metatarsal heads. Soft tissue view reveals "dumbbell"-shaped cystic mass between the right first and second metatarsal heads (*arrows*). Simple excision allowed this dancer to return to the barre in 2 weeks.

of a chronic tear of the tibialis posterior tendon is not within the scope of this chapter.) Postoperatively, a cast is applied for 2 weeks followed by a cast boot with a variable hinge. Therapy is then started. The brace is discontinued 6 weeks postoperatively.

Tendinitis or a partial tear of the *flexor hallucis longus tendon,* seen in dancers and other athletes, is treated conservatively. The tear is longitudinal. If "trigger toe" occurs it is necessary to release the tendon in the tarsal tunnel through a posteromedial incision at the ankle. The tendon is repaired with a running 5-0 polyester suture and motion is begun after the wound heals.

Acute avulsion of the *peroneus brevis tendon* from its insertion into the fifth metatarsal styloid is caused by a lengthening contraction of the muscle with plantar inversion of the foot. Treatment includes ice, elevation, a compression dressing, and a limited weight-bearing (RICE) regimen until symptoms subside, usually in 3 weeks. A foot and ankle flexibility program is begun along with use of the foot and ankle exercise board as soon as symptoms permit. Longitudinal tears of the tendon are less common and often accompany disease of the ankle, including chronic lateral instability and dislocated peroneal tendons. Treatment includes repair at the time of correction of the underlying problem.

Acute tears of the *peroneus longus tendon* are also less common, occurring in individuals over the age of 19 years. Fracture through an os peroneum requires repair. Chronic tears are associated with tears of the peroneus brevis tendon. If chronic, the tear is resected and the proximal tendon is sutured to the peroneus brevis tendon.

SPORTS SHOES

Running shoes should have cushioning to reduce impact shock. They should be designed to provide maximum shock absorption and have good heel control. Although not a cure-all, these qualities in a running shoe help prevent shin splints, tendinitis, heel pain, and stress fractures.

Walking shoes should have extra shock absorption in the heel of the shoe and under the ball of the foot. This helps reduce heel pain (plantar fasciitis and pump bumps) as well as metatarsalgia. A shoe with a slightly rounded sole or "rocker bottom" helps shift weight from the heel to the toes while decreasing the forces across the foot. Walking shoes have more rigidity in front to allow toe off distally rather than bend through them as with running shoes.

Aerobic conditioning shoes should be lightweight to prevent foot fatigue with extra shock absorption in the metatarsal area. If possible, work out on a carpeted floor.

Tennis shoes need to support the foot during quick side to side movements or shifts in weight. A shoe that provides stability on the inside and outside of the foot is an important choice. Flexibility in the sole allows repeated quick forward movements for a fast reaction. Less shock absorption is required in tennis and other racquet sports. On soft courts, softer soled shoes allow better traction. On hard courts, a sole with great tread helps in traction.

Basketball shoes need to have a thick, stiff sole. This gives extra stability when running on the court. The high top shoe provides support when landing from a jump and helps prevent ankle sprains.

Cross-training shoes, or cross trainers, combine several features that allow the athlete more than one sport. A good cross trainer should have the flexibility in the forefoot for running and the lateral support for aerobics and tennis.

SUGGESTED READING

Cimino WR. Tarsal tunnel syndrome: Review of the literature. Foot Ankle 1990; 11(1):47–52.

Distefano V, Sack JT, Whittaker R, Nixon JE. Tarsal tunnel syndrome: Review of the literature and two case reports. Clin Orthop 1972; 88:76–79.

Sammarco GJ. Turf toe. American Academy of Orthopaedic Surgeons Instructional Course Lecture. San Francisco, 1993.

Sammarco GJ. Peroneus longus tendon tears: A report of 14 cases. Foot Ankle 1994 (in press).

Sammarco GJ, Chalk DC, Feibel JH. Tarsal tunnel syndrome and additional nerve lesions in the same limb. Foot Ankle 1993; 14(2):71–77.

Sammarco GJ, Conti SF. Tarsal tunnel syndrome caused by anomalous muscles: report of seven cases. J Bone Joint Surg 1994 (in press).

Sammarco GJ, DiRaimondo CV. Chronic peroneus brevis tendon lesions. Foot Ankle 1989; 9(4):163–170.

PLANTAR FASCIITIS

JOSEPH S. TORG, M.D.

Plantar fasciitis is characterized by low-grade pain, insidious in onset, located along the medial plantar fascia just distal to the calcaneus. Pain is often felt directly beneath the calcaneus at the insertion of the plantar fascia, and at times on the medial aspect of the calcaneus. It can be felt while walking, while running, and in mild cases only after running. The pain and inflammation is a result of repeated traction on the plantar fascia at its insertion into the calcaneus. Microtears and inflammation of the plantar fascia at the calcaneus can result from limited ankle dorsiflexion due to a tight gastrocnemius soleus complex. Swelling is not a predominant symptom and yet there is likely to be tenderness. A common roentgenographic finding is a heel spur on the lateral view.

An ice massage or a slush bath for 20 minutes several times a day can help alleviate discomfort temporarily, although it may not be successful for long periods.

Rest is often an effective early treatment for overuse injuries. For the treatment of plantar fasciitis, Clancy stated that rest is to be continued until there is pain-free palpation, at which point a gradual training program can be followed. Newell also prescribed the reduction of activity. Stretching and support are used in combination with rest to provide permanent relief.

Anti-inflammatory drugs are recommended for the treatment of plantar fasciitis. The injection of steroidal medication into the calcaneal attachment can help control inflammation, but care is necessary in cases in which symptoms persist, in order to avoid local iatrogenic complications. Oral medications include naproxen (Naprosyn), Feldene, indomethacin (Indocin), and ibuprofen (Motrin).

Furey presented a study of the treatment of 116 patients with plantar fasciitis. The characteristic physical findings were pain and tenderness in the area of the calcaneal tuberosity. Patients were treated with phenylbutazone, 100 mg four times a day for 1 week, then three times a day for 1 week. Heel pads and arch supports were also used. In 71% of the patients initially treated, there were excellent or good results after an average follow-up of 5.2 years. Aspirin and other anti-inflammatory agents can be used, but none of these should be administered without close supervision.

The pain that persists in plantar fasciitis can be alleviated with an adhesive strapping known as the low dye technique. Biomechanical problems, specifically abnormal pronation of the foot, have been identified as possible causal factors for plantar fasciitis. Whitesell stated that it stabilizes the head of the first metatarsal through plantar flexion, and decreases foot pronation. Newell reported that a positive response to this strapping is indicative of mechanical problems and can be

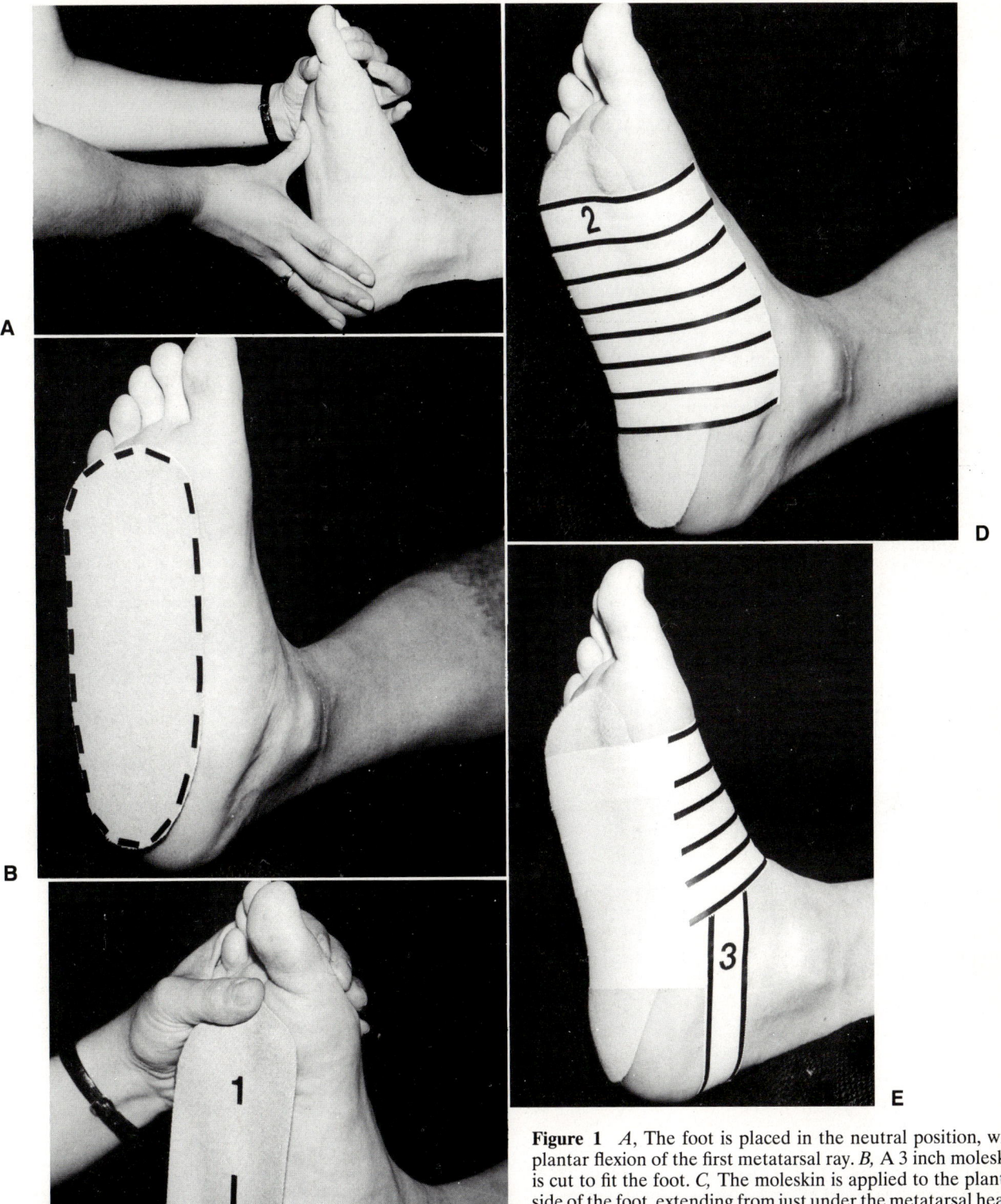

Figure 1 *A,* The foot is placed in the neutral position, with plantar flexion of the first metatarsal ray. *B,* A 3 inch moleskin is cut to fit the foot. *C,* The moleskin is applied to the plantar side of the foot, extending from just under the metatarsal heads to the calcaneus. *D,* The first piece of a 1 inch tape is applied, running upward underneath the plantar surface with equal pressure medially and laterally. *E,* Anchor strips are placed over the dorsal lateral aspect of the foot to secure the strapping. An additional anchor is placed around the posterior aspect of the calcaneus just beneath the malleoli.

used as a guide for orthotics. The use of moleskin instead of tape is suggested because it is stronger, provides more support, and wears better during exercise.

LOW DYE STRAPPING TECHNIQUE

Low dye strapping is recommended for treating conditions involving inflammation of plantar fascia, and traumatic or static sprains of the inner or outer longitudinal arches. It is also recommended for shin splints if the diagnosis is consistent with a musculotendinous inflammation along the medial border of the tibia.

Positioning. The foot is placed in a neutral position with plantar flexion of the first metatarsal ray (Fig. 1, *A*).

Materials. The materials required are 1 inch adhesive tape and 3 inch moleskin. The moleskin is cut to approximate the plantar surface of the foot from just under the metatarsal heads to the calcaneus (Fig. 1, *B*).

Instructions

Step 1. The moleskin is applied to the metatarsal head, pulled with slight tension downward through its midsection, and secured to the calcaneus (Fig. 1, *C*).

Step 2. Additional support is achieved by applying 1 inch strips of adhesive tape upward from underneath the plantar surface with equal pressure medially and laterally (Fig. 1, *D*). The length of the tape should not exceed the height of an imaginary line running just beneath the malleoli to the outer borders of the first and fifth metatarsal heads.

Step 3. To secure the strapping, the anchor strips are placed over the dorsal aspect of the foot. An additional anchor is placed around the posterior aspect of the calcaneus just beneath the malleoli (Fig. 1, *E*).

Orthotic correction is another effective method for treating plantar fasciitis. Similar in function to low dye strapping, orthotics correct the biomechanical problems responsible for the development of the injury. Refer to the chapter on orthotics.

There are several other methods for treating plantar fasciitis. Heel supports (which can be either soft or rigid: rigid when pain persists), arch supports, heel wedges, heel cups, donuts, and good running shoes are additional methods used to correct biomechanical problems.

Surgical treatment is advocated when conservative therapy fails. Clancy reported 15 patients in whom the results of surgical release of the plantar fascia were all excellent, and who returned to running in 8 to 10 weeks.

SUGGESTED READING

Bonci CM. Adhesive strapping techniques. Clin Sports Med 1982; 1:99–116.

Clancy WG. Runner's injuries. Part two: evaluation and treatment of specific injuries. Am J Sports Med 1980; 8:287–297.

Furey JG. Plantar fasciitis: the painful heel syndrome. J Bone Joint Surg 1975; 57A:672–673.

Newell SG, Miller SJ. Conservative treatment of plantar fascial strain. Phys Sports Med 1977; 68–73.

Roy S. How I manage plantar fasciitis. Phys Sports Med 1986; 11:127–131.

Whitesell J, Newell SG. Modified low dye strapping. Phys Sports Med 1980; 8:129–130.

TURF-TOE

SCOTT A. RODEO, M.D.
STEPHEN J. O'BRIEN, M.D.
RUSSELL F. WARREN, M.D.

Acute injuries of the first metatarsophalangeal (MTP) joint in football players have become a significant concern of athletes, coaches, team physicians, and trainers. Such a plantar capsule ligament sprain is commonly known as "turf-toe." The advent of artificial surfaces and lighter, more flexible shoes for use on artificial turf are suspected causes for the increasing incidence of turf-toe. Although this injury is most commonly seen among football players, it has been reported among soccer and basketball players as well. Our study of 80 active professional football players revealed that 45% of these players had incurred a turf-toe injury. Our findings also reveal a significant amount of practice time missed and game time lost due to these injuries.

ETIOLOGY

The most common mechanism of turf-toe injury is a hyperextension of the first MTP joint of a foot in a slightly dorsiflexed position. The forefoot is fixed on the ground and the heel is raised in the air. During a tackle another player falls across the dorsal surface of the player's leg, forcing the joint into hyperextension (Fig. 1). Another mechanism of injury to the plantar capsule is hyperflexion. This occurs as the ball carrier is tackled from behind when the ankle is plantar flexed. A hyperflexion injury results. A third, less common mechanism of injury reported in the literature is a valgus injury.

Our studies of turf-toe injuries have identified

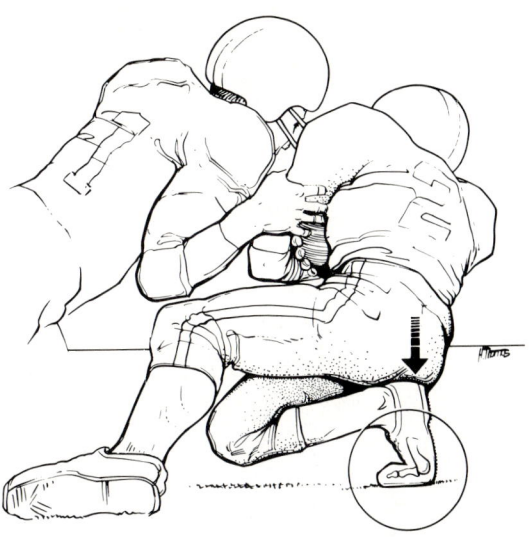

Figure 1 The most common mechanism of turf-toe injury is hyperextension of the first metatarsophalangeal joint.

several risk factors for injury. Turf-toe injuries are more common in offensive linemen, running backs, and receivers. Offensive linemen may be injured when pushing off from a stance, which forces the MTP joint into hyperextension. Running backs and receivers may be injured when tackled from behind, as the hyperextension injury usually occurs when the foot is fixed on the ground with the heel raised in the air and another player falls on the back of the player's leg, forcing the joint into hyperextension. Running backs and receivers may also suffer a hyperextension injury when making sharp cuts to change direction.

Older players and players who have had a longer professional football career also had a higher incidence of turf-toe injury, which suggests that this injury is exposure related. A greater range of ankle dorsiflexion was found to be significantly related to the incidence of turf-toe. As the ankle is usually in a slightly dorsiflexed position at the time of injury, such increased ankle dorsiflexion may allow the foot to more readily assume the position in which subsequent loading of the first MTP joint can occur. Another factor found to be related to the etiology of turf-toe was playing surface. In our survey of professional football players, 83% reported their initial injury on artificial turf. Artificial surfaces are harder and have reduced shock-absorbing characteristics compared with natural grass. As a result, such surfaces transmit the force of a tackle directly to the joint, thereby overloading the plantar capsule ligament and resulting in turf-toe.

Shoe type has also been identified in previous studies as a predisposing factor for turf-toe. The rubber-sole, multi-cleat shoe is commonly implicated in turf-toe injuries. This shoe is flexible in the distal forefoot region, unlike the conventional seven-cleat football shoe with its rigid sole. Such flexibility may fail to protect the first MTP joint from excessive hyperextension and result in plantar capsular injury.

DIAGNOSIS

The first consideration in the diagnosis of turf-toe injury is determination of the mechanism of injury. The player's presenting level of pain may vary with the severity of injury, but in all cases the pain will become more intense after several hours. Physical examination reveals a hyperemic, swollen joint. Dislocation and fracture must be ruled out. Marked tenderness to palpation is present over the metatarsal head, especially on the plantar surface where the capsular tear occurred. Passive extension of the joint is painful. Ecchymosis usually develops within 24 hours. Roentgenograms reveal only generalized soft tissue swelling unless there is concomitant fracture.

Various other forefoot and toe injuries including metatarsal and phalangeal fracture, MTP dislocation, and sesamoid stress fracture should be considered in the differential diagnosis of turf-toe. Fracture of the metatarsal or phalanx of the great toe may present similarly to turf-toe. Such injuries are relatively uncommon in athletics. Sesamoid stress fracture may be considered, but these injuries usually have an insidious onset, as opposed to acute direct trauma involved in turf-toe. Sesamoid fracture is uncommon, but has been reported in football players. Roentgenograms should be taken to aid in the correct diagnosis. Additionally, radionuclide bone scans and arthrography may aid in diagnosis.

Other less common conditions to consider in the differential diagnosis include sesamoiditis, osteochondritis, flexor hallucis brevis tendonitis, and bursitis beneath the tibial sesamoid. These injuries usually do not appear as a result of direct trauma but rather are more insidious in onset.

The diagnosis of turf-toe may involve distinguishing an acute sesamoid fracture from a multipartite sesamoid or distraction of sesamoid fragments (Fig. 2). Comparison with previous roentgenograms, if available, is helpful in assessing a change in position of pre-existing sesamoid fragments or identifying a new fracture. We have recently reported four cases of progressive diastasis of components of a multipartite sesamoid, which simulated turf-toe in terms of mechanism of injury and presentation. These players required operative repair of the plantar capsule.

We have found a passive dorsiflexion stress radiograph valuable as a provocative test for detecting diastasis of components of a bipartite sesamoid (Fig. 3). Injection of the injured joint with a local anesthetic may aid in obtaining a stress radiograph in the acutely injured player. A bone scan may be useful, especially if roentgenograms suggest a partite sesamoid rather than an acute fracture. Bone scan may show less uptake in the case of a partite sesamoid than would be seen with acute fracture.

CLASSIFICATION OF INJURY

Previous descriptions of turf-toe have not included injuries to the sesamoid complex of the first MTP joint.

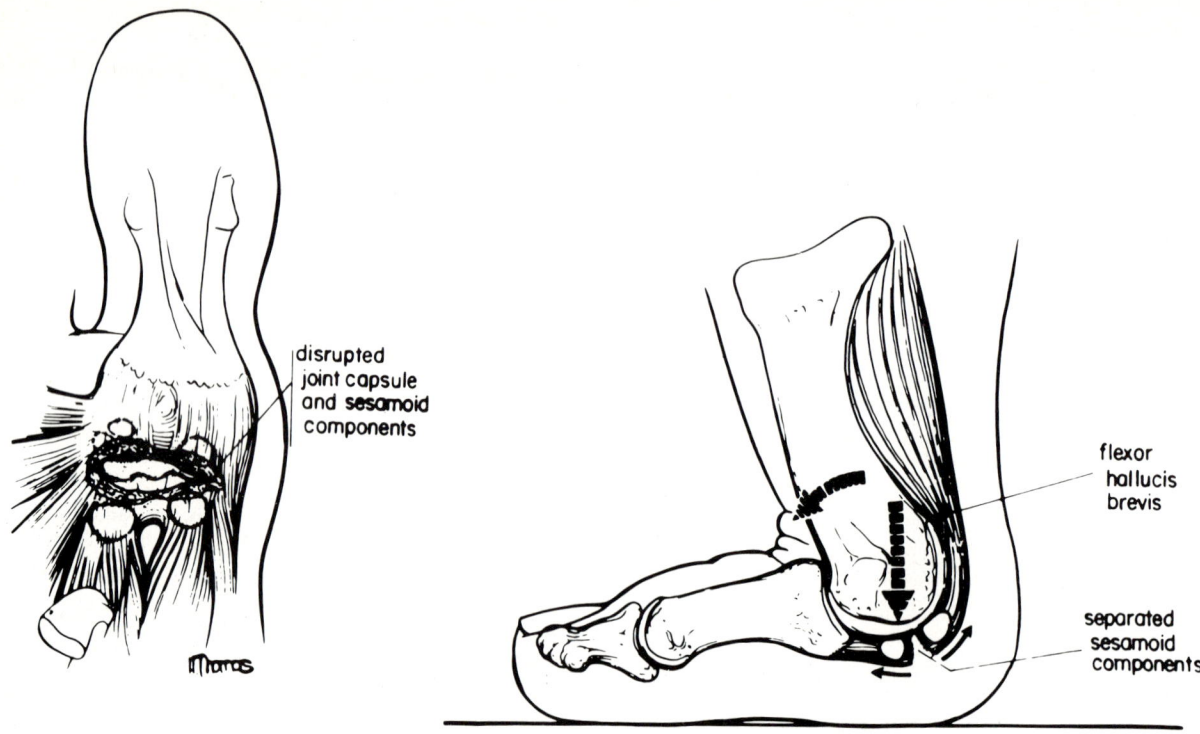

Figure 2 Hyperextension injury causing disruption of the joint capsule and the resulting separation of the sesamoid components.

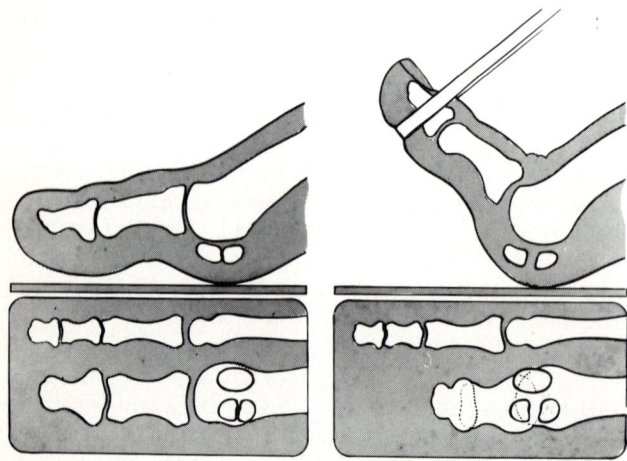

Figure 3 Our method for taking a dorsiflexion stress radiograph.

Table 1 Classification of First Metatarsophalangeal Joint Injury

Grade I: Acute sprain of plantar capsule, with localized tenderness, swelling, and pain with dorsiflexion. There is no bony pathology or joint instability. Roentgenograms are normal. Treatment is conservative.

Grade II: Actue sprain of plantar capsule with significant capsular disruption as evidenced by more extensive ecchymosis, loss of motion, painful dorsiflexion, possible diastasis of a partite sesamoid, and/or joint instability. Roentgenograms reveal no significant hallux rigidus or degenerative changes of the first MTP joint. Treatment may be surgical or conservative.

Grade III: Chronic symptoms involving the first MTP joint due to MTP joint injury, with loss of motion and significant roentgenographic changes of either hallux rigidus or degenerative joint disease. The most effective treatment is surgical.

MANAGEMENT OF TURF-TOE INJURY

In our opinion, the term turf-toe should represent the consequences of a hyperextension injury to the first MTP joint in which the volar capsule has been disrupted proximal to the sesamoid. Based on our observations of these plantar capsule injuries of the first MTP joint, we propose a classification of such injuries (Table 1). This classification represents a continuum of injury. The classification proposed is modeled after the usual clinical grading system used for joint sprains. We feel that such a classification system will aid in communication about these injuries, provide prognostic information, and direct treatment decisions.

A conservative course of therapy is initially indicated. Ice, compression, and elevation are employed to decrease the soft tissue reaction. Other treatment modalities used include ultrasound, contrast baths, and iontophoresis. The joint is taped to prevent hyperextension. A common method of taping consists of first wrapping strips of 1 inch elastic tape around the great toe such that they cross over the MTP joint in a figure-of-eight strapping fashion. Next, several strips of 1 inch adhesive tape are applied from the tip of the toe to the middle of the longitudinal arch, crossing the MTP joint. The strips are overlapped. These checkreins are secured by repeating the figure-of-eight strapping of 1 inch adhesive tape on top of the checkreins (Fig. 4). The toe may also be buddy-taped to the second toe. In addition to taping, an oval piece of foam rubber is fitted such that the metatarsal head fits into a central hole. This serves to increase the surface area of the weight-bearing region over the ball of the foot, resulting in less stress per area over the injured joint and shifting proximally the weight-bearing area of the forefoot. Crutch-walking, use of a cane, or simply walking on the heels also helps immobilize the joint. Nonsteroidal anti-inflammatory drugs are effective. Injection of steroid into the joint to mask symptoms and allow return to play is not recommended. However, it has not been determined whether this plays a therapeutic role.

Rehabilitation includes active and passive range of motion (ROM) exercises for the foot and ankle. The player's return to activity is guided by gradually increasing the weight-bearing status until the full ROM is pain free. The player starts with flat-footed walking, and then progresses to jogging and eventually to straight ahead running at full speed. Only at this point should cutting maneuvers be permitted. The player may return to play once painless extension has returned. During the return to activity the shoe is fitted with a splint to provide rigidity to the distal forefoot. Various materials have been used for such splints, such as spring steel and polyethylene.

Sesamoid diastasis injury may be managed conservatively or operatively. Conservative treatment in three of our cases resulted in increased separation of the sesamoid components associated with pain and disability, necessitating operative repair. The distal sesamoid fragment is excised, preserving distal capsule for subsequent capsular repair. The capsule is repaired by advancing the proximal capsule distally so as to position the remaining proximal sesamoid component in its proper position under the metatarsal head. If operative repair is required it is important to retain as much of the sesamoids as possible. Early repair of capsular disruption, as documented by increased separation of components of a multipartite sesamoid on stress radiography, is presently our choice in patients requiring the ability to decelerate and change directions quickly.

PREVENTION

Prevention of turf-toe injuries involves identification of predisposing factors. Turf-toe injuries are seen more commonly among running backs, offensive linemen, and wide receivers. Prophylaxis can be recommended especially for these players. Flexible, rubber-sole shoes used on artificial turf often fail to protect the first MTP joint from excessive hyperextension. Rigid shoe inserts have been designed to provide stability to the distal forefoot. The most popular inserts currently in use for this purpose are constructed of heat-sensitive plastic, (i.e., Orthoplast) or spring steel. Shoes are now available with built-in spring steel inserts in the forefoot. Players are encouraged to use a shoe that is specifically designed for use on artificial turf. Taping the first MTP joint to

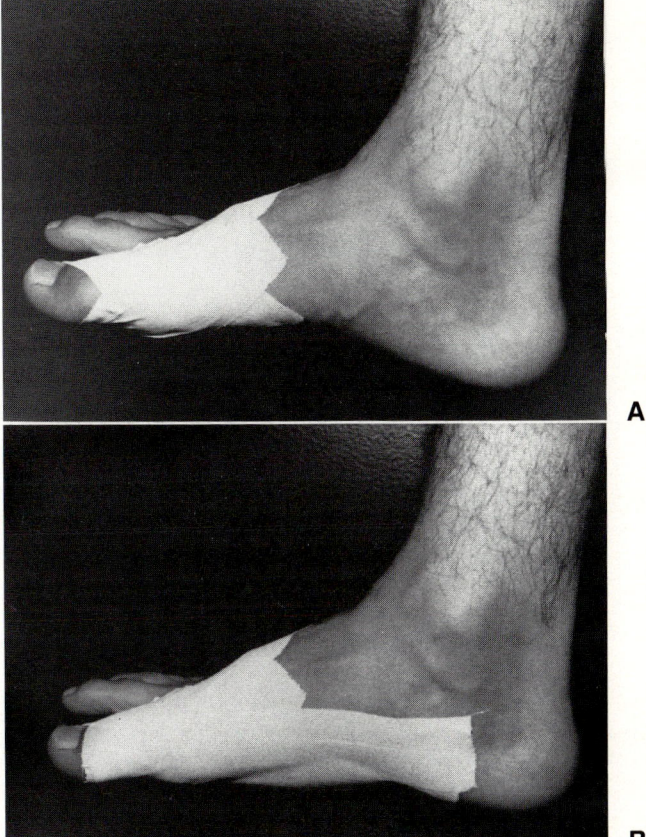

A

B

Figure 4 A technique for taping the first metatarsophalangeal (MTP) joint to prevent hyperextension. *A,* Strips of 1 inch tape cross the MTP joint in a figure-of-eight strapping fashion. *B,* Additional strips are applied from the tip of the toe to the middle of the longitudinal arch to serve as checkreins.

prevent excessive hyperextension, as described above, may also aid in prevention of turf-toe injuries.

SEQUELAE

Our studies of turf-toe injuries reveal decreased ROM at the MTP joint as a result of turf-toe. This finding demonstrates the possibility of long-term sequelae to turf-toe injury. As described above, progressive separation of the components of a multipartite seamoid may occur, with resultant pain and disability. Other possible sequelae include formation of dorsal osteophyte with progresion to hallux rigidus, progressive hallux valgus, calcification in periarticular soft tissue, and chondromalacia of the head of the first metatarsal.

SUGGESTED READING

Bowers KD, Martin RB. Impact absorption, new and old Astroturf at West Virginia University. Medicine and Science in Sports 1974; 6:217.

Bowers KD, Martin RB. Turf-toe: A shoe-surface related football injury. Medicine and Science in Sports 1976; 8:81.

Clanton TO, Butler JE, Eggert A. Injuries to the metatarsophalangeal joints in athletes. Foot Ankle 1986; 7:162.

Coker TP, Arnold JA, Weber DL. Traumatic lesions of the metatarsophalangeal joint of the great toe in athletes. Am J Sports Med 1978; 6:326.

Fahey T. Athletic training: Principles and practice. Palo Alto, Ca: Mayfield Publishing Company, 1986:410.

Nicholas JA. Football injuries. In: Nicholas JA, Hershman EB, eds. The lower extremity and spine in sports medicine. St. Louis: CV Mosby, 1986:1524.

Rodeo SA, O'Brien SJ, Warren RF, et al. Turf-toe: Diagnosis and treatment. Physician Sports Med 1989; 17:132.

Rodeo SA, O'Brien SJ, Warren RF, et al. Turf-toe: An analysis of metatarsophalangeal joint sprains in professional football players. Am J Sports Med 1990; 18:280.

Rodeo SA, Warren RF, O'Brien SJ, et al. Diastasis of bipartite sesamoids of the first metatarsophalangeal joint. Foot Ankle 1993; 14:425.

Shereff MJ, Bejjani FJ, Kummer FJ. Kinematics of the first metatarsophalangeal joint. J Bone Joint Surg 1986; 68A:392.

HAGLUND'S SYNDROME

HELENE PAVLOV, M.D.
JOSEPH S. TORG, M.D.

In 1928 Patrick Haglund established a connection between posterior heel pain, a visible and palpable "pump bump" (Fig. 1), the shape of the posterior superior border of the os calcis, and the wearing of rigid low-back shoes. He particularly emphasized the high incidence of this condition among the "Kulturmenschen" (cultured people) who wore stiff low-back shoes when playing golf or hockey.

In this chapter we (1) describe the clinical and radiologic findings of Haglund's syndrome, (2) describe an objective method for determining prominence of the bursal projection, and (3) differentiate Haglund's syndrome radiographically from other causes of posterior heel pain, including local conditions such as isolated retrocalcaneal bursitis or superficial Achilles tendon bursitis, and systemic conditions such as rheumatoid arthritis or Reiter's syndrome. Haglund's syndrome is a cause of pain in the posterior heel characterized clinically by a painful pump bump or thickening of the soft tissues at the insertion of the Achilles tendon (see Fig. 1). Patients with Haglund's syndrome range in age from young adults to the elderly, are of either sex, and have varying patterns of daily activity. The syndrome is characterized radiographically by retrocalcaneal bursitis, a loss of the lucent retrocalcaneal recess between the Achilles tendon and the bursal projection; Achilles tendinitis, an Achilles tendon measuring over 9 mm, 2 cm above the bursal projection; superficial Achilles tendon bursitis, a convexity of the soft tissues posterior to the Achilles tendon insertion; a cortically intact but prominent bursal projection; and a positive parallel pitch line (PPL).

The clinically detected pump bump is not diagnostic of Haglund's syndrome. In a controlled population, Pavlov and colleagues reported 15 patients with a pump bump that was determined radiographically to be caused

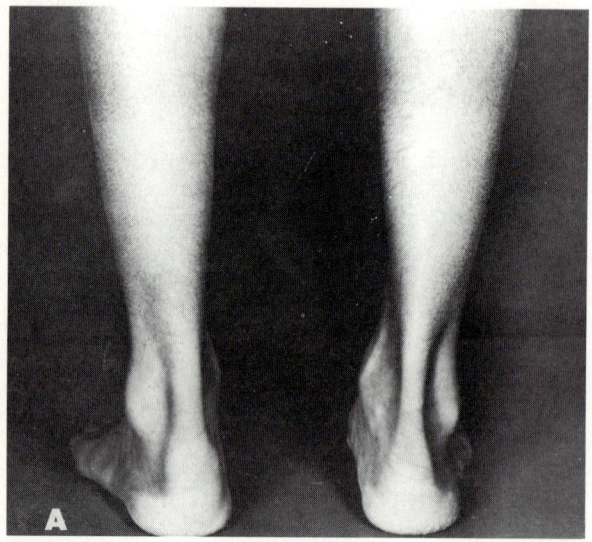
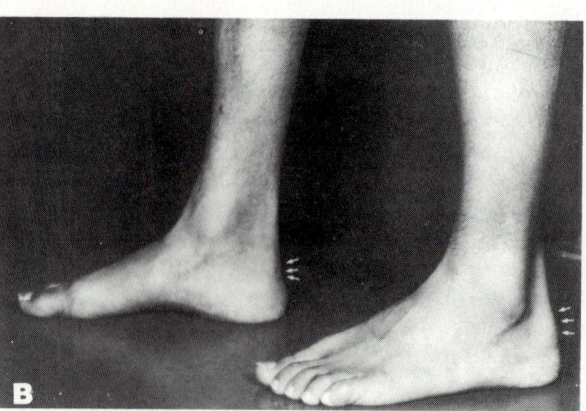

Figure 1 *A,* Clinical presentation of Haglund's syndrome. The posterior view of both heels demonstrates a soft tissue bulge at the Achilles tendon insertion on the left, compared with the normal right side. *B,* Lateral views of both feet demonstrate a pump bump on the left foot, a convexity of the superficial soft tissues. (From Pavlov H, Heneghan MA, Hersh A, et al. The Haglund syndrome: Initial and differential diagnosis. Radiology 1982; 144:93–98; with permission.)

by isolated superficial Achilles tendon bursitis in five patients, and by the posterior displacement of the soft tissues posterior to the bursal projection in 10 patients. In these latter 10 the pump bump was located at a higher level than that associated with Haglund's syndrome, posterior to the bursal projection rather than to the Achilles tendon insertion. The bursal projection was prominent, a positive PPL, in all 10 patients. These patients are predisposed to irritation of the pump bumps depending on their shoe selection.

Pump bumps also occur in association with certain systemic inflammatory articular disorders, such as Reiter's syndrome. In these patients the pump bump is more diffuse, is posterior to the Achilles tendon insertion and the bursal projection, and results from a superficial Achilles tendon bursitis and a retrocalcaneal bursitis, respectively. The cortex of the bursal projection can be eroded by the inflamed retrocalcaneal bursa; these erosions, when present, are diagnostic of an inflammatory articular process. In these patients, trauma to the external soft tissues and prominence of the bursal projection are not responsible for the pump bump, and the swelling occurs despite a negative PPL.

Determining the location of the pump bump and the prominence of the bursal projection is essential in the diagnosis and differential diagnosis of posterior heel pain. Prominence of the bursal projection is determined radiographically either by the posterior calcaneal angle (an angle greater than 75 degrees) (Fig. 2) or by the parallel pitch lines (a negative PPL) (Fig. 3). Using the PPLs, the incidence of a positive PPL was increased in patients with plantar osseous projections as compared with patients with normal plantar surfaces. A similar

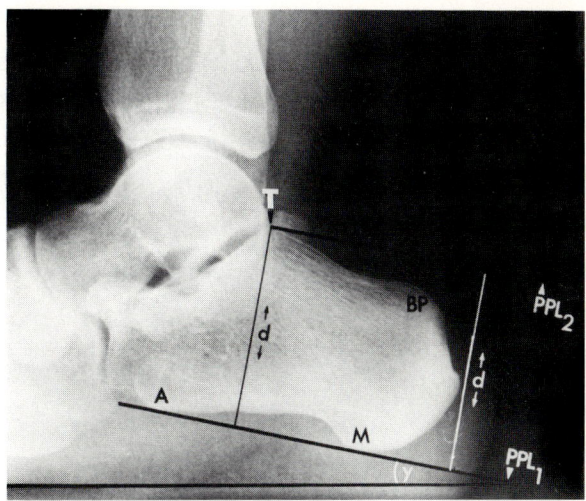

Figure 3 The parallel pitch lines (PPL) determine the prominence of the bursal projection (BP). The lower PPL (PPL₁) is the baseline, constructed as for the posterior calcaneal angle. A perpendicular (d) is constructed between the posterior lip of the talar articular facet (T) and the baseline. The upper PPL (PPL₂) is drawn parallel to the base of the distance (d). A bursal projection touching below the PPL₂ is normal, not prominent, a negative PPL. The pitch angle (y) is formed by the insertion of the baseline (PPL₁) with the horizontal. (From Pavlov H, Heneghan MA, Hersh A, et al. The Haglund syndrome: Initial and differential diagnosis. Radiology 1982; 144:93-98; with permission.)

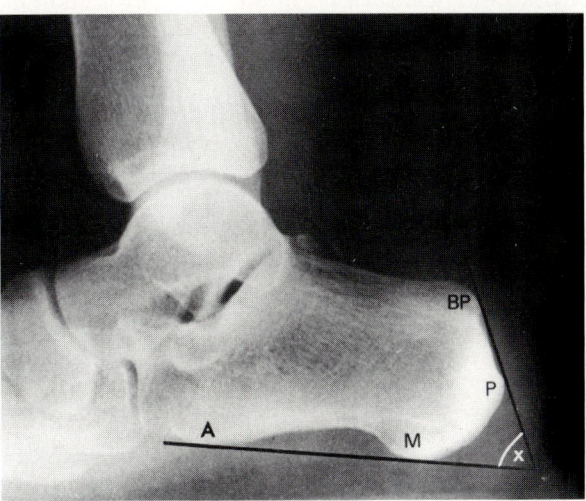

Figure 2 Quantitative evaluation of the shape and pitch of the os calcis. The posterior calcaneal angle (x) of Fowler and Philip is the angle formed by the insertion of the baseline tangent to the anterior tubercle (A) and the medial tuberosity (M) with the line tangent to the posterior surface of the bursal projection (BP) and the posterior tuberosity (P). (From Pavlov H, Heneghan MA, Hersh A, et al. The Haglund syndrome: Initial and differential diagnosis. Radiology 1982; 144:93-98; with permission.)

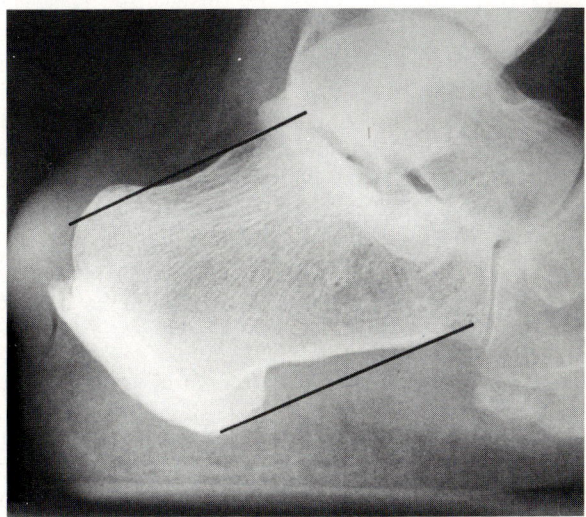

Figure 4 Haglund's syndrome is diagnosed on the lateral view of the heel by a positive PPL; a cortically intact bursal projection; loss of the retrocalcaneal recess, indicating retrocalcaneal bursitis; thickening of the Achilles tendon, measuring over 9 mm at 2 cm above the bursal projection; loss of the sharp interface between the Achilles tendon and the pre-Achilles fat pad, indicating Achilles tendinitis; and convexity of the posterior soft tissues at the level of the Achilles tendon insertion, indicating superficial Achilles tendon bursitis. Clinically, this latter finding presents as a pump bump. (From Pavlov H, Heneghan MA, Hersh A, et al. The Haglund syndrome: Initial and differential diagnosis. Radiology 1982; 144:93-98; with permission.)

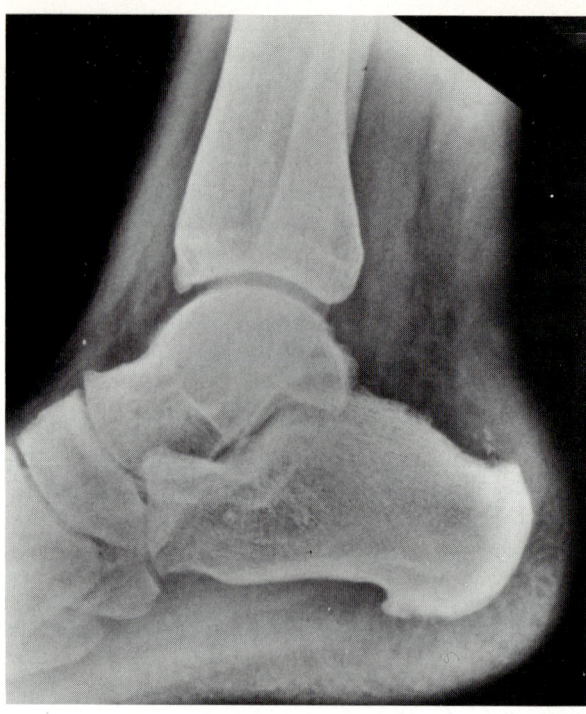

A
B

Figure 5 Preoperative (*A*) and postoperative (*B*) lateral roentgenograms of the foot, demonstrating the extent of resection of bursal projection. (From Pavlov H, Torg SS, eds. The running athlete: Roentgenograms and remedies. Chicago: Year Book, 1987; with permission.)

observation was not made by using the posterior calcaneal angle. In the series of Pavlov and colleagues, symptoms correlated statistically with a positive PPL but not with an abnormal posterior calcaneal angle. This latter discrepancy was also reported by Keck and Kelly.

The causes of a pump bump and/or heel pain at the point of contact between the heel and the shoe counter can result from Haglund's syndrome, an isolated inflammation of the superficial Achilles tendon bursa, a posterior displacement of normal soft tissues because of a prominent bursal projection, or systemic articular disorders such as Reiter's syndrome. The key to correct diagnosis is fourfold: (1) a high index of clinical and radiographic suspicion, (2) a lateral radiograph of the heel cord demonstrating soft tissue detail, (3) a careful evaluation of the cortex of the bursal projection, and (4) a working knowledge of the parallel pitch lines (Fig. 4).

Initial management of symptomatic Haglund's syndrome consists of shoe modification, heel lift, and steroid injection into the bursa. Also, an Achilles tendon stretching program is an important component of corrective management. In patients unresponsive to such a program and unable to participate in vigorous activities, surgical excision of the bursal projection may be considered (Fig. 5).

SUGGESTED READING

Keck SW, Kelly PJ. Bursitis of the posterior part of the heel. J Bone Joint Surg 1965; 47:267–273.

Nielson AL. Diagnostic and therapeutic points in retrocalcaneaobursitis. JAMA 1921; 77:463.

Pavlov H, Heneghan MA, Hersh A, et al. The Haglund syndrome: initial and differential diagnosis. Radiology 1982; 144:93–98.

Resnick D, Feingold ML, Curd J, et al. Calcaneal abnormalities in articular disorders. Radiology 1977; 125:355–366.

THE JONES FRACTURE

JOSEPH S. TORG, M.D.

Proximal fifth metatarsal fractures can be separated into two distinct types: (1) a fracture of the tuberosity and (2) a fracture of the metatarsal shaft within 1.5 cm of the tuberosity.

The latter fracture distal to the tuberosity is troublesome to manage. It requires a prolonged immobilization, has a high propensity for nonunion, and refracture after union is common after conservative treatment.

Fractures of the base of the fifth metatarsal distal to the tuberosity were first described by Jones in 1902. He reported four such fractures, including his own, which he sustained while dancing; all four healed with conservative treatment. In 1927 Carp reported 21 fractures, five of which went on to delayed union. He stated that these fractures tended to heal poorly and that a poor blood supply was the cause. In 1975 Dameron reported 20 patients, five of whom needed a surgical procedure to obtain union. He also reported prolonged healing times for 15 patients treated conservatively, but concluded that the initial treatment did not influence the final results. Dameron's surgical approach, a sliding bone graft procedure, was suggested early in the clinical course for professional athletes.

In 1978 Kavanaugh et al reported on 23 fractures of the base of the fifth metatarsal distal to the tuberosity. The average age of their patients was 20.3 years. The athletes sustaining this fracture most often were football and basketball players. Kavanaugh advised intramedullary screw fixation for young competitive athletes, selected recreational athletes, and nonathletes with nonunions. Delayed union occurred in 12 of 18 fractures treated conservatively. The fractures united in all of the 13 surgically treated patients, but in six of these patients there were complications. These included three fractured screws, two screws that missed the medullary canal, and pain in one patient that necessitated screw removal.

Kavanaugh et al also found that several patients treated with non-weight-bearing plaster casts (10 to 12 weeks) went on to nonunion, and concluded that plaster immobilization and non-weight bearing was unnecessary. Likewise, Zelko et al concluded that the clinical course did not appear to be influenced by the type of early treatment.

In 1984 Torg et al reported 46 fractures of the base of the fifth metatarsal, distal to the tuberosity, which were treated and followed for a mean of 40 months. We delineated roentgenographic criteria, which were used to define three types of fractures: (1) acute fractures, (2) those with delayed union, and (3) those with nonunion and complete obliteration of the medullary canal by sclerotic bone.

The characteristic features of the acute fractures were no history of previous fracture, although the patient

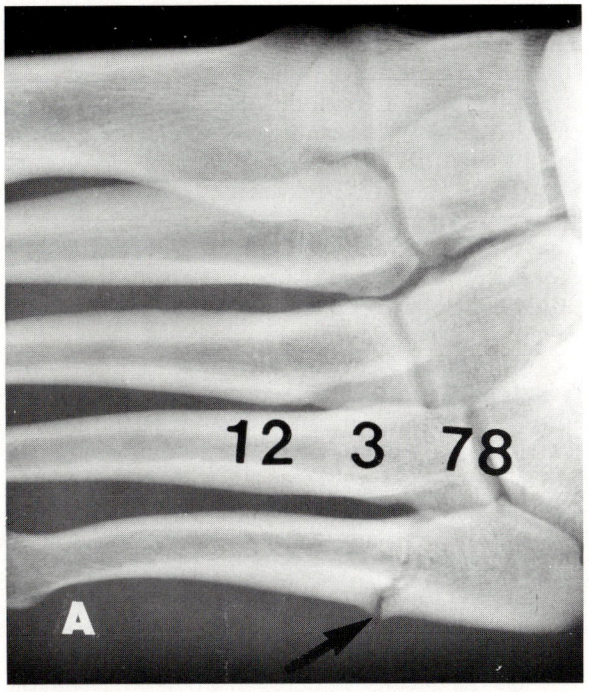 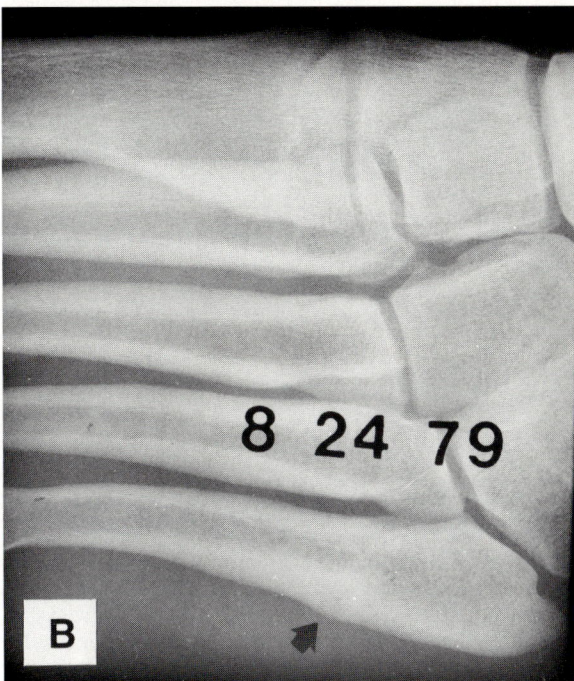

Figure 1 *A,* Oblique roentgenogram of the fifth metatarsal, demonstrating an acute fracture distal to the tuberosity. There is some cortical hypertrophy, an indicator of chronic stress, but the line is narrow, involves both cortices, and (most important) is not associated with intramedullary sclerosis. *B,* After treatment in a non-weight-bearing toe-to-knee cast for 6 weeks, there was complete healing. A roentgenogram made 9 months after the initial injury shows maintenance of fracture healing.

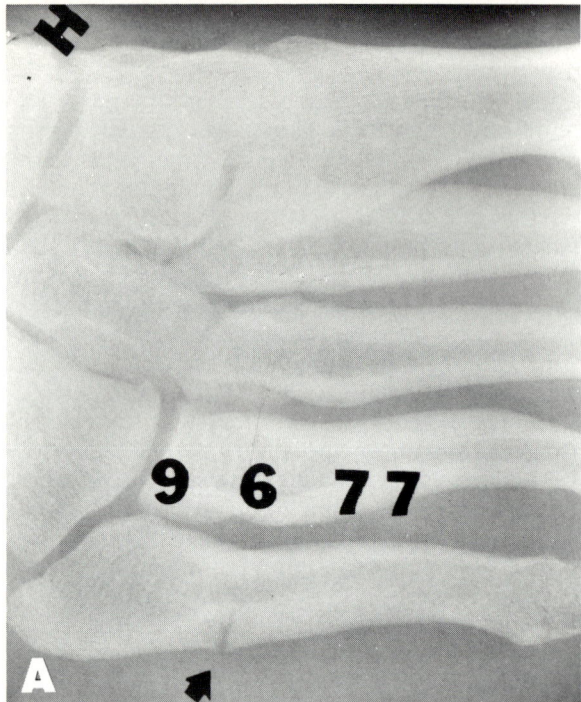

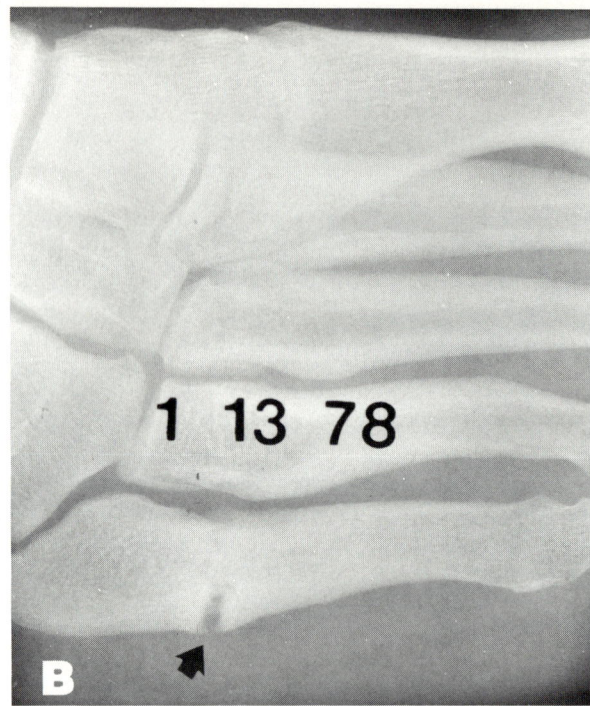

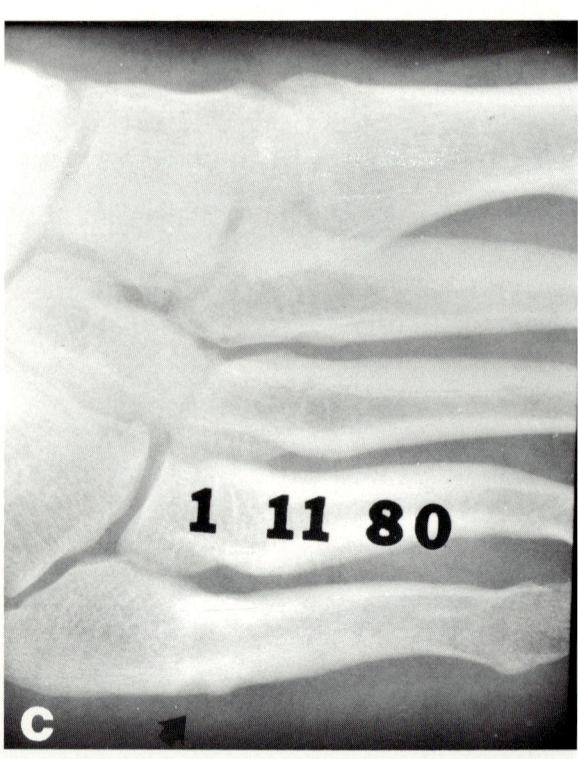

Figure 2 *A,* Oblique roentgenogram of the fifth metatarsal, demonstrating an acute fracture distal to the tuberosity. The patient was initially treated with a walking cast for 6 weeks. *B,* Four months after injury, the fracture line is seen to involve both cortices, and there is some angular deformity, a moderate degree of intramedullary sclerosis, and widening of the fracture line. *C,* Two years later, complete healing of the fracture line has occurred with minimal deformity, and there is recanalization of the medullary canal.

may have had prodromal pain or discomfort; no intramedullary sclerosis; a fracture line with sharp margins and no widening or radiolucency; and minimal cortical hypertrophy or evidence of periosteal reaction to chronic stress (Fig. 1, *A*). These roentgenographic features are not characteristic of an acute fracture in the usual sense of the term. Presumably the acute fractures in the series were located at the site of a pre-existing stress concentration or were in the lateral part of the cortex, and became disabling when they extended across the entire diaphysis. Most important was the absence of intramedullary sclerosis.

The distinguishing features of the delayed unions were a previous injury or fracture, or both; a fracture line that involved both cortices with associated periosteal bone; a widened fracture line with adjacent radiolucency due to bone resorption; and evidence of intramedullary sclerosis (Fig. 2, *B*).

The features of the nonunions were a history of repetitive trauma and recurrent symptoms; a wide fracture line with periosteal new bone and radiolucency; and a complete obliteration of the medullary canal at the fracture site by sclerotic bone, the hallmark of nonunion (Fig. 3, *A*).

Of the 25 acute fractures in our series, 15 were treated with non-weight-bearing toe-to-knee casts, and 14 healed in a mean of 7 weeks (see Fig. 1). Only four of the other 10 that were treated with various weight-bearing methods progressed to union.

Of 12 of the patients with delayed union, one refused treatment, one was treated with a bone graft, and 10 were treated initially by immobilization of the limb in a plaster cast and weight bearing. Of these 10 fractures, seven healed in a mean of 15.1 months (see

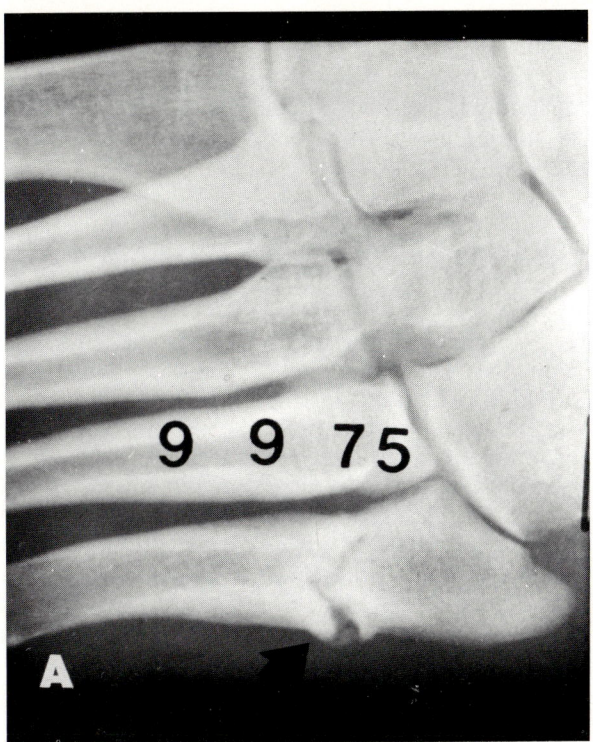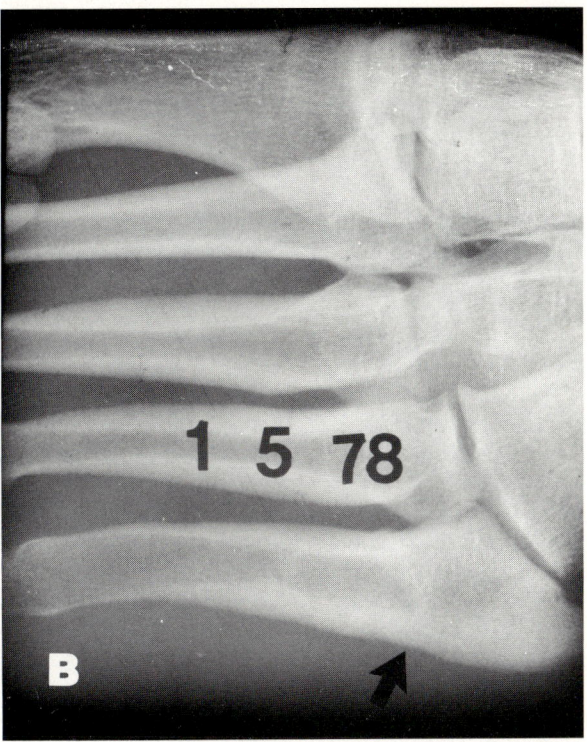

Figure 3 *A,* Oblique roentgenogram demonstrating nonunion. Note the widening of the fracture line, cortical hypertrophy, and dense intramedullary sclerosis completely obliterating the medullary canal. *B,* The fracture had demonstrated clinical and roentgenographic healing at 7 weeks. Follow-up roentgenogram 2½ years postsurgery demonstrates persistence of healed state.

Fig. 2) and three eventually required grafting for nonunion.

Of the nine nonunions in this series, which were treated primarily with medullary curettage and bone grafting, eight healed in a mean of 3 months (see Fig. 3).

Twenty fractures were treated surgically with curettage of the sclerotic bone that obliterated with intramedullary cavity and inlaid autogenous corticocancellous graft. Of these 20, 19 progressed to complete healing and one to asymptomatic nonunion. No other complications were associated with this procedure.

We concluded that the treatment of choice for acute fractures is immobilization of the limb in a toe-to-knee cast with non-weight bearing. Fractures with delayed union may eventually heal if they are treated conservatively, but in an active athlete with delayed union, medullary curettage and bone grafting are indicated. Surgery is also indicated for fractures that have progressed to symptomatic nonunion.

DeLee et al reported on 10 patients with stress fractures of the fifth metatarsal shaft. They defined stress fracture as a "spontaneous fracture of normal bone which resulted from summation of stresses, any of which, by themselves, would be harmless." Their criteria included (1) a history of prodromal symptoms over the lateral aspect of the foot prior to the acute episode that precipitated the patient's seeking medical care; (2) roentgenographic evidence of stress phenomenon in the bone, a radiolucent fracture line, periosteal reactions,

excessive callus on the lateral cortical margin, and intramedullary sclerosis that obviously preceded the acute episode of pain; and (3) no history of previous treatment for a fracture of the fifth metatarsal.

All patients in the series of DeLee et al underwent internal fixation of the fracture by insertion of a screw in the intramedullary canal of the fifth metatarsal. The average period of follow-up was 14.5 months. The authors defined clinical union as the absence of tenderness and the ability to bear weight. The average time to union was 7.5 weeks, with a range of 6 to 8 weeks. They reported no wound infections or other operative complications.

Three patients complained of tenderness over the head of the screw, and five patients complained of pain under the head of the fifth metatarsal. Four of these five patients were able to obtain relief by wearing a metatarsal pad.

DeLee et al explained this metatarsal pain as an alteration in metatarsal stiffness and/or axial alignment due to the screw. No cases of refracture were reported.

The average time to return to competitive athletics was 8.5 weeks, with a range of 7 to 14 weeks. Seven of the 10 patients required shoe modification.

Surgical procedures for delayed or nonunion fractures of the base of the fifth metatarsal distal to the tuberosity are (1) medullary curettage and inlay bone grafting and (2) closed axial intramedullary screw fixation.

MEDULLARY CURETTAGE AND INLAY BONE GRAFTING

We described obliteration of the medullary canal by dense sclerotic bone along the margins of the fracture; this bone has a tendency to progress to a nonunion. The purpose of the surgical procedure is to re-establish the continuity of the medullary canal by removing the sclerotic bone, and to facilitate healing by insertion of an inlay bone graft.

Surgical Procedure

The base of the fifth metatarsal is approached through a curvilinear dorsolateral incision. The fracture site is exposed subperiosteally, and a rectangular section of bone measuring 0.7 by 2.0 cm, centered over the fracture, is outlined by four drill holes (Fig. 4, *A*) and removed with a sharp osteotome (Fig. 4, *B*). The medullary cavity is then curetted or drilled until all the sclerotic bone has been removed and the continuity of the medullary canal has been re-established (Fig. 4, *D*). An autogenous corticocancellous bone graft measuring 0.7 by 2.0 cm is then removed from the anteromedial aspect of the distal end of the tibia through a second incision, with care taken to contour the graft with a high-speed burr so that the cortical portion of the graft fits accurately into the rectangular cortical defect and does not protrude into the medullary canal and occlude it (Fig. 4, *C*). The periosteum, subcutaneous tissue, and skin are closed sequentially in layers, and attention is turned to the graft site in the tibia. To prevent the formation of a stress raiser, the section of bone removed from the fracture site is placed in the tibial defect before the periosteum, subcutaneous tissue, and skin are closed. A non-weight-bearing plaster boot is applied, and immobilization is maintained for 6 weeks.

CLOSED AXIAL INTRAMEDULLARY SCREW FIXATION

DeLee et al reported an alternative surgical technique that does not open the fracture site and as a result of which 10 patients obtained union in an average of 7.5 weeks. These fractures met the criteria of a history of prodromal symptoms before the acute episode; radiographic evidence of a stress phenomenon (periosteal reaction, radiolucent fracture line, and intramedullary sclerosis); and no history of previous treatment. These fractures can be classified as acute injuries with an underlying stress weakness, and would be acute fractures or delayed unions according to Torg's classification.

Surgical Procedure

All patients underwent internal fixation of the fracture by the insertion of a screw into the intramedullary canal of the fifth metatarsal. After substantial changes, the technique that has evolved is as follows:

A straight incision, parallel to the plantar aspect of the foot, is used to approach the tuberosity of the fifth

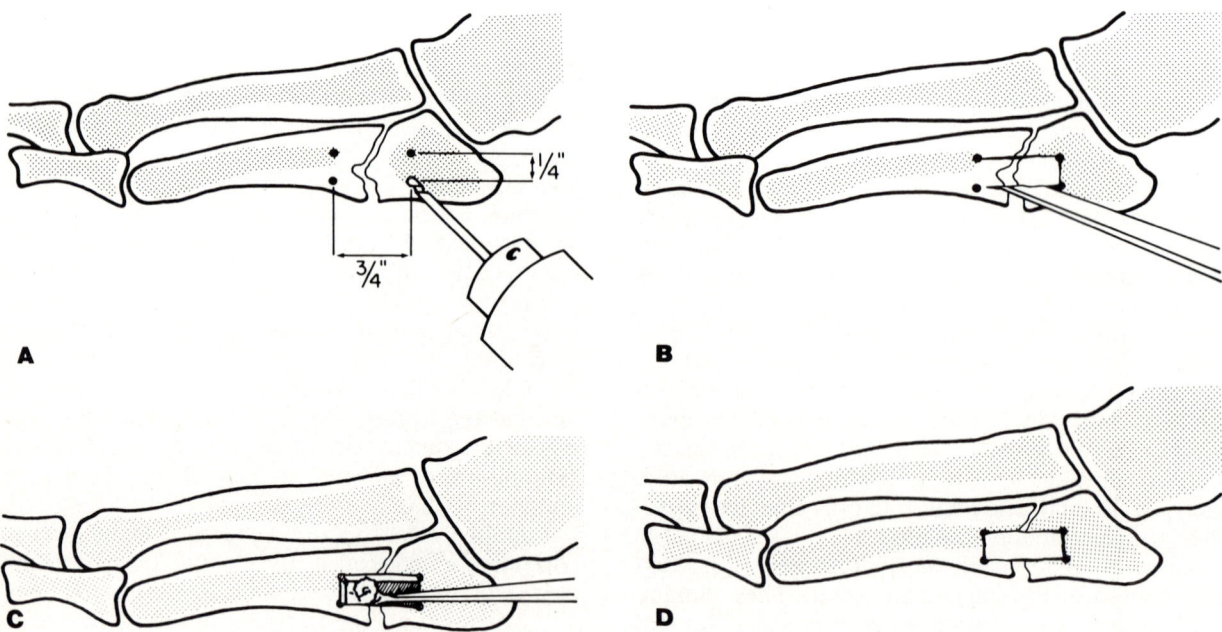

Figure 4 *A,* Subperiosteal exposure of the base of the fifth metatarsal, distal to the tuberosity, through a dorsolateral curvilinear incision reveals the fracture line and associated cortical hypertrophy. A rectangular piece of bone measuring approximately 0.7 by 2.0 cm, centered over the lateral aspect of the fracture, is outlined with four drill holes. *B,* The outlined cortical fragment is then excised with an osteotome. *C,* To re-establish the continuity of the medullary canal, the sclerotic bone in the medullary canal is removed with a curet or drill, or both. *D,* An autogenous cortical graft, obtained from the anteromedial aspect of the distal part of the tibia, is carefully contoured with a high-speed burr and placed in the previously created defect. The periosteum, subcutaneous tissues, and skin are then closed in layers, and immobilization in a non-weight-bearing toe-to-knee cast is continued for 6 weeks.

metatarsal. The interval between the peroneus longus and peroneus brevis is located, and the tuberosity of the fifth metatarsal is isolated (Fig. 5, *A*). A Kirschner wire is then inserted into the tuberosity in an effort to locate the axis of the medullary canal of the fifth metatarsal (Fig. 5, *B*). After this insertion, the location of the wire is checked roentgenographically (either with standard anteroposterior and lateral roentgenograms or under image intensification). Once correct placement of the Kirschner wire is confirmed, a sterile marking pencil is used to mark the skin in order to set the direction for screw insertion (Fig. 5, *C*). Next, a 3.2 mm Association for Study of Internal Fixation (ASIF) drill is inserted into the medullary canal in the same direction as the Kirschner wire, using the skin mark as a guide (Fig. 5, *D*). The final position of the drill in the intramedullary canal is checked roentgenographically. At this point, a 4.5 mm ASIF malleolar screw is inserted down the axis of the fifth metatarsal (Fig. 6). The longest screw that fits into

the medullary canal of the individual metatarsal is selected. Care is taken to (1) countersink the screw head so that a prominence is not present and (2) ensure that the screw threads do not cross the fracture site. At no time during the operation is the fracture site exposed or bone grafting performed.

Alternatively, a Leinbach screw is used in the medullary canal in three of the patients. The technique for insertion is similar to that used for the ASIF malleolar screw.

Following screw insertion, the patients are placed in a short-leg nonwalking cast or slipper cast for 2 weeks. The cast is then removed and the foot placed in a hard-sole shoe. Either a wooden shoe of the postbunionectomy type or a standard tennis shoe with a semiflexible steel sole insert is used to protect the foot. Gradual progression of weight-bearing is begun. The patients are allowed to return to competitive sports when pain over the fifth metatarsal and the incision is gone.

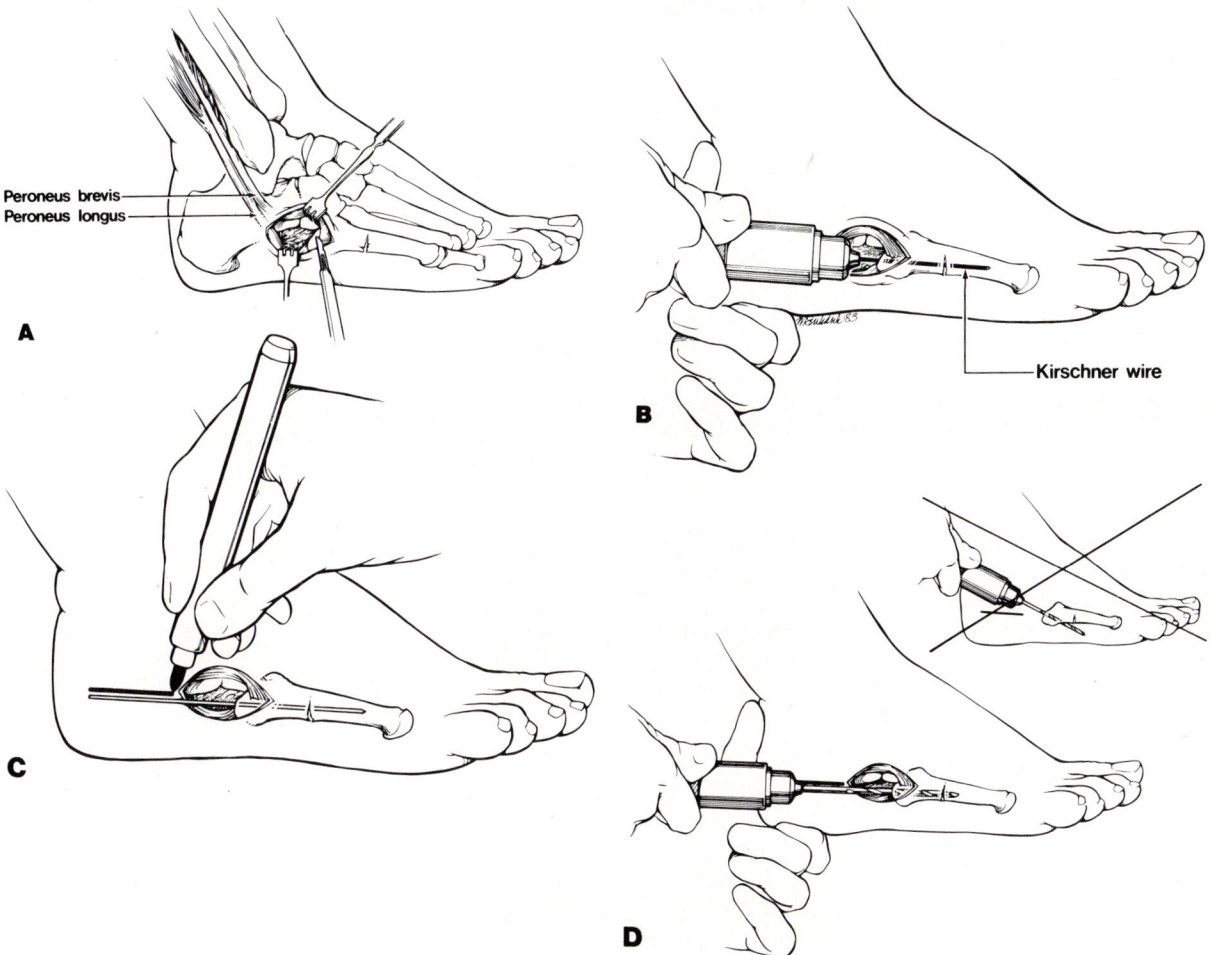

Figure 5 *A,* Surgical exposure of the base of the fifth metatarsal between the peroneus longus and peroneus brevis tendons. Minimal elevation of the peroneus brevis improves exposure. *B,* Insertion of a Kirschner wire (0.0625) into the medullary canal of the metatarsal. Adduction of the forefoot is beneficial for accurate insertion. The position is confirmed roentgenographically. *C,* A sterile marking pen is used to mark the direction of the Kirschner wire on the skin of the foot. This mark is used as a guide for insertion of the drill. *D,* Using the entrance hole of the Kirschner wire and the skin mark for alignment, a 3.2 mm ASIF drill is inserted into the fifth metatarsal. If the skin mark is not followed, the drill will penetrate the metatarsal. The drill's position is confirmed roentgenographically. A 4.5 mm ASIF malleolar screw is inserted so that the threads do not cross the fracture site.

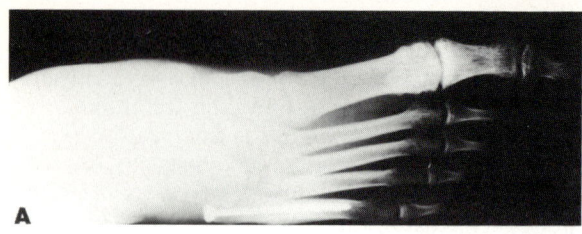
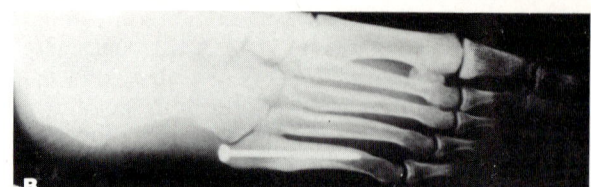

Figure 6 *A,* Anteroposterior and *B,* oblique roentgenograms of the patient 7 weeks after internal fixation. Note the trabeculae crossing the fracture site.

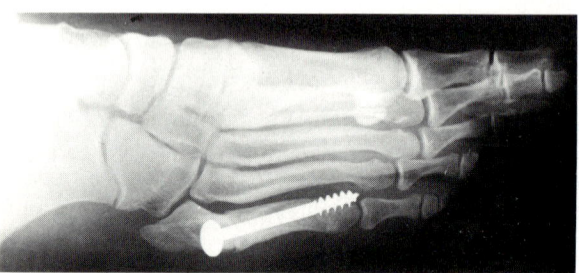

Figure 7 Complications of intramedullary screw fixation are noted and are due to failure to adhere strictly to technique. An incorrect screw is used (6.5 cancellous rather than malleolar); it is placed too distal and is too long, thereby penetrating the distal cortex.

The range of time to return to sporting activity in this series was 7 to 14 weeks.

Upon returning to activity, seven of the 10 patients used a soft shoe insert with a protective area of padding over the lateral border of the foot at the base of the fifth metatarsal, to prevent pressure on the screw head or under the fifth metatarsal head. Three patients did not require this protection.

In review of the surgical technique, the intramedullary screw procedure has the advantages of not opening the fracture site, being a shorter procedure and one that decreases healing time. This procedure is not without complications. Placement of the screw is critical and not always easily accomplished. Kavanaugh et al reported a 45% complication rate, which included screw fracture, missing the medullary canal, and complaints about the screw heads (Fig. 7). DeLee et al also reported that seven of 10 patients required shoe modification.

In conclusion, the treatment of the fracture of the base of the fifth metatarsal distal to the tuberosity should be tailored to the classification. Acute fractures should be immobilized in a non-weight-bearing plaster boot. Fractures with delayed union can be treated with non-weight bearing in a cast, but will experience a prolonged period until union. In competitive athletes, fractures with delayed union should be treated operatively, using the surgical technique with which the physician feels most competent and has experience. All fractures with nonunion should be treated operatively.

SUGGESTED READING

Carp L. Fractures of the fifth metatarsal bone, with reference to delayed union. Ann Surg 1927; 86:308–320.

Dameron TB Jr. Fractures and anatomical variations of the proximal portion of the fifth metatarsal. J Bone Joint Surg 1975; 57-A: 788–792.

DeLee JC, Evans JP, Julian J. Stress fractures of the fifth metatarsal. Am J Sports Med 1983; 5:349–353.

Jones R. Fracture of the base of the fifth metatarsal bone by indirect violence. Ann Surg 1902; 35:697–700.

Kavanaugh JH, Brower TD, Mann RV. The Jones' fracture revisited. J Bone Joint Surg 1978; 60-A:776–782.

Lehman RC, et al. Fractures of the base of the fifth metatarsal distal to the tuberosity: a review. Foot Ankle 1987; 7:245–252.

Stewart IM. Jones' fracture: fracture of the base of the fifth metatarsal. Clin Orthop 1960; 16:190–198.

Torg JS, et al. Fractures of the base of the fifth metatarsal distal to the tuberosity. J Bone Joint Surg 1984; 66-A:209–214.

Zelko RR, Torg JS, Rachun A. Proximal diaphyseal fractures of the fifth metatarsal: treatment of the fractures and their complications in athletes. Am J Sports Med 1979; 7:95–101.

STRESS FRACTURE OF THE TARSAL NAVICULAR

JOSEPH S. TORG, M.D.

Tarsal navicular stress fractures are an underdiagnosed source of prolonged disabling foot pain in young athletes. Eichenholtz and Levine, referring to all fractures of the tarsal navicular, stated that "the diagnosis is being missed with and without radiographs because this fracture is not being suspected." Towne and associates recognized the limitations of routine radiographs and, in a report of two stress fractures of this bone, suggested the need of "special roentgen views and laminography for detection," but without further elaboration. Goergen et al reported two stress fractures in runners and emphasized the importance of and difficulty involved in radiographic diagnosis. In the orthopedic literature, Torg et al described the diagnosis, fracture patterns, complications, and possible etiology of 21 tarsal navicular stress fractures in 19 patients. They emphasized the orthopedic management and stated that "the interval between the onset of symptoms and the diagnosis ranged from less than one month to thirty-eight

months (mean interval 7.2 months)" because the fracture was not evident or because it was overlooked on the routine foot radiographs.

The tarsal navicular stress fracture is notoriously misdiagnosed. Because of the ill-defined nature of the pain and the difficulty of identifying the fracture in routine radiographs, there is often a sizable delay between the onset of symptoms and correct diagnosis.

Symptoms of the tarsal navicular stress fracture include the insidious onset of vague pain over the dorsum of the medial midfoot or over the medial aspect of the longitudinal arch. The pain is an ill-defined soreness or cramping, which is aggravated by activity and relieved by rest. Usually there is a well-localized tenderness over the tarsal navicular or along the medial longitudinal arch. There is little if any swelling and no discoloration or lumps. There may be an associated decrease in dorsiflexion or subtalar motion.

Stress fractures occur commonly in the weight-bearing bones of military recruits, distance runners, and others who participate in prolonged and vigorous activity. However, the occurrence of these lesions in the tarsal navicular appears to be either rare or infrequently recognized.

The circumstances surrounding the occurrence of navicular stress fractures suggest certain features that may contribute to the development of the lesion. The patients are all very active physically. Foot abnormali-

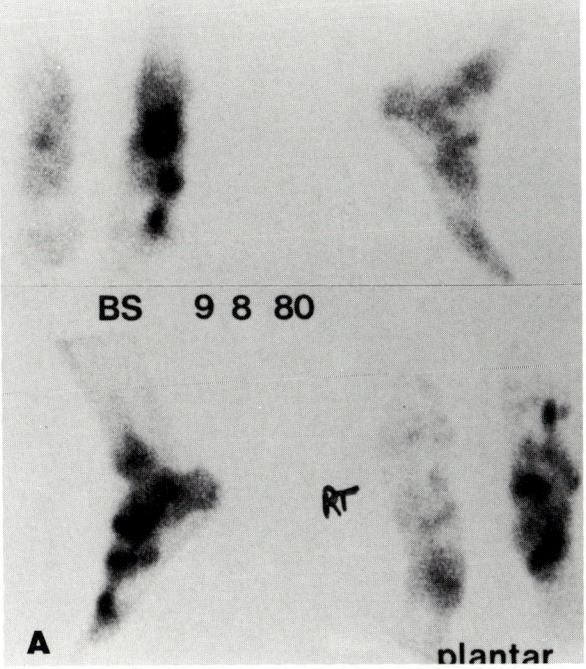
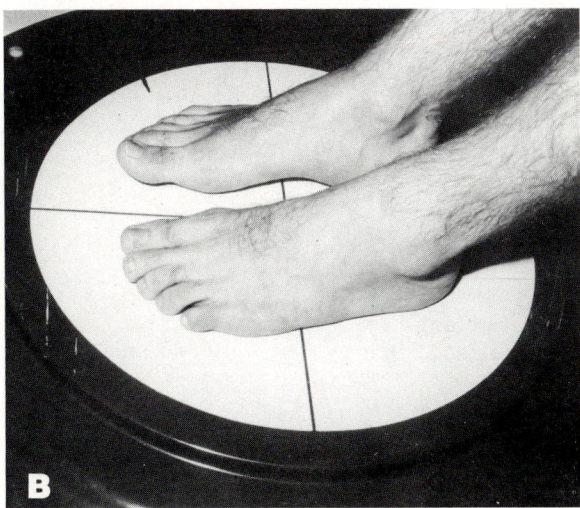

Figure 1 *A,* Radionuclide bone scanning was performed (starting in the upper left quadrant and moving clockwise) in the frontal, medial (right), plantar, and medial (left) positions. There is augmented isotope uptake in the left navicular and fourth metatarsal. In the frontal view the tarsal area is overlapped by that of the hindfoot, and it is difficult to localize the isotope uptake. On the medial (left) view the uptake is intensified in the region of the tarsal navicular; however, it is poorly localized because of other areas of augmented uptake. On the plantar view the areas of increased isotope uptake are best demonstrated and conform to the configuration of the navicular and the fourth metatarsal, respectively; stress fractures in both areas were documented. *B,* Plantar views are obtained with the soles of the patient's feet positioned on the face of the gamma camera. The patient leans posteriorly so that the isotope uptake from the body pool does not contribute to the uptake from the feet.

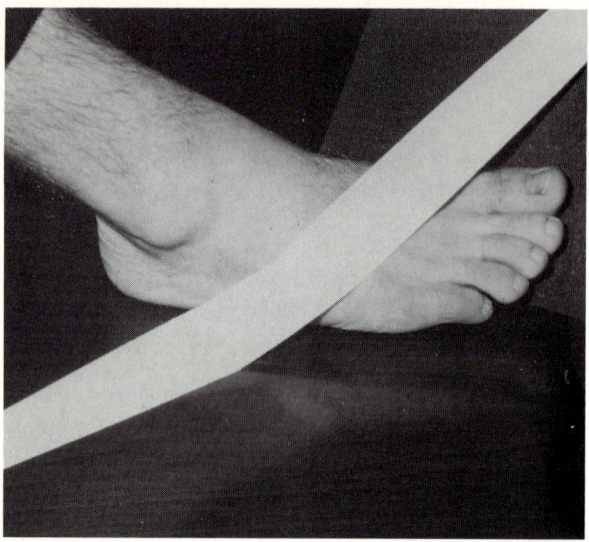

Figure 2 A foot is placed on a foam wedge and taped to the cassette in the correct position to make a so-called anatomic AP radiograph. The medial side of the forepart of the foot is elevated so that the entire foot is inverted. Fluoroscopy should be used to ensure proper positioning of the foot.

ties, including a short first metatarsal and metatarsus adductus, as well as limited dorsiflexion of the ankle or limited subtalar motion, or both, are present in some patients and may concentrate stress on the tarsal navicular. The findings of sclerosis of the proximal articular border of the navicular, narrowing of the talonavicular joint, talar breaking, accessory ossicles, and malalignment at the dorsal margins of the talonavicular and navicular-cuneiform joints in some patients may indicate the presence of some type of mechanical abnormality in the involved foot.

Microangiographic studies of the blood supply to the tarsal navicular demonstrate relative avascularity of the middle third of the bone. All these findings suggest the hypothesis that repetitive cyclic loading, associated with some as yet unidentified variations in foot structure, may result in fatigue failure through the relatively avascular central portion of the tarsal navicular.

Prompt diagnosis of tarsal navicular stress fractures requires appropriate radiographic studies. Routine standing anteroposterior (AP), lateral, and oblique radiographs of the foot should be made when a tarsal navicular stress fracture is suspected. The tarsal navicular is frequently underpenetrated on these radiographs,

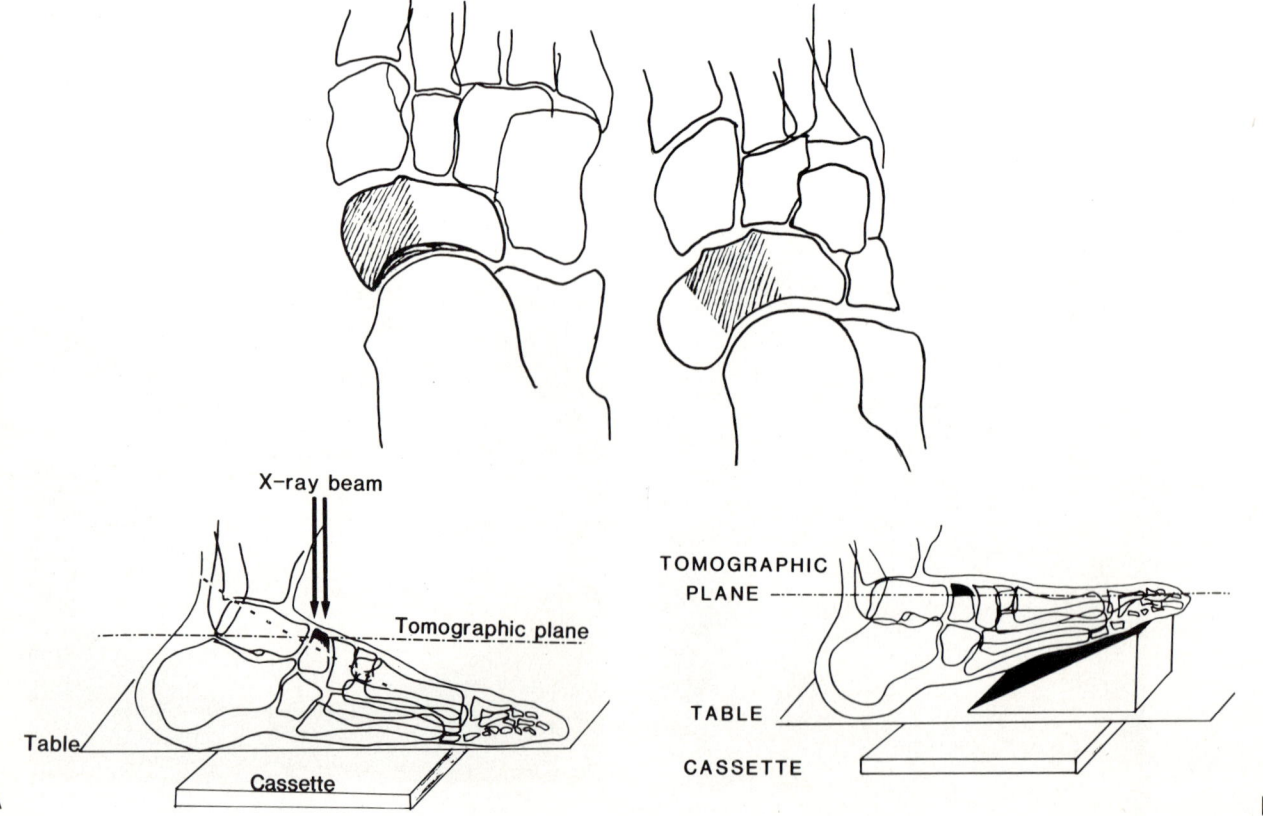

Figure 3 *A,* Standard anteroposterior (AP) tomogram position. The foot is flat on the table. *Above,* The dorsal surface of the navicular (*shaded area*) and the long axis of the talus and the navicular are oblique to the tomographic plane. *Below,* On this view the central third of the navicular (*shaded area*) is seen obliquely. Also, the undersurface of the navicular is usually seen because the x-ray beam is not tangential to the talonavicular joint. *B,* Anatomic AP tomogram position. The forefoot is lifted off the table with a wedge so that the dorsal surface of the navicular (*shaded area*) and the long axis of the talus and the navicular are parallel to the tomographic plane. *Below,* On this view the central third of the navicular (*shaded area*) is seen en face and the x-ray beam is tangential to the talonavicular joint.

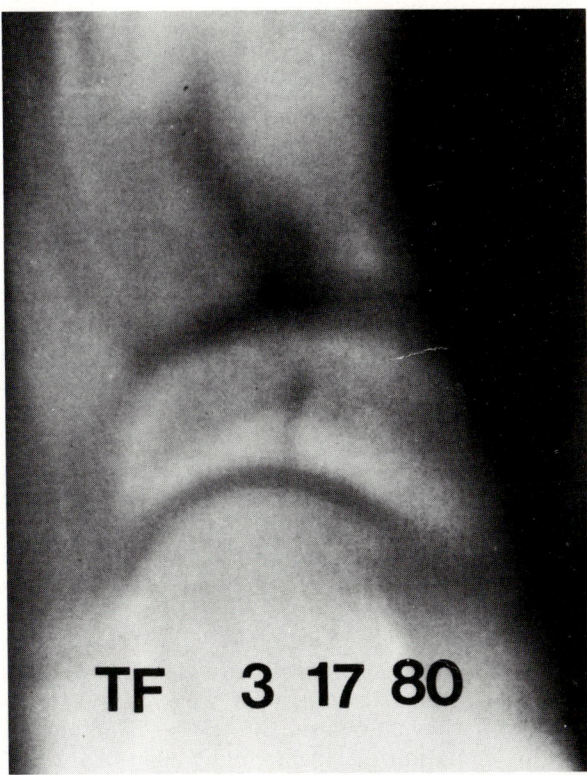

Figure 4 AP tomogram of the right foot of a 17-year-old high-school player with a partial proximal stress fracture of the tarsal navicular. The tomogram was made 3 months after the onset of the symptoms and shows a partial stress fracture involving the proximal articular border of the tarsal navicular, but the distal articular border as seen here and on comparison cuts showed no evidence of fracture. Deeper sections also showed that the fracture was limited owing to the dorsal aspect of the bone.

and a coned-down AP radiograph centered on the tarsal navicular may be required for visualization. The continuity of the cortical bone of the navicular, especially on the AP radiograph, must be carefully examined, because when there is a fracture the lateral fragment resembles a separate tarsal bone and can easily be overlooked.

If the routine radiographic examination is normal or equivocal, a radionuclide bone scan of both feet should be obtained, using technetium-99m methylene diphosphonate. Localized augmented isotopic uptake is interpreted as abnormal (Fig. 1).

When the radionuclide bone scan indicates a lesion of the tarsal navicular but the routine radiographic examination is normal, tomograms of the tarsal navicular are required. The position of the foot for the tomographic examination is critical and should be established accurately under fluoroscopic guidance. Tomograms must be made with the tarsal navicular in the true AP position. To do this, the foot should be slightly inverted until the entire medial-lateral width of the tarsal navicular is demonstrated fluoroscopically (Fig. 2). Exact positioning for the AP tomogram is important because the typical stress fracture is in the sagittal plane through the center of the bone and is obscured by even slight obliquity with respect to the x-ray beam. Also, the dorsal surface of the tarsal navicular must be parallel to the plane of the tomographic cut, because in most cases an incomplete stress fracture is confined to the dorsal aspect of the bone and can be obscured if the tomographic plane is oblique (Fig. 3).

All the fractures in the series of Torg et al were in the sagittal plane and were located in the central third of the bone. Ten of the fractures were partial, involving only the dorsal cortex, and 11 were complete. Of the partial fractures, nine involved the proximal articular border (Fig. 4) and one the distal articular border (Fig. 5). Eleven of the fractures were complete (Fig. 6); 10 were nondisplaced and one was displaced. A transverse

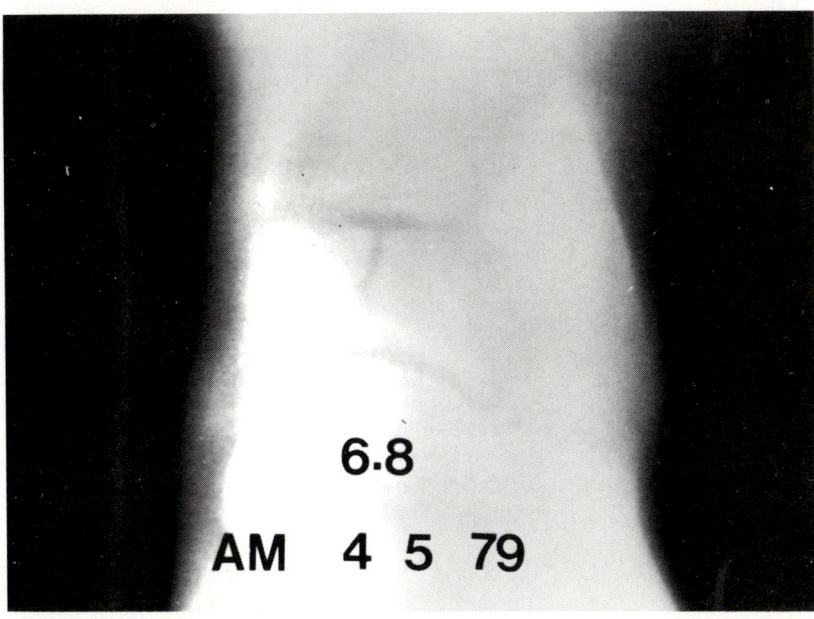

Figure 5 Tomogram of a 17-year-old middle-distance runner made 1 month after the onset of symptoms shows a partial stress fracture involving the distal articular border of the tarsal navicular. This tomogram and companion sections showed that the proximal articular border was intact. A deeper selection did not show the fracture, which indicates that it was limited to the dorsal aspect of the bone.

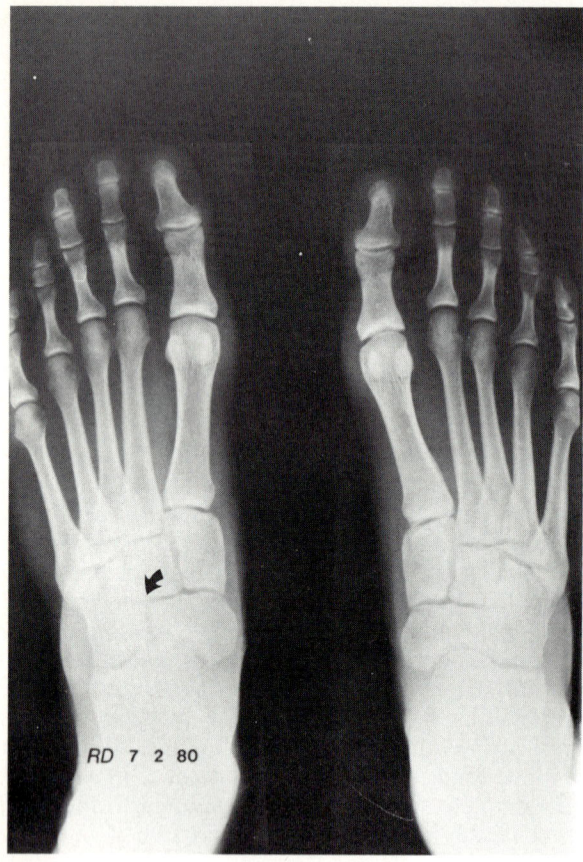

Figure 6 Complete stress fracture involving the left tarsal navicular in a 15-year-old high-school basketball player is visualized on routine AP roentgenographic views.

dorsal fracture fragment was associated with one partial fracture of the proximal articular border and with two complete fractures.

The 21 tarsal navicular stress fractures in this series could be divided into three separate groups: (1) uncomplicated fractures that went on to complete healing with treatment; (2) those in which there was a complication when they were first seen and in which treatment resulted in successful healing; and (3) those in which delayed union or nonunion developed despite treatment, or in which there was a recurrence of the fracture following treatment.

Of the 12 uncomplicated fractures that went on to successful healing, 10 were treated by immobilization in a plaster cast and non-weight bearing for 6 to 8 weeks, and two healed with only limitation of activity and continued weight bearing.

Two complicated fractures, one with acute displacement of the fragments and the other with an established nonunion and aseptic necrosis of the lateral fragment, were treated surgically at the outset, the first by open reduction and internal fixation and the second by medullary curettage and autogenous bone grafting (Fig. 7). Both fractures were immobilized in a non-weight-bearing cast for 6 weeks postoperatively, and both healed (Fig. 8).

In seven patients the result of treatment was either a delayed union, a nonunion, or a refracture after healing. All seven had been permitted to continue weight bearing during the initial treatment. In two of these seven fractures, union was delayed, but healing occurred after immobilization in a non-weight-bearing cast for 8 weeks in one and 18 weeks in the other. A third fracture, initially treated in a weight-bearing cast for 8 weeks, went on to nonunion, which was successfully treated by an inlay bone graft and internal fixation, followed by immobilization in a non-weight-bearing cast for 8 weeks. The other four patients were disabled and unable to participate in sports activity as a result of the fractures. One patient was a professional basketball player with a complete, nondisplaced fracture associated with a dorsal transverse fragment. Initially he attempted to continue playing on the injured foot, but eventually the fracture was immobilized in a series of partial-weight-bearing casts. The fracture healed, but marked osteoporosis accompanied by pain developed. Subsequent attempts to return to playing basketball resulted in recurrence of the fracture and continued disability 42 months after the initial injury.

The other three fractures that resulted in disability were partial, proximal, undisplaced fractures, one having an associated dorsal transverse fragment. One was treated with a weight-bearing plaster cast, and the other two with limitation of activity and weight-bearing. Of these three patients, the first, a professional basketball player whose treatment consisted of limitation of activity and continued weight bearing, had a refracture at 12 months and was still disabled at 24 months. The second, a recreational distance runner who was similarly treated, had delayed union and was still disabled at 16 months. The third, a recreational tennis player who was treated with a weight-bearing cast, had a nonunion and was still disabled at 30 months.

TREATMENT GUIDELINES

On the basis of the above experience, I recommend the following guidelines for management of tarsal navicular stress fractures:

1. Uncomplicated partial fractures and nondisplaced complete fractures of the tarsal navicular should be treated by immobilization in a plaster cast with non-weight bearing for 6 to 8 weeks. The decision to allow a return to weight bearing and activity should be guided by the patient's clinical picture as well as roentgenographic evidence of the union.
2. Complete displaced fractures can be treated with either immobilization in a plaster cast with non-weight bearing for 6 to 8 weeks or open reduction and internal fixation, followed by immobilization and non-weight bearing for 6 weeks.
3. Fractures complicated by delayed union or nonunion should be treated with medullary curettage

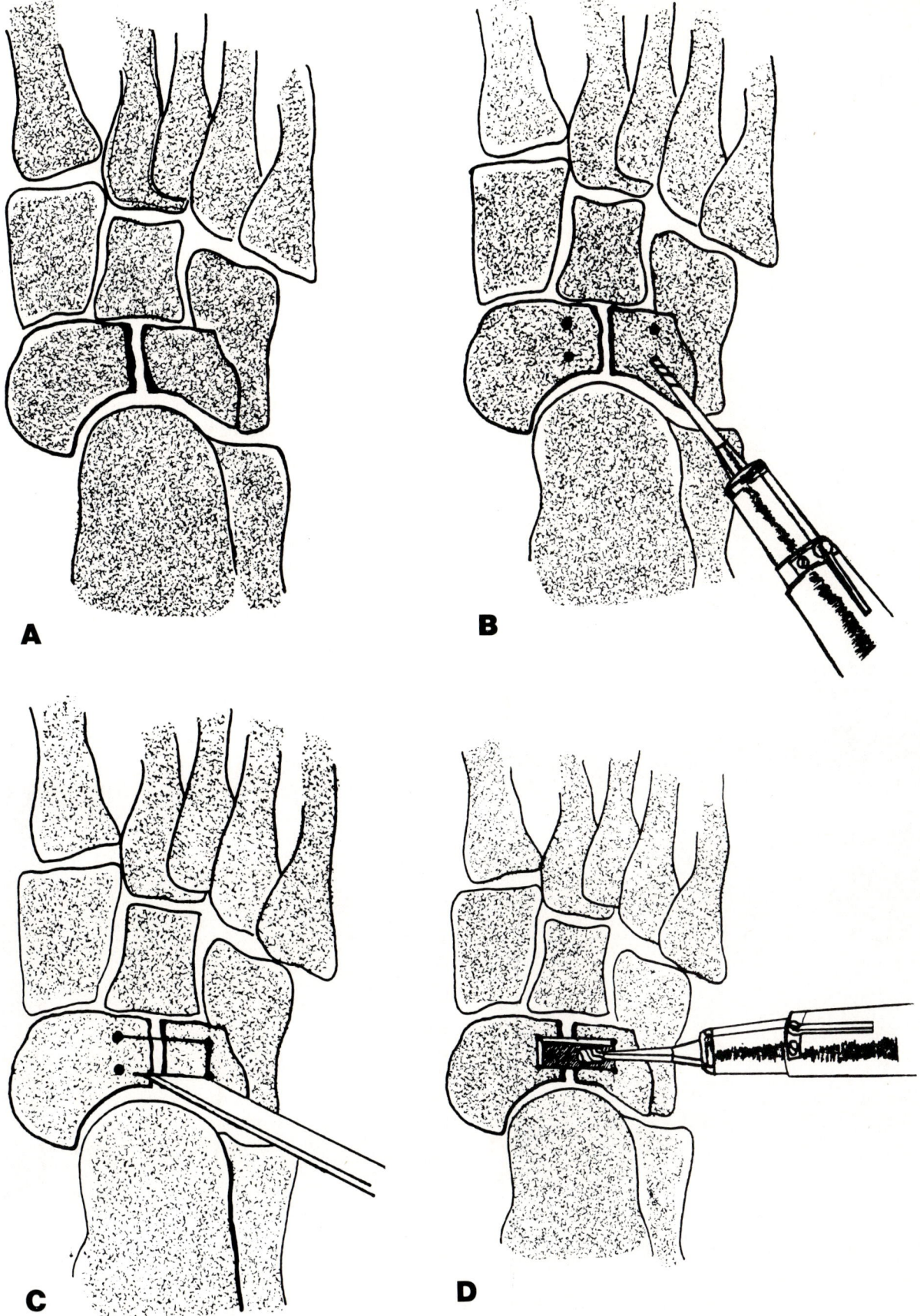

Figure 7 *See legend on next page.*

Continued.

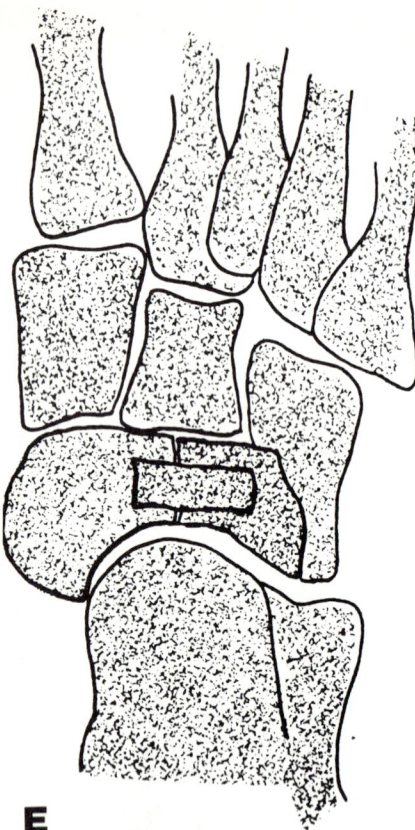

Figure 7 *A,* In instances of established nonunion of a tarsal navicular stress fracture, with or without aseptic necrosis of one of the fragments, medullary curettage and inlaid bone grafting is indicated. If a fibrous union exists, do not attempt to reduce the fracture. Do not excise sclerotic fragments. If there is motion, internal screw fixation is indicated. *B,* A rectangular piece of bone measuring approximately 0.7 by 2.0 cm, centered over the fracture, is outlined with four drill holes. *C,* The outlined cortical fragment is then excised with an osteome. *D,* The sclerotic bone in the medullary canal is removed with a drill. *E,* An autogenous cortical graft, obtained from the anteromedial aspect of the distal part of the tibia, is carefully contoured with a high-speed burr and placed in the previously created defect. The periosteum, subcutaneous tissues, and skin are then closed in layers, and immobilization in a non-weight-bearing toe-to-knee cast is continued for 6 weeks.

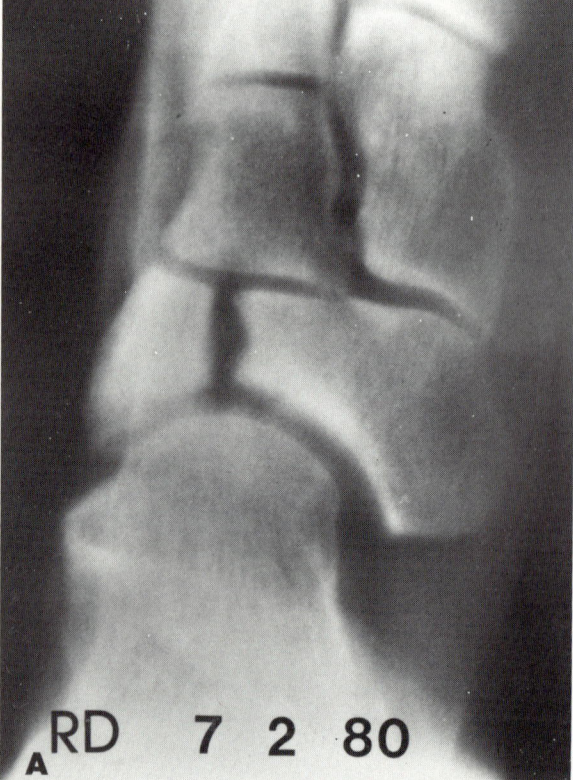

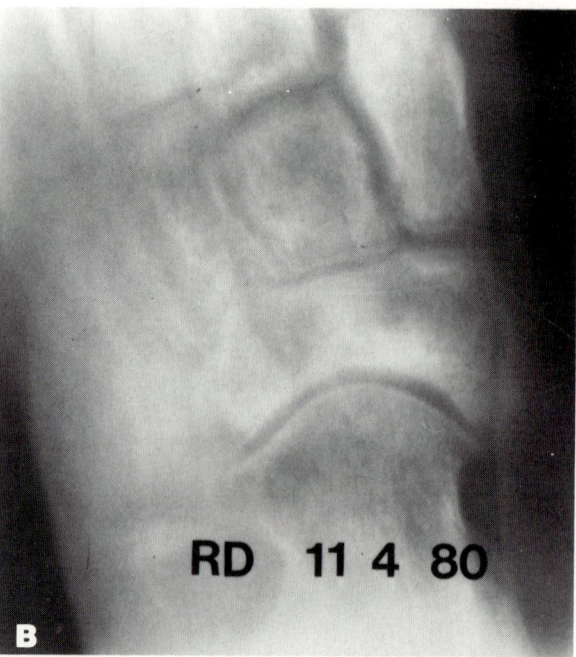

Figure 8 *A,* Nonunion of a stress fracture of the tarsal navicular with aseptic necrosis of the lateral fragment. *B,* Roentgenograms following medullary curettage and inlaid bone graft without attempt at reduction of fracture demonstrate complete healing.

and inlaid bone grafting. In these situations, a fibrous union may exist and no attempt should be made to reduce the fragments. If the fragments are mobile, internal fixation should be effected using a malleolar screw. After medullary curettage and inlaid bone grafting, with or without internal fixation, the patient should be placed in a non-weight-bearing short-leg cast for 6 to 8 weeks. Again, mobilization and return to activity should depend on clinical and roentgenographic evidence of healing. It should be noted that in fractures treated by bone grafting, the healing course may be protracted and firm bony union may not occur for 3 to 6 months.

4. Partial fractures complicated with a small dorsal transverse fracture may require excision of the dorsal fragment.

5. Complete fractures complicated by a large dorsal transverse fracture will go on to union with immobilization but may require excision of the fragment.

6. Associated dorsal talar beaks should be excised. Apart from these and the small dorsal transverse fragments, sclerotic fragments associated with delayed union and nonunion should not be excised, but treated with medullary curettage and inlaid bone graft as indicated.

SUGGESTED READING

Eichenholtz SN, Levine DB. Fractures of the tarsal navicular bone. Clin Orthop 1964; 34:142–157.

Goergen TG, Venn-Watson EA, Rossman DJ, et al. Tarsal navicular stress fractures in runners. Am J Roetgenol 1981; 136:201–203.

Pavlov H, Torg JS, Freiberger RH. Tarsal navicular stress fractures: radiographic evaluation. Radiology 1983; 148:641–645.

Torg JS, Pavlov H, Cooley LH, et al. Stress fractures of the tarsal navicular. J Bone Joint Surg 1982; 63-A:700–712.

Towne LC, Blazina ME, Cozen LN. Fatigue fracture of the tarsal navicular. J Bone Joint Surg 1970; 52-A:376–378.

CUBOID SUBLUXATION IN CLASSICAL DANCERS

PETER MARSHALL, M.A., P.T.
WILLIAM G. HAMILTON, M.D.

Foot injuries are common in classical ballet dancers. Repetitive foot movements through extreme ranges of motion, a vocabulary that requires maximum external hip rotation, and the ballistic nature of dance are responsible for creating an environment conducive to foot injuries. Cuboid subluxations were recently reported to have been responsible for over 17% of the foot and ankle injuries that required physical therapy at American Ballet Theatre during a 3 week performance schedule and a 3 week rehearsal period. This chapter presents a method of detection, treatment, and prevention of what we consider to be a frequently misdiagnosed and overlooked syndrome.

ETIOLOGY

Male dancers typically sustain cuboid problems as they land from a series of big jumps. Foot and ankle pronation that occurs in these landings is thought to be a major factor in the development of cuboid subluxations. Indeed, the etiologic factors hypothesized by Newell and Woodie for the development of this syndrome in athletes may play an important role in male classical dancers as well. Newell and Woodie felt that excessive pronation allowed the peroneus longus to pull the lateral border of the cuboid dorsally, causing the medial border to subluxate in a plantar direction. Certainly, the muscle belly of the peroneus longus becomes tight after a cuboid subluxation and must be relaxed with deep message before reduction is attempted.

Cuboid subluxations occur much more frequently in female dancers and appear to be of a different type than in males. While cuboid problems usually occur acutely in male dancers, they are generally seen as part of an overuse syndrome in females. Anyone who has seen a ballerina bourré (move across the stage on full pointe) or perform fouettés (rapid spinning movements combined with relevés from foot-flat to full-pointe) can appreciate some of the extreme stresses placed on the ballerina's foot as she performs pointe work. Indeed, cuboid subluxation in female dancers may be secondary to dorsal ligamentous laxity associated with hypermobility of the joints of the midfoot, which is common in these dancers.

Further stress is directed to the midfoot when pointe work is performed incorrectly. This can occur when a valgus attitude of the maximally pointed (plantar-flexed) foot is assumed. This technical error is often seen after an inversion sprain of the lateral ankle as the dancer seeks security by "leaning" on the strong deltoid ligament. Also, some dancers compensate for inadequate plantar flexion by assuming a valgus position when attempting pointe work (Fig. 1). These repetitive forces may gradually decrease the stability of the

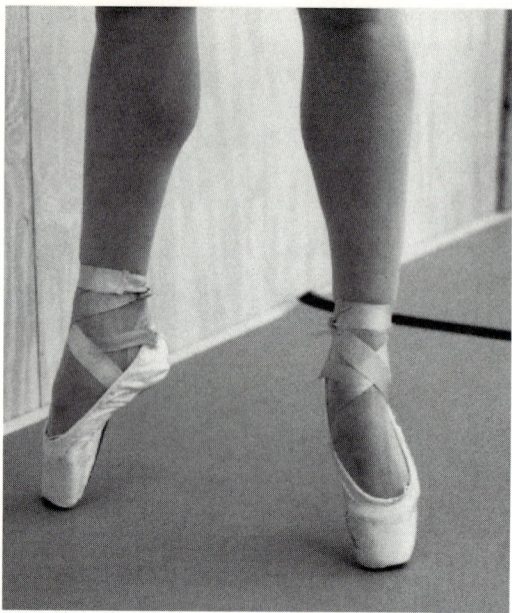

Figure 1 Dancers with less than optimal plantarflexion will compensate by assuming a valgus position when en pointe.

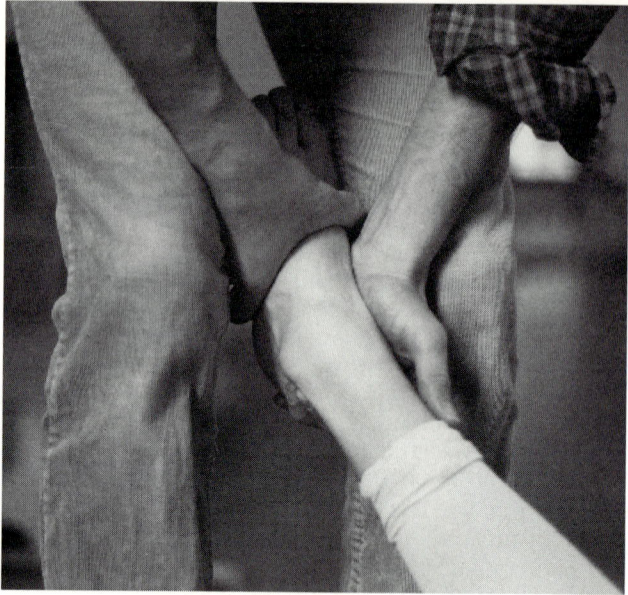

Figure 2 To realign an abducted midtarsal joint, the patient's foot is positioned between the clinician's knees. The medial foot is contacted at the distal talus and the lateral foot at the lateral aspect of the cuboid. An adduction force is then applied by the therapist's hands and knees. (From Marshall P, Hamilton WG. Cuboid subluxation in ballet dancers. Am J Sports Med 1992; 20:169–175; with permission.)

midfoot, predisposing some dancers to cuboid subluxations. Cuboid subluxation can also result from a traumatic sprain of the lateral foot. This is particularly true of a sprain involving the dorsal calcaneocuboid ligament and the dorsal cuboid-forth or cuboid-fifth metatarsal ligament. Cuboid subluxations that occur secondary to such acute sprains should be recognized and managed carefully if one is to prevent a chronic condition from developing.

CLINICAL PICTURE

A dancer with a cuboid subluxation will present with a chief complaint of sharp lateral foot pain and weakness in push-off. The dancer frequently reports an inability to "work through the foot" when moving from foot-flat to demi or full pointe. Vigorous dancing and leg jumps are difficult or impossible due to pain. Careful physical examination will show that the cuboid's minimal dorsal/plantar joint play is markedly reduced or absent when compared to the uninvolved foot. Dorsally directed pressure on the plantar aspect of the cuboid will be sharply painful. Visual inspection may suggest slight midfoot abduction. Unfortunately, the diagnosis is subjective. Repeated attempts to confirm the diagnosis by roentgenograms, computed tomography (CT) scans, or magnetic resonance imaging (MRI) studies have failed to document the pathology—due to the normal variations seen in these studies between the cuboid and its surrounding structures, and the minimal amount of subluxation that often occurs. (Other widely accepted syndromes, such as subluxation of the glenohumeral joint and tarsometatarsal joints, are also diagnoses that

are based solely on the history and physical examination.)

Cuboid subluxation secondary to a sprain of the lateral foot or ankle is often difficult to detect because of the presence of injured soft tissues. Effusion and ecchymosis make determination of the cuboid's joint play confusing, and it is difficult to assess the implications of a pain response when pressing dorsalward on the plantar aspect of the cuboid. However, lingering symptoms and disability may indicate that cuboid subluxation has occurred and, as sprained soft tissue structures heal, careful clinical examination as outlined previously will help determine the presence or absence of cuboid subluxation.

TREATMENT

There are a variety of effective techniques that will reduce the cuboid. Before any of these techniques are attempted, it is important to relax the peronei with deep massage and attempt to correct an abducted midtarsal joint if present (Fig. 2). Until recently, the most frequently employed approach was the "cuboid whip," which is performed with the patient in the prone position. The clinician is positioned at the patient's feet and holds the forefoot with his or her fingers while the thumbs are on the plantar surface of the cuboid. The foot is then whipped forcefully into plantarflexion; simultaneously, the thumbs deliver a dorsally directed reduction

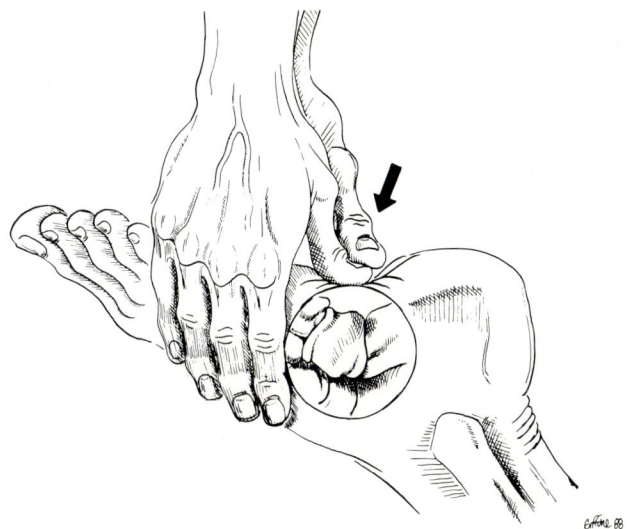

Figure 3 The correct position, hand placement, and direction of the reduction force for performing the "cuboid squeeze." (From Marshall P, Hamilton WG. Cuboid subluxation in ballet dancers. Am J Sports Med 1992; 20:169–175; with permission.)

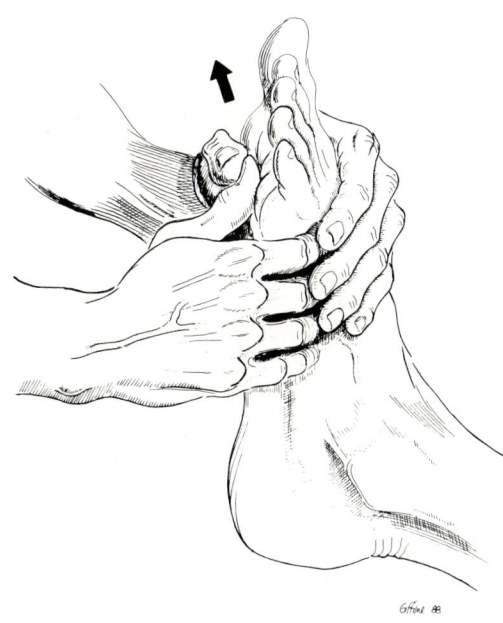

Figure 4 The examiner "hangs" the patient's injured foot by grasping the fourth metatarsal. Cuboids are reduced with a distraction force in the direction of the arrow. (From Marshall P, Hamilton WG. Cuboid subluxation in ballet dancers. Am J Sports Med 1992; 20:169–175; with permission.)

force to the cuboid. Marshall has described an adaptation of this technique and labeled it the "cuboid squeeze." The cuboid squeeze uses the same positioning and hand placement as the cuboid whip. In the cuboid squeeze, however, the clinician gradually stretches the foot and ankle into maximum plantarflexion. When the dorsal soft tissue structures have completely relaxed, the cuboid is reduced with a final squeeze from the thumbs (Fig. 3). Unlike the cuboid whip, none of the reduction force is absorbed by dorsal soft tissue structures in the foot and ankle and the direction and intensity of the reduction force is completely controlled by the clinician. In our experience, the cuboid squeeze yields significantly better results and is tolerated much better than the cuboid whip. Another extremely effective technique has the therapist at the foot of the treatment table and the patient supine. The clinician then grasps the fourth metatarsal and lifts the patient's foot and leg from the table. This allows gravity and the weight of the extremity to help distract the cuboid-fourth metatarsal articulation and requires the patient's complete relaxation. The cuboid is then reduced by delivering a distraction force in the direction of the long axis of the fourth metatarsal (Fig. 4).

Another successful technique again has the patient supine and the therapist at the foot of the table. The therapist then maximally everts the forefoot on a neutrally positioned rearfoot and delivers the reduction force with the lateral aspect of the second metacarpal of the other hand (Fig. 5). An adaptation of this technique has the clinician maximally evert the rearfoot on a neutrally positioned forefoot before attempting a reduction.

Successful reduction is almost always audible and, in

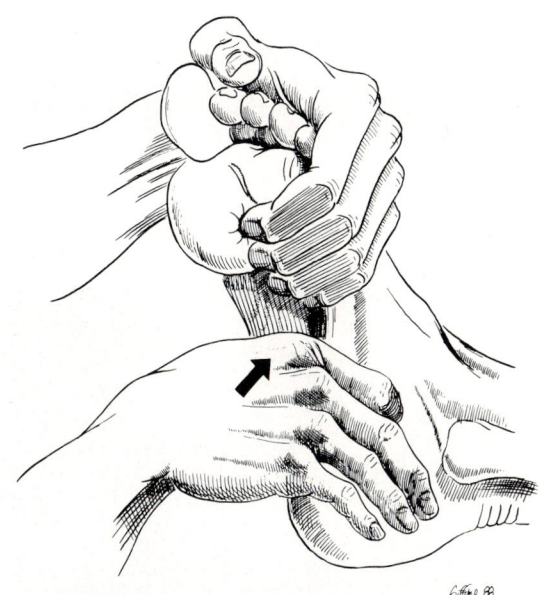

Figure 5 The clinician reduces the cuboid using the lateral aspect of the second metacarpal. The forefoot is maximally pronated on a neutrally positioned hindfoot before delivering a reduction force. A useful adaptation of this technique has the hindfoot maximally everted on a neutrally positioned forefoot before attempting the reduction. (From Marshall P, Hamilton WG. Cuboid subluxation in ballet dancers. Am J Sports Med 1992; 20:169–175; with permission.)

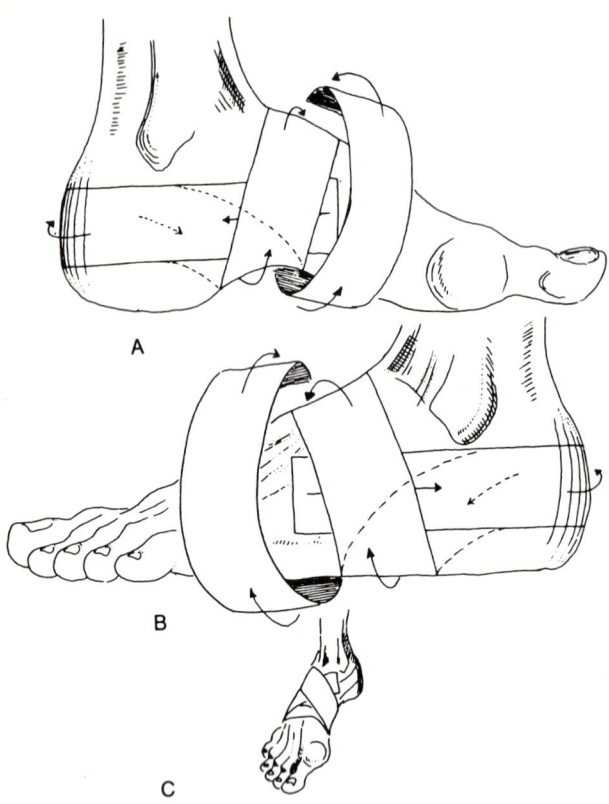

A

B

C

Figure 6 A minimal three-piece taping method is used to maintain reduction of the cuboid subluxation. Begin taping from the medial aspect of the foot (*A*), and continue from the lateral aspect (*B*). The final step (*C*) secures the foot. (From Marshall P. The rehabilitation of overuse foot injuries in athletes and dancers. Clin Sports Med 1988; 7:175–191; with permission.)

cases handled within 24 hours of onset, produces immediate and complete resolution of pain and dysfunction. Individuals who have had a cuboid subluxation for long periods of time will have immediate resolution of sharp pain and dysfunction, but may complain of dull, achy pain for a day or two that we feel is due to prolonged capsular irritation.

Ideally, dancers should rest for 2 to 3 days after a successful reduction to ensure its maintenance. However, a rest period is often a luxury that dancers ignore and financially strapped dance companies can ill afford. Indeed, cuboid subluxations are often reduced during a 20 minute intermission. In such instances we recommend the following:

1. Have the dancer relevé on one leg up to 10 times to see if the reduction will hold.
2. If the subluxation seems to have occurred with the foot in the plantargrade position, place a one-eighth inch felt pad beneath the cuboid on the plantar aspect of the foot.
3. Secure the midfoot by using the taping method outlined in Figure 6.

Cuboid subluxation following a varus sprain of the lateral foot challenges the diagnostic acumen and clinical skills of the medical team. It is difficult to ascertain whether a cuboid subluxation has occurred in an acute injury, due to the expected presence of effusion, ecchymosis and pain in the lateral aspect of the midfoot. However, complaints of pain exceeding that expected by the traumatized soft tissues, or sharp pain and dysfunction that persists for a prolonged period may signal the presence of a cuboid subluxation. When a cuboid subluxation is suspected after a lateral foot sprain, the therapist should refrain from attempting a reduction for 3 to 7 days or until the effusion and ecchymosis have significantly diminished and the possibility of a fracture

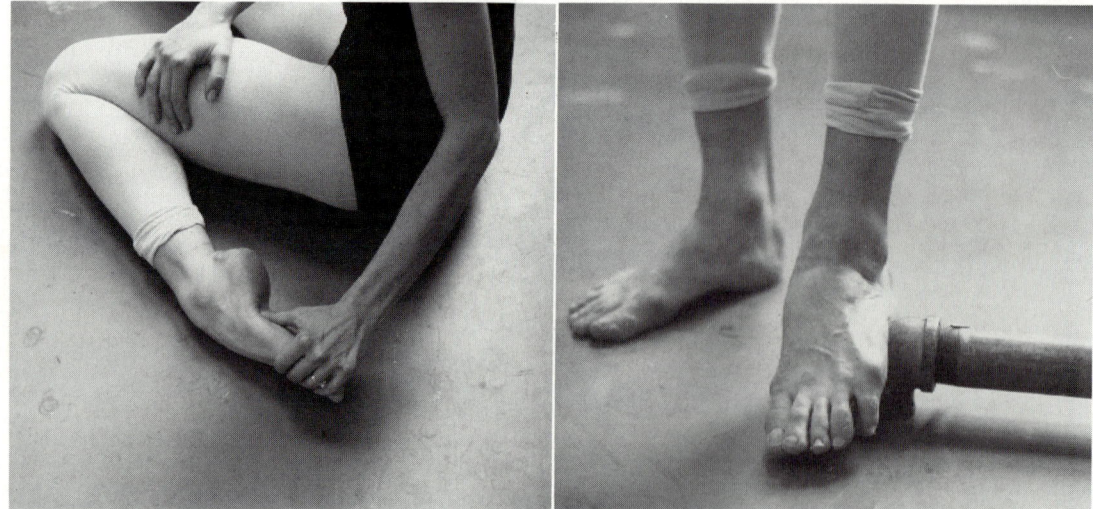

A   B

Figure 7 Self-mobilization techniques for cuboid subluxation. The dancer provides a reduction force via the cuboid squeeze (*A*) or by the base of the ballet barre (*B*). (From Marshall P, Hamilton WG. Cuboid subluxation in ballet dancers. Am J Sports Med 1992; 20:169–175; with permission.)

has been ruled out. A cautious reduction can then be attempted; however, the cuboid squeeze is not recommended if positioning the patient for the reduction is painful. Successful reduction should be maintained with tape as described previously. A recurrent subluxing cuboid following a lateral midfoot sprain may indicate that the affected joint capsule and ligaments have not healed adequately to maintain the reduction and repeated reductions should be avoided. A minimum of 2 and 3 days is recommended before attempting another reduction.

Dancers who present with chronically subluxing cuboids should be instructed in the self-mobilization techniques shown in Figure 7. These techniques are particularly successful in individuals who reduce easily when the cuboid squeeze is performed. It is imperative that dancers and physical therapists reduce chronically subluxing cuboids only when absolutely necessary in order to prevent further laxity.

Given the subjective nature of the diagnosis, if severe pain is present, one should obviously evaluate the foot for an acute fracture before manual reduction is attempted. In cases where cuboid subluxation is suspected but treatment is unsuccessful, other diagnosis should be considered:

- Unrecognized fracture or stress fracture.
- Subluxation of the talonavicular joint.
- Anterior impingement of the talocrural joint.
- Fracture of the anterior process of the calcaneus.
- Subtalar joint sprain.
- Sinus tarsi syndrome.
- Distal fibular hypomobility.

SUGGESTED READING

Hiss JM. Establishing a foot practice. J Am Osteopath Assoc 1928; 27:536–541.

Hiss JM. Functional foot disorders. Los Angeles: Oxford Press, 1949:295.

Marshall P. The rehabilitation of overuse foot and ankle injuries in athletes and dancers. Clin Sports Med 1988; 7:175–191.

Marshall P, Hamilton WG. Cuboid subluxation in ballet dancers. Am J Sports Med 1992; 20:169–175.

Newell SG, Woodie A. Cuboid syndrome. Phys Sports Med 1981; 9:71.

Taplin GC. Foot technique. J Am Osteopath Assoc 1928; 27:606–608.

TARSAL TUNNEL SYNDROME

DAVID L. JACKSON, M.D.
BRETT C. HYNNINEN, M.D.

Foot pain and paresthesias has been a topic of discussion in the literature for many years. However, it was not until 1962 that the identification of a specific tarsal tunnel syndrome was noted in the literature, by Keck in the United States and Lam in Great Britain. In Keck's description of bilateral tarsal tunnel syndrome in a boot camp army recruit, evidence of entrapment of the posterior tibial nerve (under the flexor retinaculum behind the medial malleolus) was documented at operative decompression.

Tarsal tunnel syndrome is not a common cause of foot pain in athletes, but if unrecognized it can result in prolonged discomfort and limited activity in these individuals. Endurance athletes (especially runners) are at increased risk for overuse injuries of the lower extremities. The foot and ankle is the second most common location for overuse injuries in runners with achilles tendinitis and plantar fasciitis the most common diagnoses. However, because of its location and vulnerability, the posterior tibial nerve in the tarsal tunnel is at risk for injury in these individuals and must be considered.

ANATOMY

The tarsal tunnel is a fibro-osseous tunnel, roughly comparable to the carpal tunnel, the floor of which is formed by the talus and calcaneus bones and the tibialis posterior, flexor digitorum longus, and the flexor hallucis longus muscles. The roof is formed by the flexor retinaculum, also known as the lancinate ligament, a fan-shaped thin sheet of fibrous tissue extending from the medial malleolus to the calcaneus and to the proximal border of the abductor hallucis muscle. Distally the tunnel is at its narrowest and blends into the superficial and deep fascia of the abductor hallucis muscle.

The tibial nerve is one of the two major divisions of the sciatic nerve. It travels inferior to the medial malleolus, anterior to the Achilles tendon, and through the tarsal tunnel, which, as previously described, is an inelastic, fixed space covered by the flexor retinaculum. At the distal end of the tarsal tunnel the tibial nerve branches. The actual location of these branches is variable although it is generally agreed that the branching takes place beneath the flexor retinaculum or soon after the nerve exits the tunnel. The medial calcaneal branch of the posterior tibial nerve arises beneath the flexor retinaculum or proximal to it, and exits at the distal edge of the flexor retinaculum (or pierces it) to supply the skin of the heel and portions of the calcaneus. The medial plantar nerve is the largest terminal branch of the posterior tibial nerve and runs superior to the abductor hallucis muscle belly supplying motor branches to the abductor hallucis, the flexor digitorum brevis, and the first lumbrical muscles; and, it supplies sensory cutaneous branches to the plantar aponeurosis, the sole of the foot and the first, second, third, and medial fourth toes (similar to the median nerve in the hand). The lateral plantar nerve branch courses obliquely forward between the third and fourth muscle layers of the foot, deep to the abductor hallucis and flexor digitorum muscles and superficial to the quadratus plantar muscle, emerging between the flexor digitorum brevis and abductor digiti minimi muscles. The lateral plantar branch of the posterior tibial nerve extends motor branches to the remaining muscles of the plantar aspect of the foot, superficial to the third plantar and fourth dorsal interosseous muscles and deep to the lateral two or three lumbrical and remaining interosseous and both heads of the adductor hallucis muscle. It also provides cutaneous sensory nerve branches to the lateral half of the fourth and fifth toes (similar to the ulnar nerve in the hand).

In general, entrapment of a nerve may occur anywhere the anatomic configuration allows compression of a nerve or continued inflammation after trauma. Any condition that promotes inflammation or compression at the level of the tarsal tunnel may result in tarsal tunnel syndrome due to the tunnel being particularly inelastic.

Although it may occur at any point from the proximal edge of the flexor retinaculum to the distal branchings of the nerve, most commonly entrapment occurs at the anterior, inferior aspect of the tarsal tunnel where the nerves wind around the medial malleolus. The lateral plantar nerve branch is more frequently affected than the medial plantar nerve branch.

Some authors limit the definition of the tarsal tunnel to that portion under the flexor retinaculum. The proximal and distal borders of the retinaculum, however, are often difficult to define as they blend proximally with the deep fascia of the leg and distally with the dorsal aponeurosis of the foot. With this broader definition of the tarsal tunnel, compressive lesions observed proximal to the flexor retinaculum, under the deep fascia of the leg, and, distally, under the abductor hallucis muscle may be considered as tarsal tunnel syndrome.

PATHOPHYSIOLOGY

Peripheral nerve injuries are most commonly related to ischemic changes either from compression or tension, with the sensory nerves more susceptible to injury than motor nerves. Since the posterior tibial nerve is confined in a fixed fibro-osseous tunnel, tarsal tunnel syndrome may occur when the contents of the tunnel are compressed either intrinsically or extrinsically. In addition, tarsal tunnel syndrome may occur when the cross-sectional area of the tunnel is compromised (e.g., in varus deformities of the ankle) or when the nerve is placed on tension (e.g., in valgus deformities of the ankle).

Intrinsic compression of the nerve may occur with any space occupying lesion within the tarsal tunnel. The most common reported in the literature include: ganglions, varicosities, lipomas, neurilemmomas, and a bony prominence associated with talocalcaneal coalition. Other factors listed in the literature are hypertrophic flexor retinaculum, hypertrophic or accessory abductor hallucis muscle, joint hypermobility, rapid weight gain or fluid retention, chronic thrombophlebitis, and proliferative synovitis (e.g., rheumatoid arthritis).

Systemic diseases also play a role in the development of tarsal tunnel syndrome with peripheral vascular diseases (especially venous insufficiency) and metabolic dysfunction (hyperuricemia, diabetes mellitus, hypothyroidism) being the most common. Frequently, in these situations, there is a condition referred to as "double crush." What this means is the nerve is initially damaged by the systemic effects of a disease (e.g., diabetes), the first insult or "crush," and subsequently the nerve is damaged again by local mechanical compression (e.g., tarsal tunnel syndrome) resulting in the second "crush." This is especially important to remember in athletes with systemic diseases that may affect the peripheral nervous system.

In the athletic population, foot and/or heel pain can be due to tarsal tunnel syndrome, but is most commonly related to soft-tissue overload, such as plantar fasciitis. Abnormal foot/ankle mechanics may place an athlete at risk for development of tarsal tunnel syndrome. The repetitive nature of running associated with abnormal or excessive pronation would place the posterior tibial nerve "on stretch" and at risk for injury. In fact, Rask described a condition he called "jogger's foot," in which excessive valgus or external rotation of the foot during running puts excessive stretch on the medial plantar nerve, resulting in tarsal tunnel syndrome. Henricson and Westlin presented a report of runners with chronic heel pain caused by compression or entrapment of the calcaneal branch of the posterior tibial nerve, all of whom responded well to surgical decompression. Tanz also described an entrapment syndrome of the calcaneal branch. He felt the pain was due to a dynamic compression of the nerve by the abductor hallucis muscle when stretched, as would occur with excessive pronation. The possibility of tenosynovitis of one of the tendons running through the tarsal tunnel (i.e., flexor hallucis longus, flexor digitorum longus or tibialis posterior) causing swelling and compression of the posterior tibial nerve must also be considered.

Other causes of tarsal tunnel syndrome in athletes include those related to cumulative trauma and acute direct trauma. Tight or ill-fitting boots (e.g., ski boots) can result in direct compression of the posterior tibial nerve at the level of the medial malleolus. Acute trauma, such as a severe medial ankle sprain or fracture, can result in immediate direct injury to this nerve. In fact, in one review of 87 cases of tarsal tunnel syndrome, trauma was the leading cause. The most commonly reported injuries were fractures, sprains, and surgical trauma.

Table 1 Signs and Symptoms of Tarsal Tunnel Syndrome

> Burning or tingling pain in the toes and foot
> Worsens at night or with walking (activity)
> Radiation of pain to the calf
> Weakness of toe flexion
> Loss of two-point sensory discrimination
> Tinel test may be positive at medial malleolus
> Pain may worsen with forced dorsiflexion and eversion

Table 2 Differential Diagnosis of Tarsal Tunnel Syndrome

> Plantar fasciitis
> Calcaneal stress fracture
> Foot sprain or strain
> Arthritis
> Peripheral vascular disease
> S_1-Radiculopathy

CLINICAL FINDINGS (TABLE 1)

The exact incidence of tarsal tunnel syndrome is unknown. In our experience, there seems to be a slight female predominance, which is supported by the literature. The history is very important as it may alert the clinician to a previous soft tissue injury, fracture, or systemic arthritis. In addition, most patients complain of intermittent dysesthesias or paresthesias that is worse with activity or at the end of the day. Patients may describe relief with removal of shoes, massage, elevation, and walking. Most athletes with tarsal tunnel syndrome complain of discomfort with activity.

In the classic description of tarsal tunnel syndrome by Lam and by Keck, symptoms include pain at the medial malleolus radiating to the sole of the foot, the heel, and the calf at times; paresthesias, dysesthesias, and hypesthesias; worsening of symptoms at night, with walking, or with dorsiflexion of the foot; weakness of toe flexion; increased fatigue of the foot; and trophic changes of the foot and nails. Since this description other symptoms have been noted including numbness and burning paresthesia on the plantar aspect of the foot and in the toes, which also may radiate up the leg. Sensory losses may occur in any of the three branches of the posterior tibial nerve in any combination. An early sign is felt to be loss of two point discrimination. Later signs are motor loss or paralysis and proximal radiations. Pain is often poorly localized but reproduced by tapping over the nerve, producing Tinel's sign. Tenderness distal or proximal to the area of entrapment may be present, and this is referred to as Valleix sign. Forced dorsiflexion and valgus of the ankle causing pain and palpable fusiform swelling over the course of the nerve may also be present. Symptoms may be intermittent initially but may become more constant over time. In addition to pain and sensory changes, weakness of the intrinsic musculature of the foot may be present but is, of course, difficult to evaluate and is a later finding than the sensory symptoms.

DIFFERENTIAL DIAGNOSIS

Tarsal tunnel syndrome is considered by some to be underdiagnosed. Its recent appearance and improved electrodiagnostic techniques and documentation have increased the frequency of diagnosis, although the actual incidence of the syndrome is not known. The diagnosis should be entertained in the differential of almost all infirmities of the foot and in some systemic illnesses presenting with symptoms in the foot as previously described (Table 2). Heel and foot pain may be due to plantar fasciitis as seen in runners, pressure on the medial anterior heel pad as from the shoe in soccer players, rheumatologic disease, ankylosing spondylitis, Reiter's disease, gout, or acute foot strain. Other possible causes of similar symptoms are interdigital neuroma, metatarsalgia, plantar callosities, longitudinal arch sprain, localized rheumatoid disease, sciatica, peripheral neuritis, peripheral vascular disease, and S_1 radiculopathy.

In order to accurately determine the etiology of pain or paresthesia in the foot it is important to consider the specific symptoms and presence of associated illnesses.

In the running athlete it is fairly easy to differentiate between plantar fasciitis and achilles tendinitis, but it may not be as easy to differentiate between tarsal tunnel syndrome and plantar fasciitis (Table 3).

In plantar fasciitis, symptoms start insidiously as a slow dull ache and may only be associated with running. Eventually the pain becomes sharp and well localized and worse when the area is cold or contracted, such as first getting up out of bed or first starting a run, with gradual improvement during the run.

The symptoms in tarsal tunnel syndrome are different but may be in the same location as plantar fasciitis. The pain usually starts as numbness or tingling sensation at the medial malleolus or heel and sole of the foot. This may worsen to a "burning" sensation with loss of sensation or weakness in the foot. The pain tends to be worse at night (especially if one has been standing all day or done a lot of running) and may radiate up the calf. There is less pain in the morning when one first gets out of bed, which is completely opposite of plantar fasciitis.

DIAGNOSTIC TESTS

Diagnosis of tarsal tunnel syndrome has most commonly relied upon history and physical examination. Electrodiagnostic studies can be helpful in confirming the diagnosis or excluding other diagnoses (e.g., radiculopathy), and plain radiographs should be obtained to rule out any bony abnormalities (degenerative changes, old fractures, bony spicules, and accessory ossicles) in the area. Recently, the use of magnetic resonance imaging (MRI) in the diagnosis and management of tarsal tunnel syndrome has been reported.

Electrodiagnostic studies are extremely important in the work-up of a patient with suspected tarsal tunnel syndrome as it may help confirm the diagnosis, rule out other diagnoses, and help determine prognosis. Initial electrodiagnostic criteria for tarsal tunnel syndrome

Table 3 Differentiating Signs and Symptoms in Tarsal Tunnel Syndrome and Plantar Fasciitis

Tarsal Tunnel Syndrome	Plantar Fasciitis
Paresthesias sole and toes	Medial calcaneal pain
Nocturnal pain	Morning pain
Radiation into calf	Point tender at origin
Sensory deficit	Loss of Gastroc-Soleus flexibility
Excessive pronation	Excessive pronation
Abnormal electrodiagnosis	Calcaneal spur on x-ray film

Table 4 Treatment of Tarsal Tunnel Syndrome

Rest
NSAIDs
Orthotics
Corticosteroid injection
Surgical decompression

were established by Goodgold and co-workers in 1965 for the medial and lateral plantar motor nerves. Johnson and Oritz in 1966 also reported the results of distal motor latencies in 100 normal patients and six patients with tarsal tunnel syndrome confirmed surgically. They felt that the distal motor latency was the most sensitive parameter and that the lateral plantar nerve was affected to a greater extent than the medial plantar nerve. Using the distal motor latency for the diagnosis of tarsal tunnel syndrome has unfortunately resulted in less than acceptable findings in the literature. Edwards and colleagues studied 19 patients with tarsal tunnel syndrome and only three had abnormal distal latencies. Linscheid and co-workers had electrodiagnostic data on 23 of 34 patients with tarsal tunnel syndrome and only 10 had increased motor latencies and eight had completely normal studies. It is felt that analysis of the distal motor latency of the medial and lateral plantar nerves is not adequate in the evaluation of tarsal tunnel syndrome.

In analysis of electrodiagnostic results in populations of patients with documented tarsal tunnel syndrome at operative decompression, sensory nerve conduction velocities were more likely to be abnormal than motor nerve conduction velocities at the level of mean $\pm$ 2 SD. In Oh's series, 52.4% or 11/21 cases had abnormal motor nerve conduction velocities. However, 90.5% or 19/21 patients exhibited abnormal sensory nerve conductions or absent potentials.

Electromyographic studies of the lower extremities must also be performed in the assessment of tarsal tunnel syndrome. Several studies have shown that frequently the motor conduction may be normal in the plantar nerves while the electromyelogram (EMG) reveals denervation of the tibial-innervated muscles in the foot. In addition, EMG findings in the muscles supplied by the tibial nerve above the tarsal tunnel would help differentiate between a radiculopathy, sciatic nerve entrapment, and tarsal tunnel syndrome. All patients being evaluated for tarsal tunnel syndrome must have a careful, needle examination study of the foot, leg, and back, in addition to nerve conduction studies. The presence of denervation potentials only in the distribution of the tibial nerve distal to the flexor retinaculum helps confirm the diagnosis of tarsal tunnel syndrome.

For purposes of diagnosis of tarsal tunnel syndrome, electrodiagnostic testing must include both motor and sensory studies of the medial and lateral plantar nerves, as well as needle EMG of the foot, leg, and back muscles.

MRI provides excellent detail of the bones, soft-tissue contents, and boundaries of the tarsal tunnel. It is most helpful in surgical planning by indicating the extent of decompression required. MRI is useful for localizing lesions in the tarsal tunnel, determining the lesions extent and its relationship to the posterior tibial nerve. We do not use MRI as a diagnostic study for tarsal tunnel syndrome as a good history and physical examination generally provides that for us. Regardless, one study showed abnormal findings on 88% of patients with a diagnosis of tarsal tunnel syndrome. Unfortunately, the same study found 25% of asymptomatic feet to have significant findings on MRI. Therefore, we reserve MRI of the tarsal tunnel for those patients with a questionable diagnosis or in operative candidates.

One additional diagnostic test for tarsal tunnel syndrome can also be therapeutic. A tarsal tunnel block with a mixture of lidocaine and a corticosteroid should bring immediate temporary relief of pain as well as some prolonged relief of symptoms.

TREATMENT

While the treatment of tarsal tunnel syndrome follows many of the same guidelines as for soft-tissue injuries (relative rest, ice, anti-inflammatories, flexibility, strengthening, and correction of biomechanical abnormalities), there are a couple of differences that will result in a more successful outcome (Table 4). Conservative management is generally considered to include treatment with a nonsteroidal anti-inflammatory agent, local steroid injection, and well-fitting shoes and orthotic devices to improve biomechanics and decrease inflammation. If conservative management fails to provide symptomatic relief, release of the flexor retinaculum and resection of connective tissue bridges where possible is suggested, with dissection of both plantar branches beyond the compression but retaining all muscles whole. Symptoms unrelieved by surgical release are felt to be due to insufficient release distal to the impingement. Repeat release is indicated in this instance. In the running athlete, abnormal foot mechanics appear to be the major etiologic factor in the development of tarsal tunnel syndrome. Therefore, unless the clinician addresses this aspect of treatment, correcting the excessive pronation, the condition will be difficult to control.

Corticosteroid injection into the tarsal tunnel can result in significant improvement in symptoms in many athletes. A mixture of 40 mg of methylprednisolone in 1% lidocaine or procaine is injected into the tunnel using a 25 gauge needle. We inject into the tunnel from above, about 1.5 cm proximal to the most prominent aspect of the medial malleolus. A distal injection can also be done.

SUGGESTED READING

Dellon AL, Mackinnon SE. Tibial nerve branching in the tarsal tunnel. Arch Neurol 1984; 41:645–646.

Edwards WG, Lincoln CR, Bassett FH, et al. The tarsal tunnel syndrome: Diagnosis and treatment. JAMA 1969; 207:77.

Frey C, Kerr R. Magnetic resonance imaging and the evaluation of tarsal tunnel syndrome. Foot Ankle 1993; 14:159–164.

Goodgold J, Kopell HP, Spielholz NI. The tarsal tunnel syndrome: Objective diagnostic criteria. N Engl J Med 1965; 273:742–745.

Grumbine NA, Radovic PA, Parsons R, Scheinin GS. Tarsal tunnel syndrome: Review of 87 cases. J Am Pod Med Assoc 1990; 9:457–461.

Henricson AS, Westlin NE. Chronic calcaneal pain in athletes: entrapment of the calcaneal nerve? Am J Sports Med 1984; 12:152–154.

Jackson DL, Haglund BL. Tarsal tunnel syndrome in athletes: Case reports and literature review. Am J Sports Med 1991; 19:61–65.

Johnson EW, Ortiz PR. Electrodiagnosis of tarsal tunnel syndrome. Arch Phys Med 1966; 47:776–780.

Keck C. The tarsal tunnel syndrome. J Bone Joint Surg 1962; 44A:180–182.

Kibler WB, Goldberg C, Chandler JT. Functional biomechanical deficits in running athletes with plantar fasciitis. Am J Sports Med 1991; 19:66–71.

Lam SJS. A tarsal tunnel syndrome. Lancet 1962; 2:1354–1355.

Linscheid RL, Burton RC, Fredericks EJ. Tarsal tunnel syndrome. South Med J 1970; 63:1313.

Oh SJ, Sarla PK, Kuba T, et al. Tarsal tunnel syndrome: Electrophysiological study. Ann Neurol 1979; 5:327–330.

Rask MR. Medial plantar neuropraxia (jogger's foot). Report of 3 cases. Clin Orthop 1978; 134:193–195.

Takakura Y, Kitada C, Sugimoto K, et al. Tarsal tunnel syndrome: Causes and results of operative treatment. J Bone Joint Surg 1991; 73B:125–128.

Tanz SS. Heel pain. Clin Orthop 1963; 28:169–178.

ORTHOTIC DEVICES: INDICATIONS

R. CHARLES BULL, M.D., B.Sc. (Med), F.R.C.S.(C), F.A.C.S., F.I.C.S.

Ortho is derived from the Greek word "orthos," denoting straight. Thus, orthotics means a pursuit of straightening or correcting. An orthotic device, or orthosis, is similar to a brace or splint, but connotes an attempt to limit, straighten, or assist the body in an alignment problem. Orthotic devices for the feet attempt to align the entire lower extremity structurally in order to take pressure off the foot, ankle, shin, knee, hip, and possibly back. The orthotist spends as much time trying to line up the knees and hips as he does correcting the abnormality of the feet. Thus, if he can line up the great toe, patella, and anterior superior spine and have uniform spacing between the ankles and knees, he feels successful. An attempt is made to toe out the foot slightly by 15 degrees. This is accomplished through the foot rather than through external rotation of the tibia, and a correction of the valgus or inturned heel is also attempted when the orthotic device is made. The exact location of the mechanical axis of the ankle corresponding to the subtalar joint, allowing for tibial torsion, is a key factor in fashioning orthoses.

These orthoses are basically inserts that can be interchanged from shoe to shoe, but more positive control is possible with caliper bracing, ankle joint stirrups, and spring-loaded rods with a ring attachment to the knee.

Orthoses can be prefabricated (ready-made off the shelf) or tailor-made. Most are made of plastic or a Neoprene type of material, although they have been made of metal, stainless steel and aluminum, hard plastic, hard and soft rubber, and stiffened felt components. Prices vary from a few dollars to as much as $400. The orthoses made by an orthotist under the direction of a physician and molded to the patient's foot at the time of fabrication are inexpensive and continue to be effective for at least 2 years. The podiatrist's orthoses are more sophisticated and more expensive, and they tend to be more effective in difficult cases. They are smaller and better fit the running shoe.

The ready-made orthotics from Spenko or Dr. Scholl (soft, rubbery-type material) can be satisfactory, although they usually are not. The more substantial plastic skeleton types are better, but do not naturally correct all types of foot abnormalities. The soft, tailor-made orthotic with Sorbothane or PVT tends to be a little bulky. It needs a deeper shoe to hold the orthosis and to keep the wearer from falling out of the shoe, but it usually does a very satisfactory job.

The podiatrist's orthosis made by Langer Laboratories of Deerpark, New York can be made from a casting of the runner's foot. The cast is made with care to maintain the foot in neutral position and align with the hind foot in a similar neutral position, with some pressure under the fourth and fifth metatarsal heads and the talonavicular joint. This creates a negative impression of the plantar surface of the foot; Langer then makes a positive plaster cast and fashions the plastic orthosis to that cast. An acrylic heel and anterior post are bonded to this case, and the initial pronation or longitudinal abnormality is corrected. More posting or correction can be done once the orthosis is fitted to the runner by the podiatrist.

We have compared video tapes of runners running with normal foot structure and pronated feet with tapes of runners wearing custom-made orthoses that (1) fit correctly, (2) are undercorrective, or (3) are overcorrective. It is difficult to draw an accurate conclusion from this type of study, but the correction of the pronation usually has to be very accurate or the running gait is made appreciably worse by an incorrect orthotic device.

The orthotic device is of most benefit for foot, ankle, and knee overuse problems such as fasciitis and tendinitis. We doubt that it does much for a true hip problem, and the effect on the back certainly is minuscule. Commonly the patient has pronated feet and valgus heels and knees.

Excess weight, poor running style, and inexperience all contribute to an altered footplant. The constant repetitive incorrect plant in running causes accumulated stress on the entire lower limb. Runners made up 58% of the patients receiving orthoses in our sports clinic.

It is important to see an abnormal wear pattern on the running shoe. I set the running shoe itself on a flat surface to see how much it is falling inward. The ideal running shoe should either be neutral or fall outward slightly if the runner plants properly.

I also have patients stand facing me with feet parallel and approximately 1 foot apart to see how much of an arch there is and then have them turn around to see how much valgus deformity there is to the heels. The Achilles tendon should be completely vertical when the patient is standing relaxed. Then the patient lies face down with heels out over the end of the bed and again the degree of valgus deformity is measured, and forefoot and rearfoot pronation are noted.

The mere presence of flat feet does not necessitate orthotic correction. There are hundreds of runners with flat feet and no symptoms, many of whom have won major races in the United States. It may be a racial or ethnic factor—most blacks and North American Indians tend to have flat feet, for instance. These people do not need correction unless they are having symptoms of overuse.

PLANTAR FASCIITIS

The plantar fascia is an inflexible band of tough tissue that is prone to inflammation where it originates from the calcaneus. The point is a central focus for maximal stress, and the inflammation often is localized.

Initial treatment with a felt pad or heel lift or with a Sorbothane heel lift is often beneficial, but if the patient has significant pronation that causes an increased stretching and strain on the plantar fascia, suitably designed orthoses probably help decrease the problem. Elevation of the heel in this type of correction distributes more of the forces toward the forefoot. Initially, we were taught that the pressures were distributed, with 50% of the force of walking or running taken in the heel, and then that the force fanned out, the hallux taking two units of force and each of the other four metatarsals taking one. This concept has changed as a result of biomechanical sensor studies. The consensus is that the heel actually takes more than 50% of the weight, and the load transfers down through the second and third metatarsals, leaving less weight or pressure on the first, fourth, and fifth metatarsal areas. Thus, the dynamics of correcting plantar fasciitis involve getting a lot of that weight off the heel or area of plantar fascia origin. These patients should be encouraged to wear their orthoses all day long. In difficult cases appropriate physiotherapy, medications, injections, and even surgery are indicated along with the orthosis.

ACHILLES TENDINITIS

This inflammation, which accounts for approximately 11% of all the running injuries seen in our clinic, is attributed to microtears in the tendon causing inflammation of the adjacent tendon structures (i.e., the vestigial sheath), which can become chronic and even calcifies in rare cases.

Initial treatment consists of rest, cycling, and swimming (but no running); anti-inflammatory agents; and elevation of the heel with felt or Sorbothane pads. The wearing of moderately high heels, such as cowboy boots, may help by (1) causing relative shortening of the Achilles tendon, (2) causing absorption of forces transmitted to the tendon, and (3) resting the tendon and allowing the microtears to heal.

Varus deformities of the feet have been recognized in runners by the use of high-speed films. The average runner lands on the outer heel, and the forces transfer to the outer side of the foot through the midstance phase. If he or she overpronates through this phase, the Achilles undergoes a "whip-like" action in its sequence. Obviously this initiates, aggravates, and perpetuates the tendinitis. Orthotic correction reduces this type of motion. The gait has more of a light productive force, and less stress is transferred to the Achilles.

Once the tendinitis has subsided, the tendon is stretched and the gastrocnemius-soleus complex is strengthened. With this additional strength and flexibility, the runner should be able to plant better and, after a year or two, dispense with the orthosis. I want to emphasize that many orthoses can be used temporarily. At least 6 months is required to settle an acute problem, and many people improve their running style, strength, and flexibility and thus can dispense with the orthosis after a year or two. This is particularly true in the mature, high-quality runner who has functioned for years without injury; the orthotic device can be used on a temporary basis, and eventually a shoe with a good support, especially a strong heel support, will suffice.

TIB POSTERIOR TENDINITIS

This inflammation occurs at the junction of the posterior tibial muscle and tendon in the midportion of the medial aspect of the leg. It is the most common type of "shin splint" and its most likely cause is "pronated feet." "Shin splints" or inflammation of the shin area (common in runners) can occur in the tib posterior or the periosteum overlying the free tibial border (the classic location), or in the anterior (lateral) compartment. All three types usually benefit from the use of orthotics.

The muscle functions to help maintain the arch of the foot and to supinate the foot so that it can roll out after footplant. A pronated foot stretches the tendon and muscles, and as the foot pronates through the midstance phase an increased force is transmitted to the musculotendinous junction and into the muscle origin along the tibia. Microtears result and create inflammation (tendinitis).

An orthotic device shortens the muscle tendon complex and lessens the need to maintain the arch and supinate the foot. Thus, there is less strain as the foot pronates through the midphase of the running motion. Correction of foot pronation is probably the most important step in relieving the initial inflammation and preventing recurrence. In some cases, if it is left uncorrected, the condition progresses to periostitis, a compartment syndrome, or even a stress fracture.

PATELLOFEMORAL SYNDROME

This is the most common problem seen in our sports clinic. The etiology, reason for pain, management, response to treatment, and long-term sequelae are all controversial.

The most realistic cause is a "malalignment phenomenon." The patella travels in the femoral groove, and as the knee flexes beyond 135 degrees or a quarter squat, the compression between surfaces increases.

Ideally the patella tracks symmetrically, but in chondromalacia there appears to be asymmetry. This causes abnormal wear and tear on the patellar surface and thus a softening or roughening, which is manifested clinically by a grating when the patella is moved on the femoral surface. This situation is particularly uncomfortable when the patella is held against a strong quads contraction. What is incomprehensible is that some of the worst clinical cases exhibit minimal signs arthroscopically. Other clinical signs are a widened Q angle, noticeable infacing or squinting of the patella, a broad pelvis, femoral anteversion, genu valgus, external tibial rotation, and pronated feet. A correction of the pronated feet by an orthosis will alter the alignment of the leg. This is relative, similar to eyeglasses correcting shortsightedness. Basically, the malalignment returns when the orthoses are not used. Thus, tracking is more efficient, causes less irritation on the patellar articular surface, and thereby reduces the pain. Adjunctive treatment includes vastus medialis strengthening and the use of a knee brace for patellar stabilization.

OTHER KNEE PROBLEMS

Pes tendinitis is an inflammation of the pes, which is a confluence of three tendons on the medial aspect of the knee. Because these tendons mesh together so congruently at the knee, they are relatively prone to tendinitis, particularly in the presence of genu valgus. An orthotic device tends to transfer the forces laterally and take the pressure off this medial compartment of the knee. Conversely, iliotibial band and popliteus tendinitis are helped by a lateral wedge, which eases the lateral forces

in the knee. In many cases, an orthotic device makes this type of problem worse.

VAGUE KNEE PAINS

The best treatment for fat pad syndrome, synovitis, plicae, internal derangement of the knee (IDK), and patellar tendinitis is alteration of the running schedule, i.e., decreased hills, decreased speed, new shoes, quadriceps-hamstring exercises to correct an imbalance, increased flexibility, and anti-inflammatory medications.

In a resistant case it is worthwhile to watch patients run. If they tend to pronate, throw their feet in or out, or have a heavy wide-track Pontiac style, orthoses may help. It is hard to correct the running style in a master athlete. The orthotic devices alter the style subtly and thereby help to decrease the problem.

CAVUS FOOT

This is almost a contraindication to running. The relatively spastic, high-arched foot is very uncomfortable with ordinary walking. It can become unbearable with running. An orthotic device can cushion the impact but usually cannot create a good mobile running foot.

SUCCESS RATE AND COMPLIANCE

In our study of soft orthotic devices in which 100 patients were reviewed after 1 year, 89% felt that the orthoses were of definite benefit; 38% limited the use of their orthoses to sports shoes only, while the rest used them in all their shoes; 21% stopped using them because the problem had been solved; 69% were still using them after 1 year; 10% stopped using them because they were of no benefit; and 47% returned for a check of their orthoses. It is important to check these at 3 or 4 weeks and again after 3 or 4 months to ascertain that correction is satisfactory. Minor adjustments can make the world of difference in their use. In the same series, 9% sought the advice of a podiatrist after receiving their orthoses. Probably 10% to 20% of runners use orthotic devices. We have prescribed over a thousand in the past 10 years. We wanted to know (1) whether this was necessary and (2) whether the patient used them. In our series, 69% of the 100 patients still used them after 1 year, and 21% discarded them because their problem was solved. Thus, we feel orthoses have been beneficial.

Soft orthotic devices are much less expensive than those prescribed by the podiatrist and can be more comfortable. We believe they can be used on a long-term basis to correct a biomechanical problem.

Studies of the hard orthotics prescribed by the podiatrist often cannot delineate a correction of pronation when the runner is filmed or studied biomechanically. However, orthotic devices do work. Podiatrists have been a definite boon to the runner, often eliminating the pain experienced in running. Obviously, the development of quality running shoes has also helped to prevent running injuries.

Orthotics can be applied to other sports. Certainly the use of orthoses in ski boots has been helpful in some cases. Ski boots can also be canted extrinsically to correct a pronated foot. This basically serves the same purpose as an orthosis. Most stop-and-start sports, such as squash and tennis, do not require an orthosis, as the unremitting footplant that occurs in running creates a more serious problem. Thus, orthotic devices are used in racquet sports, but are not as necessary or popular.

The principle of orthosis construction, patient selection, and the biomechanical studies of different sports will change markedly in the next few years. Orthotic devices can be beneficial for specific problems, but should be used in conjunction with other methods of treatment. Certainly, strengthening programs for the entire lower limb should be instituted when the orthoses are prescribed. In my experience, careful patient selection is the key to proper orthosis use. If patients are made aware of the exact indications for orthoses and are observed closely and instructed in their use, the vast majority should improve. It is only the rare patient with a cavus foot, for instance, who continues to have disability after using the orthoses and cannot tolerate them. Old-time runners from the 1950s and 1960s, who had one pair of shoes that they discarded when the sole fell off, were guaranteed to have blisters, missing toenails, and general aches and pains, which they did not acknowledge to anyone. Modern runners complain if the workout is less than 100%. They make use of sports clinics, podiatrists, orthoses, and coaches, and probably run a lot longer, farther, and faster in comfort. In many cases this is because of the use of orthotic devices.

ORTHOTIC DEVICES: FABRICATION

JOSEPH S. TORG, M.D.

Overuse injuries involving either the feet or other areas of the lower extremities can often be effectively treated with orthotic devices. Orthotics can correct "biomechanical abnormalities" that, when combined with overtraining, create excessive or unusual stress on various weight-bearing structures.

The purpose of these devices is to place the subtalar joint in its neutral position during the midsupport phase of the running cycle. This usually consists of maintaining both the forefoot-heel alignment and the leg-heel alignment. Forefoot-heel alignment is normal when the forefoot, at the metatarsal level, is perpendicular to the heel. Leg-heel alignment is present when the subtalar joint is in neutral and the heel is parallel to the distal one-third of the leg.

When these alignments are not "normal," the variations can cause stress on various parts of the musculoskeletal system. If the plane of the forefoot shifts so that the medial side lifts above the neutral plane, supination, or varus (inversion, abduction, and plantar flexion), is observed. Pronation, or valgus (eversion, adduction, and dorsiflexion), occurs when the medial side drops below the neutral plane. Pronation and supination can stress structures of the foot as well as those of the lower leg and knee.

Orthotics are indicated for the treatment of symptomatic pronation, plantar fasciitis, "runner's knee" (chondromalacia), popliteal tendinitis, posterior tibial tendinitis, "shin splints," and Achilles tendinitis.

Plantar fasciitis is an example of injury to the foot caused by either abnormal pronation or supination. In the case of excessive pronation or pes planus, the plantar aponeurosis stretches and causes fascial strain. Orthotics will correct this. For pes cavus, orthotics alleviate the "windlass" effect in which the fascia is tight and there is strain on the calcaneal insertion. If untreated, the stress on plantar fascia can lead to the formation of calcaneal bone spur. Orthotics serve to maintain the subtalar joint in neutral and the midtarsal joint in stable pronated position.

Abnormal pronation is also a contributing factor to the development of "runner's knee." With this injury the relationship between a biomechanical problem in the

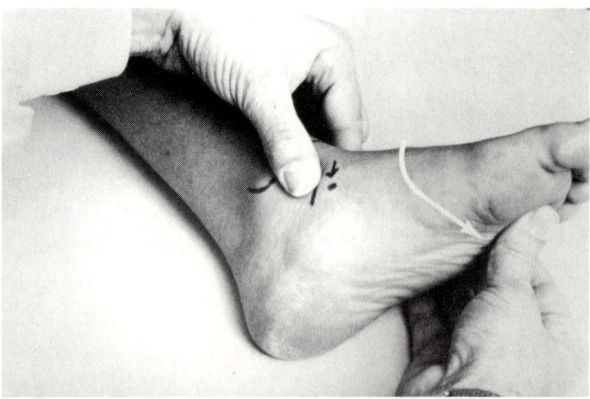

Figure 1 Positive casting for running orthotics should be taken with the subtalar joint in a neutral position; i.e., no eversion and no inversion should be present. Presumably, this is determined by ascertaining talonavicular joint congruity. This is done by palpating the medial and dorsolateral aspects of the talonavicular joint with the thumb and forefinger of one hand, then supporting the forefoot in a neutral position with pressure under the fourth and fifth metatarsal heads as demonstrated.

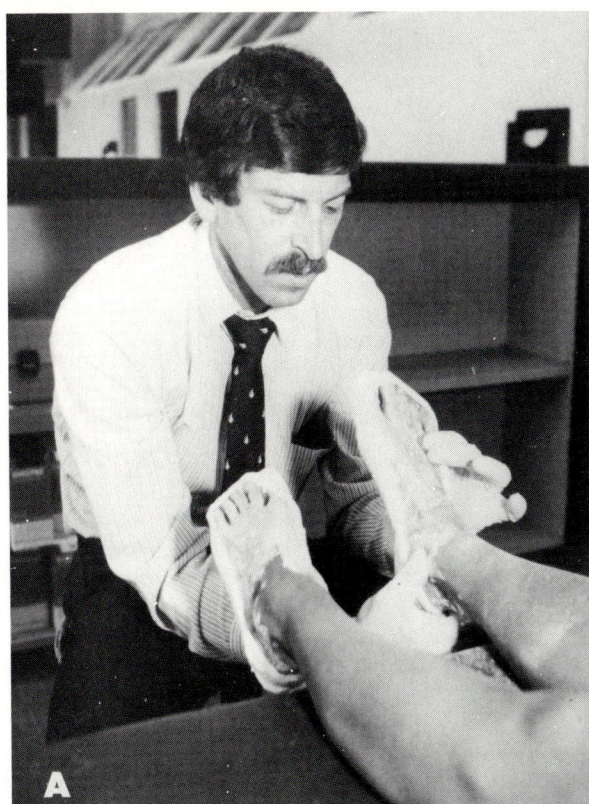
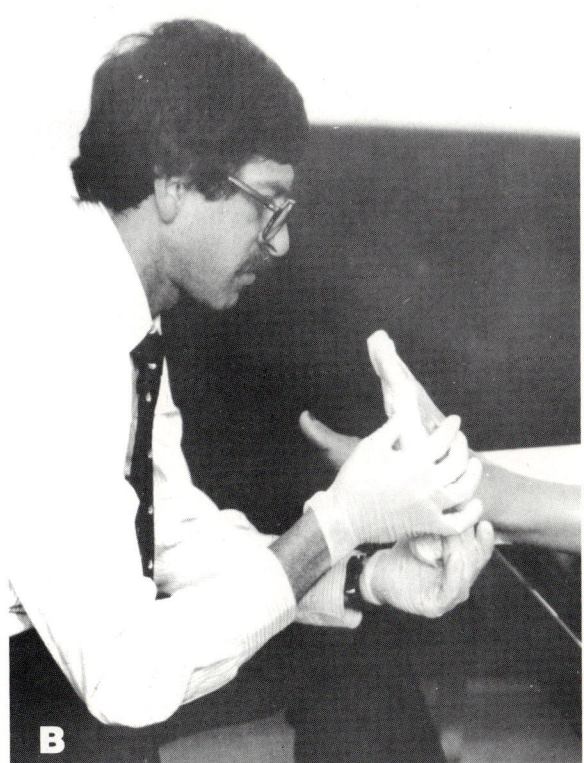

Figure 2 *A,* Casting for runner's orthotics necessitates palpating the talonavicular joint and maintaining it in a neutral position. *B,* With congruity of the talonavicular joint, the forefoot is maintained in a neutral relationship with the hindfoot by exerting pressure under the fourth and fifth metatarsal heads.

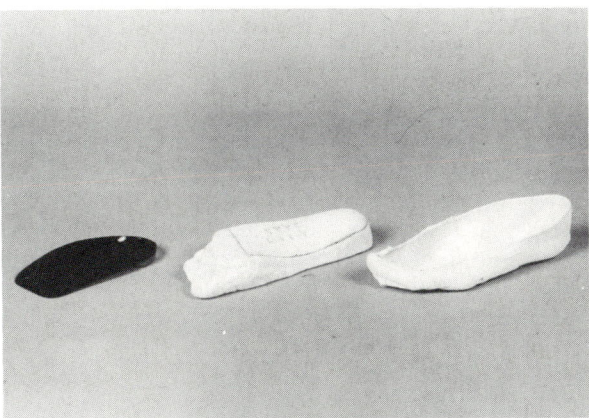

Figure 3 From the positive casting (*right*), a negative impression of the plantar surface of the foot is obtained (*center*). From this an acrylic rigid orthosis is fabricated (*left*).

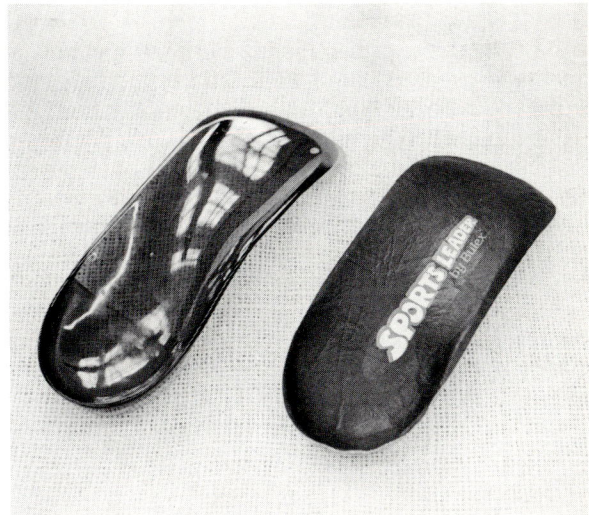

Figure 4 A rigid orthotic (*left*) is used primarily in non-athletic footwear. The sport orthotic (*right*) is more flexible and used for athletic participation.

foot and an injury elsewhere in the body is evident. The patellofemoral joint receives an unusual amount of stress when, owing to abnormal pronation in the foot, there is excessive internal rotation of the entire leg. Lateral displacement of the patella can occur and chondromalacia develops.

A similar scenario is observed in the case of popliteal tendinitis. Hyperpronation causes excessive internal rotation, which stresses the lateral compartment of the knee and the femoral attachment of the popliteal tendon.

A fourth injury resulting from excessive pronation is posterior tibial tendinitis. Krissoff located the pain characterizing this injury behind the medial malleolus

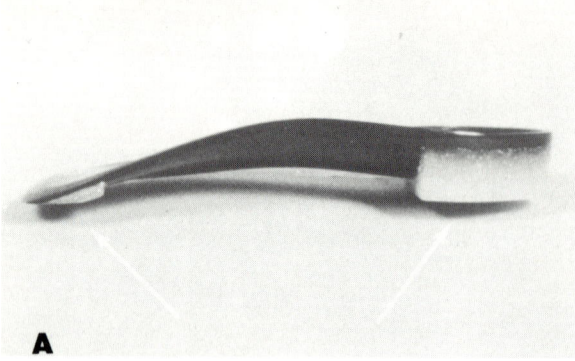 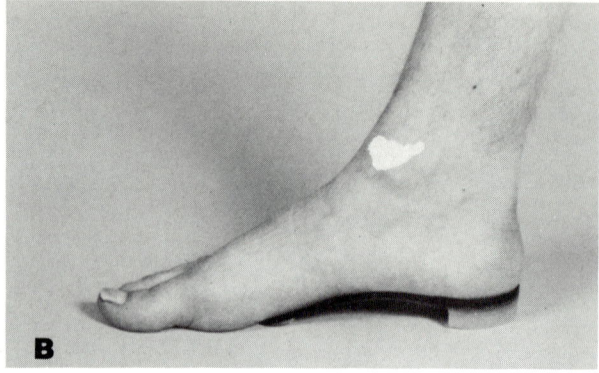

Figure 5 *A,* Viewed from the medial aspect, an anterior and heel post is bonded to the acrylic member. *B,* The runner's orthotic serves two functions: it presumably maintains the subtalar joint in a neutral posture, and it provides support for the medial longitudinal arch.

and on the posterior medial border of the tibia. Orthotics are the most effective means of treating this injury.

Anterior and posterior "shin splints" develop when various muscles in the leg become overused through attempts to compensate for biomechanical problems. In the case of anterior shin splints the tibialis anterior can be overused if there is forefoot imbalance. This muscle works as a decelerator during heel strike and prevents "heel slap" during the midstance phase. Abnormal pronation can place excessive demands on the posterior tibial longus, flexor digitorum longus, and flexor hallucis longus units, and posterior shin splints can develop. Fatigue tears of the fibers of the tibialis posterior muscle at its insertion into the periosteum of the tibia are common.

Stress reactions and stress fractures are other overuse injuries in which biomechanical difficulties are contributory factors. Supination can lead to tibial stress fractures, and pronation to fibular stress fractures.

Orthotics can also be used to treat Achilles tendinitis. Smart reviewed the etiologic mechanism involved in this condition. The biomechanical factor designated is also that of prolonged pronation. Slow-motion, high-speed cinematography has enabled researchers to identify a whipping action or bowstring effect of the Achilles tendon produced by prolonged pronation, which could possibly lead to microtears. It is speculated that degenerative changes of the tendon are related to torsional forces transmitted through the tendon during pronation. Orthotics work to shorten the phase of pronation during the support phase of running.

A variety of ready-made arch supports are available in shoe stores and sporting goods stores. However, the erudite and sophisticated runners of today usually settle for nothing less than a pair of custom orthotic devices, which cost approximately $275 for their prescription and fabrication.

The semirigid and rigid runner's orthosis requires positive plaster casting or mold of the patient's foot taken with the subtalar joint in neutral position. Presumably, this occurs when the talonavicular joint and forefoot are also in a neutral relationship; i.e., no eversion and no inversion should be present (Figs. 1 and 2). Leg-heel and forefoot-heel alignments, described previously, should also be assessed, and corrections for any deviations from neutral made. The plaster positive mold is then sent to the orthotic laboratory. From the positive casting, a negative impression of the configuration of the plantar surface is obtained. From this, an acrylic rigid orthosis is fabricated (Figs. 3 and 4). The orthosis, in addition to providing rigid support for the medial arch and midfoot, is "posted" anteriorly and posteriorly in such a manner as to support the subtalar joint in a neutral position (Fig. 5).

ACUTE TEAR OF THE MEDIAL HEAD OF THE GASTROCNEMIUS

CLARENCE L. SHIELDS, Jr., M.D.
L.T. JOHNSON, M.D.

DIAGNOSIS

Acute tears of the medial head of the gastrocnemius typically occur in middle-aged individuals, although tears have occurred in the third decade. Patients frequently describe a sudden, sharp pain and a feeling of having been hit in the calf by an object or by another person. While the pain initially seems relatively innocuous, it quickly becomes more severe with tenderness and swelling. Over the next several hours to days, discoloration may occur. Some patients report a prodrome of dull pain for several weeks prior to the acute tear. Patients have a palpable defect at the tear site within 2 weeks of the injury. Patients are typically unable to perform a single-legged toe raise. The patients deny any numbness or tingling. The foot is held in equinus and patients have pain on passive and active dorsiflexion of the ankle.

Acute rupture of the medial head of the gastrocnemius is sufficiently rare to cause confusion to the examiner who sees an occasional athletic injury. Such disorders as thrombophlebitis, acute vascular occlusion, compartment syndrome, popliteal cyst rupture, cellulitis, direct blunt trauma, and popliteal artery aneurysm are among the more commonly confused entities. Thrombophlebitis demands early assessment and decision making. Ultrasonic venography is a noninvasive method of determination and, when confusion subsequently continues to exist, an intravenous contrast venogram remains the gold standard. Both tests can be done on an out-patient basis.

Compartment syndrome can accompany the acute rupture and surgical decompression is done on an emergency basis. Vascular compression conditions are frequently secondary to the anomalous conditions affecting the gastrocnemius and/or the popliteal vessels. A history of intermittent claudication can help rule out vascular compression syndromes. Acute symptoms of a giant popliteal cyst, such as might be seen in a patient with rheumatoid arthritis, are diagnosed by history and an ultrasonic study of soft tissues should help establish continuity of the gastrocnemius. The diagnosis of such disorders as acute hemorrhage in bleeding diatheses, direct blunt trauma, cellulitis, and referred neurogenic pain and acute vascular embolization are aided by an appropriate history and physical examination. Popliteal aneurysm is a rare consideration.

ANATOMY

The gastrocnemius, which is the most superficial of the posterior crural muscles, has two heads. The two heads arise from the posterior capsule of the knee and also the femoral condyles. Embryologically the medial head migrates from the lateral femoral condyle to the medial femoral condyle. After this migration, the fibers of the medial head and belly tend to go in a more oblique than vertical direction while the lateral fibers are more vertically oriented with only a slight oblique angulation. The lateral head is usually smaller and arises from the lateral femoral condyle slightly inferior to the medial head origin. The muscle bellies merge into a broad aponeurosis that tapers and unites with the soleus tendon to form the Achilles tendon. The blood supply is derived from the sural branches of the popliteal artery and the nerve is from the tibial nerve, termed S_1 and S_2.

ETIOLOGY

In considering the cause of these ruptures, it is helpful to understand the biomechanics of the musculotendinous junction. Tensile strength of the muscle is less than 50% of the tensile strength of the tendon. In fact, more than 50% of a healthy tendon must be severed for contraction of the associated muscle to cause tendon rupture. Diseased, atrophied, and injured musculotendinous units are more likely to rupture with little force. Even well-trained musculotendinous junctions will rupture under appropriately severe loads. Severe opposing forces applied to a muscle tendon junction while the muscle contraction is eccentric, places the junction at risk. Since the gastrocnemius muscle crosses two joints, the combination of hyperextension of the knee and dorsiflexion of the ankle can lead to failure. The medial head is more prone to rupture because of its larger size and more oblique fiber orientation.

PREFERRED TREATMENT

Once the diagnosis is confirmed and more serious differential diagnoses are eliminated, the patient is encouraged to elevate the affected limb to decrease swelling as often as necessary and to use ice decrease hemorrhage. Crutches combined with a short leg cast splint may be required for severe cases of swelling and muscle spasm. A snug fitting uniform circumferential pressure bandage is applied using an ACE wrap or Neoprene sleeve. This helps decrease bleeding and is comfortable. A 10-day course of oral, nonsteroidal anti-inflammatory drug is prescribed if there are no medical contraindications. Muscle relaxants and oral analgesics may be helpful. A one-half inch felt pad is placed in the heel of the shoe to relax the injured muscle.

Early functional rehabilitation can begin after 72 hours when acute bleeding has stopped. Hot and cold contrast baths are added. The patient is then encouraged to begin passive towel stretching of the posterior calf musculature with the knee extended in order to help decrease stiffness and contracture. Isometric ankle dorsiflexion and plantar flexion exercises are also initiated. These are performed to tolerance. At approximately 2 weeks, the patient begins to perform standing stretch maneuvers. The patient then begins active resistive exercises against an elastic band with dorsiflexion and plantar flexion. These are advanced as tolerated to toe raises with weight. The patient can expect a full strength return in 4 to 6 weeks. An isokinetic evaluation of plantarflexion strength is useful to gauge the restoration of the muscle unit.

PREVENTION

In most instances the injury occurs at an age of declining physiologic resilience. Stiffness of joints and less than completely supple soft tissues are common. All athletes, professional and recreational, require longer periods of warm up and stretching with advancing years. Maintenance of good lower extremity strength, including toe raises with weight, and agility along with proper activity-specific training techniques is important. Conditioning to the requirements of the activity can be expected to decrease the incidence of injury.

SUGGESTED READING

Arner O, Lindholm A. What is tennis leg? Acta Chir Scand 1958; 116:73–75.
Anouchi YS, Parker RD, Seitz WH. Posterior compartment syndrome of the calf resulting from misdiagnosis of a rupture of the medial head of the gastrocnemius. J Trauma 1987; 27:678–680.
Durig M, Schuppisser JP, Gauer EF, Miller W. Spontaneous rupture of the gastrocnemius muscle. Br J Accident Surgery 1977; 9:143–145.
Fleiss DJ. To the editor—correspondence. J Bone Joint Surg 1992; 74:792.
Froimson AI. Tennis leg. JAMA 1969; 209:415–416.
McClure JG. Gastrocnemius musculotendinous rupture: A condition confused with thrombophlebitis. South Med J 1984; 77:1143–1145.
McMaster PE. Tendon and muscle ruptures. J Bone Joint Surg 1933; 15:705–722.
Menz MJ, Lucas GL. Magnetic resonance imaging of a rupture of the medial head of the gastrocnemius muscle. J Bone Joint Surg 1991; 73:1260–1262.
Miller WA. Rupture of the musculotendinous juncture of the medial head of the gastrocnemius muscle. Am J Sports Med 1977; 5:191.
Perri JA, Rodnan GP, Maukin HJ. Giant synovial cysts of the calf in patients with rheumatoid arthritis. J Bone Joint Surg 1968; 50:709–719.
Shields Jr CL, Redix L, Brewster CE. Acute tears of the gastrocnemius. Foot Ankle 1985; 5:186–190.
Smith MJ. Muscle fiber types. Orthop Clin North Am 1983; 14:403–411.
Strackley D, Jones WW. Acute compartment syndrome (anterior, lateral and superficial posterior) following tear of the medial head of the gastrocnemius muscle. Am J Sports Med 1986; 14:96–99.
Sutro CJ, Sutro WH. The medial head of the gastrocnemius: A review of the basis for partial rupture and for intermittent claudication. Bull Hosp Jt Dis 1985; 45:150–157.
Zarins B, Ciullo JV. Acute muscle and tendon injuries in athletes. Clin Sports Med 1983; 2:167–182.
Zarins B, Ciullo JV. Biomechanics of the musculotendinous unit: Relation to athletic performance and injuries. Clin Sports Med 1983; 2:71–86.

STRESS FRACTURE OF THE ANTERIOR TIBIAL DIAPHYSIS

RODNEY K. BEALS, M.D.

Stress fractures of the anterior tibial diaphysis are an uncommon but important cause of tibial pain in athletes because they do not heal promptly or surely with rest. Seventeen percent of all stress fractures occur in the tibia. Only 5% of these are anterior stress fractures.

This entity was described in 1956 by Jackson Burrows who observed a "fatigue infraction of the middle of the tibia" in four ballet dancers. He considered the infraction to be caused by leaping and to be an incomplete fracture due to tension stress on the convex anterior surface of the tibia. His concept of the pathogenesis is supported by the subsequent observations that most affected patients are high-performance leaping athletes and that stress on the anterior tibial cortex during running is known to be a tension stress.

The diagnosis is based on an appropriate history, physical, and radiographic findings. The pain is localized over the anterior middle-third of the tibia. Patients are often mildly symptomatic for months before seeking medical attention. The pain is aggravated by use and improved with rest. There may be a palpable and tender swelling of the anterior tibia.

Radiographs demonstrate a transverse fissure in an hypertrophied anterior tibial cortex (Fig. 1). The defect is usually a single cleft but there may be multiple small clefts and it may be bilateral especially in runners (Fig. 2). When typical symptoms, signs, and radiographic findings are present, further diagnostic studies are not required. Occasionally a bone scan showing localized increased update will help establish the diagnosis or differentiate it from shin splints. A tomogram will occasionally be required to demonstrate the cleft. The pathology shows fibrous tissue in the cleft and often demonstrates nonviable cells in the adjacent bone. This is in contrast to most stress fractures that demonstrate active remodelling of laminar bone.

A complete mid-tibial fracture that occurs without major trauma in a leaping athlete may be the first presentation of a tibial stress fracture. A clue to diagnosis may be the fracture pattern, which is an anterior transverse fracture with an oblique or butterfly extension posteriorly. A retrospective history of pain

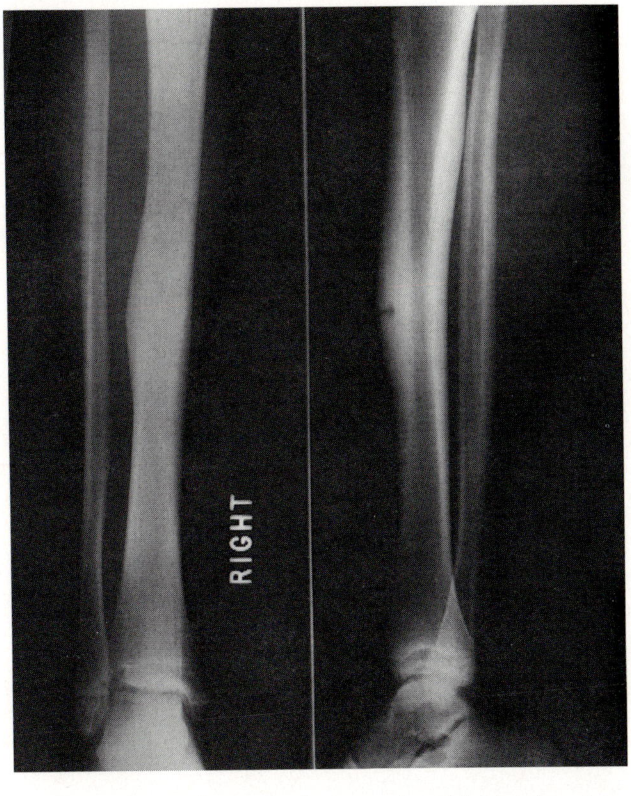

![Figure 1 radiograph showing RIGHT]

Figure 1 The radiograph of an anterior tibial tension stress fracture in a gymnast demonstrates the classic thick anterior cortex and transverse cleft. (From Beals RK, Cook RD. Stress fractures of the anterior tibial diaphysis. Orthopedics 1991; 14:869–875; with permission.)

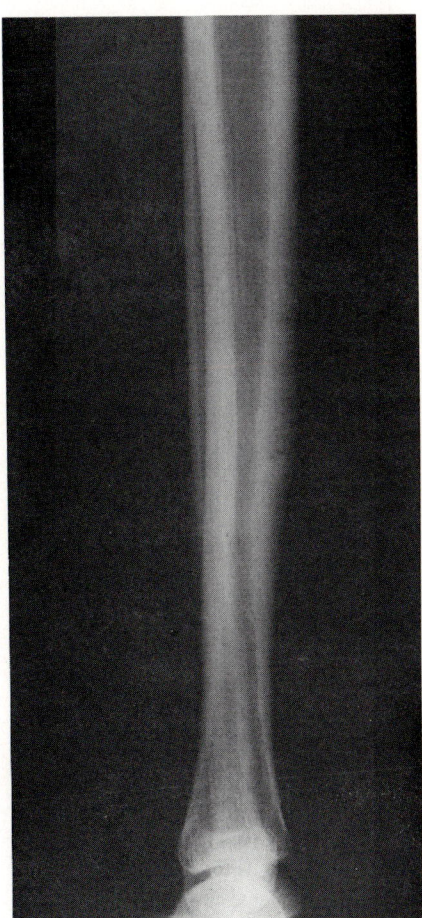

Figure 2 The radiograph of a runner with anterior tension stress fracture demonstrates a thickening of the anterior cortex, a cleft traversing half of the cortex, and the residue of multiple healed clefts.

with activity, a thick anterior tibial cortex, and additional transverse stress fissures may confirm the diagnosis.

The differential diagnosis includes compression stress fractures, which are usually on the posterior cortex, intracortical bone abscess (Brodie's abscess), Garre's sclerosing osteomyelitis, or metaphyseal osteomyelitis. It also includes Paget's disease, osteogenic sarcoma, and especially osteoid osteoma. Although both osteoid osteoma and tension stress fractures are common in young males, the quality of pain, relation to activity, and radiographic features should distinguish stress fractures from osteoid osteoma. Tension stress fractures exhibit pain proportional to activity. The cleft of a stress fracture is at right angle to the cortex at the site of maximum thickness, may be multiple, and may be bilateral. Osteoid osteoma is characterized by pain not related to activity and by the presence of an oval or round lucent nidus and surrounding increased bone

density and classic histologic features. When osteogenic sarcoma is a diagnostic consideration, a computed tomography scan is helpful as stress fractures usually involve the medullary canal and osteogenic sarcoma usually does not.

A review of 46 patients with anterior tibial stress fracture revealed that most were young, many were professional athletes, and that males predominated (39/46). The sport most often involves leaping, basketball being by far the most common (Table 1).

The untreated natural history is not precisely known. Of eight affected patients who were allowed full activity, five incurred a complete fracture. When this type of stress fracture was treated by modified activity in 20 patients, only eight (38%) were able to return to full activity after 1 to 14 months of modified activity. It is clear that these fractures do not heal promptly with rest.

Table 1 Etiology of Anterior Tibial Stress Fracture in 46 Patients

Sport	No. of Cases
Basketball	20
Track and Field	8
Ballet	6
Football	3
Other	5
Unknown	4
Total	46

TREATMENT

It is reasonable to assume that all anterior tibial stress fractures occurring in normal individuals will heal spontaneously if rest is enforced and prolonged. There may be circumstances where this is the preferred treatment. Because those affected are often high-performance athletes who are in a narrow window of opportunity for their sports, prolonged rest with uncertain results is often not desirable.

For those with persistent symptoms associated with the typical tibial defect the recommended treatment is

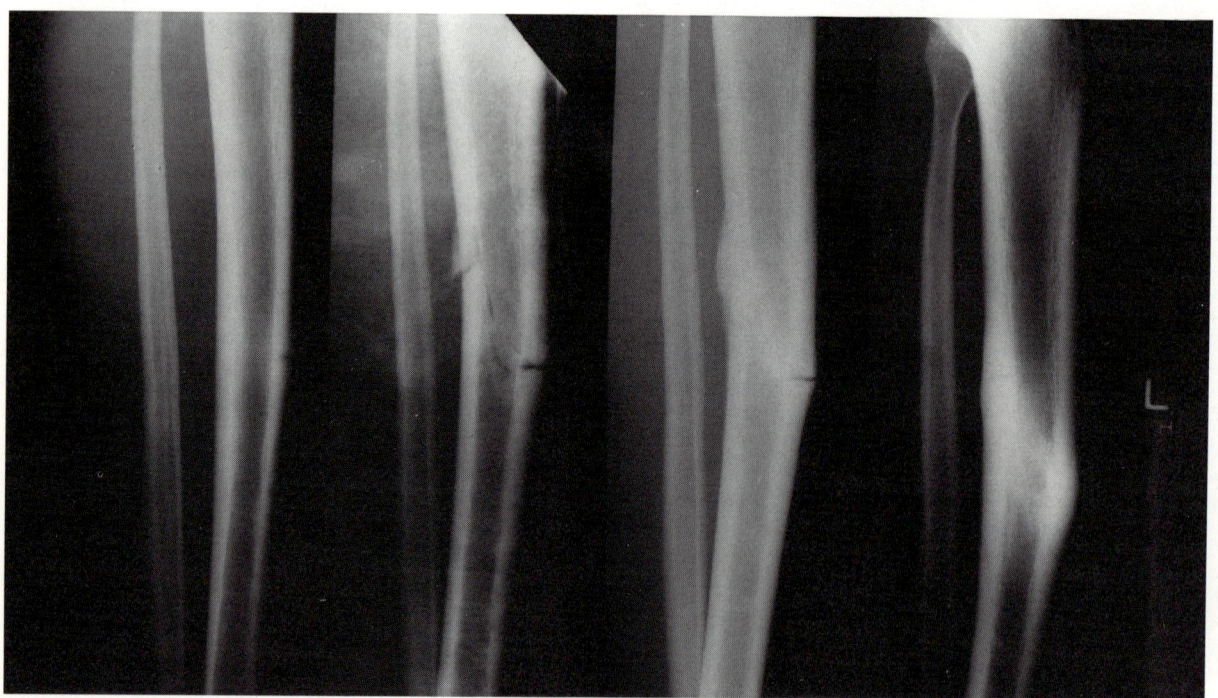

Figure 3 Radiographs of a complete fracture of the tibia in a patient with anterior tension stress fracture treated in a cast demonstrates normal fracture healing with an increased anterior bow and persistence of the tension stress fracture. (From Beals, RK, Cook RD. Stress fractures of the anterior tibial diaphysis. Orthopedics 1991; 14:869–875; with permission.)

excision of the debris in the fissure, multiple transverse drilling of the bone, and cancellous graft in and around the defect. Following this procedure professional athletes have been able to return to their sport in as soon as 4 months. The criteria to return to full activity whether treated nonoperatively or surgically should include resolution of the defect as well as pain relief. Review of the literature suggests that excision alone or excision and graft are not as effective as when transverse drilling is added. The use of electrical stimulation may be beneficial but it has not yet been shown to allow a prompt and predictable return to sports.

The use of an intramedullary rod to allow healing of the fissure and to prevent fracture may also be considered. This treatment has been demonstrated to produce healing of the anterior cleft, presumably by decreasing the tension stress. Cautions in the use of a rod include the possibility of eccentric reaming and increased heat with drilling because of the thick anterior cortex of the tibia and irritation of the infrapatellar tendon by the rod.

In complete fractures, open reduction with bone grafting is recommended. Internal fixation is not required, but plates or rods have been successfully used with excellent results. Closed treatment leads to fracture healing in a normal length of time, but these fractures are prone to have a small increase in anterior bowing that increases the anterior tension stress and the fissure defect often persists after healing of the fracture (Fig. 3).

Prevention of stress fractures during training or participation in high performance sports is clearly desirable. Gradual increase in activity level and cross training may allow increase in bone strength without producing bone loss. The use of cushion shoes and a resilient playing surface would intuitively seem beneficial. Stretching of joints and muscles, and the development of strong muscles assist in attenuation of stress on the bones. Cyclic training has shown promise in preventing stress fractures, but at this point there is not a firm science regarding training techniques to prevent stress fractures generally or the anterior tension stress fracture of the tibia.

SUGGESTED READING

Barrick EF, Jackson CB. Prophylactic intramedullary fixation of the tibia for stress fracture in a professional athlete. J Orthop Trauma 1992; 6:241–244.
Beals RK, Cook RD. Stress fractures of the anterior tibial diaphysis. Orthopedics 1991; 14:869–875.
Burrows HJ. Fatigue infraction of the middle of the tibia in ballet dancers. J Bone Joint Surg 1956; 38B:83–94.
Margulies JY, Simkin A, Leichter I, et al. Effect of intense physical activity on the bone-mineral content in the lower limbs of young adults. J Bone Joint Surg 1986; 68A:1090–1093.
Orava S, Hulkko A. Stress fracture of the mid-tibial shaft. Acta Orthop Scand 1984; 55:35–37.
Rettig AG, Shelbourne KD, McCarroll JR, et al. The natural history and treatment of delayed union stress fractures of the anterior cortex of the tibia. Am J Sports Med 1988; 16:250–255.
Scully TJ, Besterman G. Stress fracture — a preventable training injury. Military Medicine 1982; 147:285–287.

CHRONIC RUPTURE OF THE ACHILLES TENDON

ROGER A. MANN, M.D.

The effects of a chronic rupture of the Achilles tendon are directly proportional to the weakness that is present. Obviously, there are an infinite number of injuries to the tendon, ranging from an acute rupture to chronic degeneration, that can cause weakness of the Achilles tendon complex.

When discussing the Achilles tendon it is always important to reflect upon the normal biomechanics of the posterior calf muscles. The Achilles tendon, which originates from the gastroc-soleus muscle complex, is the largest, strongest posterior calf muscle by a factor of almost four. The basic function of the posterior calf is to control the forward movement of the tibia over the fixed foot. When there is significant weakness of the muscle group, there is an element of sagittal plane instability at the ankle joint. This results in more rapid dorsiflexion at the ankle joint as the body moves over the fixed foot, resulting in a shortened contralateral step length. It may also result in easy fatigability, and from an athletic standpoint, would certainly diminish the pushoff power of the affected extremity.

The physical examination demonstrates significant loss of the muscle belly mass of the posterior calf. Single toe rise testing demonstrates either insufficient strength to complete this maneuver or the patient fatigues quickly on the involved side when compared to the uninvolved side.

Depending on the etiology, one might look on this condition as presenting three basic types. The first would be residual of an acute rupture in which the tendon healed in a lengthened position, resulting in chronic weakness of the tendon. The other two conditions represent a degenerative process of the tendon itself, either within the mid-substance of the tendon or at its insertion into the calcaneus.

The patient who presents with the residual of an acute rupture that has healed in a lengthened position can either be treated conservatively with an ankle-foot orthosis, giving the patient increased stability of the ankle-foot complex, or undergo surgical correction of the problem. This is in contrast to the patient who presents with an active degenerative process either within the substance of the Achilles tendon or at its insertion. This patient may respond to conservative treatment such as the use of a short-leg walking cast for a period of 8 to 16 weeks. After immobilization, if the reaction about the tendon has subsided, then the patient may be treated with an ankle-foot orthosis for several more months until the symptom complex completely subsides and the tendon once again becomes more functional and less painful. In the patient with an active degenerative problem, often there is inhibition of function due to pain rather than a chronic lengthening of the tendon. If the degenerative process can be stabilized by a prolonged period of immobilization, this is certainly preferable to any type of reconstructive procedure.

PHYSICAL EXAMINATION

Careful palpation of the Achilles tendon can be quite revealing in patients with tendon dysfunction. The patient that has the residuals of an old rupture may demonstrate some thickening and nodularity along the tendon, even a palpable defect, but as a rule there is little or no pain along the course of the tendon. In the patient who has a degenerative process, there may be a moderate degree of swelling and warmth around the involved area of the tendon. I tend to believe that this demonstrates that the degenerative process is active and probably still ongoing, as compared to the patient in which there is thickening but no significant evidence of inflammatory response.

PRINCIPLES OF RECONSTRUCTION

One of the basic principles in reconstruction of the Achilles tendon is creation of a substitute tendon by using an intact musculotendinous unit.

The tendon that I have chosen is the flexor digitorum longus (FDL), although others have claimed a similar result can be obtained utilizing the flexor hallucis longus (FHL). These two tendons are somewhat expendable. The FDL, I believe, is more expendable than the FHL, and this is why I prefer to use it. Others have advocated using a peroneal tendon which, unfortunately, may create a certain element of instability of the ankle joint.

When looking at the relative strengths of the muscles of the posterior calf, the work of Silver et al points out that the gastroc-soleus has a relative strength percentage of 49.1 units, compared to 11.6 units for all of the remaining plantar flexors. Obviously, based on this marked difference in muscle strength, any attempted reconstructive procedure must of necessity attempt to re-establish the continuity between the muscle mass of the gastroc-soleus group and the calcaneus. This is the only way that one has a chance to re-establish adequate strength.

By using a normal musculotendinous unit to establish the new resting length of the posterior calf muscles, the remainder of the Achilles tendon can be developed around it in such a way so as to span the gap between the muscle and the calcaneus. Cross-suturing of the reconstructive portion of the Achilles tendon to the intact musculotendinous structure, namely the FDL, allows the vascularity of the muscle mass associated with the transfer tendon to help in the revascularization of the reconstructed Achilles tendon.

TECHNICAL PROBLEMS

When carrying out a major reconstructive procedure around the Achilles tendon there are several significant technical problems that may arise that make one's approach to this procedure a very cautious one. First and foremost is the fact that the skin along the area of the Achilles tendon and posterior calcaneus, unfortunately, is rather nonyielding and has a significant tendency to slough, particularly if previous surgical scars are present. It is therefore imperative that all skin flaps be full thickness and carried down directly to the tendon sheath of the Achilles tendon both proximally and distally. At times, depending on the nature of the problem, particularly if there has been an old, untreated rupture of the Achilles tendon, it may be difficult to mobilize the mid-portion of the tendon because of the marked scarring that has occurred. To overcome this problem the proximal and distal ends of the tendon are identified and then, working from distal to proximal and proximal to distal, the old bed of the Achilles tendon is identified so that the reconstructed tendon can be placed into it. While doing this, one must also be mindful of the neurovascular bundle, which is usually out of harm's way, but one should approach the dissection with due caution.

The next technical problem that arises is wound closure. When the Achilles tendon and the transfer tendon are pulled down under tension in order to re-establish some semblance of normal musculotendinous length against the retracted gastroc-soleus muscle mass, tenting of the structures occurs. As a result, closure may be difficult and the possibility of a slough is once again increased.

TECHNICAL FACTORS

The mobilization of the Achilles tendon may be carried out in several ways, depending on the clinical presentation. If dealing with an old-acute, mid-substance rupture that went untreated one may only need to plicate the tendon by creating a long, oblique incision in the tendon itself, overlapping and cross-suturing the tendon side-to-side. This can then be reinforced with the FDL or FDH transfer.

If the tendon pathology is at the insertion of the

tendon, in which the distal portion is resected, then the FDL or FHL is used to set the tension, and the remaining proximal Achilles tendon is lengthened and inserted into the calcaneus.

If the tendon pathology is in the middle of the tendon, one has to decide if it should be completely resected or if it could be left intact, with the central portion removed, and uninvolved tendon advanced across this area. Then the FDL or FDL may be utilized to support the construct.

The decision about how much tendon needs to be resected is always difficult. Precisely where the pathology starts and stops is not always well defined. The guide I use is that of resecting enough of the pathologic appearing tendon until the normal fibril structure of the tendon is present. This is usually where the tendon is no longer abnormally thickened and there is no color change noted. Usually the involved tendon will be thicker and whiter than the uninvolved tendon. As a rule, 3 to 5 cm of tendon may need to be excised.

The lengthening of the remaining Achilles tendon is carried out in several ways, depending on the nature of the proximal tendon structure. Most commonly, there is a large, central, thick tendinous structure that can be lengthened by mobilizing the mid portion, advancing it into a drill hole in the calcaneus, and then closing the defect side-to-side. On occasions this large, central tendon structure is absent and a long, proximal V-Y advancement is made, anchoring the distal end into the calcaneus. Following this the proximal defect is closed.

There are times when the advancement of the remaining Achilles tendon requires some ingenuity of the surgeon, but I have presented the basic techniques that can be used. It is critical, however, that the distal stump be embedded into the calcaneus and the tension of the posterior calf be pre-set by suturing the FDL or FHL into a drill hole in the calcaneus.

SURGICAL APPROACH

The surgical approach for reconstruction of the Achilles tendon is divided into three parts. The first is the surgical approach that exposes the proximal and distal portion of the Achilles tendon. Second is obtaining the FDL or FHL from the plantar aspect of the foot. The third part is securing the FDL or FHL tendon into the calcaneus and securing the lengthened Achilles tendon into the calcaneus.

With the patient in a prone position and a tourniquet around the thigh, the initial skin incision is made along the posterior medial aspect of the calf, starting at approximately the mid portion of the leg, and carried distally, almost bisecting the interval between medial border of the gastrocnemius and the posterior-medial tibia. The incision is continued distally, and at about the mid portion of the calcaneus it's brought lateralward across the midline for about 1 cm.

The incision is deepened directly down through the subcutaneous tissue and fat to expose the medial aspect of the gastroc-soleus muscle and the sheath of the Achilles tendon proximally and distally. At the inferior portion of the wound the medial and lateral aspect of the calcaneus is exposed. Caution is taken not to traumatize the skin edges.

Isolation of the pathologic portion of the Achilles tendon determines where the maximum area of scar is located. Generally speaking, proximally and distally the sheath can be readily opened and the two incisions are worked towards each other in order to expose the tendon. It is important to remember that the neurovascular bundle lies just along the anterior-medial aspect of the tendon.

Once the tendon has been freed circumferentially, one must decide whether or not the problem is the result of an old rupture of the mid substance, in which case, as mentioned above, a long oblique incision can be made and the tendon plicated. If one is dealing with a degenerative portion of the tendon at the insertion of the calcaneus, resection of the distal portion of the Achilles tendon is required. If one is dealing with pathology in the mid substance of the tendon, then one must decide whether or not this segment needs to be completely or partially resected. Partial resection leaves a portion of the Achilles tendon intact and hence retains the proper tension.

Once the tendon and the pathology has been exposed, the FDL or the FHL tendon needs to be harvested.

1. The skin incision is made along the medial aspect of the foot after carefully palpating the posterior tibial tendon. The incision starts just plantar to the tendon and is carried along the top of the abductor hallucis muscle to about the distal third of the first metatarsal.
2. Once the posterior tibial tendon is exposed, the next tendon sheath plantar to this is the FDL. The tendon sheath is opened and by sharp and blunt dissection the FDL is traced distally into the plantar aspect of the foot.
3. The tendon passes lateralward, beneath the master knot of Henry, which is carefully released along with the origin of the flexor hallucis brevis muscle. In the mid portion of the foot where the FDL and FHL cross each other, the two tendons are sutured together and the FDL harvested. If one is going to utilize the FHL, it is harvested and the FDL is left intact. There is often significant cross-connection between these two tendons, sometimes suturing them together is not necessary.
4. Returning into the proximal portion of the wound, the deep fascia enveloping the neurovascular bundle and tendons is carefully split. Just anterior to the neurovascular bundle lies the FDL and just posterior to this the FHL. The overlying fascia is split for the full length of the skin incision so that there will be no tethering of the muscle belly against a sharp fascial edge.
5. The harvested tendon is then delivered into the proximal wound and the foot incision is closed.

The next part of the procedure involves the attachment of the tendon into the calcaneus, the development of the Achilles tendon, and securing the tendon into the calcaneus.

1. A transverse drill hole of adequate size is now made approximately 2 cm plantar to the dorsal aspect of the posterior portion of the calcaneus.
2. If it is necessary to advance the Achilles tendon into the calcaneus by lengthening it, a hole of adequate size is now made in the superior aspect of the calcaneus, either splitting the remaining stump of the Achilles tendon or placing the hole just anterior to it. It should be about 1 cm in depth.
3. Two small drill holes are made into the larger hole through which suture can be passed in order to secure the Achilles tendon into the calcaneus.
4. The Achilles tendon is now lengthened either by developing the central portion of the tendon, as described previously, or developing a large V-Y flap.
5. The FDL or FHL tendon is brought through the calcaneus and, with the knee flexed to 90 degrees, is secured so that the ankle joint is held in about 10 degrees of plantar flexion. One gently pushes on the metatarsal area in order to see how much tension is being placed into the tendon transfer, and it should be secured so that the ankle is held in about 5 to 10 degrees of equinus. This, I believe, will re-establish satisfactory muscle tension.
6. The developed portion of the Achilles tendon is advanced into the hole in the calcaneus. It is secured in the hole with the sutures that are brought out through the small drill holes placed through the bottom of the large hole as described above. After this is done, an attempt is made to advance the remaining portion of the gastrocsoleus and Achilles tendon, as a unit, in order to try to re-establish satisfactory musculotendinous tension. Care should be taken that the Achilles tendon is not over-lengthened when doing this portion of the procedure.
7. At this point there should be a moderate amount of tension both in the reconstructed Achilles tendon and in the FDL or FHL. As the ankle is now brought up towards neutral, there should be just about equal tension in the FDL and Achilles tendon. The Achilles tendon is now sutured into the FDL to secure the transfer.
8. After thoroughly irrigating the wound, it is closed in layers over a Hemovac drain. As the skin is closed it is usually necessary to leave the foot in maximum equinus in order to relax the transfer, which would be tenting the skin if the ankle was brought up towards neutral position. At times a vertical mattress of relaxing suture is required, particularly in a thin patient.
9. Once the wound has been closed, a compression dressing is applied, incorporating plaster splints.

The foot is kept in almost full equinus at this point in order to minimize the tension along the margin of the incision.

POSTOPERATIVE MANAGEMENT

The surgical dressing is changed after approximately 10 days, at which time if the wound is healed in a satisfactory manner the foot is placed into a short-leg non-weight-bearing plaster cast with the ankle in approximately 10 degrees of equinus. It is kept in this position for 2 months, after which gentle range of motion (ROM) exercises are begun, but the immobilization is continued. The patient is placed into a removable weight-bearing cast with the foot in neutral position at 3 months, and permitted to gently work on ROM exercises using an elastic band, but no unprotected weight bearing is permitted.

By 4 months, depending on the "feel" of the tendon, the patient may be permitted out of the cast around the house. Whether activities are permitted without the cast at this time is dependent on the degree of reaction that is still present around the Achilles tendon. If there is still a great deal of swelling and warmth, then unprotected weight bearing is not permitted. If the swelling and warmth subside and there starts to be definition of the tendon once again, then the level of activities is gradually increased. Most patients are immobilized for approximately 5 to 6 months, after which if there is any question about the stability of the transfer and reconstruction, the patient is placed into a polypropylene ankle/foot orthosis with an articulated ankle with about 10 degrees of dorsiflexion being permitted.

As the area over the surrounding Achilles tendon gradually matures with less warmth and swelling, and the definition of the underlying tendon occurs, the patient is permitted to gradually increase his or her exercise regime. This should consist of progressive resistant exercises, both eccentric and concentric. As the area becomes more mature, increased activities are permitted. Rarely is running permitted before 6 months, at which time the patient is started on treadmill exercises and then progressed from there as tolerated.

RESULTS

In a report utilizing this procedure in seven patients with an average follow-up of 39 months, four believed their results were excellent in that they had no pain, limitation of activity, or postoperative wound problems. These four patients had normal dorsiflexion and excellent strength with independent tiptoe stance. Two patients had a good result, were pain free, and had dorsiflexion to neutral, but were unable to return to their preinjury level of activities or had a postoperative problem with their wound. One patient had a fair result since she required a local rotational flap due to an area of wound necrosis. She eventually returned to preinjury activities. Subsequent to this report, approximately eight more patients have been treated, with the same satisfactory long-term results.

SUGGESTED READING

Mann RA, Holmes GB, Seale KS, Collins DN. Chronic rupture of the Achilles tendon: A new technique of repair. J Bone Joint Surg 1991; 73A:214–219.

Silver RL, DeLaGarza J, Rang M. The myth of muscle balance. A study of relative strengths and excursions of normal muscles about the foot and ankle. J Bone Joint Surg 1985; 67B:432–437.

Turco VJ, Spinella AJ. Achilles tendon rupture – peroneus brevis transfer. Foot Ankle 1987; 7:253–259.

Wapner KL, Allardyce T, Shea J, Hecht P: Anatomic basis for tendon selection in reconstruction of ruptures of the Achilles and posterior tibial tendon. Presented at AOFAS Summer Meeting, Napa, Calif., July, 1992.

FUNCTIONAL POSTOPERATIVE TREATMENT OF ACHILLES TENDON REPAIR

THOMAS R. CARTER, M.D.

The operative versus the nonoperative treatment of Achilles tendon ruptures has historically been and continues to be a controversial issue. Advocates of surgical treatment cite the lower incidence of rerupture and increased function with operative treatment. The increased medical costs and high rate of complications with surgical repair are noted by the proponents of nonoperative treatment.

The final decision to treat Achilles tendon tears operatively or nonoperatively must be individualized, for neither treatment is ideal in all cases. The age of the individual, activity demands, general medical condition, and the time period since the tear occurred are several factors that need to be considered. Elderly patients with low activity demands who have the tear treated early (within the first week) are considered the most appropriate candidates for nonsurgical treatment. Conversely, young active individuals are the prime candidates for surgical repair.

Regardless of the method of treatment, there has been a general consensus that a period of casting is required after the injury. However, immobilization is not innocuous and affects essentially all tissues of the musculoskeletal system in a deleterious manner. The orthopedic literature abounds with studies supporting this statement with complete discussion beyond the scope of this chapter. A brief summary for the reader's information of the ill-effects does warrant mention. Those wishing further details are referred to the Suggested Reading.

Due to the visible difference, muscle atrophy is the most readily apparent sequelae of cast treatment. Studies have shown that with 6 weeks of immobilization after Achilles tendon repair, the calf musculature decreases on average approximately 20%. Just as the muscle is "stress shielded" the intracapuslar and ligamentous structures are similarly affected, which can lead to random association of the collagen within these tissues. This in turn leads to weakness of the supportive structures as well as joint stiffness. Osteoporosis of bone has also been noted to occur with the lack of stress.

With the absence of motion, fibrofatty connective tissue proliferation within the joint occurs within the first few weeks and can cause adhesions between the articular surfaces. If there is forceful movement of the joint subsequent to the adhesions, superficial tearing of the articular surfaces can occur. In addition, partial necrosis develops at the point of the cartilage-cartilage contact, while atrophy of the cartilage can occur in the unopposed areas.

The reparative process of the torn ligament itself is also negatively affected by cast treatment. The scar tissue laid down during the healing phase is done so in a random manner when a joint is immobilized. This in turn causes delay of the normal tensile properties. If motion is present during the healing phase, collagen is laid down in an organized manner in response to the stresses applied upon it. This subsequently leads to accelerated return to normal tensile strength. In addition, motion diminishes the prevalence of scar tissue adherence of the healing tendon to the surrounding tissues, which if present can affect the normal gliding mechanism of the Achilles.

With the many negative effects of joint immobilization, it would seem prudent to maintain motion during the healing process to prevent these sequelae. Early motion is obviously not compatible with nonoperative treatment as the torn ends would not be held in direct apposition. The proponents of surgical treatment meanwhile have been hesitant to implement motion after surgery because of the concern of compromising the repair and leading to a higher rerupture rate.

Early motion following Achilles tendon repair is not a new concept; the initial study was reported by Marti and Weber in 1974. Their postoperative regimen involved immobilizing the foot in a relaxed equinuus position for the initial few days after surgery. Once the postoperative dressing was removed, the patient was encouraged to move the ankle ad lib. When the ankle was able to be brought to neutral, usually in 1 to 3 days, a short leg cast was applied and maintained for approximately 6 weeks. Since their report, other authors have implemented similar postoperative treatment protocols. Their findings confirm that of Marti and Weber in that early controlled motion can be used safely without increased risk of rerupture. These studies have also shown that the patient is able to return to normal activities at an earlier time period than standard postoperative casting.

The less restrictive use of a "mobile cast" following Achilles tendon repair was reported in 1988 by Cetti. His postoperative regimen entailed placing the patient in a cast that limited the foot to 20 degrees short of neutral in regard to dorsiflexion and allowed unlimited plantar flexion. There was a metal extension bar on the bottom of the cast that prevented the patient from directly applying pressure to the foot when ambulating. The report of his results were similarly very good regarding return to function without increased risk of rerupture.

While these studies demonstrate that early motion after an Achilles tendon repair can be beneficial, both protocols still impose notable restrictions. In the case of Marti and Weber, 6 weeks of casting was part of their treatment, while in the latter program, range of motion (ROM) and weight bearing were both notably limited.

PREFERRED PROTOCOL

The postoperative protocol that I currently implement further raises some of these restraints. A total of 30 patients have been followed to date, with the original 21 patients studied retrospectively and reported in the American Journal of Sports Medicine in 1992. The latter nine patients have been studied prospectively with there being only a slight modification in regard to their postoperative treatment.

The 30 patients included 21 males and nine females with the average age of injury being 36.8 years (range 19 to 65). The dominant leg was involved in 16 patients; the nondominant leg in 14 patients. The preinjury level of activity of the patients was varied, ranging from the professional athlete to the homemaker. The activity at the time of injury was similarly diverse.

The same standard surgical repair was performed on all patients. All but one was performed acutely (within 3 weeks). A longitudinal medial incision was used to avoid damage to the sural nerve. The repair was performed end-to-end using Bunnell or modified Kessler suturing. The ankle was put through a ROM prior to closure of the wound with each being able to be brought to neutral or beyond in regard to dorsiflexion without compromising the repair. No fascial flaps or grafts were used, and no reinsertion into the calcaneus were performed.

A bulky compressive dressing was applied postoperatively and maintained for 3 to 5 days. During this time, toe-touch weight-bearing crutch ambulation was permitted. On the initial postoperative visit the dressing was discontinued and a brace subsequently used. The initial 21 patients wore a custom-made Plastizote dorsal

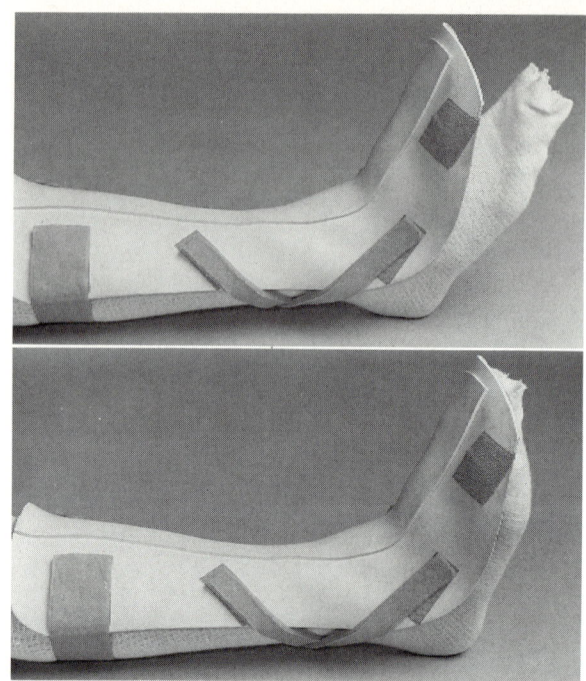

Figure 1 Postoperative orthosis demonstrating ROM permitted.

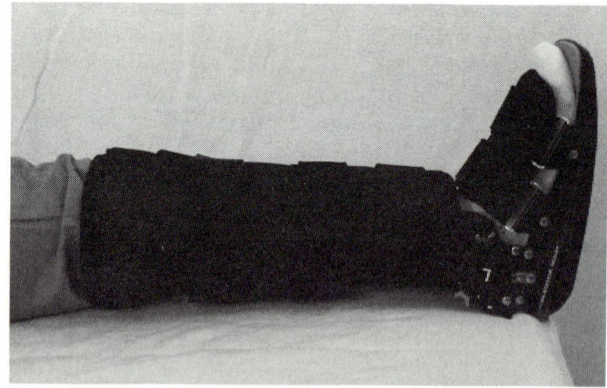

Figure 2 Postoperative walking boot.

extension block orthosis. The device allowed unlimited plantar flexion and blocked dorsiflexion to neutral (Fig. 1). Due to the patients noting the brace being somewhat cumbersome at night, the prospectively studied group wore a walking boot during the day (Fig. 2). At night a posterior fiberglass splint keeping the ankle at neutral and held in place with an Ace wrap was worn. The initial few patients wore the orthosis for 8 weeks, but as experience was gained this was reduced and continues to be 6 weeks duration. Weight bearing on the involved extremity was allowed as tolerated, with all patients full weight bearing before discontinuation of the brace. No heel lifts or other devices were used once the device was discontinued. After the use of the brace, the patients were encouraged to swim, bicycle ride, and walk ad lib. Further activities were progressed as tolerated but running and strenuous athletic endeavors were avoided until the patient had full confidence in the leg and no gross signs of weakness. Routinely the patient returned to full activities at 3 to 4 months postoperative. It should be noted that while most patients did attend physical therapy as part of their postoperative treatment, not all had supervised rehabilitation for a variety of reasons.

RESULTS

The results of this treatment regimen have been most encouraging. Of the 30 patients only one was not pleased with the result. The patient noted weakness in the extremity that caused him to walk with an antalgic gait by the end of the day. Twenty-five of the 30 patients felt they returned to their preinjury level of activity. On reviewing the orthopedic literature, these results compare favorably to previously reported studies. Most authors report a 90% to 95% rate of patient satisfaction, with the current series being 97%. A return to preinjury level of activity of 80% to 90% is routinely noted, with 83% in this group.

The patients noted few difficulties with abiding by the protocol. As noted previously, the main complaint was that the initial orthosis was cumbersome at night. Since switching to the current use of walking boot during the day and posterior splint at night, no problems have been noted by the patients. Seven of the patients previously wore casts for a variety of reasons, and all stated strongly that they would prefer brace treatment to casting if they had the option.

Objectively the calf circumference and ROM were not statistically different when comparing the operatively treated leg to the contralateral limb at a minimum 2 year follow-up. On average, plantar flexion was unchanged and dorsiflexion increased only 2 degrees.

Three complications directly related to surgical repair were present in the group. Two involved superficial wound infections that healed without sequelae, and the third involved scar adherence of the skin to the tendon. This correlates to a complication rate of 10%, which compares well to the average of approximately 20% reported in the literature. It should be noted though that studies done more recently report a complication rate similar to this series.

Isokinetic evaluation was performed on every patient and revealed no statistical differences in the strength, power, or endurance of the involved leg when compared to the unaffected side. For dorsiflexion the average strength, power, and endurance of the repair side were 91%, 95%, and 90%, respectively. Plantar flexion strength, power, and endurance as a percent of "normal" were 97%, 97%, and 93%, respectively. These results, again, compare favorably to previously reported studies.

In summary, while there has been much hesitation to implement early controlled motion after Achilles tendon repair, recent research has shown that it can be a safe and effective form of postoperative treatment. Patient compliance is of utmost importance and it should not be universally implemented following Achilles tendon repair. However, due to early controlled motion avoiding the effects of immobilization and expediting recovery, it should be strongly considered in reliable patients when trying to return them to the playing field or to gainful employment.

SUGGESTED READING

Akeson WH, Amiel D, Abel MF, et al. Effects of immobilization on joints. Clin Orthop 1987; 219:28.

Carter TR, Fowler PJ, Blokker C. Functional postoperative treatment of Achilles tendon repair. Am J Sports Med 1992; 20:459.

Cetti R. Ruptured Achilles tendon—preliminary results of a new treatment. Br J Sports Med 1988; 22:6.

Enwemeka CS, Spielholz NI, Nelson AJ. The effects of early functional activities on experimentally tenotomized Achilles tendons in rats. Am J Phys Med Rehab 1992; 71:33.

Inglis AE, Scott WN, Sculco TP, et al. Ruptures of the tendo Achilles: An objective assessment of surgical and non-surgical treatment. J Bone Joint Surg 1976; 58A:990.

Marti RK, Weber BG. Achillessehnenruptur-funktionelle Nachbehandlung. Helv Chir Acta 1974; 41:293.

Nistor L. Surgical and non-surgical treatment of Achilles tendon rupture: A prospective randomized study. J Bone Joint Surg 1981; 63A:394.

Renstrom P, Ledbetter WB. Tendinitis: I—Basic concepts. Clin Sports Med 1992; 11.

Willis CA, Washburn S, Caiozzov V, et al. Achilles tendon rupture: A review of the literature comparing surgical vs. non-surgical treatment. Clin Orthop 1986; 207:156.

RUPTURE OF THE POSTERIOR TIBIAL TENDON

LEE C. WOODS, M.D.

The key to management of posterior tibial tendon injury in athletes is the proper index of suspicion in order to make the diagnosis in its early stages. Individuals with a flattened arch are predisposed. Similarly, a typical case of posterior tibial tendon rupture is that of a middle-aged woman who may have hypertension, obesity, or diabetes mellitus. However, we have experience with younger athletes who have sustained acute posterior tibial tendon injury. We have found that some of these individuals have not had a pre-existing flat foot deformity or systemic disease. They had a normal foot architecture, reflected in the absence of excessive heel valgus or depression of the mid-longitudinal arch. Therefore, it must be recognized that posterior tibial tendon rupture can occur as a traumatic sports-related injury.

The onset of posterior tibial tendon injury may be heralded by the insidious progression of mid-tarsal pain and swelling related to sports activities. With progression, the symptoms may occur during normal ambulation, without the stress of sports activities. The pain can originate at the navicula tuberosity, plantar to the medial malleolus, or just posterior to the medial malleolus and radiating proximally into the mid leg. With prolonged stress, the posterior tibial tendonitis can progress to complete rupture in athletes. This posterior tibial tendon injury can then result in unilateral acquired flat foot deformity, heel valgus, medial midfoot sag, medial hindfoot swelling, posterior tibial tendon pain, and inability to push-off at terminal stance phase. Unopposed function of the peroneus brevis tendon is thought to contribute to this process.

In this setting, posterior tibial tendon repair may be required, for loss of posterior tibial tendon function is a devastating injury to the athlete. The posterior tibial tendon is critical as a dynamic stabilizer of the hindfoot against eversion forces at push-off. The tibialis posterior function is essential at all levels of activity, from routine ambulation to vigorous sports activity. Its malfunction is debilitating for athletes and nonathletes alike.

POSTERIOR TIBIAL TENDONITIS

Because synovitis may be a forerunner of disruption, it should be considered in any discussion of the management of posterior tibial tendon injury. Many of these individuals may have chronic posterior tibial tendonitis, which often does not present with acute pain and swelling.

Management is initiated with a thorough physical examination, which includes examination of the entire lower extremity, beginning with evaluation of hip range of motion (ROM) for associated sources of rotational abnormality, including femoral anteversion and retroversion. The knee is examined for genu varum and valgum, as other sources of rotational abnormality, resulting in hindfoot valgus, subsequent overuse, and pain of the posterior tibial tendon. Heel cord tenderness and tightness are evaluated with the foot fully supinated in order to completely reduce the calcaneus beneath the longitudinal axis of the tibia. Dorsiflexion of the supinated foot, short of the neutral position, indicates heelcord tightness. The sinus tarsi is palpated in order to rule out sinus tarsi pain in those individuals who have progressed to severe hindfoot valgus deformity with lateral impingement pain. In severe cases, the first ray and great toe are pronated, with elevation of the first ray, hypermobility of the first ray, and a plantar transfer lesion of the second metatarsophalangeal joint, manifested by severe metatarsalgia.

The foot is also examined in the standing position, in order to evaluate hindfoot valgus, loss of arch height, functional ankle ROM, and the windlass mechanism. The windlass mechanism (Fig. 1), which includes the great toe proximal phalanx, metatarsal head, and the plantar aponeurosis, is tested in order to evaluate the flexibility of the longitudinal arch. Extension of the great toe in the standing position externally rotates the leg, plantar flexes the first ray, shortens and inverts the foot, and elevates the longitudinal arch in a flexible foot. Inability to stimulate the windlass maneuver and elevate the longitudinal arch indicates a rigid flat foot deformity. Individuals with flexible feet are supported more suc-

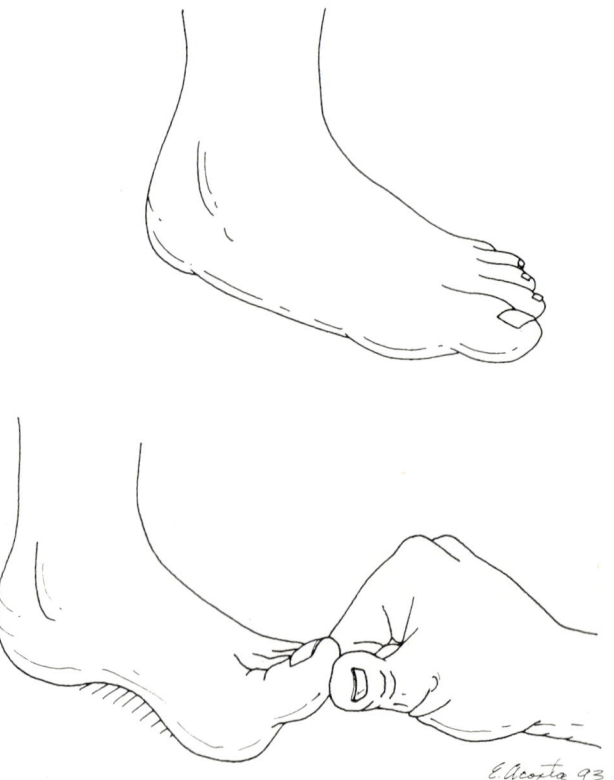

Figure 1 Windlass mechanism.

cessfully with orthotics than those with rigid longitudinal arches.

The integrity of the posterior tibial tendon is confirmed with palpation just posterior to the medial malleolus and continuing to its insertion into the navicula. The posterior tibial tendon is palpated for localized tenderness, which may radiate from its insertion in the navicula, proximally posterior to the medial malleolus and into the leg, to the mid calf. The single limb heelrise test of Johnson is performed with difficulty in those individuals with posterior tibial tendonitis. Inability to perform this test is an infallible manifestation of posterior tibial tendon rupture. In the weight-bearing position, the "too many toes sign" is seen in the posterior standing view of the acquired flat foot deformity. In severe cases, a pelvic obliquity exists in conjunction with functional limb shortening as a result of loss of arch height and depression of the medial malleolus in the weight-bearing position. Manual muscle testing of the posterior tibial tendon is performed with resistance against the fully everted foot in order to isolate posterior tibial tendon function.

Management

Those individuals who have not progressed to posterior tibial tendon rupture with an isolated posterior tibial tendonitis benefit from conservative management, which begins with proper custom made orthoses. The orthotics must be of a tolerable, semi-rigid material that provides the patient with adequate relief and simultaneous support. These orthoses are tailored to the individual, preferably by a ped orthotist. Individuals without severe valgus deformity may achieve relief with a semi-rigid custom orthotic such as that of custom made Pelite and PPT materials. These closed-cell polyethylene foam material orthotics are rigid, yet flexible and comfortable enough to be well tolerated for sports activities. Hygienically, they also are preferable to the open-cell foam materials.

In conjunction with the orthotics, we stress the use of well-structured and soled, lace-up, rigid hind counter sports shoewear for routine use. These orthotic devices should otherwise be worn in high-top shoewear, in order to fully support the ankle and hindfoot. Adolescents, in particular, with painful flexible flat feet, will find relief with a custom polypropylene University of California Biomechanical Laboratory (UCBL) orthotic worn in high-top shoewear (Fig. 2).

Individuals who have posterior tibial tendonitis with a flexible flat foot, manifested by an intact windlass mechanism, routinely find relief with custom orthotics. In severe cases, the management of both flexible and rigid flat foot deformities begins with UCBL orthotics. This provides adequate functional relief for many individuals to perform sports activities without pain. The UCBL device is cumbersome and inflexible, which can result in poor compliance. In those cases in which the UCBL is not tolerated or the device is too cumbersome for sports activity and shoewear, a standard, custom-fitted, semi-rigid orthotic is prescribed (Fig. 3).

Physical therapy assists in strengthening of the posterior tibial tendon. Anti-inflammatory medication is given to reduce inflammation. The primary treatment modality, though, is the orthotic. With an intact posterior tibial tendon and a flexible foot, an orthotic often provides complete relief. An inability to adjust to orthotic wear is indication for hindfoot reconstruction, including possible flexor digitorum longus (FDL) tendon transfer and calcaneal osteotomy.

The patient with posterior tibial tendonitis often does not have the acute pain and swelling experienced by patients with Achilles tendonitis. Those with chronic posterior tibial tendonitis suffer the gradual development of foot deformity, including hindfoot valgus, forefoot pronation, abduction, and a severe flatfoot deformity. For patients with chronic posterior tibial tendonitis unresponsive to conservative management, surgical release of the tendon sheath and debridement of the tendon may be required. Transfer of the FDL to the posterior tibial tendon, recommended by Mann and Thompson and by Johnson, is indicated in those individuals with disruption of the posterior tibial tendon. With this procedure, there is probable relief of pain and return of modest posterior tibial tendon function, but the flat foot deformity remains. Limitation of push-off persists, creating awkwardness while attempting a quick step. I therefore perform this procedure in conjunction with a varus calcaneal osteotomy and internal fixation (Fig. 4). This procedure assists in restoring arch height and function at push-off.

Radiographic Evaluation

Radiographs should be taken in the standing position in order to demonstrate acquired abnormality, including flat foot deformity. The anteroposterior view

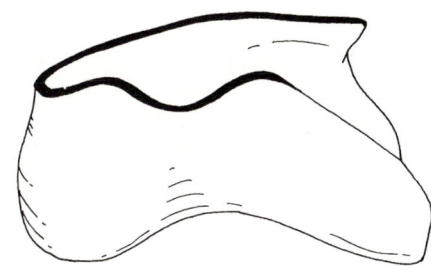

Figure 2 The University of California Biomechanical Lab (UCBL) orthotic.

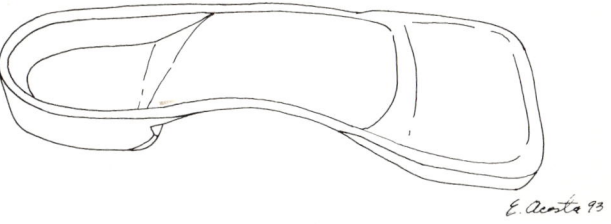

Figure 3 Custom-fitted semi-rigid orthotic comprised of closed-cell foam.

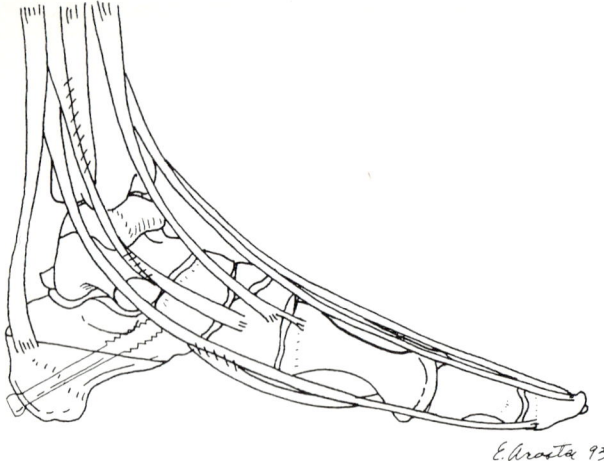

Figure 4 Transfer of flexor digitorum longus to posterior tibial tendon with varus calcaneal osteotomy and internal fixation.

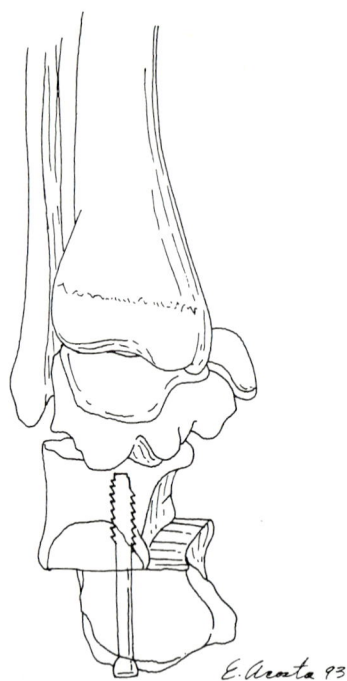

Figure 5 Harris semiaxial view of varus calcaneal osteotomy with internal fixation.

demonstrates an increased talocalcaneal angle, with medial displacement of the talar head, from the talonavicular articulation. The lateral view may also demonstrate plantar displacement of the talonavicular or naviculocuneiform joints. The Cobey view standing radiograph, posterior roentgenographic technique demonstrating the relationship between calcaneus, tibia, talus, and forefoot, confirms hindfoot valgus deformity.

Although the diagnosis of posterior tibial tendon injury is primarily a clinical diagnosis, magnetic resonance imaging (MRI) is utilized as an adjunctive diagnostic technique. The MRI study is sensitive to the integrity of the tendon injury. When properly read, MRI can provide the information necessary to appropriately stage the tendon injury and plan surgical intervention.

ACUTE POSTERIOR TIBIAL TENDON RUPTURE

Acute posterior tibial tendon rupture in the athlete requires surgical intervention. When surgery is undertaken shortly after injury (i.e., while the integrity of the posterior tibial tendon is maintained with a good arch), the outcome is excellent. In those instances where the posterior tibial tendon has ruptured and the patient has developed a flattened longitudinal arch and pronated foot, the patient's condition can improve. They may be able to return to activity. All of these individuals require a custom orthotic postsurgery in order to provide continuous support for the foot and prevent recurrent tendonitis and pain.

In all populations, young and old, acute rupture is rarely recognized because of its limited clinical signs. A typical individual having sustained a posterior tibial tendon rupture can often retrospectively recall a specific episode of injury or onset of pain with the subsequent, gradual progression of symptoms and deformity. In those cases where it is recognized, immediate exploration is in order.

Surgical Approach

The approach is made through a longitudinal incision, just posterior to the medial malleolus in order to expose the posterior tibial tendon sheath. The incision is carried inferiorly to the insertion of the posterior tibial tendon at the navicula. The tendon sheath is opened. In those cases with rupture in continuity or partial rupture, just proximal to the navicula attachment, the tendon can be reattached to the navicula through drill holes and oversewn onto itself. The tendon sheath is generally found to be thickened and the tenosynovium hypertrophied and inflamed. Dense, fibrous tissue in continuity with the proximal tissue, and the more distal navicular tendon attachment, can be found. The fibrous tissue and tenosynovium are resected.

In Johnson's Classification System, those with avulsion injury just proximal to the navicula are classified as group I. Mid substance tears between the medial malleolus and navicula insertion are classified as group II. These require excision of the collagenous scar tissue. The FDL is utilized for transfer in these cases. In this situation, the previously described mid-longitudinal medial foot incision is utilized. The FDL is exposed; its distal segment is sutured to the flexor hallucis longus at the Knot of Henry in order to retain phalangeal function. The FDL is then released just proximal to this junction at the Knot of Henry, rerouted through the posterior tibial tendon sheath, through a drill-hole in the navicula, and sutured back onto itself. The proximal posterior tibial tendon is then attached to the FDL. Johnson Classification group III ruptures are those in continuity without complete transection of the tendon. Group IV includes those patients with synovitis only.

In patients with severe hindfoot valgus, a varus calcaneal osteotomy (Fig. 5) is performed through a lateral calcaneal incision that originates at the superior and lateral aspect of the calcaneus, radiating laterally to the base of the fifth metatarsal, approximately 2.5 cm inferior to the lateral malleolus, avoiding the sural nerve. The lateral cortex of the calcaneus is exposed. An oblique osteotomy of the calcaneus is performed. The proximal portion is shifted medially. Approximately 12 to 15 mm of displacement can be achieved. This is held in position with K-wires while rigid internal fixation with a cannulated compression screw is performed through a transverse posterior heel incision just above the weight-bearing surface.

The patients are treated in a short-leg inversion cast, non-weight bearing for 6 weeks. A vigorous posterior tibial tendon rehabilitation program is initiated, including strengthening of the posterior tibial tendon and active-assistive to active ROM exercises in order to avoid loss of subtalar motion. Within 4 to 6 months after surgery, athletic individuals may resume activity. Individuals who return to athletic activity usually do so at a lesser level than prior to tendon rupture. More often than not, a very extreme, intense physical therapy program is necessitated, particularly in those individuals who have developed a fixed hindfoot deformity with limited subtalar motion.

Results

Our surgical cases consisted of one group I case, two group II cases, and three group III cases in Johnson's Classification System. Those individuals who return to activity, usually do so at a lower level than prior to their injury. However, with early surgical intervention in those cases in which deformity has not yet occurred, presurgical running capacity can be regained.

SUGGESTED READING

Cobey J. Posterior roentgenogram of the foot. Clin Orthop 1976; 118:202–207.

Conti S, Michelson J, Jahss M: Clinical significance of magnetic resonance imaging in preoperative planning for reconstruction of posterior tibial tendon ruptures. Foot Ankle 1992; 13:208–214.

Funk DA, Cass JR, Johnson KA. Acquired adult flatfoot secondary to posterior tibial tendon pathology. J Bone Joint Surg 1986; 68A: 95–102.

Henderson WH, Campbell JW. UCBL shoe insert: casting and fabrication. University Calif Biomech Lab Rep Ser 53, August 1967.

Hicks JH. The mechanics of the foot: II. The plantar aponeurosis and the arch. J Anat 1954; 88:25–30.

Holmes GB, Mann RA. Possible epidemiological factors associated with rupture of the posterior tibial tendon. Foot Ankle 1992; 13:70–78.

Jahss MH. Spontaneous rupture of the tibialis posterior tendon: Clinical findings, tenographic studies and a new technique of repair. Foot Ankle 1982; 3:158–166.

Johnson KA: Tibialis posterior tendon rupture. Clin Orthop 1983; 177:140–147.

Leach RE. Pathologic hindfoot conditions in the athlete. Clin Orthop 1983; 177:116–121.

Lysholm J. Injuries in runners. Am J Sports Med 1987; 15:168–171.

Mann RA. Acquired flatfoot in adults. Clin Orthop 1983; 181:46–51.

Mann RA. Principles of examination of the foot and ankle. In: Mann RA, Coughlin MJ, eds. Surgery of the foot & ankle. 6th ed. St. Louis: Mosby-Year Book, 1993:49.

Mann RA, Thompson FM. Rupture of the posterior tibial tendon causing flat foot. J Bone Joint Surg 1985; 67A:556–561.

Simpson RR. Posterior tibial tendon rupture in a world class runner. J Foot Surg 1983; 22:74–77.

Trevino S: Surgical treatment of stenosing tenosynovitis at the ankle. Foot Ankle 1981; 2:37–45.

Woods LC, Leach RE. Posterior tibial tendon rupture in athletic people. Am J Sports Med 1991; 19:495–498.

ANTERIOR COMPARTMENT SYNDROME OF THE THIGH: CONSERVATIVE TREATMENT

DROR ROBINSON, M.D., Ph.D.
NAHUM HALPERIN, M.D.

The rationale for conservative management of anterior compartment syndrome of the thigh in athletes is presented here as well as methods of treatment and results.

RELEVANT ANATOMY

The thigh contains three compartments that are contained by fascia. The anterior compartment contains the quadriceps muscle, the femoral nerve, and the lateral and medial femoral cutaneous branches. The medial compartment contains the adductor muscles as well as the major vascular bundle of the limb and the saphenous nerve. The posterior compartment contains the hamstrings and the sciatic nerve as well as the deep femoral artery. Thus, each of the compartments contains both muscles, allowing motor function evaluation and at least one sensory nerve, allowing sensory function evaluation. When acute trauma to the soft tissues of the thigh occurs, the importance of the sensory evaluation increases, as pain inhibition could lead to an unreliable assessment of motor function.

PATHOPHYSIOLOGY

A compartment syndrome (CS) is essentially a situation in which microcirculation through soft tissue is stopped due to increased pressure in the tissue as compared to the intravascular pressure. Only in the late stages is macrocirculation (i.e., arterial pulses) also diminished. Thus, the classical "P" signs of CS (pallor, lack of pulses, paralysis) often occur late, if at all. Indeed early on in the detection of CS only pain and increased interstitial pressure are reliable. However, the limita-tions of both signs should be understood. Paresthesia might occur due to direct contusion of a nerve without any evidence of CS. Probably the most well-described example is paresthesia of the lateral femoral cutaneous nerve (meralgia paresthetica). Another commonly in-jured sensory nerve in the thigh is the medial femoral cutaneous nerve, which is often transitionally paralyzed by direct trauma. Increased tissue pressure is the most reliable clue for diagnosis. Tissue pressure can be measured either by using a central venous pressure system or more reliably by a dedicated instrument (such as the intracompartmental pressure monitor system by Stryker Surgical, which we use). The limit of normal tissue pressure is somewhat controversial. Some of the literature suggest an arbitrary level of 40 mm Hg, while others have tried to relate the limit to mean arterial pressure.

Consequences of an undiagnosed CS include muscle necrosis and nerve damage. Due to the large muscle mass, muscle necrosis in the thigh often leads to significant myoglobinemia with subsequent myoglobin-uria and renal damage. Chronic complications include scarring down of the quadriceps to the bone and shortening of the rectus femoris muscle due to fibrosis. Both complications lead to limited knee flexion.

ETIOLOGY

Anterior CS of the thigh often occurs after direct blunt trauma. Handball and football tackling injuries are frequently responsible. However, similar contusions are caused during road accidents.

Femoral fractures with the ensuing massive hemor-rhage can also cause a CS. Due to the proximity of the profunda femoris artery to the bone, a posterior CS is often associated. It should be noted that even if the fascial barriers are ruptured, in cases of massive hem-orrhage, the skin can reach the limit of its stretching capacity, resulting in increased pressure. In such cases, a mixed syndrome affecting all muscle groups of the thigh could result.

An additional cause is bleeding from a pelvic fracture or operation. This could lead to a massive hematoma in the thigh. Unfortunately this component of the injury is often ignored, due to the life-threatening nature of the pelvic trauma.

Knee arthroscopy in which pressurized irrigation

fluid system is used can also cause a CS. In such situations the suprapatellar pouch is sometimes ruptured by the pressure, allowing leakage of massive amounts of fluid into the anterior compartment of the thigh. In our experience this occurs more often in older patients with osteoarthritic knees, perhaps due to scarring-down of the suprapatellar pouch. A less common iatrogenic cause may be the poor positioning of the patient on an operating table, causing direct pressure on a limited area (most often of the medial compartment). Another iatrogenic reason for CS of the thigh is misapplication of a pneumatic tourniquet (i.e., without padding) or of MAST trousers. Rarely, infection of the thigh muscles, especially with gas forming bacteria, can cause sufficient elevation of pressure within the limb. Such patients are often critically ill, and the CS is often ignored. It is difficult to separate the effects of the CS from those caused by direct toxicity of the microbes.

DIAGNOSIS

An important clue in conscious patients is severe pain, often out of proportion to the injury. This is of course difficult to appreciate in patients with femoral fracture and impossible to evaluate in unconscious patients.

As most of the muscle groups in the thigh are subcutaneous, it is often possible to palpate the muscles and notice the unnatural firmness within. It has been our experience that this sign is highly reliable.

The definitive test is the pressure in the limb. This should be measured in a sterile fashion (to prevent infection of the hematoma), and the point of measurement as well as the angle of the needle and depth of penetration should be clearly noted. This allows repeated measurements from the same spot. This is particularly important in atypical cases in which only part of a compartment is involved (such as CS due to direct pressure). We do not leave the needle inside for prolonged periods as it could act as a conduit for bacteria.

TREATMENT

Compartment Syndrome Due to Blunt Trauma

The option of operative treatment is discussed in the next chapter. The major disadvantage of surgery is a high infection rate in open fasciotomy due to necrotic tissue. Aggressive debridement during the primary operation might well prevent infection, but will require removal of large amounts of tissue, because early on it is difficult to distinguish between dead muscle and ischemic muscle, which can recover. Both types will not twitch in response to a nerve stimulator and both might look cyanotic. As mentioned above, subcutaneous fasciotomy in the thigh might not be enough, as the intact skin can act as barrier keeping interstitial pressure elevated. Other disadvantages of surgery are the resultant scar, the frequent need

for skin grafting, and the high cost. Thus, conservative treatment may be preferable. Percutaneous evacuation of the hematoma might not be successful due to blood clots. It probably increases the risk of infection, and we no longer attempt it.

The patient should be hospitalized, placed supine, with the leg at heart level. No circular wraps of any kind should be placed on the limb. Ice packs are placed to slow the bleeding. The patient should be well hydrated. Antibiotic treatment is instituted to prevent secondary infection of the hematoma (we currently usually use cefonicid 1 g/day). Analgesic drugs are prescribed as needed.

The condition of the skin as well as sensory function should be assessed hourly. The size of the hematoma can be monitored by repeated measurements of limb circumference. A more high-tech (and more expensive) method is by repeated ultrasound examinations. The advantage is that the size of the hematoma itself can be assessed, and furthermore the presence of active bleeding into the hematoma can be determined by Doppler examination. The use of computed tomography scans or magnetic resonance imaging scans is probably unwarranted due to the prohibitive cost as well as the need to transfer the patient to the radiology suite.

If active arterial bleeding is found during sonography, angiographic embolization of the vessel can be performed. If a decision is made to manage a CS conservatively, careful monitoring of several laboratory parameters is essential. These include tests of kidney function (creatinine clearance, urinalysis) and repeated determinations of creatine phosphokinase (CPK) levels in order to follow the degree of muscle destruction. Hemoglobin levels should also be monitored frequently as bleeding can be massive. Intracompartmental pressure should be monitored frequently. We currently use a protocol in which pressure is measured in several spots every 12 hours during the first day, and every day subsequently.

RESULTS

We have treated eight patients with anterior CS of the thigh due to blunt trauma. In all patients intracompartmental pressures were above 50 mm Hg (range 55 to 95 mm Hg). Elevation of pressure above 40 mm Hg persisted for 3 to 5 days, peaking usually on the second day after injury. On admission, two patients complained of minimal paresthesia in the distribution of the medial femoral cutaneous nerve. As the lesion appeared to be localized and partial (i.e., no anesthetic region) and quadriceps function was present (due to pain inhibition only slight flickering was elicited), these patients were carefully followed and conservatively managed. In none of the patients was deterioration of neurologic function observed. Had it occurred, such a finding would, in our opinion, constitute an indication for operative treatment.

CPK levels increased an average of 50%, usually on the second day after injury. In none of the patients was renal function affected. All patients returned to the previous sport activities after an average period of 5 weeks (range 3 to 8 weeks). During a follow-up examination 1 year later, none of the patients demonstrated evidence of rectus femoris shortening, and the Elly test was negative. Thigh circumference was similar to that of the contralateral side. No limitation of joint motion or weakness of the quadriceps was observed.

Thus, in selected young patients in whom an isolated anterior CS of the thigh occurs, conservative treatment seems to yield superior results to fasciotomy, as no infections or scarring was observed.

Compartment Syndrome After Arthroscopy

Two factors may cause CS of the thigh after arthroscopy, tourniquet misapplication and infusion of large amounts of irrigation fluid into the thigh. We became aware of this syndrome after a rather unfortunate case in which CS developed with ensuing complications of myoglobinuria and renal shut-down. Since then we have had several patients in whom high intracompartmental pressures developed after arthroscopy. All were operated on without a tourniquet, thus limiting the cause to leakage of irrigation fluid into the thigh. The treatment protocol we currently use is similar to that described for hematomas. Ultrasonography is not useful because no collection of fluid is found. Rather, the fluid infiltrates the interstitium. This treatment protocol also prevents aspiration of the fluid.

Intracompartmental pressures usually peak immediately (pressures up to 100 mm Hg were measured) and remain elevated for 12 to 24 hours. In none of the patients, who were carefully followed, was either renal dysfunction or muscle fibrosis observed.

In order to better investigate the time course of pressure elevation, an animal model was developed. Anesthetized rabbits were used. Their thigh muscles were injected using a fine (27 F) needle. Various volumes of different fluids (Ringer's lactate, saline solution, distilled water, hypertonic saline, 5% glucose in water) were used. In order to relate the volumes used to the humans, the volume of the thigh was measured using a water bath and data expressed as volume of fluid injected per total thigh volume. It appears that in order to cause an increase in anterior compartment pressure, at least in the rabbit, a volume equal to thigh volume should be injected in a gradual fashion. The gradual nature of the process appears to be critical as immediate injection of a large volume would cause tear of the fasciae and decompression of the muscles. The minimal period for injection, in order to cause a sustained pressure elevation, is 30 minutes. The time course of pressure relief following such an injection is similar to all fluids examined (Fig. 1). Histologic examination of the muscle did not demonstrate fibrosis or necrosis of the fibers.

In another study, intracompartmental pressures were measured during arthroscopy in patients. Peaks of up to 160 mm Hg were measured. A pneumatic tourniquet placed over the proximal thigh can cause pressure elevation in the anterior compartment of the

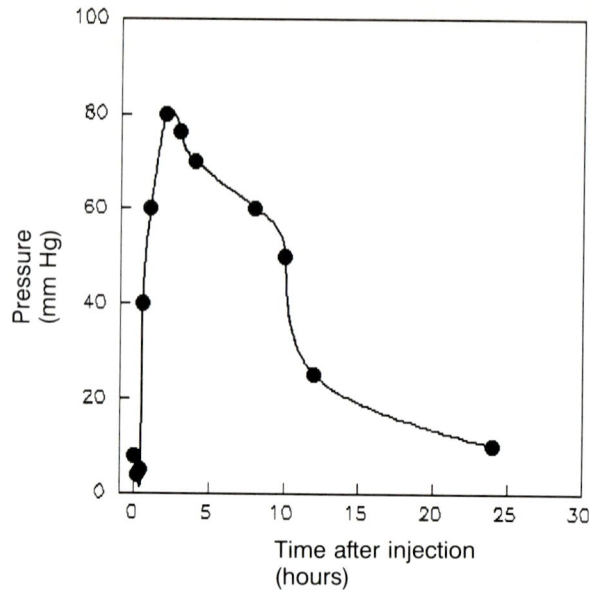

Figure 1 Elevation and subsequent relief of pressure after fluid injection.

distal thigh of up to 300 mm Hg during arthroscopy. However, if leakage of fluid does not occur, the pressure is diminished immediately after release of the tourniquet.

CONTRAINDICATIONS

The following factors contraindicate conservative management:

1. Evidence of myoglobinuria or renal damage.
2. Deteriorating neurologic status (mostly based on sensory examination).
3. Skin blisters.
4. Lack of facilities to carefully observe these patients.

SUGGESTED READING

Allen MJ, Stirling AJ, Crawshaw CV, Barnes MR. Intracompartmental pressure monitoring of leg injuries: An aid to management. J Bone Joint Surg 1985; 67:53–57.

Connoly J. Acute compartment syndrome in the thigh. J Orthop Trauma 1987; 1:265.

Editorial. Compartment syndrome of the thigh. Lancet 1989; II: 485–486.

Matsen FA. A practical approach to compartmental syndromes: Part I—definition, theory and pathogenesis. In: McCollister EC, ed. Instructional course lectures. Vol. 32. St. Louis: CV Mosby, 1983:88.

Mubarak SJ. A practical approach to compartmental syndromes: Part II—diagnosis. In McCollister EC, ed. St. Louis, CV Mosby, 1983:92.

Robinson D, On E, Halperin N. Anterior compartment syndrome of the thigh in athletes—indications for conservative treatment. J Trauma 1992; 32:183–186.

Rooser B. Quadriceps contusion with compartment syndrome: evacuation of hematoma in 2 cases. Acta Orthop Scand 1987; 58:170–172.

Rothwell AG. Quadriceps hematoma. A prospective clinical study. Clin Orthop 1982; 171:97–103.

ANTERIOR COMPARTMENT SYNDROME OF THE THIGH: SURGICAL MANAGEMENT

ANGELO J. COLOSIMO, M.D.

Although contusions of the thigh are common in all sports and athletic competition, a compartment syndrome (CS) of the thigh from a closed, blunt, traumatic blow, without associated femur fracture, is extremely rare. Trauma to the quadriceps musculature during athletic competition can result in contusions of varying degrees of severity. Loss of playing time, reinjury, muscle weakness, and possible formation of myositis ossificans are common. Because of larger, more compliant osteofascial compartments in the thigh, thigh CS is rare in the athletic population, mainly because athletes are rarely exposed to the severe trauma necessary to cause it. It is more frequent in the multitrauma patient with associated fracture. Most cases of thigh CS are associated with multitrauma, gunshot wounds, prolonged external compression, postischemic swelling secondary to revascularization, or intermedullary rodding of the femur. Only 22 cases of thigh CS have been described as resulting from a closed, blunt, traumatic episode, without fracture, during athletic participation.

Although a rare entity, CS of the thigh does exist and, if not appreciated and rapidly diagnosed, serious predictable morbidity can be expected. Despite some controversy, the standard of care remains immediate fasciotomy of the involved compartment, draining of the hematoma, ligation of any vascular perforators, and delayed primary closure of the skin. CS should be considered if a single, blunt, traumatic blow to the thigh causes massive swelling, limited knee range of motion (ROM), and a progressive increase in pain unresponsive to the usual clinical modalities of elevation, ice, non-weight bearing, and analgesics.

ANATOMY

The anatomy of the thigh is quite different from that of the lower leg or forearm. Because of the larger compartments and thick protective musculature, neurologic deficits are rarely seen; however, sensory deficits over the saphenous nerve distribution, as well as the anterior femoral cutaneous nerve, have been reported. The femoral nerve transverses the anterior lateral compartment, innervates the quadriceps muscle, and is responsible for knee extension. Sensation to the anterior medial thigh and lower leg is supplied by the anterior femoral cutaneous nerve and saphenous nerve, respectively (Fig. 1). The thigh is separated into three major compartments by thick fascial septa. These divisions are the anterior (quadriceps), medial (adductor), and posterior (hamstring) compartments. The lateral intermus-

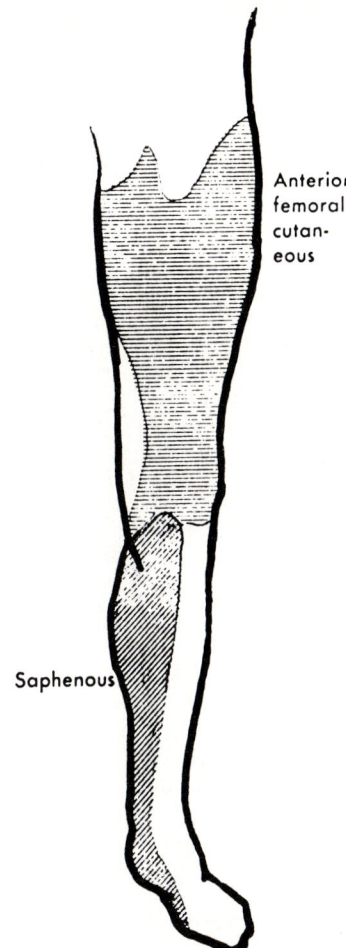

Figure 1 Sensory distribution of femoral nerve.

cular septum appears to be the thickest of the three (Fig. 2). The large thigh compartments allow for larger volume expansion, increased compliance, and a greater degree of swelling before reaching the critical pressures necessary for the development of a full blown CS commonly seen in the lower leg.

Although CS has been described in all three compartments of the thigh, most cases associated with athletic participation are limited to the anterior quadriceps compartment. In contact sports such as football, the anterior compartment is most commonly exposed to injury from a direct blow. CS of the posterior compartment has been reported, and is usually associated with massive rupture of the hamstring musculature.

PATHOPHYSIOLOGY

CS may occur in any compartment of the body in which significant trauma, compression, or bleeding creates soft tissue swelling or fluid within a given finite rigid osteofascial compartment. Swelling within a compartment can result from rupture of a perforating vessel, with subsequent hematoma, or swelling from increased capillary permeability, with resulting third-space fluid in

451

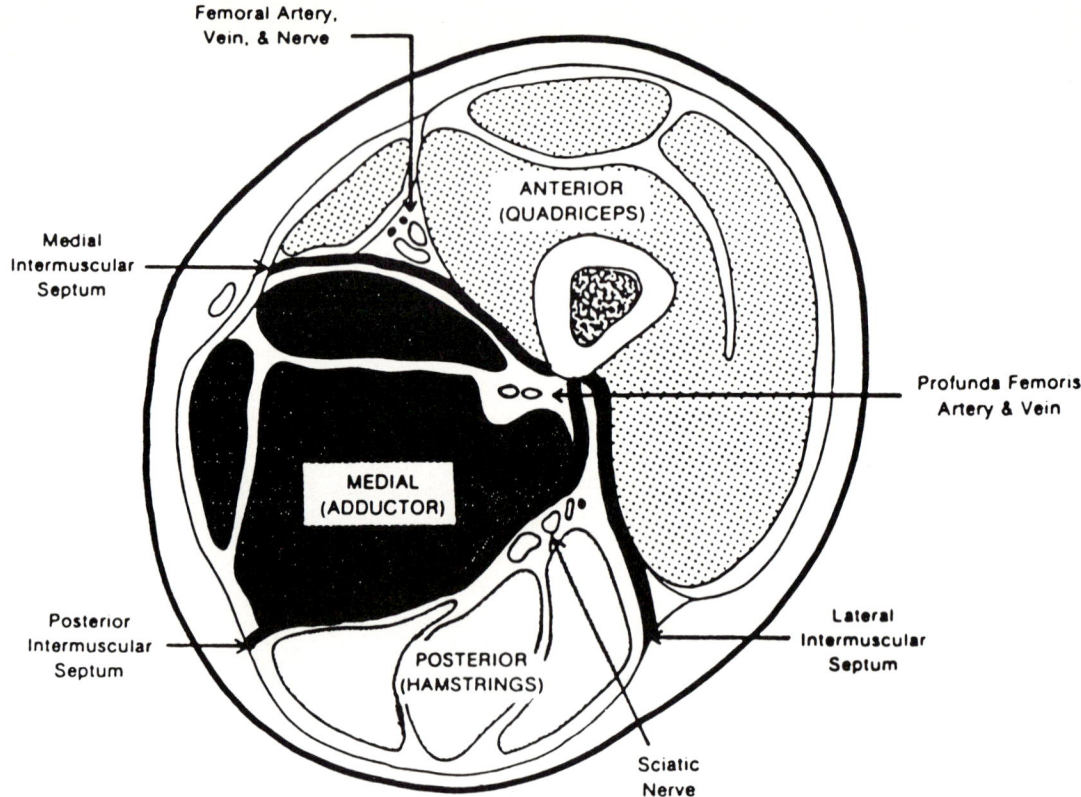

Figure 2 Cross-section of thigh, showing its three major compartments.

the damaged muscle compartment. In either case, the pathophysiology is the same for all compartment syndromes. Increased compartment pressures lead to muscle ischemia, metabolic and ultrastructural deterioration, and necrosis of the skeletal muscle with cellular acidosis. In cases of misdiagnosis or prolonged definitive treatment, as in drug overdose or in an unconscious patient, muscle necrosis can lead to eventual myoglobinuric renal failure and systemic involvement. Local complications include Volkman's ischemic contracture and myositis ossificans, both of which can be prevented with early diagnosis and appropriate treatment.

DIAGNOSIS

CS is defined as an increased tissue pressure in a closed fascial compartment, compromising the circulation to the nerves and muscles. Pressures are measured using the Stryker handheld intracompartmental monitoring system or the conventional wick catheter method. Controversy still exists as to the actual pressures within a compartment that warrant surgical intervention. Normal tissue pressures lie within the 0 to 8 mm Hg range. Through the work of Whitesides it has been accepted that decompression should be performed when compartment pressures lie within 10 to 33 mm Hg of the systemic diastolic blood pressure. Rather than using absolute values, this method takes into consideration the variable pressure tolerances in a given clinical situation, based on factors such as systemic hypotension, where higher

compartment pressures are less well tolerated. Factors that must be considered when measuring pressures are the height of the measured pressure, the duration of time the increased pressures are maintained, and the systemic blood pressure. It should be emphasized that the diagnosis of CS is not based solely on the measurement of compartment pressures, but rather on the entire clinical situation.

Compartment pressure must be measured whenever CS is clinically suspected. On examination, the classic "five Ps" (pain out of proportion to the injury, pain on passive motion of associated joints, pulselessness, paresthesias, and pallor) must be evaluated. The last three are usually late symptoms in which irreversible damage may have already occurred. They are rarely seen in thigh CS.

The indication for measurement of compartment pressures is based solely on clinical impression. Absolute indications include patients who are uncooperative, have closed head injuries, are unresponsive, and have known vascular or nerve deficits. However, it should be emphasized that pressure measurements are only relative indicators of the need for decompression. The patient's overall physical condition, tissue profusion, and clinical findings must be considered.

Differential Diagnosis

Thigh contusions can be extremely painful and debilitating to the athlete, but must be distinguised from thigh CS. Patients can present with mild contusions

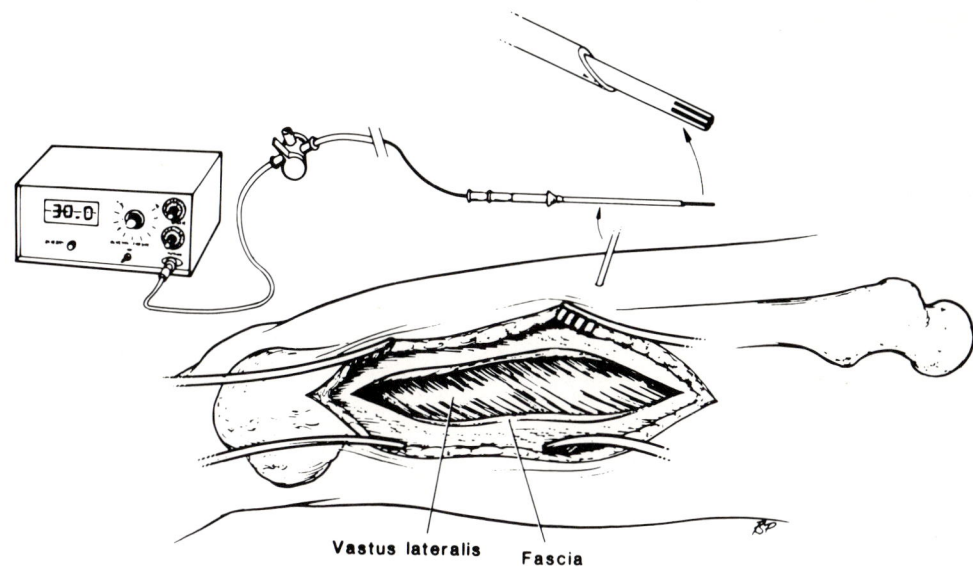

Figure 3 Exposure of fascia overlying vastus lateralis. Procedure is performed under intercompartmental pressure monitoring.

Vastus lateralis   Fascia

characterized only by local tenderness in the quadriceps with minimal loss of knee ROM and no alteration of gait. A moderate contusion is slightly more severe with a swollen, tender thigh, and less than 90 degrees of active knee motion. Passive stretch of the quadriceps as in knee flexion is extremely painful, and quadriceps muscle contraction is inhibited. The patient is relatively comfortable and pain tolerable.

The severe quadriceps contusion is sometimes the most difficult to separate from a true CS. The patient with a severe quad contusion usually has massive swelling of the thigh, has difficulty ambulating, and is extremely apprehensive about any motion of the knee. Knee motion is usually limited to less than 45 degrees. The thigh is firm and swollen and quadriceps muscle contraction is nonexistent. By contrast, a patient who has a thigh CS presents with a severely swollen, rock-hard thigh. The pain is unbearable and the patient usually does not find comfort in icing, elevation, or nonsteroidal anti-inflammatories. Thigh girth measurements should be made at the time of the injury, as well as sequentially, in order to evaluate progressive swelling. Further neurovascular signs of CS result from bleeding or increased capillary permeability with third-space fluid accumulation and acidosis. Except in the presence of major arterial injury, peripheral pulses are usually palpable and intact in the thigh CS. Rupture or tearing of the vascular perforators, usually branches of the profunda femoral artery, have also been seen. Pressures within the compartment are rarely high enough to compress a major vessel. The presence of paresthesias of the knee and medial aspect of the lower leg is difficult to interpret in cases of suspected CS. Such findings can be associated with pain from direct bruising, or actual muscle ischemia, secondary to the trauma. They could also represent compression of the anterior femoral cutaneous and saphenous nerve from elevated compartment pressures. Knee effusions are common. Therefore, thorough initial and follow-up knee examinations should be performed to rule out any associated ligamentous

knee damage. The major difference between a full blown thigh CS and a severe quad contusion lies within the level of pain and the amount of swelling and firmness in the anterior lateral thigh. Roentgenograms should always be obtained to rule out femoral fracture.

TREATMENT

When the clinical picture is confirmed by intercompartmental pressure measurements consistent with a CS, immediate surgical decompression is the treatment of choice.

Under intraoperative compartmental pressure monitoring, a 6 to 8 cm incision is made directly over the anterior lateral aspect of the thigh, over the vastus lateralis. The fascia overlying the vastus lateralis is then exposed (Fig. 3). The fascia is opened in line with the initial incision and extended proximally and distally subcutaneously until the entire anterior compartment has been decompressed. An immediate decrease in the intracompartmental pressures will be observed. Careful observation of the quadriceps musculature should be performed. Usually, the quadriceps musculature, and especially the vastus lateralis, is pale upon initial incision, but becomes red and viable after decompression (Fig. 4). The muscle should contract on stimulation, either manual or electrical. Careful exploration for small vascular perforators, usually branches of the profundus femoris artery or venous bleeders, should be identified and ligated. All clotted blood and hematoma should be evacuated. The wound is then abundantly irrigated, packed with gauze soaked in povidone-iodine, and dressed loosely. The patient is returned to the operating room within 48 hours for repeat irrigation, debridement, and delayed primary closure of the subcutaneous tissues and skin. The fascial layer is left open. Careful examination and evaluation of the knee, especially when knee effusion is present, should be performed at the time of delayed primary closure.

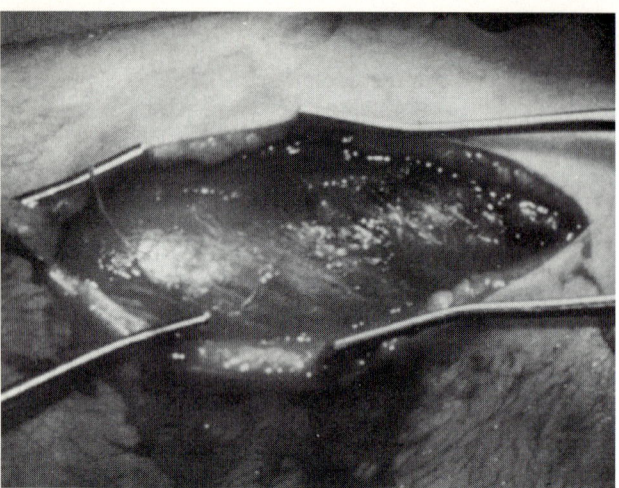

Figure 4 View of exposed quadriceps musculature.

Postoperatively, patients experience dramatic relief of pain. CPM should be started directly after the delayed primary closure, along with an active and active-assisted knee motion protocol. Partial weight bearing is allowed as soon as tolerable and indomethacin is used postoperatively for 6 weeks to prevent the formation of myositis ossificans.

There is a trend to attempt to treat thigh compartment syndromes in the athlete conservatively, without surgical decompression. This involves hospitalization, with careful, serial tissue pressure measurements, thigh girth measurements, evaluation of renal function, and close monitoring of creatine phosphokinase (CPK) levels. Advocates of conservative treatment cite surgical morbidity rates of up to 50% as reason for conservative treatment, although these high rates of morbidity have not been our experience.

We currently favor surgical decompression for acute thigh CS in the young athlete. The success of surgical decompression is based on accurate early diagnosis and early decompression. If decompression is performed later, after attempts at conservative treatment, irreversible damage may occur. The risk of possibly developing a permanent Volkman's contracture and quadriceps scarring due to delay far outweigh the risk of surgical incision.

Formation of myositis ossificans appears to be one of the most serious complications with severe thigh contusion and thigh CS. Up to 70% of patients with severe to moderate thigh contusions have been noted to develop myositis ossificans. Although only a few patients with thigh CS have been described in the literature, none that were surgically decompressed ever developed myositis ossificans. From these small number of cases, we cannot say definitely that surgical decompression prevents the formation of ectopic bone, but this has been our observation.

SUGGESTED READING

Colosimo AJ, Ireland ML. Thigh compartment syndrome in a football athlete: A case report and review of the literature. Med Sci Sports Exerc 1992; 24:958–963.

Heppenstall RB, Scott R, Sapega A, et al. A comparative study of the tolerance of skeletal muscle to ischemia. J Bone Joint Surg 1986; 68:820–827.

Jackson DW, Feagin JA. Quadriceps contusions in young athletes. J Bone Joint Surg 1973; 55:55–105.

Matson FA, Winquist RA, Krugmire RB. Diagnosis and management of compartmental syndromes. J Bone Joint Surg 1980; 62A:286–291.

Mubarak SJ, Owen CA, Hargens AR, et al. Acute compartment syndromes: Diagnosis and treatment with the aid of a wick catheter. J Bone Joint Surg 1978; 60A:1091–1095.

On HS, Simpson MJ, Gayle S, Jackson WT. Acute anterior compartment syndrome of the thigh: A case report and review of the literature. J Orthop Trauma 1987; 1:180–182.

Robinson D, On E, Halperin N. Anterior compartment syndrome of the thigh in athletes: Indications for conservative treatment. J Trauma 1992; 32:183–186.

Rooser B. Acute compartment syndrome from anterior thigh muscle contusion: Report of eight cases. J Orthop Trauma 1991; 5:55–59.

Schwartz JT, Brumback RJ, Lakatos R, et al. Acute compartment syndrome of the thigh. J Bone Joint Surg 1989; 71A:392–400.

Winternitz WA, Metheny JA, et al. Acute compartment syndrome of the thigh in sports related injuries not associated with femoral fractures. Am J Sports Med 1992; 20:476–477.

ASPIRATION OF BLUNT TRAUMA HEMATOMAS WITH LIPOSUCTION APPARATUS

RICHARD V. DOWDEN, M.D., F.A.C.S.

Closed trauma from sports injuries frequently produces soft tissue hematomas, with or without fractures. Hematomas can lead to necrosis of the overlying skin, in addition to being quite painful. The mechanisms for this skin necrosis are still under study, but it is known that pressure obstructs blood flow, leading to thrombosis, and also that hematomas release free radicals of iron that are toxic to skin. Such necrosis can greatly complicate the patient's problems, may lead to infection, and will prolong convalescence and delay return to sports and other activities.

PREVENTION

Prevention of a hematoma is difficult due to the vascular pressures involved in an injury. The standard measures for injured extremities are appropriate, including elevation, immobilization, and compression. The presence of a hematoma may not be obvious at first due to diffuse swelling. As the swelling subsides, the hematoma is evidenced by persistent painful localized swelling, most likely with discoloration of the skin. As time passes, the overlying skin may darken, en route to necrosis. The sports medicine specialist needs to be aware of the methods of treatment of such an established hematoma.

TREATMENT

The traditional methods of treating a hematoma have been either open evacuation or aspiration using a needle and syringe. Opening the hematoma is effective, but is a major procedure, while aspiration may be ineffective due to viscosity of the hematoma. The equipment and techniques that were developed for liposuction in plastic surgery can be used to deal with such hematomas, regardless of viscosity.

The plastic surgical technique of high-vacuum liposuction has proven extremely safe in the hands of those adequately trained to perform it. It has been used for aspiration of facelift hematomas, fat necrosis, removal of free silicone gel, and the hematomas under discussion here.

Equipment

The liposuction technique requires a vacuum pump capable of generating a strong negative pressure close to 29 inches of Hg, which means that wall suction is inadequate. The apparatus also comprises rigid transparent tubing, a collection bottle, and a trap to keep the aspirated material from entering the pump. The design of the cannula is critical, and the standard liposuction cannula has been found ideal. The cannula has a blunt tip for penetration through tissue without injuring any but the smallest vessels or nerves. The aperture of the cannula is not at the tip but along its side, and the edges of the opening are not sharp. These requirements mean that *the cannulae used in arthroscopy are totally unsuitable for this purpose.*

Technique

The procedure should be done as soon as the diagnosis is established. Ideally this would be immediately upon initial evaluation, but diffuse swelling and pain may make an early diagnosis difficult. Typically, several days elapse, at which time the skin may show discoloration, and localized swelling may indicate the hematoma.

The aspiration is done under sterile conditions in an operating room. Local anesthesia should suffice. The incision is situated near the edge of the hematoma in healthy skin that is neither compromised nor infected, with due consideration for nerves, tendons, and vessels. Local anesthetic is infiltrated only in the region of the skin incision and the proposed tunnel, with no attempt to anesthetize the hematoma and its surroundings.

With the suction pump off (otherwise the vacuum could impede passage through the subcutaneous tissue), the small cannula, about 4 mm, is advanced, tunnelling through subcutaneous fat into the hematoma cavity. This is then followed by the larger diameter 6 or 8 mm cannula. Penetrating the hematoma should be easy, as no fibrous capsule will have formed around a fresh hematoma.

After the cannula has entered the hematoma cavity, the vacuum pump is turned on. After about 10 seconds the pump is usually down to working pressure; if not the connections need to be checked. The cannula can then be maneuvered within the cavity as needed. The opening at the tip of the cannula should face toward the sides or the roof of the cavity, and not downward against the highly vascular muscle or fascia (this is the opposite of liposuction, where the opening faces downward). Care should be taken when facing the opening up toward the skin, where it could further damage the subdermal vascular network. This also is different from the technique described for facelift hematomas, where there is already a surgically-defined subdermal plane. The vacuum should be maintained as the suction cannula is withdrawn.

Neither irrigation nor chemical clot dissolution have been required. Drains should not be required, unless active bleeding is noted. Pain relief has been prompt and dramatic. A compression bandage is applied, and the patient should elevate the extremity until the edema resolves.

COMPLICATIONS

The potential complications of this method theoretically include infection, persistent hemorrhage, further injury to the overlying skin vasculature with necrosis, nerve or tendon injury, and unintentional passage of the cannula into adjacent areas. Proper training in liposuction, and the modifications of the liposuction technique outlined here, should make these complications quite unlikely. It is probably not worthwhile to purchase the liposuction equipment just for aspiration of the occasional hematoma, as most hospitals have the equipment and a plastic surgeon trained in its use.

RECOMMENDATIONS

This technique is highly recommended for evacuation of persistent viscous or coagulated subcutaneous hematomas after blunt trauma. When compared with open evacuation techniques, this method appears to be faster, easier, less expensive, less disfiguring, less painful, and safer. After trying it once, it will be apparent why a controlled randomized study has never been done, because there are no apparent advantages to the older techniques. I have not used this technique for hematomas occurring around a closed fracture; it would no doubt be effective, but one then is converting to an open fracture situation.

SUGGESTED READING

Dowden RV, Bergfeld JA, Lucas AL. Aspiration of hematomas with liposuction apparatus. J Bone Joint Surg 1990; 72A:1534.
Gerut ZE. Effective treatment of intraoperative breast prosthesis rupture: new use of the suction-assisted lipectomy machine (Letter). Plast Reconstr Surg 1987; 80:645.
Haddad J Jr, Angel MF, Abramson M. Reduction of hematoma-induced necrosis by deferoxamine. Surg Forum 1986; 37:564.
McEwan CN, Jackson IT, Stice RC. The application of liposuction for removal of hematomas and fat necrosis. Ann Plast Surg 1987; 19:480–481.

SOFT TISSUE INJURY TO THE HIP AND THIGH

R. CHARLES BULL, M.D., B.Sc. (Med), F.R.C.S.(C), F.A.C.S., F.I.C.S.

HEMATOMAS

In hockey the missed hip check resulting in a thrust of the knee at a fleeting opponent can often inflict an unpenalized and unrecognized serious injury. The blow taken on the central lateral midthigh area produces a hematoma with moderate initial pain. The injured player is often able to continue to participate and in so doing effectively pumps more blood into the hematoma. He can even take an additional injury, compounding the problem. Then, after the 10 minute intermission, he is unable to walk or skate. Untreated, this injury may lead to the complication of myositis ossificans, which may leave the individual sidelined with a partially mobile knee for as long as 1 year in some cases.

Initial Management

The measures that constitute immediate local management—RICE (spelled by the first letter of each measure)—are as follows:

1. *Rest* (R) with the leg on a bench or on pillows at 90-90 degree position of hip and knees. The important thing is to have the foot elevated well above the heart.

2. *Ice pack* (I) in a towel over the hematoma, on the area of maximal pain because there is not usually any bruising initially. The ice pack should be removed every 20 minutes for 20 minutes and then reapplied (20 minutes on, 20 minutes off), and continued to a lesser extent for at least 72 hours. *Do not apply heat.*

3. *Compression* (C) with two or three 6-inch, tightly applied tensor bandages. Be careful not to compromise the circulation; monitor the circulation by checking the peripheral pulses frequently. Just elevate the leg. Do not massage it or otherwise exercise it.

4. *Elevation* (E), with the foot elevated well above the heart, for 72 hours. The patient should remain totally off the feet for this period.

Medications

The use of Papase (*Carica papaya* enzymes) has never been proved effectual and should be abandoned.

Anti-inflammatory medications should be given as early as possible, particularly within the first 24 hours, to reduce the swelling and muscle spasm. The antiprostaglandins, such as Anaprox (naproxen sodium), are probably the most effective preparations—two tablets immediately and then one tablet three times daily for 7 to 10 days. Antiprostaglandins are recommended because a large amount of prostaglandin is released immediately at the time of injury, and this is a major factor in causing the initial swelling. Muscle relaxants do not work and theoretically can cause more bleeding in the relaxed muscle. (Alcohol is also contraindicated for the same reason.)

The most important initial management is recognition of the serious nature of the problem. Thus, rest, crutches, bed rest, ice, and elevation should be followed by a surgical assessment.

An initial soft tissue radiograph delineates a hematoma in one-third of the cases and is worthwhile. One should probably try to grade these hematomas as first, second, and third degree, as determined by pain, lack of mobility, degree of swelling, and response to rest.

First- and second-degree hematomas permit 90 degree movement and straight leg raising. Third-degree hematomas restrict movement to less than 90 degrees and permit *active* knee flexion, but not straight leg raising. These patients have severe pain in spite of medication and should be hospitalized.

The very serious third-degree injuries usually are fairly obvious. There is severe pain, immobility of the knee in particular, as well as the hip, and swelling that increases by 1 ½ to 2 inches (4 to 5 cm) the girth of the quadriceps by actual measurement. A very tense, large swollen area, 6 to 8 inches in diameter (15 to 20 cm), can often be felt bulging beneath the fascia lata. It feels "different," not truly fluctuant but much tenser than normal muscle, and there is often an associated large, tense synovial effusion in the knee. This can be mistaken for an intrinsic knee problem, but is actually a sympathetic response and the knee itself is normal.

Wydase (hyaluronidase), steroids, or local anesthetics have been injected into these hematomas in the first 72 hours, but this practice is contraindicated because of (1) increased tendency to infection and (2) their alteration of the defense mechanism and production of collagen fibers, which in essence would delay healing rather than enhance it.

At 72 hours the repair stage starts, and patients with first-degree hematoma should be fairly comfortable. Some swelling is noted, but there should be moderately good mobility and, at this stage, fairly extensive bruising in the classic cases.

The muscle fibers are crushed or torn and the hematoma can be very extensive. The most frequent problem is an *inter*stitial or *inter*muscular hematoma in which the muscle sheath ruptures and the blood and bruising tracks up or down the leg. These are the "good ones," although they do look bad because of extensive bruising.

The "bad ones" are the *intra*muscular hematomas, in which the muscle sheath remains intact and thus the hematoma remains isolated. Absorption is much more difficult. In these cases the periosteum also is often damaged and osteoblasts become available to convert the subperiosteal or intramuscular hematomas into myositis ossificans.

Physiotherapy can push the "good ones" (intermuscular), but the "bad ones" have to rest to prevent further bleeding and enlargement of the hematomas. Cool whirlpool, range-of-motion exercises, light cycling, light weights, springs and pulleys, and early walking progressing to light jogging and early skating can be instituted in the good ones.

The third-degree injuries are worse at the end of 72 hours, with unremitting severe pain and increasing immobility, and these should be operated on. Under general anesthesia, a satisfactory 4 inch (10 cm) incision is made laterally through the fascia lata. Careful probing with a Kelly hemostat is then undertaken, and as soon as blood and clot are released the incision is opened more widely by blunt dissection.

The hematoma usually lies right on top of the bone and can be evacuated and completely removed with the assistance of copious irrigation with gentamicin sulfate (Garamycin) solution. The fascia lata, the subcutaneous tissue, and the skin are then closed and a Jones bandage is applied from toes to groin. Once the clot has been evacuated, treatment can be the same as for a first-degree injury over the next 7 to 10 days — physiotherapy, ice, sound, progressing to range of motion, but no massage.

Second-degree injuries are puzzling, but when in doubt they should be treated as third-degree injuries. A long 16 or 14 gauge needle introduced into the hematoma in an attempt to aspirate blood seems a sensible procedure, but is not. It is usually hard to find the exact fluctuant area, and often the clot cannot be aspirated. Furthermore, the needle is likely to introduce an infection; once the hematoma is infected, a systemic problem exists, requiring surgical drainage and systemic antibiotics and increasing the danger of long-term complications. Therefore, the hematoma is either decompressed satisfactorily in the operating room or treated conservatively.

A missed third-degree injury may come to light at the 7 to 10 day mark, as indicated by a swollen painful thigh and an immobile hip and knee. These injuries are often treated with hot baths and are the most likely to develop into myositis ossificans.

I still surgically explore these on occasion. I also prescribe physiotherapy to try to mobilize these people with gentle pool therapy, ultrasonography, and management to decrease the swelling, but again no massage, no faradism to stimulate the muscle or increase bleeding, and no isokinetic or isotonic weight program.

The first radiologic signs of ossification, the typical "sandstorm" appearance, are visible about 3 weeks after the injury. As this matures, an anvil-shaped lesion appears. The full-blown myositis ossificans, verified radiographically (Fig. 1), need no treatment other than rest. Swimming and cycling are permitted, but no running, skating, and the like.

It can take up to 6, even 12, months for this problem to settle completely. I never operate on a fully developed myositis ossificans (fully calcified) because the ossification tends to recur.

The fully developed quiescent case of myositis ossificans allows a normal return to unlimited sports.

Prevention consists of

1. *Better conditioning* to avoid the missed hip check.
2. *Better warm-ups.*
3. *Stretching exercises* starting from the neck and working down literally to the Achilles tendon, feet, and toes. These form part of the basis of a sensible warm-up program.
4. *Equipment* that fits properly; this should be used

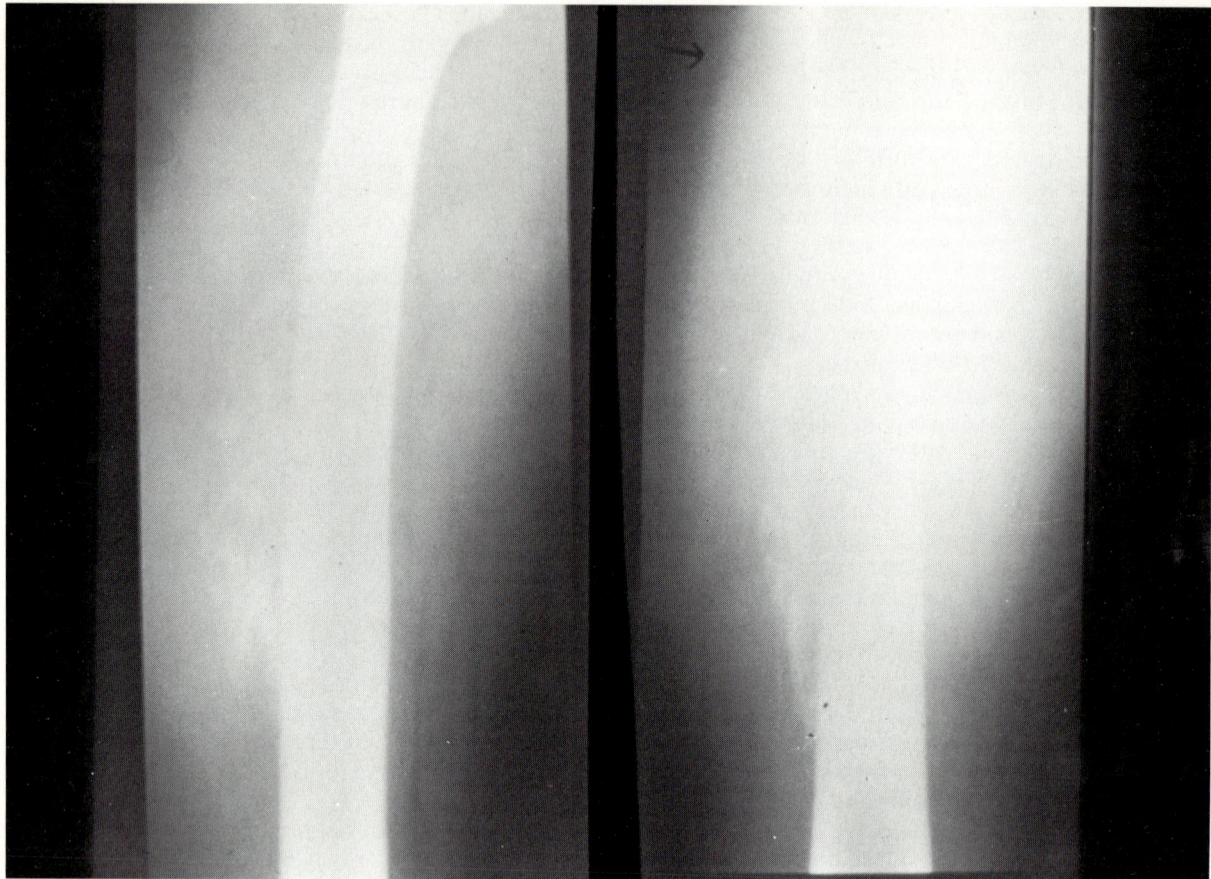

Figure 1 Myositis ossificans subsequent to thigh hematoma.

even during light practice. The Cooperall reduces hematomas because of its uniform fit and total body padding (Fig. 2).

5. *Following the rules.* Kneeing, spearing, and crosschecking rules all have to be enforced by the coach as well as the referee.

6. *Protective taping or adhesive,* tensor bandage, or bracing. This is beneficial on a weakened joint or limb. In current use are "pro" type neoprene sleeves or even pantaloon leg sleeves, for thigh hematomas in particular, which are effective but expensive.

7. *Cautious return.* Beware of further trauma. Basically, the player can skate in a straight line at first, but must not push, twist, or pivot; gradually he progresses to these activities as strength returns.

8. *Caution regarding massage.* Trainers, physiotherapists, and masseurs must be very careful in the active phase not to prolong or initiate bleeding or augment tissue damage.

9. *Avoiding other methods* of treatment. Ethylchloride spray (which is probably of no benefit), analgesic balm, and DMSO are contraindicated as they only remove the pain. Pressure or trigger point injection, acupuncture, and TNS Probe are advocated by some and may have some

benefit, although to date this has not been proved.

10. *Strengthening.* After severe injury it takes at least 6 weeks to get into the remodeling phase with additional strength. This can be graded clinically from 1 to 6 by the physiotherapist or physician, but it is more realistically graded by Cybex isokinetic equipment. This gives a computerized assessment of the exact strength deficiency and compares it with the opposite leg, as well as quadriceps to hamstrings and fast-twitch to slow-twitch muscle strength. In our clinics, results of these Cybex tests should be 90% of normal before the patient returns to the sport.

11. *Additional overall strength training.* Isokinetic training is best, and in the case of the thigh it should be not only the gastrocnemius and hamstrings, but also the adductors and abductors, evertors and invertors with stereotactic training (jumping over sticks or boxes), and thus the athlete is less apt to restrain the injured limb. This is different from conventional weight training, which is strictly isotonic. The isokinetic strengthening also develops the fast-twitch fibers and creates more overall strength in the limb. This type of training has not been emphasized enough in the past.

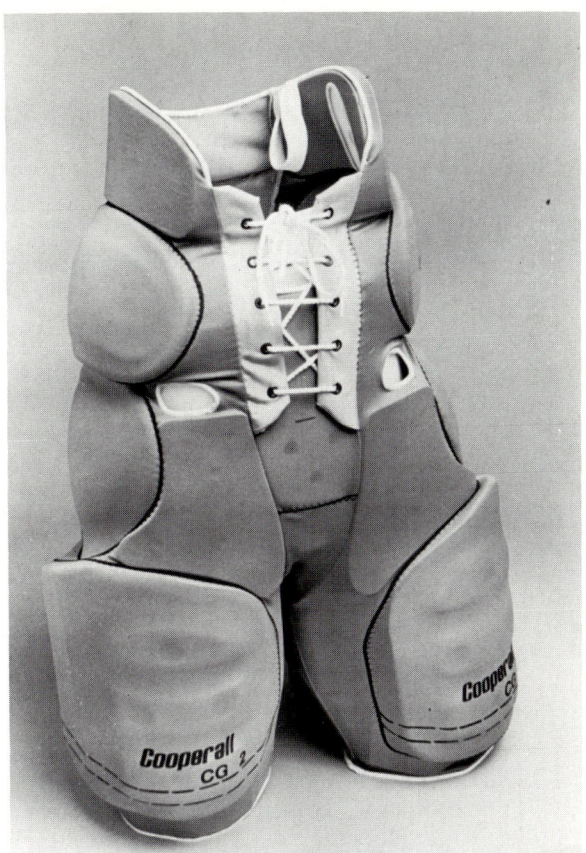

Figure 2 Protective equipment, such as the Cooperall, greatly reduces the incidence of thigh hematoma.

HIP POINTERS

Hip pointers are more likely to be self-inflicted by a fall into the boards or goalpost or, less often, a hard crosscheck, in lacrosse for instance. Specifically, a collection of blood forms beneath the periosteum in the area adjacent to the iliac crest, and involves the muscles and soft tissues above the crest. The hip pointer is a very painful localized swelling with significant localized bruising. However, it is never as serious on a long-term basis as the previously discussed hematomas.

Because long-term problems are very unusual, treatment can be a little less aggressive. However, the same principles apply: (1) RICE and (2) immediate physiotherapy with sound or interferential, no injections, and usually no operation.

X-ray studies should be performed to rule out a fracture or displaced epiphyseal fracture, which requires a much longer immobilization process (6 to 8 weeks). In an uncomplicated hip pointer, a large protective doughnut-type pad can be fashioned over the hip, and in many cases the player can return in 7 to 10 days, although I have known some to take as long as 2 months.

Better warm-up and conditioning are the best preventive measures, and better equipment (e.g., the Cooperall) is second in importance.

MUSCLE STRAINS

Muscle strains can result from indirect or direct injuries. Muscles commonly affected are antagonist or checking muscles, such as the hamstrings or adductors, and the condition can occur anywhere in the muscle tendon unit. It is most likely to affect the muscle origin or insertion, but a muscle tendinous junction, muscle belly, or tendon sheath can be involved.

The resultant inflammatory response (tendinitis), in the case of the adductors, causes the "pulled groin." Psoas and rectus muscle involvement are alternative forms of the "pulled groin." In the hamstrings the tendinitis-periostitis picture at the ischial tuberosity characterizes the "pulled ham."

The isolated inner-body muscle strain in the midportion of the hamstrings or adductors is usually more responsive to treatment, and with successful therapy athletes return to their sport in approximately half the time. The same principles of early recognition and caution regarding reaggravation apply. The cause is often some new stretching exercise or a sport or drill unrelated to the major sport, e.g., off-ice drills such as dancercize or running as an adjunct to hockey. The essential management is to stop the off-ice activities.

Physiotherapy is the key here, and a good physiotherapist (massage therapist) can initially decrease a lot of the muscle spasm. Then, a strong rehabilitation strengthening program with springs, pulleys, surgical tubing, stair stepping, and side stepping should be added. Progress in the final remodeling-strengthening phase through isokinetic equipment is very worthwhile. (The adductor-abductor machine, for instance, can be used for both speed and endurance.)

Aquabics or pool therapy—running in water, doing the alphabet in water, kicking in water—is quite worthwhile in early phases, but should be followed by a return to short-stride activities such as skating without stretching out the stride or slow running without lifting the leg. *Pain should be your guide,* and obviously anything that hurts should be avoided.

Muscle strains are endemic in quality runners, and are usually due to the drills. Hard interval training, such as repeat 50s, 100s, and 200s with unsatisfactory rest breaks, is the culprit. Many national sprinters warm up for 1 hour before doing their interval work.

The A and B drills, which require a hard goose-step kicking out very quickly, or a high-stepping, very quick knee elevation like that of a majorette, can cause these muscle strains and should be done only after a 20 minute basic warm-up, and deemphasized when any type of injury has been sustained.

These muscle and ligament strains can also be satisfactorily classified as first, second, and third degree. The first-degree strains, particularly in sprinters, are often just a type of muscle spasm or strain, and in some cases the sprinter can compete the same day. Calcium lack is a possible cause, and calcium (Sandoz, 4 ml or 1 teaspoon daily) is sometimes a good prophylactic medication.

The second-degree strain is usually an overuse,

overtraining injury that can respond quickly to a training alleviation or alteration, e.g., substituting cycling and swimming for running.

The third-degree conditions give the athlete pain before, during, and after the sport. They interfere with life-style and everyday activities and are probably associated with a true tear in the muscle, muscle tendon junction, or insertion into the periosteum. Treatment consists of complete rest for as long as 6 to 8 weeks, and in cases of severe adductor or hamstring tendinitis, some quality athletes are kept away from sport as long as 3 to 6 months; running is prohibited, but judicious cycling and swimming are allowed.

Return to competition should be determined by leg strength. Cybex evaluation can indicate when drills such as cuts, pivots, figure-of-eights, hard striding, jumps, and full stretching work-outs can be resumed.

A person who is subject to repeated muscle strains needs to have the training schedule reevaluated. Some athletes experience a "true overuse syndrome," in which the resting pulse is elevated. They are agitated and restless, literally owing to total body exhaustion. They are prone to muscle strains and pulls.

Complete blood work, a zeta sedimentation rate (ZSR) and serum ferritin determination may show altered chemistry and should be repeated in athletes who are trying to "peak" and are not succeeding.

Principles

1. *It is hard to strain a hot muscle.* Therefore, warm up. Olympic sprinters warm up for more than 1 hour to run a 50 or 100 meter run.
2. *You cannot tire a young athlete.* Some of the tennis greats can run for half an hour, skip for half an hour, and play for half an hour before the match. A proper warm-up will not tire you; it enhances performance and prevents injuries.
3. *Sensible drills.* The only person who has to do Olympic weight training is an Olympic weight lifter. Thus, sensible drills to strengthen and tone up muscles with realistic weights—three sets of 10 or three sets of 30—are indicated. Isokinetic work-outs, beating the clock (for instance, 20 times in 20 seconds), are also good, but the muscle has to be exercised short of excess fatigue or exhaustion. There is no point in wearing out a muscle. The principle is to strengthen it.
4. *The best training is the sport itself.* Skating is for hockey players, gymnastics for gymnasts. They are most apt to get hurt in alternative sports or repetitive drills, e.g., repetitive jumping and dunking in basketball or running with ankle weights on.
5. *Routine medications and diet supplements.* Vitamin C is probably needed by individuals in hard training to improve the biochemical environment and regeneration of constantly strained muscles. Calcium can be used in certain cases to decrease muscle cramps. Emphasize a balanced diet, and no other regular medications or supplements are needed.
6. *Avoid muscle overload.* Strengthen muscles, reduce load, alter equipment, improve style.
7. *Chronic problems.* Heat before playing, aspirin before playing, massage with liniment, ultrasonography, whirlpool as necessary.
8. *Trigger points* for massage. Good athletic trainers can often remove some of the muscle knots and spasms before competition.
9. *Stretch throughout the day,* four times daily for 10 to 15 minutes, to keep muscles relaxed and in tone.
10. *Bone scans* can be used to elucidate the magnitude of the muscle-periosteal injury in some cases, but usually are not indicated.
11. *Other medications.* Spreading or dispersal agents and oral proteolytic enzymes are ineffective. Muscle relaxants usually have no place in muscle strains of the hip and just tire a young athlete. Local anesthesia to freeze the area of muscle strain or spasm to allow the athlete to play is too risky. It is almost guaranteed to increase the injury (to convert a first-degree to a third-degree injury).
12. *Steroids.* Local steroids can be used if there is an isolated trigger point or a localized point, such as the adductor tendon origin strain. The steroids are then injected around the pubic tubercle and cautiously instilled beneath the spermatic cord. Steroids should not be introduced into the tendon itself or into the cord, but injected judiciously along the periosteum with a small 25-gauge needle. This can be done in resistant cases and repeated on three occasions 1 month apart. This must be augmented by physiotherapy. Oral steroids basically are never used in my practice. Topical agents are ineffectual. However, some benefit may be derived from iontophoresis with 5% hydrocortisone cream and 5 amps of electronic stimulation placed over a gauze pad for 20 minutes, administered at 2 day intervals.
13. *Anabolics.* Oral anabolics are considered to have some effect in the healing of a torn muscle, but they are used so indiscriminately for muscle strengthening and training that these nontherapeutic uses of anabolic steroids, or even growth hormones, make their therapeutic use questionable. Thus, even if therapeutic uses are beneficial, one should probably avoid these medications.
14. *Surgery.* I have operated on the adductor tendon to release it from its insertion into the pubis. This is a full adductor tendon release; it is similar to a tennis elbow release in that it allows the pressure to be removed from that area, but results have not been proved. In my hands it has been beneficial in the long-term, very resistant case.

Differential Diagnosis

Lumbar disc herniation with resultant nerve root irritation and sciatica may be mistaken for muscle strain, as may stress fracture of the pubic ramus. Strained rectus femoris muscles can be confused with a stress fracture of the femur or an intrinsic pathologic condition in the hip joint itself.

Around the hip joint two major bursal complexes are subject to inflammation in response to athletic activity. The gluteal bursa in the buttock, and the trochanteric bursa over the greater trochanter, may both be the sites of a very troublesome bursitis.

The trochanteric bursa is inflamed from repetitive slipping back and forth across the trochanter of the tensor fascia lata. Common in runners, dancers, and gymnasts, it may also trouble racquet sports players with pain during activity; local tenderness to pressure may prevent lying on the affected side. The deep gluteal bursae when inflamed are associated with a deep-seated buttock discomfort, which may simulate referred pain from the back and has to be distinguished from a lumbar disc problem or piriformis syndrome in which the sciatic nerve is irritated at its emergence through the greater sciatic notch.

Modification of activity is the mainstay of treatment; physiotherapy with deep heat or ultrasonography, anti-inflammatory medication, and local steroids also has a place. Occasionally, surgical release of the tensor fascia is necessary in refractory cases of trochanteric bursitis, and on occasion a piriformis release is necessary in patients with a piriformis syndrome, but care has to be taken to rule out a lumbar spine problem absolutely.

PARTICIPANT CHARACTERISTICS AND SPORTS PARTICIPATION

Guidance in the selection of a suitable sport for an individual should be an important factor in pregame physicals. Obviously, people who are much too stiff and inflexible should not be allowed to participate in sports in which pulled muscles and tendons are a problem. Similarly, individuals with undue joint laxity may be at risk in contact sports. Judicious guidance to the player from the coach, doctor, or parent may help prevent many of these injuries. There should also be avenues for immediate medical referral and satisfactory physiotherapy of an immediate nature, followed by long-term complete rehabilitation and counseling regarding reinjury if the morbidity rate of these common soft tissue injuries is to be reduced.

TRAUMATIC SUBLUXATION OF THE HIP

DANIEL E. COOPER, M.D.

In contrast to the well-known entity of traumatic subluxation of the athlete's shoulder, traumatic subluxation of the hip has only recently been recognized. Although this is certainly rare, the lack of awareness of this injury pattern has probably contributed to the infrequent clinical diagnosis or case report. Because of the potentially significant sequelae of this injury, it is important for the sports medicine clinician to be aware of this hip injury and its potential complications.

In a previous report we documented the clinical and radiographic course of a 23-year-old healthy, black, male, professional running back who was injured when tackled during a scrimmage. The injury was witnessed by the team physician, and the mechanism of injury was a direct blow to the anterior knee with the hip positioned in flexion and adduction. Subsequent aseptic femoral head necrosis was documented. It was the intent of this case report to heighten the awareness of the clinician to this entity.

More recently, the injury sustained by Bo Jackson has directed a great deal of attention toward the diagnosis of traumatic subluxation of the hip. This increased awareness is likely to lead to increasing frequency of occurrence of this injury due to accurate diagnosis.

DIAGNOSIS

Pain out of proportion to the usual soft tissue injury should lead to suspicion that a more significant osseous hip injury may be present. The liberal use of plain radiographs should be employed, and Judet rotational views of the pelvis can reveal posterior acetabular fractures that might otherwise go unnoticed. Additionally, review of game films or videos can confirm the exact injury mechanism.

Computed tomography (CT) provides additional sensitivity in detecting posterior acetabular lesions (Fig. 1). Magnetic resonance imaging (MRI) is exquisitely sensitive and may potentially identify pathology that would otherwise go unnoticed. However, it may reveal radiographic abnormalities such as bone bruises, which

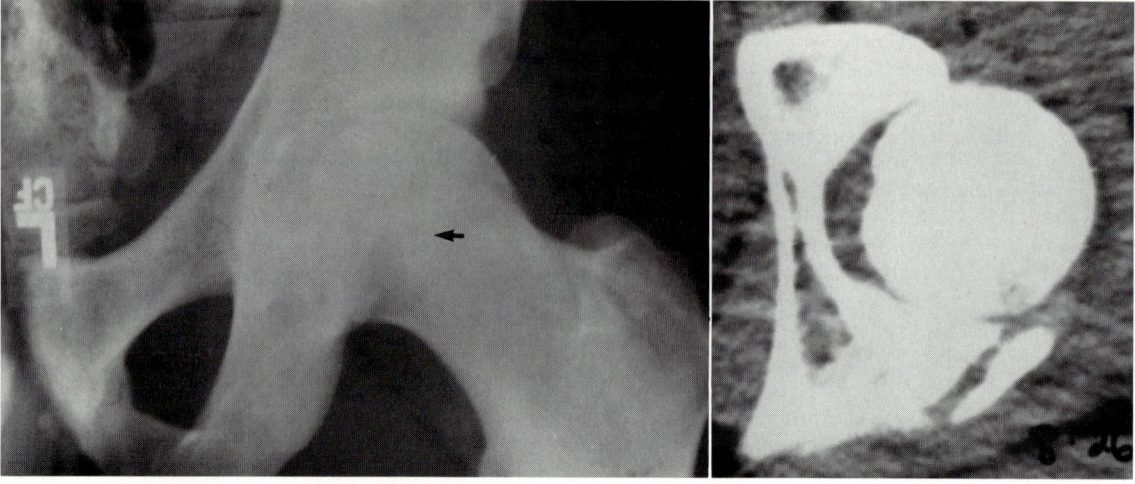

Figure 1 *A,* Initial anteroposterior radiograph of the left hip after injury, demonstrating a subtle rim fracture of the posterior acetabular wall. *B,* CT scan of the left hip, demonstrating a rim fracture of the posterior acetabular wall, which is analogous to the Bankart type fracture in the shoulder. (From Cooper DE, Warren RF, Barnes R. Traumatic subluxation of the hip resulting in aseptic necrosis and chondrolysis in a professional football player. Am J Sports Med 1991; 19:322, 323; with permission.)

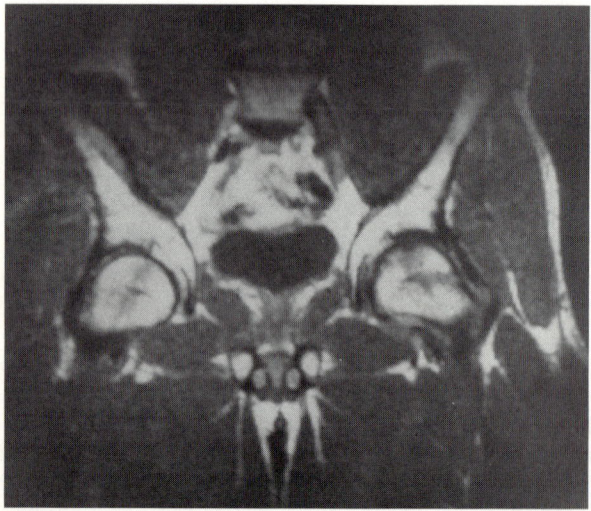

Figure 2 MR image (TR = 0.5, TE = 40) demonstrating the focal pattern of aseptic necrosis in the left femoral head. In addition, the hemarthrosis is well demonstrated. (From Cooper DE, Warren RF, Barnes R. Traumatic subluxation of the hip resulting in aseptic necrosis and chondrolysis in a professional football player. Am J Sports Med 1991; 19:323; with permission.)

may be clinically insignificant. Therefore, MRI is not routinely used in the early workup of hip injuries in the athlete. However, with persistent pain and limp, it is a useful imaging modality.

The MRI appearance of avascular necrosis (AVN) is well known. Segmental AVN has been associated with traumatic subluxation of the hip, as opposed to more diffuse pattern of AVN that may result from complete dislocation (Fig. 2). The limited number of available cases makes this trend somewhat anecdotal.

INJURY PREVENTION

It is more relevant to discuss the prevention of adverse sequelae, rather than prevention of the injury itself. Since the full contact nature of many sports precludes the elimination of this injury mechanism, it is imperative that the injury be recognized and treated appropriately by the sports medicine clinician.

With early diagnosis and appropriate avoidance of participation, subsequent deterioration due to unawareness of the diagnosis is avoided. Although the radiographic findings may be subtle, traumatic subluxation is usually a much more painful injury to the hip than the usual muscle strain and ligament sprains common in sports. This should heighten the clinician's suspicion in this setting.

TREATMENT

The early treatment for traumatic subluxation of the hip is protected weight bearing with crutches and avoidance of participation in sports. The athlete should be in a toe-touch, weight-bearing status. Unless the diagnosis of a posterior acetabular rim fracture is made, it is difficult to document this diagnosis. If clinical suspicion is great enough, I recommend treating the patient in the same manner. Because of the potential consequences, any traumatic posterior subluxation of the hip associated with an acetabular rim fracture should be treated as would a complete hip dislocation after reduction of the dislocation. Therefore, protective weight-bearing status should be maintained for 6 weeks. CT is useful for evaluating the presence of intra-articular osteochondral fragments. Should this exist, an arthrotomy would be necessary for removal. Unless the posterior acetabular rim fragment is large, the treatment for this fracture is nonoperative.

COMPLICATIONS

Chondrolysis

Chondrolysis is a poorly understood, post-traumatic entity in the hip. It may be seen after drill or pin penetration into the hip, as well as after slipped capital femoral epiphysis in a child. Chondrolysis is a rapid dissolution of cartilage that may be related to an inflammatory synovial-like membrane over the cartilage. This has not been studied in traumatic subluxation of this hip, but has been reported to occur in association with this entity (Fig. 3).

Joint space narrowing after traumatic subluxation may be due to the initial trauma of the injury with subsequent cartilage necrosis. It may also be that the rapid destruction of articular cartilage is due to an inflammatory process similar to chondrolysis. It is well known that recurrent intra-articular hemorrhage, as in hemophilia, leads to enzymatic destruction of articular cartilage. Although it is possible that the hemarthrosis that was present after the initial injury may be a contributing factor to the rapid destruction of articular cartilage, this seems to be an unlikely mechanism based on a single episode.

Aseptic Necrosis

Aseptic necrosis of the hip has many etiologies. Atraumatic etiologies include corticosteroid use, alcoholism, hemoglobinopathies, and idiopathic causes. The less common post-traumatic aseptic necrosis of the hip generally occurs after complete dislocation of the hip. Its incidence varies from 15% to 20% and increases with delay in reduction. These numbers do not reflect routine use of MRI technology in diagnosis. However, most cases of post-traumatic aseptic necrosis occur within the first year after injury. The true incidence of aseptic necrosis after traumatic subluxation of the hip is not known.

In underlying conditions such as alcoholism and steroid use, the pathophysiology is the subject of much debate. However, post-traumatic aseptic necrosis has been clearly shown to be due to interruption of the blood supply to the femoral head. This commonly occurs as a result of posterior dislocations that disrupt the superior retinacular vessels. Any blood supply remaining through the ligamentum teres is also disrupted in a dislocation. It was not previously recognized that this complication might result from traumatic subluxation alone. In fact, our report was the first in the English literature.

When considering aseptic necrosis as a possible complication of dislocation of the hip, the time between dislocation and reduction is a critical prognostic factor. In traumatic subluxation the hip congruity is only instantaneously disrupted, whereas in a complete dislocation the femoral head is often left unreduced for hours. If the time factor alone is considered, it follows

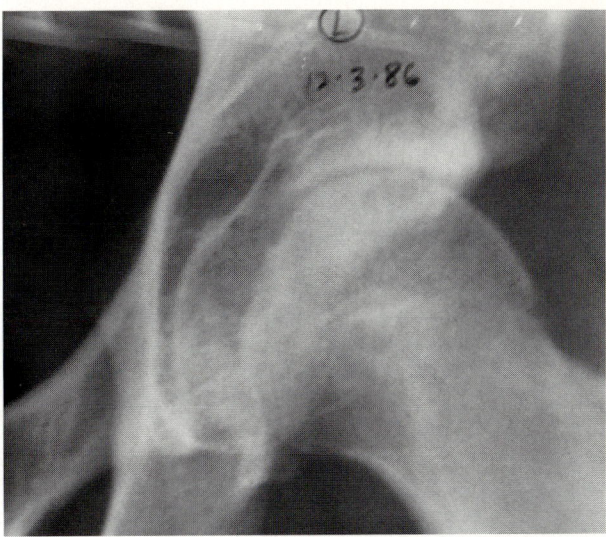

Figure 3 Radiograph of the left hip 4 months after injury, demonstrating the rapid destruction of articular cartilage and loss of joint space. (From Cooper DE, Warren RF, Barnes R. Traumatic subluxation of the hip resulting in aseptic necrosis and chondrolysis in a professional football player. Am J Sports Med 1991; 19:323; with permission.)

that post-traumatic aseptic necrosis after subluxation might be less extensive than after complete dislocation. This segmental pattern of necrosis, which was evident in the case that we have reported, may be due to only segmental compromise of intraosseous blood flow as opposed to the more diffuse pattern commonly seen after disruption of the superior retinacular vessels. This, of course, is only a conjecture based on current knowledge of the disease process.

RETURN TO SPORT

Prior to return to sport there should be a full, painless motion of the involved hip. I recommend that return to contact sports be avoided for 3 months after injury. Repeat hip radiographs are useful to screen for joint space narrowing suggestive of chondrolysis. In any athlete, but particularly an elite athlete, it is prudent to obtain an MRI scan before return to sport to rule out aseptic necrosis. A 3 month delay in obtaining an MRI has the advantage of allowing resolution of less significant MRI diagnoses such as bone bruises. Should aseptic necrosis be diagnosed by MRI, it would be imprudent to allow the athlete to return to sport until the revascularization phase is complete. Because of the potential for collapse during the revascularization phase, running and contact sports would cause an increased risk of collapse and post-traumatic arthrosis.

The decision regarding the return to sport is pivotal on the existence of the diagnosis of aseptic necrosis, or chondrolysis. Should one of these diagnoses be present, the return to sport would be greatly delayed. Additionally, the athlete should be informed in detail of the inherent risks of return to such sport with this diagnosis. It is best for the longevity of the hip in this setting to avoid impact sports.

SURGERY

In the acute setting, surgery is indicated if there is an intra-articular osteochondral loose body or a large posterior acetabular wall fracture. Arthrotomy and, in certain instances, hip arthroscopy will be needed for the former, and open reduction and internal fixation for the latter. However, intra-articular loose bodies are more frequently found after a complete dislocation and subsequent reduction.

Surgery to address the complication of severe post-traumatic hip arthrosis falls into two categories; arthrodesis and arthroplasty. Although the former is no longer frequently performed, there is no better indication than unilateral hip arthritis in a young active patient. Total hip arthroplasty in a young active patient is more controversial, and in spite of the short-term performance of the one known elite athlete with a prosthesis implanted for the purpose of returning to sport, there is a great deal of scientific evidence to suggest that such a prosthesis will be subject to very early aseptic loosening. Though neither procedure is conducive to elite athletics, arthrodesis is the most durable for the young patient who wishes to remain physically active. The patient who does not want an arthrodesis must be willing to accept a sedentary life-style prior to my recommending hip arthroplasty.

SUGGESTED READING

Cooper DE, Warren RF, Barnes R. Traumatic subluxation of the hip resulting in aseptic necrosis and chondrolysis in a professional football player. Am J Sports Med 1991; 19:322–324.
Cruess RL. Osteonecrosis of bone. Current concepts as to etiology and pathogenesis. Clin Orthop 1986; 208:30.
Duncan CP, Shim SS. Blood supply of the head of the femur in traumatic hip dislocation. Surg Gynecol Obstet 1977; 144:185–191.
Epstein HC. Posterior fracture-dislocations of the hip. J Bone Joint Surg 1961; 43A:1079–1098.
Epstein HP. Traumatic dislocations of the hip. Clin Orthop 1973; 92:116–142.
Ficat RP. Idiopathic bone necrosis of the femoral head (review article). J Bone Joint Surg 1985; 67B:3.
Gregory CF. Early complications of dislocation and fracture-dislocation of the hip joint. AAOS Instructional Course Lectures 1973; 22:150–153.

FEMORAL NECK STRESS (SHEAR) FRACTURE

LeROY R. FULLERTON, Jr., M.D.

Femoral neck stress fractures were first reported in significant numbers in military runners. The common factor in the hip region lesions and stress fractures elsewhere was repetitive impact. The vigorous training history continues to be the setting for this injury in athletes. Understanding the causes and diagnostic features is the key to a program of prevention and to the sometimes controversial treatment recommendations.

ETIOLOGY

The history of repetitive lower extremity stress, usually over a 2 to 4 week period, is common. In athletes this type of training occurs early in pre-season endurance conditioning. It also can be found in mid-season increased intensity or abrupt changes in the exercise routine. Examples of the latter would be a runner conditioned for 10 km races pushing too rapidly to prepare for his first marathon. Another common setting is the change from flat, especially resilient, terrain to a more hilly course or harder running surface. The military experiences seem to accelerate conditions leading to these injuries to the hip. In this situation, group rather than individual conditioning is the norm. Forced marching or running can produce muscle fatigue. The loss of the efficiency of the hip muscles as shock absorber intensifies the stress loads seen by the bony structure of the femoral neck. A third factor that contributes, at least in theory, is the harmful effect of an altered running gait. This change in mechanics can come from multiple causes, but blisters, foot or knee injuries, different stride lengths, and structural abnormalities are all factors to consider at the start and throughout training in running sports. Finally, the body's response to mechanical impact stress seems to play a central role. When the training program does not allow the osteoblastic or bone-rebuilding activity to keep pace with the osteoclastic or bone resorbing response, then the conditions are there for mechanical damage to the hip. Important differences in susceptibility to the injury have long been known. Women runners have a higher incidence than men, and amenorrhiac female runners are at even greater risk. In addition, whites are more susceptible to hip stress fractures than blacks. Finally, while it might seem that older runners might be at greater risk because of gradually increasing osteoporosis, there are only isolated case reports of this injury in runners over 40.

PREVENTION

Preparticipation screening is the first stage in prevention. Any abnormalities in hip, knee, or ankle, or lost range of motion indicates a higher risk. In addition, any gait abnormalities should be carefully assessed. Finally, a history of congenital, metabolic, or endocrine abnormalities (such as menstrual irregularities) should be noted. Those with increased risk factors should then be followed more closely for the symptoms of hip stress fracture.

Training programs should be based on the etiologic theories just listed. Prevention of mechanical overuse is the hallmark of all conditioning efforts. The most successful methods have been a graduated increase in distance and speed. The program should be flexible enough to bring individuals who are most vulnerable along at a slower rate. This type of program is most straightforward in an individual sport such as in mid-distance track athletes and tri-athletes. It is more complex in team or group conditioning where there are differences in age, sex, race, and height (stride length differences).

An additional component of a preventive training program is an emphasis on the hip shock absorber—the supporting musculature. Combining hip muscle strengthening with endurance training gives added protection to the underlying bone. Finally, an alteration or cycling in the intensity of the conditioning gives added protection. Clinical trials have shown that a switch from an intensive running program to low impact conditioning reduces the incidence of this injury. The physiologic bone strengthening or osteoblastic response seems to lag behind after 2 weeks. A change to a nonimpact conditioning such as biking, swimming, ski-track exercises, or a weight program (avoiding squats and military presses) that does not overload the femoral neck, has decreased the incidence of this injury in intense military conditioning programs such as Officer Candidate School.

DIAGNOSIS

The earliest symptom of femoral neck stress injuries is groin pain, which can occur both during the run and at rest. Some athletes report night pain in the hip region, but this is not common. Hip pain at the extremes of passive range of motion is the earliest sign of a femoral neck stress fracture. An antalgic gait usually follows.

The diagnosis is confirmed by radiographs or special studies. The initial anteroposterior and lateral hip radiograph may not be positive, especially if the activity change or the injury is less than 2 weeks old. Plain radiographs will usually show sclerosis, which is the osteoblastic healing response if the symptoms are detected early. If the injury has progressed, a crack in the cortex with or without callus is often seen.

If the initial radiographs are negative, serial radiographs should be taken. Once a week is enough unless symptoms increase.

In those cases where the initial plain films are negative and early confirmation of the diagnosis is critical, special studies are indicated. Technetium bone scanning has been the more reliable technique. Increased uptake in the symptomatic femoral neck is for all practical purposes diagnostic in an athlete. It is important to note that there have been reports of false negative early bone scans. Milgram reported a normal scan at 5 days that later became positive. With this in mind, magnetic resonance imaging (MRI) has the capability of determining early edema and early bone response—endosteal and periosteal.

TREATMENT

As with other fractures, classification schemes are intended to help guide treatment. There are two frequently referenced classifications. Devas has a biomechanical description based on whether the changes are on the compression or tension side of the femoral neck. Blickenstaff and Morris base their classification on the anatomic description of the fracture. After evaluating a series of 54 femoral neck stress fractures, I have found that a modification of both older classifications is helpful in guiding treatment of the athlete. This scheme has three types of hip stress fractures: Compression side (Fig. 1, *A*), tension side (Fig. 1, *B*), and displaced (Fig. 1, *C*). The modifiers are the stage at presentation: acute symptoms (1 to 2 weeks), subacute (3 to 8 weeks), and chronic (over 8 weeks).

Whichever classification is used, the fact that this is an athletic injury must be recognized. The individual competitive nature of the patient and the added pressures of being part of a team make definitive diagnosis and treatment essential. It is my feeling that the common response in most athletes is to attempt to maximize every allowable rehabilitative exercise, to try to resume the activity that caused the injury as soon as possible, and to take risks in order to return to competition. Based on these assumptions, I use the modified classification system to guide treatment recommendations.

With the exceptions of the femoral neck stress fractures that are diagnosed by acute displacement, these injuries present with normal or abnormal radiographs. This is where the treatment decisions must begin.

Symptoms of Femoral Neck Stress Fracture with Normal Radiographs

In this case, a presumptive diagnosis of hip stress reaction is made. The goal is to prevent a hip stress fracture. The athlete should be placed on touch-down weight bearing with crutches. Radiographs are taken at weekly intervals for 6 weeks (increased pain is an indication for more frequent radiographs). If there are no radiographic changes, the athlete progresses to full weight bearing with crutches until there is no pain with activities of daily living or on examination. This usually takes 6 to 8 weeks. At that point a walk-run program is begun under the daily supervision of the trainer, therapist, or doctor. Once the patient is running without symptoms and has a normal examination, a final radiograph is taken. If it is still normal or if the fracture has healed, the athlete may return to competition. If pain persists or if the athletic situation requires the earliest possible confirmation of the daignosis, bone scintigraphy or MRI is appropriate.

Symptoms of Femoral Neck Stress Fracture with Positive Radiograph

If the history, examination, and radiographs are all positive, if the radiographs progress from negative to positive, or if bone scan or MRI are positive, the diagnosis of hip stress fracture can be confirmed. The treatment is then based on the classification of the radiographs.

Nondisplaced tension side and compression side fractures that present with sclerosis but without any visible cortical disruption are treated aggressively but nonoperatively. The patient is placed on crutches (touch-down weight bearing) immediately. Radiographs are taken weekly. If there is increased pain, immediate repeat radiographs are done. Crutches are used until the patient has no symptoms and no pain on full passive range of motion and stable callus on the radiograph at that time. Supervised protected conditioning (swimming, exercise biking) is begun. After 12 weeks a

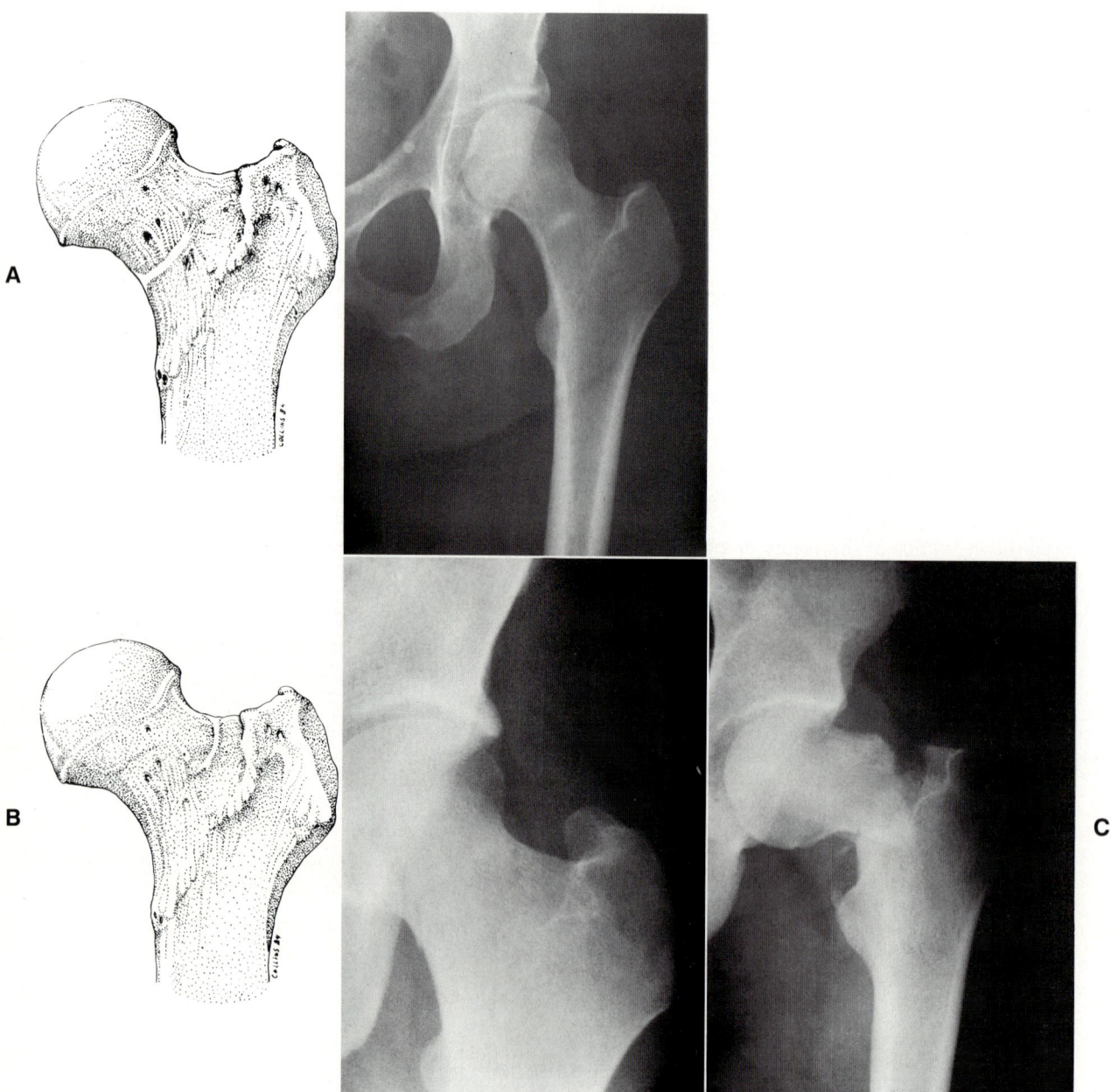

Figure 1 Types of femoral neck stress fracture. *A,* Compression. *B,* Tension. *C,* Displaced.

walk-run program is begun. A check radiograph is taken prior to release to competition.

Nondisplaced fractures that present with a visible crack in the cortex represent a significant progression toward displacement. The athlete is placed at bedrest. Semi-emergent stabilization is performed to prevent displacement (Fig. 2). Threaded cannulated type hip screws are used. Return to sports is based on fracture healing. As there is concern about stress risers from the screw holes in the cortex and the bone volume defect (especially if a large compression type screw was used), the hardware is normally left in place. In those instances when fixation devices have been removed, the hip must be protected until the fracture fixation defects have filled in and no longer serve as stress risers.

Fractures that are displaced at presentation are treated by emergent reduction and fixation (Fig. 3). I have used a compression screw and side plate for strength and a cannulated cancellous screw to help prevent rotation. There is a high complication rate in this setting, making the prognosis of returning to athletic competition guarded.

COMPLICATIONS

While the largest series of femoral neck fractures reported that only 5% presented as displaced fractures, the consequences of displacement are great. In Protzman's 1976 series of high energy femoral neck fractures in young adults the incidence of avascular necrosis was 86% and of nonunion was 49%. Other series support the frequency of such problems. These consequences dictate that the overriding principle of treatment is to follow a

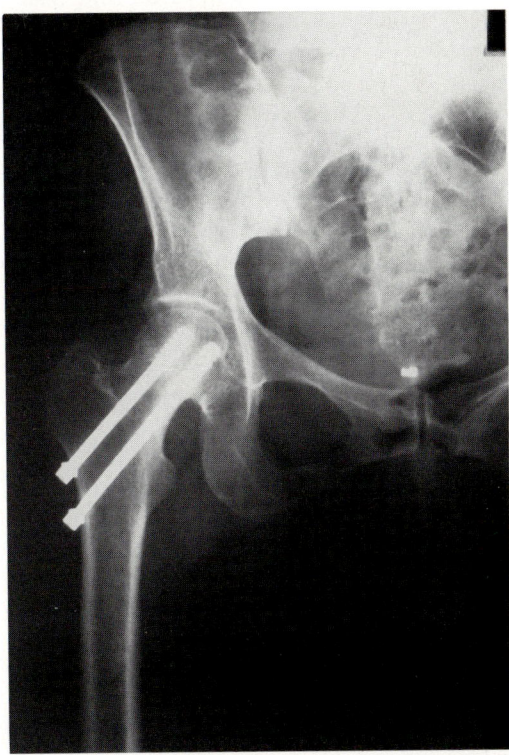

Figure 2 Cannulated pin fixation of a femoral neck stress fracture.

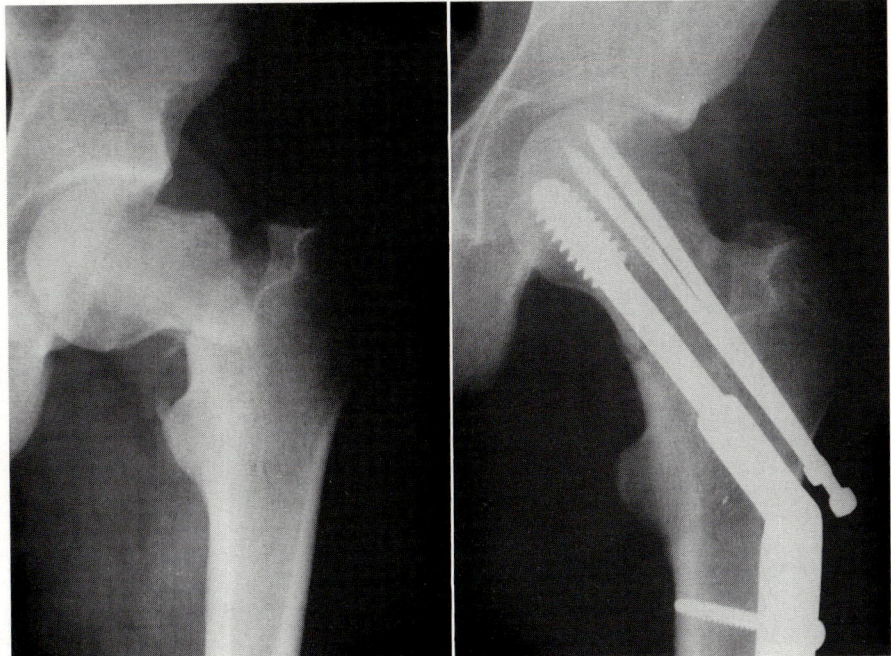

A   B

Figure 3 Treatment of a displaced femoral neck stress fracture with a compression screw/side plate and an antirotation cancellous screw.

prudent protective course, erring on the safe side in every instance.

CONTROVERSIES

The athlete often presents with a healing femoral neck stress fracture. The pain has improved but the initial radiograph shows evidence of fracture healing. In the semi-acute phase, which I usually accept as 3 to 8 weeks, I individualize the treatment based on the examination and radiographs. This involves the same treatment as the acute phase explained earlier. The time on crutches and rehabilitation is shortened accordingly. The sub-acute nondisplaced tension side fracture is an important exception. Because of the increased biomechanical forces on the tension side, the high complication rate if displacement occurs and the competitive nature of most athletes, I feel that fixation with multiple cannulated screws is indicated, even in the semi-acute stage. I have treated several of this type fracture at bedrest without surgery, but I am less likely to accept this risk with the low morbidity and the reliability of image intensifier directed cannulated screws.

The presence of retained fixation hardware at the time of release to competition is often a question. I have returned patients to running both with the hardware in and after removing it. The indications to remove fixation are mechanical irritation and significant exposure to re-fracture. The disadvantage of hardware removal is the potential for stress risers in the cortex and the volume defect of the cancellous bone. Documentation of healing by radiograph or MRI should be done before return to competition. When these fractures present sub-acutely or chronically, one advantage of nonoperative treatment is avoiding the potential of hardware problems.

PROGNOSIS

The prognosis of a nondisplaced hip stress fracture in an athlete is reasonably good. Discomfort for up to a year has been reported and the time to return to sports may be delayed by this prolonged remodeling. Because of the significant incidence and type of complications, the overriding factor in decision making in this injury should be conservative.

SUGGESTED READING

Blickenstaff LC, Morris JM. Fatigue fracture of the femoral neck. J Bone Joint Surg 1966; 48A:1031–1047.
Blum GM, Crues JV III, Sheehan W. MR of occult bony trauma: The missing link. Applied Radiology.
Devas MB. Stress fractures of the femoral neck. J Bone Joint Surg 1965; 47B:728–738.
Ernst J. Stress fractures of the neck of the femur. J Trauma 1964; 4:71–83.
Fullerton L, Snowdy H. Femoral neck stress fractures. Am J Sports Med 1988; 16:365–377.
Mendez A, Joseph J, Kaufman E. Stress fractures of the femoral neck following hardware from healed intertrochanteric fractures. Orthopaedics 1993; 16:822–826.
Milgram C, Chisin R, Giladi M, et al. Negative bone scans in impendial titial stress fractures: A report of three cases. Am J Sports Med 1984; 12:488–491.
Protzman RR, Burkhalter W. Femoral neck fractures in young adults. J Bone Joint Surg 58A:689–694.

FRACTURE OF THE PELVIS AND FEMUR

JAMES F. KELLAM, B.Sc., M.D., F.R.C.S.(C)

THE PELVIS

The pelvis is composed of two innominate bones and the sacrum. These bones in isolation represent no stability. In order for the pelvis to perform its function, the innominate bones must be firmly fixed to the sacrum and to themselves. This fixation is obtained posteriorly with the anterior sacroiliac ligaments and the posterior sacroiliac ligaments. The posterior sacroiliac ligaments running from the posterior tubercle of the ilium to the sacrum are the largest and strongest ligaments in the body. The anterior structures of the ilium and the two innominate bones are joined through the symphysis pubis, which is a strong fibrous junction. Pelvic stability is also maintained by strong ligaments running from the sacrum to the ischial tuberosity (the sacrotuberous ligament) and to the ischial spine (the sacrospinous ligament). The lumbar spine also participates in pelvic stability with the iliolumbar ligaments, which run from both transverse processes of the fifth lumbar vertebra to the posterior iliac spines. With these ligaments intact, the pelvis is thus a stable structure able to withstand the forces of weight bearing through the acetabulum, up the strong thick cancellous and cortical bone of the posterior ilium, and through the sacrum and along the vertebral column. The anterior structures, the pubic rami and ischial rami and symphysis, do not participate significantly in the weightbearing forces, but act as a strut to maintain the pelvis in its normal anatomic configuration and to protect the pelvic contents in massive pelvic disruptions because they are frequently injured and can lead to bladder, urethral, nerve, and (particularly) acute hemorrhagic problems.

Pelvic stability is defined as the ability of the pelvis

to withstand physiologic forces applied to it. This means that the posterior ligamentous complexes must remain intact. Pelvic instability represents disruption of the posterior osseous ligamentous complex. This may occur by fractures through the sacrum, sacroiliac dislocations, or a combination of fracture-dislocations of the ilium and sacroiliac joint as well as fractures through the posterior iliac wing. This stability can be represented as a spectrum and must be assessed in each individual case.

Stress fractures appear to occur more commonly in women than in men. This may be due to the fact that female bones are somewhat more slender and the pubic symphysis shallower, and to several other anatomic differences that really do not effectively explain this difference. Gait differences between male and female during running may account for some mechanistic differences. The female runner tends to rely on hip extension forces to a greater extent than does the male, so that the female pelvis would be more acceptable to tensile stresses. It is interesting to note that stress fractures in the pelvis appear to be secondary to exposure to tensile stress rather than compression stress. This is because of the medial position of the fractures in the pubic or ischial ramus where muscle pulls are occurring during hip extension. This would account for a single fracture occurring in a winglike structure. The other interesting difference in pelvic stress fractures is that they do not appear to be associated with the usual changes in technique, equipment, or surfaces of running. They do appear to occur within a specific time after high-intensity activities, which may represent failure from excessive repetition of muscle contraction.

Incidence of Pelvic Fractures

In order for major pelvic disruptions to occur, high energy must be transmitted through the pelvic ring. This is normally seen in motor vehicle and motorcycle accidents in the civilian population. It may also be noted after falls from heights. Sports are not known for the production of major pelvic disruptions. It is obvious that such high-energy sports as motorcar racing, motocross, and rodeo lead to the potential for major pelvic disruptions. However, in most sports the participant is well protected and does not suffer massive pelvic disruption. Stress fractures or stable pelvic fractures are more common.

Clinical Presentation

Pelvic fractures can be divided into two groups: stress fractures and major pelvic fractures.

With the major pelvic fracture, the mechanism of injury is obviously one of a high-velocity, high-energy transfer. This acute injury occurs as a sudden event. When first seen, the patient generally is unable to bear weight and is in significant pain in the region of the pelvic girdle. The history should point to the mechanism of injury. Pelvic fractures occur from anteroposteriorly directed forces, forces directed laterally to the pelvis such as a blow over the buttock or greater trochanteric region, and the vertical shear forces that occur in falls. Further questioning of the patient should bring to light symptoms of associated intra-abdominal or intrapelvic injuries, such as abdominal pain, an inability to void, and neurologic symptoms of numbness, tingling, or weakness in the lower extremities.

Stress fractures generally occur as a sudden onset of discomfort, usually related to the pelvic region. They are seen in runners or people who are doing repetitive activities that place significantly high stresses across the pelvis over a prolonged period. It is important to inquire into the training regimen of the athlete: whether there has been a sudden increase in mileage, a change in technique, or a change in training surfaces and location. It is also important to know when the discomfort occurs: whether with weight bearing such as walking or only during the athletic event or training.

Physical examination of the pelvis determines the stability of the injury as well as associated injuries. It is imperative to remember that the acute pelvic fracture is often accompanied by hypovolemic shock. The initial evaluation of the patient requires the physician to remember the priorities of resuscitation. Examination of the airway, breathing, and circulatory status of the patient should be done before the pelvic examination. Stabilization of the patient in hypovolemic shock or with airway problems is imperative. Intra-abdominal bleeding should also be evaluated.

The assessment of the pelvis begins with inspection. One should look for areas of swelling and bruising. Major pelvic disruptions are noted in patients with large flank hematomas, scrotal hematomas, and large hematomas posteriorly over the sacroiliac complex. Deformity of the lower extremity may also be noted. A lateral compression pelvic fracture causes an internal rotation deformity of the lower extremity, and an anteroposterior displaced fracture results in increased external rotation of the lower extremity. A vertical shear fracture causes a discrepancy in leg length, the shorter side being on the fracture side. Palpation of the pelvic ring, both posteriorly over the posterior sacroiliac complex and anteriorly over the pubic rami and symphysis, is imperative to determine areas of tenderness and discomfort. Manual compression of the pelvis by placing the hands on the anterosuperior iliac spines and forcing the pelvis inward will reveal an instability or discomfort posteriorly or anteriorly, depending on the fracture; forcing the pelvis outward also shows instability. The urethra is inspected for blood, an indication of urethral disruption. In addition, a rectal examination is made in males to determine the position of the prostate. A high-riding prostate or one that is mobile is another indication of urethral tears. Catheterization should not be attempted in these patients until cystourethrography has been performed to evaluate the urethra. If it is intact, a catheter may then be passed. Further evaluation of the lower extremities for neurologic involvement and vascular involvement should also be done at this time.

Investigations

In order to assess the pelvis radiographically, three views are required. The pelvis is approximately 40 degrees oblique to the long axis of the body. Consequently, an anteroposterior (AP) film of the pelvis represents an oblique view of the pelvis. This view is necessary to provide an overview of the pelvis and its structures. Two further views at right angles to each other can be obtained. The inlet view is done with the patient supine and the x-ray beam directed from cephalad to caudad at 45 degrees to the long axis of the body. This view permits assessment of posterior displacement, of rotation (whether internal or external), and of the sacrum for fractures. The outlet view, or tangential view, is done at 45 degrees to the long axis of the body with the tube directed from caudad to cephalad. This view allows assessment of the sacrum, sacral foramina, and superior rotation as well as superior migration of the pelvis. These two views, at right angles to each other, fill the criteria of fracture evaluation, especially that of stress fractures. Because of overlap in the AP view, it may be difficult to determine the exact structure that is injured in a stress fracture with only the AP view.

Bone scanning is particularly useful in the athlete who complains of a potential stress fracture. The bone scan is particularly sensitive to areas of increased bone turnover, as occur in stress fracture. If radiographs do not demonstrate a fracture, bone scanning is the next step. The stress fracture is demonstrated on the scan as a well-localized area of increased activity in the area of fracture.

Computed tomography (CT) is another useful technique for assessing the pelvis and its displacement, but more so in acute pelvic fractures than in stress fractures.

Tomograms of the pelvis may also be useful in the delineation of stress fractures.

Management

Once a pelvic fracture is diagnosed in an athlete, the major decision in management concerns the stability of the pelvic ring. Stability depends on the degree of disruption of the posterior bony, ligamentous complex of the pelvis. A clinical impression of instability can be verified radiographically. Significant displacement posteriorly in the femoral sacral arch around the sacroiliac joint region of greater than 5 mm to 1 cm represents significant instability. Evidence of avulsion fractures of the transverse process of L5, of the spinous process of the ischium, and occasionally of the origin of the sacrotuberous and sacrospinous ligaments from the sacrum also represents potential instability. The type of fracture pattern is also helpful in determining instability. Impacted fractures in cancellous bone represent a stable situation, whereas a shear fracture or a fracture through cancellous bone in which a gap is noted is potentially unstable. Stable pelvic fractures can be managed on bed rest until comfort is achieved. At this point the patient may be mobilized on crutches, non-weight bearing on the involved side. During this period, functional rehabilitation involving the cardiovascular system and the uninjured side may be carried out within the limits of discomfort for the patient. Pelvic fractures take approximately 6 to 8 weeks to become relatively solid, so that partial weight bearing may occur. This time period should be judged clinically with the assessment of each individual athlete. A stable pelvic fracture may be well united and early rehabilitation of the athlete may be possible within 6 weeks in some circumstances, provided lower extremity deformity, such as rotation or shortening, is not significant.

In the unstable pelvic fracture, AP compression injuries disrupt the symphysis and open the pelvis like a book. With less than 2.5 cm of disruption through the symphysis, these fractures remain relatively stable and may be managed with some method of closing the book—by internal fixation, external skeletal fixation, or a pelvic sling. A minimum of 6 weeks (more likely 3 months) is required for union to occur with this type of treatment. External skeletal fixation of the pelvis in an anteroposterior stable compression injury is ideal in that it allows functional rehabilitation. The patient may be up with crutches, non-weight bearing on the involved side, and be able to participate in upper extremity activities. Most lateral compression injuries are stable and may be managed with appropriate bed rest and mobilization. The vertical shear injury is an unstable injury. The end point of all mechanisms results in an unstable fracture that follows the pattern of a vertical shear injury. With a posterior instability, evaluation must be made as to how significant this is. Control of posterior instability is not possible with external skeletal fixation frames, but requires open reduction and internal fixation of the posterior bony ligamentous complex. This type of internal fixation of the pelvis is not without complications. Infection, gluteal muscle necrosis, and impingement of the sacral roots with internal fixation devices into the sacrum have occurred. This type of surgical intervention should be done by a surgeon experienced in pelvic fracture treatment. Other methods of treatment of the unstable fracture are combinations of external skeletal fixation and traction. This type of treatment usually requires 3 months of bed rest, with 6 to 8 weeks of traction followed by another 6 weeks of recumbency for union of the fracture to occur.

Stress fractures are managed symptomatically. If they occur during weight bearing and walking, crutch walking or pool therapy may be helpful. If they occur during training, this must be either slowed down or abandoned and other forms of maintenance of the athlete must be instituted. Evaluation of technique, environment, and equipment should be undertaken by consultation among physician, coach, and athlete in order to ascertain why this occurred and what can be done to correct it. The presence of a stress fracture should alert one to other potential problems, such as primary or secondary malignant disease.

Athletes should not return to competitive sports until they are pain-free and have regained strength, endurance, and agility. Otherwise, they are at significant risk for recurrent or new injury.

THE FEMUR

Fractures of the femur are a serious problem to an athlete. The femur, the largest bone in the body, is subject to the greatest stress and is surrounded by the major musculature of the lower extremity. At either end of the femur are the two major weight bearing joints required in all athletic activities: the hip and the knee. The hip is important in that stress fractures of the femoral neck may occur in athletes and thus lead to significant problems if missed or treated inadequately. If femoral shaft fractures are not treated properly, the thigh musculature cannot be maintained in good condition and ultimately affects knee function, through weakness, fibrosis, or secondary joint stiffness. Fractures in or above the knee are discussed elsewhere in this text.

Fractures of the femoral neck, which usually are stress fractures but may be incurred during high-energy sporting activities, can lead to several difficulties, the most serious being the development of avascular necrosis of the femoral head. This blood supply to the femoral head comes from a circle of vessels around the greater trochanteric region, courses up the posterior retinaculum of the femoral neck, and dives into the femoral head at the articular cartilage margin. Fractures of the femoral neck may disrupt this blood supply and thus lead to avascular necrosis and its attendant complications if late segmental collapse of the femoral head occurs. Nonunions and malunions also may occur. The hip requires an anatomic reduction in order that the biomechanics of gait, particularly for running, are maintained. Therefore, if a nonunion or malunion does occur, the athlete will be hindered.

The femoral shaft is enclosed within the major musculature of the lower extremity. Anteriorly the quadriceps, the major extensor of the knee as well as one of the major components of the patellofemoral mechanism, can be injured. Posteriorly, the hamstring groups of muscles are also involved as well as the sciatic nerve. Thus, femoral shaft fractures involve some form of muscle injury, particularly anteriorly to the quadriceps, and ultimately lead to knee problems through the weakness or loss of function of the quadriceps. Depending on the treatment of femoral shaft fractures, knee stiffness may result. This stiffness, along with shortening and malunion, may be a particular problem to athletes who require their lower extremities for repetitive and power activities. In addition to fractures of the femoral shaft caused by high velocity, stress fractures of the shaft, neck, and proximal area have been reported.

Incidence

Femoral fractures in athletes are extremely uncommon. The usual causes of stress fracture are overuse and change, particularly in marathon runners. It generally occurs in the beginning of training or after a sudden intensification of activity, such as a long run. Nonstress fractures or acute fractures of the femoral shaft have been documented in different contact sports. In a series of hockey injuries, only one of 108 fractures reviewed was to the femur. In other reviews, contact sports or high-velocity sports do not involve significant femoral shaft fractures, although they do occur sporadically.

Clinical Presentation

The acute femoral neck fracture or femoral shaft fracture usually occurs in isolated incidents with the sudden onset of acute discomfort and pain after a significant transfer of energy to the extremity. This may be through contact or can occur simply through twisting activities. The patient is unable to bear weight and complains of pain at a specific site.

Stress fractures of the femoral neck or medial aspect of the proximal femur usually are gradual in onset. The patient develops pain and discomfort, normally during activity or during a long run. This pain persists and is aggravated by increased activity. It is relieved by rest or non-weight bearing. This fracture occurs as an acute episode and is not preceded by chronic discomfort. Pain in the knee region, particularly on the medial aspect of the knee, may be indicative of hip joint disease. It also appears that stress fractures of the femur occur in the early part of a training routine, because increased stress is placed on the bone before the bone is able to withstand it.

Physical examination of an acute fracture usually shows the patient lying with an externally rotated leg, with acute pain and discomfort on motion and crepitus at the fracture site. With femoral shaft fractures, significant blood loss may occur, although it is uncommon. In a patient with a stress fracture, the leg usually has normal alignment, but on range-of-motion examination of the hip there are decreases in the range owing to pain with rotation and flexion. Pain usually occurs at the extremes. There may be tenderness at the region of the fracture.

Investigations

The first study consists of an AP and lateral roentgenogram of the hip or femur. It is important that both the joint above and that below the fracture be examined radiographically, particularly in the acute fracture. Because a stress fracture may not be visible on initial examination of the films, a high index of suspicion is necessary. One should also be aware of other diagnoses that may cause pain in this region (tumors or infection). A stress fracture may be one of two types and it is important to make the distinction. The compressive type, which usually is noted at the lower border of the femoral neck, is demonstrated radiographically as increased radiodensity along the fracture site or sclerosis at the fracture line. This type of fracture is rarely displaced unless continued stresses are placed on it. The second type of stress fracture, the distraction fracture, is transverse in direction, is seen in older individuals, and usually occurs at the superior aspect of the neck with a radiolucency. The fracture line develops at right angles to the line of stress, and displacement is common.

Acute fractures of the femoral neck are obvious. It

is important to determine the amount of displacement. The greater the displacement of the femoral neck fracture, the greater is the risk of avascular necrosis and the greater the necessity for an accurate anatomic reduction.

Acute fracture of the femoral shaft should also be assessed. It is important to determine the type of comminution present and thus whether the fracture is stable or unstable. Fractures of the femoral shaft that have more than 50% of the cortex intact on both the distal and proximal fragment are stable fractures. The two fragments can be lined up to prevent any axial displacement such as shortening. Comminution is particularly important in the proximal and distal portions. Although 50% of the cortex may be intact in the distal fracture, comminution may allow the fracture to slip, depending on the treatment, and thus shorten. If there is less than 50% cortical contact between both fractures, the fracture is considered unstable.

Bone scan may be indicated. Radionuclide images of the femoral shaft or femoral neck may be diagnostic in individuals in whom stress fractures are expected but not visualized on the plain radiographs. Tomography may also be necessary to delineate the fracture. This study may be necessary for diagnosis or to determine the extent of the fracture, particularly in the femoral neck, i.e., whether the fracture is completely across the neck or incomplete.

Management

In managing the acute fracture, one should initially ascertain that the patient is stabilized. If this fracture has occurred in a high-velocity situation, other associated injuries may be present. Priorities of resuscitation should be honored before treatment of the fracture is begun. This is not a particular problem with stress fractures.

Treatment of a stress fracture involving the femoral neck is based on the nature of the fracture. Compression fractures of the femoral neck, as mentioned, rarely cause displacement if the stresses are removed by appropriate non-weight bearing, either by crutches or by bed rest. The distraction stress fracture of the femoral neck usually is displaced and should be internally fixed. Any displaced fracture of the femoral neck should undergo internal fixation to allow for anatomic reduction. Most stress fractures are minimally displaced or may be reduced anatomically by means of a closed method using a fracture table. After this maneuver, they may be internally fixed by means of an appropriate device. Fractures in which anatomic reduction cannot be obtained should be considered for open reduction.

There are many techniques for the fixation of femoral neck fractures. The principle of internal fixation of these fractures requires a technique that allows for controlled impaction of the fracture, usually by means of a sliding compression screw system. Multiple pin fixation, using smooth pins or cancellous screws, is also a useful technique for the minimally displaced or anatomically reduced stress fracture of the femoral neck. After reduction and internal fixation of the fracture, the vascularity of the femoral head should be evaluated. It is probably best done at this time by a bone marrow scanning technique using technetium-99m sulfur colloid. It may also be adequately performed with one of the currently used bone scanning agents incorporating technetium-99m. If the femoral head is viable, no further treatment should be considered. However, if the bone scan demonstrates an avascular head, consideration should be given to a muscle pedicle bone graft using the quadratus femoris-based bone-block technique. This may increase the chances of revascularization of the femoral head and fracture union.

After operative or nonoperative treatment, weight bearing should not be allowed for approximately 6 weeks. This should be guided basically by the radiographic evidence of fracture union. As the fracture unites, gradual weight bearing may be reinstituted. Cardiovascular fitness may be maintained by activities that do not allow stresses to be placed across the femur (e.g., swimming or waist-deep water walking or running). These should be incorporated into the treatment as the clinical course permits. Most patients with stress fractures of the femoral neck can resume activities about 6 months after injury.

The treatment of acute femoral shaft fractures should preserve and encourage as much functional return as possible as quickly as possible. The technique of closed intramedullary nailing of long bone fractures is ideally suited for this fracture. This technique, developed by Gerhard Küntscher, is based on his principles of fracture care. The first and foremost principle was the restoration and preservation of function, which is imperative in the athlete. This was accomplished by a technique that allowed for fracture immobilization until healing occurred, but at the same time avoided assault on the fracture site, thus eliminating significant muscle dissection and devascularization of fracture fragments. This technique also encouraged healing by secondary bone union, particularly with its own internal bone graft from reamings.

The technique is performed with a closed reduction of the femoral shaft fracture. When this has been completed on the fracture table, through a small incision over the greater trochanteric region, the greater trochanter is entered in line with the axis of the medullary canal, a guide wire is passed across the fracture site, and the medullary canal of the femur is reamed with reamers of progressively increasing size. This allows for the internal aspect of the medullary canal to be made into a tube of a specific size, to permit passage of a nail large enough to immobilize the femur without bending and to allow for impingement between the nail and the internal aspect of the femur. This elastic impingement, which occurs as the nail is driven into the bone, provides the stability if associated with a stable fracture pattern. However, only fractures that are transverse or short oblique in nature are amenable to this closed technique because the nail is a weight-sharing device. It allows the fracture to participate in bone healing and weight-bearing stresses. Because it is close to the central axis of the femur, very few stresses are placed on the nail as far as tension or bending are concerned. There is minimal change in the cortical bone of the femur, and thus the problems of removal of the nail are minimal for recovery.

The indications for this technique have been extended by the development of a locked intramedullary nail, which is a cloverleaf nail that has holes at the proximal and distal ends. Through specially designed siting devices, these holes may be filled with locking screws. Unstable fractures (i.e., comminuted fractures, fractures in the distal and proximal third of the femur) may also be treated by the closed intramedullary nailing technique, as may any fracture of the shaft of the femur from within approximately 2 to 3 cm of the lesser trochanter to within 5 cm of the adductor tubercle.

This method of treatment of femoral shaft fractures allows for immediate mobilization of the athlete. The first day postoperatively the athlete may begin quadriceps setting exercises and be encouraged in straight leg raising. Once straight leg raising has been accomplished, there is sufficient quadriceps control for the patient to be mobilized onto crutches in a non-weight bearing or partial weight-bearing mode, depending on fracture stability. If a locking nail has been used and it has been necessary to lock this at both ends, i.e., a static locked nail, weight bearing is delayed until bridging callus is noted between the fracture fragments. This usually occurs at 3 months, at which point one of the sets of screws may be removed and full weight bearing may be commenced to mature the callus. Range-of-motion exercises of the knee are begun immediately. Usually by 3 weeks 90 degrees of motion has been obtained, and in stable fractures full weight bearing may be commenced. Union is rapid with this technique. During the initial 6 weeks, cardiovascular fitness may be obtained by non-weight bearing exercises such as swimming, walking in waist-deep water, and bicycling. Once the fracture has consolidated adequately, further rehabilitation may be started. Usually by 12 months the fracture has fully consolidated and healing has matured to allow removal of the nail. Nail removal should be undertaken in patients under the age of 50. This is a simple operation requiring several days of hospital admission. After this, the patient may recommence activities in a protected fashion until comfortable, usually within 3 to 6 weeks. Removal of the implant should be timed with the sporting activities. As long a period as possible should be observed between nail removal and the recommencement of highly stressful activities. Usually in 6 to 9 months the femur has regained its strength and full activities can be allowed.

Reports of the closed intramedullary nailing technique have shown that a 99% union rate with a less than 1% infection rate in closed femoral shaft fractures has been obtained. These results are similar to the early results of the locked intramedullary nailing technique. Other methods of femoral fracture treatment are associated with problems that may be particularly difficult for the athlete to overcome. The treatment of femoral shaft fractures in traction is usually associated with significant quadriceps atrophy and weakness, as well as a decrease in the range of motion of the knee. Cast bracing of fractures may, as with traction, allow for some decreased quadriceps power, range of motion of the knee, and occasional shortening and malunions. Plate fixation of femoral fractures allows for an anatomic reduction, but requires an open procedure with stripping of the muscle, particularly the quadriceps, which may lead to decreased range of motion and quadriceps weakness. Plate fixation is also associated with refracturing, particularly at the time of plate removal. Although the incidence of this is low if the fracture is united, there is evidence that the bone underneath the plate may undergo cancellization or become weakened owing to the weight-relieving aspects of a plate. To avoid this requires protection of the patient for a 12 month period before stressful activities are resumed.

With femoral shaft fractures, knee ligament injuries and internal derangements of the knee may also occur. This has been noted in up to 25% of patients with femoral shaft fractures. Once the fracture has been stabilized, examination of the knee is imperative. If significant knee injuries have occurred, these should be treated appropriately. In this situation, it is imperative that the femoral fracture be fixed in order that a knee reconstructive procedure and rehabilitation can be undertaken.

Finally, as far as treatment is concerned, return of athletes to full activity depends on their ability to regain strength, endurance, and agility.

REHABILITATION

PRINCIPLES OF STRENGTH TRAINING

JOSEPH J. VEGSO, M.S., A.T.C.

Muscular strength is a very important factor in athletic performance. After injury or surgery, a significant portion of the rehabilitation program must be devoted to regaining strength in the muscle groups that have been injured or immobilized. In addition, one must not lose sight of the loss of strength in the other muscle groups that help to support and stabilize the injured joint, or the muscles affected by simple disuse.

In recent years there has been a tremendous increase in the variety of devices available for strengthening muscles. Despite the overabundance and variety of equipment, the basic principles of muscle strengthening have remained unchanged.

Muscle strength is defined as the maximal force that a muscle can exert in a single contraction. Strength can be further defined as being static or dynamic. Static strength is commonly associated with a muscular contraction that does not produce joint movement (i.e., isometric), whereas dynamic strength involves a contraction with associated joint movement. Furthermore, a muscular contraction can be concentric or eccentric in nature.

Concentric muscular contraction is defined as muscle contraction with associated shortening of the muscle and joint movement (e.g., the biceps muscle contracts concentrically as it flexes the elbow). Eccentric muscular contraction is defined as muscle contraction with associated lengthening of the muscle and joint movement (e.g., after a concentric contraction of the biceps muscle, it goes through an eccentric contraction as it controls or resists elbow extension). An important aspect of the eccentric contraction is that a muscle can produce more tension during this phase than during the concentric phase.

There has been and continues to be considerable debate regarding the advantages of eccentric methods of strengthening versus traditional, concentric methods. The advocates of eccentric strengthening methods cite the fact that because a muscle is able to produce more tension eccentrically, a heavier training load will result in a more intense stimulus for greater strength gains.

Research comparing the eccentric method with other methods (concentric-isotonic, isometric, variable resistance, and isokinetics) has not demonstrated a significant advantage. It has shown, however, that eccentric methods of training are as effective in producing gains in strength as the other methods.

ISOMETRIC EXERCISE

Isometric exercise is typically defined as being a muscular contraction without associated movement of the joint or limb on which the muscles act. Simply put, the force a muscle produces is less than or equal to the resistance being applied. The effectiveness of isometric exercise in increasing strength first became popular in the 1950s as a result of the work of Hettinger and Muller. The most recognizable and popular way to exercise a muscle is to contract it for 6 seconds at a minimum of two-thirds maximal effort. The number of repetitions can be varied, depending on the phase of rehabilitation and the condition of the muscle.

There are several considerations for the use of isometric strengthening exercises in a rehabilitation setting. Isometric strengthening is most effective (1) in the very early stages of rehabilitation when joint motion is limited or inadvisable, (2) when the force that a muscle produces is insufficient for the use of weights or other resistance equipment, and (3) for patients with conditions that do not permit strengthening through an isotonic method.

One of the significant limitations of isometric exercise is joint angle specificity. Strength gains are produced at the specific angle of exercise, with minimal carry-over into other angles in the range of motion.

Isometric exercise is an effective method of increasing strength, particularly in a rehabilitation setting. It is convenient and advantageous because it requires minimal equipment and supervision.

ISOTONIC EXERCISE

Isotonic exercise is defined as a strengthening exercise in which the muscle shortens and the joint moves through a range of motion against a constant resistance or weight. This is easily accomplished through the use of a barbell, a sandbag, a weight bench, or other sophisticated equipment such as a universal gym.

As the weight is lifted, the muscle fatigues. Ideally a weight (resistance) is selected that causes the muscle to fatigue within a maximum of six to 10 repetitions. Over time, the muscle adapts and increases in strength. When this occurs, it becomes easier to lift the weight, and additional weight is added to overload the muscles again. This cycle is referred to as "progressive resistance exercise" (PRE). Developed by DeLorme in the 1940s, it is the hallmark of muscle-strengthening programs. Since that time, many variations on the theory have been introduced, but the basic principle has remained unchanged. The amount of weight lifted must be increased progressively in order to increase muscle strength.

Typically, a minimum of three sets of six to 10 repetitions of each exercise are performed during each rehabilitation or exercise session. In many instances, an injured athlete can perform strengthening exercises every day.

When isotonic exercises are used for rehabilitation, it is important to monitor the patient on a regular basis (daily if possible) to ensure that the exercise program is not aggravating the injury. Swelling, discomfort, pain, effusion, and loss of motion are important warning signs that the athlete is not ready for an isotonic strengthening program or is progressing too rapidly.

VARIABLE RESISTANCE

A variation of the isotonic strengthening method that has become popular in recent years is variable resistance exercise. As in isotonics, the joints or muscle groups move through a range of motion against resistance. Unlike isotonics, however, the resistance changes in an attempt to mimic or reproduce the mechanical advantages of the muscle and joint, so that the muscle must work at a near-maximal resistance throughout the range of motion.

In theory, variable resistance exercise should produce strength gains superior to those obtained from constant resistance methods. Unfortunately, objective research has not shown variable resistance training to be more advantageous. Despite the lack of definitive answers, variable resistance equipment has become the most widely used exercise equipment for strength training, thanks in large part to its ease of use and wide availability in health clubs and rehabilitation facilities.

ISOKINETIC EXERCISE

Isokinetic exercise is dynamic in nature, as are the isotonic and variable resistance methods. The aspect of isokinetic exercise that distinguishes it from the other forms of dynamic exercise is maximal accommodating resistance. The equipment provides resistance equivalent to that which the athlete exerts throughout the entire range of motion for every repetition. This is accomplished by controlling the speed at which the exercise is performed, usually through an electrohydraulic system. Typically, the athlete exerts maximal effort on every repetition.

Isokinetics have become the single most popular form of exercise used in rehabilitation today, partly because of the versatility (one piece of equipment can be used for all extremities), multiple exercise potentials (concentric, eccentric, isometric, and isokinetic), and recording and research ability of the equipment. The expense of isokinetic equipment seems to deter very few clinicians from purchasing it.

Like other methods of strength training, isokinetic methods have been scrutinized extensively. Two basic questions remain: what is the optimal training speed, and do strength increases at one particular speed carry over to other speeds? Available data have yet to answer these questions completely. Moderately slow-speed training seems to be more effective than either high-speed or very-slow-speed training for improving strength and carry-over effect.

Without question, isokinetic strengthening techniques will continue to be the most popular method of strengthening for rehabilitation, for the reasons cited and in view of the continuing advances in technology.

MANUAL RESISTANCE

Often overlooked, manual resistance is a very effective method of strengthening muscles in a rehabilitative setting. It requires no equipment, is an excellent method of isolating specific muscles, and can produce isokinetic or near-maximal accommodating resistance. Typically, exercise regimens follow a pattern similar to that of isotonics or isometrics. However, this may vary with the speed of exercise. At faster rates of speed, more repetitions are performed to provide a sufficient workload.

COMMENTS

The best method of strengthening muscles after injury is not easily defined. Factors such as postinjury condition, the availability of equipment, and the knowledge and familiarity of the trainer or therapist with various methods all play an important role in determining the best approach. Therefore, the physician must rely on the basic philosophy of increasing strength along with range of motion, and allow the methods to be dictated by the patient's needs and the equipment available. The most important factor related to the improvement of strength is the intensity of the load. Heavy loads produce the greatest stimulus for strength gain, but maximal loading does not necessarily produce maximal gains. A variety of factors must be considered when selecting the appropriate method of muscle strengthening. For rehabilitation, a combination of methods based on healing time and patient tolerance seems appropriate.

SUGGESTED READING

Atha J. Strengthening muscle. Exerc Sport Sci Rev 1981; 9:1–73.
DeLorme TL, Watkins, AL. Techniques of progressive resistance exercise. Arch Phys Med 1948; 29:263–273.
DeVries HA. Physiology of exercise for physical education and athletics. Dubuque: Brown, 1980.
Fleck SJ, Kraemer WJ. Designing resistance training programs. Champaign, IL: Human Kinetics Books, 1987.
Gettman LR, Pollock ML. Circuit weight training: a critical review of its physiological benefits. The Physician and Sport Medicine 1981; 9:44–60.
Gonyea WJ, Sale D. Physiology of weight-lifting exercise. Arch Phys Med Rehabil 1982; 63:235–237.
Torg JS, Vegso JJ. Rehabilitation of athletic injuries: an atlas of therapeutic exercise. Chicago: Year Book, 1987.

PRINCIPLES OF STRETCHING

JOSEPH J. VEGSO, M.S., A.T.C.

Flexibility and range of motion (ROM) are frequently considered synonymous. By definition, however, there are several differences. Flexibility is an integral component of ROM.

Flexibility most often is defined as the ability of muscles to elongate as a joint or body segment moves through a ROM. From a physiologic basis, it is a component of physical fitness related to athletic performance. Flexibility can increase through specific exercises or decrease through inactivity and disuse. Flexibility can be body part-specific and sport-specific (e.g., gymnasts require excellent overall flexibility, whereas swimmers need excellent shoulder and upper body flexibility).

ROM refers to the movement of a specific joint. This motion is influenced by a variety of factors, including bone congruence, the joint capsule, ligamentous structures, and the flexibility of the muscle-tendon units acting on the joint. In addition, injury, surgery, or immobilization may affect one or more of these structures, thereby reducing or totally restricting ROM and flexibility.

Full ROM and flexibility are essential for normal activities of daily living and athletic performance. In many activities such as gymnastics, karate, diving, and ballet, hyperflexibility is the norm for high-level performance. Consequently, most health care professionals, physical educators, and coaches have advocated a regimen of stretching exercises as an integral component of physical conditioning programs and warm-up activities. As a result, attention has been focused on the physiologic basis of stretching and its relationship to injury prevention and athletic performance.

Human contractile tissue is elastic. This elasticity is directly affected by tissue temperature and blood saturation of the muscle. At higher temperatures, contractibility is improved because the internal viscosity of muscle protoplasm is reduced. This phenomenon is reversed when muscle tissue is cooled. It is common in cold weather to hear individuals complain of feeling stiff or that they need more time to warm up. Recent reports also indicate that muscle contracture is more rapid and forceful when the muscle temperature is slightly elevated. This can be attributed to the increase in muscle elasticity and to the increased sensitivity and conductivity rate of the nervous system associated with a temperature increase. In addition to the effects on muscle tissue, joint range of motion is also enhanced at higher temperatures owing to an increase in extensibility of ligaments, tendons, and other connective tissue. As a result of this knowledge and several clinical studies on animals that demonstrated similar increases in flexibility and joint range of motion associated with higher tissue temperature, it has become a common practice for athletes to warm up before stretching.

Typically, a precompetition regimen includes three components: (1) a warm-up period consisting of jogging or moderate calisthenics for 5 to 10 minutes to raise body temperature to a level that produces mild to moderate sweating; (2) a period of generalized stretching, to loosen muscle and joint tissue, progressing to specific stretches to enhance flexibility and ROM for the particular sport or position; and (3) agility exercises for body coordination and proprioceptive warm up.

INJURY PREVENTION

Several authors have described flexibility as a component of fitness that is health related rather than performance related. It is difficult to separate the two; an athlete who has a tight muscle group certainly cannot perform at an optimal level without risk of injury. As stated previously, a joint that is unable to move through its full ROM because of joint capsule or muscle inelasticity is certainly more susceptible to sprains and strains if forced to move beyond its available motion. Loss of flexibility and range of motion in the lower extremities can have a significant effect on normal gait and running patterns, followed by a decrease in performance and conditioning.

When soft tissue temperature increases, several other changes occur in addition to increased elasticity. Muscle contraction tends to be more rapid and forceful with slight rises in temperature. Nerve function is also affected at higher tissue temperatures. The sensitivity of nerve receptors is enhanced and nerve impulse transmission is improved. Theoretically, these changes could improve the athlete's ability to perform complex sensorimotor tasks, thereby reducing the risk of injury.

Early research in the area of flexibility indicated that stretching exercises done on a regular basis may help to improve the tensile strength and elasticity of ligaments and fascia. This concept appears to make sense, in that connective tissue responds to stress by organizing itself along the axis of that stress. Therefore, after injury, stretching can have a significant effect on the healing of connective tissue. As new collagen is formed and placed under stress, it organizes itself in the direction of tension, thereby creating stronger and more elastic tissue and reducing the chance of reinjury.

STRETCH REFLEX MECHANISM

Neurologically, muscle elasticity is controlled by the stretch reflex mechanism. It is a neurophysiologic phenomenon controlling the length-tension relationship within a muscle. Two types of nerve receptors within a muscle respond to changes in muscle length: the muscle spindle and the Golgi tendon organ. The latter also responds to changes in muscle tension.

When a muscle is stretched, the muscle spindle reacts by sending a signal to the spinal cord. In response, the spinal cord informs the muscle that it should contract, thereby resisting the stretch. Secondarily, if the stretch continues for longer than 6 seconds, the Golgi tendon organ reacts to the change in length and tension by signaling the spinal cord. The spinal cord responds by sending a message to the muscle to relax. The coordinated response by both receptors acts as a protective mechanism to allow for controlled extensibility of muscle units.

TYPES OF STRETCHING

Recommendations for a stretching program must be guided by the needs of the individual patient or athlete. After injury or surgery a rehabilitation program may include several types of exercises to regain joint ROM and maintain or increase muscle flexibility. An athlete should perform routine stretching exercises as part of the warm-up procedure.

Further refinement of the definition of flexibility and ROM can lead to a clearer understanding of how the therapeutic needs of the patient can be met through the various methods of stretching. There are two types of flexibility: static and dynamic. Static flexibility usually refers to passive movement of a joint. Hence, passive stretching activities are most frequently associated with improving joint range of motion and muscle extensibility after injury or immobilization, whereas dynamic flexibility refers to movement of a joint resulting from active muscle contraction.

These two types of flexibility must be considered when designing a stretching program. In the early phase of rehabilitation, passive ROM must be developed with the aid of a therapist or athletic trainer. As the athlete recovers and begins to resume athletic activities, more dynamic exercises must be incorporated into the rehabilitation program.

Static Stretching. This is the most popular and safest method of stretching. The techniques used in performing this type of stretching involve moving a joint or muscle to the extreme of comfortable motion and holding the position for a given period, normally 10 to 30 seconds or longer. Several repetitions should be performed (five to 10), depending on the need for improvement.

In therapeutic settings, static stretching should be preceded by the application of a heat modality such as a hydrocollator pack or warm whirlpool. Athletes should perform some type of warm-up activity as described previously before stretching.

Ballistic Stretching. This utilizes repetitive contractions of an agonist muscle or muscles to produce a quick, active stretch of the antagonist muscle(s). An example is a "bouncing" toe-touch exercise to stretch the hamstrings. Although this method of stretching can be effective, it is not widely used for therapeutic purposes because of the potential risk of overstretching. It is, however, widely used as a type of warm-up for multiple muscle groups to simulate specific skill activities such as a golf or baseball swing.

Proprioceptive Neuromuscular Facilitation (PNF). This technique has gained widespread popularity in sports medicine and physical therapy facilities as a versatile way to improve flexibility, range of motion, and proprioception. Several techniques are used in PNF: slow-reversal-hold, contract-relax, and hold-relax. Each involves alternating a muscle contraction with relaxation in order to produce an increase in motion. Typically, the contraction is held for 10 seconds followed by 10 seconds of relaxation (stretch). All three techniques require a partner (therapist or trainer) to assist the athlete.

In the *slow-reversal-hold* technique, the partner passively moves the joint into a position of stretch. The athlete then contracts the antagonist muscles that are to be stretched against the resistance being applied by the partner for 10 seconds. After the 10 second contraction the athlete relaxes the antagonist muscle(s) and actively contracts the agonist muscle as the partner attempts to move the joint further into the range of motion. This sequence is usually repeated three to five times.

The *contract-relax* and *hold-relax* techniques are similar. In both techniques the partner passively moves the joint into a position of stretch. The athlete then contracts the antagonist muscles that are to be stretched against the resistance of the partner. In the contract-relax method the contraction is isotonic; in the hold-relax method it is isometric. After the contraction phase in either method, the partner again passively stretches the antagonist muscles while the athlete relaxes both the antagonist and agonist muscles.

In conclusion, several types of stretching have been proven effective in increasing flexibility and range of motion. However, in terms of safety and injury prevention, the ballistic method has received much less support from the medical community. A variety of factors can influence flexibility: activity, inactivity, the type of injury, immobilization, growth, the type of athletic activity, and tissue temperature. All must be considered when evaluating an individual with poor flexibility.

Finally, it is important to recognize that increasing flexibility is a slow process. Clinicians must emphasize this to help patients avoid the frustrations of slow progress.

SUGGESTED READING

Anderson B. Stretching. Bolinas, CA: Shelter Publications, Inc., 1980.

Lehmann JF, Masock AJ, Warren CG, et al. Effect of therapeutic temperatures on tendon extensibility. Arch Phys Med Rehabil 1970; 51:481–487.

Sapega AA. Advances in nonsurgical treatment of joint contracture: a biophysical perspective. In: post graduate advances in sports medicine. Vol. 3. Lesson 1. Berryville, VA: Forum Medicum Inc., 1988.

Sapega AA, Quedenfeld TC, Moyer RA, et al. Biophysical factors in range of motion exercises. The Physician and Sports Medicine 1981; 9:57–65.

Torg JS, Vegso JJ. Rehabilitation of athletic injuries: an atlas of therapeutic exercise. Chicago: Year Book, 1987.

PHYSIOLOGY, BIOMECHANICS, AND ENVIRONMENT

EXERCISE, FITNESS, AND HEALTH

ROY J. SHEPHARD, M.D., Ph.D., D.P.E., F.A.C.S.M.

Sports physicians frequently use the terms exercise, fitness, and health. These terms are central to the discipline of Sports Medicine, but there is a lack of unanimity on their meaning, and it is unclear whether health is related to the amount of activity that is undertaken, or to the level of fitness that is realized. In June 1988 an attempt was made to establish an international consensus on interactions between physical activity, fitness, and health. It was quickly agreed that the three variables were closely inter-related. However, each was also influenced by heredity, lifestyle, the physical and social environment, and personal attributes. Moreover, many intervening variables modified the impact of physical activity on fitness and fitness on health. Most sports physicians are conditioned to think in terms of positive relationships, but it is important to note that the interactions can also be negative. For example, excessive physical activity, whether undertaken by an athlete or a patient, can lead to a deterioration in both fitness and health, and sometimes to untimely death (see the chapter *Sudden Cardiac Death*).

We here define the three terms briefly, look at their inter-relationships, and summarize the evidence to consider when deciding which types of sport and exercise programs have a beneficial impact on fitness and health.

PHYSICAL ACTIVITY

Physical activity may be considered as a body movement produced by the skeletal muscles that results in an appreciable increase over resting energy expenditure. Some types of physical activity are more effective than others in achieving fitness and health. A distinction is commonly drawn between occupational, leisure, and other types of physical activity, although all can influence both fitness and health.

Occupational Physical Activity

Early epidemiologic studies pioneered by investigators such as Jeremy Morris and Ralph Paffenbarger demonstrated the value of occupation as a source of regular, vigorous, and health-giving physical activity. Because work is performed up to 8 hours per day, "heavy," health-giving occupational activity corresponds to a lower energy expenditure than "heavy" leisure activity. Nevertheless, the number of jobs that make significant energy demands has been progressively decreasing with automation. Patients may still claim to work in heavy industry, but the number who actually perform heavy work is now quite small. Thus in the future, an unhealthy population must look to its leisure hours for health-giving physical activity.

Leisure Physical Activity

Leisure physical activity is undertaken voluntarily, in a person's discretionary time. The element of choice is critical, and because many people would prefer to do things other than exercise, they will plead "lack of time." However, most people have a reasonable amount of freedom to modulate both the extent and the characteristics of their leisure activity to meet personal goals and interests, altering the impact of leisure pursuits upon fitness and health.

Examples of leisure activity include exercise (where the patient has a specific predetermined objective such as an improvement of personal health), sport (in Europe, this term implies most types of physical activity, but in North America it is restricted to activities where pleasure is sought in vigorous competition or rapid body movement), training (where the objective is the development of physical fitness or the improvement of physical performance through repetitive bouts of a specific exercise over an extended period), and dance (where a person is seeking the aesthetics of graceful body movement or social interaction, although a gain of health may be a useful by-product).

Other Types of Physical Activity

There are other less voluntary categories of physical activity that can influence fitness and health, for example domestic chores, gardening, and "do it yourself" activities around the home. Women usually have more of such activities than men and, unless a careful activity history is taken, their level of activity may be underestimated. Children also participate in required school programs of gymnastics and sport (at least in certain grades), and for a small segment of the population there is personal involvement in commercial sport.

Pattern of Physical Activity

When a physician prescribes exercise, the required pattern of physical activity is usually defined in terms of its type, frequency, duration, intensity, and amount. Each of these variables can modify the impact of the prescription upon fitness and health.

Type

The type of physical activity is an important variable, whether the activity occurs at work or in leisure time. A broad distinction may be drawn between rhythmic movements where there is little increase of muscle tension (*"isotonic"* activity), and rigidly opposed efforts where there is little movement (*"isometric"* activity). Rhythmic activity is generally most effective in developing cardiovascular fitness, but heavily loaded contractions are needed for the conservation of muscle mass and thus body strength as a person ages.

It is advisable to discuss whether there is a shortening (*concentric* activity) or a lengthening (*eccentric* activity) of the muscle as it contracts (the latter situation is well illustrated by running downhill). If musculoskeletal injuries are to be avoided, eccentric contractions must be held to a minimum.

A distinction must also be drawn between *continuous* and *intermittent* bouts of activity. If the activity is intermittent, it is important to consider the duration of both active and recovery periods, and the nature of the recovery interval (whether complete rest or light activity). A short active phase and a long recovery interval are desirable to avoid a progressive accumulation of anaerobic metabolites.

Finally, thought should be given to the *distribution* of the activity and the *posture* that is required. Is there a relatively uniform involvement of the body muscles or is the effort sustained mainly by a few small muscle groups? Does the associated body posture help or hinder perfusion of the active tissues? The use of small muscles in an awkward body position may induce a dangerous rise of blood pressure, particularly in a hypertensive patient.

Frequency

The patient usually reports the frequency of physical activity as the number of sessions of activity undertaken in a recent week, but a better picture is obtained if the patient discusses participation in physical activity over a month or even a year. It is important to allow for seasonal variations in the frequency of activities caused by extremes of climate or (in the case of children) with the passage of the school year.

Duration

The duration of a typical physical activity session should be noted in minutes. Patients commonly exaggerate the duration of their activity. It is therefore important to distinguish the time involved in travel, preparation, changing clothes, and socializing from the minutes allocated to actual physical activity. Likewise, the peak intensities of effort reported for some heavy occupations are rarely sustained throughout an entire eight-hour working day.

Intensity

The intensity of physical activity may be reported and prescribed in either absolute or relative terms. Physiologists often express the absolute intensity of sustained, aerobic activity as a rate of energy expenditure (kJ per minute) or as an equivalent oxygen consumption (1 L per minute equals some 21 kJ per minute), but most physicians find it easier to consult tables that show the energy cost of exercise as a ratio of resting metabolic rate (METS). This last type of unit has the advantage of minimizing differences in the cost of a given activity between patients of differing body mass. Laboratory workers express the absolute intensity of muscular activity as units of force (Newtons) or as the torque developed at a specified rate of movement (Newton-meters), but the average doctor can get useful information by asking about function—for example, the heaviest load that the person normally carries.

The relative intensity of activity is inversely related to the fitness of the individual. It also depends on the volume of muscle that is activated. In the exercise-testing laboratory, aerobic activity is expressed as a percentage of the individual's maximal aerobic power, but in daily life intensity can be monitored as the corresponding fraction of maximal heart rate or heart rate reserve. If the peak rate of energy production is measured in METS, and due allowance is made for the influence of age, then the absolute and relative approaches can be reconciled (Table 1). Laboratory tests report the relative intensity of muscular activity as a percentage of the maximal force or torque that can be developed by the muscle group in question, and in general practice one can think in terms of the percentage of the load that can be displaced by a single maximal effort.

Amount

The total amount of physical activity is critical to the control of obesity and the optimization of lipid profiles. The nutritionist summarizes the weekly energy expenditure in kilojoules, either as a gross value or as an excess over resting energy expenditure. For the average, sedentary patient, the most important element in the gross total is the basal metabolic rate, so a small change

Table 1 Relative and Absolute Intensity of Aerobic Activity at Selected Ages, Evaluated from the Viewpoint of Fitness

Categorization	Relative Intensity (% Maximal Effort)	Absolute Intensity (METS)			
		Young (20 yr)	Middle-aged (40 yr)	Old (60 yr)	Very Old (80 yr)
Rest		1.0	1.0	1.0	1.0
Light	< 35	< 4.5	< 3.5	< 2.5	< 1.5
	> 35	< 6.5	< 5.0	< 3.5	< 2.0
Moderate	> 50	< 9.0	< 7.0	< 5.0	< 2.8
Heavy	> 70	> 9.0	> 7.0	> 5.0	> 2.8
Maximal	100	13.0	10.0	7.0	4.0

in the rate of basal metabolism (for example, a delayed effect of vigorous exercise) can have an important effect on the total weekly energy expenditure. Voluntary physical activity is the most variable component in the total energy usage, but small effects can also arise from the thermic effects of ingested food. It has been suggested that a part of the problem in the obese patient is that the long-term thermic effects of eating and exercise are depressed.

The basal metabolic rate is commonly expressed per unit of heat-dissipating body surface area. Values vary with age and sex. Depending on the age and fitness of the individual, a fourfold to twentyfold increase over basal metabolism can be sustained for a few minutes of exercise, and a healthy young adult can maintain a fivefold to eightfold increase over basal values throughout an eight-hour day of vigorous physical activity.

There appears to be a dose-response relationship between the total amount of physical activity undertaken by an individual and that person's biologic response in terms of improvements in both health and physical performance. There is probably a threshold dose of exercise below which little or no adaptation occurs. Then there is a zone of increasing effect, and finally a ceiling is reached; beyond this ceiling, there is no further improvement of health, and signs of overdosage such as injuries or deranged immune function begin to appear.

Details of the dose-response relationship depend on the type of activity that is undertaken, the benefit that is sought, and the fitness and age of the individual. For example, the development of aerobic fitness requires more intensive activity than does a program designed to induce stress relaxation. Aging narrows the margin between an effective and an excessive or dangerous amount of exercise, so activity must be prescribed more carefully for older individuals. The short-term effects of a single dose of activity (such as a local increase of protein synthesis) may persist for several hours or days. It is therefore important to understand the interaction between intensity, frequency, and duration when designing an optimal exercise prescription.

PHYSICAL FITNESS

Physical fitness has been defined by the World Health Organization as "the ability to perform muscular work satisfactorily." The components, including cardio-respiratory endurance, muscular strength and endurance, body fat, flexibility, and bone health, are determined by a combination of habitual physical activity level, diet, heredity, and general health.

In general, fitness implies that the individual concerned has characteristics that permit a good performance of a physical task in a specified physical, social, and psychological environment. However, fitness may be viewed in Darwinian terms, as a means to performance, or as a means to health.

Darwinian Fitness

Darwinian fitness implies a matching of inherited personal characteristics with environmental demands. The individual thus gains an advantage in the quest for reproduction and colonization of a specific habitat. For instance, a high level of fitness might allow a person to undertake additional physical activity in a harsh environment, thus finding enough food for survival of the family unit. Anthropology suggests that humans have adapted, over many centuries, to the moderate but sustained activity associated with a hunter/gatherer life-style, and health should therefore be optimized if the modern city-dweller develops a similar pattern of physical activity.

Performance-Related Fitness

Performance-related fitness reflects the ability to perform particular motor tasks. It is generally more important to the high-performance athlete than to the average patient (although loss of functional abilities can also threaten the happiness and independence of older individuals). Many school fitness tests primarily assess performance using a simple battery of field tests (for example, a standing broad jump and a 50 meter run). Scores are intended to assess muscular strength, capacities, and powers, but the results are heavily influenced by body build, motivation, immediate environmental conditions, and recent practice of the required skills. The data bear only a limited relationship to the long-term health of the individual, and in some cases children who are quite fit and healthy may be discouraged because teachers have reported poor scores using such evaluations.

Health-Related Fitness

Health-related fitness comprises morphologic, physiologic, and metabolic components. In addition to laboratory measures of cardiorespiratory performance such as the peak power output or the maximal oxygen intake (determined on a treadmill or cycle ergometer), body composition, body fat distribution, blood pressure, ECG characteristics, glucose tolerance, insulin sensitivity, blood lipid levels and lipoprotein profile, immune function, perceived health, and stress tolerance should be noted.

From the viewpoints of both health and performance, certain values are plainly more desirable than others. For example, neither very high nor very low blood pressure readings are desirable from the viewpoints of fitness and health.

HEALTH

Health should be viewed as much more than the mere absence of disease. Health has physical, social, and psychological dimensions. Each of these aspects of health is characterized by positive and negative poles. The patient with positive health or well-being has a capacity to enjoy life and to withstand environmental challenges, while the patient in a negative state of health has an increased risk of morbidity and premature mortality.

Increases in both physical activity and fitness have been linked to improvements of health, although part of the association may be indirect, through a mutual dependence on a healthy life-style. Health in turn has an important influence on both the physical activity patterns and the physical fitness of a patient.

Wellness

Wellness or well-being is a holistic concept. It describes a positive state of physical, social, and psychological health, and in contrast to some traditional medical models it focuses on the quality of the patient's life rather than on the quantity. An increase in the quality of life is a much more powerful argument for exercising than a mere extension of lifespan.

Morbidity

Morbidity has traditionally been defined in terms of specific diseases, but it should be defined as any departure, subjective or objective, from a state of complete physical, social, or psychological well-being, short of death.

Potential indices of morbidity include (1) the number of persons reporting any loss of wellness per unit of population per year (that is, the incidence of overall morbidity), (2) the number of persons found to be unwell per unit of population (that is, the prevalence of overall morbidity), (3) the incidence or prevalence of specific morbid conditions, (4) the average duration of poor health resulting from specified morbid conditions, and (5) the cumulative loss of years of positive health (allowing calculation of a quality-adjusted lifespan).

Mortality

Mortality is much easier to measure than morbidity, and many of the traditional evaluations of exercise programs have looked at the impact on mortality rates. Mortality is often expressed as the death rate for an age- and sex-specific population sample. Alternative measures are the average life expectancy of the population, the average loss of productive years relative to a healthy population, or an appraised age based on the patient's chances of death from common conditions over a specified period such as the next 10 years. This last statistic is a useful way of presenting a change in risk status to a patient. We found that men who became involved in an employee fitness program quickly reduced their appraised age by more than 2 years.

Life-style

Personal life-style is an important and neglected component of any patient history. It covers all of the many individual behaviors, actions, and habits that can affect personal health. Negative characteristics include smoking and an excessive consumption of alcohol; positive characteristics include regular physical activity and adoption of a low-fat diet. There is some evidence of a linkage between various types of life-style behaviors; for example, endurance exercise is sometimes helpful in encouraging cessation of smoking. On the other hand, sports with a strong social connotation may encourage smoking and an excessive consumption of alcohol, particularly in middle-aged members of a sports club.

VARIABLES INTERVENING BETWEEN ACTIVITY, FITNESS, AND HEALTH

Personal Attributes

Personal attributes may affect the impact of physical activity and fitness on health. Sociodemographic and psychological variables such as age, sex, socioeconomic status, personality, and motivation must be considered. For example, the recommendation of a sport requiring costly equipment and clothing may be badly received by a patient who has only minimum-income employment.

Heredity

The importance of inheritance is still strongly debated, but it is probably an important intervening variable. It may be genotypic or cultural.

Differences of intracellular DNA from one patient to another provide the molecular basis for genetic variations in both the observed physical characteristics of the individual and the ability of that individual to respond to deliberate changes of life-style such as an increase of physical activity.

Cultural inheritance is not mediated directly by genes, but is transmitted rather by common patterns of education, home conditions, and other environmental factors. Thus, if the parents are obese, physically inactive, and heavy smokers, the children are likely to follow this example.

Both types of inheritance contribute to interindividual differences in personal life-style, physical fitness, and health. They can also influence responses to changes of life-style, particularly altered patterns of nutrition and habitual physical activity. Thus one patient will respond well to a controlled program of diet and exercise, but another who is exposed to the same regimen will show a disappointing response.

Environment

Physical activity, fitness, and health status are all influenced by the physical and chemical environment in which a patient lives. Relevant factors influencing both the acute response to exercise and the success of training include conditions of temperature, humidity, altitude, and air quality. For example, hot weather supplements the normal effects of cardiorespiratory training, although it can also lead to a dangerous rise of core temperature if the activity is prolonged.

Social, cultural, political, and economic factors—friendships, poverty, and community attitudes—towards a healthy life-style also affect the patient's acceptance of a given activity prescription, and thus fitness and health.

EVIDENCE

Much of this volume will discuss the benefits of exercise in various medical conditions. It is therefore important to offer a few comments about the quality of available evidence about relationships among exercise, fitness, and health. Scientists are increasingly moving to a stratification of reports in terms of their technical quality, particularly when attempting to reconcile conflicting studies. Inferences may be drawn from various sources, including population data, clinical studies, epidemiologic studies, and experimental studies.

Population Data

Population data must be obtained on a representative sample of the group for which generalizations are to be made. For example, activity patterns might be measured on an age and sex stratified subsample of an Inuit community to show that a high level of habitual activity in that community contributed to the unusually high levels of physical fitness seen in that same population. Unfortunately, it is difficult to recruit representative samples, and data are often biased because the most active people in a community volunteer to complete surveys or to participate in fitness tests. In contrast, smokers are notoriously difficult to recruit for such investigations.

Clinical Studies

Clinical studies often provide the groundwork for hypotheses that are later tested by more sophisticated means, and the general practitioner should recognize that many of the important pieces of medical knowledge were gathered through careful observation of individual patients.

The types of clinical evidence include anecdotes such as the 80-year-old patient who progresses from a sedentary life-style to climbing Mount Rainier, detailed case studies such as the linkage between gains of muscle strength and improved aerobic power in patients undergoing rehabilitation following cardiac transplantation, case-control studies where the experience of active individuals is compared with that of carefully matched control patients, and intervention studies where some type of treatment has been applied.

Epidemiologic Studies

Epidemiologic studies explore relationships among physical activity, fitness, and health in a large and representative sample of the population. For example, Dr. Jeremy Morris found better cardiovascular health in active, London bus conductors than in their sedentary peers who drove the buses, suggesting the practical value of occupational activity. Epidemiologic studies may look at the incidence or the prevalence of a particular condition in relevant segments of the population, and an attempt is usually made to control statistically for differences in other variables relevant to the disease process.

In general, epidemiology shows associations rather than cause and effect relationships; for example, in the study of bus drivers, there was an association between inactivity and heart disease, but a part of this association arose because obese individuals elected the job of driver rather than that of conductor. An attempt can nevertheless be made to draw causal inferences from epidemiologic data, using a specific set of rules first proposed by Bradford Hill; application of this approach has provided relatively convincing evidence that a low level of physical activity causes an increased risk of cardiovascular disease.

Experimental Studies

In theory, the best evidence comes from experimental studies. These involve the random assignment of appropriately stratified groups of subjects to an intervention and a placebo treatment.

It is unfortunately difficult to suggest an appropriate placebo for physical activity, and patients are often unwilling to be assigned to active or sedentary groups on a long-term basis. We attempted a randomized control trial of exercise following myocardial infarction, but the benefit of exercise was obscured because many of the control subjects began exercising, and quite a number of the exercisers failed to maintain their prescribed physical activity. Nevertheless, statisticians maintain that randomized studies are needed before we can definitively attribute causes and define the mechanisms of the benefit that are attributed to exercise.

Other Evidence

Other analytic tactics include correlational studies and meta-analyses. The latter have found considerable application to studies of physical activity and health. In essence, meta-analyses pool data from several laboratories. Such an approach may be justified if the exercise protocols are similar from one center to another, because it is difficult for any one laboratory to accumulate data on a sufficient number of randomly assigned and compliant individuals to draw valid conclusions.

SUGGESTED READING

Bouchard C, Shephard RJ, Stephens T, et al. Exercise, fitness and health: A consensus of current knowledge. Champaign, Ill: Human Kinetics Publishers, 1990.

Bouchard C, Shephard RJ, Stephens T. Physical activity, fitness and health: Consensus statement. Champaign, Ill: Human Kinetics Publishers, 1993.

Bouchard C, Shephard RJ, Stephens T. Physical activity, fitness and health: International proceedings and consensus statement. Champaign, Ill: Human Kinetics Publishers, 1994.

Shephard RJ. Physical activity, aerobic fitness and health. Champaign, Ill: Human Kinetics Publishers, 1993.

RESPONSES OF THE CARDIOVASCULAR SYSTEM TO EXERCISE AND TRAINING

ROY J. SHEPHARD, M.D., Ph.D., D.P.E., F.A.C.S.M.

Sustained rhythmic exercise depends on delivery of adequate quantities of oxygen to support the metabolic conversion of stored energy (mainly glycogen and fat) to a form that allows muscular work (ATP). Table 1 lists the main components of both oxygen delivery and utilization. Delivery is also influenced by pulmonary function and the binding and release of oxygen by hemoglobin. However, this chapter focuses on the acute and chronic effects of exercise on the heart and circulation, since these are the most important determinants of oxygen delivery when a healthy patient performs large muscle exercise.

ACUTE CARDIOVASCULAR EFFECTS OF RHYTHMIC EXERCISE

Table 2 summarized typical acute cardiovascular changes observed in healthy, young adults during maximal steady-state rhythmic exercise.

Cardiac Output

In the healthy human, the amount of oxygen delivered to the working muscles during rhythmic exercise depends largely on an increase in cardiac output. Cardiac output increases (1) by an increase in heart rate and (2) by an increase in stroke volume.

Clinicians have traditionally expressed the resting cardiac output per square meter of body surface area (total 1.5 to 1.6 m^2 in women, 1.8 to 1.9 m^2 in men), the so-called "cardiac index." There are statistical objec-

Table 1 Main Factors Influencing Oxygen Delivery and Utilization

Delivery	Utilization
Ambient oxygen pressure	Basal metabolic rate
Respiratory minute volume	Respiratory work rate
Dead space-alveolar ventilation	Cardiac work rate
Pulmonary diffusing capacity	Core temperature
Ventilation-perfusion matching	and BMR
Intracardiac shunts	Muscle metabolism
Cardiac output	O_2 debt repayment
Hemoglobin level, oxygen affinity	
Distribution of blood flow	
Capillary/fiber ratio	
Capillary patency	
Tissue enzyme activity	

Table 2 Acute Cardiovascular Changes During Rhythmic Exercise (Typical Findings for Healthy Young Men)

Variable	Rest	Maximal Exercise
Cardiac output (L/m^2/min)	3.5	15
Heart rate (beats/min)	70	195
Stroke volume (ml, upright)	80	110
Blood pressure (mm Hg)	120/80	190/90
Myocardial O_2 cons. (ml/min)	70	420
Arteriovenous O_2 diff. (ml/L)	40	140

tions to the use of a simple ratio of this sort when the relationship does not necessarily proceed in linear fashion from its origin, but the cardiac index does allow comparisons between individuals who differ somewhat in body size. Resting values are typically about 3.5 L/m²/min, but in maximal rhythmic exercise values may reach 10-20 L/m²/min, depending on age, sex, and physical condition.

Heart rate (HR) increases during rhythmic exercise (and the anticipation of such exercise) due to a centrally-mediated modulation of parasympathetic and sympathetic nerve activity. As exercise becomes more vigorous, there are effects attributable to peripheral vasodilatation and the chronotropic action of circulating catecholamines.

The resting HR is typically 70 to 80 beats/min, but it is increased 5 to 10 beats/min by cigarette smoking, and drops to 50 to 60 beats/min in the well-trained endurance athlete. A few very well-trained individuals have had values as low as 30 beats/min. There have been suggestions that the exercise-induced increase of HR becomes disproportionately larger in relation to oxygen consumption once the anaerobic threshold has been passed, but this does not seem a very reliable index of anaerobic activity, at least under laboratory conditions.

If maximal rhythmic large-muscle activity is sustained for a few minutes, HR rises to a peak value that has often been characterized as 220 minus the person's age in years. Higher values (up to 250 beats/min) have been observed momentarily (for instance, during the vigorous isometric contractions associated with a tight turn in downhill skiing), but the traditional formula for calculating the peak HR reading is certainly appropriate for children and young adults who are performing endurance sport. On the other hand, some 65-year-old adults seem capable of peak readings of 170 rather than 155 beats/min while exercising on a laboratory treadmill. If a smaller muscle mass is activated (for instance, during arm ergometry), the HR is higher for any given submaximal oxygen consumption, but effort tends to be limited by peripheral muscular fatigue, so the peak HR is lower than during a large muscle task. It is important to take account of these differences if HR is used to prescribe exercise.

Stroke volume (SV) increases via three possible mechanisms: (1) increased preload, (2) increased contractility, and (3) decreased afterload. The primary mechanism for the increase of SV during exercise is an increased preload. Venous return to the heart is boosted by muscle and respiratory pumping. The left ventricle therefore receives an increased volume of blood from the pulmonary veins and the left atrium during diastole. This larger volume increases both end-diastolic volume (EDV) and pressure, and by the Frank-Starling effect distension of the left ventricle stimulates it to a more forceful contraction, thus ejecting a larger SV (although not necessarily a larger fraction of the ventricular contents).

The second mechanism for the increase of SV is an increase of myocardial contractile state that is independent of the Frank-Starling effect. This enhancement of contractility typically first appears as exercise becomes more vigorous; it results from an increased sympathetic nerve discharge and the effects of circulating catecholamines. A larger volume of blood is then pumped for a given combination of EDV and pressure. There is little increase of end-systolic volume but the ejection fraction (EF) nevertheless increases from perhaps 50 percent at rest to as much as 70 percent during vigorous exercise.

The third mechanism for an increase of SV is a decreased afterload. In simple terms, this means that there is less impedance to blood flow, allowing the left ventricle to eject a larger volume of blood with each contraction. This mechanism depends on peripheral vasodilatation. Often, rhythmic exercise involves some isometric component, and then the systemic blood pressure (BP) rises, increasing rather than decreasing the impedance to cardiac ejection. In older adults (particularly if there is poor myocardial contractility due to occult coronary insufficiency), SV and EF may thus decrease somewhat as peak effort is approached. If the function of the cardiac pump is poor (as in congestive heart failure), there may also be a peripheral vasoconstriction that adds to afterload. Such patients may be helped by the administration of ACE inhibitors such as captopril (Capoten, Capozide).

The relative contribution of the three mechanisms to the exercise response varies with the circumstances. Much clinical exercise testing involves light or submaximal effort and it is often carried out with the patient lying supine or semisupine. Under such conditions exercise has little effect upon venous return and SV remains relatively constant at a value of about 110 ml in a sedentary person and 140 ml in an endurance athlete. Under the more common natural conditions of seated or standing physical activity the pre-exercise cardiac SV is about 80 ml in a sedentary adult and perhaps 110 ml in an endurance athlete. Furthermore, if the patient is erect, SV increases progressively with exercise intensity to match the values seen in the supine position at about 50% of the individual's maximal oxygen intake. In the young adult SV remains relatively constant from 50 to 100% of maximal effort but, as previously noted, older individuals may have difficulty in sustaining SV as they approach maximal aerobic effort.

Blood Pressure

The systolic blood pressure (SBP) increases progressively over the course of vigorous rhythmic exercise, with a potential to reach final levels of 180 to 200 mm Hg in normal adults and even higher figures in those with labile hypertension. The diastolic pressure is difficult to measure by sphygmomanometer during exercise because the Korotkov sounds become indistinct during vigorous work. In general, there seems to be little change of diastolic pressure in response to rhythmic muscle contractions.

The primary cause of the rising SBP is a local restriction of blood flow to muscles that are contracting at a large fraction of their maximal voluntary force. This leads to an accumulation of potassium ions and other metabolites in the working muscles, with a reflex stimulation of the cardiovascular centers in the brain. Sometimes the effects of centrally-induced vasoconstriction also exceed the counterinfluence of local vasodilator metabolites. Failure of the BP to rise with an increase in the intensity of exercise is an adverse sign of failing left ventricular function, and generally it is an indication to halt exercise immediately.

The body temperature rises substantially with vigorous exercise (sometimes by as much as 3 to 4°C), causing a progressive relaxation of the capacity vessels (particularly the large veins of the legs). If a person remains standing after exercise the loss of muscle pumping reduces venous return; there may thus be a sudden drop in BP during the recovery period. This may provoke a loss of consciousness, a vasovagal attack, myocardial ischemia, and abnormalities of heart rhythm including ventricular fibrillation. Appropriate precautions include a gradual warm-down (for instance, the conclusion of an endurance exercise prescription by a 5 minute period of slow walking), sitting down while changing, and avoidance of hot showers immediately after vigorous activity. Particular care is needed in patients with a history of myocardial ischemia or sudden attacks of loss of consciousness and in those who are taking hypotensive medications.

Myocardial Oxygen Consumption

The heart consumes substantial amounts of oxygen in pumping blood around the circulation, perhaps 70 ml/min at rest and as much as 420 ml/min in vigorous exercise.

The double product (HR × SBP) provides a simple clinical estimate of cardiac work-rate and thus myocardial oxygen need. In keeping with the figures already cited, the double product shows a fivefold to sixfold increase during maximum rhythmic exercise.

The coronary oxygen extraction is virtually complete even at rest (an arteriovenous oxygen difference (A-V_{O_2}) of 180 ml/L or more). The meeting of myocardial oxygen demand during vigorous exercise is therefore critically dependent on the ability of the coronary blood vessels to dilate. Because normal vascular control lies in the arterioles, and vascular impedance is proportional to the fourth power of vessel radius, a coronary arterial obstruction of 50 to 70% is needed to have a clinically significant impact on myocardial oxygen delivery.

Peripheral Oxygen Consumption

Delivery of oxygen to the working tissues depends on the product of cardiac output and A-V_{O_2}. At rest, the A-V_{O_2} is 40 to 50 ml/L of blood but in vigorous exercise this figure rises to 120 to 160 ml/L, peak values being largest in fit young men.

The arterial oxygen content depends on hemoglobin concentration and arterial oxygen saturation. The hemoglobin level normally averages about 156 g/L in men and 138 g/L in women. Low values have sometimes been described in athletes of both sexes; suggested explanations include a poor iron uptake (due to both dietary fads and a high fat intake), an increased iron loss in the sweat, impaired red cell formation, intestinal or vesical hemorrhage, and increased hemolysis. However, the main reason why somewhat low values are seen in well-trained individuals is probably an increase of plasma volume and thus "dilution" of a normal total hemoglobin content.

Each gram of hemoglobin can carry about 1.34 ml of oxygen if fully saturated with oxygen and free of interfering substances (for instance, the carbon monoxide found in cigarette smokers). Arterial saturation in a healthy lung usually reaches near 100%, but occasionally athletes may develop such a large cardiac output that the transit time through the pulmonary capillaries is inadequate to allow a full saturation of blood. Low arterial oxygen saturations are also seen with poor matching of ventilation and perfusion or a frank venous-arterial shunt such as can develop through a small atrial or ventricular septal defect during vigorous exercise.

Venous oxygen extraction is relatively complete in the working muscles. The main factor modifying the oxygen content of mixed venous blood is therefore the proportion of the cardiac output that is directed to other parts of the body such as the skin and the kidneys (where oxygen extraction is relatively incomplete). As the intensity of exercise is increased, blood flow is increasingly redirected from inactive muscles, skin, and the viscera to the working muscles. However, an obese person dissipates heat less readily and therefore must direct more blood flow to the skin; for this reason, such individuals have a low peak A-V_{O_2}.

ACUTE CARDIOVASCULAR EFFECTS OF RESISTANCE EXERCISE

Table 3 lists the main acute effects of resistance exercise. The primary features of resisted exercise are a rapid increase of HR and BP while the contraction is maintained, the mechanism being a local accumulation of potassium ions and a reflex stimulation of cardiovascular centers in the brain.

The rise of HR and BP inevitably lead to a substantial increase of myocardial oxygen consumption, with a risk of provoking various manifestations of myocardial ischemia. The rise of BP with a maximal isometric effort can be sufficiently dramatic that older people were once warned against undertaking any form of resistance training. However, the rise of pressure depends on both the fraction of maximal voluntary contraction force (MVC) that is exerted and the period for which effort is sustained. A local restriction of muscle blood flow begins if effort exceeds 15 percent of MVC and occlusion of the muscular vasculature is complete at efforts exceeding 70% of MVC.

It is currently agreed that there is little danger of an excessive rise of BP during brief contractions (2 to 3 sec), provided that adequate recovery intervals are allowed to disperse the accumulating metabolites. Indeed, programs of resistance exercise have been prescribed very successfully for both nonagenarians and cardiac pa-

Table 3 Acute Cardiovascular Effects of Resistance Exercise

Variable	Effect
Heart rate	Rapid rise, proportional to percent of maximal voluntary contraction
Stroke volume	Temporary fall, particularly if Valsalva maneuver adopted
Blood pressure	Rapid rise of both systolic and diastolic pressure, proportional to fraction of maximal voluntary contraction
Myocardial O_2 consumption	Large increase
Arteriovenous O_2 difference	Small increase

Table 4 Chronic Cardiovascular Adaptations that Occur with Rhythmic Exercise

Left ventricular function:	
Resting heart rate	Decreased
Submaximal heart rate	Decreased
Maximal heart rate	Unchanged or small decrease
Peak stroke volume	Increased
Peak end-diastolic volume	Increased
Peak ejection fraction	Increased
Myocardial contractility	Sometimes increased
After-loading	Small decrease
Submaximal cardiac output	Decreased
Peak cardiac output	Increased
Left ventricular structure:	
Wall thickness	Increased
Blood pressure:	
Resting	Small decrease
Peak	Increased
Myocardial oxygen consumption:	
Resting	Decreased
Submaximal	Decreased
Peak	Increased
Oxygen delivery	Increased
Peripheral oxygen delivery:	
Hemoglobin	Unchanged
Plasma volume	Increased
Arterial oxygen	? small decrease
Venous oxygen	Decreased
Muscle flow	Relative increase

tients. Nevertheless, prolonged straining, particularly against a closed glottis, is to be avoided.

CHRONIC CARDIOVASCULAR EFFECTS OF RHYTHMIC EXERCISE

Rhythmic exercise training increases an individual's peak oxygen consumption through adaptations in the general oxygen delivery system, and possibly through local changes at the tissue level (extraction and utilization of oxygen by the working muscle). Table 4 summarizes the cardiovascular and muscle tissue adaptations that occur in response to training.

The extent of the response to rhythmic training is determined by the initial fitness of the individual and the intensity of the precribed activity relative to initial working capacity. The traditional recommendation has been to undertake three to five 30 to 60 min bouts of large muscle exercise per week, each session reaching an intensity of effort demanding at least 60 to 70% of the individual's maximal oxygen intake. Such a regimen augments the maximal oxygen intake of a sedentary person by 20 to 30% over the course of 2 to 3 months, the speed of response being somewhat faster if the intensity of training is adjusted upward as the condition of the individual improves.

More recently it has been recognized that in older subjects and in cardiac patients the frequent repetition of less vigorous bouts of rhythmic exercise can also have a useful training effect. For such individuals, fast walking is more practicable than running or jogging and is less likely to induce either musculoskeletal or cardiovascular problems. The recommendation has therefore been broadened to 20 to 60 min at 50 to 70% of maximal oxygen intake, a longer duration of exercise compensating for a lower intensity.

Training-induced Changes in Left Ventricular Function

Heart Rate

The most obvious cardiovascular effect of rhythmic training is a decrease of HR at rest and during submaximal exercise. However, there is relatively little change of peak HR, so the heart rate reserve (the difference between resting and peak HR) is increased in a trained subject.

Stroke volume

Regular rhythmic exercise also leads to a 20 to 30 ml increase in peak SV, with an increase of both EDV and EF. The main factor accounting for the increment of SV is probably an expansion of plasma volume, and therefore an increase of cardiac preloading. There may also be some increase of ventricular contractility and there is often a small decrease of systemic BP and thus after-loading of the heart. A strengthening of the skeletal muscles may contribute to the reduction of after-loading in a number of types of patient with chronic debility.

Cardiac Output

Training has little effect on the resting cardiac output but, because of a more effective distribution of blood flow, there may be a small decrease of cardiac output at a given submaximal work-rate. Given the absence of change in peak HR and a training-induced increment of peak SV, there is an equivalent 10 to 20% increase of peak cardiac output.

Changes in Left Ventricular Structure

Early research stressed the large heart of the athlete as seen on PA chest radiographs, although it was vigorously debated whether this was a positive or a negative consequence of training. Recent echocardiographic studies have clarified that the large radiographic shadow reflects both an increase of left ventricular muscle mass (up to 30% in endurance competitors) and an increase of EDV.

Adherence to an intense and prolonged training regimen frequently induces an increase in the thickness of the ventricular wall. The practical consequence is that a given intraventricular pressure can be sustained while developing a lesser force per unit cross-section of the myocardium.

The interventricular septum commonly participates in the training hypertrophy, and there is some evidence that excessive thickening of the septum increases vulnerability to abnormalities of heart rhythm.

Blood Pressure

Most reports suggest that endurance training leads to a small (5 to 10 mm Hg) but clinically useful decrease of resting BP both in normal subjects and in those with some hypertension. Taking account of poor compliance with drug therapy and the complications caused by many hypotensive drugs, a regular exercise program may be the treatment of choice for many individuals with mild hypertension.

The BP also tends to be lower at a given submaximal work-rate after training. However, a combination of several factors (greater ventricular preloading, increased wall thickness, and augmented ventricular contractility) may allow a patient to reach a higher peak BP after training. This is particularly likely if peak effort is limited by myocardial ischemia prior to training.

Myocardial Oxygen Consumption

The training-related decrease of HR and BP lowers the myocardial oxygen demand both at rest and in submaximal effort. On the other hand, the unchanged maximal HR and the potential increase of peak SBP imply a small increase of peak myocardial oxygen consumption after training.

There is an associated increase of coronary blood flow after training. The main mechanism for this is a relative lengthening of the diastolic phase of the cardiac cycle. Left ventricular blood flow occurs mainly during the diastolic phase of the cardiac cycle, so that the training-induced lengthening of diastole facilitates coronary perfusion. Some animal experiments have suggested that regular exercise encourages the development of collateral vessels but, perhaps because of an inadequate intensity of effort or difficulty in visualizing small vessels, there has to date been no convincing demonstration of such a response in humans.

Ventricular hypertrophy is a further possible factor enhancing coronary flow. Such hypertrophy reduces the ventricular wall tension, allowing perfusion of the subendocardial tissues via the perforating coronary vessels. The lower wall tension also reduces the oxygen demand of unit volume of the heart muscle. On the other hand, unless there has been a parallel development of myocardial capillaries, ventricular hypertrophy lengthens the oxygen diffusion pathway within the myocardium. The net effect of ventricular hypertrophy may therefore be little change of local oxygen supply.

Peripheral Oxygen Delivery

Hemoglobin concentrations are unchanged or may show a small decrease after training because of plasma volume expansion. Any training-related increase of peripheral oxygen delivery therefore reflects an increase of A-V_{O_2}.

The arterial oxygen saturation remains close to 100 percent after training (with the exception that in very highly-trained athletes, the pulmonary diffusing capacity may be inadequate to match their large cardiac output). However, the mixed venous oxygen content is decreased, so that the A-V_{O_2} is broadened, perhaps from an initial value of 140 to 160 ml per liter.

Muscle biopsy studies have shown an increase in the activity of aerobic enzymes in the working muscles after training, and some authors have argued that this change is responsible for the increased local oxygen extraction. During vigorous exercise, however, the oxygen content of blood draining from the active muscles is very low even in sedentary subjects, so training is unlikely to induce much further increase of oxygen extraction in the working tissues. Any specificity of training probably reflects rather local muscle hypertrophy; the strengthened muscles contract at a smaller fraction of their maximal voluntary force and thus offer a lower impedance to perfusion.

There is little or no change in the blood flow demands of the viscera with rhythmic training. However, a decrease of subcutaneous fat and an increase of sweating may reduce the need for subcutaneous blood flow, particularly in a warm climate. But even with no change in skin or visceral perfusion, if there is an increase of total cardiac output, then a larger proportion of this blood flow is inevitably directed to the working muscles, with an increase of the overall peak A-V_{O_2}.

CHRONIC CARDIOVASCULAR EFFECTS OF RESISTANCE EXERCISE

Table 5 summarizes the chronic effects of resistance training. The primary change is an increase of peak muscular force. This initially reflects better coordination of individual motor units, but as exercise is continued there is also an increase of muscle bulk. A given muscle force can consequently be developed with a smaller force per unit cross-section of muscle. This, in turn, reduces the intramuscular compression of blood vessels, with favorable effects on the cardiovascular response to acute bouts of exercise.

Table 5 Chronic Cardiovascular Effects of Resistance Exercise

Variable	Change
Peak muscle force	Increased
Muscle bulk	Slower increase
Left ventricular function	
Resting heart rate	Little change
Exercise heart rate	Decreased
Resting stroke volume	Little change
Exercise stroke volume	Better sustained
Left ventricular structure	Little change
Blood pressure	
Rest	Little change
Exercise	Slower rate of rise
Myocardial oxygen consumption	
Rest	Little change
Exercise	Reduced
Peripheral oxygen delivery	
Hemoglobin	Sometimes increased
Arteriovenous O_2 difference	Unchanged

Heart Rate

There is little change of resting HR with resistance training, but a given muscle force can be developed with a smaller and less rapid increment of HR.

Stroke Volume

Resistance training has little effect on the resting SV. As the muscles become stronger there is less tendency to hold the breath while producing a given effort, so there is less tendency to reduce venous return and SV during isometric activity.

Changes in Left Ventricular Structure

Left ventricular hypertrophy is a response to sustained overload, as occurs during prolonged rhythmic exercise. Resistance training is generally ineffective in inducing such changes because the increments of BP are maintained for only a few seconds at a time.

Blood Pressure

Resistance training generally has little effect on the resting BP. However, because contractions are produced at a smaller fraction of MVC, the rate of rise of blood pressure is smaller after training.

Myocardial Oxygen Consumption

The reduction of exercise HR and BP lead to a substantial decrease in the myocardial oxygen cost of undertaking a given isometric effort. At the same time, the slower heart rate facilitates myocardial perfusion. Resistance training can therefore make a useful contribution to an overall exercise prescription in an older person with some compromise of the coronary circulation, and a good training program includes at least 2 days of resisted exercise per week.

Table 6 Current Recommendation for Exercise Prescription

Warm-up. Exercise should begin with a warm-up, 5-10 minutes of walking at increasing speed.

Flexibility component. The main joints of the body should be taken through their full range of motion, with gentle stretching at the end of the range of motion. Warm-up and flexibility exercises should precede rapid and vigorous physical activity.

Aerobic component. The aerobic component should involve the major muscles of the body (walking, jogging, running, cycling, vigorous dancing, cross-country skiing, swimming, skating, rope-skipping, stair-climbing, rowing, or endurance sports) and it should be carried out at least three and preferably four or five times per week. Individual sessions should be of 20–60 min duration at 50–85% of maximal oxygen intake. If a low intensity is thought advisable in view of the patient's general condition, then the duration of sessions should be prolonged.

Muscle strengthening component. Muscle strengthening exercises should be performed at least twice per week. They should include a circuit of 9–10 exercises, involving the main muscle groups of the body. At each station, subjects should perform one set of 8–12 repetitions at 50–60% of peak muscle force for a single effort.

Warm-down. The program should finish with a deliberate warm-down—at least 5 minutes of walking at decreasing speed.

Peripheral Oxygen Delivery

Muscle hypertrophy is sometimes accompanied by an increase of hemoglobin levels, particularly in athletes who have been abusing androgenic steroids. However, there is no reason to anticipate that resistance training will induce any increase of A-$\dot{V}o_2$ and thus peripheral oxygen delivery, except insofar as the hypertrophied muscles are more readily perfused during subsequent rhythmic activity. This response seems largely responsible for reports of a regional specificity of endurance training.

RECOMMENDATIONS

A well-designed exercise program includes elements of both rhythmic activity, aerobic activity, and resisted exercises. The type of program currently favored by the American College of Sports Medicine is summarized in Table 6.

SUGGESTED READING

Shephard RJ. Aerobic fitness and health. Champaign, Ill: Human Kinetics Publishers, 1993.

Shephard RJ, Åstrand PO. Endurance in sport. Oxford: Blackwell Scientific Publications, 1992.

Shephard RJ, Miller HS. Exercise and the heart in health and disease. New York: Marcel Dekker, 1992.

MATHEMATICAL MODELING OF HUMAN MOTION

MICHAEL RAYMOND PIERRYNOWSKI
PAUL WILLIAM STRATFORD

The computer simulations of the mathematically oriented biomechanician sometimes seem far removed from the practical needs of the sports physician. This chapter illustrates how such techniques can help in designing a safe and effective rehabilitation program after injury or surgery to the knee.

Injury to the knee joint results in significantly greater atrophy of the quadriceps (Q) muscle compared to the hamstrings (H) muscles. Furthermore, it is the rate of recovery of the quadriceps muscle strength, rather than the knee's range of motion (ROM) or the patient's ability to ambulate without aids, that dictates the duration of rehabilitation and ultimately the patient's ability to return to the normal activities of daily living. Since vigorous strength training occurs when a muscle is required to produce a high force, exercise techniques that maximally stress a muscle should be identified and prescribed, provided they do not traumatize the compromised anatomic structures.

In the human body, each active striated muscle generates force ($\mathbf{F}$)* acting at a patient specific distance and direction ($\mathbf{P}$) from the joint center of rotation. This force in turn generates a torque (the moment of force, $\mathbf{M}$). The $\mathbf{M}$ generated by any $\mathbf{F}$ acting at the point $\mathbf{P}$ from the axis of rotation can be calculated as the vector cross product of application point $\mathbf{P}$ and force $\mathbf{F}$. If $\mathbf{P}$ and $\mathbf{F}$ lie on the XY plane, with components in the x and y directions of P_x, P_y, and F_x, F_y, respectively, then:

$$M_z = P_x F_y - P_y F_x \qquad (1)$$

where M_z is the moment of force about an axis through the point of rotation perpendicular to the XY plane (the Z direction).

At each joint in the body, the sum of the moments of force acting around that joint must sum to zero when the joint is in static equilibrium. Application of external moments of force ($\mathbf{M}^E$) must be actively resisted by the sum of the muscle moments of force ($\mathbf{M}^M$) acting at that joint. The overall $\mathbf{M}^M$ can be conceived as composed of two parts: a positive ($\mathbf{M}^{M+}$) and a negative ($\mathbf{M}^{M-}$) moment of force. Therefore, to stress a muscle maximally, producing $\mathbf{M}^{M+}$ at a joint, one must maximize $\mathbf{M}^E$ and $\mathbf{M}^{M-}$. At the knee joint, if one considers extension to be positive, one must maximize a negative sum of $\mathbf{M}^E$ and $\mathbf{M}^H$ (both of which tend to flex the knee) to strengthen the quadriceps muscle maximally by maximizing the moment produced by the quadriceps, $\mathbf{M}^Q$.

We have implied that $\mathbf{M}^Q$ does not generate actions other than those needed to resist $\mathbf{M}^E$ and $\mathbf{M}^H$; however, $\mathbf{M}^Q$ also translates the tibia, because of the location and orientation of the patella ligament ($\mathbf{P}^Q$) and $\mathbf{F}^Q$ often has a component in the anterior direction. This anterior shearing force is resisted by the anterior cruciate ligament (ACL) and other secondary restraints.

In patients with ACL deficient knees, or in patients who have had reconstructive surgery of the ACL, strengthening of the quadriceps muscle poses a special challenge, since $\mathbf{F}^Q$ stresses the weakened ACL and the secondary restraints. In recognition of this problem, the rehabilitation community has responded by devising two potential approaches to strengthen the quadriceps in patients with ACL deficient knees.

The first method proposes a non-weight-bearing resisted knee extension exercise, with $\mathbf{F}^E$ applied at the mid-leg position, rather than at the more traditional distal pad placement. The rationale for this exercise is that by using a more proximal pad position, a greater $\mathbf{F}^E$ is required in order to maintain the same $\mathbf{M}^E$. Accordingly, this greater $\mathbf{F}^E$ will directly oppose any forces tending to displace the tibia anteriorly. Johnson initially provided the biomechanical rationale supporting this argument and Jurist and Otis experimentally showed a change in the direction of tibial displacement for selected joint angles from the anterior direction (with a distal pad placement) to posterior (with a more proximal pad placement).

The alternative method advocates a weight-bearing resisted knee extension exercise in the form of a partial squat, since $\mathbf{F}^Q$ with $\mathbf{F}^H$ (co-contraction) occurs during this exercise. Thus, the $\mathbf{F}^H$ resists the anterior tibial displacement produced by $\mathbf{F}^Q$. However, the anterior-posterior component of $\mathbf{F}^Q$ and $\mathbf{F}^H$ varies as a function of knee angle. The anatomy of the knee suggests that $\mathbf{F}^H$ is more favorably placed to resist anterior shear forces at the knee while the knee is flexed. Ohkoshi and colleagues studied the effect of varying knee joint angle and $\mathbf{F}^Q$ and $\mathbf{F}^H$ co-contraction while weight bearing on the anterior-posterior shear forces at the knee joint. They reported $\mathbf{F}^Q$ and $\mathbf{F}^H$ co-contraction and that the shear force at the knee was in a posterior direction and increased with greater knee flexion angles.

Our review of the literature located one paper by Yack et al that presents tibial displacement data during a squatting exercise and during a resisted knee extension (distal pad placement) in ACL deficient and normal knees. The $\mathbf{M}^E$ was determined for the squatting maneuver and then matched to the extension exercise. Significantly greater anterior tibial displacements in the knee extension group were observed between 10 and 66 degrees of knee flexion. However, there are three important limitations to this work. First, a distal pad placement was used and this does not reflect clinical practice in this patient population. Second, Yack and associates matched the knee extensor $\mathbf{M}$ to the squat. Presumably, maximum knee extension $\mathbf{M}$ will be greater

---

*Bold faced symbols represent vectors; normal faced symbols represent vector components or constants.

than the squat resistance **M** obtained as a result of body weight without external resistance. Accordingly, the work of these investigators does not address either the feasibility or the outcomes of applying maximal loads during the squat and knee extension exercises. Third, their measurement of anterior tibial displacement assumed that the patella did not move in an anterior-posterior direction while the knee goes through a ROM.

In this chapter, we illustrate the type of information that can be obtained from a mathematical simulation of the anterior translation at the knee. This translation is proportional to the posterior shear force, as affected by: (1) knee angle (θ^K), (2) the ratio of hamstring to quadriceps force (H/Q), (3) the point ($\mathbf{P}^E$) and (4) the direction (θ^E) of external force application. These relationships are explored (1) while the quadriceps is generating maximum force and (2) under conditions of constant external force application. The combinations of external force application simulate resistive kick and squatting activities. Overall, the search is for those conditions that minimize anterior tibial displacement, since these are the types of activities best prescribed to patients with ACL deficient knees.

SIMULATION MODEL

In this chapter we examine the effect of θ^K, H/Q, $\mathbf{P}^E$, and θ^E on anterior translation at the knee joint by a computer simulation. In order to perform these calculations, one must define (1) a mechanical/mathematical model of the system, (2) appropriate dimensions, and values for that system, and (3) a set of constraints that define the boundary conditions of the problem. These are outlined below.

A sagittal (XY) plane free-body diagram of a rigid lower leg and foot is constructed showing the quadriceps and hamstring muscle forces ($\mathbf{F}^Q$, $\mathbf{F}^H$) acting at locations ($\mathbf{P}^Q$, $\mathbf{P}^H$) and direction (θ^Q, θ^H), an external force ($\mathbf{F}^E$) acting at location $\mathbf{P}^E$ and direction θ^E the weight of the leg and foot ($\mathbf{F}^W$) acting at location $\mathbf{P}^W$ and direction θ^W, and a reaction force resolved into x and y components ($F_x{}^K$, $F_y{}^K$) acting at the knee ($\mathbf{P}^K$). The +X direction is directed anteriorly from the tibial plateau, +Y is is directed proximally and all angles are measured from the X axis in a counterclockwise direction (+Z rotations). Partitioning the forces into components along each of these axes the moment of force about the Z axis and the anteriorly directed force (X) about $\mathbf{P}^K$ can be stated mathematically as follows:

$$\Sigma M_Z = M_Z^Q + M_Z^H + M_Z^E + M_Z^W = 0 \qquad (2)$$

$$\Sigma F_X = F_X^Q + F_X^H + F_X^E + F_X^W + F_X^K = 0 \qquad (3)$$

where M_Z^* is given by equation (1) and

$$F_X^* = F^* \cos \theta^* \qquad (4)$$

$$F_Y^* = F^* \sin \theta^* \qquad (5)$$

the asterisk representing Q, H, E, W, or K. We define θ^H as equal to θ^K, and after Draganich et al.,

$$\theta^Q = 59.54 + 0.47 \, (\theta^K - 90) \qquad (6)$$

The location of the center of mass and the mass of the combined leg and foot segment are assumed to be 52.4% of leg length and 44.6 N respectively. This weight is always directed downwards relative to the seated (horizontal thigh) or squatting (ankle always below hip) patient simulated by the model. Additionally, $\mathbf{P}^Q$ and $\mathbf{P}^H$, relative to $\mathbf{P}^K$, are defined as (0.036, -0.042) and (-0.017, -0.042) meters in the X and Y directions respectively (Pierrynowski, 1994). Lastly, θ^E is set at 180 degrees for the resistive kick condition, and

$$\theta^E = ATAN \, \frac{-\cos \theta}{\sin \theta + 1} + 90 \qquad (7)$$

for the squat condition. This latter calculation assumes that $\mathbf{F}^E$ is directed from the ankle to the hip joint and the length of the thigh and lower leg are equal to 0.35 m (see Cappozzo et al, 1985).

The boundary conditions for the simulations are set as follows: θ^K ranges from 90 to 180 degrees (full extension to 90 degrees flexion), the H/Q ratio from 0 to 0.5, and $\mathbf{P}^E$ from 20% to 100% of the lower leg length. To examine the magnitude of the anterior shear force when the quadricep muscle was maximally activated, $\mathbf{F}^Q$ is set at 7,500 N, a value approximately equal to its maximal output in a healthy average-sized male individual (Pierrynowski, 1994). In order to simulate when a constant external force is applied, $\mathbf{F}^E$ is set at 75 N, a value attainable when the quadriceps are weak. Finally, $\mathbf{F}^E$ is set at 750 N, a value approximating a one-legged squat.

In making these various calculations, we used a microcomputer equipped with MathCad 4.0 software. An appropriate series of numerical and graphical checks were incorporated to verify the appropriateness of the simulations.

FINDINGS FROM SIMULATIONS

The effects of changes in θ^K, $\mathbf{P}^E$ and H/Q on $F_x{}^K$ during the resistive kick simulations with constant values of $\mathbf{F}^E$ (75 N and 750 N) and $\mathbf{F}^Q$ (7,500 N) are presented in Figures 1, 2, and 3, respectively. Knee angles (θ^K) ranging from full extension (0 degrees) to 90 degrees flexion are plotted along the abscissae, potential points of external force application ($\mathbf{P}^E$) ranging from 20% to 100% of lower leg length are plotted along the ordinates, and possible ratios of hamstring to quadriceps co-contraction (H/Q) of 0%, 20%, and 40% are plotted in the left, middle, and right-hand Figures, respectively. Within each plot, constant force lines are drawn at 100 or 1,000 N intervals; these lines join conditions that produce the same anterior shear force ($F_x{}^K$) at the knee. Negative values indicate loading in structures that exert a backwardly directed force on the tibia. In individuals

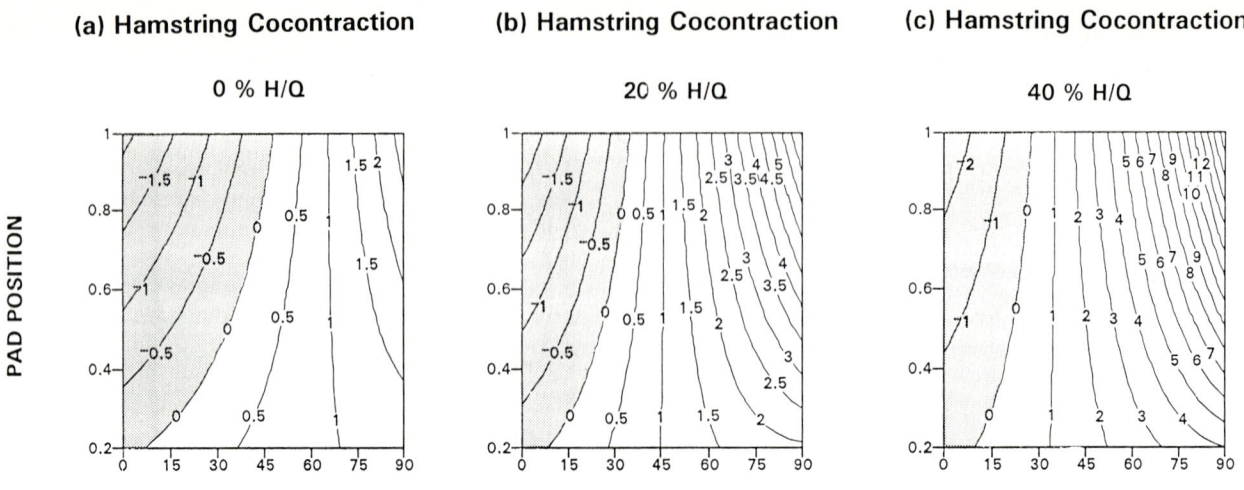

Figure 1 The effect of knee angle (θ^K), pad position ($\mathbf{P}^E$), and hamstring/quadriceps co-activity (H/Q) on the anterior shear force during a resistive kick with a constantly applied 75 N resistance. Constant force lines are plotted at 100 N intervals. The shaded area indicates the clinically dangerous region where the anterior cruciate ligament and secondary restraints are loaded.

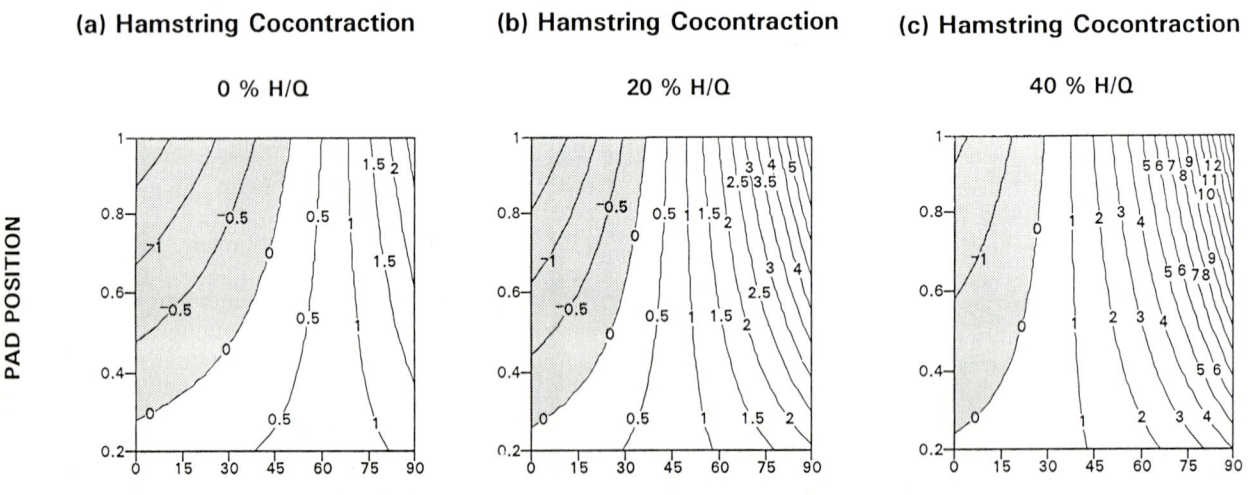

Figure 2 The effect of knee angle (θ^K), pad position ($\mathbf{P}^E$), and hamstring/quadriceps coactivity (H/Q) on the anterior shear force during a resistive kick with a constantly applied 750 N resistance. Constant force lines are plotted at 1,000 N intervals. The shaded area indicates the clinically dangerous region where the anterior cruciate ligament and secondary restraints are loaded.

with weakened ACL or secondary restraints at the knee, these regions must be avoided.

The simulations show nonlinear relationships between all these variables. However, in order to keep F_x^K positive (thereby avoiding the undesired loading of the ACL), one must increase θ^K (flex the knee), apply the external force ($\mathbf{F}^E$) close to the knee, and maximize H/E (hamstring-quadricep co-contraction). These results support the findings of Johnson, Jurist and Otis, Ohkoshi et al, and Yack et al. Additionally, our simulation

suggests that an exercise with knee flexion angles less than 30 degrees, proximal pad placements, and a constant $\mathbf{F}^E$ will displace the tibia anteriorly.

The analogous effects of θ^K and H/Q on F_x^K during simulated squats are presented in Figure 4 for the constant $\mathbf{F}^E$ (750 N) and $\mathbf{F}^Q$ (7,500 N) conditions, respectively. As in the resistive kick exercise, a nonlinear relationship exists between these variables. In order to maximize F_x^K, one must increase θ^K and maximize H/E. The results also suggest that constant $\mathbf{F}^E$ exercises

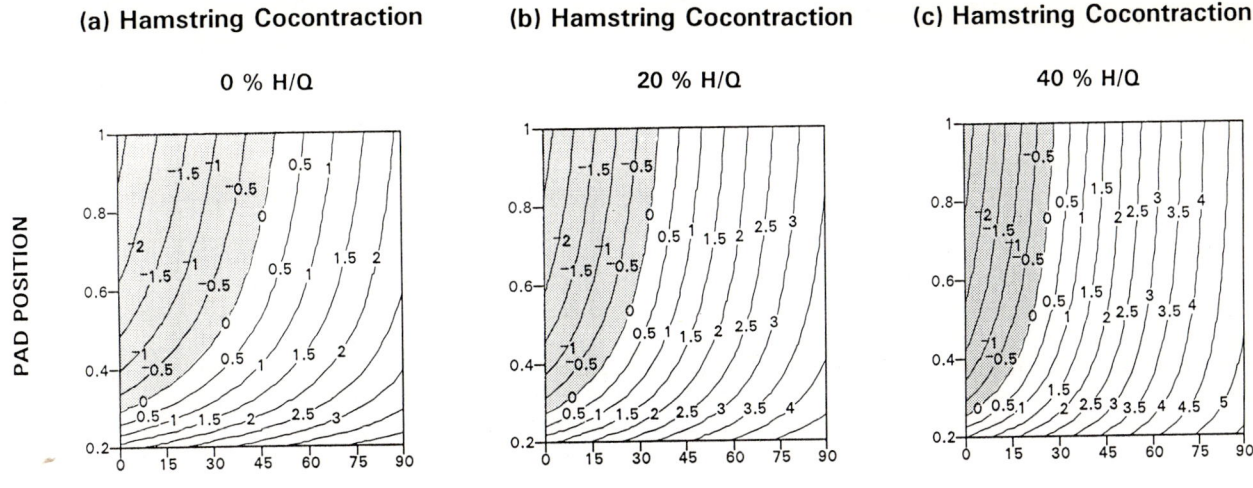

Figure 3 The effect of knee angle (θ^K), pad position ($\mathbf{P}^E$), and hamstring/quadriceps coactivity (H/Q) on the anterior shear force during a resistive kick with a constant quadriceps force of 7,500 N. Constant force lines are plotted at 1,000 N intervals. The shaded area indicates the clinically dangerous region where the anterior cruciate ligament and secondary restraints are loaded.

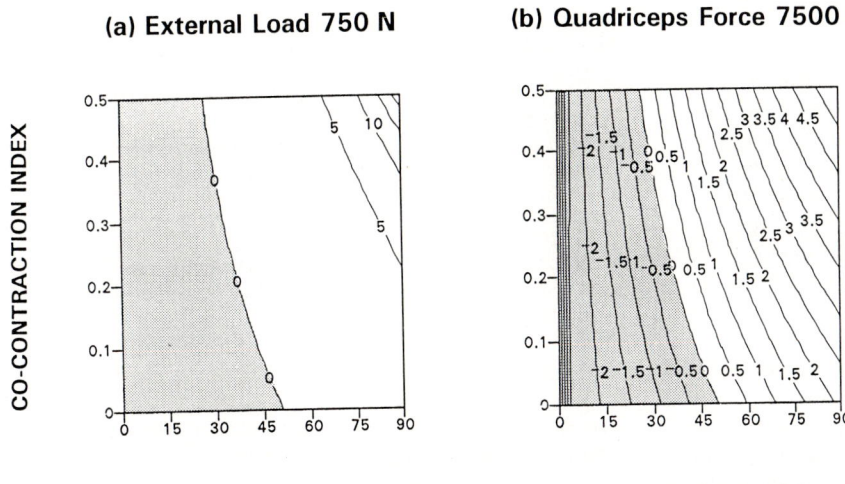

Figure 4 The effect of knee angle (θ^K), and hamstring/quadriceps coactivity (H/Q) on the anterior shear force during a squat with a constant external load of 750 N (*left*) and a constant quadriceps force of 7,500 N (*right*). Constant force lines are plotted at 1,000 N intervals. The shaded area indicates the clinically dangerous region where the anterior cruciate ligament and secondary restraints are loaded.

reduce anterior tibial displacements at low levels of cocontraction.

IMPLICATIONS OF FINDINGS

Kick Exercise

1. A more proximal pad placement provides greater ACL protection for any given quadriceps force and knee joint angle.
2. A greater flexion angle also provides greater ACL protection for any given quadriceps force and pad placement.
3. When a proximal pad placement (0.3) is used, a greater external resistance force provides greater protection. This does not hold true for more distal pad placements.
4. When a mid to proximal pad placement is used and the joint is near terminal extension, the relative amount of co-contraction has little effect on the shear forces (i.e., the amount of co-contraction does not appreciably expand the protected ROM).

Squat

Protection is offered at knee flexion angles greater than 30 degrees when the co-contraction index is 0.5. Protection is still observed beyond 50 degrees, even when the co-contraction index is 0.

CLINICAL RELEVANCE

In order to illustrate the potential impact of these findings on the clinical practice of sports medicine and rehabilitation, we will consider a typical case scenario that follows a subject from the time of injury to a return to full activity.

Case Scenario. The subject is a 20-year-old male who sustained a partial tear of the ACL while playing basketball 2 days earlier. Specifically, he twisted his knee and fell to the floor in significant discomfort. There was immediate swelling and he was unable to continue play. Roentgenograms were negative, but physical examination revealed discomfort and increased anterior laxity when performing the Lachman test. An end-point was present.

In addition to applying ice, compression, elevation, rest, and crutches (partial weight bearing), one immediate goal in the management of such a patient is to initiate quadriceps exercises in order to minimize muscle atrophy. How can this goal best be achieved? Because the patient is allowed only partial weight bearing, the squat is not a viable choice. The results of the kick simulation show that any magnitude of resistance can be applied without stressing the ACL, provided knee flexion is within the range 35 to 90 degrees, and a mid to proximal pad placement is used.

The next important clinical decision must be made some 2 weeks later, when the swelling has subsided and the patient is progressed to full weight bearing without an ambulatory aid. Over the next several months, the goal of rehabilitation is to strenghten the quadriceps efficiently while minimizing the stress on the ACL. When a proximal pad placement (0.3 of tibial length) is chosen for the kick exercise, the safe ACL strengthening extends from 20 to 90 degrees (75 N load), and from 5 to 90 degrees (750 N load). These values are based on a co-contraction index of 0. The effect of a co-contraction index greater than 0 would be to expand the safe exercise ROM towards 0 degrees of flexion. The safe exercise window for the squat exercise varies significantly, depending on the co-contraction index. For example, an index of 0.5 allows a safe exercise range of 30 to 90 degrees of flexion, whereas a co-contraction index of 0 provides a safe range only from 50 to 90 degrees of flexion. The safe ROM estimates for the squat do not vary appreciably for constant load (750 N) or constant quadriceps force (7,500 N) conditions.

In summary, the computer simulations of knee mechanics provides valuable clinical information. It shows that both kicks and squats can be used to strengthen the quadriceps muscle, while at the same time avoiding tensile loading to the anterior stabilizers of the knee. Furthermore, the simulations suggest that if the resistive kick exercise is performed with a proximal pad placement, this provides a greater protected ROM. From a practical perspective this finding is encouraging for several reasons: (1) training can begin even when weight bearing is still contraindicated; (2) external resistance can be progressed easily, and when the external resistive torque is generated by an isokinetic device, the resistance torque profile will match the patient's generated torque profile; and (3) unlike the squat, the resistance force with the kick can be applied safely and uniquely to the knee.

SUGGESTED READING

Cappozzo A, Felici F, Figura F, Gazzani F. Lumbar spine loading during half-squat exercises. Med Sci Sports Exer 1985; 17:613–620.

Draganich LF, Andriacchi TP, Andersson GBJ. Interaction between intrinsic knee mechanics and the knee extensor mechanism. J Orthop Res 1987; 5:539–547.

Johnson D. Controlling anterior shear during isokinetic knee extension exercise. J Orthop Sports Phys Ther 1982; 4:23–31.

Jurist KA, Otis JC. Anteroposterior tibiofemoral displacements during isometric extension efforts. J Orthop Sports Phys Ther 1985; 13:254–258.

Ohkoski Y, Yasuka K, Kaneda K, et al. Biomechanical analysis of rehabilitation in the standing position. Am J Sports Med 1991; 19:605–611.

Pierrynowski MR. Analytic representation of muscle line of action and geometry. In: Allard P, Stokes IAF, Blanchi JP, eds. Champaign, Il: Human Kinetics Publishers, 1994.

Yack HJ, Collins CE, Whieldon TJ. Comparison of closed and open kinetic chain exercise in the anterior cruciate ligament deficient knee. Am J Sports Med 1993; 21:49–53.

SKELETAL MUSCLE FIBERS: TYPES AND DISTRIBUTION

JAN MELICHNA, Ph.D.
CHRISTIAN W. ZAUNER, Ph.D.

Muscle fiber typing is increasingly used by sports medicine laboratories to assess the inherent aptitude of athletes for particular types of competition, to moderate training programs, and to evaluate the "nature versus nurture" controversy. In the last 20 years, improved techniques of muscle biopsy and development of superior methods for the histochemical and biochemical analyses of muscle tissue have led to a much better understanding of the structure and function of muscle cells and more precise typing in the individual competitor. This chapter focuses in part on continuing methodologic problems in fiber typing and in part on the more fundamental processes governing the regulation and differentiation of skeletal muscle fibers.

BIOPSY TECHNIQUES

Duschenne took the first muscle biopsy samples from human subjects in 1868. He did so from patients presenting with apparent muscular dystrophy and utilized a special biopsy needle. The next major advance was in 1975, when Bergström developed a highly improved biopsy instrument that can provide not only samples for clinical purposes, but also for physiologic and biochemical investigations. At present, several types of modified muscle biopsy needles exist.

The selection of the muscle to be biopsied depends not only upon the athlete's event, but also upon muscle size, presence or absence of large blood vessels, and/or the proximity of important nerves to the proposed sampling site. However, the degree to which the muscle contributes to the physical activity patterns of the competitor is of prime importance. For instance, the gastrocnemius may be a likely candidate for sampling in the runner, the vastus lateralis in cyclists, and in weight lifters the biceps may be a logical choice. In comparative or genetic studies, the muscle used is typically the vastus lateralis.

Sampling of muscle tissue is a minor procedure. It takes place under aseptic conditions, after administration of a local anesthetic. An incision about 1 to 2 cm long is made through the skin and subcutaneous fat and the biopsy needle is introduced through it into the underlying muscle. A segment of muscle tissue can be excised by a quick closing maneuver of the biopsy needle sleeve, the leading edge of which is formed from sharpened surgical steel. The resulting sample has a mass of 15 to 25 mg. Exerting negative pressure through the core of the needle by means of a syringe and connective tubing maximizes sample size; using such an approach, one can obtain tissue samples of 50 to 100 mg. This technique eliminates the need to perform repeated biopsies for histochemical studies, since a sample so obtained will include a minimum of 500 fibers.

Current muscle biopsy technique, although invasive and with some risk of minor complications, is fast, relatively simple, and results in minimal trauma. The procedure is contraindicated in those with eczema, allergic diseases, inflammatory blood vessel diseases, or varicose veins. Furthermore, restraint from physical activity is advised for at least 48 hours after skeletal muscle biopsy.

HISTOCHEMICAL METHODS

For purposes of histochemical analysis, the sample must be mounted on a metal block with adhesive in such a manner as to assure that subsequent cross-sections of the tissue will be made perpendicular to the longitudinal axes of the fibers. After the sample is fixed in proper perspective on the block, it is frozen in isopentane cooled by liquid nitrogen. The sample is then sectioned in series to 10 μm thickness, using a refrigerated microtome at $-20°$ C. The serial cross-sections are now ready for incubation at various pHs and subsequent staining for different enzyme activities. The number of enzymes that can be demonstrated histochemically now exceeds 70.

Histochemical methods can be used to differentiate fast twitch glycolytic (Type IIb), fast twitch oxidative-glycolytic (Type IIa), and slow twitch oxidative (Type I) muscle fibers. Furthermore, such techniques can demonstrate the structural changes such as hypertrophy and atrophy that are associated with training and detraining, and they can show a deficit or depletion of specific enzymes and substrates.

After histochemical staining and typing of specific muscle fibers, it is possible to express the relative size of the various fiber types as fiber areas or diameters. Either hand-operated or computerized planimetry can be employed to estimate muscle fiber area, although the former is very tedious. Bloomstrand et al have discussed the main questions concerning calculation of muscle fiber areas, and Song et al have delineated a method for assessing fiber diameter. Although both measures express similar concepts, area is more commonly reported since the advent of computer software for planimetry.

BIOCHEMICAL TECHNIQUES

For biochemical studies, the muscle sample need not be mounted, but is rather quickly frozen in liquid nitrogen, freeze-dried, and weighed. It is then placed in an extractor buffer and homogenized. The enzyme activities or substrate contents are determined spectrophotometrically, usually using kits based upon NAD-

NADP coupled reactions. Through microdissection of freeze-dried fiber fragments, followed by appropriate biochemical and chromatographic analyses, it is possible to quantify certain enzyme activities and substrate levels in the various fiber types.

TECHNICAL PROBLEMS

It is well known that a number of muscle fiber categories exist and that their histochemical profiles are correlated to muscle contraction times and resistance to fatigue. However, histochemically derived morphological data are often not completely compatible with the functional characteristics of the intact muscle. One explanation for the observed discrepancies could be that there are variations in fiber type populations at different depths within a muscle. Thus, a single biopsy sample may be a poor estimator of fiber type proportions in the muscle as a whole. In order to restrict the possibility of such error, Lexell et al recommended counting fibers in three separate biopsy samples, taken at different depths from the muscle in question, with each sample containing more than 150 fibers. If fewer than three biopsy samples are examined, there is risk of a substantial sampling error.

Another general technical problem concerns the matter of taking samples from the same individual before and after some experimental intervention such as a specific training program. It is critical that all samples be taken from essentially the same site within the muscle that is being studied. Although one can readily identify the prior incision site, there is a danger that the muscle depth from which samples are taken will vary. It thus becomes impossible to be certain whether the differences observed over time are due to the treatment (e.g., training or detraining) or whether they merely reflect differences in depth of sampling.

When one athlete is compared with another, even though the same muscle may be sampled, the matter of site is again critical. Anatomic landmarks allow a fairly close approximation relative to surface site. For instance, when sampling from the vastus lateralis, one can use a fixed percentage of the distance between the distal end of the femur and the greater trochanter. However, this approach fails to address the matter of sampling depth, a problem that is complicated by the fact that the vastus lateralis has varying thicknesses in different competitors.

Details of the freezing process can also influence muscle fiber size, whether this be expressed as fiber area or diameter. Furthermore, the selection of fibers for size assessment can compromise the validity of the estimate. We recommend that at least 20 fibers of each type be randomly selected for measurement. The selected fibers must be without artifacts, show no evidence of a longitudinal cut, have distinct borders, and not be in close proximity to the edge of the sample. Furthermore, the period between removal of the muscle sample and its freezing should be no more than 2 to 4 minutes.

MUSCLE FIBER DIFFERENTIATION

As long ago as 1678, Lorenzini reflected on the observation that intact, unstained mammalian skeletal muscles ranged in color from nearly white to dark red. He thus suggested that muscles be described as either white or red in type. Ranvier, in 1870, was the first to note that the red muscles of the rabbit contracted more slowly than the white ones. Early histochemical studies revealed that mammalian skeletal muscles are usually heterogeneous, that red fibers are usually thin, dark, and with many mitochondria, whereas white muscle fibers are thicker, with fewer mitochondria and fat droplets than the red fibers.

The present-day histochemical identification of muscle fiber types depends on an analysis of oxidative and glycolytic enzymes. Type I fibers are fatigue resistant and have a relatively slow contraction speed. They demonstrate rather little ATPase reaction, but considerable reactivity of the oxidative enzymes succinic dehydrogenase (SDH) and NADH diaphorase. On the other hand, Type II fibers are rich in ATPase but show little reaction for SDH and NADH diaphorase. Type II fibers may be assigned to one of two subclassifications; Type IIb and Type IIa. Although members of both Type II subgroups show relatively fast contraction speeds, Type IIb is easily fatigued whereas Type IIa is somewhat fatigue resistant. Type IIa muscle fibers always show a higher reactivity for the oxidative enzymes than do Type IIb fibers.

Barany associated specific activity of myosin ATPase with the contraction time of skeletal muscle. Fibers with a high myosin ATPase activity have the shortest contraction times. The Ca^{++}-activated myosin ATPase activity of Type II fibers is approximately 2.5 times that of Type I fibers. Burke et al examined the effects of repetitive stimulation, noting a decline in muscle tension with repeated stimulation. He termed this property *fatiguability*, and found it developed more slowly in Type I as opposed to Type II muscle fibers. Thus, of the fiber types, Type I shows the greatest resistance to fatigue. However, because of relatively rapid contraction velocities, Type II fibers generate the greatest power per contraction.

Biochemically, Type I muscle fibers react strongly to most indicators of oxidative metabolism. Type IIb fibers depend chiefly on anaerobic carbohydrate metabolism for energy release and Type IIa fibers have moderate to high levels of markers for both oxidative and anaerobic metabolism.

Specific morphologic characteristics are associated with the various skeletal muscle fiber types. Type I fibers in humans are generally the smallest and Type IIa fibers are typically the largest in diameter. The local blood supply (expressed as the capillary to fiber ratio) and the mitochondrial volume is greatest among Type I fibers.

Unfortunately, the literature still demonstrates a variety of nomenclature for muscle fiber types. Two systems are commonly used. One applies alphabetical letters symbolizing the predominant characteristics of the individual fibers, and the other relies mainly on

Roman numerals. In the first system, fibers that contract relatively slowly and depend on oxidative metabolism are referred to as SO (slow oxidative) fibers. Fast-contracting glycolytic fibers are symbolized as FG and fast fibers with both oxidative and glycolytic enzyme pathways are symbolized as FOG. The second system has been utilized throughout this chapter. In this latter classification, Type I fibers are synonymous with SO fibers, Type IIb with FG, and Type IIa with FOG muscle fibers. Classification is further complicated by the existence of a Type IIc skeletal muscle fiber, commonly considered as embryonic in type. It is also rather common to refer to the Type IIa (FOG) fiber as an intermediate fiber.

In 1966 Dubowitz described three phases of human muscle fiber differentiation. Undifferentiated (Type IIc) fibers were predominant through 20 weeks of gestation. From 20 through 26 weeks, most fibers were Type II, with high myosin ATPase activity. Complete differentiation of Type I and Type II fibers was not evident until after 30 weeks of gestation.

Although the ultimate number of muscle fibers is approached during prenatal development, the number of fibers continues to increase for a short period after birth. Even though Type IIc is the most common fiber through 20 weeks of gestation, at birth only about 20% of fibers are of this type. By age 1 year, the percentage of Type I fibers is about the same as in adults and Type IIc fibers are practically nonexistent. At age 6 years, the distribution of Types I, IIa, and IIb is practically identical to that of adults. This implies that an optimal decision regarding involvement in power or endurance sport can be reached at an early age.

The average muscle fiber diameter at birth is approximately 15 μm, whereas in adults this value approaches 60 μm. At the age of 1 year, the fiber diameter is about 30% of that seen in the adult, and by 5 years, 50% of the adult value has been achieved. Muscle mass increases from about 23.6% of body mass at birth to approximately 40% at adulthood. In absolute terms, muscle mass increases from close to 0.78 kg at birth to about 28 kg at maturity. These increases in muscle fiber size and muscle mass are due to fiber hypertrophy (an enlargement of existing fibers) rather than hyperplasia (the formation of additional fibers).

Growth in muscle tissue is thus characterized by an increase in the protein to DNA ratio. The ratio is greater in boys than in girls, and is positively related to age. Elevations in protein to DNA ratio are particularly marked at the time of the adolescent spurt in growth of muscle mass. Muscle fiber thickness continues to increase until about the eighteenth year and in males is greatly facilitated by the increase of testosterone secretion that accompanies sexual maturation. Finally, mitochondrial size and volume are greater in children aged 1 month to nearly 13 years than in adults.

In boys 11 to 15 years of age, the activity of the glycolytic enzyme phosphofructokinase is only about one-third of that observed in adults and the mitochon-drial enzyme succinic dehydrogenase is somewhat greater in children as opposed to adults. Although young boys have similar concentrations of muscle adenosine triphosphate and creatine phosphate, glycogen content is lower than in adults. Such differences may influence both immediate performance and responses to training.

The muscle distribution in homogeneous muscles varies greatly from one individual to another, the proportion of a given fiber type ranging from 10% to 95%. For instance, top ranked endurance athletes have a high percentage of Type I fibers in their leg muscles, but top-ranked sprint runners are characterized by a preponderance of Type IIb fibers in the same muscles. Studies of monozygous and dizygous twins suggest that such differences in muscle fiber patterns are the result of inheritance rather than training, an important argument supporting the view that athletes should exploit their constitution, rather than try to prepare themselves for an event which does not match their fiber distribution.

SUGGESTED READING

Barany M. ATPase activity of myosin correlated with speed of muscle shortening. J Gen Physiol 1967; 50:197–218.

Bell RD, Macdougall JD, Billeter R, Howald H. Muscle fiber types and morphometric analysis of skeletal muscle in six-year-old children. Med Sci Sports Exerc 1980; 12:28–31.

Bloomstrand E, Ekblom B, Newsholme EA. Maximum activities of key glycolytic and oxidative enzymes in human muscle from differently trained individuals. J Physiol 1986; 381:111–118.

Burke RE, Levine DN, Zajac FE, et al: Mammalian motor units: physiological–histochemical correlation of three types in cat gastrocnemius. Science 1971; 200:709–712.

Cheek DB. Growth and body composition. In: Cheek DB, ed. Fetal and postnatal cellular growth: hormones and nutrition. New York: John Wiley & Sons, 1975:389.

Close RI. Dynamic properties of mammalian skeletal muscle. Physiol Rev 1972; 52;129–197.

Colling-Saltin A-S. Skeletal muscle development in the human fetus and during childhood. In: Berg, et al, eds. Children in exercise IX 1980. Baltimore: University Park Press, 1980:193.

Dubowitz V. Diseased muscle: a histochemical study. SIMP Research Monograph No. 2. Leicester, England: Heineman Medical Books Ltd., 1968.

Dubowitz V, Brooke MH. Muscle biopsy: a practical approach. 2nd ed. Philadelphia: WB Saunders, 1985.

Eriksson BO. Physical training, oxygen supply and muscle metabolism in 11-13 year old boys. Acta Physiol Scand 1972; 384(suppl):1–48.

Essen-Gustavsson B, Henriksson J. Enzyme levels in pools of microdissected human muscle fibers of identified type. Adaptive responses to exercise. Acta Physiol Scand 1984; 120:505–551.

Gollnick PD, Armstrong RB, Saltin B, et al. Effect of training on enzyme activities and fiber composition of human skeletal muscle. J Appl Physiol 1973; 34:107–111.

Gollnick PD, Armstrong RB, Saubert CW, et al. Enzyme activity and fiber composition in skeletal muscle of untrained and trained men. J Appl Physiol 1972; 33:312–314.

Jerusalem F, Engel AG, Peterson H. Human muscle fiber fine structure: morphometric data on controls. Neurology 1975; 25: 127–134.

Komi PV, Karlsson J. Physical performance, skeletal muscle enzyme activities and fiber types in monozygous and dizygous twins of both sexes. Acta Physiol Scand 1979; 462(Suppl.):1–43.

Lexell J, Taylor C, Sjostrom M. Analysis of sampling errors in biopsy techniques using data from whole muscle cross sections. J Appl Physiol 1985; 59:1228–1235.

Mackova EV, Melichna J, Novak J, et al. Histochemical and metabolic characteristics of athletes of different kinds of sports. In: Tsopanakis, Poortmans, eds. Physiological biochemistry of exercise and, training. Athens: Olympic Sports Center of Athens, 1987:155.

Malina RM. Growth and muscle tisssue and muscle mass. In: Falkner, Tanner, eds. Human growth 2. Postnatal growth. New York: Plenum Press, 1978:273.

Saltin B, Gollnick PD. Skeletal muscle adaptability: Significance for metabolism and performance. In: Peachey, et al, eds. Handbook of physiology: Skeletal muscle. Baltimore: Williams & Wilkins, 1983: 555.

Song SK, Shimada N, Anderson PJ. Orthogonal diameters in the analysis of muscle fiber size and forms. Nature 1963; 200:1220–1221.

Stein JM, Padykula JV. Histochemical classification of individual skeletal muscle fibers of the rat. Am J Anat 1962; 110:103–123.

BIOCHEMICAL RESPONSES TO ENDURANCE TRAINING

PETER M. TIIDUS, Ph.D.

Elite athletic performance depends on a multitude of physiologic, biochemical, and psychological factors. A high maximum ability to consume oxygen ($\dot{V}o_2max$) has commonly been regarded as a primary factor in the success of world class endurance athletes. While elite marathon runners do exhibit much higher $\dot{V}o_2max$ values than nonelite runners, several other factors may be at least as important to their overall success. For example, Frank Shorter (the 1972 Olympic marathon gold medallist) and Derek Clayton (the first man to run a marathon under 2:10:00) both had treadmill-determined $\dot{V}o_2max$ values of approximately 70 $ml \cdot kg^{-1} \cdot min^{-1}$. While these values are high compared to untrained individuals or recreational athletes, they are unremarkable among endurance athletes. Middle-distance runners generally have higher $\dot{V}o_2max$ values than marathoners, yet their times for a marathon race would be significantly slower. Measurements made on elite-distance runners in the 1930s indicated $\dot{V}o_2max$ values very similar to those reported in the endurance athletes of today, despite significant improvements in competitive performance. Running efficiency and psychological motivation are only two of many other components required for long-distance running success. However, this chapter concentrates on the importance of the adaptations in muscle biochemistry that occur as a result of extensive endurance training and how they may influence performance and fuel selection in long endurance-related athletic events.

TRAINING EFFECTS ON $\dot{V}o_2max$, MUSCLE MITOCHONDRIA AND ENDURANCE PERFORMANCE

Intramuscular biochemical responses to the repeated contractions that occur in exercising muscle vary, depending on numerous factors. There are acute and transient biochemical changes that take place during or immediately after an exercise bout that reverse themselves shortly postexercise. There are also more long-lasting biochemical adaptations that occur in response to chronic exercise of various intensities, durations, or frequencies. When young and sedentary, but otherwise healthy adults are endurance trained for 3 to 6 months they may improve their $\dot{V}o_2max$ by only 20%, yet still increase running time to exhaustion at 70% of their pretraining $\dot{V}o_2max$ by up to 300 to 400%. A significant portion of this improved endurance capacity can be attributed to the long-term enhancement of their muscular oxidative enzyme activities and mitochondrial concentration, both of which can increase by approximately 100% from pretraining levels.

ADENOSINE TRIPHOSPHATE UTILIZATION AND REGENERATION

When muscle is stimulated to contract, the immediate energy source for this contraction is adenosine triphosphate (ATP). During repeated bouts of muscular contraction, ATP is hydrolyzed to adenosine diphosphate (ADP) and inorganic phosphate. This hydrolysis is catalyzed mainly by ATPase enzymes on (1) the head of the myosin molecule (to power crossbridge movement between the thick and the thin muscle filaments), (2) the sarcoplasmic reticulum (to power calcium reabsorption) following crossbridge formation and (3) the sarcolemma (to maintain cellular sodium/potassium homeostasis during repeated depolarization of the muscle). The biochemical pathways that couple energy liberation with ATP formation are closely regulated by the local ADP concentration [ADP]. The rate of ATP utilization by ATPase enzymes will therefore be intimately linked with ATP regeneration in order to minimize disturbances of cellular ATP homeostasis throughout a range of exercise intensities. Decreases to muscular [ATP] exceeding 30 to 40% are intimately associated with muscular fatigue. During endurance exercise, the vast majority of ATP regeneration occurs by a mitochondrial process of oxidative phosphorylation.

ROLE OF CARBOHYDRATES IN ENDURANCE EXERCISE

Carbohydrate, in the form of muscle and liver glycogen, is of primary importance in ATP regeneration during any type of exercise. Not only is it a more efficient fuel source than fat (approximately 21.1 kJ or 5.05 kcal versus 19.5 kJ or 4.65 kcal of energy liberated per liter of oxygen consumed), but oxidation of fat cannot occur without a minimum obligatory oxidation of carbohydrate. This is likely because carbohydrate breakdown may also support the obligatory reformation of intermediate compounds that are broken down during the Krebs cycle of oxidative metabolism. Additionally, since the central nervous system (CNS) relies on blood borne glucose as its primary fuel source, any compromise in blood glucose availability will limit CNS function and thus severely restrict the individual's work capacity. Limitations to marathon running performance may therefore be related (along with other factors) to the ability of the competitor to maintain muscle and liver glycogen stores when the demand for intramuscular ATP regeneration is high for an extended time period.

Training-induced elevations in muscle mitochondrial content will effectively improve endurance performance at a given submaximal work-rate by (1) decreasing the rate of muscle glycogen oxidation, (2) increasing the oxidation of alternative fuels (intramuscular and adipose lipids), (3) lowering the muscle and blood lactate concentrations, and (4) promoting uptake rather than release of lactate by exercising muscle. These adaptations will occur mainly due to an increase in the mitochondrial metabolic rate at any given substrate concentration and its resultant effect in decreasing glycolytic flux. Performance improvements in the endurance-trained individual are due in part to the ability to conserve the limited muscle glycogen store during intense endurance exercise.

BIOCHEMICAL FACTORS IN ENDURANCE TRAINING ADAPTATIONS

Since training does not significantly affect muscle blood flow or $\dot{V}O_2$max at any absolute submaximal work-rate, training-related elevations in fat oxidation and decreases in carbohydrate utilization and lactate production by the working muscles cannot be attributed to increased circulatory lipid delivery or oxygen availability. Instead, these changes can be attributed almost entirely to the increased muscle concentrations of mitochondrial oxidative enzymes that are induced by endurance training. A theoretical model of the training process, based on Henri-Michaelis-Menten kinetics, was first suggested by Gollnick and Saltin in 1982. This model proposed a biochemical explanation for why training-induced increases in muscle mitochondrial concentration caused the above adaptations in fuel selection and lactate production. Considerable empirical data have subsequently emerged to support the scenario that they proposed.

To understand how the biochemical concomitants of training happen, it is important first to review some of the basics regarding general enzyme kinetics. Reactions between most of the enzymes of the Krebs cycle, the electron transport chain and their substrates can be described by what biochemists term "zero order"

kinetics. This means that the rate of enzyme-substrate formation and its subsequent dissociation into enzyme and end-product is limited by the rate of random contact between the enzyme and its substrate. Random contact increases nearly linearly with increasing substrate concentration; however, as the amount of free enzyme declines at higher substrate concentrations, a nonlinear relationship results, and the maximum reaction velocity (Vmax) is only reached at inordinately high substrate concentrations (Fig. 1).

Every enzyme has a characteristic substrate concentration that induces an activity equal to half of its Vmax. This is known as its *Michaelis constant* (Km) and is independent of enzyme concentration. Therefore, if the concentration of an enzyme were for example doubled, this would not only approximately double its Vmax, but would also double its reaction rate at Km (or at any other submaximal substrate concentration). This reaction characteristic greatly enhances the precision of control of enzyme activity at the low substrate concentrations that tend to prevail in vivo.

In particular, a higher post-training muscle mitochondrial concentration will be more sensitive to changes in the [ATP]/[ADP] concentration ratio. Mitochondrial respiration is regulated primarily by the intracellular ADP concentration. ADP is the substrate for the mitochondrial adenine nucleotide translocase enzymes, and ultimately for the phosphorylation process that occurs on the F_1 complexes of the mitochondrial inner membrane. Reaction rates between cytosolic ADP and the mitochondrial enzymes can also be described in terms of "zero order" kinetics, whereby increasing [ADP] through the ranges that occur in vivo will result in near linear increases in mitochondrial respiration. Therefore, if endurance training results in a doubling of muscle mitochondria, any [ADP] will induce twice as much mitochondrial respiration as would have occurred prior to training.

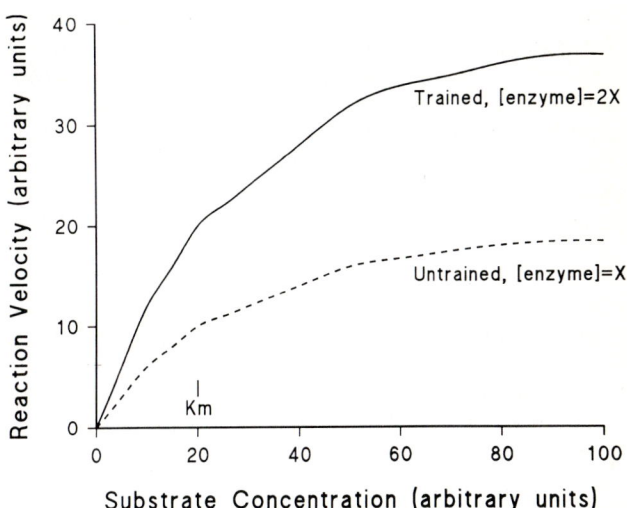

Figure 1 Reaction velocity at an arbitrary mitochondrial enzyme concentration (X = untrained, 2X = trained), illustrating increased sensitivity to substrate concentration in the trained condition.

If we view this effect in practical terms, we know that (other factors being equal) the ATP turnover rate for an endurance-trained individual will be the same as that for an untrained individual who is exercising at the same work-rate. Since the trained individual is likely to have twice the muscle mitochondrial concentration of the untrained individual, they will also be capable of incurring twice the rate of ATP regeneration via mitochondrial oxidative phosphorylation at any cytosolic [ADP]. Conversely, a much smaller increase in cytosolic [ADP] will be required to induce the same amount of mitochondrial respiration ($\dot{V}O_2$) and ATP regeneration. This will result in the maintenance of a higher cytosolic [ATP]/[ADP] ratio at any given $\dot{V}O_2$. It will also significantly reduce the time required to increase $\dot{V}O_2$ to steady state levels following the onset of exercise, thereby further limiting the increase in cytosolic [ADP].

BIOCHEMICAL EFFECTS ON ENDURANCE PERFORMANCE

[ADP] is a major regulator of the key enzymes in the glycolytic pathway. Reducing cytosolic [ADP] at submaximal work-rates significantly reduces glycolytic flux. This has several positive repercussions for endurance performance. Of primary importance is the diminished rate of muscle glycogen and blood borne glucose usage that delays the time to muscle and liver glycogen depletion and resultant fatigue. Additionally, a reduction of [ADP] curtails the production of pyruvate and glycolytic NADH.

This has two important ramifications. First it reduces the substrate available for the enzyme lactate dehydrogenase (LDH), thereby limiting lactate production. It is now well accepted that muscle lactate production does not occur only as a result of anaerobiosis. Lactate production can occur in fully oxygenated muscle and during submaximal exercise as a result of an imbalance between the potentially very high enzyme activities of the glycolytic pathway and the relatively slower rates of mitochondrial oxidative phosphorylation pathways. When activated by increased cytosolic [ADP], glycolysis produces pyruvate and NADH at rates faster than they can be utilized by the mitochondria. However, if glycolytic flux is reduced by limiting the build up of cytosolic [ADP] during submaximal exercise, glycogenolysis and lactate generation, which contribute relatively little to ATP resynthesis during this type of work, are significantly diminished.

The decreased glycolytic flux also diminishes the availability of pyruvate as a source of acetyl units; this enhances the entry into the Krebs cycle of acetyl-CoA units derived from beta-oxidation of fatty acids. Since the enzymes needed for beta-oxidation of fatty acids are located within the mitochondrial matrix, endurance training increases the presence of these enzymes and hence their kinetics at low substrate concentrations. Delivery to and uptake by muscle of circulating fatty acids at similar submaximal work-rates is not significantly enhanced by endurance training. Once in the

muscle cell, the entry of fatty acids into the mitochondria is limited by the abiilty of the enzyme carnitine palmityl transferase (CPT) to translocate such compounds across the mitochondrial membrane and also by the availability of the transporter molecule carnitine. Training-induced increases in the concentration of CPT and carnitine enhance mitochondrial fatty acid entry and oxidation. An increased muscle mitochondrial concentration thus increases the utilization of fatty acid oxidation as a fuel source for ATP resynthesis while simultaneously decreasing the subject's reliance on glycogen and glucose.

Muscle and blood lactate accumulation occurs when the rate of lactate production exceeds its rate of removal. The primary mechanism for lactate removal during endurance exercise is oxidation in the mitochondria of muscle and liver. Lactate is more readily produced during exercise in the more glycolytic (Type II) muscle fibers. During long distance running, the Type II muscle fibers (which are used less extensively during endurance exercise) tend to release lactate; this lactate can then be taken up and oxidized by the more oxidative (Type I) muscle fibers, particularly if their mitochondrial concentration has been increased by training. Not only does this mechanism reduce blood lactate accumulation, but it also provides the Type I fibers with an alternative source of glucose equivalents, thereby further reducing reliance on their endogenous glucose supply.

ONSET OF BLOOD LACTATE ACCUMULATION

Fatigue during endurance exercise can be caused by numerous factors other than lactate accumulation, and blood lactate levels do not necessarily accurately reflect muscle lactate levels. Nevertheless, there seems to be a

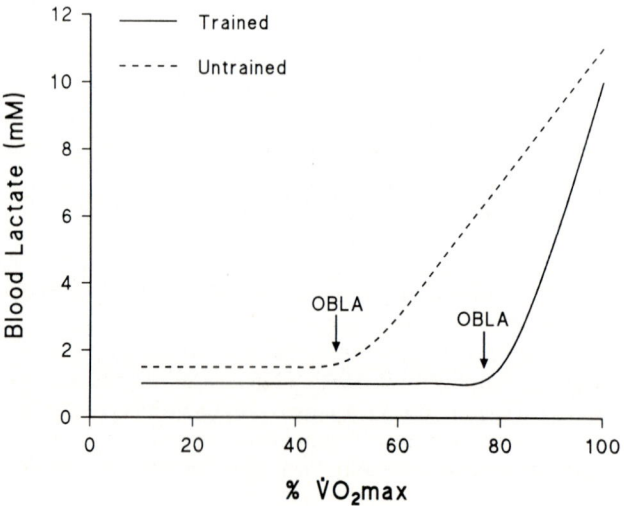

Figure 2 Relationship between $\dot{V}O_2$max and blood lactate concentrations in a trained and an untrained individual. Onset of blood lactate accumulation (OBLA) occurs at approximately 50% and 80% of $\dot{V}O_2$max in the untrained and the trained individual, respectively. The absolute $\dot{V}O_2$max value for the trained individual would be approximately 20% higher than that of the untrained individual.

strong temporal relationship between the so called threshold for the "onset of blood lactate accumulation" (OBLA) and endurance performance. The relationship between exercise intensity and blood lactate accumulation is not linear (Fig. 2). Instead, an increase of treadmill running velocity (and $\dot{V}O_2$) result in a lactate threshold; accumulation occurs exponentially, but only after a distinct threshold has been passed. In relatively untrained individuals, OBLA occurs at approximately 50 to 60% $\dot{V}O_2$max, whereas elite marathon runners may not reach their OBLA until they use approximately 90% $\dot{V}O_2$max. Running at velocities significantly above the OBLA threshold cannot be sustained long enough to complete an endurance sports event. Thus, marathon runners attempt to run at speeds that are highly correlated with their OBLA.

All of the biochemical factors associated with endurance-training induced augmentation of muscle mitochondrial concentration contribute to the ability of marathoners to sustain exercise at very high percentages of their $\dot{V}O_2$max. Training-induced changes in $\dot{V}O_2$max are probably limited by central and peripheral circulatory adaptations and are unrelated to adaptations in muscle mitochondria. In fact, the running velocity at OBLA seems a much better predictor of marathon running performance than the $\dot{V}O_2$max.

Many physiologic, biomechanical, and psychosocial factors determine an individual's final marathon performance, but the importance of cellular biochemical adaptations (only some of which have been described in this chapter) cannot be overlooked. An understanding of these mechanisms contributes to our appreciation of the complexity and interdependence of the workings of the human body and how it adapts to the stress of chronic endurance training.

SUGGESTED READING

Gollnick PD, Riedy M, Quintinskie JJ, Bertocci LA. Differences in metabolic potential of skeletal muscle fibres and their significance for metabolic control. J Exp Biol 1985; 115:191–195.
Gollnick PD, Saltin B. Significance of skeletal muscle oxidative enzyme enhancement with endurance training. Clin Physiol 1982; 2:1–12.
Hochachka P. Fuels and pathways as designed systems for support of muscle work. J Exp Biol 1985; 149–164.
Joyner MJ. Physiological limiting factors and distance running: Influence of gender and age on record performances. In: Holloszy JO, ed. Exercise and sport sciences reviews. Baltimore: Williams & Wilkins, 1993:103.
Powers SK, Howley ET. Exercise physiology: Theory and application to fitness and performance. Dubuque: WC Brown Publishers, 1990.
Saltin B, Åstrand PO. Free fatty acids and exercise. Am J Clin Nutr 1993; 57:752S–758S.
Stainsby WN. Biochemical and physiological bases for lactate production. Med Sci Sports Exerc 1986; 18:341–343.

HUMORAL FUNCTIONS AND EXERCISE

ATKO VIRU, D.Sc.

Body fluids, including the blood, have a great variety of functions. These can be summarized by the term *humoral functions*. Various humoral functions (including metabolic, transport, defense, and homeostatic functions) are discussed in other chapters. In this chapter, the main object of discussion is the humoral regulatory function, bearing in mind that the latter influences metabolic, transport, defense, and homeostatic functions.

PRINCIPLES OF HUMORAL REGULATION

Humoral regulatory functions operate via (1) hormones and other bioactive substances, and (2) metabolites that are transferred into body fluids from the intracellular compartment as a result of their intensive production in metabolic processes.

Hormones are secreted into the blood stream by endocrine glands (and to a limited extent by endocrine-active cells localized far from the corresponding gland). In the blood, most hormone molecules are bound to plasma proteins. The bound hormone is a transportation form. It avoids metabolic degradation of the hormone and also penetration of the hormone through the vascular membrane into the interstitial fluid. The amount of a hormone reaching the tissues therefore depends not only on the rate of hormone secretion by the gland, but also on the ratio between bound and unbound hormones in the blood, and on the bound⇌unbound transition processes. In most instances, pronounced increases in hormone secretion result in a rise of hormone concentration in the blood to a level that exceeds the binding capacity of blood proteins. Thus the amount of free unbound hormone increases, with a corresponding increase of the inflow of hormone to the tissues.

A part of the hormone molecules that reach the cell will be bound by specific proteins (hormone receptors), localized for various hormones on the cellular membrane, in the cytoplasm, or in the cellular nucleus. A great binding affinity for "their" hormone is common among such proteins. However, their binding capacity is limited. A considerable fraction of the hormone molecules is also bound nonspecifically by other proteins and by enzymes catalyzing metabolic degradation of the hormone. The metabolic effect of a hormone is initiated only by hormone-receptor complexes; that is by hormones that have been specifically bound to their receptors. The more hormone-receptor complexes there are, the higher is the hormone metabolic effect. An increased hormone inflow favors the formation of a greater number of hormone-receptor complexes, until the maximum binding capacity of the hormone receptor proteins is reached. However, the hormone inflow is not the only factor determining the metabolic effect. Both the number of binding sites for the hormone (the density of hormone receptors) and the affinity of the hormone receptors may be either up-regulated or down-regulated. Consequently, the hormonal regulation of metabolism is achieved by the production of signal molecules and the reception of these molecules on the target cells.

The autoregulation of metabolic processes within a cell is governed by the ratio between substrates and products of a metabolic pathway. Metabolites accumulating in the extracellular compartment may participate in the regulation of body function by the following mechanisms:

1. a direct influence of metabolites on the smooth muscles of blood vessels, as a result of which the blood supply to a tissue is regulated according to its metabolic activity.
2. an influence of metabolites on chemosensitive receptors in the tissues (metaboreceptors).
3. an influence of blood metabolites on chemosensitive receptors in the blood vessels.
4. a direct influence of blood metabolites and blood pH on nervous centers.
5. a direct influence of blood metabolites and blood pH on the endocrine glands.
6. a direct influence of blood metabolites and blood pH on metabolism in various tissues and on the function of some organs.

NEED FOR HORMONAL REGULATION

Exercise demands a general mobilization of energy and protein resources to sustain muscle activity. Exercise also requires homeostatic adjustments in order to avoid exaggerated shifts in those parameters of the internal milieu that determine the optimal activity of enzymes. Both of these tasks are accomplished largely by hormonal regulation.

The overall mobilization of cellular and bodily resources requires the interference of hormonal regulation in cellular autoregulation. In such situations as muscular activity, the task of hormonal regulation may run counter to that of cellular autoregulation. Cellular autoregulation is directed toward immediate satisfaction of cellular needs, on the one hand, and avoidance of pronounced changes in the cellular compartment on the other hand. It is important in the resting state, but does not provide a suitable basis for an overall mobilization of cellular and bodily resources. This is because a drop in the substrate-product ratio causes an inhibition of enzymes catalyzing product formation and stimulates enzymes catalyzing the opposing metabolic pathway. The main aim of hormonal regulation is to adjust metabolic processes to levels that correspond with the actual needs of life activities, and to counter opposing influences that may be originating in cellular autoregulation. This aim is achieved through the action of hormones on enzymes. Hormones either induce transition of enzymes from an inactive to an active form (or vice-versa), or alter the rate of synthesis of enzyme molecules.

EXERCISE-INDUCED HORMONE RESPONSES

Many studies have examined changes in blood hormone levels during exercise. Analysis of the accumulated results has established the main characteristics of hormonal responses as well as discriminating the main determinants of hormone responses during exercise and factors modulating the changes induced by the main determinants.

Triggering of Hormone Response

At least a part of the hormonal changes are triggered by the "central motor command" at the beginning of exercise. The actual amplitude of the hormone response is further adjusted by impulses arising from the proprioreceptors and metaboreceptors in muscles. A certain role belongs also to direct influences of metabolites on either the endocrine glands or the nervous centers controlling their activity. Glucostatic regulation has an essential role, based on changes in glucose availability and actualized through the central glucoreceptors. During sustained exercise, hormonal responses are also significantly influenced by receptors sensing temperature, intravascular volume, oxygen tension, and osmotic pressure.

Threshold Intensity of Exercise

There are no serious doubts about the dependence of hormone responses on the intensity of exercise; a certain threshold of exercise intensity triggers the hormonal responses. Both of these features have been convincingly demonstrated in regard to catecholamine responses. Up to a relative exercise intensity of 50 to 70% $\dot{V}o_2$max, the catecholamine changes are only modest and may not even be detectable. A pronounced increase in epinephrine concentration follows further increases in exercise intensity. An increase in the blood cortisol, corticotropin and β-endorphin concentration is displayed if the intensity of exercise exceeds 60 to 90% of $\dot{V}o_2$max. Simultaneous determination of lactate levels suggests that the threshold intensity for these hormone responses is closely related to the "anaerobic threshold".

The existence of a threshold intensity of exercise for a growth hormone response and its dependence on exercise intensity have been shown in several studies. Comparison of the effects of various exercises have demonstrated that the threshold intensities eliciting a somatotropin increase or a drop in blood insulin are lower than the anaerobic threshold.

Threshold Duration of Exercise

There is a threshold duration of exercise as well as a threshold intensity. The evidence is as follows: (1) in exercise below threshold intensities, hormonal responses may still appear when a certain amount of work has been performed; (2) in 2 hours of exercise, the most frequent variant of corticotropin, cortisol, and β-endorphin dynamics is a biphasic increase in their concentrations, with increases during the first 10 to 20 min and again at the end of exercise; (3) the hormonal responses may be more pronounced if exercise is more prolonged but less intensive (Fig. 1).

Training Effects

A large body of data claims that training reduces or eliminates increases in catecholamine, cortisol, glucagon, and growth hormone concentrations during submaximal exercise. The decrease in the blood insulin level also becomes less pronounced. These alterations are related to changes in the individual threshold intensity for induction of endocrine responses to exercise. After training, the threshold intensity, measured in units of power output, is shifted to a higher level. Therefore, exercises that were initially above the threshold, are brought below the threshold after training.

Training also increases the capacity of endocrine glands to secrete hormones. Consequently, the magnitude of blood catecholamines, cortisol, corticotropin, and growth hormone responses to supramaximal exercise is increased. Training also induces changes in hormone receptor density. As a result, the sensitivity of tissues to hormonal actions is enhanced.

During strenuous exercise the hormonal responses are determined by an integration of exercise intensity and duration, as well as by the performance capacity of the subject. Responses are triggered by exercise intensity. An additional stimulus arises from exercise duration. The actual magnitude of the response also depends on the functional capacities of the endocrine systems.

Homeostatic Needs

Vasopressin and renin-angiotensin-aldosterone complexes contribute to the renal and sweat gland retention of fluid and sodium, as well as to the regulation of the peripheral vascular tone. Aldosterone increases the excretion of potassium. The secretion of vasopressin and aldosterone increases during exercise in order (1) to avoid or to reduce dehydration and sodium loss due to intensive sweating, and (2) to avoid hyperkalemia due to a release of potassium into the extracellular compartment as a result of the degradation of glycogen and proteins, also as an insufficient function of the Na,K-pump on the membranes of the muscle fibers.

The responses of these hormones depend on the water and salt supply and the environmental temperature. Virtually no increase in plasma renin activity and aldosterone and natriuretic peptide concentrations are observed after salt loading. During prolonged exercise in

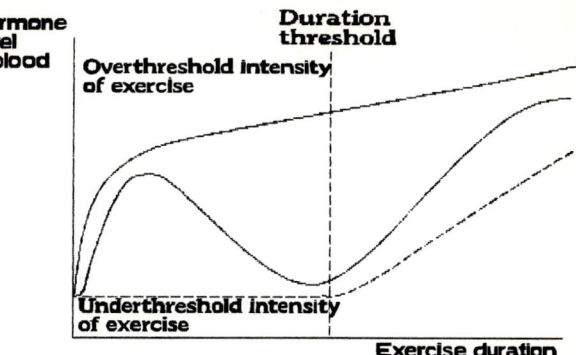

Figure 1 Threshold duration for triggering hormonal responses. Hormonal dynamics in exercise above the threshold intensity is indicated by solid lines, and in exercise below the threshold intensity by interrupted lines. When the threshold duration is reached, then at intensities above threshold a further increase in hormonal response occurs, or a second rise in hormone concentration is seen. However, at subthreshold intensities, the hormonal response may only appear after the threshold duration has been passed.

the heat, renin and angiotensin increases can be significantly reduced by the administration of a sodium-potassium solution in amounts equivalent to the subject's sweat loss. The plasma volume loss and subsequent increase in vasopressin and renin-angiotensin levels during 4 hours of exercise can also be prevented by progressive rehydration.

Modulating Influences

In situations of emotional stress, adrenocortical activation occurs with exercise of less than threshold intensity. In subjects with a high trait-anxiety or pronounced emotional liability, there are more pronounced catecholamine responses to exercise. Accordingly, the same exercise activates the sympathoadrenal system and suppresses the blood insulin level more in competition than in training. Tennis players who exhibited a good mood and self-assurance were shown to have a higher testosterone level before competition. After the match the winners exhibited a further elevation of testosterone level, whereas a decrease was observed in the losers.

Hypoxic conditions not only change the basal blood levels of hormones but also enhance hormonal responses to exercise. A blood cortisol response is seen below the usual threshold intensity. In contrast, hyperbaric conditions reduce norepinephrine concentration during exercise.

The concentrations of noradrenaline, cortisol, somatotropin, and glucagon are higher when exercising in a hot environment. Conversely, catecholamine and somatotropin responses are inhibited if exercise is performed at 4° to 10°C.

A carbohydrate-rich diet or glucose administration reduces the responses of hormones related to mobilization of energy reserves. Instead of the expected drop in insulin level, an increase occurs. The opposite effect is peculiar to a low carbohydrate and lipid-rich diet, fasting, and conditions where glycogen stores are decreased.

HORMONAL CONTROL OF MOBILIZATION OF ENERGY AND PROTEIN RESOURCES

The metabolic effects of hormones during exercise are summarized in Figure 2.

Muscle Glycogenolysis

A release of acetylcholine and an increase of cytoplasmic calcium, necessary for the initiation of muscular contraction, concomitantly stimulate glycogen breakdown. However, these actions are not sufficient to maintain glycogenolysis at the required level during exercise; additional stimulation by epinephrine is essential. The effect of epinephrine is mediated by a chain of events: binding with β-adrenoceptors → activation of adenylate cyclase → accumulation of cAMP → conversion of inactive glycogen phosphorylase-b to the active form, phosphorylase-a. The essential role of epinephrine in the stimulation of muscle glycogenolysis suggests that this hormone has significance in mobilization of the anaerobic working capacity.

Hepatic Glucose Output

It was once assumed that the hyperglycemia at the beginning of exercise was related to epinephrine-induced glycogenolysis in the liver. However, more recently there has been convincing evidence that blood-epinephrine plays a negligible role in increasing the glucose output of the liver during exercise. Actually, this response is caused in part by a direct autonomic influence on the liver. The main factor is a change in the insulin/glycogen ratio. After the first 10 to 15 min of exercise, the ratio increases due to a reduction of blood insulin concentration. At the end of the first hour of exercise an increase in the blood glucagon level additionally supports the stimulation of hepatic glycogenolysis.

Blood Glucose

The glucose uptake of the muscle cells is stimulated by insulin as well as by muscular contraction. The exercise-induced drop in blood insulin concentration

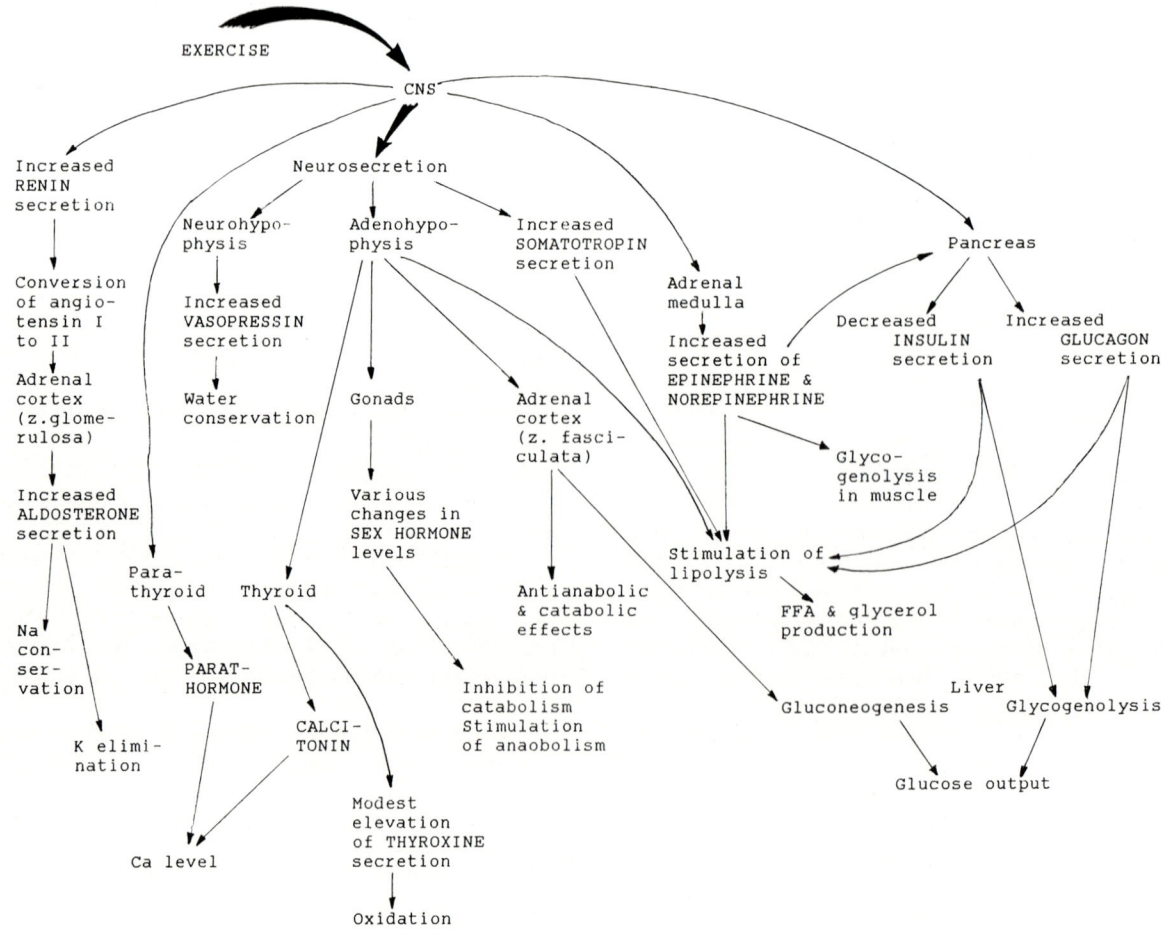

Figure 2 Schema showing the metabolic effects of hormones during exercise.

does not preclude glucose uptake by the muscle cells. Indeed, the reduced insulin level augments the transport of glucose to the muscle cells. It is thought that the regulatory role of the decrease in insulin level consists in (1) conserving blood glucose for nerve cells (glucose transport across the cellular membrane of the neurons is independent of insulin), (2) stimulation of hepatic glucose output, and (3) encouraging a transition from carbohydrates to lipids as the substrate for oxidation (see below).

During prolonged exercise, euglycemia is maintained by an increase in the hepatic glucose output that precisely balances the increased glucose utilization of various tissues. When changes in insulin and glucagon are prevented (by infusion of insulin and somatostatin respectively), plasma glucose concentration falls over a 1 hour exercise. In this case, hepatic glucose output does not compensate for the increase in glucose uptake, associated with an elevated rate of glucose oxidation.

Gluconeogenesis

Approximately 70 to 75% of the hepatic glucose output is derived from glycogenolysis and the remainder from gluconeogenesis. The precursor substrates available for conversion to glucose are lactate, pyruvate, glycerol, and glucogenic amino acids. Among the amino acids, alanine makes the largest contribution, accounting for 5 to 8% of the total glucose output and 20 to 25% of gluconeogenic components. During prolonged exercise, which increases the hepatic glucose output twofold, the relative contribution of gluconeogenesis to the overall hepatic output increases from 25 to 45%.

The role of alanine in gluconeogenesis is related to the glucose-alanine cycle. The anaerobic degradation of blood-borne glucose or muscle glucogen in muscle cells leads to the formation of pyruvate. A part of the pyruvate combines with amino groups, released in the deamination of amino acids before their oxidation. The result is alanine formation. Blood transports alanine to the liver, where its deamination takes place. The nitrogen-free residue of alanine is now used in the process of gluconeogenesis. Thus, formation of alanine avoids the accumulation of NH_3 in the muscles. At the same time a quantity of carbohydrate has been returned to the liver in the form of the carbohydrate skeleton of alanine.

The glucose-alanine cycle and overall gluconeogenesis is stimulated by cortisol and inhibited by insulin. Thus both exercise-induced hypercortisolemia and hypoinsulinemia promote gluconeogenesis.

Lipid Mobilization

The main link in the mobilization of lipid resources is the activation of lipases. Hormone-sensitive lipase is the rate limiting enzyme in the lipolytic process. For its activation, adipocytes possess β-adrenoceptors that are stimulated by epinephrine. Growth hormone, glucagon, thyroxin, and corticotropin also exert a lipolytic action through activation of the hormone-sensitive lipase. The action of epinephrine and other lipolytic hormones is supported by the permissive influence of cortisol. Insulin possesses a direct antilipolytic action, excluding the effect of lipolytic hormones. Consequently, hypoinsulinemia is a decisive factor in the mobilization of lipid resources and in the transition from carbohydrate oxidation to lipid oxidation during prolonged exercise.

Mobilization of Protein Resources

Exercise typically suppresses protein synthesis and increases protein degradation. Both of these processes take place mainly in less active muscles. The catabolic response extends to the smooth muscles of the gastrointestinal tract, lymphoid tissue, liver, and kidney. Both antianabolic and catabolic effects are tools for the mobilization of protein reserves. As a result, an increased pool of free amino acids is available for protein synthesis, but it is used as "building material" only to a minor extent. The free amino acids are used mainly as an additional energy source for the contracting muscles.

The most essential factor controlling antianabolic and catabolic responses is the increased level of blood cortisol. The action of cortisol is opposed by hypertestosteronemia. However, the exercise-induced increase in blood testosterone concentration is not a common response.

HUMORAL FUNCTION IN THE MECHANISM OF TRAINING EFFECTS

Evidence is accumulating that an intensive protein turnover provides a background for adaptive changes, favoring the synthesis of proteins most responsible for exercise performance. This change in protein metabolism takes place a certain time after training sessions. Increased function activates the genetic apparatus of the cell through an intracellular mechanism. A specific stimulation of protein synthesis (adaptive protein synthesis) is the result. It has been hypothesized that the metabolites accumulated within the cell determine the specific choice of proteins (both structural and enzyme proteins) for the adaptive protein synthesis. Hormones amplify this adaptive synthesis. Testosterone amplifies the action of metabolites on the synthesis of myofibrillar proteins after resistive exercises. Data have also been obtained pointing to the role of thyroid hormones in the amplification of the action of metabolites on mitochondrial proteins in skeletal muscles after endurance exercise. The translatory process may be supported by growth hormone and insulin. Cortisol is essential for creating the pool of free amino acids used as the building materials of protein synthesis.

SUGGESTIONS FOR TESTING ENDOCRINE FUNCTION

The testing of endocrine function is meaningful when valid methods are used for hormone determination. However, the use of precise and highly specific radioimmunomethods is complicated by their high cost. For this reason, the widespread testing of endocrine functions in athletes is not advised. The following approach to the testing of endocrine function is suggested:

1. Determine the concentration of various hormones during incremental exercise. The most significant result is the determination of the intensity threshold — the minimal exercise intensity triggering a significant hormonal response. The shortcomings are: (1) a delayed response to one exercise step may interfere with the response to the next exercise step and (2) the highest possible exercise intensity may not cause the greatest hormonal response: the highest response is usually found when a comparatively high (not the highest) intensity coincides with a certain duration of exercise.
2. Evaluate exercise performed at the highest possible rate for 5 to 7 min. The most significant result is a characterization of opportunities for mobilization of the various endocrine functions. The most informative results are obtained if the type of test exercise is close to the competitive exercise.
3. Evaluate exercise sustained for 30 to 40 min at intensities above the "anaerobic threshold." In this case, the highest possible hormonal responses can be recorded.
4. Have patient perform specific exercise for a long period of time to test the functional stability of the various endocrine systems.
5. Evaluate exercise tests at various temperatures and in various states of hydration to evaluate hormonal responses and compare them with changes in water and electrolyte balances. These tests allow an evaluation of the efficiency of hormones in homeostatic regulation.
6. Measure the hormonal changes induced by training sessions, in order to assess whether the training regimen induces the hormonal changes needed to amplify adaptive protein synthesis. The main problem concerning this approach is when to take the blood samples. The essential thing may not be the hormone level immediately after a training session, but at some later point in the course of recovery.
7. Monitor training by a determination of blood hormone concentrations. The main benefit of this approach is the possibility of assessing changes in adaptivity of the organism and to determine the conditions preceding overtraining.
8. Test for the sensitivity of tissues to hormonal actions in order to characterize the alterations at the hormone receptor level.

SUGGESTED READING

Fortherby K, Pal SB, eds. Exercise endocrinology. Berlin, New York: W. deGruyter, 1985.

Galbo H. Hormonal and metabolic adaptations to exercise. Stuttgart: Thieme Verlag, 1983.

Galbo H. Exercise physiology: humoral functions. Sport Sci Rev 1992; 1:65–93.

Kjaer M. Regulation of hormonal and metabolic responses during exercise in humans. Exerc Sport Sci Rev 1992; 20:161–184.

Urhausen A, Kindermann W. Biochemical monitoring of training. Clin J Sport Med 1992; 2:52–61.

Viru A. Hormones in muscular activity. Vol. 1. Hormonal ensemble in exercise. Boca Raton, Fl: CRC Press, 1985.

Viru A. Plasma hormones and physical exercise. Int J Sports Med 1992; 13:201–209.

EXERCISE, INFECTION, AND IMMUNE FUNCTION

DAVID C. NIEMAN, Dr.P.H., F.A.C.S.M.

In a classic 1932 review, Dr. Anna M. Baetjer of The Johns Hopkins University indicated that the prevailing view at that time was "that muscular fatigue lowers resistance and is a predisposing factor to infectious diseases, especially with regard to respiratory infections." This viewpoint is still prevalent, especially among elite athletes and coaches. For example, Liz McColgan blamed overtraining "which led to a cold and two subsequent illnesses," for her poor performance in the 1992 World Cross Country Championships. During the Winter and Summer Olympic Games, it has been regularly reported by clinicians that "upper respiratory infections abound" and that "the most irksome troubles with the athletes are infections."

On the other hand, there is a common belief that regular exercise confers resistance against infection. For example, a 1989 *Runner's World* subscriber survey revealed that 61% of 700 runners reported fewer colds since beginning to run, while only 4% felt they had experienced more.

The Centers for Disease Control has estimated that over 425 million colds and influenzal infections occur annually in the United States, resulting in $2.5 billion in lost school and work days, and the costs of immediate medical care. The National Center for Health Statistics reports that acute respiratory conditions (primarily the common cold and influenza) have an annual incidence of 90 per 100 persons. Understanding the relationship between exercise, infection, and immune function has potential public health implications and, for the athlete, may mean the difference between being able to compete, performing at a subpar level, or missing the event altogether because of illness.

EXERCISE AND UPPER RESPIRATORY TRACT INFECTION IN HUMANS

The relationship between exercise and upper respiratory tract infection (URTI) may be modeled in the form of a "J" curve (Fig. 1). This model suggests that although the risk of URTI may decrease below that of a sedentary individual when one engages in moderate exercise training, the risk may rise above average during periods of excessive, high-intensity exercise.

Much more research, using larger subject pools and improved research designs, is necessary before this model can be wholly accepted or rejected, but there is compelling evidence to suggest the model offers a useful clinical guideline. Table 1 summarizes studies investigating this model.

Does Heavy Exertion Increase URTI Risk?

Several epidemiologic reports suggest that athletes engaging in marathon-type events and/or very heavy

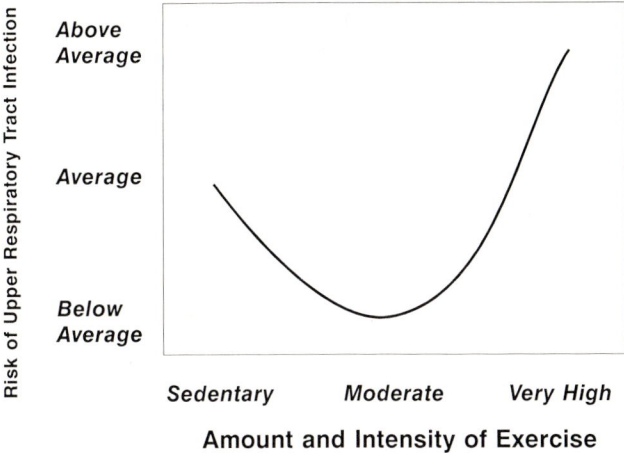

Figure 1 The "J" curve model of the relationship between upper respiratory tract infection and exercise workload.

Table 1 Research on the Relationship Between Exercise and Upper Respiratory Tract Infection (URTI)

Investigators, Country, Year Published	Subjects	Research Design	Major Finding
Peters & Bateman, South Africa, 1983	141 South African marathon runners vs 124 live-in controls	2 wk recall of URTI after 56 km race in Capetown; retrospective	URTI incidence twice as high in runners after race vs controls (33.3% vs 15.3%)
Linde, Denmark, 1987	44 Danish elite orienteers vs 44 matched nonathletes	12 mo prospective; runners kept daily log of symptoms	Orienteers vs controls had 2.5 vs 1.7 URTIs during year
Nieman et al, USA, 1989	294 California runners	2 mo before, 1 wk after March 5 km, 10 km, 21.1 km races; retrospective	Training 42 vs 12 km/wk associated with lower URTI; no effect of race on URTI
Nieman et al, USA, 1990	2,311 Los Angeles marathon runners	2 mo before, 1 wk after March 42.2 km race; retrospective	Runners training ≥97 vs <32 km/wk at higher URTI risk; odds ratio 5.9 for runners in race vs those not, 1 wk after
Peters, South Africa, 1990	108 marathon runners vs 108 controls	2 wk recall of URTI after 56 km race in Pretoria; retrospective	28.7% of runners sick vs 12.9% of controls
Nieman et al, USA, 1990	36 mildly obese, inactive women	Subjects randomized to walking, sedentary control groups; five 45 min walking sessions/wk for 15 wk, late January to May	Walking group reported fewer days with URTI symptoms than controls (5.1 vs 10.8)
Heath et al, USA, 1991	530 runners, South Carolina	12 mo prospective; runners kept daily logs of symptoms	Increase in running distance positively related to increased URTI risk
Peters et al, South Africa, 1993	84 long-distance runners vs 73 nonrunner controls	2 wk recall of URTI after 90 km race; 21 days before, 600 mg/day vitamin C supplement, random, double-blind, placebo	URTI incidence lowest in runners taking vitamin C (33%) vs placebo runners (68%) and controls (49%)
Nieman et al, USA, 1993	32 inactive and 12 highly conditioned elderly women	Subjects randomized to walking, sedentary control groups; five 37 min walking sessions/wk for 12 wk, September to November	Incidence of URTI 8% in highly conditioned, 21% in walkers; 50% in controls

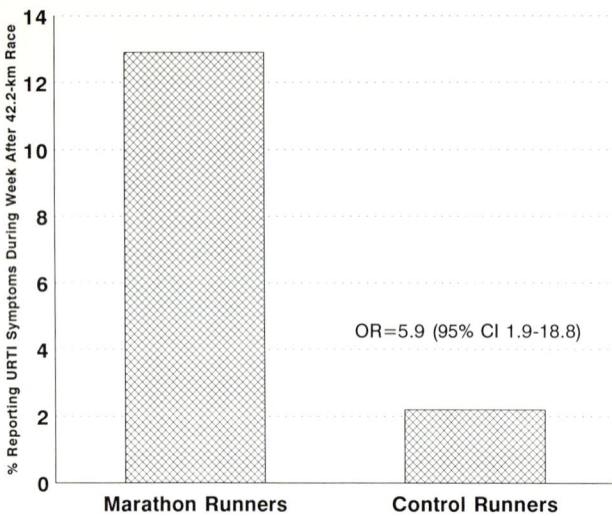

Figure 2 During the week after the 1987 Los Angeles Marathon, runners who ran were nearly six times more likely to report an upper respiratory tract infection than runners not participating in the race event.

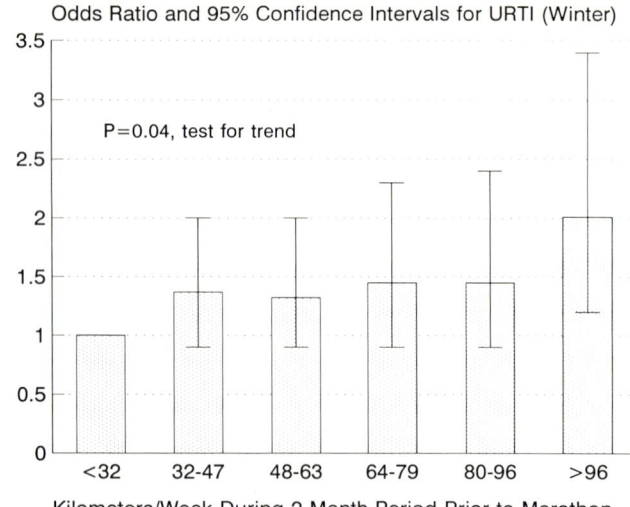

Figure 3 During the 2 month period prior to the 1987 Los Angeles Marathon, runners training more than 96 km/wk were twice as likely to report an URTI than runners training less than 32 km/wk.

training are at increased risk of URTI (Table 1). In one study, the incidence of URTI was surveyed in a group of 2,311 marathon runners who varied widely in running ability and training habits. Runners retrospectively self-reported demographic, training, and URTI episode and symptom data for the 2 month period before and the 1 week period immediately after the 1987 Los Angeles Marathon.

Some 12.9% of Los Angeles Marathon participants reported an infectious episode during the week after the race, in comparison to 2.2% of similarly experienced runners who had applied but did not participate in the race (for reasons other than sickness). Controlling for important demographic and training data by logistic regression, the odds were 6 to 1 in favor of sickness for the marathon race participants versus the nonparticipants (Fig. 2). Forty percent of the runners reported at least one URTI during the 2 months before the race. Controlling for important confounders, runners training more than 96 km/wk doubled their odds for sickness compared to those training less than 32 km/wk. The lowest odds of sickness were in the less than 32 km/wk group, but the odds ratio did not increase significantly until 96 km/wk were exceeded (Fig. 3).

Several other epidemiologic studies support these findings. Researchers from South Africa led by Dr. Edith Peters compared the incidence of URTI in 150 randomly selected runners who took part in a 56 km Cape Town race versus matched controls who did not run. Symptoms of URTI occurred in 33.3% of runners compared with 15.3% of controls during the 2 weeks following the race; complaints were most common in those who achieved the faster race times. Sore throats and nasal symptoms were most prevalent; moreover 80% of the symptoms lasted longer than 3 days, suggesting an infectious origin. Two subsequent studies from this group of researchers confirmed these findings (see Table 1).

Together, these epidemiologic studies suggest that heavy acute or chronic exercise is associated with an increased risk of URTI. The risk appears to be especially high during the 1 or 2 weeks following marathon-type races. Among runners varying widely in training habits, the risk of URTI is slightly elevated for those covering the greatest distances, but only when there is control of several confounding factors.

Does Moderate Physical Activity Lower URTI Risk?

What about the common belief that moderate physical activity decreases URTI risk? Very few studies have been carried out in this area, and more research is certainly warranted.

No published epidemiologic reports have compared incidence of URTI in large groups of moderately active and sedentary individuals, either retrospectively or prospectively. Several epidemiologic studies have compared URTI incidence rates among runners training over varying distances, but these studies are more useful for determining whether heavy versus moderate training has a negative effect.

Two randomized experimental trials using small numbers of subjects have provided important preliminary data in support of the viewpoint that moderate physical activity may reduce URTI symptoms. As summarized in Table 1, in one randomized, controlled study of 36 women (mean age 35 years), exercised subjects walked briskly 45 minutes, 5 days a week, and experienced one-half as many days with URTI symptoms during a 15 week period as did a sedentary control group (5.1 ± 1.2 vs 10.8 ± 2.3 days, $p = 0.039$).

In a recent study of elderly women, the incidence of the common cold during a 12 week period in the fall was lowest in highly conditioned, lean subjects who exercised moderately for about 1.5 hours each day (8%). Elderly subjects who walked 40 minutes, 5 times a week had an incidence of 21%, as compared to 50% for the sedentary control group.

EXERCISE AND EXPERIMENTALLY INDUCED INFECTIONS IN ANIMALS

Since the beginning of this century, investigators have studied the effects of varying exercise workloads on the course of experimentally induced infections in laboratory animals. Early studies seemed to suggest that one or two periods of exhausting muscular exercise following inoculation of the animal with foreign organisms led to a more frequent appearance of infectious disease, more commonly and more rapidly fatal, whereas moderate exercise before inoculation tended to improve host resistance to infection.

However, it now appears that the influence of any exercise intervention is pathogen specific, and dependent on the species, age, and sex of the animals selected for study, and the type of exercise paradigm. For example, the virulence of tetanus toxin, pneumococcus, streptococcus, *Toxoplasma gondii,* or *Francisella tularensis* seems to be unaffected in various animals undergoing heavy and fatiguing exertion.

On the other hand, there are many reports that the virulence of the coxsackievirus B3 is markedly augmented by intense exercise in animals; increased replication of the virus in heart muscle leads to cell necrosis and commonly to death of the animal. Heavy exertion after injection with *Trypansoma cruzi* or the influenza or poliomyelitis viruses is also associated with a poor prognosis. For example, in 1945, in response to many anecdotal reports that exhausting exercise had preceded the onset of poliomyelitis in humans, researchers demonstrated in a series of studies with rhesus monkeys that swimming to exhaustion (usually 2 to 3 hours) markedly lowered their resistance during the incubation period of an experimental poliomyelitis infection.

Few investigators have studied whether moderate exercise improves resistance to experimentally induced infections. In one study, mice randomly assigned to cages with activity wheels for 2.5 weeks survived intraperitoneal injections of *Salmonella typhimurium* much better than sedentary controls (44% versus 29%).

MANAGEMENT OF THE ATHLETE DURING INFECTION

Various clinicians have suggested that if an athlete experiences a sudden and unexplained deterioration in performance during training or competition, viral infection should be suspected, in addition to other factors. Various measures of physical performance capability are reduced during an infectious episode. Several case histories have demonstrated that sudden and unexplained deterioration in athletic performance can sometimes be traced to either recent URTI or protracted subclinical viral infections. A mild fever has a marked adverse effect on the ability and/or willingness of some individuals to perform both cardiorespiratory and musculoskeletal exercise.

Should athletes exercise when they have a viral infection? It has been known for several decades that many types of viral infections can produce myocarditis and/or pericarditis. Respiratory infections, including the "common cold" and "flu" syndromes are potentially serious, because (although rare) the sick athlete who exercises intensely may develop cardiac damage and sudden death through an acute arrhythmia. Patients who develop viral cardiomyopathy are usually previously healthy young people who have stressed themselves with vigorous and prolonged physical exercise at the height of a viral infection, or soon thereafter. Furthermore, these subjects usually have continued with stressful exercise, ignoring the early onset of dyspnea, palpitation, weakness, fatigability, and general malaise—all warning symptoms and signs observed in persons suffering cardiac damage.

For these reasons, most clinicians recommend that if an athlete has symptoms of a common cold with no constitutional involvement, regular training may be resumed safely a few days after symptoms resolve. Mild exercise during a common cold does not appear to be contraindicated, but there is insufficient evidence at present to say one way or the other. However, if there are symptoms or signs of systemic involvement (e.g., fever, extreme tiredness, muscle aches, swollen lymph glands), 2 weeks should be allowed before resumption of intensive training. Seemingly innocent infections have led to severe cases of myocarditis, and there is no way to predict which sick athlete will develop viral myocarditis, cardiomyopathy, pericarditis, or valvulitis.

Elite athletes devote years of intensive training and preparation for major competition, and are often extremely nervous about acquiring a cold or flu infection around the time of a major event. Several precautions may help reduce their risk of URTI (Table 2). Two environmental factors, improper nutrition and psychological stress, can compound the negative influence of heavy exertion on the immune system. The athlete should thus be urged to eat a well-balanced diet, keep other life stresses to a minimum, avoid overtraining and chronic fatigue, obtain adequate sleep, and space vigorous workouts and race events as far apart as possible. Immune function appears to be suppressed during periods of inadequate energy intake and weight reduction, so if weight loss is necessary, the athlete should be advised to accomplish this slowly during the phase of noncompetitive training. Regular sleep habits also appear to be important. Total sleep time, sleep efficiency, and the duration of nonREM sleep have each been correlated with natural killer (NK) cell activity. Cold viruses are spread by both personal contact and breathing air near sick people. Therefore, if at all possible, athletes should avoid being around sick people before and after important events. If the athlete is competing during the winter, influenza vaccination is recommended.

Table 2 Recommendations for Athletes to Lower Their Risk of Upper Respiratory Tract Infections

Develop habits that reduce the risk of self-innoculation (e.g., keep hands away from face, wash hands frequently).
Before important events, avoid sick people and crowded living and working arrangements. Flu shots are recommended.
Eat a well-balanced diet, and avoid low caloric intake and rapid weight loss (associated with immune suppression).
Keep other life stresses to a minimum (stress has been consistently linked to an increased risk of the common cold).
Maintain regular sleep habits (abrupt change in sleep habits has been linked to immune suppression).
Avoid overtraining, chronic fatigue, and excessive muscle soreness. Space vigorous workouts and race events as far apart as possible—keep "within yourself."

ACUTE AND CHRONIC EFFECTS OF EXERCISE ON THE IMMUNE SYSTEM

If heavy and fatiguing exertion leads to an increased risk of URTI, various measures of immune function should be negatively affected. Conversely, if moderate exercise decreases URTI risk, some aspect of immune function should be chronically or at least transiently improved. Despite intensive investigation during the last 10 years, there is no clear consensus on this issue. The wide variety of research designs, exercise protocols, subject characteristics, and methodologies combined with the innate complexity of the immune system have made the interpretation of published findings extremely formidable and equivocal.

Acute Immune Response to Exercise

A growing number of reports on exercise immunology provide evidence that the immune system is profoundly effected by acute exercise. However, the clinical significance of these large but transient alterations is disputed.

High-intensity, endurance exercise is associated with a biphasic perturbation of the circulating leukocyte count. Immediately post exercise, total leukocytes increase 50% to 100%, represented evenly by lymphocytes and neutrophils with a small contribution from monocytes. After prolonged endurance exercise such as a marathon race, the increase can be even larger (200% to 300%). Within 30 minutes of recovery from exercise, the lymphocyte count dips 30% to 50% below pre-exercise levels, remaining low for 3 to 6 hours. There is no clear consensus on the tissue site to which the blood lymphocytes are transferred, some investigators providing evidence that peripheral lymphoid tissues (e.g., the thymus and spleen) are also depleted. Eosinophils also vacate the blood in large numbers, while basophils are largely unaffected. Meanwhile, there is a marked and prolonged neutrophilia (Fig. 4). Moderate-intensity exercise induces a much smaller leukocytosis, lympho-

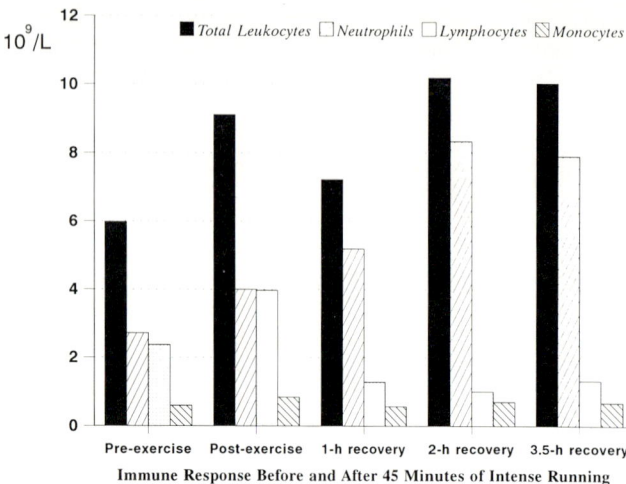

Figure 4 After intense exercise, circulating concentrations of neutrophils rise strongly for several hours while lymphocytes show a marked decrease.

cytosis, neutrophilia, and lymphocytopenia. The extent and duration of the alterations in leukocyte subset counts depend on exercise-induced changes in epinephrine and cortisol, which begin to increase strongly when the exercise intensity rises above 60% of $\dot{V}O_2$max.

Of the three major lymphocyte subpopulations (T, B, and NK cells), NK cells are by far most responsive to exercise. NK counts typically increase 150% to 300% within minutes of initiating high-intensity exercise, contributing substantially to the overall lymphocytosis. Circulating numbers of T cytotoxic/suppressor cells also increase markedly (50% to 100%) after high-intensity exercise, but T helper/inducer and B cells are relatively unaffected. Changes are transient, and within 30 minutes, lymphocytes from each of the subpopulations exit the circulation in large numbers under the influence of cortisol.

Immediately after high-intensity but not moderate-intensity exercise, mitogen-stimulated proliferation of separated mononuclear cells is decreased 35% to 50%, but it returns to pre-exercise levels within 2 hours. The clinical importance of this observation has been challenged, because the decrease may merely reflect a redistribution of various lymphocyte subsets, and not an actual decrease in the ability of T cells to function normally. Some investigators believe that even though the function of each T cell may be unaltered by intense exercise, the blood and peripheral lymphoid compartments may have less T cells than normal for several hours after exercise, which may have the same impact on host protection as having fewer soldiers on the front lines of a battlefield. Research to settle this issue is warranted and may improve our understanding of the acute immune response and its link with epidemiologic findings.

Investigators have also consistently reported that immediately after high-intensity exercise, NK cell cytotoxic activity (NKCA) is increased by 40% to 100%, although it falls 25% to 35% below pre-exercise levels by

1 hour and 2 hours of recovery. Most researchers agree that the immediate postexercise increase in NKCA is due to the recruitment of NK cells into the circulation, but they disagree on the reasons for the transient NKCA decrease during recovery. Some investigators reason that the drop in NKCA can be ascribed to numerical shifts in NK cells, and others report that prostaglandins from activated monocytes and neutrophils or elevated stress hormone levels suppress the ability of NK cells to function appropriately. This issue requires further investigation. Nonetheless, most researchers agree that the NKCA of the blood compartment is significantly reduced for several hours after heavy exertion, primarily because of the transfer of NK cells to other tissues.

Neutrophils, one of the body's most effective phagocytes, are a part of the innate functional division of the immune system (as are NK cells), acting as a first line of defense against infectious agents. There is growing evidence that both moderate and intense endurance exercise are associated with a prolonged improvement in the killing capacity of blood neutrophils and peritoneal macrophages. In contrast, immediately after a 20 km race, neutrophils in a nasal lavage taken from 12 male runners were less able to ingest bacteria, an effect that lasted for 3 days. Prolonged impairment of lung neutrophil antimicrobial function has also been reported in race horses after participation in a single strenuous event. Although blood neutrophils are easier to study, data from these two studies suggest that the exercise response of neutrophils from the respiratory area may differ from that of cells in the blood.

There is no convincing data that exercise-induced changes in T-cell function, NKCA, or neutrophil/macrophage function explain the increased risk of URTI suggested by epidemiologic data. Researchers disagree on the mechanistic interpretation of their findings, and none have provided follow-up data of large numbers of subjects to determine if the various changes in immune function translate to altered host protection. Further research is needed to settle these issues, and to determine if the large but transient perturbations in leukocyte cell concentrations in both blood and peripheral lymphoid tissue (which often underlie reported in vitro functional alterations) are important from a clinical viewpoint.

Immune Response to Chronic Exercise

Several studies have made cross-sectional comparisons between the immune systems of athletes and nonathletes, or have followed sedentary individuals as they initiated exercise programs, comparing pre-exercise and postexercise training immune measures relative to control groups. Most of these studies have failed to demonstrate any important effects of regular exercise training on circulating concentrations of total leukocytes or lymphocytes or on their various subpopulations. Most researchers have also reported that the resting serum immunoglobulin levels of trained athletes are within the normal reference range and similar to those of sedentary

controls. Research on the effect of regular exercise on resting neutrophil and T cell function is contradictory, with more research needed to resolve several methodologic issues. Several studies on animals and humans have shown significant improvements in NKCA with exercise training, although researchers disagree on the clinical implications.

RECOMMENDATIONS

Because of the lack of agreement among published findings, there are no recommendations at present for conducting laboratory tests of immune function to ascertain when an athlete is at increased risk of an infectious episode due to overtraining. However, if an athlete experiences a sudden and unexplained deterioration in performance during training or competition, viral infection should be suspected. Additionally, if signs and symptoms indicate that a viral infection is impending, the athlete should greatly reduce the volume and intensity of training to allow the immune system to give full attention to combating the illness.

SUGGESTED READING

Baetjer AM. The effect of muscular fatigue upon resistance. Physiol Rev 1932; 12:453–468.

Cannon JG. Exercise and resistance to infection. J Appl Physiol 1993; 74:973–981.

Chao CC, Strgar F, Tsang M, Peterson PK. Effects of swimming exercise on the pathogenesis of acute murine *Toxoplasma gondii* Me49 infection. Clin Immunol Immunopathol 1992; 62:220–226.

Ferry A, Rieu P, Le Page C, et al. Effect of physical exhaustion and glucocorticoids (dexamethasone) on T-cells of trained rats. Eur J Appl Physiol 1993; 66:455–460.

Fitzgerald L. Overtraining increases the susceptibility to infection. Int J Sports Med 1991; 12(suppl 1):S5–S8.

Gabriel H, Schwarz L, Born P, Kindermann W. Differential mobilization of leucocyte and lymphocyte subpopulations into the circulation during endurance exercise. Eur J Appl Physiol 1992; 65:529–534.

Heath GW, Macera CA, Nieman DC. Exercise and upper respiratory tract infection: Is there a relationship? Sports Med 1992; 14:353–365.

Jokl E. The immunological status of athletes. J Sports Med 1974; 14:165–167.

MacNeil B, Hoffman-Goetz L. Chronic exercise enhances in vivo and in vitro cytotoxic mechanisms of natural immunity in mice. J Appl Physiol 1993; 74:388–395.

Nieman DC. Physical activity, fitness and infection. In: Bouchard C, Shephard RJ, eds. Exercise, fitness, and health: A consensus of current knowledge. Champaign, Il: Human Kinetics Books, 1993.

Nieman DC, Henson DA, Gusewitch G, et al. Physical activity and immune function in elderly women. Med Sci Sports Exerc 1993; 25:823–831.

Nieman DC, Nehlsen-Cannarella SL. Effects of endurance exercise on immune response. In: Shephard RJ, Astrand PO, eds. Endurance in sport. Oxford: Blackwell Scientific Publications, 1992.

Pedersen BK. Influence of physical activity on the cellular immune system: Mechanisms of action. Int J Sports Med 1991; 12(suppl 1):S23–S29.

Peters EM, Goetzsche JM, Grobbelaar B, Noakes TD. Vitamin C supplementation reduces the incidence of postrace symptoms of upper-respiratory-tract infection in ultramarathon runners. Am J Clin Nutr 1993; 57:170–174.

DIETARY REQUIREMENTS OF THE ATHLETE

GAIL BUTTERFIELD, Ph.D., R.D.

Optimal performance by professional or recreational athletes is a consequence of maximizing genetic endowment by appropriate training and nutrition. Failure to attend to the last two factors may obviate any advantage provided by the first. And failure to attend to the last factor may make the second sporadic and ineffective. Thus, optimum nutrition for the elite or recreational athlete is essential to making the most of workouts and attaining the best performance.

However, much of the information we have about nutrient requirements is derived from the experience of sedentary and lightly active individuals, not the athlete who is engaged in training or competition. Thus, the active individual, in an attempt to optimize performance, relies on what may be inappropriate sources of dietary information. Especially in those circumstances where training and genetics combine to produce an exceptional athlete, the individual runs the risk of becoming pray to much misinformation in the quest for "the edge" in performance. Fortunately, the field of sports nutrition has blossomed over the last 10 years and there are now Registered Dietitians (R.D.s) who specialize in sports nutrition and dispense accurate information about the nutrient needs of the athlete. These individuals are becoming an important link in the athlete's optimization of performance.

The primary focus of recent research has been the timing and composition of meals to ensure a continued ability to train, so that the person's genetic potential can be fully expressed. Emphasis has been placed on the type, amount, and timing of carbohydrate intake, and on protein requirements to maintain and augment muscle tissue. Frequent attempts to investigate the ergogenic nature of vitamins and trace minerals have led to the conclusion that as long as intake meets the basic needs of the general population, as outlined by the National Research Council (Recommended Dietary Allowances for Americans) and Health and Welfare, Canada (Recommended Dietary Allowances for Canadians), no performance advantage is provided by increasing the intake of these nutrients.

Thus, on one level, the "problem" related to the dietary requirements of athletes is similar to that of the general population, i.e., obtaining a sufficient nutrient intake to perform the required tasks while maximizing the intake of carbohydrate and minimizing the intake of fat. Athletes, however, face an additional challenge in that the primary nutritional concern, energy (kilojoules or kcal), is required in greater than normal amounts, and due to the competing demands of training schedules and competitions, food cannot be consumed in great quantities at any one time. Female athletes, especially those desiring to maintain low body weights (gymnasts, ballerinas), must obtain sufficient nutrients despite only a moderate energy intake consumed over an activity-packed day. An individually appropriate composition pattern can lead to decreased feelings of fatigue and a decreased risk of over-training injuries.

ENERGY REQUIREMENT

Energy is the first nutritional concern in any diet. Without a sufficient energy intake, the body energy stores will be used to accomplish the activities of the day. Not only are fat stores tapped, but body proteins are utilized to provide a substrate for hepatic gluconeogenesis. The consequent increase in circulating levels and excretion of protein by-products (urea) may result in fatigue and loss of appetite. Continued loss of body protein may also result in muscle weakness. Unfortunately, most athletes cannot afford to lose muscle mass, and many have only marginal fat stores as well. Thus, matching a person's energy intake with the energy expended in the activities of choice becomes very important to maintenance of the tissue most involved in the performance.

Often sports nutritionists working with athletes are confronted by the opinion of the coach, usually through the athlete, that low body weight is the primary nutritional goal for the athlete. Somewhere in the mythology of sport, the idea that the weight to power ratio is best accomplished by decreasing weight has become the dogma. Especially with young female athletes who are engaged in weight-bearing exercise such as dancing, running, or field events, the focus of dietary intervention is often intended to be weight loss. The goal of optimal weight for optimal performance is ignored. Thus, in working with young, talented athletes (both male and female), a training period is required for both coaches and athletes where their focus must shift from a minimization of body weight to a maximization of performance. Acknowledgment of the coach's attitude by the nutritionist, and a willingness to work with the athlete in dealing with the pressure that such an attitude imposes are important in maintaining an effective relationship with the athlete.

In the case of an athlete who needs to lose weight, the emphasis must remain on a maximization of performance. First, body fat mass must be assessed to determine whether the athlete really has any "weight" to lose. Then, weight loss goals should be met during the "off season," so that the nutrient intake can meet energy requirements during training, thus maximizing the opportunity that training will lead to the desired improvement in performance.

As in the general population, energy conservation mechanisms may come into play when the energy intake of athletes is restricted, and these mechanisms may permanently compromise future attempts to maintain a constant and appropriate body mass. A decline in basal metabolic rate in weight loss has been documented in nonathletes and exercise seems unable to counter this phenomenon in many cases. In addition, there is some evidence, although controversial, that physical activity is associated with development of a mechanism of energy conservation in some men and women, leaving the total energy requirement for such individuals equal to that of sedentary individuals of the same size and body composition. To guard against the initiation of any possible permanent energy conservation mechanisms, the sports nutritionist should work with the athlete to ensure the greatest energy intake possible within the confines of the other requirements for performance.

Finally, there is some evidence that stress fractures and other over-use injuries are related to an inadequate total energy intake. When energy intake is low, the incidence of these injuries may increase. Thus, it is important to maintain a high energy intake to allow continued training.

CARBOHYDRATE REQUIREMENT

To replenish muscle and liver glycogen stores depleted during a strenuous work-out an athlete must consume carbohydrate (CHO) before, during, and after the training period. The total CHO intake recommended is about 8 g/kg of body mass per day. This should be spaced over the day, but if taken in association with workouts, it can help to maximize performance.

Consumption of CHO just before a workout has been eschewed until very recently, based on experiments in which blood glucose fell at the beginning of an exercise bout when CHO had been consumed within 45 minutes of the event. Subsequent data have shown that such a fall in blood sugar is common when an individual has eaten anything within 45 minutes of an exercise bout, but that the decline in blood sugar is not associated with hypoglycemic symptoms in most instances. In fact, the blood glucose after an hour or so of work is higher when the individual has been fed before than when he or she has not. Low blood glucose is a major determinant of fatigue, and it may be responsible for truncating a workout if it is not maintained. Thus, regimens that maintain this vital blood parameter are useful, especially

for training. Athletes should not skip breakfast because a training session is "too close" to the time they arise. The training session will be improved if a meal high in carbohydrate is consumed, thus providing fuel to replenish the liver glycogen supplies depleted during the overnight fast, and ensuring a mechanism for delivering blood sugar during the training session. Recommendations for pre-event CHO consumption range from 50 to 100 g, taken 30 to 60 minutes before initiation of exercise. Such a CHO intake can be accomplished by consuming foods selected from Table 1.

Provision of a liquid food supplement during the training session will assist in maintaining blood glucose and proper hydration and, thus, the ability to thermoregulate. These topics are discussed in another chapter. The recommendation made is that 10 g of CHO be consumed in 150 ml of liquid every 15 minutes.

Finally, eating at least 50 g of CHO within 30 minutes after cessation of exercise provides the best replenishment of muscle glycogen stores used during the exercise bout. A second 50 g dose of CHO, taken 1 to 2 hours after exercise adds additional advantage. Inclusion of a small amount of protein in the postexercise meal increases insulin secretion and commensurate glycogen storage. Such a dietary regimen immediately after exercise also helps to maintain lean body mass. The 24-hour postexercise urea excretion, an indicator of protein utilization, decreases when individuals are fed immediately after exercise.

The optimal type of CHO to be consumed is also a subject of some controversy. Unfortunately, most CHO foods of significant nutritional value also contain significant amounts of fiber (fruits, vegetables, whole grains). Thus, gastrointestinal (GI) distention may decrease appetite and discourage an adequate CHO intake over the day. The consumption of CHO around the time of the exercise training sessions increases the likelihood that the recommended level will be consumed, but foods must be chosen carefully to ensure a comfortable workout. CHO sources that enter the blood stream quickly ("high glycemic index food" such as breads, cereals, and fruits like bananas) are sometimes recommended for consumption before and during exercise,

Table 1 Food Providing About 50 g Carbohydrate (CHO) Per Serving

Foods	CHO Content (g)	Protein Content (g)
Bagel and 8 oz. fruit juice	60	7
2 slices of bread and 8 oz LF milk	50	12
English muffin, 1 Tbsp jam, 8 oz LF milk	50	12
Fruit yogurt (1 cup) and corn tortilla	60	14
Popcorn (4 cups) and 8 oz fruit juice	50	4
Cold cereal (1 cup), 8 oz LF milk, piece of fruit	50	8+*
Pasta (1 cup) and marinara sauce (1 cup)	50	8
Pancakes (3 large) and syrup (2 Tbsp)	50	6
Pretzels (1 oz) and 8 oz fruit juice	50	2
Rice (0.5 cup) and beans (0.5 cups) and corn tortilla	50	13
Thick pizza (1 slice) and 12 oz soda	60	15
Graham crackers (1 large) and 8 oz LF milk	40	10
Rice (1 cup) and broccoli (1 cup)	50	8

LF = low fat
*Cereals are highly variable in protein content

whereas foods that enter the blood more slowly ("low glycemic index foods" such as pastas with sauce or beans) are best consumed after exercise. There does not appear to be any inherent advantage to a liquid form of CHO as compared to a solid, except that the liquid format provides another limiting nutrient, water, in conjunction with the CHO. During and immediately after exercise, a liquid concoction is more easily consumed. The formulation of special performance drinks and foods has become a lucrative business. Although these products are well-formulated and effective, they hold little advantage over regular foods with the exception of convenience of delivery and the *mystique* of being "athletic" foods.

PROTEIN REQUIREMENTS

Recent evidence suggests that endurance athletes working out at high intensities, and perhaps also individuals performing strength programs, require at least 25% more protein than prescribed by the National Research Council for sedentary people (0.8 g/kg of body mass per day). When these requirements are converted to recommendations (by adding two standard deviations to the basic requirement to accommodate the needs of 97.5% of the population), the intakes are almost 50% more than those recommended for sedentary people. The recommendation now made for endurance athletes and for the maintenance of lean tissue in individuals performing resistance exercise either alone or as a part of an overall training program is thus about 1.2 to 1.4g/kg of body mass per day. Some researchers recommend higher protein intakes for individuals who want to increase their lean mass, but such high protein intakes may lead to the accretion of fat as well as lean tissue. Consumption of the maintenance level with sufficient energy intake to allow for growth (an extra 800 kilojoules, 200 kcal per day) and an increased stimulus to synthesis (as provided by increased workouts) will allow a significant accretion of lean tissue without an accumulation of fat.

Although the optimum protein intake is still controversial, the usual intake of North American athletes exceeds even the highest recommendation. Protein intakes, even in the nonathletic community, often average 2 g/kg of body mass per day, or about 25% above the highest recommended intake for those performing endurance or resistance exercise. Thus, deliberate supplementation of protein intake is unnecessary for most athletes.

A notable exception to the adequacy of protein intake may be the female athlete who has a very low energy intake. In such a person, the protein intake may approach only the recommendations for a sedentary individual (0.8 g/kg), but the actual requirement may be elevated because the total energy intake is low. Thus, in such circumstances we have found protein requirements are about 1.1 g/kg, with a recommendation of 1.6 g/kg. Under circumstances of a low energy intake and an increased need, the protein intake must be carefully monitored to ensure an adequate replenishment of daily losses. Intakes as high as 16% of the total energy intake may be required. If the CHO recommendations indicated above are also to be followed, there will be little room for fat in the diet of such athletes.

VITAMIN AND MINERAL SUPPLEMENTATION

As stated earlier, there is no conclusive evidence that vitamin and mineral intakes above the recommendations for sedentary individuals can provide significant ergogenic benefit. However, two minerals (iron and calcium) are of special concern to the female athlete.

Iron is necessary for the production of iron-containing cytochromes and hemoglobin. Due to the loss of this nutrient with the menses, and a low nutrient density in the general food supply, iron intake may be marginal in women with a low energy intake. In such circumstances, iron status should be evaluated, especially if the athlete complains of fatigue or poor performance, and an appropriate diet (or iron supplementation) arranged as necessary.

The protein intake necessary to maintain lean tissue mass in female athletes consuming a low total energy (1.6 g/kg) may be associated with significant urinary calcium loss. Although exercise may protect somewhat against this loss, the calcium intake may also be compromised due to the low total energy intake. Thus, attention should be given to ensuring a calcium intake of at least 800 mg/d in these individuals (1,200 mg/d if they are under 25 years) to increase the probability that they will realize their maximal potential during their young adult years.

WATER

Although covered in great detail in other chapters in this book, the importance of an adequate fluid intake should be noted. The ability of the athlete to thermoregulate depends directly on the maintenance of blood volume, and especially under circumstances of training in the heat, fluid depletion may be life threatening. Because the thirst mechanism is inadequate to maintain fluid balance, athletes frequently exercise in a state of moderate dehydration. Proper hydration can be assured if athletes weigh before a workout and are required to regain their preworkout weight before training is undertaken on a subsequent day. The fluid to be consumed may be water, although a fluid and electrolyte replacement containing some sodium and potassium may conserve the thirst mechanism better than water, thus increasing fluid intake and improving fluid balance. The flavor of the fluid supplement may also increase its palatability and thus total consumption.

PREFERRED APPROACH

I. First interview of athlete by sports nutritionist (Registered Dietitian)

A. Assess
  1. Health history and current health status
  2. Overall activity pattern—training schedule, other activities performed (cycling to class, recreational sports activities)
  3. Overall food and energy intake and attitude toward same—requires careful handling if they are to remain interested in nutritional advice
      a. Watch for symptoms of eating disorders in *both* male and female athletes
          1. Obsession about body weight rather than performance that is generated from outside (coach)
          2. Overtraining
      b. Body fat—to determine availability of stores to be modified
  4. Pattern of food intake relative to workouts—many athletes skip breakfast because of the timing of morning training sessions, and fail to eat immediately after exercise because food is not available
  5. Present food and CHO intake, in general (see food patterns in Houtkooper, 1992)
  6. Assess whether athlete knows what a "carbohydrate" food is (see Moses and Manore, 1991)
  7. Attitude toward performance—are they doing well or is a poor overall performance part of why they are seeking counsel?
  8. Potential problems in attaining desired CHO or energy intake in general and on days of performance
  9. Preferred CHO-containing foods
B. Counseling
  1. Commend athlete for positive practices
  2. Answer all questions that arise (of which there will be many, because the athlete is very interested in any claim made for any potion that claims to improve performance)
  3. Encourage eating around workouts (Table 2)
  4. Request a 3 to 4 day food record, including training sessions and assessment of performance
  5. If necessary and the athlete is receptive, recommend interaction with a professional trained to handle disordered eating
II. Second interview of athlete by sports nutritionist (minimum interaction should be two meetings; three to six is optimum to accomplish significant changes in eating patterns)
  A. Evaluate food record
      1. Estimate energy requirements of athlete based on height, body mass, age, and activity pattern
          a. Harris-Benedict equation is a good first approach to determine basal needs (Basal Energy Expenditure, BEE)

Men: BEE = 66.47 + 13.75M + 5.0H − 6.76A
Women: BEE = 655.1 + 9.56M + 1.85H − 4.68A
where M = body mass in kg, H = height in cm,
A = age in years

Table 2 Eating Plan Around Workouts

Pre-event meals (may be breakfast)—to be consumed within an hour of workout
  Goal: 50–100 g Carbohydrate + 8–16 g Protein
    Men—choose 2 from Table 1
    Female—choose 1 from Table 1
During event feeding
  Goal: 10 g Carbohydrate and 150 ml fluid every 15–20 minutes
    Commercial fluid replacements
    Dilute fruit juice
Post-event meals—immediately after exercise; again after 1–2 hours
  Goal: 50–100 g Carbohydrate + 8–16 g Protein
    Men—choose 2 from Table 1
    Female—choose 1 from Table 1

Table 3 Energy Expenditure at Various Activities

Activity	Energy Expenditure (kcal*/kg body mass/hour)
Basketball	8.3
Boxing	13.3
Rowing (race)	6.3
Cycling (8.8 km/hr)	7.1
Cycling, racing	10.2
Dancing	8.0
Field Hockey	8.0
Football	7.9
Gymnastics	4.0
Running (3.7 min per km)	16.7
Running (3.1 min per km)	18.0
Skiing, level, moderate speed	7.2
Skiing, uphill, maximum speed	16.4
Squash	12.7
Swimming, backstroke	10.2
Swimming, breast stroke	9.7
Swimming, fast crawl	9.4
Tennis	6.6
Volleyball	3.0

Modified from Brooks G, Fahey T. Exercise physiology: Human bioenergetics and its applications. New York: John Wiley and Sons, 1984.
*1 kcal = 4.16 kilojoules

      b. Maintenance energy requirements = 1.5 × BEE for women, 1.7 × BEE for men
      c. Training activities must be added to this requirement, using estimates of energy expended during these activities (see Table 3 for examples). Caution should be taken to subtract maintenance values during the time spent performing activities, or the estimated energy requirement will be too high.
      d. Take seriously a claim that energy intake must be curtailed to maintain weight. Such claims may flag an eating disorder that could markedly effect performance, or may represent the truth for an athlete who has become extremely energy conservative. In

any event, if the comment is not taken seriously, it will hamper further relations, because the changing of attitudes about weight versus performance as the outcome variable of importance *takes time*.

   e. How closely does the reported energy intake come to estimated need (keep in mind that most food records underreport intake by as much as 20%)

2. Evaluate the CHO intake
   a. Does it meet the recommendation of 5 to 8 g/kg of body mass per day?
   b. What are the main sources?
   c. What is the fat content of the diet?
   d. Test the athlete's knowledge of CHO foods
3. Evaluate the timing and composition of meals relative to workouts
   a. Does the athlete eat before a workout?
   b. Does the athlete eat soon after a workout?
4. Evaluate the fluid intake—this should be sufficient to replace daily losses, bringing body mass back to the pre-exercise value before the next workout
5. Evaluate the overall quality of the diet—does it meet the recommendations for other nutrients and food groups?
   a. Protein intake—this is of special concern in women athletes with a low energy intake
   b. The calcium and iron are also of concern especially in women athletes

B. Counseling
1. Commend the athlete for positive changes
2. Assist the athlete in choosing CHO-rich foods that are liked and tolerated before, during, and after exercise bout
   a. Acquaint the athlete with the CHO content of fruits and vegetables
   b. Encourage monitoring the quality of workouts relative to eating pattern

3. If weight loss is appropriate, assist in determining what foods are high in fat and can be limited or eliminated
4. Discuss strategies for ensuring energy and CHO intake on days of performance when anxiety is high
   a. Concentrate on "favorite foods"
   b. Consume foods as fluids—these are easily consumed and are absorbed quickly
   c. Adopt a high CHO, low fat diet so that transit time is minimized

III. Additional Meetings
   A. Continue to commend athlete on positive habits
   B. Continue to evaluate the CHO and energy intake and the timing of meals relative to workouts and the effect on performance
   C. Minimize the focus on body weight whenever possible
   D. Continue to answer questions asked.

SUGGESTED READING

American Dietetic Association and Canadian Dietetic Association. Position of the American Dietetic Association and the Canadian Dietetic Association: Nutrition for physical fitness and athletic performance for adults. J Am Dietetic Assoc 1993; 93:691–696.

Berning JR, Steen SN, eds. Sports nutrition for the 90's. Gaithersburg, Md: Aspen Publishers, 1991.

Clark N. Sports nutrition guidebook: Eating to fuel your active lifestyle. Champaign, Ill: Leisure Press, 1990.

Coleman E. Eating for endurance. Palo Alto, Ca: Bull Publishing, 1992.

Houtkooper L. Food selection for endurance sports. Med Sci Sports Exerc 1992; 24:S349–S359.

Moses K, Manore MM. Development and testing of a carbohydrate monitoring tool for athletes. J Am Dietetic Assoc 1991; 91:962–965.

Sports and Cardiovascular Nutritionists, American Dietetic Association. In: Benardot D, ed. Sports nutrition: A guide for the professional working with active people. 2nd ed. Chicago: American Dietetic Association, 1993.

FLUID AND ENERGY REPLACEMENT DURING PROLONGED EXERCISE

TIMOTHY D. NOAKES, M.B., Ch.B., M.D., F.A.C.S.M.
JOHN A. HAWLEY, Ph.D., F.A.C.S.M.
STEVEN C. DENNIS, Ph.D.

The first studies showing that carbohydrate (CHO) ingestion during prolonged exercise lasting more than 90 minutes enhanced endurance performance and prevented hypoglycemia were conducted on runners in the 1920s and 1930s. However, these findings were largely ignored by the athletic community. So, too, were the early investigations showing the importance of adequate fluid replacement during prolonged exercise in the heat.

One of the first references to fluid replacement during long-distance running can be found in the 1953 International Amateur Athletic Federation (IAAF) Handbook controlling marathon (42 km) races (Table 1). That handbook stated that "refreshments shall (only) be provided by the organisers of a race after 15 km. No refreshments may be carried or taken by a competitor other than that provided by the organisers." As water was the *only* drink available to runners, it was clear that the IAAF had little knowledge of the benefits of CHO ingestion during prolonged exercise.

In the 1960s the IAAF modified their rules slightly, so that by 1967 refreshments were available after only 11 km of a race. Presumably the term *refreshments* again referred only to water.

For the next decade, the idea that water was more important than CHO replacement during exercise gained the ascendancy, in part because of studies showing that runners who were the most dehydrated after distance races had the highest postrace rectal temperatures. This observation promoted the belief that the rises in rectal temperature and dehydration were causally related, so that water, in large volumes, should be ingested to prevent heat exhaustion. This hypothesis is only partially correct; the major determinant of the rise in rectal temperature during exercise is the metabolic rate, which also determines the sweat rate and, hence, the level of dehydration. The level of dehydration does, however, have an additional rather smaller independent effect on the rectal temperature during exercise.

Nevertheless, the belief that fluid replacement alone was of primary importance for optimizing performance during prolonged exercise was promoted to such an extent that CHO ingestion was actively discouraged; it was believed to slow the rate of gastric emptying and hence the rate at which fluid could be replaced during exercise. As a result of the perceived importance of fluid replacement, the IAAF again altered their rules in 1977 to allow competitors to ingest fluids (water) earlier and more frequently during competition (see Table 1).

The question of whether water or CHO replacement should be emphasized during prolonged exercise was not fully resolved until the mid to late 1980s, when commercial interests in America revived research into the value of CHO ingestion during exercise. These more carefully controlled studies confirmed the findings of some 50 years earlier, demonstrating that the ingestion of CHO-containing solutions enhanced performance and endurance during prolonged exercise. Hence, the consumption of CHO-electrolyte beverages is currently advocated by the IAAF in all races of 10 km and longer (see Table 1). The exact amounts that should be consumed to provide sufficient fluid, CHO, and electrolytes to replace sweat and energy losses during exercise remain to be established.

FLUID LOSS AND REPLACEMENT

Fluid loss during exercise is determined principally by sweat rate, which is proportional to the athlete's metabolic rate. The principal ions lost in sweat are sodium and chloride ions from the extracellular compartments; their concentration depends on an individual's level of fitness and heat acclimation. Estimated sweat rates calculated in endurance athletes, along with their rates of fluid intake and measured weight losses are shown in Table 2. An early study conducted in the 1960s reported very low rates of fluid intake during a 32 km

Table 1 Evolution of the International Amateur Athletic Federation Rules Governing Fluid Intake During Marathon Running

Year	Beverage	First Drink (km)	Interval (km)
1953	Water	15	5
1967	Water	11	5
1977	Water	5	2.5
1990	Water + CHO + Electrolytes	3	3

Note: Interval, the distance between refreshment stations; CHO, carbohydrate.

Table 2 Rates of Fluid Loss and Fluid Ingestion During Various Long Distance Running Races

Race Distance (km)	Fluid Intake (L/hr)	Estimated Sweat Rate (L/hr)	Weight Loss (kg)
32	0.15	1.35	2.4
42*	0.4 ± 0.2	1.1 ± 1.1	2.4 ± 0.3
56	0.5	0.9	2.0
67	0.4	0.8	2.4
90	0.5	0.85	3.5

The total fluid intake of runners was determined as the sum of their individual intakes, as reported at various recording points during a race. Sweat rate was estimated from the rate of water loss, minus estimated respiratory losses. Total weight loss was determined as the sweat loss, plus metabolic fuel loss plus fluid intake minus urine output.

*42 km (marathon) values are the means ± SD of the average values from seven studies on male subjects. Female sweat rates were lower than those for males over distances of 42 km (0.6 L/hr versus 1.1 L/hr) and 67 km (0.5 L/hr versus 0.8 L/hr).

race (0.15 L/hr), with resultant weight losses of 2.4 kg and elevated postrace rectal temperatures. On the basis of this finding it was subsequently recommended that runners needed to drink "at least 900 ml of fluid per hour during competition in order not to collapse from heat stroke." However, most runners voluntary ingest no more than 0.5 L/hr during exercise. In contrast, sweat rates are invariably around 1 L/hr, resulting in an average weight loss of around 2.5 kg during exercise lasting 2 or more hours.

One explanation for the failure of athletes, especially runners, to meet their fluid requirements during exercise is that they develop symptoms of "fullness" when they attempt to drink fluid at high rates. Feelings of abdominal fullness may be due to limited rates of fluid absorption. Duodenal and jejunal perfusion studies have shown the maximum rate of water absorption occurs from isotonic solutions containing glucose, but that the maximum rate is only 0.8 L/hr. Similarly, in studies in which sufficient fluid was ingested to match fluid losses during exercise, not all of the ingested fluid appeared in the extracellular or intracellular fluid pools. Thus, the maximum rate of fluid absorption by the small bowel during exercise may be less than the high rates of fluid loss incurred by some athletes during more intensive exercise, leading to progressive ("involuntary") dehydration.

Alternatively, unlike other mammals, humans may develop progressive dehydration during exercise because they lose sodium chloride (NaCl) in sweat. Sodium losses decrease the rise in serum osmolality during exercise-induced dehydration in humans. Since thirst is regulated by changes in both serum osmolality and plasma volume, dipsogenic drive in dehydrated humans ceases before either fluid or sodium losses are fully replaced if serum osmolality is returned to normal values by water ingestion. Ingestion of NaCl solutions also terminates drinking prematurely by restoring plasma and extracellular volumes before intracellular fluid losses have been replaced. Hence, whether dehydrated humans drink plain water or NaCl solutions, they tend to stop drinking before they are fully rehydrated. These complex interactions may explain why some humans are unable to prevent the development of "involuntary" dehydration during prolonged exercise. Additionally, the rapid alleviation of the symptoms that initiate drinking, such as dryness of the mouth, may also cause premature cessation of drinking before full rehydration has occurred.

Depending on the type and intensity of exercise, and the posture adopted, plasma volume falls to varying extents in the first 5 to 10 minutes of exercise. Thereafter, further falls in plasma volume and resultant increases in the activity of the renin angiotensin-aldosterone axis are determined by the amount of fluid ingested during exercise; changes are reduced if the rate of fluid ingestion equals the rate of fluid loss. Falls in plasma volume during exercise are perhaps best prevented by the ingestion of an isotonic CHO-electrolyte solution. At rest, the ingestion of such solutions produces the highest rates of fluid absorption. Another advantage of adding

NaCl to the ingested solutions is that palatability is increased and drinking is promoted. The ingestion of sodium-containing solutions during exercise may also limit the fall in plasma volume by reducing the movement of sodium from the extracellular space into the unabsorbed fluid in the small bowel. Serum sodium concentrations and hence serum osmolality fall when large quantities of plain water are ingested during exercise, perhaps due to this sodium movement into a "third space." Such a movement would be expected to decrease the extracellular fluid volume.

With severe dehydration, rises in serum sodium concentration, serum osmolality, and antidiuretic (ADH) activity correlate with the increase in esophageal temperature and may be a stimulus for the reduction in sweating that develops at advanced levels of dehydration.

An important goal of fluid ingestion during exercise may be to prevent rises in serum osmolality or serum sodium concentrations, thereby maintaining rates of skin blood flow that are high enough to maximize evaporative and convective heat losses.

With sufficient fluid ingestion, rises in rectal or esophageal temperature are attenuated. However, the magnitude of this effect is not great. Most studies indicate that a 2 to 4 L fluid loss increases rectal temperature by less than 1°C, whereas the rise in metabolic rate associated with high-intensity exercise can increase the rectal temperature by 3 to 4°C.

Perhaps the greatest effect of fluid ingestion is on the perception of effort during exercise. The increases in performance observed with fluid ingestion correlate better with improvements in ratings of perceived exertion than with any other physiologic variable currently measured. Indeed, even partial fluid replacement has a significant effect on the perception of effort and performance during high-intensity exercise in the heat at very modest (i.e., 1.1 to 1.3 L) levels of dehydration.

CARBOHYDRATE INGESTION AND OXIDATION DURING EXERCISE

Although the addition of high concentrations of CHO to fluid replacement beverages may impair intestinal fluid absorption, inadequate CHO ingestion may impair performance by limiting CHO oxidation late in exercise; recent attention has thus focused on methods to optimize the rate of CHO ingestion during prolonged exercise. Gastric volume may be a more important determinant of the rate of gastric emptying during exercise than either solute energy content or osmolality, particularly when solutions are ingested repeatedly during exercise.

Thus, the maximum rate at which CHO and water can be delivered to the intestine from an ingested solution is strongly influenced by the average volume of fluid in the stomach; this, in turn, is governed by the drinking pattern of the athlete. The principal findings of studies that have simultaneously measured rates of gastric emptying and the oxidation of CHO solutions that have been ingested in repeated doses during exercise are that (1) the amount of solutions containing a variety of mono-, di-, and oligosaccharides emptied from the stomach is at least double the amount that is oxidized by the active muscles, and (2) irrespective of the ingestion regimen, peak rates of ingested CHO oxidation rise to ~ 1 g/min after 70 to 90 minutes of exercise. Hence, the rates of ingested CHO oxidation must be limited *either* by the release of the CHO into the systemic circulation *or* the rate of glucose oxidation by the working muscles. In order to distinguish between these two possibilities, we recently compared the rates of oxidation of ingested or infused U-^{14}C labeled glucose. Both the ingested and infused glucose were eventually oxidized at 1 g/min under euglycemic conditions whereas much higher rates were achieved when the infusion rate was increased to produce hyperglycemia. This proves that the physiologic plasma glucose and insulin concentrations present during prolonged exercise regulate the rate at which the ingested CHO is oxidized by the active muscles. Because all CHO solutions that are ingested during exercise maintain blood glucose concentrations at 5 mmol/L, the maximum rates of ingested CHO oxidation will also be limited to approximately 1 g/min.

RECOMMENDATIONS FOR THE OPTIMAL FLUID-REPLACEMENT BEVERAGE DURING EXERCISE

The principal aims of fluid ingestion during prolonged exercise are (1) to limit any dehydration-induced decreases in plasma volume and skin blood flow, (2) to prevent any rise in serum sodium osmolality or serum osmolality, (3) to diminish progressive rises in rectal temperature, (4) to decrease the subjective perception of effort and, (5) to improve athletic performance.

Although it has been assumed that the optimum rate of fluid ingestion is the rate that equals the rate of fluid loss, the precise composition of the solution that will optimize electrolyte and fluid replacement of the extracellular space has not been established. Furthermore, the rates of fluid ingestion needed to replace the high (~1 L/hr) sweat rates typically induced during prolonged exercise, may exceed the maximal intestinal absorptive capacity for water. Most people only achieve such fluid intakes with great difficulty. However, fluid consumption can be maximized by attention to a number of factors, including the temperature and palatability of the drink and the addition of electrolytes, particularly sodium, to the beverage.

CHO ingestion during exercise can be recommended whenever the exercise is of sufficient duration or intensity to deplete endogenous CHO stores. If CHOs are ingested frequently enough and in appropriate volumes it appears that (1) the type of CHO consumed does not greatly influence the rate of gastric emptying of equicaloric solutions; (2) there are no physiologically important differences in the rates of CHO oxidation

resulting from the repeated ingestion of a variety of mono-, di-, and oligosaccharides during exercise; and (3) all ingested CHOs are oxidized at a rate of ~1 g/min after the first 70 to 90 minutes of exercise. This last phenomenon probably arises because the physiologic concentrations of glucose and insulin normally present during prolonged, moderate-intensity exercise set the upper limit for the rate of glucose uptake and oxidation by skeletal muscle. The ingestion of highly concentrated (i.e., 15 to 20 g/100 ml) CHO beverages in the first 75 minutes of prolonged, exhaustive exercise should probably be avoided. Such beverages attenuate fat oxidation and accelerate CHO utilization, potentially causing premature fatigue.

The following practical guidelines are suggested for athletes participating in prolonged, moderate-intensity exercise of up to 6 hours duration:

1. Immediately before exercise or during the warm-up the athlete should ingest up to 300 ml of cool (10°C) flavored water.
2. For the first 60 to 75 minutes of exercise, the athlete should ingest 100 to 150 ml of a cool, dilute (5.0 g/100 ml) glucose polymer solution at regular (10 to 15 minute) intervals. It seems unwarranted to consume CHO in amounts much greater than 30 g during this period, as only 20 g of ingested CHO are oxidized in the first hour of moderate-intensity exercise, irrespective of the type of CHO consumed or the drinking regimen.
3. After 75 to 90 minutes of exercise, the concentration of the ingested glucose polymer solution should be increased to 10 to 12 g/100 ml, to which 20 mEq/L of sodium should be added. Higher sodium concentrations, although possibly promoting rapid intestinal fluid absorption, are not palatable to most athletes. Potassium, which may facilitate rehydration of the intracellular fluid compartment, could be included in the replacement beverage in small amounts (2 to 4 mEq/L). For the remainder of the race, the athlete should consume 100 to 150 ml of this solution at regular (10 to 15 minute) intervals. Such a drinking regimen will ensure optimal rates of both *fluid* and *energy* delivery, thereby limiting any dehydration-induced decreases in plasma volume, and maintaining the rate of ingested CHO oxidation at ~1 g/min late in exercise.

SUGGESTED READING

American College of Sports Medicine. The prevention of thermal injuries during distance running. Med Sci Sports Exerc 1987; 19:529–533.

Coggan AR, Coyle EF. Carbohydrate ingestion during prolonged exercise: effects on metabolism and performance. Exerc Sports Sci Rev 1991; 19:1–40.

Coyle EF, Hamilton M. Fluid replacement during exercise: effects on physiological homeostasis and performance. In: Gisolfi CV, Lamb DR, eds. Perspectives in exercise science and sports medicine. Vol 3. Fluid homeostasis during exercise. Carmel, Ind: Benchmark Press, 1990:281–308.

Hawley JA, Dennis SC, Noakes TD. Oxidation of exogenous carbohydrate ingested during prolonged exercise. Sports Med 1992; 14:27–42.

Montain SJ, Coyle EF. Influence of graded dehydration on hyperthermia and cardiovascular drift during exercise. J Appl Physiol 1992; 73:1340–1350.

Noakes TD. Fluid replacement during exercise. Exerc Sports Sci Rev. 1993; 21:297–330.

Noakes TD, Adams BA, Myburgh KH, et al. The danger of an inadequate water intake during prolonged exercise. Eur J Appl Physiol 1988; 57:210–219.

EXERCISE TESTING AND PRESCRIPTION FOR SEDENTARY ADULTS

SCOTT G. THOMAS, Ph.D.

Increased emphasis is being placed on the role of health professionals in health promotion. Exercise is believed to have positive health effects. Substantial evidence has accumulated that body composition, aerobic fitness, and muscular strength and endurance are important to health. Epidemiologic studies have established the importance of adiposity and lack of aerobic fitness to morbidity and mortality. Muscle strength and endurance have also received increased recognition as important health determinants. It has proven more difficult to establish whether flexibility influences health, but some research data and considerable anecdotal evidence suggest that flexibility is important to injury-free function. Health professionals who want to improve their clients' health need to know what exercise recommendations should be made and how to assist the client in making the required behavioral changes.

This chapter starts by considering strategies to increase the probability that a client will continue a regular exercise program. Next, the components of fitness and methods to assess those components are examined. Finally, the prescription of exercise for each component is outlined. It is assumed that the clients are apparently healthy adults who want to assess their current physical status and perhaps change their physical fitness. The apparently healthy adult can be identified using a health history and simple questionnaires such as the PAR Q (Fitness Canada, 1986). The American College of Sports Medicine (ACSM) has published further guidelines for relative and absolute contraindications to exercise.

Provision of exercise assessments and prescriptions requires skill in communicating with the client as well as expertise in the physiologic and behavioral aspects of exercise. A sedentary adult who requests assistance in starting an exercise program has made a crucial first step toward improving health. You must ensure that the exercise assessment and prescription that you provide are accurate, appropriate to the client's needs, and clearly communicated. The low prevalence of regular exercise in the population, despite clear evidence of its benefits, suggests that effective exercise prescriptions must be coupled with an understanding of the methods available to assist clients in modifying their behavior.

MOTIVATIONS AND GOALS

The starting point in any exercise assessment and prescription process must be the client's motivations and goals. These goals are often ill-defined; for example, a client may want "to increase energy" or to "feel better." As a health professional you can assist in defining such goals, in breaking a long-term goal into a series of short-term goals, and finally in cooperatively devising a strategy to achieve those goals. Assessment of your client's goals requires time to establish rapport, so that they will be willing to discuss openly issues such as dissatisfaction with body image or decreasing ability to meet the physical demands of work.

STRATEGIES TO PROMOTE REGULAR EXERCISE

Effective strategies are required to increase the incidence of physical activity participation in the population and to maintain participation once started. Approximately two-thirds of men and women in North America do not exercise regularly and approximately 50% of people drop out within 12 months of starting exercise programs. Some authors suggest that an emphasis on physical fitness, which the public finds unpalatable, reduces participation. Public health initiatives are being refocused on increasing physical activity in the least active rather than increasing physical fitness in more active people. However, the interests of an individual client are, most often, best served by increasing both physical activity and physical fitness.

Sallis and Hovell have argued that to be more effective we must consider the determinants of behavior at each stage in the natural history of exercise. The stages are adoption, maintenance, drop-out, and resumption of physical activity. Critical factors that health professionals can modify in the first stage include exercise self-efficacy, health knowledge, exercise knowledge, and attitudes toward exercise.

Exercise self-efficacy is the client's belief that he or she can perform the exercise. Exercise testing has proven effective in raising the exercise self-efficacy of heart patients. To increase health and exercise knowledge, you may choose to talk with the client and/or rely on brochures and posters that are available through various agencies. Attitudes toward exercise may be influenced through role models and peer support.

In the maintenance stage, adherence to the exercise program is facilitated by behavioral skills, spousal support, and the client's perception that time is available to do the activity. Strategies that may be effective in aiding the client to maintain an exercise habit are suggested in Table 1. Clients may be assisted by goal-setting, feedback regarding progress, and self-monitoring. Exercise assessments can play a critical role in improving adherence to exercise, by defining reasonable fitness goals, providing objective feedback on progress, and assisting clients in developing self-monitoring skills. Self-monitoring is aided if clients are given daily or weekly diaries to record exercise intensity and duration. Heart rate monitoring instructions or devices and assistance in using perceived exertion scales also assist clients in self-monitoring.

Program factors may influence a client's continued participation in an exercise program. Recent studies have suggested that properly organized and monitored home programs are as effective in maintaining an exercise routine as exercise programs in a supervised facility. A biweekly or monthly telephone call by exercise program personnel will increase adherence to home exercise regimens. Structured exercise programs are more successful if they are (1) convenient in terms of time, location, and mode of exercise (little preparation required, e.g., jogging versus skiing); (2) enjoyable (exercise tailored to client's preference, program includes fun activities and encourages group camaraderie); and (3)

injury free (low initial intensity and slow increase in intensity of exercise).

Unanticipated disruptions in routine can end a regular exercise program. Anticipation and planning for disruptions will assist the client in resuming an exercise routine after illness or work or family pressures have required a temporary halt to activity. Clients should be reassured that a brief interruption in training, or an decrease in the frequency of training, will not seriously reduce their physical capacity. The factors that influence the probability of clients resuming participation in an exercise program after a lengthy absence have not yet been identified.

COMPONENTS OF EXERCISE ASSESSMENTS AND PRESCRIPTIONS

Information obtained from a physical activity history and assessment of the components of physical fitness can be used to establish an exercise plan, monitor progress with a plan, and educate a client regarding her or his physical capacities. Recent publications have distinguished health-related assessment from performance-related assessment. Health-related assessments stress measurement of risk factor related items such as adiposity and blood pressure. Performance-related assessments may stress the measurement of work- or sport-related components such as aerobic power, strength, or muscular endurance. However, for many client groups, such as the elderly, the distinction is moot. The World Health Organization definition of health as a resource for living suggests that an improved ability to perform physically has a positive impact on health. An improved physical capacity provides clients with a resource for a healthier life.

If the client has clearly defined fitness and health goals, you may be able to limit the assessment of physical capacity to one relevant fitness component. More often, assessment of several or all fitness components (body composition, aerobic fitness, flexibility, muscular strength, and muscular endurance) may be necessary to provide the information that is required to develop fitness goals with the client. As a health professional, you may wish to use a comprehensive assessment to identify any "weak links" in the client's physical fitness profile.

As Table 2 illustrates, each component of fitness

Table 1 Strategies for Increasing Exercise Adherence

Identify the client's objectives
Assist the client in making these objectives as realistic as possible
Provide access to and use various techniques to increase self-efficacy
Provide exposure to alternative self-control or self-management strategies
Instruct exercise supervisors in the use of motivational techniques
Incorporate social support systems into the exercise program
Ensure rapid feedback of gains in fitness
Provide follow-up visits after graduation from a fitness class

Data from Dishman R. Exercise adherence: Its impact on public policy. 1991

Table 2 Assessing the Components of Physical Capacity

Level	Body Composition	Aerobic Fitness	Muscular Strength	Muscular Endurance	Flexibility
Simple	Height, body mass, BMI	Submaximal prediction of $\dot{V}o_2max$	Maximal handgrip force	Repetition to failure e.g., pushups against body mass	Sit and reach test (Wells Dillon)
Moderate	Skinfold thickness, bioelectric impedance	Maximal prediction of $\dot{V}o_2max$	1 RM, several muscle groups	Fatigue index	Gravity dependent flexometer
Complex	Hydrostatic measure of body density	Direct measurement of $\dot{V}o_2max$	Force/velocity curve	Fatigue index at specific speeds	Radiography, biomech. modeling & analysis

may be assessed using simple field tests, that have moderate validity, or using sophisticated laboratory tests that may be regarded as the "gold standard." Sophisticated assessment of each physical function component would involve a daunting cost (in money, time, and effort) for most sedentary adults. As a result, your task is to select judiciously the assessment tools that will provide the required information without overburdening the client. In making that judgement, you should consider whether the additional information, obtained from a sophisticated assessment, will have a significant impact on the exercises you prescribe to achieve the client's goals.

Your selection from among the alternative methods of assessing each component of fitness should be based on the characteristics of the measurement tool (validity, reliability, responsiveness), the cost (time, effort, money) and the benefit (importance of information) derived from the assessment. This chapter emphasizes simple and moderate complexity measures, since these are more accessible to most health professionals. Details of testing protocols are available from other sources (see Suggested Reading).

METHODS OF ASSESSMENT

Physical Activity History

Information about the clients' exercise habits will assist you in evaluating how responsive they may be to exercise and may suggest activity preferences. Clients who are currently very active will be able to exercise more intensively but will observe less change in fitness than clients who are initially inactive. The probability of adopting and maintaining an activity that was enjoyed in the past is higher than for novel activities. A recent study that compared 10 physical activity questionnaires suggested that all were highly reliable. The ability of the questionnaires to assess high-intensity activities was generally good, but their ability to quantify participation in low- and moderate-intensity activities was limited.

Body Composition

Epidemiologic studies have linked total adiposity and fat distribution to health risks. Fat deposits on the trunk (the typical male pattern of deposition) increase health risks more than fat deposits on the limbs and buttocks (the female pattern). In addition, adiposity should be assessed because clients are often motivated to exercise by a desire to reshape their bodies.

The body may be logically divided into components, using a variety of schemes. The simplest division into fat tissue and fat free tissue (lean body mass) has been used extensively in fitness assessment. The use of more complex divisions into several compartments has been confined largely to research settings.

The simple measurement of total body mass can be misleading, since fat and lean body mass may change in opposite directions. Advice to a client should be based on an assessment of body composition, not on the measurement of body mass. The average Body Mass Index (BMI = body mass[kg]/height^2 [m^2]) is a useful measure of adiposity for population studies. However, the BMI is much less useful in following the progress of a specific client in exercise programs that increase lean body mass and decrease adipose tissue mass. The ratio of waist to hip girths is used in population and clinical studies as a rough indicator of fat distribution. A high ratio indicates that a high proportion of fat is deposited on the trunk.

In the hands of a skilled appraiser, the assessment of subcutaneous fat by caliper measurement of skinfold thickness is a valid and reliable indicator of adiposity and fat distribution. The percentage of body fat may be predicted to within 3% to 5% of the actual value from skinfold and girth measures, using general or population specific equations. However, many appraisers have rejected the idea of predicting the percentage of body fat and report their adiposity measure directly in terms of the sum of skinfold measures or compare the sum of skinfold measures with population values. This approach avoids making tenuous assumptions about the relationship between skinfold thickness measurements and total body fat content. However, your client may find a percentile ranking less satisfying than a percent body fat value. Skinfold measures from the trunk can be compared to normative values to assess the health risk attributable to a male pattern of fat deposition.

Bioelectrical impedance is used with increasing frequency to assess body composition. Assessment of adiposity with this method depends on the relative resistance and reactance of fat free tissue and fat tissue to a high frequency electric current. Guidelines for eating, drinking, exercise, and diuretics must be followed when making such measurements, since changes in hydration affect the estimate of body composition. If test procedures are followed carefully, the percentage of body fat can be estimated to within 3% to 4% for most populations. However, this method provides no information about the distribution of fat.

Aerobic Fitness

Aerobic fitness, which is often assessed because of its relation to cardiorespiratory health and to performance of activities such as running, cycling, and swimming, depends on the integrated functioning of the pulmonary and cardiovascular systems and the ability of muscle tissue to generate energy aerobically. It is determined largely by habitual physical activity, but genetic inheritance explains about 25% of the variation in aerobic fitness, as well as a considerable part of the response to physical training.

Choices in testing include which response measure to report, use of a submaximal or maximal test, exercise mode (e.g., walking, running, cycling, arm cranking) and specific test protocol. Direct measurement of maximal oxygen consumption $\dot{V}O_2max$) during treadmill running is the "gold standard" measure of aerobic fitness. The intraindividual, day to day variation of $\dot{V}O_2max$ is approximately 5%. Estimates of $\dot{V}O_2$max from submaximal tests generally rely on assumptions of a linear relationship between heart rate (HR) and oxygen uptake, a constant mechanical efficiency, and a consistent maximum HR for a given age. These assumptions result in predictions of $\dot{V}O_2$max that are usually within 10% of the actual value.

Aerobic fitness may be quantified using submaximal indices such as the Physical Work Capacity (expressed in Watts) at a given HR (for example, PWC_{150}), or HR response at a given oxygen uptake (for example $HR_{1.0}$, commonly reported as a heart rate at a $\dot{V}O_2$ of 1.0l/min). Use of these indices avoids assuming a particular age-predicted maximal HR. Submaximal measures generally demonstrate lower reliability but higher responsiveness compared with direct measures of $\dot{V}O_2$max. Training of a previously sedentary adult typically produces a 10% to 40% change in maximal oxygen uptake. Training-induced change in submaximal endurance will range from 20% to 80%.

The choice of exercise modality for the assessment of aerobic fitness is based on the client's activity preferences and available equipment. The smaller the muscle mass employed in testing (for instance, arm vs leg exercise), the lower the $\dot{V}O_2$max and the more likely a peripheral (muscle vasculature or tissue) versus central (cardiac output) limit to test performance. If a peripheral limit is reached, the test results will be specific to exercise with that muscle group.

Muscular Strength and Endurance

The ability to exert force during a single maximal contraction (muscular strength) and the ability to exert a large, but submaximal force repeatedly (muscular endurance) are distinct but closely related aspects of physical capacity. Maximum voluntary contraction (MVC) and muscular endurance measures depend on client motivation. A small coefficient of variation over repeated trials indicates that each effort was maximal. Performance on tasks demanding muscular strength and endurance is determined by the amount of muscle available (the effective cross-sectional area) and the ability to activate the muscle effectively. Effective activation of the muscle by the motor control system is the most labile and task specific determinant of muscle strength. Complete activation of the muscle depends on the client's willingness to make a maximum effort.

Ideally, the examiner can identify the demands of important functional tasks and select a test that matches those demands. Matching of the test measure to the task may be in terms of the type of contraction (concentric, eccentric, isometric, isotonic, or isokinetic), the velocity of contraction, and the muscle groups that are active. Unfortunately, we seldom have the requisite task description, and less often the ability and time to match the task demands carefully. As a result, strength is often assessed using simple isometric or isotonic measures.

Isometric measures, such as the handgrip, and manual muscle testing require careful specification of the joint angle that has been used for testing, because of the force-length relation for muscle. If the joint angle is changed, the muscle length will be altered and its ability to generate force changed. Isometric strength is joint angle specific, yet it correlates moderately well with the corresponding isotonic measure.

Isotonic tests with free weights require a larger component of motor skill than tests with weight equipment. As a result, practice and learning produce initial increases in scores. Client safety may be less with free weights than with a weight stack and lever arm system such as the Universal Gym.

The ability to continue generating a given force (absolute muscular endurance) is greater in those with greater strength. The ability to keep generating force at a given fraction of MVC (relative muscular endurance) is the same or less in individuals with greater strength than in those with lesser strength. Muscular endurance tests may look at the number of repetitions the client can complete before failure, or they may assess the decrease in force generated after a fixed number of repetitions (15 to 60) have been completed. Simple tests such as pushups record the number of repetitions before failure to lift a portion of body weight.

Flexibility

Flexibility depends on the structure of a given joint and the status of the soft tissues (muscles and connective tissues) around the joint. It is largely dependent on the habitual activity of the client, rather than on age, gender, or body type. Flexibility may be assessed using angular measures of range of motion (ROM) about a joint, or indirect measures such as the linear distance reached from a specific starting position. Flexibility measures may be active (the client moves to the position) or passive (the appraiser moves the client's limbs into position), and they depend on the compliance of the soft tissues, which is affected by temperature. The tissue temperature is changed by prior activity and by environmental conditions; therefore, these factors must be consistent between repeated measurements.

As with muscular strength, flexibility is joint and muscle specific. As a result, measurement at a single joint does not necessarily provide a good representation of a client's flexibility. Two approaches to this problem may be used. A measure that requires movement across several joints may be used to obtain an "overall" measure, or the flexibility at each of several joints of particular relevance may be assessed. The sit and reach, or Wells and Dillon test, requires movement through the back and hips. Although some appraisers have used it as an indicator of back flexibility, it appears to depend largely on the extensibility of the hamstrings.

Goniometers measure the angular distance between adjacent body segments. Good measurements depend on standardized protocols, which ensure accurate placement of the center of the goniometer at the axis of rotation for the movement. Flexometers (e.g., Leighton) measure movement relative to gravitational force and may provide a superior, if slightly more expensive, alternative to goniometers. Anatomic landmarking of the flexometer position increases measurement reliability, but the axis of rotation does not have to be identified. However, movements must be in the gravitational plane.

For the apparently healthy adult who wants to be more active or more physically fit, the simplest of assessment methods are appropriate. The Canadian Standardized Test of Fitness (CSTF) provides simple tools for assessing all components of fitness. This test battery may be used with clients across a wide range of ages (15 to 69 years). Extensive testing of the aerobic component of the package indicates that it has good reliability and validity. A further advantage of the CSTF package is a normative table for each measure. The client's results can be compared to an age and gender specific distribution of values. The client will then know in what category or percentile ranking their results currently fall.

EXERCISE PRESCRIPTION

As emphasized earlier, an exercise prescription is useful only if it is well formulated and clearly communicated. The client and the appraiser must agree on the goals of the program and the means to achieve those goals. The assessment should serve as a guide in formulating the program and as a tool for educating and motivating the client.

The principles underlying exercise prescription are specificity, overload, progression, and reversibility. Gains in physical capacity are specific to the type of exercise employed in the training program. Training responses are specific because the physiologic adaptations that permit increased performance or decreased disturbance of homeostasis are specific to the tissues (muscle and connective tissues) that are trained, and to the biochemical systems that produce the energy required for a particular activity.

To induce a physiologic adaptation, the training stimulus must exceed the normal demands placed on the system. The overload must be followed by a rest period, during which the adaptive response occurs. As the client adapts to the exercise, the training stimulus must be progressed in order to ensure it remains an overload. Typically, a sedentary client will start a program with exercises at a low intensity and short duration; the duration will be increased first and then the intensity. A period of improvement in capacity ensues, lasting for weeks or months. Eventually, physical capacity reaches a plateau that is difficult or impossible to exceed. Although the time course varies somewhat with the particular adaptation, training adaptations are gained and lost over roughly the same time period. The reversibility of training requires a lifelong commitment to exercise if the client is to maintain lifelong benefits.

Body Composition and Aerobic Fitness

Changes in body composition are effected when the balance between the energy consumed and the energy expended is disrupted. Regular aerobic exercise can play a critical role in decreasing adiposity by increasing the client's energy expenditure. A client's strongest exercise motivation may be to change body fatness. The health professional who recognizes that an increase in aerobic activity and fitness would be beneficial to the client's health can thus couple the client's interest in fat loss with a prescription for aerobic activity.

Energy expenditure is increased during exercise, and to a variable degree after exercise has been completed. The importance to fat loss of the postexercise increase in metabolic rate has not yet been clearly established. Exercise may attenuate the decrease in metabolic rate observed with dietary restriction. Several studies indicate that a combination of dietary restriction and aerobic exercise decreases fat weight while maintaining lean body mass. The optimum program for fat loss is one that the client can accept and continue over a lifetime. Weight loss programs that include exercise appear to have higher long-term success rates than dietary restriction alone. Recent research suggests that resistance training (weight training) may be effective in decreasing adiposity but further confirmation of these findings is required.

Aerobic exercise prescriptions are described using the FITT principle. As indicated in Table 3, a wide range of *Frequency* (number of sessions per week), *Intensity,* and *Time* (duration of an exercise session) may be used in developing an aerobic prescription as long as the *Type* of exercise employs a large muscle mass in rhythmic activities (i.e., running, cycling, rowing, or walking). Selection of a combination of frequency, intensity and time is based on the client's goals and current physical capacity. As the range in Table 3 indicates, fat loss is enhanced with moderate intensity, longer duration exercise. This occurs primarily because the total energy expenditure is markedly greater in moderate intensity, long duration exercise than in high intensity, moderate duration exercise. For example, the total added energy expenditure is 33% higher in a 60 minute exercise session at 50% of $\dot{V}o_2max$, compared to a 30 minute session at 75% of $\dot{V}o_2max$.

All clients should be encouraged to start their training programs with low intensity (50% to 60% of HR_{max}), short duration (10 to 15 minutes) exercise sessions. The client who is interested in fat loss should hold intensity constant, increase the exercise time per session, and perhaps increase the number of sessions per week. Clients whose primary concern is enhancement of aerobic fitness should increase the exercise duration to 30 minutes over 3 to 4 weeks and then increase exercise intensity.

Exercise training intensity is often set relative to the client's $\dot{V}o_2max$. If individuals of the same age, but differing $\dot{V}o_2max$, exercise at the same percentage of their maximal capacity, they experience similar physiologic responses (HR, redistribution of blood flow) and sense of effort (rating of perceived exertion). Thus, setting exercise intensity relative to $\dot{V}o_2max$ helps to standardize exercise responses. Exercise intensity is rarely set in terms of oxygen uptake, because the monitoring of oxygen demands during training is diffi-

Table 3 Exercise Prescription for Fat Loss and Aerobic Fitness Gain

	ACSM Recommendations	*Fat Loss Emphasis*	*Aerobic Power Emphasis*
Frequency	3–5 sessions/week^{-1}	5–7 sessions/week^{-1}	3–5 sessions/week^{-1}
Intensity	60–90% HR_{max}	50–70% HR_{max}	70–90% HR_{max}
	50–85% HR reserve	40–60% HR reserve	70–90% HR reserve
Time	20–60 min/session^{-1}	30–80 min/session^{-1}	20–40 min/session^{-1}

Table 4 Exercise Prescription for Muscular Strength and Endurance

	ACSM Recommendations	*Muscle Strength Emphasis*	*Muscle Endurance Emphasis*
Frequency	2+ sessions/week^{-1}	2–3 sessions/week^{-1}	2–3 sessions/week^{-1}
Intensity	60–80% MVC	80–100% MVC	50–70% MVC
Total	8–12 reps/set^{-1}	4–6 reps/set^{-1}	15–30 reps/set^{-1}
	1–2 sets/session^{-1}	1–2 sets/session^{-1}	2–3 sets/session^{-1}

cult. As a consequence, HR is usually monitored as an indicator of physiological strain. As indicated in Table 3, the training HR may be set relative to the measured or the age-predicted maximum HR or relative to the range between resting and maximum HR.

Medications, other substances such as caffeine and pathologies that disrupt the normal relationship between HR and physiologic strain reduce the usefulness of HR as an indicator of training intensity. Ratings of perceived exertion provide an alternative. Two forms of the Borg Scale (6 to 20, and 0 to 10) are both useful methods of encouraging clients to attend to their body's feedback regarding exercise intensity. Client use of the Borg scale is facilitated by using the scale during exercise testing.

Muscular Strength and Endurance

Muscular strength and endurance are important in maintaining the ability to function independently. Furthermore, the strain experienced during occasional activities that require strength is much reduced through regular resistance training, which increases muscular strength and endurance. Work-place injuries are less frequent in stronger workers. Resistance training increases the strength of ligaments and increases the thickness of articular cartilage. Resistance training may also increase bone density and may influence the profile of blood lipids favorably.

The principles of specificity, overload, progression, and reversibility that were discussed in relation to aerobic training also apply to resistance training. Responses are specific to the muscle groups used in training and the speed and range of motion employed in the training sessions. Isometric exercise may be used in the presence of an existing pathology (i.e., rheumatoid arthritis) and for rehabilitation, but it is less desirable for general conditioning, since it is joint angle specific. To enhance muscular fitness, the major muscle groups of the body must be exercised through their full ROM, at a low to moderate speed.

Resistance training programs are described in terms of their Frequency, Intensity, and Total volume of training (the number of repetitions and sets) (Table 4). The balance between intensity and total volume depends on whether the client wants to emphasize muscular strength (high intensity, low volumes) or muscular endurance (low intensity, high volume). An intermediate program, such as that recommended by the ACSM, increases both muscular strength and endurance. Muscle hypertrophy is greater with muscular strength programs.

Muscular strength initially increases due to more effective neural activation of the muscle. Subsequent increases are due to muscle hypertrophy and occur at a slower rate. In clients with low initial fitness, muscle strength and endurance initially change rapidly in response to resistance training. Reassessment of the one repetition maximum may be required, in order to readjust training intensity and thus maintain a training overload. Muscular fitness can be developed with two to three training sessions per week and maintained with one to two sessions per week. The order in which the various muscles are trained should ensure that the same muscle group is not exercised twice in sequence. For example, exercise with the knee extensors should be followed by exercise with the biceps brachii rather than with a military press exercise.

Concentric exercises produce less muscle soreness and injury than eccentric resistance exercise. However, eccentric training appears to decrease the probability of subsequent eccentric exercise injury. Eccentric exercise may be employed, with caution, if protection from injury during a required eccentric task is desirable. Most often clients use concentric resistance exercises, which may have a small eccentric component.

Flexibility

As indicated earlier, flexibility is joint specific. Enhancement of flexibility depends on increasing the compliance of the soft tissues around a joint. This is best accomplished when the tissues are at an elevated temperature. Therefore, flexibility exercises should be performed following the warm-up preceding either aerobic or resistance training and on completion of the aerobic or resistance session. The specificity of flexibility implies that the ROM for a given joint can only be increased if stretch training is performed at that joint. How long flexibility training effects last has not yet been defined. However, flexibility may decrease at a faster rate than other aspects of fitness.

Static positioning or Proprioceptive Neuromuscular Facilitation (PNF) are the preferred methods of stretching. Ballistic stretching is not recommended, because of a high incidence of damage to the muscle-tendon junction. In static stretching, the client is instructed to stretch to a position that does not produce pain and then to hold the position for a minimum of 10 seconds. The duration of the hold may be increased to 60 seconds as the client becomes accustomed to such stretching. PNF stretching involves assuming a stretched position, performing an isometric contraction, relaxing the muscle and then contracting the antagonist muscle. Flexibility gains may be greater with this method, but the research is not yet conclusive. Clients who feel pain with this method should be encouraged to use static stretching.

COMMENTS

The sedentary adult who wants to exercise faces a formidable challenge. Assisting the client make the behavioral changes required to become a regular participant in physical activity is a most important task for the expert in sports medicine. You can assist your client by providing relevant, factual information about the client's current physical capacities, the activities that will produce the desired change, and the size of change that may be expected. Providing your clients with evidence that they are capable of exercising, feedback on their progress, and with tools to overcome any setbacks all increase the probability that they will stay with the exercise prescription that you have carefully and individually formulated for them.

SUGGESTED READING

American College of Sports Medicine. Recommended quantity and quality of exercise for developing and maintaining cardiorespiratory and muscular fitness in healthy adults (1990).
American College of Sports Medicine. Resource manual for guidelines for exercise testing and prescription. Philadelphia: Lea & Febiger, 1988.
Bouchard C, Shephard RJ, Stephens T, et al. Exercise fitness and health. A consensus of current knowledge. Champaign, Ill: Human Kinetics, 1990.
Dishman RK. Exercise adherence: Its impact on public policy. 1991.
Fitness Canada. Canadian standardized test of fitness operations manual. 3rd Ed. Ottawa: Govt of Canada, 1986.
Heyward VH. Advanced fitness assessment and exercise prescription. 2nd Ed. Champaign, Ill: Human Kinetics, 1991.
Hubley-Kozey CL. Testing flexibility. In: MacDougall JD, Wenger HA, Green HJ, eds. Physiological testing of the high-performance athlete. 2nd Ed. Champaign, Ill: Human Kinetics, 1991.
Sale DG. Testing strength and power. In: MacDougall JD, Wenger HA, Green HJ, eds. Physiological testing of the high-performance athlete. 2nd Ed. Champaign, Ill: Human Kinetics, 1991.
Sallis JF, Hovell MF. Determinants of exercise behavior. Exerc Sport Sci Rev 1990; 18:307–330.
Stefanick ML. Exercise and weight control. Exerc Sport Sci Rev 1993; 21:363–396.

OVERTRAINING

DONALD C. McKENZIE, M.D., Ph.D.

Most coaches and sport scientists believe that it is necessary to induce significant physical stress in order to develop the physiologic and mental characteristics of a high-performance athlete. Fatigue is a familiar complaint in elite athletes and there are many valid medical reasons for this condition. Illness, anemia, and iron deficiency are all common in this population and the Sports Medicine practitioner must be cognizant of the special medical issues that accompany individuals involved in high-performance sport. In the absence of a readily discerned cause, fatigue that is out of proportion to the training stimulus is often explained as a manifestation of overtraining. This diagnosis is usually achieved through the process of exclusion and it provides the clinician with a satisfactory explanation that also has some measure of acceptability for the athlete and the coach. Unfortu-

nately, there is no diagnostic tool that can readily confirm the condition and the clinician must be cautious not to offer the diagnosis of overtraining without ruling out other valid medical causes for fatigue. Once the diagnosis has been made, the clinician must be ready to offer a treatment plan to overcome the condition, together with advice to avoid recurrence. Most cases are difficult to deal with and, because of the lack of simple clinical markers of overtraining, the physician will be intellectually challenged to provide specific guidelines for recovery and return to competition.

No uniform terminology has been adopted to describe overtraining and a wide spectrum of adjectives has been used to report on the clinical picture. Two particular kinds of overtraining have been distinguished, parasympathetic and sympathetic, each with their own constellation of symptoms (see Fry et al, 1991). Other descriptive terms have been used to describe the overall condition or some portion of it: "over-reaching" and "staleness" represent attempts to give a measure of precision to the analysis of athletic fatigue but, in the absence of clinical or laboratory methods of confirmation, such attempts merely add confusion to an already complex area of medicine. Much of the confusion surrounding terminology results from authors using the various possible descriptors indiscriminately. A wide range of biochemical, hematologic, and physiologic markers have been reported as associated with overtraining, yet there are little scientific data to support the relationships. A great deal of the literature on overtraining is anecdotal.

The mere fact of a visit by the athlete to the clinician for an assessment regarding overtraining indicates that there has been a failure in the training monitoring system. In an ideal program, overtraining does not occur. However, errors in training are common and the coach should recognize the early signs of this condition. The full-blown clinical picture of the overtrained athlete is relatively easy to recognize, but detection of the subtle symptoms and signs that mark an athlete who is developing the overtrained state represent a major challenge for the Sports Medicine practitioner. One must be aware that other medical conditions can coexist and that overtraining is usually the result of the accumulation of many different stressors. Recovery from the established overtraining syndrome always takes weeks and often months of modified training. Clearly, prevention is the preferred strategy.

CLINICAL PICTURE

The classic symptoms of overtraining are presented in Table 1. The most frequent clinical complaints are fatigue, mood change, a decreased resistance to infection, and poor performance. Poor performance is a necessary symptom of overtraining. The clinical presentation is frequently vague and nonspecific. The physician must take a thorough history that includes the physical demands of the sport and the associated training program. Many athletes keep a detailed diary; this will often provide useful information regarding their training program and other stressors that could be contributing to the medical problem. Functional inquiry may elicit other features of the overtraining syndrome: insomnia, poor appetite, night sweats, muscle and joint discomfort, and reactive depression. Physical examination, with few exceptions, is unrewarding. Cervical or inguinal lymphadenopathy is present occasionally but the clinical significance of this finding and its relationship to overtraining has yet to be determined.

Table 1 Common Symptoms Associated with Overtraining

Decreased performance
Fatigue
Injury
Diffuse pain in joints and muscles
Frequent URTI
Sore throat, gland enlargement
Neuropsychiatric symptoms
Insomnia, irritability
Poor attitude toward training, depression
Confusion, anger

PATHOGENESIS

The exact etiology of overtraining remains unclear, but there is some good information suggesting that functional alterations in the hypothalamic-pituitary axis are responsible for the syndrome. A common focus for consideration of the condition has been the General Adaptation Syndrome (GAS) proposed by Hans Seyle in the 1930s. Many clinicians feel that the concept of the GAS can be applied, albeit with some limitations, to the overtraining syndrome. Thus, overtraining can be viewed as the resultant of many stressors, both physical (related to the training program), and nonphysical (emotionally taxing situations apart from training that have arisen both inside and outside the sport).

DETECTION

Although the literature abounds with anecdotal reports of methods that can be used to detect overtraining, there is no single laboratory measurement that can determine with certainty whether an athlete is overtrained. The plasma ratio of free testosterone to cortisol (T/C ratio) has met with some success as a means of confirming the clinical picture in an athlete who has the classical features of overtraining. However, such tests tend to be expensive, and are not available in all laboratories. Moreover, if the findings are to be useful, baseline measurements are necessary. Unfortunately, confirming the diagnosis does little to help the athlete; once the T/C ratio has dropped significantly, it is unlikely that the athlete will be able to return quickly to top level competition. Detection of overtraining has academic and medical significance but prevention of overtraining must be the goal of the coach and support staff.

PREVENTION

Overtraining appears to reflect failure to adapt to a training stimulus. This may be because the training load is too high or too little time is allowed for recovery and adaptation. Nontraining stressors can play a major role in the development of overtraining; they must therefore be recognized and minimized. The primary method of preventing overtraining is to develop a training program that is based on achievable goals and adopts a reasonable approach to application of the training stimulus. Virtually all coaches are familiar with the concept of periodization and training programs that plan for a progressive enhancement of performance over several years. Stressors, training and nontraining, must be monitored in a longitudinal fashion throughout such conditioning programs. Regular supervision of the training program and attention to issues such as sleep and nutrition will pay dividends to both the athlete and the coach. Recognition of the cumulative nature of physical and mental stressors is often overlooked, but the cumulative stress can be followed with a monitoring tool that has been developed, revised, and used for several

Athlete   Monitoring

Name:_____   Date: _____
Heart Rate (am): _____   Wt: _____

Mark the point (**X**) on the line that best describes your status at this moment!

		none or minimal	relative to yesterday <- better worse ->	unable to train

1. Generalized fatigue

2. Muscle/joint pain

3. Sore throat, fever, cough, etc.

4. Change in sleep pattern

positive,   average   very low,
very high   consistent problems

5. How do you feel about yourself
    (confidence in training and
    competition, ability to focus,
    level of annoyance & frustration)

6. How do you feel about canoeing
    (satisfaction with training and
    relationships with individuals
    inside the sport: other paddlers,
    coaches, support staff)

7. How do you feel about situations
    outside of canoeing (school, $,
    individuals not involved in
    canoeing: boyfriends, girlfriends,
    spouse etc)

easy   average   hard

8. How does your training program
    feel to you

no   yes,   yes,
                      no effect   affects training

9. Irregular diet

10. Time zones travelled (#)

Figure 1   Athlete monitoring form.

years by different Canadian national sports teams. A generic version of this monitoring tool is presented in Figure 1.

The athlete completes a one-page questionnaire consisting of 10 items; responses can be completed by the athlete within 60 seconds. It is therefore a practical device that can be completed daily during the phases of training leading to major games, and once or twice weekly in less stressful parts of the season. It attempts to acknowledge the stressors that contribute to the overtraining syndrome and its primary achievements are to highlight the stressors that exist inside and outside of sport, and to remind the coach to be watchful for this condition.

This questionnaire is scored from zero to four, and the results can be recorded in a log book or on a computer data base. As the questionnaire is divided into different segments, the respondent is creating a stressor index for medical, psychological, training, and miscellaneous conditions. The sum of these segments represents the total stressor index. It is possible to plot the different stressors plus the total stressor index versus time, thus giving a visual display of the status of each athlete. Figure 2 is an example of an athlete who was followed daily for a 45 day period leading up to a major competition. A higher score indicates more stress and the likelihood of a decrease in performance. It is possible to keep a copy of the daily stressor questionnaire, and thus to review responses for individual days, examining the causes for any disturbance in the stressor index. Clearly there are "normal" stress levels for any given athlete and these will be reflected in the baseline measures. The perception of stress varies enormously between individuals and therefore this monitoring tool is only valid as a means of following individual athletes. Several issues contributed to the observed changes in Figure 2. On day 16, the stressor index was high, due to an increase in the medical score. In fact, the athlete had developed a sore throat over the preceding 2 days and this was being treated with increased fluid intake. On day 33, there was an overseas trip that covered six time zones. The index was very low on that day, but subsequently there was a significant and prolonged increase in the total stressor index. The medical index moved higher, due to alterations in sleep pattern, and there was an increase in the psychological stress perceived by this athlete. It took 6 to 7 days for this athlete to overcome the effects of travel. Coaches frequently expect athletes to recover within 2 to 3 days following travel such as this but clearly, in this particular case, recovery would be incomplete with such a short period of adjustment.

Although it is difficult to generalize, one consistent observation has been that athletes who develop the overtraining syndrome show a change in their stressor index. Reviewing athletes who complained of symptoms of overtraining and demonstrated poor performance, it was apparent that the psychological stressor index

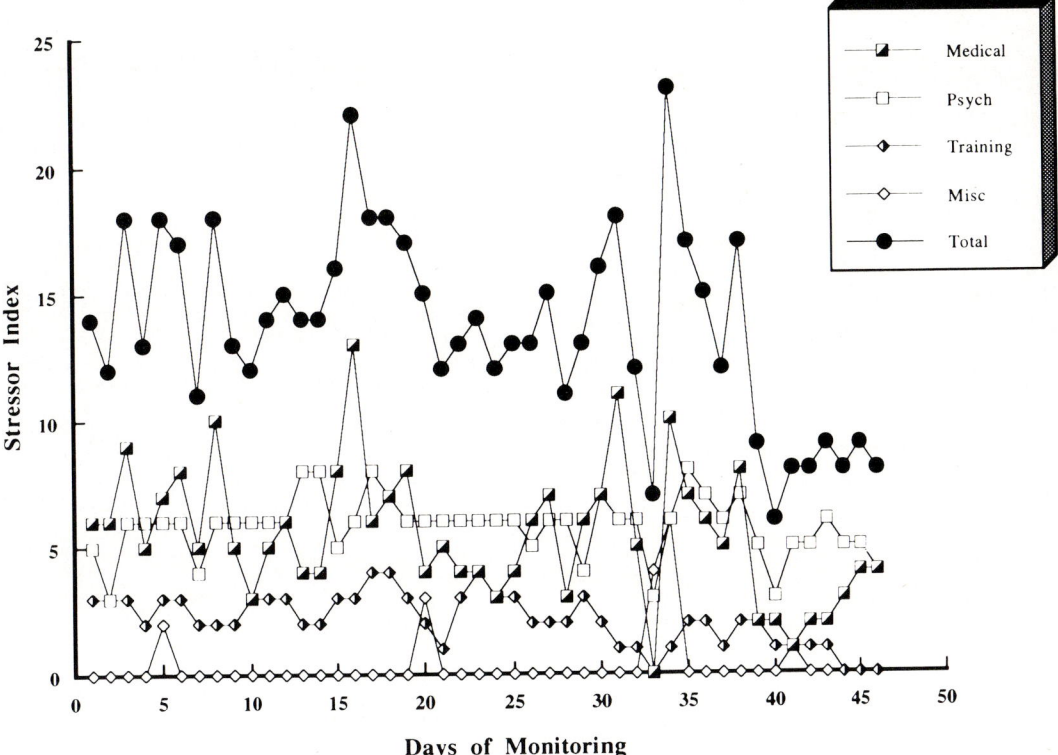

Figure 2 Example of the monitoring program used to follow athletes at risk of overtraining. In this case the daily stress questionnaire response has been plotted against time. Individual lines reflect the medical, psychological, training, miscellaneous, and total stressor index.

changed before any deterioration in performance. Symptoms of insomnia, an URTI, increased fatigue, or muscle or joint discomfort next caused the medical index to rise. Performance indicators usually remained unchanged. If the condition persisted unchecked, performance began to decrease within a few days. The pattern of decrement seems to be, in order, psychological status, medical condition, and then performance. The perception of training does not seem to play a major role in the development of this condition. The monitoring tool can be used effectively to follow athletes and it allows interventions designed to prevent the overtraining syndrome from developing fully.

As demonstrated in the example, one contributor to the overtraining syndrome is the stress of long-distance travel. This factor often precedes a major competition and when it spans three or more time zones, it significantly augments the stressor index. The anxiety of impending competition, exposure to the media, and other changes in the training program are also present concurrently with travel. Alterations in sleep patterns, exposure to individuals with URTIs, and less than optimal nutrition are all common features of international travel and, in my opinion, contribute substantially to the development of overtraining.

The initial form of intervention need not always be related to the physical training program, and does not always require a reduction of training intensity or volume. If an increase in the stress index can be traced to interpersonal difficulties between team members, the appropriate intervention is to resolve the conflict. In such a case, the physical demands of training need not be modified.

HEART RATE MONITORING

The use of portable telemetric heart rate monitors is routine in the physiologic assessment of high-performance athletes. Portable computers and computer-heart rate monitor interfaces permit the coach or support staff to record the heart rate daily during every workout. This has many advantages and several observations warrant comment when dealing with the possibility of overtraining. Assessment of morning heart rate has been cited frequently in the literature as the gold standard for the identification of overtraining. This parameter has considerable variability and the observation of an increase in resting heart rate, associated with

symptoms of overtraining, is not a consistent finding. Only one study that recorded sleeping heart rate consistently demonstrated increased heart rates. The slope of the recovery heart rate following a maximal exercise task has also failed to demonstrate a consistent pattern that could serve as an index of overtraining.

A decline in maximal heart rate is a very common finding in athletes who are showing signs of overtraining and alterations in questionnaire scores. I have been impressed with the reproducibility of this observation. The maximal heart rate obtained during periods of intense training will drop by 10 to 15 beats per minute (bpm). For example, an athlete who routinely obtains a heart rate of 195 bpm during an interval workout will demonstrate a peak rate of approximately 180 bpm during an identical workout if the subtle symptoms of overtraining and a change in the stressor index are present. Performance currently remains unaffected. The advantage of recording the heart rate during workouts is emphasized and the computer interface assumes added importance, as these observations would often be missed unless computerized monitoring was available to the athlete and the coach. The heart rate changes are often quite dramatic and can occur over the course of 7 to 10 days. The maximal heart rate rises slowly as the stressor index returns toward baseline values. Following the athlete with these two monitoring tools, as they prepare for competition, offers clearer insight into responses to any adjustments in the training program and clarifies the impact of other stressors that may be influencing performance adversely.

SUGGESTED READING

Barron GL, Noakes TD, Levy W, et al. Hypothalmic dysfunction in overtrained athletes. J Clin Endocrin Metab 1985; 60:803–806.

Fry RW, Morton AR, Keast D. Overtraining in athletes: An update. Sports Med 1991; 12:32–65.

Fry RW, Lawrence SR, Morton AR, et al. Monitoring training stress in endurance sports using biological parameters. Clin J Sports Med 1993; 3(6):6–13.

Karvonen J. Overtraining. In: Karvonen J, Lemon PWR, Iliev I, eds. Medicine in sports training and coaching. Med Sport Sci Basel Karger, 1992; 35:174–188.

Kuipers H, Keizer HA. Overtraining in elite athletes. Review and directions for the future. Sports Med 1988; 6:79–92.

Morgan WP, Brown DR, Gaglin JS, et al. Psychological monitoring of overtraining and staleness. Br J Sports Med 1987; 21:107–114.

Ryan AJ, Brown RL, Fredrick EC, et al. Overtraining in athletes; a round table discussion. Physician Sportsmed 1983; 11(6):93–110.

Seyle H. The stress of Life. New York: McGraw-Hill, 1956.

EXERCISE AND TRAINING RESPONSES IN THE HEALTHY CHILD

ROY J. SHEPHARD, M.D., Ph.D., D.P.E., F.A.C.S.M.

Much of our current knowledge of normal responses to exercise has been obtained from observations of young adult males. When carrying out exercise screening, testing, and prescription in children, it is therefore important to recognize that both the acute and the chronic responses to exercise differ between children and mature adults. This chapter examines the nature of these differences, looking at the course of normal growth and development and discussing gender differences.

NORMAL GROWTH AND DEVELOPMENT

Children do not grow at a uniform rate throughout their development. There is a particularly rapid increase in height followed (particularly in boys) by a rapid increase in body mass during puberty (the pubertal "growth spurt"). Further, there are substantial interindividual differences in biologic age at any given calendar age, with corresponding variations in the timing and magnitude of the pubertal growth spurt. These factors have important implications for the sports physician in terms of appropriate procedures for the standardization of test data and the matching of contestants to ensure fair and safe competition.

Data Standardization

The simplest method of adjusting exercise test data for individual differences in body size is to express findings as a ratio to body mass. For example, a subject's maximal aerobic power may be expressed in units of ml/[kg · min]. Using a test score to assess a child's potential performance in an endurance event may be effective, since most such competitions involve the displacement of body mass against gravity, and the oxygen cost of a sustained physical task is usually roughly proportional to the individual's body mass. If, however, the intent is to compare fitness scores from one age category to another, the choice of units becomes more controversial. When aerobic power is expressed per kilogram of body mass, scores commonly decrease over much of childhood, with the rate of loss accelerating at puberty (Fig. 1). This has led at least one investigator to infer that because of insufficient or inadequate school programs of physical education, aerobic fitness deteriorates once a child sits behind a classroom desk.

However, there is no fundamental biologic reason why maximal oxygen intake should develop as a constant linear function of a child's body mass. Indeed, some

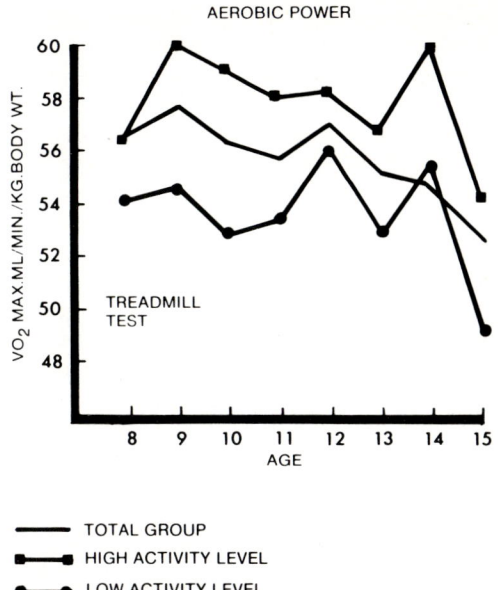

Figure 1 Relationship between maximal oxygen intake (expressed per kilogram of body mass) and age. Longitudinal observations on Saskatchewan boys arbitrarily divided into active and sedentary categories. The authors concluded from their investigation that there was a progressive deterioration of fitness over the period of school attendance. (Based on the data of Bailey DA. Exercise, fitness and physical education for the growing child. In: Orban WAR, ed. Proceedings of the National Conference on Fitness and Health. Ottawa: Health and Welfare Canada, 1974:13.)

dimensional theorists have argued that there are good reasons for anticipating that aerobic power would increase in proportion to height^2, or (body mass)$^{2/3}$. If the height^2 assumption is made, the data set used to calculate Figure 1 would show aerobic power as remaining relatively stable throughout childhood, and schools would no longer stand accused of causing a decrease in fitness among their pupils.

A third possible approach to data standardization is to measure physiologic variables throughout childhood, and to determine empirically how values develop in relation to height. Fitting logarithmic equations to our data, we have found height exponents in the range 2.50 to 3.0, a relationship that is close to the per kilogram assumption.

Competitive Matching

Competitive matching is important in growing children, both to ensure fair contests and to avoid unnecessary injuries. Participants in team competitions such as ice-hockey are commonly classified by age group. This is not a satisfactory approach, given that there are substantial interindividual differences in body size at any given calendar age. Particularly around the time of puberty, children may find they are playing against others who are much larger, stronger and heavier than themselves. In consequence, small and late-maturing children are at a substantially increased risk of physical injury if they participate in contact sports. A combination of such hazards with the discouragement of unsuccessful competition leads to a high drop-out rate from age-category sports leagues, with selective retention of a minority of tall, heavy, early maturers in the ice-hockey leagues (Fig. 2).

An alternative option is to base the classification of players on body mass, as is already done for some individual contests such as wrestling, boxing, and rowing. Unfortunately, weight-based systems of classification have stimulated drastic precompetition reductions of body mass by restriction of food and fluids, heat exposure, the wearing of impermeable garments during training, the administration of diuretics, and even blood donation, with such abuses beginning early during high school competition.

Given the fairly close cubic relationship between standing height and body mass, the individual's stature provides a simple method of classification with little potential for abuse. It is commonly used for commercial assessments of age (for instance, the determination of eligibility for children's bus fares), but to date has had surprisingly little use in the classification of sports contestants.

Maximal Oxygen Intake in Children

It is not easy to make good laboratory determinations of maximal oxygen intake in prepubertal children. Many young subjects are unwilling to push themselves into oxygen deficit, and probably for this reason a substantial proportion of those who are tested fail to reach the classical definition of an oxygen consumption plateau (an increase in oxygen consumption < 2 ml/[kg·min] with a substantial increase of power output). It may also be difficult to assess the quality of a subject's peak effort from the subsidiary criteria of heart rate and blood lactate concentration that would be applied in an adult. Anxiety in the test situation can give a young child a heart rate that approximates theoretical maxima during vigorous submaximal exercise. Likewise, peak lactate levels are substantially lower than in adults, although it is unclear how far this reflects physiologic maturity and how far it indicates unwillingness to sustain anaerobic effort.

Most authors have described peak heart rates of around 195 to 200 beats/min, much as in young adults, although there have been occasional reports that with strong encouragement, children can attain peak readings as high as 210 to 215 beats/min. The cardiac output for a given absolute oxygen intake is apparently somewhat less in a child than in an adult (the so-called "hypokinetic circulation"), but there seems no other physiologic reason for the difference in peak heart rate between children and young adults. The consensus ceiling of 195 to 200 beats/min is therefore probably realistic for an average child. The peak oxygen intake observed at heart rates of 195 to 200 beats/min has consistently been 48 to 50 ml/[kg·min] in urban boys, and around 40 ml/[kg·min] in urban girls. Scores are currently somewhat lower in rural than in urban communities, probably

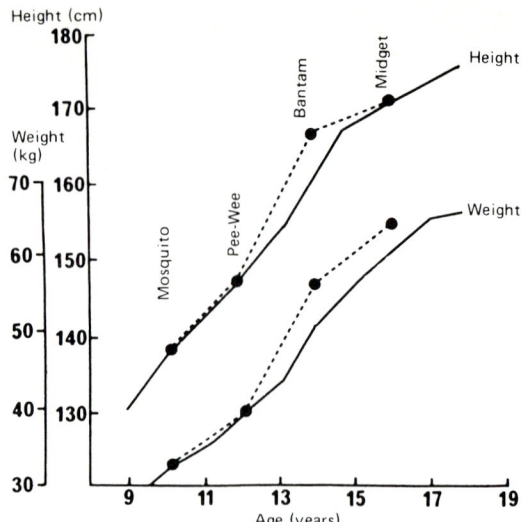

Figure 2 The influence of competitive selection on the physical characteristics of boys participating in an ice-hockey league categorized by chronologic age. The solid lines illustrate the normal growth of height and weight in Canadian children, and the interrupted lines show the characteristics of the ice-hockey players. (From Shephard RJ, Lavallée H, Larivière G. Competitive selection among age-class ice-hockey players. Br J Sports Med 1978; 12:11–13; with permission.)

because rural children are now taken to school by bus and have less facilities for active recreation than do their urban peers. However, values as much as 20% above the urban average have occasionally been observed in very active populations, such as the traditional circumpolar community of Inuit children that we studied in 1969/70. It would therefore appear that the average North American prepubescent child is no longer active enough to develop full cardiorespiratory potential. Support for this view is provided by the long hours that young children now devote to sedentary pursuits such as watching television and playing video games, the 10 to 20% improvements in the physical working capacity of Canadian school-aged children that have followed community-wide fitness campaigns, and the recently observed decline of fitness among circumpolar children as television programs and video stores have reached the far north.

For any given maximal oxygen intake, physical performance is somewhat poorer in a child than in a young adult, because most tasks from running to competitive sports are performed with a lower mechanical efficiency. This is due in part to shorter limb length and in part to poorer coordination of body movements. It is important to take account of such differences when translating the distance covered during a timed run into an approximation of aerobic power (Table 1).

Anaerobic Capacity and Anaerobic Power

Local reserves of oxygen and energy rich phosphagens per unit of muscle mass are very similar in children and adults, but if the much smaller muscle mass is

Table 1 Estimation of Aerobic Power from the Distance Covered in a 12 Minute Run. A Comparison of Normal Values for a Young Adult, with the Values Derived from the Energy Cost of Running in 9–12-Year-Old Children

	Estimated Aerobic Power (ml/[kg · min])		
Distance Run (km)	Adult	Girl	Boy
1.6	28	39	41
2.0	34	47	48
2.4	42	55	56
2.8	52	63	64

Data from Cooper K. Aerobics. New York: Evans, 1968, and Shephard RJ, et al. Union Médicale 1974; 103:1767-1777.

considered, the total anaerobic power of a young child is much smaller than that of an adult. Scores on a test of relative anaerobic power (the Margaria staircase sprint) increase progressively from 8 through 20 years of age, although the observed gains in performance probably reflect an improvement of coordination as much as a true increase of anaerobic power.

Blood lactate levels of prepubescent children commonly peak at 8 to 10 mmol/L during bouts of exhausting effort, as compared with 10 to 12 mmol/L in a young adult. The peak oxygen deficit (an average of 63 ml/kg of body mass in boys and 47 ml/kg in girls) is also less than the figure (70 to 75 ml/kg) that might be expected in an adult. The child thus has less ability to undertake sustained anaerobic activities. This has been attributed to an immaturity of physiologic and biochemical systems, particularly low concentrations of glycolytic enzymes in the skeletal muscles. Another important consideration is that the total muscle mass is smaller relative to blood volume. A lower peak blood lactate concentration would thus be expected, even if the peak muscle lactate concentrations were identical with those seen in a young adult. Finally, it is more difficult to persuade young children to sustain maximal anaerobic effort to biochemical exhaustion. In one study, we found terminal blood lactate figures as high as 12 mmol/L in that third of children who were judged to have made a strenuous effort.

Training Response of Children

The optimal age of beginning serious training remains a controversial issue, with particular implications for the training of international-class competitors. Some authors have argued that it is difficult to induce gains of either aerobic fitness or muscle strength in the prepubescent child through physical education or training programs. This has been attributed either to a high inherent level of physical activity or to an immaturity of biochemical systems.

Several pieces of evidence now support the view that gains of aerobic condition are possible during the primary school years: (1) in the Trois Rivières regional experiment, the addition of an hour per day of vigorous physical education to the normal primary school curriculum was enough to induce 10 to 15% gains of

maximal oxygen intake in students 8 years of age and older (Fig. 3); (2) blind students who attended a residential school with a strong physical education program developed a high level of aerobic fitness, but this was lost during the summer vacation months when they returned to their homes; and (3) highly active young Inuit children living in a rigorous circumpolar environment had a high level of aerobic fitness when they were first tested in 1969/70, but this advantage was lost as television and video rentals became available to the community. Earlier negative reports may reflect such factors as training programs that were too short in duration or intensity, compensating reduction of "free" activities, and the neglect of seasonal variations in physical condition.

In the case of strength training, it is also becoming clear that peak muscle force can be increased before puberty. A newborn child has about 2% large type I fibers, 50 to 60% normal type I fibers, 20% type IIa fibers, 3 to 5% type IIb fibers, and 15 to 20% undifferentiated fibers (see the chapter *Skeletal Muscle Fibers: Types and Distribution*). In contrast, at maturity there are no large type I fibers and very few undifferentiated fibers. Considerable differentiation of fibers must therefore occur over the course of normal human development. The total number of muscle cells seems fixed early in infancy, however, and any subsequent increase of muscle dimensions occurs by hypertrophy (the growth of existing fibers) rather than by hyperplasia (the development of new fibers). It was once thought that prepubescent children could not respond to resistance training because of low concentrations of circulating androgens. Several reports have now shown that demanding programs can induce gains of voluntary strength in the prepubescent age group, although the response occurs more slowly than in an adult who is exposed to a similar volume of training. A training response develops in the absence of significant muscle hypertrophy. Presumably, it is attributable to such factors as an increase of muscle-excitation coupling, improved motor skills, and increased motor unit activation.

Exercise Guidelines for the Healthy Child

Participation in vigorous sport and physical activity establishes patterns of behavior that, if pleasurable, are likely to continue into adult life. Many school programs of physical education unfortunately fail to establish a lifelong interest in physical activity. A substantial part of the class period is often occupied by changing clothes and listening to instructions, and the time allocated to vigorous movement may be too little to have any useful training effect. The program may also fail to arouse the interest of the student, so that exercise ceases abruptly once the program is no longer a required part of the curriculum. Failure to pursue activity into adult life seems particularly likely where children have allocated many hours per day to intensive competitive training, neglecting their normal social development in the hope of success in international competition.

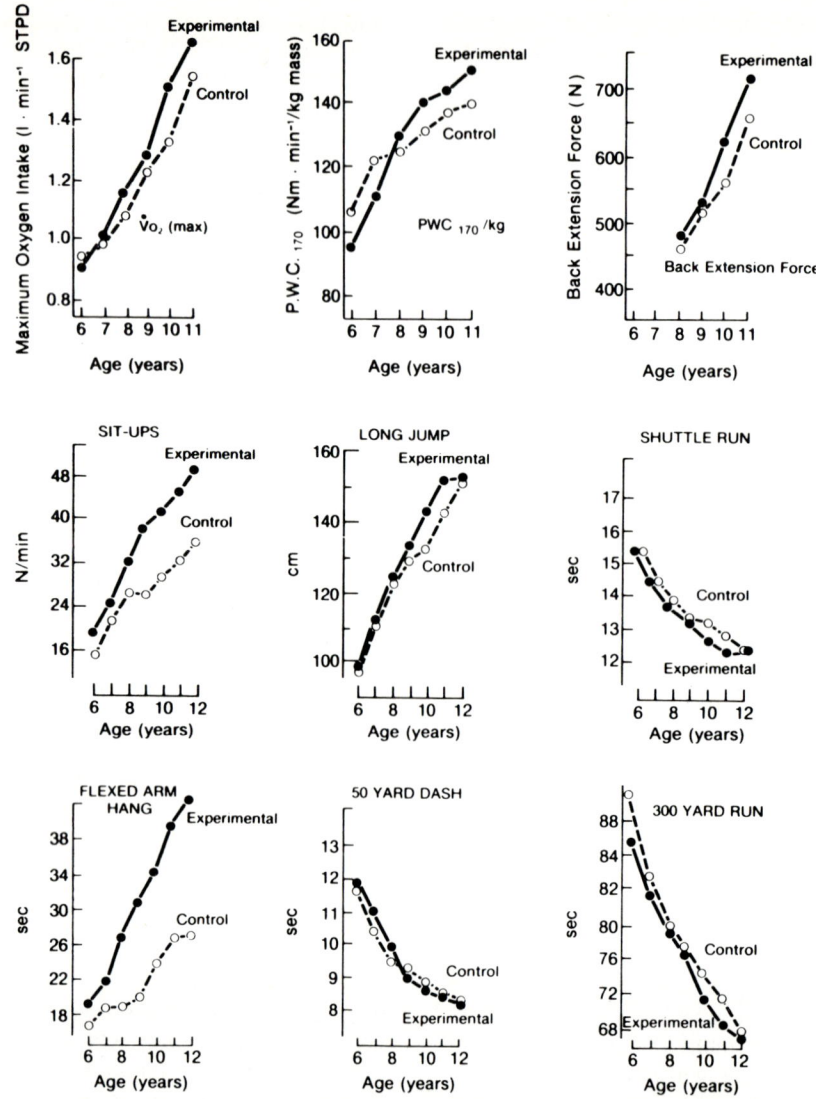

Figure 3 Influence of an hour per day of required physical activity on the fitness of primary school students. Data from the Trois Rivières regional experiment. (Based on the data of Shephard and Lavallée, 1977; from Shephard RJ. Physiology and biochemistry of exercise. New York: Praeger Publishers, 1982; with permission.)

Nevertheless, there are important advantages to the introduction of a regular, moderate, well-disciplined, and well-designed program during the growing years. Initially the program should focus on instruction in the basic motor skills. From the age of 7 to 8 years coordination is sufficient for the child to progress to vigorous pursuits that will develop cardiorespiratory stamina and muscle strength. In the final years of primary school the child can also be introduced to a variety of team games. The physical education curriculum should be broad enough that every child can discover pursuits in which he or she can excel. A particular emphasis should be given to "carry over" pursuits that can later be followed as a family, and it may be helpful to increase the interest in long-distance hiking, canoeing, and cross-country skiing by linking such activities to the study of fauna, flora, and geology.

An ideal curriculum offers as much as a nominal hour of physical activity per day. Our studies in Québec have demonstrated that the primary school student can engage in such periods of exercise without any negative impact on the learning of academic subjects. Each class session should offer stimulus to the main muscle groups, and 20 to 30 min of varied aerobic exercise in the classical training zone (for children, a heart rate of 150 to 160 beats/min). Both the American Academy of Pediatrics and the American Orthopedic Society for Sports Medicine have concluded it is acceptable for prepubescent children to undergo strength training. However, care must be taken to avoid over-use injuries. Problems are particularly likely in events where there is a repeated strong reaction from the ground (for example, the epiphysitis of the tibial tubercle that develops from running excessive distances and excessive jumping) or from equipment (for example, medial epicondylitis in the baseball pitcher who is encouraged to throw an excessive number of "curved" balls).

Athletic Participation and Menarche

Participation in top-level gymnastics, figure skating, and prolonged endurance events is frequently associated with delayed menarche. The affected athlete is often dissatisfied with her current body image; the individual concerned thus has an inadequate intake of food energy and a very low percentage of body fat. In sports such as gymnastics, which favor the petite competitor, the deliberate selection of late maturers by coaches is a further factor contributing to late menarche. In a few unfortunate instances there may have been rumors of a deliberate delaying of normal maturation by "doping" procedures.

The onset of irregular menstruation or the development of a temporary amenorrhea are common concomitants of heavy training, particularly when such training is associated with a negative energy or nitrogen balance and the stress of intense competition. Normal menstruation is usually resumed when training is moderated or the food intake is increased. A weakening of bone structure is one possible negative consequence of such menstrual disturbances, and it is as yet unclear whether any resulting lack of bone mineralization can be made good after heavy training has ceased. If menstruation becomes irregular the sports physician should first rule out causes other than exercise (including pregnancy!). If an exercise-induced energy deficit is responsible for the irregularity, a normal cycle can usually be restored by a combination of counseling, a 10 percent reduction of training volume, and an increase of food intake sufficient to induce a modest (2 kg) increase of body mass. If anovulation or amenorrhea persist for longer than 3 to 6 months, medroxyprogesterone can be administered 14 days monthly, and calcium intake should also be increased to 1500 mg/day to minimize the risk of bone demineralization.

ISSUES OF GENDER

Sociocultural Influences

The extent of inherent physiologic differences between boys and girls is an extremely controversial issue, with important practical implications for the coaching of young athletes.

Some feminists have argued that much if not all of the commonly described gender differences in body form, physiologic characteristics, and athletic performance are not biologically determined, but are rather the result of substantial, gender-determined differences in opportunities and encouragement to practice physical activity and sport from an early stage in childhood. Attention has been drawn to the shrinking gap between male and female records in many types of competition, and it has been suggested that the currently available range of events favors male dominance. Further, it has been claimed that the time will soon arrive when young women outperform male competitors in a number of types of athletic competition.

More cautious analysts have recently noted that the rate of progress of female records is slowing down as a higher proportion of all girls and young women become involved in competition, and that it is looking less likely that the males will eventually be overtaken. Realists have pointed to the handicaps to endurance performance that emerge in the female competitor at puberty, particularly the added burden of fat and lower hemoglobin concentration. Nevertheless, it is also true that the average girl could realize much more of her potential with appropriate encouragement, and there remains much scope to persuade both schools and parents to give developing girls the equality of access to sport and physical education programs that they need and deserve.

Development of Morphologic Differences

With the specific exception of the sex organs, there are only minor differences of anthropometric characteristics between girls and boys through to the age of puberty. Girls tend to be a little fatter than boys from an early age, but it is hard to be certain that this does not reflect merely a lesser encouragement to a physically active lifestyle.

Girls commence their pubertal growth spurt 1 to 2 years earlier than the boys, around 9 to 10 years of age, thus complicating gender comparisons of physical performance between older school-age children. For a short period, the girls are taller than boys of a similar age, favoring their performance on many tests of physical skill. However, growth also tapers and ceases several years earlier in the girls, so their ultimate height is 10 to 15 cm less and their body mass 10 to 15 kg less than that of the boys.

At puberty girls also show a substantial increase in body fat, particularly in the breasts and around the hips and thighs. In males the dominant change is an increase of muscle, although there is also some increase of subcutaneous fat over the abdomen and chest. At maturity the males have a substantially larger muscle mass and greater cardiac dimensions than the female. However, there do not seem to be any consistent sex differences in the relative proportions of slow and fast twitch muscle fibers.

The mature female has a smaller thorax, a larger abdomen, a broader and shallower pelvis, shorter legs, and a lower relative center of gravity than the male. In part because of the nature of the games that have been played, and in part because of these biomechanical differences, girls show more graceful and better coordinated movements than boys. However, the broader hips increase their likelihood of patellar tracking problems and the shorter limb length limits stride frequency and thus peak running speeds.

All of the bones are smaller and lighter in girls, reducing the average density of the lean body compartment (a key figure in hydrostatic determinations of body fat). Some of the female fat accumulation of puberty is culturally imposed, but the minimum quantity of fat associated with good health is substantially larger in the female than in the male (10 to 12% rather than 3% of body mass). There has been an excessive emphasis on a slender physical appearance in some female sports (particularly figure skaters, ballet dancers, gymnasts, and baton twirlers), and participants have pursued this goal through a negative energy balance that sometimes progresses to frank anorexia nervosa. It is therefore useful to be able to estimate a patient's minimal desirable body mass. Katch and Katch have suggested that this can be calculated as Mass (kg) = 1.11 (Height, m) $\times$ $(D/33.5)^2$, where D is the sum (in centimeters) of twelve diameters (biacromial, chest, bi-iliac, bitrochanteric, right and left knees, right and left ankles, right and left elbows, and right and left wrists).

Problems of Data Standardization

A major problem in comparing the performance of older boys and girls is a lack of agreement on appropriate methods for data standardization. As previously noted, values such as peak muscle forces and maximal oxygen intake could be expressed per unit of $height^2$, per $height^3$, per kilogram of body mass, or per kilogram of lean mass. Total body mass is the usually adopted criterion, but this immediately places older girls at a disadvantage, since a higher proportion of the body mass is fat in postpubertal females. Again, many measurements of muscular performance examine torque (the product of muscle force and the length of the lever arm) rather than force itself, so gender-related differences in limb length become an issue as well as differences in muscle bulk.

Aerobic Power

Even before puberty there are commonly substantial differences of peak power output and maximal oxygen intake between average girls and boys. However, such discrepancies seem due almost entirely to sociocultural factors.

The gender discrepancy in aerobic power widens at puberty. Given that the absolute value for peak oxygen transport is a power function of body size, the greater height of the males could account for at least 30% of their ultimate advantage. A second important factor is a gender difference in blood hemoglobin concentration (typically 13.8 g/dL in a maturing young woman, but 15.6 g/dL in an adolescent boy). The lower values of the female apparently arise from a combination of a menstruation-related iron loss, lower blood levels of androgenic steroids, and in some cases deliberate dietary restriction. For every liter of blood that is pumped by the heart, a typical male can carry to the working tissues a 13% greater quantity of oxygen than a female subject. It is therefore particularly important to carry out regular checks of hemoglobin level and iron saturation in maturing female competitors. The smaller skeletal muscles of the female are an added handicap; the weaker muscles tend to contract at a larger fraction of their maximal voluntary force. Thus, at any given absolute work rate the cardiac after-load is greater in the female than in the male. After puberty, the absolute aerobic power as measured on a treadmill or cycle ergometer is at least 30-40% smaller in a female than in a male subject of similar age. Gender-related differences in the peak oxygen transport during aerobic arm exercise are of a similar order.

The substantial physiologic disadvantages of the female competitor are offset by a lighter body mass. She therefore performs a smaller total amount of work in any task that involves a displacement of body mass. If maximal oxygen intake values are expressed per kg of body mass, the gender discrepancy narrows to less than 20%. However, claims that there is no gender difference in the aerobic power of highly-trained postpubertal endurance athletes seem unwarranted. Oxygen transport is closely related to muscle mass and gender differences of aerobic power are smallest if data are expressed per kg of lean tissue mass. However, the practical significance of oxygen transport per kg of lean mass is unclear. Weight-supported tasks demand a certain level of absolute aerobic power and weight-dependent tasks require a specific oxygen transport per kg of total body mass. Depending on the activity to be performed, the aerobic power of male and female subjects should therefore be compared either in absolute units or per kg of body mass.

Anaerobic Power and Capacity

An individual's anaerobic power reflects mainly local stores of phosphagen energy in the active muscles. Because older girls are less muscular than boys, a substantial disadvantage of anaerobic power might be envisaged. Estimates based on tests such as all-out cycle ergometry (the Wingate test) and peak blood lactate readings suggest that the average female attains only 68 to 73% of typical male values. Much of this disadvantage disappears, however, if the anaerobic task is performed against body mass (for example, the Margaria staircase sprint). The ventilatory threshold is also reached at a similar fraction of maximal oxygen intake in both sexes.

Strength

After puberty the absolute muscular strength shows a 20 to 30% difference, but values for leg extension and quadriceps force become almost independent of gender if expressed per kilogram of body mass. The gender difference is smallest for the hip flexors and extensors. The discrepancies are larger for the muscles of the chest, shoulders, arms, and forearms. Young women are able to increase their muscle strength somewhat by resistance training, but they show little of the increase in muscle bulk seen when male adolescents engage in a similar regimen.

Perhaps the most striking gender difference is in the time required to reach peak force. Although female subjects have a higher proportion of fast twitch fibers, it

Table 2 Chromosome Patterns and Resulting Clinical Syndromes

Chromosome Pattern	No. of Barr Bodies	Clinical Syndrome
XY	0	Normal male
XX	1	Normal female
XO	0	Turner's syndrome (short, web-necked female)
XYY	0	Aggressive male (tall, sometimes psychopathic)
XXX	2	"Super-female" (low fertility, mental retardation)
XXY	1	Klinefelter's syndrome (tall, thin, eunuchoid appearance, poor coordination)
XXXXY	3	Klinefelter's syndrome (more severe variant)

still takes them almost twice as long to reach 70% of peak muscle force.

Flexibility and Coordination

Females have a substantial advantage of flexibility and fine motor skills, although it has been suggested that this is due largely to differences in play patterns that are imposed from an early age. Other factors contributing to the better coordination of the female are the lower center of gravity and the shorter average limb length. Reaction times of the female are similar to those of male peers but, because of shorter limb lengths and less powerful muscles, movement times are substantially slower in female subjects.

Determination of Gender

Because of the morphologic and physiologic differences previously discussed, the typical male has a significant advantage over the typical female in certain categories of athletic competition, particularly events calling for high levels of strength and explosive force. On occasion, the sex of competitors has therefore been disputed (for example, if there has been masculinization of appearance secondary to abuse of anabolic steroids). Pseudohermaphrodites with normal chromatin material but endogenous hormonal disturbances, rare variants of normal chromosome patterns (Table 2), and true hermaphrodites (with a mosaicism of the XY chromosomes) may also figure in such challenges.

Determination of the sex of athletes is normally based on an examination of cells scraped from the buccal mucosa, supplemented where necessary by blood tests and a gynecologic examination. Some 20 to 50% of cells in female subjects show darkly staining Barr bodies, formed by attachment of the second X-chromosome to the inner edge of the cell nucleus.

SUGGESTED READING

American Academy of Pediatrics. Weight training and weight lifting: Information for the pediatrician. Phys Sportsmed 1983; 11: 157–161.

Bar Or O. Pediatric sports medicine. New York: Springer, 1983.

Drinkwater BL, Bruemmer B, Chestnut CH. Menstrual history as a determinant of current bone density in young athletes, JAMA 1990; 263:545–548.

Fasting K, Tangen JO. The influence of traditional sex roles on women's participation and engagement in sport. In: Borms J, Hebbelinck M, Venerando A, eds. The female athlete: A socio-psychological and kinathropometric approach. Basel: S. Karger, 1980:41.

Frisch RE, Wyshak G, Vincent L. Delayed menarche and amenorrhea in ballet dancers. N Engl J Med 1980; 303:17–19.

Greendorfer SL, Brundage CL. Gender differences in children's motor skills. In: Adrian MJ Sports women. Basel: S. Karger, 1987; 125.

Prior JL. Reversible reproductive changes with endurance training. In: Shephard RJ, Åstrand PO, eds., Endurance in sport. Oxford: Blackwell Scientific Publications, 1992: 365.

Ramsay JA, Blimkie CJR, Smith K, et al. Strength training effects in prepubescent boys. Med Sci Sports Exerc 1990: 22:605–614.

Shephard RJ. Physical activity and growth. Chicago: Year Book Publishers, 1981.

Shephard RJ. Effectiveness of training programmes for the prepubescent children. Sports Med 1992;13:194–213.

Shephard RJ, Lavallée H, LaBarre R, et al. On the basis of data standardization in prepubescent children. In: Ostyn M, Beunen G, Simons J, eds. Kinanthropometry II. Basel: S. Karger, 1980: 306.

EXERCISE PRESCRIPTION FOR CHILDREN WITH CARDIO-RESPIRATORY DISORDERS

ROY J. SHEPHARD, M.D., Ph.D., D.P.E., F.A.C.S.M.

The principles of exercise for the healthy child have been discussed in a previous chapter. Here, some general recommendations are made for the child with various categories of cardio-respiratory disorder. Because of overprotection by parents, teachers, and even physicians, most such children fall far below their physiologic potential. Considerable gains of physical condition can thus accrue by authorizing a period of residence at a summer camp away from the parents, where the staff are familiar with both the disability and its potential response to a progressive conditioning regimen.

CONGENITAL HEART DISEASE

In a few forms of congenital heart disease, it is dangerous to encourage exercise (Table 1). Rare incidents of sudden death in school athletic programs have usually been traced to an anomalous origin of the coronary arteries. The heart is perfused with venous blood, and although the normal venous oxygen content (about 140 ml/L) may meet the needs of the resting heart, a fivefold to sixfold increase in myocardial oxygen consumption and a decrease of mixed venous oxygen content (to about 60 ml/L) quickly lead to myocardial ischemia during vigorous exercise.

The pressure gradient across an aortic or pulmonary valvular stenosis increases as the cardiac output rises. A lesion that is well tolerated at rest can quickly provoke myocardial ischemia during heavy exercise.

A large left-to-right intracardiac shunt provokes structural changes in the pulmonary vasculature. Pulmonary arterial pressures are higher than normal, even under resting conditions, and during vigorous exercise they may exceed systemic pressures. The consequence is a sudden reversal of the intracardiac shunt. Sometimes, the drop in arterial oxygen saturation is sufficient to cause a loss of consciousness, which can be dangerous in a number of sports. Loss of consciousness is also possible if a septal defect damages the normal mechanism for the conduction of electrical impulses in the heart.

Most major cardiac anomalies are now corrected surgically at an early age. Assuming a successful operation, such children can be encouraged to pursue a normal sports program. Minor lesions such as a small left-to-right interventricular shunt or a minor narrowing of the pulmonary outflow tract are not normally contraindications to an active life-style. Nevertheless, such

Table 1 Absolute and Relative Contraindications to Vigorous Exercise in Children with Congenital Heart Disease

Absolute contraindications
  Aortic stenosis (peak gradient >40 mm Hg)
  Pulmonary stenosis (RV pressure >80 mm Hg)
  Pulmonary hypertension (mean pressure >30 mm Hg)
  Large ventricular septal defect (Q_p/Q_s >2.5)
  VSD + Pulmonary stenosis, RV pressure >80% of LV
  Tetralogy of Fallot (prior to operation)
  Transposition of great arteries
  Hypertrophic cardiomyopathy
  Congestive cardiomyopathy
  Ebstein's anomaly
  Anomalous left coronary artery
  Uncorrected cyanotic heart disease
  Myocarditis
  Marfan's syndrome with aortic dilatation
Relative contraindications
  Postoperative coarctation or tetralogy of Fallot
  Moderate atrial septal defect
  Inoperable pulmonary atresia

conditions can lead to a progressive right ventricular hypertrophy and, if the coronary blood supply does not keep pace, there may be a growing tendency to right ventricular ischemia. It is therefore important to monitor the right ventricular dimensions of such individuals periodically by radiography and/or echocardiography, and to test for exercise-induced abnormalities in the ST segment of the electrocardiogram, making recordings over the surface of the right ventricle (V_1, V_2 leads).

Most children who have had congenital heart disease are restricted in their physical activity due to parental fears. It is therefore important to encourage exercise to the limits permitted by a knowledgeable physician.

ASTHMA

Depending on the rigor of diagnostic criteria, 4 to 10 percent of children have asthma. Most are vulnerable to exercise-induced bronchospasm (EIB). Such spasm may create a fear of physical activity in the affected child and/or the parents, resulting in below average levels of physical activity and physical fitness. In the great majority of cases, the exercise-induced attack is dramatic, but has little long-term health significance. The spasm typically wanes over 30 to 60 minutes of recovery. Although there are physiologic precipitants of asthma, there is also a strong psychogenic component. Both allergen- and exercise-precipitated attacks are reduced if the child is separated from the parents and sent to a summer camp that includes a vigorous physical activity program.

There are several physiologic reasons why exercise can precipitate bronchospasm. When ventilation exceeds about a third of the peak ventilatory effort, mouth breathing begins, thereby exposing the bronchi to cold, dry, and unfiltered air. Possibly, the mouth opens even earlier in a young child, because of the smaller size of the nasal passages. Once mouth breathing begins, heat is lost from the bronchial airways in an attempt to warm and humidify the inspired air. This causes a release of histamine from the mucosal mast cells, initiating bronchospasm. Equally, the process can be prevented by ingestion of cromolyn sodium before strenuous exercise; this medication stabilizes the mast cells.

A narrowing of the small peripheral airways leads to an uneven distribution of inspired gas. During expiration, there is also a steep pressure gradient along the intrathoracic airways, increasing the likelihood that the air passages will collapse if a forceful expiration is attempted.

Exercise typically causes unpleasant breathlessness if ventilation exploits more than 50 percent of the vital capacity range, although there is much interindividual variation. At the breathing rate adopted in vigorous exercise (40 to 50 breaths/min, with more rapid expiration than inspiration), much of the potential flow/volume curve is exploited with every breath. EIB is diagnosed if the one-second forced expiratory volume (FEV_1) is decreased by 15% or more, and one would anticipate at least a corresponding decrease in the threshold of unpleasant breathlessness. The likely consequence of EIB is a sudden halting of activity, and even if this does not occur, the intensity of voluntary activity will be moderated at least sufficiently to compensate for the bronchospasm.

In mild cases, reassurance, avoidance of cold, dry air, and prophylactic cromolyn sodium may allow a normal exercise schedule. In more severe cases, it may be useful to undertake special exercises to strengthen the inspiratory muscles; this then allows the child to take a rapid inspiration, followed by a slow expiration, avoiding expiratory collapse of the airway.

CYSTIC FIBROSIS

Cystic fibrosis (CF) affects several body systems. Lung function may be impaired by chronic bronchial infection, with a restriction of both vital capacity and FEV_1 that limits peak ventilatory efforts, and a poor distribution of inspired gas that leads to large increases in dead space ventilation. Associated pancreatic lesions lead to poor digestion and absorption of food, with resulting muscular weakness. The disorder may also affect the sweat glands; thermoregulation seems unimpaired, but salt losses are larger than anticipated, so that generous quantities of salt must be provided in hot weather.

Many children with CF are unwell, with low levels of physical fitness. Nevertheless, their functional capacity, and thus their quality of life, can be substantially increased by exercises designed to strengthen major muscle groups, increase ventilatory endurance, and develop cardiovascular fitness. In 1984, three Norwegian teenagers with CF successfully completed the New York Marathon.

SCOLIOSIS AND KYPHOSIS

There are many causes of spinal curvature, and in some instances the primary disorder (for example, cerebral palsy) may have more functional significance than the spinal deformity. A moderate spinal curvature is quite compatible with a normal level of fitness; however, severe scoliosis leads to a substantial reduction of aerobic power.

The primary impact is on the respiratory system, a stiffening of the rib cage increasing the work of breathing and decreasing lung volumes. A rapid and shallow pattern of breathing leads to a poor distribution of inspired gas, with an enlarged physiologic dead space, and an increase of the alveolar-arterial oxygen tension gradient. The pulmonary arterial pressure is often increased, due to a combination of hypoxic vasoconstriction and secondary proliferation of the vascular media.

A severe spinal curvature also tends to give an awkward gait and thus a high cost of ambulation. Partly because of these physical problems and partly because of embarassment at personal appearance, the habitual physical activity of such individuals is commonly limited, exacerbating their poor inherent fitness levels. A training program can improve physical condition in those with moderate curvature, but care must be taken in exercising individuals where pulmonary hypertension has already developed.

SUGGESTED READING

Bar-Or O. Pediatric sports medicine for the practitioner. New York: Springer Verlag, 1983.

Cumming GR. Exercise therapy in pediatric cardiology. In: Torg J, Welsh P, Shephard RJ, eds. Current therapy in sports medicine. 2nd ed. Philadelphia: BC Decker, 1990:39.

Godfrey S. Exercise induced asthma. In: Clark TJH, Godfrey S, eds. Asthma. London: Chapman & Hall, 1977.

Jones NL. Dyspnea in exercise. Med Sci Sports Exerc 1984; 16:14–19.

Lindh M. Energy expenditure during walking in patients with scoliosis: the effect of surgical correction. Spine 1978; 3:122–134.

Orenstein DM, Nixon PA. Exercise in cystic fibrosis. In: Torg J, Welsh P, Shephard RJ, eds. Current therapy in sports medicine. 2nd ed. Philadelphia: BC Decker, 1990:26.

Shephard RJ. Exercise-induced bronchospasm: A review. Med Sci Sport 1977; 9:1–10.

Shephard RJ. Exercise for the asthmatic patient: A brief historical review. J Sports Med Phys Fitness 1979; 18:301–307.

Shneerson JM. Pulmonary artery pressure in thoracic scoliosis during and after exercise while breathing air and pure oxygen. Thorax 1978; 33:747–754.

Schneerson JM, Madgwick R. The effect of physical training on exercise ability in adolescent idiopathic scoliosis. Acta Orthop Scand 1979; 50:303–306.

Stoboy H. Exercise tolerance in scoliosis. In: Welsh P, Shephard RJ, eds. Current therapy in sports medicine 1985–1986. Burlington, Ont: BC Decker, 1985:114.

EATING DISORDERS IN ATHLETES

CAROLINE DAVIS, Ph.D.
SIDNEY H. KENNEDY, M.D.

Anorexia Nervosa or Bulimia Nervosa

↟

Continuous Subsyndromal Form of Either Disorder

↟

Intermittent Abuse of Unhealthy
Weight Control Methods

↟

Intermittent Dieting Related to
Specific Competitive Events

↟

Healthy Eating Habits and Body Image

Figure 1 Suggested spectrum of disturbed eating patterns in athletes.

In sports such as gymnastics, dance, and synchronized swimming, success is determined not only by technical prowess, but also by grace and physical appeal. Therefore, an ultra-slender form confers an important performance advantage in such activities. In many other sports, a weight that is greater than a healthy minimum limits speed, endurance, and agility, and contributes to increases in fatigue. Thinner is faster, up to a point! As a consequence, the typical female athlete confronts body image pressures at a number of levels, from those performance-related pressures reinforced by coaches and trainers, to those inherent in the judging criteria that give physically attractive athletes "the winning edge". In recent years, we have also seen the widespread and vigorous promotion of regular exercise, weight control, and low-fat diets for the putative purposes of disease prevention, and an increase of physiologic and psychological well-being. Together, these influences convey a powerful message to the competitive female athlete, and provide strong incentives for her preoccupation with food intake and her efforts to reduce body mass.

Indeed, a number of studies have found that female athletes frequently employ extraordinary, and often extreme, methods to reduce body fat in order to improve both appearance and performance. Estimates of the proportion of female athletes who have employed at least one pathogenic weight-loss technique have varied from 30% to over 60%, depending on the sport(s) being examined. As a consequence, many experts believe that female athletes are at greater than normal risk of developing a serious clinical eating disorder. In the general population, about 4% of young women in the 15 to 35 years age range are affected by *anorexia nervosa* or *bulimia nervosa,* and up to 10% may have a partial form of either disorder. Typically, only 5% of cases seen at most specialized clinics are male. Figure 1 suggests a spectrum of disturbed eating patterns among athletes.

Despite the evidence that female athletes show greater weight concerns and problems with body image than one would expect among age-matched nonathletes, definitive large-scale prevalence studies have yet to be done. However, in a recent study of hospitalized eating disordered patients, undertaken at a major treatment center, and sampled over a 2 year period, we found that approximately 60% of the women had been involved in competitive athletics or dance before the onset of their disorder—a finding that supports the view that prevalence rates are substantially higher than in the general population. Of particular interest was our finding that a number of the athletic patients developed the clinical disorder only *after* terminating participation in their sport. A common theme emerged: When the patient stopped training, usually as a result of injury or conflicting scholastic pressures, she developed a strong fear of weight gain. Reasoning that food intake should be restricted if little energy was being expended, she then began seriously to restrict her food intake. Regrettably, it seems that the institutionalized preoccupation with body weight and slenderness that characterizes most female sports has consequences that reach beyond the competitive arena.

The diagnostic criteria for anorexia nervosa, as defined in the American Psychiatric Association *Diagnostic and Statistical Manual*—III (Revised), are a body mass less than 85% of the population average and, in women, at least 3 months of amenorrhea, associated with an uncompromising desire to be thin, and a disturbance in the self-perception of one's body. The bulimia nervosa syndrome may occur at an average or above average body mass, and in all cases is associated with strong body image disparagement. Criteria of bulimia nervosa include the presence of at least two binge-eating episodes a week for at least 3 months, accompanied by some attempt to reverse the effects of energy intake. This usually takes the form of self-induced vomiting and/or laxative abuse, but may also involve intense exercising or fasting.

Few medical disorders have attracted as diverse a range of etiologic theories. How women are presented in the media and by the fashion industry (e.g., the pairing of sexual attractiveness and career success with thinness) is seen as an underlying factor predisposing all women to the disorder. However, the preoccupation with weight and diet does not develop simply because there are social pressures on women to conform to a very slender standard of female beauty. Nor can we assume that these attitudes occur among female athletes merely because there are strong performance and competitive advantages to very low levels of body fat. Considerable research indicates that certain psychological characteristics are associated with eating pathologies. Unduly low self-esteem, high anxiety, and perfectionism are the most commonly reported premorbid personality characteristics of anorexic and bulimic women. These factors may drive the competitive athlete in her quest for "success" through external approval by coaches, admiration by peers, or better performances. Additional social factors are believed to contribute to the risk profile for eating disorders. Some women have experienced traumatic childhood events, whereas others perceive rejection or strong criticism by their families or their peers. Typically, the decision to boost self-esteem through dieting and attempts at altering external appearance is the first step to a severe eating disorder.

For the past decade or so, the concept of "compulsive exercising," or "exercise addiction" has been the subject of discussion both in the popular press and the academic literature—in particular because of claims that overexercising is a variant of anorexia nervosa, and that both syndromes have a similar etiology and similar psychological characteristics. In fact, the frequency with which a severe restriction of food intake and excessive physical activity coexist, offers some support to this theory. In our research, we found that 78% of a patient sample could be described as excessive exercisers during the acute phase of their eating disorder. Nevertheless, the nature of the relationship between self-starvation and hyperactivity is not entirely clear. Although most authorities have concluded that overactivity is simply a purging behavior, others have proposed that it occupies a more central role in the etiology of the eating disorder.

One theory that is highly relevant to the subculture of competitive athletics proposes that for many patients anorexia is not a *nervosa*, but represents a physiologically mediated outcome that occurs when dieting is combined with strenuous physical activity, whereby the two behaviors potentiate one another and become self-perpetuating. The impetus behind this theory of *activity-induced anorexia* has come from a body of well-controlled animal research. Experimental rats with voluntary access to an activity wheel begin to run when their daily food supply is restricted. They exhibit decompensated eating behavior within 1 week, with exponentially increasing running and decreasing food intake. In the original experiments, the animals literally ran themselves to death. On the other hand, control rats, with no access to a running wheel, learn to eat sufficient food in the restricted time frame to remain in energy balance. We found a remarkable parallel between these results and the pattern of exercising and dieting seen in our patients. Seventy-five percent of the patients reported an inverse relationship between physical activity and food intake, similar to that seen in the experimental animals, during the period of their maximum weight loss. Comments such as "the more I restricted food intake, the more I exercised"; "all I was doing was exercising"; and "the lower my weight got the more energy I had" were pervasive.

A complementary theory postulates that both self-starvation and excessive exercising are variants of an obsessive-compulsive disorder and are behavioral reflections of a dysregulation of the serotonergic system in the brain. In the light of this hypothesis, it is especially important to consider the large proportion of our patients (>90%) for whom exercising had, indeed, become a compulsive and ritualized behavior, who described their need to be physically active as "beyond my control," "driven to exercise," and "nothing would prevent me from exercising." The reports of these women left no doubt that their hyperactivity was not entirely determined by voluntary cognitive choice—it clearly resembled a compulsive activity.

TREATMENT OF ANOREXIA NERVOSA

Because of the potentially serious and irreversible complications associated with anorexia nervosa, there is an increasing emphasis on early detection and treatment. "Prevention packages" that provide information about the hazards associated with dieting are being evaluated among school children as young as 9 years old, although it may be equally important to reach other family members in an attempt to influence approaches to eating and weight regulation.

Patients referred to our center with a diagnosis of anorexia nervosa have been ill for an average of 7 years and have often failed to respond to various forms of treatment or have relapsed. In contrast to patients with most of the other conditions discussed in this book, it cannot be assumed that the anorexic patient is fully committed to recovery if this means the restoration of a healthy eating pattern and reversal of weight loss. The first step is to define a balance between "medical management" of the consequences of starvation with or without various forms of purging (see Table 1 for a summary of the most frequently reported complica-

Table 1 Complications of Anorexia Nervosa and Bulimia Nervosa

Cardiovascular	Endocrine	Metabolic
Peripheral cyanosis	Amenorrhea	Hypokalemia
Bradycardia	Hypothermia	Hyponatremia
Hypotension	Increased growth hormone levels	Increased serum amylase
Arrhythmias	Increased cortisol levels	Edema
Cardiomyopathy	Decreased T3, T4	Increased blood urea nitrogen
Dermatological	Musculoskeletal	Hypercholesterolemia (?)
Dry skin and nails	Delayed bone maturation	Decreased trace element levels
Thinning scalp hair	Reduced stature	Gastrointestinal
Lanugo hair	Osteoporosis	Dental caries
Carotene pigmentation	Hematologic	Parotitis
Callus formation on hands	Mild anemia	Bloating/early satiety
Irritation at corners of mouth	Low WBC count	Constipation
Neurologic	Low ESR	Diarrhea
Seizure	Thrombocytopenia	Esophageal or gastric dilation or rupture
Reversible cortical atrophy		Pancreatitis

tions), and the development of a trusting "therapeutic alliance."

We use structured assessment instruments to obtain detailed information about behavior and attitudes associated with both anorexic and bulimic disorders. The diagnosis is not one that is made by exclusion; rather, the cardinal features described earlier must be elicited. Out-patient treatment can be carried out by an individual therapist, provided that he or she is willing and able to manage both physical and psychological care. Under other circumstances, a physician may take responsibility for weight management (we aim for a weight gain of 0.5 to 1 kg/week for out-patients) often in association with a dietician, while a psychotherapist attempts to explore the developmental issues associated with low self-esteem, as well as the factors that are perpetuating the disorder. A target weight range is chosen, based on historical information about premorbid weight and weight at the time of last menstrual function; the target Body Mass Index (weight[kg]/height[m^2]) should generally equal or exceed 19. The menses may not return until the percentage of body fat is about 10% higher than its level prior to the onset of amenorrhea. Measures of weight, electrolytes, and electrocardiogram should be taken frequently if there is clinical concern.

If weight loss or further metabolic disturbances continue, despite several months of out-patient therapy, we admit patients to an intensive in-patient or day hospital therapy program. In both settings, supervised meals and steady increases in energy intake (from 6 megajoules [1500 kcals] up to 4 megajoules [3500 kcals] per day) are essential components of treatment. Various group and family therapy sessions are also part of these programs. It is not unusual for a patient to remain hospitalized for 14 to 16 weeks in order to reach the target weight, although more and more we are encouraging outside passes as well as participation in social sports activities (in contrast to the previous solitude of the compulsive anorexic exerciser). Using indices such as weight maintenance, menstrual regularity, ability to work or attend school, and "interpersonal connectedness," about 50% of the anorexic patients treated in this unit have a good outcome, with 30% in intermediate and 20% in poor outcome categories after a 3 to 5 year follow-up.

Patients with anorexia nervosa receive drug treatment for three main reasons. The significant relationship between anorexia nervosa and osteoporosis has caused us to consider estrogen replacement therapy as early as possible. We prescribe antidepressants only after weight gain and when a clear-cut depressive syndrome coexists. Preliminary evidence suggests that fluoxetine, at lower doses than are recommended for the treatment of bulimia nervosa, may reduce the obsessive component of anorexic behavior and make weight gain or maintenance easier. This awaits further confirmation. We rarely prescribe neuroleptic drugs such as chlorpromazine, although this was formerly considered to be a cornerstone of pharmacotherapy in anorexia nervosa. There is certainly no definitive antianorexia nervosa drug therapy at this time.

Table 2 Psychoeducational Themes in the Treatment of Bulimia Nervosa

Dieting predisposes to binge eating
Giving up vomiting decreases binges
Medical complications of bingeing and purging
Effect of these behaviors on mood and vice versa
Faulty beliefs about food, weight, and shape
Relationship between self-worth and bulimia nervosa
Setpoint and the regulation of body weight
Relative ineffectiveness of weight control

TREATMENT OF BULIMIA NERVOSA

We now rarely admit patients with bulimia nervosa to the in-patient unit unless there is an added complication such as failure to gain weight in pregnancy or uncontrolled diabetes mellitus. For most bulimic patients treated in our program, the deciding factors about where they receive treatment include the severity of the symptoms, as well as their need and willingness to take time off work or school in order to attend an intensive 5 days a week "day hospital" as opposed to a once-weekly group therapy program. The least intensive intervention involves a "psychoeducational" approach. Principles of psychoeducation are listed in Table 2. Up to 30% of the least severely ill bulimia nervosa population show a significant improvement with this treatment alone.

Individual cognitive-behavioral psychotherapy is the next level of treatment. A pathologic belief that alteration of weight and shape will lead to happiness, enhanced self-esteem, and self-control is challenged as a self-monitoring of weight and food intake is promoted.

There is more evidence to support specific pharmacologic interventions in bulimia nervosa either alone or preferably in combination with cognitive behavioral strategies. Fluoxetine (60 mg daily) has significant benefits in reducing both binge and vomit episodes. Other antidepressants including desipramine (Norpramin, Pertofrane), imipramine (Tofranil), and monoamine oxidase inhibitors such as phenelzine (Nardil) and isocarboxazid (Marplan), are also helpful, although side effects tend to be more limiting than with fluoxetine. Recently, the combined use of desipramine for 24 weeks with cognitive behavioral therapy was reported as being more effective than either treatment alone.

SUGGESTED READING

Brownell, KD, Rodin J, Wilmore J. Eating, body weight and performance in athletes. Philadelphia: Lea & Febiger, 1992.
Davis C, Kennedy SK, Ralevski E, Dionne M. The central role of physical activity in the development and maintenance of eating disorders. Psychol Med (in press).
Epling WF, Pierce WD. Solving the anorexia puzzle. Toronto: Hogrefe & Huber Publishers, 1992.
Kaplan AS, Garfinkel PE. Medical issues and the eating disorders: The interface. New York: Brunner/Mazel, 1993.

EXERCISE AND THE TREATMENT OF OBESITY

JANET WALBERG-RANKIN, Ph.D.

DIAGNOSIS

The point at which weight loss is medically recommended for someone who is currently above average weight has been controversial. Experts gathered by the National Institutes of Health in 1985 gave guidance in this regard by developing a definition of obesity based on the body mass index (BMI $= kg \cdot m^{-2}$). A BMI greater than approximately 27 was considered to be the point where obesity typically posed an increased health risk.* An example of an individual who would have a BMI of 27 would be someone who is 5 feet 8 inches tall and 186 pounds. A BMI in this range is comparable to the definition of obesity used by the American Medical Association in 1988 — an individual who is 20% or more above the "desirable weight" for their height. Preliminary analysis of the data from the recent U.S. nation-wide, NHANES III study suggests that the percentage of Americans considered to be obese has increased from 27% to 34% of the population over the last 10 years. Since obese individuals have three times the risk of diabetes and hypertension, and two times the risk of hypercholesterolemia, this represents an important focus for preventive medical efforts.

Another classification to look at when deciding who is most in need of weight loss is the pattern of body fat distribution. Those with fat in the abdominal region are at greater risk than those with fat primarily in the buttocks and thigh regions. Measurement of the waist to hip circumference ratio has been used to classify such risk. Those with a ratio greater than 0.95 or 0.8 (for men and women, respectively) are considered at increased risk. Recent evidence also suggests that the compartmentalization of abdominal fat as visceral or subcutaneous is important in predicting risk. Those individuals with high amounts of visceral fat appear to have the highest risks of hypertension, insulin resistance, and hyperlipidemia.

ETIOLOGY

Human obesity has been shown to have a genetic component through studies on twins and on adoptees. Heritability of body fat has been estimated to account for as much as 25% of the variance in population data. Genetic factors might be involved via an effect on metabolic rate. For example, a study of a group of southwest-ern American Indians that has a high proportion of obese individuals, suggests that their extremely high incidence of obesity may be linked with a genetic tendency towards a low metabolic rate. The weight gain in a group of these Indians over a 4 year interval was predicted by their metabolic rates; those with the lowest metabolic rates when first measured had the largest weight gains.

Environmental factors such as access to palatable foods can also play a role in the development of obesity. Research comparing the diet of obese and lean individuals has shown that the percent fat is often higher in the diets of obese individuals. A sedentary life-style is another risk factor for obesity. A recent report from the U.S. Centers for Disease Control showed a link between habitual physical activity and body mass in a sample of over 18,000 men and women. Obesity was most common in those who were inactive and uncommon in those who were active.

RATIONALE FOR EXERCISE

Dietary modifications, including a reduction in energy and fat intake, are an intrinsic part of an obesity treatment program. However, this chapter focuses on the role that exercise plays in treatment of obesity.

Many obese individuals want to avoid exercise. Why is it important to encourage them to exercise? Exercise appears to have health and psychological benefits. For some people, it is easier to add a new, positive behavior than to deprive themselves by changing their eating behavior. They get positive feedback and a feeling of accomplishment about their increased physical activity, regardless of any change in body mass.

Other benefits include an increased body fat loss compared to the same energy deficit induced by dieting. The hormonal changes that are induced by exercise stimulate a release of fat from the adipose cells and enhance the utilization of this fat by the working muscles. With aerobic exercise training, the capacity of the muscles to use fat during exercise increases. Thus, the drain on body fat during exercise increases as the individual's training status improves.

Perhaps the most compelling reason to incorporate exercise into a weight loss regimen is the evidence that continued exercise is one of the most consistent predictors of maintained body weight loss after cessation of a formal treatment program. Relapse is common in weight reduction programs, but several research groups have found that those who had most success in maintaining weight loss were more likely to report that they were still exercising than those who regained the lost weight.

SCREENING

Is everyone in a weight loss program a candidate for exercise? Most people who are recruited to such programs could begin low- to moderate-level exercise without sophisticated and expensive exercise stress testing. The exception is that those with known disease, such as

---

*Editor's Note: When applying the BMI to *individuals* rather than populations, it is important to recognize that some categories of athlete have a high BMI because of a muscular body build rather than obesity.

cardiovascular, pulmonary, or diabetes mellitus should always undergo an exercise test supervised by a physician before beginning any exercise program. Individuals with at least two cardiovascular risk factors (hypertension, hypercholesterolemia, smoking, diabetes mellitus, family history of premature heart disease, or apparently healthy men and women who are above 40 and 50 years of age, respectively) should undergo an exercise test only if they are planning to participate in vigorous exercise ($>60\%$ $\dot{V}o_2max$). In order to stratify individuals as suggested above, the use of health history questionnaires and basic clinical evaluations is appropriate. If their history or clinical examination suggests latent disease, they should be referred for a more detailed medical evaluation before participation in exercise.

MOTIVATION

How can one motivate an obese individual to exercise? Reports estimate that only 22% of all adult Americans exercise at the level recommended for health improvement. It seems likely that a much smaller percent of the obese population is currently exercising. The first step in encouraging an increase in physical activity is to determine the barriers to exercise participation. A Gallup Poll of over 1,000 U.S. citizens, conducted in 1985, reported that the top reason given by those surveyed who did not exercise was "lack of time"; several large surveys of Canadians have reached similar conclusions. A counselor should undertake a time analysis for these people, to see where exercise could most logically fit into a normal day. There may be a misconception that exercise requires commitment of a large block of time. A study from Stanford University found that 10 minutes of exercise, repeated three times per day, was almost as effective as one 30 minute session. Thus, someone might gain the necessary exercise by taking a short walk before work, during lunch, and after work. Also among the top seven reasons given by people surveyed in the Gallop Poll for not exercising was "not necessary." Individuals with such an opinion need to be informed about the multiple, confirmed benefits of exercise for things like a reduction in the risks of cardiovascular disease and cancer, preservation of bone strength with delay or prevention of osteoporosis, and possible reductions in back pain and injury due to a strengthening of the supporting musculature.

The impact of a physician recommending an increase in physical activity to a patient cannot be underestimated. A 1989 survey found that most of the individuals reporting 2 days or less of exercise per week would consider more exercise if this had been recommended by a physician.

EXERCISE PRESCRIPTION

Once the individual is mentally ready to begin an exercise program and has been sufficiently screened to rule out contraindications, the exercise prescription should be developed. This prescription should define the type, frequency, intensity, and duration of the exercise sessions.

Type

Type includes the decision about the mode of activity. Most exercise programs for the treatment of obesity emphasize aerobic activity, since such exercise tends to utilize the most energy as well as the most body fat. Walking, jogging, swimming, and cycling are common activities that qualify as aerobic. One advantage of walking and jogging is that such activity can be pursued anywhere, without a need for special facilities or equipment. Also, little skill training is likely to be necessary for such activities. The decision whether to walk or to jog is largely determined by the individual's fitness level. Walking is excellent for an initial exercise program, but it may provide an insufficient stimulus for continuing fitness gains and energy consumption once the individual's fitness improves. One advantage of walking over jogging is that stresses on the feet are diminished and the potential for injury is correspondingly reduced.

Swimming requires a basic level of skill before this can be used as a means of weight reduction. Since obese individuals are very buoyant, they expend little energy to remain on the surface of the water. Most of the energy expenditure comes from propulsion through the water. It is especially important to monitor the intensity of exercise, using heart rate measurements, when swimming, in order to ensure a significant energy expenditure. An additional point regarding intensity is that the heart rate is lower during water exercise than a corresponding intensity of land exercise. Thus, the target heart rate must be modified downward by about 10% when giving a swimming exercise prescription.

Stationary exercise on a cycle ergometer can be useful for overweight individuals, since the body weight is then supported, reducing the stress on the joints. Boredom may be reduced by using distractions such as music or videos.

Resistance weight training is not typically included in an exercise prescription for the overweight individual. However, the theoretical benefits of this type of exercise include an increase in lean body mass and possibly an increase of metabolic rate. Recent research using resistance weight training along with very-low-energy diets ($\sim$3.4 megajoules, $\sim$800 kcal/day) has not found complete protection against a loss of lean body mass. However, muscle biopsies showed hypertrophy of the muscle fibers that have been involved in the weight training. This shows that muscle growth is possible even during periods of relatively rapid weight loss. A study using a more modest energy restriction ($\sim$5 megajoules, 1,200 kcal/day) actually found an increase in total lean body mass in women who were participating in weight training. Our laboratory has used weight training with success in a weight reduction program for obese women. The initial prescription we used was 15 repetitions at

50% to 60% of the measured maximum strength for five lifts. Additional exercises and sets were added over the 12 week program, until participants were completing three sets of 8 to 12 repetitions at 70% to 85% of maximal force. Positive aspects of a weight training program include a rapid feedback of improvements in strength, an increase in self-esteem, and a reduced sense of effort during daily activities, due to increased muscle strength. The negative aspects of including a weight training program in an exercise prescription are that equipment is required, initial skill training is necessary, and injuries are possible.

Another important issue is whether the individual should participate in a supervised exercise program or whether they can exercise on their own. Some people may require the constant encouragement involved in a supervised setting, whereas others may find it too inconvenient to attend a supervised program. Both settings can be effective. Cost, convenience, personality, skill, and risk level are important when determining the appropriateness of supervised or unsupervised programs.

If a supervised exercise program is recommended, who should be doing the supervision? Exercise leaders certified by national organizations such as American College of Sports Medicine (ACSM) have the knowledge and skills to lead an exercise program safely. These leaders should also be certified in CPR and prepared to handle any emergencies that may arise. One of the most important characteristics of a good exercise leader is enthusiasm. One of the most frequently listed strengths of our weight loss exercise programs in written evaluations has been the "enthusiasm of instructors."

Frequency and Duration

We typically have our participants exercise at least 4 days per week, but 3 days per week should be considered a minimum for weight loss. Exercising at the same time each day helps to develop the exercise as a habit and a routine part of a normal day. Duration should be emphasized as time permits, since more prolonged exercise increases the utilization of body fat. We typically begin with 20 minutes and work up to 40 minutes per session. An appropriate goal is to expend 800 to 1,200 kilojoules (200 to 300 kcal) per session. Certainly, frequency and duration can be overemphasized to the point that overuse injuries arise. To prevent this, both the frequency and the duration of exercise should be increased gradually. The individual should also be reminded to reduce training if pain or discomfort arise.

Intensity

In the past, ACSM stated that a minimum intensity of 60% of maximal heart rate is required to benefit from aerobic exercise. However, more recent research has led them to modify this recommendation. It is now suggested that benefits such as a reduced mortality accrue even from low levels of activity, as compared to a sedentary life-style. So, it is likely that any exercise, even if discontinuous and of low-intensity, is beneficial for the sedentary individual. But, to maximize energy usage and a resultant metabolism of body fat, a moderate intensity of aerobic exercise (at 60% of maximal heart rate) might be a suitable goal for those who can tolerate this. As fitness increases, the intensity should be increased as tolerated, but not to the extent that the duration and frequency of effort are compromised.

Education

Many obese individuals avoid exercise and thus do not have the skills or the knowledge to participate in certain activities. Thus, education is an important component of a program that includes exercise. Topics to be covered could include: appropriate clothing, safety issues, handling minor injuries, environmental conditions and fluid consumption, description of what happens to the body during exercise, and teaching of new physical skills (e.g., weight training). This information could be provided just before the time of supervised activity or on a rest day. For example, we have used a regimen of 4 days exercise and a 1 day education session for each week of formal treatment.

Maintenance

Initiation of exercise behavior is important in enhancing the loss of body weight and fat during a weight control program. But, maintaining the exercise behavior is a bigger challenge. Relatively simple procedures such as keeping a personal record of diet and activity may increase the patients' awareness of changes in their behavior. Goals and rewards could be planned, based on these records. Encouraging development of a social support network may also help people to initiate and to sustain exercise behavior. For example, exercising with a spouse, a friend, or a group is likely to increase compliance with the physical activity program.

Program counselors may contribute to maintenance of exercise through intermittent contact with participants after the formal program has been completed. Monthly phone contact from program personnel following formal treatment enhanced weight loss maintenance in a study conducted at Stanford University. The program counselors may aid maintenance by emphasizing certain topics during the intervention period—for instance, problem solving and handling high-risk situations. Thus, a participant who is involved in a regular outdoor walking program may be asked how they would handle a day when the weather was inclement.

Finally, sporadic reassessment of fitness, body composition, or other health-related factors may provide some motivation to continue an exercise program. These tests allow individual feedback concerning the patient's progress.

An increase in physical activity can help obese individuals to reduce their body fat content as well as to improve their general health. Following screening to rule out contraindications to exercise, an aerobic exercise prescription should be developed. The emphasis should be on duration and frequency of physical activity, with intensity being moderate and comfortable. Recent evidence suggests that weight training has psychological as well as physical benefits for the overweight individual. However, adequate initial skill training and supervision are required to make this an effective component of the program. Individuals attempting to lose weight should be told that continued exercise is one of the most consistent predictors of sustained weight loss.

SUGGESTED READING

American Medical Association. Treatment of obesity in adults. JAMA 1988; 260:2547–2551.

Burton BT, Foster WR. Health implications of obesity: an NIH consensus development conference. J Am Diet Assoc 1985; 85: 117–121.

Donnelly J, Sharp T, Houmard J, et al. Muscle hypertrophy with large-scale weight loss and resistance training. Am J Clin Nutr 1993; 58:561–565.

Kayman S, Bruvold W, Stern JS. Maintenance and relapse after weight loss in women: behavioral aspects. Am J Clin Nutr 1990; 52:800–807.

King AC, Frey-Hewitt B, Dreon DM, Wood PD. Diet vs exercise in weight maintenance; the effects of minimal intervention strategies on long-term outcomes in men. Arch Intern Med 1989; 149: 2741–2746.

Methods for voluntary weight loss and control: NIH technology assessment conference panel. Ann Intern Med 1992; 116:942–949.

Walberg JL. Aerobic exercise and resistance weight-training during weight reduction: implications for obese persons and athletes. Sports Med 1989; 7:343–356.

EXERCISE AND THE FEMALE ATHLETE

CHARLOTTE F. SANBORN, Ph.D.
CATHERINE M. JANKOWSKI, M.S.

The rigors of training and competition are similar for today's male and female athlete. Likewise, the responses and adaptations to training are virtually the same in both sexes. The physiologic differences between elite male and female athletes are actually smaller than within the general population. Special issues for the female athlete correspond to the gender-specific physiologic changes that occur during puberty. Maximal aerobic power ($\dot{V}O_2$max) is an excellent example to use when examining the impact of these physiologic changes. Prepubescent girls and boys have similar aerobic power values. Then, between the ages of 16 and 20 years, absolute $\dot{V}O_2$max peaks and the difference between genders becomes approximately 50%. The developing discrepancies in aerobic power can be attributed primarily to sex differences in body composition and the oxygen transport system. Other specific issues for the female athlete are a high prevalence of primary and secondary amenorrhea, disordered eating, and premature osteoporosis—the female athlete triad. This chapter highlights the major physiologic considerations, athletic amenorrhea, and the female athlete triad.

PHYSIOLOGIC CONSIDERATIONS

Cardiorespiratory Capacity

Aerobic Power

The major factors that affect $\dot{V}O_2$max are peak cardiac output and oxygen carrying capacity, body mass and body composition, and oxidative capacity of the skeletal muscles. Women have a smaller heart (volume) than men, resulting in a smaller stroke volume. At the same oxygen consumption ($\dot{V}O_2$), women have a higher heart rate (HR) than men. Women have a smaller left ventricular mass than men, whether expressed in absolute terms or relative to lean body mass. Women generally have a lower oxygen carrying capacity than men because of a lower hemoglobin concentration. The large 52% differences in absolute $\dot{V}O_2$max (L/min) between the genders decreases to 20% to 30% when expressed relative to body mass ($\dot{V}O_2$ ml/[kg · min]) and then to approximately 15% when calculated relative to fat free mass ($\dot{V}O_2$ ml/[kg FFW · min]).

If the intensity of exercise is prescribed using a range of percent heart rate max (% HRmax), this assumes a direct and proportional relationship between $\dot{V}O_2$ and HR. The HRmax method is valid for women performing such exercises as walking, jogging, running, and cycling. However, an adjustment needs to be made for aerobic dance when using the HRmax method. The HR response during aerobic dance is disproportionately high relative to an equivalent treadmill effect; therefore, 75% to 80% HRmax is needed to achieve an aerobic training effect by this type of activity.

Heat Tolerance

The following adaptations of exercise response occur with heat acclimatization: decreased HR, decreased rectal temperature, increased plasma volume, and increased sweat rate. Heat tolerance depends more on the cardiovascular fitness of an individual than on gender. Young girls are less tolerant of exercise in hot dry climates than are adult females because a larger surface area to body mass ratio increases heat gain from the environment, the onset of sweating is slower, and the sweating rate is smaller than in an adult. The phase of the menstrual cycle also has an impact on thermoregulation in women. During the luteal phase of the menstrual cycle, the resting core temperature is approximately 0.4°C higher than during the follicular phase. The threshold core temperature for the onset of sweating is also elevated in the luteal phase. Thermoregulation, therefore, may be compromised during prolonged exercise or heat exposure in the luteal phase. Thermoregulation during exercise can also be altered by estrogen replacement therapy. Women who are receiving estrogen replacement therapy have a lower set-point temperature for the initiation of sweating and vasodilation during exercise than when they are not taking such therapy.

Body Composition

Precise, individualized assessment of human body composition can only be made by dissection and analysis of cadavers under controlled conditions of humidity. Indirect methods must be used to assess body composition in the living. Though each method of estimating body composition has its advantages and disadvantages, all methods are subject to substantial error, even in the hands of the most experienced technician. The magnitude of error when predictions are based upon skinfolds is shown in the study by Lohman and associates. Sixteen female, college basketball athletes were measured at five skinfold sites. Four experienced investigators used four different types of caliper (three research calipers and one plastic "field" caliper). The percentage of body fat was estimated from five different skinfold-density equations, yielding estimates of mean body fats that ranged from 14% to 28%! "At present, however, different equations, investigators, and instruments make the estimates of body composition in female athletes unreliable for accurate assessment of weight loss and especially inappropriate to those inexperienced with the limitations of this anthropometric approach."

Body Fat

Body fat is classified as storage fat or essential fat. The absolute amount of storage fat is similar in men and women, but women have a larger relative amount of storage fat than men. Because of sex-specific fat, the percentage of essential fat is higher in women (9% to 12%) than men (3%). Overall, adult women have 8% to 10% more body fat than men. Most female athletes have less body fat than sedentary college-aged women (23% to 27%). Further, many female athletes, especially runners, gymnasts, and ballet dancers, have a lower percentage of body fat than average college-age men (15% to 18%).

Muscle Tissue

The muscle fiber area and the total muscle cross-sectional area of women average 60% to 85% of male values, with the relative proportion of fast-twitch (glycolytic) and slow-twitch (aerobic) fibers being similar in the two sexes. The differences in absolute strength between sexes are virtually eliminated if strength is expressed relative to fat-free mass. Thus, the differences in muscle strength between trained women and men appears to be explained by muscle mass. Weight (resistance) training elicits similar relative gains in strength and similar muscle hypertrophy in women and men. Resistance training should be a high priority when prescribing a fitness program for women. An increase in strength enhances athletic performance, and also maintains or slows the loss of muscle mass in elderly and dieting women.

ATHLETIC AMENORRHEA

Etiology

Athletes have a high prevalence of both primary and secondary amenorrhea. However, there are large discrepancies in reported prevalence between studies, stemming in part from the lack of a consistent definition of amenorrhea. The most probable site of menstrual dysfunction in the athlete is at the level of the hypothalamus or above, based on pituitary and ovarian hormonal responses to gonadotropin-releasing hormone (GnRH) stimulation tests. The highest frequency of amenorrhea is seen among ballet dancers and runners, leading to the most popular theory, the "fat hypothesis." Overall, the mean percentages of body fat are similar in amenorrheic and regular menstruating athletes, with a wide range of values within and between groups. The question remains whether each athlete has her own critical level of body fat; however, on average the percentage of body fat does not differentiate between the two groups. Although the etiology remains unknown, the two current hypothesis are: (1) adrenal axis activation during exercise inhibits the hypothalamic GnRH pulse generator, or (2) a negative energy balance due to both an inadequate food intake and an increased daily energy expenditure results in an "energy drain."

A surprising finding has been the low total energy intakes reported by many female athletes, regardless of their menstrual status. The mean total energy intake of female athletes has been reported to be as low as 5,325 kilojoules/day (1,272 kcals/day) to as high as 10,000 (2,400 kcals/day). Most athletes appear to incur an energy deficit. Therefore, the question arises, whether a negative energy balance or "energy drain" is a possible explanation of athletic amenorrhea? The hypothesis postulates that the athlete expends more calories than she is consuming, thus providing too little energy to maintain the endocrine reproductive system. Overall, the amenorrheic athlete tends to consume less energy per day than the regularly menstruating athlete; however, the differences between the two groups have not always been significant, because of large individual variations. Conflicting findings have been reported, one explanation being a compensatory reduction of resting metabolic rate and the other being an under-reporting of food, or restricting energy intakes. To date, the validity of the energy deficit hypothesis remains unclear.

Two questions of utmost importance to the female

athlete are whether athletic amenorrhea is reversible and whether there are any harmful effects. Preliminary findings suggest that athletic amenorrhea is not a permanent problem to fertility. The finding of osteopenia (premature osteoporosis) in amenorrheic athletes is alarming. In addition, extreme competitive pressures to achieve a low body fat content have resulted in a high prevalence of disordered eating among athletes. A new question then arises: is the amenorrhea related to exercise or is the amenorrhea a symptom of an eating disorder?

Disordered Eating and Athletic Amenorrhea

Many similarities exist between amenorrheic athletes and patients with anorexia nervosa: ritualized dietary habits, compulsive behavior, a low food intake, a heightened energy expenditure, and amenorrhea. In 1987 we examined the possible parallel between athletic amenorrhea and preoccupation with diet and minimal body weight. Ninety minute psychiatric interviews of 13 amenorrheic and 19 regularly menstruating runners were conducted. The two groups were similar in age, menarche, kilometers of training per week, height, and percentage of body fat. Based upon DSM III criteria, 62% ($n = 8$) of the amenorrheic runners had eating disorders versus none of the regularly menstruating runners. Further, only among the amenorrheic runners (23%) were there any diagnosis of major affective disorders.

A word of caution is needed regarding the body mass of amenorrheic athletes and DSM III criteria for the diagnosis of anorexia nervosa. In the above study, the body mass of the amenorrheic runners averaged 49 kg, which is higher than patients with anorexia nervosa (44 kg). The body mass of the amenorrheic athlete may also be higher than the DSM III criterion of 15% below normal weight for age and height because of the athlete's greater than average lean muscle mass. The amenorrheic athlete would have weighed substantially less without the increased musculature that she has developed through training and if sedentary would have displayed the emaciated appearance associated with anorexia nervosa. Further, some athletes who have significant symptoms and the pathology of eating disorders nevertheless have not met the strict *DSM-III-R* criteria for the diagnosis of either anorexia nervosa or bulimia nor have they been identified by a standard eating disorder questionnaire (Eating Attitudes Test). Whether disordered eating is the underlying etiology of athletic amenorrhea therefore remains unknown, but it appears that at least a subset of amenorrheic athletes represent a variant of anorexia nervosa or bulimia nervosa.

Athletic Amenorrhea and Premature Osteoporosis

Amenorrheic athletes have low bone mineral densities. The hypogonadal state offsets the potentially beneficial effect of exercise on bone mass. Drinkwater et al found that lumbar bone mineral density was 14% lower in amenorrheic women than in the regularly menstruating athletes. The lower bone mass was observed despite the fact that amenorrheic women ran a greater distance per week than the regularly menstruating athletes (67.1 versus 40.0 km, respectively).

The finding of osteopenia (reduced bone mass) is alarming because these women are losing bone mass at a time when bone should become denser. Optimal levels of peak bone mass may not be reached in such individuals, predisposing them to premature osteoporosis. Is the decrease in bone mineral density (BMD) seen in the amenorrheic athletes a premature and irreversible loss? Resumption of ovarian function is associated with a significant increase in vertebral BMD. Although increases in BMD can occur during the first 2 years after resumption of menses, densities may remain below age-related values.

Stress fractures are of concern for the amenorrheic athlete with low bone mass. Female athletes who develop stress fractures have lower lumbar and femoral BMD than control athletes. Other factors associated with stress fractures include late menarche, oligo/amenorrhea, low body fat, non use of contraceptives, and low dietary calcium.

Prevention

Female athletes are under intense pressure to maintain a low body fat content not only to enhance performance but also to improve physical appearance. This pressure is compounded by society's emphasis on a svelt look, and the psychological profile of an elite athlete, which tends to be goal oriented and perfectionist. The outcome is an athlete who is vulnerable to disordered eating, which may in turn lead to the cascading problems of menstrual irregularities, amenorrhea, premature osteoporosis, and injuries. The snowball begins with the emphasis on low body weight. Prevention involves de-emphasizing a low body fat content, and implementing appropriate nutrition education programs, a coordinated team approach involving the athlete, coach, parent, physician, athletic trainer, and nutritionist.

De-emphasize Low Body Fat

One common rationale for athletes to become thin is the misconception of a highly negative correlation between physical performance and the percentage of body fat. The coach and athlete translate this relationship to mean that performance is optimal at the lowest percent body fat. The athlete keeps striving or is required to be leaner and leaner, and either no minimal limit is set, or too low of a value is established. In fact, there is only a mild to moderate negative association between body fat content and performance ($r = -0.40$ to $r = -0.68$). The percent body fat accounts for only 16% to 46% of the variation in performance. Further, the studies that have reported moderate rather than weak correlations ($r = -0.60$ to -0.68) have included nonathletes who typically had a wide range in body mass, for example from 52 to 100 kg.

Table 1 Clinical Evaluation of Menstrual Dysfunction in the Female Athlete

History
    Menstrual history—age of secondary sexual characteristic development, menarche, current and past menstrual pattern, oral contraceptives, sexual history, pregnancy history
    Physical training history—age at onset of training, intensity, amount, frequency, type(s), injuries
    Nutritional history—eating habits, calcium/caloric intakes, disordered eating patterns (binging, fasting, use of laxative or diuretics)
    Body composition—weight history: high and low, perceived body image, desired body weight/body fat, fear of becoming obese?, mandated body weight/body fat by coach?
    Psychosomatic complaints—insomnia, fatigue, depression, coping with injury
    Family history—menstrual history of mother & sister(s), osteoporosis, family dysfunction
    Medications
Physical Exam
    Height, weight, blood pressure, pulse
    Secondary sex characteristics—breasts and pubic hair development, signs of androgen excess (hirsutism, clitoromegaly, severe acne)
    Pelvic exam
Delayed Menarche
    Consider hormonal therapy to effect pubertal development
    Discuss with patient/parent
    Concern development of peak bone mass
Luteal Phase Dysfunction
    No treatment required unless pregnancy desired
    Treatment:
    • reduction in training (athlete usually opposed to this option)
    • individualized therapeutic alterations such as clomiphene citrate, progesterone suppositories, or gonadotropin therapy
Oligomenorrhea and Amenorrhea
    Laboratory tests:
    • pregnancy test and vaginal smear on initial exam (assess estrogen effect)
    • FSH, LH, prolactin, TSH, cortisone, testosterone (? androgen excess)
    • progestin challenge test
    • bone mineral density (lumbar and femur)—may provide leverage for athlete opposed to hormonal therapy
    Treatment of anovulation—offer several options:
    • monthly progestin therapy
    • oral contraceptives
    Treatment of hypoestrogenic amenorrhea:
    • oral contraceptives
    • cyclic estrogen-progestin therapy
    • 1,500 mg/day calcium

Based on information from Highet R. Athletic amenorrhoea: An update on aetiology, complications and management. Sports Med 1989; 7:82–108, and Shangold M, Rebar R, Wentz A, Schiff I. Evaluation and management of menstrual dysfunction in athletes. JAMA 1990; 263:1665–1669.

Another fallacy is that every sport has an "ideal percent body fat." One coaching manual states that the ideal percent body fat for female gymnasts is 5% to 10%, but uses the higher value of 10% for calculation of ideal body weight! Where are the facts to support this assertion? It seems there are none. Low percentages of body fat are also suggested for male and female nonathletes. For example, a table of standard values indicates 20% to 28% body fat as average for women aged 20 to 29 years, but recommends the lowest, 20%. Further problems arise when percent body fats are broken down into categories labeled as poor, fair, average, good, and excellent. In this resource, the "excellent" rating for women aged 20 to 29 years is <15% body fat, and for men the corresponding figure is <10%. No women, especially female athletes, want the acceptable classification of average; they desire the standard of excellent. Not only are the quoted values extremely low, but "less than" (<) implies that an even lower body fat is the ideal goal. Such tables perpetuate the belief that the lowest possible body fat is best.

The association between body fat and performance needs to be individualized and viewed as a parabola, with a wide range of optimal body mass or relative body fat for each athlete. There is certainly a point at which an athlete weighs too much, so that performance is compromised or the athlete is at an increased risk of injury. There is also a point at which the athlete's weight and body fat content is too low, so that performance declines and the athlete is at an increased risk of eating disorders, injury, and health problems.

Nutrition Education Programs

Nutrition education is an essential element of an athlete's training. The value of sound dietary habits must be emphasized by the athlete's most influential figure, her coach. Since nutrition is not, typically, part of a coach's expertise, a cooperative effort is required, involving the coach, parent, athletic trainer, sports nutrition expert, physician, and athlete. The goals of such a program are to (1) replace nutrition myths with facts; (2) educate athletes as to nutrient-dense food choices within the context of their environment (i.e., home, dormitory, or "on the road"); (3) provide hands-on practice of food preparation; and (4) promote dietary habits that will reduce the risk factors for both disordered eating and long-term health problems such as cardiovascular disease, hypertension, and osteoporosis.

Treatment

Athletes have a greater prevalence of luteal phase deficiency, oligomenorrhea, amenorrhea, and delayed menarche than nonathletes. It is tempting to assume that strenuous training caused the menstrual disorders; however, many other conditions could also produce the same result. Thus, the first step toward treatment of an athlete with menstrual dysfunction is a very careful history. Clinical evaluation is recommended if any female athlete has not experienced menarche by the age of 16 years, or has not menstruated for 3 to 6 months. Luteal phase deficiency may be suspected if the athlete menstruates frequently (every 21 to 23 days). Although uncommon among athletes, hyperprolactinemia, hyperandrogenism, hypothyroidism, and premature ovarian failure should not be overlooked as possible causes of the menstrual dysfunction. If disordered eating is suspected, the athlete should be evaluated further by a nutritionist and a psychiatrist. A therapeutic approach to menstrual dysfunction is shown in Table 1. Detailed evaluation, treatment, and management have been described elsewhere.

Acknowledgment. We thank Dr. Nancy DiMarco and David L. Nichols for their review of the manuscript.

SUGGESTED READING

Brownell KD, Nelson Steen S, Wilmore JH. Weight regulation practices in athletes: analysis of metabolic and health effects. Med Sci Sports Exerc 1987; 19:546–556.

DeSouza MJ, Metzger DA. Reproductive dysfunction in amenorrheic athletes and anorexia patients: a review. Med Sci Sports Exerc 1991; 23:995–1007.

Drinkwater B, Nilson K, Chestnut C, et al. Bone mineral content of amenorrheic and eumenorrheic athletes. N Engl J Med 1984; 311:277–281.

Lohman TG, Pollock ML, Slaughter MH, et al. Methodological factors and the prediction of body fat in female athletes. Med Sci Sports Exerc 1984; 16:92–96.

Loucks AB. Effects of exercise training on the menstrual cycle: existence and mechanisms. Med Sci Sports Exerc 1990; 22:275–280.

Loucks AB, Horvath SM. Athletic amenorrhea: A review. Med Sci Sports Exerc 1985; 17:56–72.

Loucks AB, Vaitukaitis J, Cameron J, et al. The reproductive system and exercise in women. Med Sci Sports Exerc 1992; 24:S288–S293.

Sanborn CF. Fact and fat of body composition in sports nutrition. In: Berning JR, Steen SN, eds. The health professionals handbook. Rockville, Md: Aspen Publishers, 1991.

Shangold MM, Mirkin G. Women and exercise: Physiology and sports medicine. Philadelphia: FA Davis, 1988:279.

Wells CL. Women, sport, & performance. 2nd ed. Champaign, Ill: Human Kinetics Books, 1991:367.

Williford HN, Scharff-Olson M, Blessing DL. Exercise prescription for women. Sports Med 1993; 15:299–311.

EXERCISE AND PREGNANCY

LARRY A. WOLFE, Ph.D., F.A.C.S.M.
MICHELLE C. AMEY
MICHAEL J. McGRATH, M.D., F.R.C.S.(C)

The risks and benefits of participation by pregnant women in occupational and recreational physical activity have been the subject of intensive historic debate. The need for reliable information on this topic has become particularly urgent in the 1990s, due to increased involvement of young women in vigorous fitness programs, competitive sports, and employment in occupations that require strenuous exertion (e.g., military service, police work, fire fighting, and construction). Thus, it is important for personal physicians and obstetricians to be able to advise pregnant patients on safe and beneficial types and intensities of exercise at different stages of gestation. This should be done on an individual basis, as an integral part of prenatal medical surveillance. The advice given should take into account the woman's age, medical and obstetric history, life-style factors, past exercise participation, and other relevant information.

PHYSIOLOGIC ADAPTATIONS TO PREGNANCY

Anatomic and physiologic adaptations to pregnancy are initiated by ovarian and placental hormones. The purpose of these changes is to nourish and protect the developing fetus in addition to satisfying maternal biologic needs. Pregnancy-induced changes in the operation of maternal physiologic control systems are powerful and highly integrated, resulting in sufficient adaptive reserve to accommodate maternal and fetal needs in a variety of physiologic circumstances, including moderate exercise. Specific changes during pregnancy that can alter maternal responses to exercise and physical conditioning are described below.

Total weight gain during pregnancy averages approximately 12 kg, and includes fetal body mass (3.5 kg), uterine enlargement (1.0 kg), breast enlargement (1.5 kg), placental growth (0.7 kg), amniotic fluid (0.8 kg), additional fluid (2.0 kg), and increased maternal adiposity (2.5 kg). Increased adiposity is promoted by hyperinsulinemia. This develops in early pregnancy and promotes maternal energy storage during the first two pregnancy trimesters. In late gestation, insulin resistance caused by other gestational hormones (e.g., human chorionic somatomammotropin) causes a reduction in maternal adiposity and helps to protect fetal glucose availability from the maternal blood glucose pool.

Cardiovascular changes include a 40% to 50% increase in maternal blood volume; a lesser percentage increase in red cell volume results in a state of relative anemia. The increase in blood volume is partly accommodated by an increase in venous capacitance. Resting heart rate (HR) increases abruptly in early pregnancy and then rises moderately until term. Cardiac output increases with advancing gestational age as a result of a higher HR and stroke volume. The change in cardiac output is balanced by a reduction in peripheral vascular resistance, so that arterial blood pressure is similar to or slightly lower than in the nonpregnant state. In late gestation, women may experience hypotension in the supine posture, due to aortocaval obstruction by the gravid uterus.

Pulmonary ventilation increases at rest. This is in part the result of an increase in resting metabolic rate, which by term reaches 20% to 30% above that of the nonpregnant state. More importantly, there is a progesterone-mediated increase in respiratory sensitivity to carbon dioxide. This results in an increase in the ventilatory equivalent for oxygen ($\dot{V}_E$:$\dot{V}o_2$), a substantial reduction in arterial carbon dioxide tension, and a moderate increase in arterial oxygen tension. The resultant tendency toward respiratory alkalosis is partly compensated by renal excretion of bicarbonate and the arterial pH rises to approximately 7.46. Dyspnea is a common complaint, both at rest and during exercise.

MATERNAL PHYSIOLOGY OF EXERCISE

As a result of the previously described changes in metabolic and cardiorespiratory control, physiologic responses to exercise are substantially different from those of the nonpregnant state. As might be expected, the energy cost of weight-bearing exercise (e.g., walking or jogging) rises in proportion to maternal weight gain. However, the energy cost of weight-supported exercise (e.g., stationary cycling) is reported to be either unchanged or only slightly increased.

Cardiorespiratory adaptations to standard submaximal exercise are generally similar to those observed at rest, and include increases in absolute values for HR, pulmonary ventilation and the ventilatory equivalent for oxygen, and significant reductions in alveolar and arterial carbon dioxide tensions. Oxygen uptake kinetics at the beginning of a submaximal exercise bout also appear to have a faster time constant than in the nonpregnant state.

Available evidence suggests that the onset of blood lactate accumulation (OBLA) is not altered significantly by pregnancy. However, very little information is available on maternal responses to exercise intensities above OBLA. Since blood buffering capacity is reduced, there is some concern that pregnant women may be more prone to metabolic acidosis during strenuous exercise. However, some evidence also suggests that maternal ability to utilize carbohydrate and produce lactate may also be reduced in late gestation. Studies of maximal oxygen uptake (L/min) in pregnancy have not provided conclusive results and may be complicated by problems in obtaining a true maximal effort in the face of a reduced ability to utilize carbohydrate. More information is also needed on maternal responses to prolonged submaximal exercise (>30 minutes duration).

An integrated view of maternal HR responses to exercise appears in Figure 1. As previously described, HR is elevated at rest and during submaximal exertion. However, the degree of HR elevation due to pregnancy decreases with increasing exercise intensity and some evidence suggests that maximal HR is reduced in late gestation. The net result of these changes is a blunted HR response to graded exercise and a reduced maximal HR reserve. In contrast, the relationship between relative exercise intensity and perception of effort does

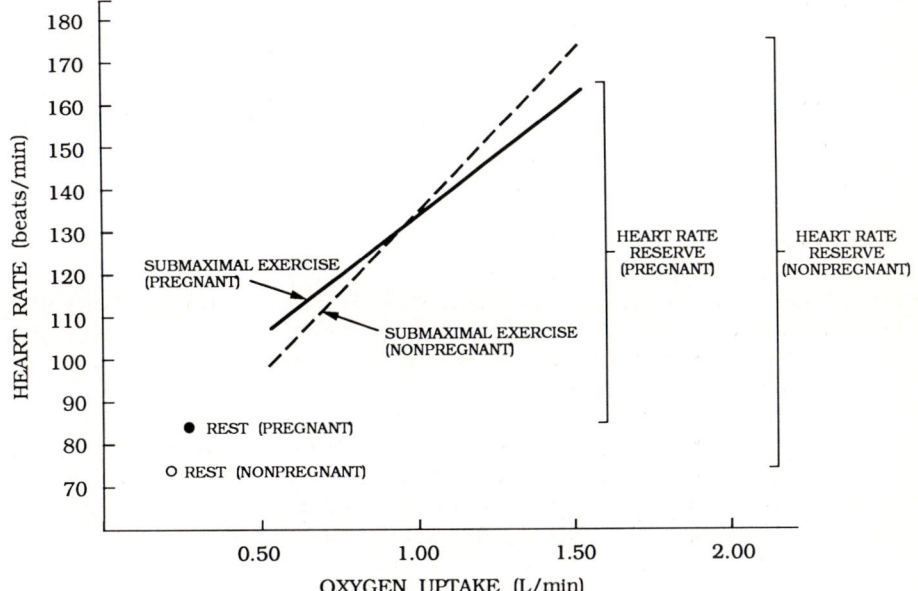

Figure 1 Effects of pregnancy on maximal heart rate reserve. (From: Wolfe LA, Mottola MF. Aerobic exercise in pregnancy: an update. Can J Appl Physiol 1993; 18: 119–147; with permission.)

not appear to change significantly with advancing gestational age.

Completed studies have identified similarities and differences in the responses of pregnant and nonpregnant women to physical conditioning. Findings from studies of moderate aerobic conditioning have included evidence for improved maximal oxygen uptake (L/min), an increase in work rate at OBLA, evidence for attenuation of insulin resistance that develops in late gestation, and preservation of the ability to utilize carbohydrate and produce lactate during strenuous exercise. In contrast to the nonpregnant state, maternal adiposity (as reflected by skinfold thicknesses) may be maintained rather than reduced by moderate aerobic conditioning in late gestation, since insulin resistance is attenuated by such exercise.

Another important finding from recent studies is that resting HR does not appear to be reduced by moderate aerobic conditioning. In nonpregnant subjects, development of bradycardia during training is attributed to augmented vagal/parasympathetic cardiac effects. Thus, it appears that the endocrine and/or hemodynamic factors that increase resting HR during pregnancy prevent or override the vagal/parasympathetic cardiac effects of aerobic conditioning in the resting state. Recent research further suggests that exercise HR is reduced following aerobic conditioning, but changes become more prominent with increasing work rate. Apparently, afferent signals from trained maternal skeletal muscle become more influential at higher exercise intensities.

FETAL EFFECTS OF MATERNAL EXERCISE

Available information on fetal responses to acute maternal aerobic exercise suggests that the fetus experiences mild hypoxia, due to a reduced uterine blood flow. However, this appears to be well tolerated by normal human fetuses. The most common fetal reaction appears to be a moderate increase in fetal HR, which is proportional to both the intensity and duration of exercise. However, transient fetal bradycardia is also occasionally observed, particularly in the immediate recovery period following strenuous exercise. Presumably this is a reaction to reduced venous return, maternal hypotension, and reduced uterine blood flow during early recovery from intense maternal exertion. The fetal HR responses described above appear to be normal protective reflexes that are not associated with altered fetal development or perinatal morbidity when experienced by healthy women during a normal pregnancy.

It is clear from human epidemiologic studies that strenuous physical work combined with nutritional stress can result in fetal growth retardation. However, existing research supports the viewpoint that moderate prenatal physical conditioning regimens (including an aerobic conditioning component) do not result in an increased risk of premature labor, intrauterine growth retardation (IUGR), or altered fetal development. Moderate reductions in infant birth weight have been reported in recreational athletes who continued to perform regular strenuous exercise in late gestation. However, evaluation of neonatal morphometrics indicated that this was due primarily to reduced adiposity.

BENEFITS AND RISKS OF EXERCISE DURING PREGNANCY

The traditional medical belief that pregnant women should rest has been called into serious question as a result of research findings published since the mid-1980s. The most important concerns have been that chronic maternal overexertion may cause premature labor, IUGR, or altered fetal development. However, a growing body of evidence supports the viewpoint that a carefully prescribed and monitored prenatal exercise program does not increase the risk of these complications. Conversely, it is apparent that regular exercise can preserve or increase maternal metabolic and cardiopulmonary capacities. Other benefits may include facilitation of labor (especially in primiparas), promotion of good posture, prevention of gestational low back pain and diastasis recti, and wide-ranging psychological benefits. Recent evidence also supports the value of regular aerobic-type exercise to prevent and treat gestational diabetes mellitus.

It is also important to consider the potential risks of maternal physical inactivity. These may include reduced metabolic and cardiopulmonary reserve and fetoprotective capacities, excessive weight gain, deterioration of glucose tolerance, greater risk of deep vein thrombosis and varicose veins, excessive bone loss due in turn to high circulating estrogen levels, urinary incontinence, and a greater risk of musculoskeletal problems (e.g., low back pain and diastasis recti).

MEDICAL CLEARANCE AND ONGOING SURVEILLANCE

For the majority of pregnant women, the most important question is not whether they should participate in regular physical activity, but rather what types and how much physical activity is most appropriate for each individual? Pregnancy is often a good time to establish permanent healthy life-style habits—including regular moderate physical activity. However, it is prudent for some women with serious health problems or a poor obstetric history to forego physical activity throughout pregnancy or at specific stages of gestation.

The most efficient way for physicians to provide medical clearance for prenatal exercise participation is to ensure that the individual does not have contraindications to exercise in pregnancy. Various authorities have identified such contraindications. General agreement exists that these should include: clinically significant cardiopulmonary disorders (e.g., ischemic or valvular heart disease; uncontrolled hypertension; peripheral vascular disease; chronic obstructive pulmonary disease), which may compromise maternal cardiac output;

uterine blood flow or arterial oxygen saturation; serious or uncontrolled metabolic disorders (e.g., Type I diabetes mellitus or thyroid disease); infectious diseases (e.g., mononucleosis or hepatitis); obstetric problems in previous pregnancies (e.g., incompetent cervix or a significant history of preterm delivery); multiple pregnancy; and conditions such as eating disorders, poor nutrition, or very low maternal adiposity, which may compromise maternal-fetal energy exchange. Other important factors that should be considered include use of medications that may alter maternal metabolic and cardiopulmonary capacities, smoking, alcohol and caffeine consumption, and previous physical activity. Pregnant women should be strongly advised to avoid smoking and alcohol consumption and to limit their caffeine intake. Women with Type II diabetes mellitus may benefit from a carefully prescribed and monitored exercise regimen.

Medical clearance for exercise should be withdrawn if serious obstetric problems or symptoms arise. These include: multiple pregnancy; evidence of IUGR; placenta previa; ruptured membranes or premature labor; development of pre-eclampsia/eclampsia or abnormal glucose tolerance; and development of clinically significant pubic or low back pain. It is important to note, however, that appropriately prescribed exercise may be useful to prevent or treat gestational diabetes mellitus, low back pain, or pregnancy-induced hypertension.

Exercising pregnant women and prenatal fitness instructors should be aware of the signs and symptoms of common obstetric problems indicating the need for medical intervention. These include evidence of bleeding; fluid discharge from the vagina suggesting premature rupture of membranes; sudden swelling of the extremities; unexplained abdominal pain; absence or decrease in fetal movements; persistent uterine contractions suggesting the onset of premature labor; insufficient weight gain; and other symptoms including persistent headaches, visual disturbances, dizziness, or general fatigue.

EXERCISE PRESCRIPTION

Over the past decade, numerous authorities have published specific guidelines and advice for exercise during pregnancy. As described in recent reviews, widespread agreement exists in many areas, but significant controversy remains in others. However, a growing body of evidence supports the wisdom of using an individualized common sense approach when selecting appropriate exercise modalities, intensities, and durations.

Muscular Conditioning

There is general agreement that properly-executed muscular stretching, strengthening, and relaxation exercises can be beneficial to maintain muscular fitness, promote good posture, and prevent conditions such as gestational low back pain, diastasis recti, and urinary incontinence (Table 1). Such exercises may also strengthen muscles involved in the active stage of labor. Participation in weight-training programs is probably safe, provided that precautions are taken to avoid physical injury or overexertion. Special considerations for muscular conditioning in pregnancy include modification of specific exercises to accommodate changes in maternal body mass and biomechanics; avoidance in late gestation of exercises performed in the supine posture (to prevent maternal aortocaval obstruction and hypotension); avoidance of Valsalva's maneuver during strengthening exercises; and avoidance of overstretching ligaments and tendons that may have increased laxity caused by gestational hormones.

Aerobic Conditioning

Existing research strongly supports the existence of a dose-response effect for the quantity and quality of maternal aerobic exercise. Too little exercise may be ineffective to induce the beneficial effects described. Conversely, exercise that is too intense may result in reduced uterine blood flow and impaired fetal oxygen delivery, temporary reduction in fetal glucose availability from the maternal glucose pool, or fetal exposure to hyperthermic conditions. Thus, it is very important to avoid chronic maternal overexertion.

The area of greatest controversy in maternal aerobic exercise prescription has been the use of maternal HR to monitor exercise intensity. A safe upper limit of 140

Table 1 Muscular Strengthening Exercises for Pregnant Women

Category	Purpose	Example
Upper back	Promotion of good posture	Shoulder shrugs, shoulder blade pinch
Lower back	Promotion of good posture	Pelvic tilts, pelvic rocks
Abdomen	Promotion of good posture, prevent low-back pain, prevent diastasis recti, strengthen muscles of labor	Abdominal tightening, abdominal curl-ups
Pelvic floor ("Kegels")	Promotion of good bladder control, prevention of urinary incontinence	"Faucet", "wave", "elevator"
Upper body	Improvement in muscular support for breasts	Shoulder rotations, arm circles
Buttocks, lower limbs	Facilitation of weight bearing, prevention of varicose veins	Pelvic tucks, pelvic tilts, pliés, standing leg lifts

From Wolfe LA. Pregnancy. In Skinner JS, ed. Exercise testing and exercise prescription for special cases: Theoretical basis and clinical application. 2nd Ed. Philadelphia: Lea & Febiger, 1993; with permission.

Table 2 Suggested Heart Rate Target Zones for Aerobic Exercise in Pregnancy*

Maternal Age (Years)	Heart Rate Target Zone
Less than 20	140–155
20–29	135–150
30–39	130–145
Greater than 40	125–140

Values apply to most healthy pregnant women. Women should exercise at the lower part of the recommended heart rate range at the beginning of a new exercise program and in late gestation.

Adapted from Wolfe LA. Pregnancy. In Skinner JS, ed. Exercise testing and exercise prescription for special cases: theoretical basis and clinical application. 2nd Ed. Philadelphia: Lea & Febiger, 1993; with permission.

Table 3 Example of Gradual Increase in Aerobic Exercise Quantity During the Second Trimester for a Previously Sedentary Woman

Week of Gestation	Duration (Minutes/ Session)	Frequency (Sessions/ Week)
Do not begin a new exercise program or increase habitual quantity and quality prior to the 15th week.		
16	15	3
17	17	3
18	19	3
19	21	3-4
20	23	4-5
21	25	3-4
22	26	4-5
23	27	3-4
24	28	4-5
25	29	3-4
26	30	4-5
27	30	3-4
28	30	4-5
Do not increase exercise duration or frequency after the 28th week of gestation. If necessary, reduce exercise quantity and quality to avoid chronic fatigue in late gestation.		

Adapted from Wolfe LA. Pregnancy. In Skinner JS, ed. Exercise testing and exercise prescription for special cases: theoretical basis and clinical application. 2nd Ed. Philadelphia: Lea & Febiger, 1993; with permission.

beats/min has been recommended by the American College of Obstetricians and Gynecologists. In our experience, this is too low to produce optimal changes in fitness for many pregnant women. However, it may also be too high for others, depending on maternal age, physical fitness, stage of pregnancy, and other individual factors. Accordingly, we have suggested a series of age-adjusted maternal pulse rate target zones for healthy pregnant women (Table 2). Since maximal HR reserve is reduced in late gestation, these target zones are narrower (15 vs 20 beats/min) and have lower upper limits than the usual pulse rate prescriptive zone recommended for healthy nonpregnant adults.

Recognizing that pulse rate is less dependable as an index of exercise intensity in the pregnant versus nonpregnant state, it is prudent to use other practical methods to prevent overexertion. In our experience, perception of effort-work rate relationships are not altered significantly by pregnancy and do not change significantly during the course of gestation. Therefore, rating of perceived exertion (RPE) scales are recommended for use in addition to pulse rate target zones modified for pregnant women. The usual prescriptive zone for healthy nonpregnant adults is between 12 and 16 on Borg's 15-point (6 to 20) RPE scale. Accordingly, a range of 12 to 14 is suitable for most pregnant women. A final method to protect against overexertion is to caution pregnant women against exercising at an intensity that precludes carrying on a verbal conversation (the "talk test").

It is well established that the physiologic stress of physical conditioning depends on the intensity, duration, and frequency of exercise sessions. There is agreement that pregnant women should not increase the intensity or duration of habitual physical activity prior to the 15th week of gestation, in order to avoid the possibility of fetal teratogenic effects caused by exposure to exercise-induced hyperthermia during closure of the neural tube. It is also unwise to increase maternal exercise intensity, duration, or frequency after the 28th week, when fetal demands for fuel substrates and oxygen delivery are highest. However, there is good scientific support for the concept that previously inactive women can safely increase the quantity and quality of aerobic exercise between approximately the 16th and 28th week of gestation, when both the discomforts of pregnancy and risks of conflicting maternal-fetal physiologic demands are low (Table 3).

The choice of an appropriate modality for aerobic exercise is very important. It is clear that pregnant women should avoid activities with a risk of falling, physical injury, or exposure to hyperbaric or hyperthermic environmental stress. Also, participation in activities such as walking, stationary cycling, and low impact aerobics is preferable to involvement in exercise that involves repetitive weight-bearing movements (e.g., running) and an accompanying risk of overuse orthopedic injury. Aquatic activities (swimming, aquafit classes) are often recommended, since maternal body mass is supported by the buoyancy of water and metabolic heat loss will be encouraged if water temperature is lower than skin temperature. Note, however, that the pulse rate and RPE targets recommended above for land exercise may not be valid for application to exercise in the water.

The best method to avoid excessive increases in maternal-fetal body temperature is to restrict aerobic exercise to reasonable intensities and durations and to avoid exercising in warm and/or humid environments. Periodic rest periods and drinking water before and after exercise sessions can also help to avoid maternal-fetal hyperthermia.

It is particularly important for pregnant women involved in aerobic exercise programs to be aware of the basic principles of good nutrition during pregnancy and to adjust daily energy intake to satisfy the additional energy requirements of regular physical activity in addition to those of pregnancy itself. The combined effects of an appropriate exercise prescription and adequate nutritional intake will help to ensure that maternal fitness is improved, without creating an energy drain that could lead to fetal growth retardation.

Acknowledgments. The following agencies have given financial support for exercise/pregnancy research at Queen's University: Health and Welfare (Canada), Canadian Fitness and Lifestyle Research Institute, Ontario Ministry of Culture, Tourism and Recreation, Ontario Ministry of Health, and Ontario Thoracic Society.

SUGGESTED READINGS

American College of Sports Medicine. Pregnancy. In: Pate RR, Blair SN, Durstine JL, et al, eds. Guidelines for exercise testing and prescription. 4th Ed. Philadelphia: Lea & Febiger, 1991:180.

Artal Mittelmark R, Wiswell RA, Drinkwater BL, eds. Exercise in pregnancy. 2nd Ed. Baltimore: Williams & Wilkins, 1991.

McMurray RG, Mottola MF, Wolfe LA, et al. Recent advances in understanding maternal and fetal responses to exercise. Med Sci Sports Exerc 1993; 25:1305–1321.

White J. Exercising for two. What's safe for the exercising pregnant woman? Physician Sportsmed 1992; 20:179–184, 186.

Work JA. Is weight training safe during pregnancy? Physician Sportsmed 1989; 17:257–259.

Wolfe LA. Pregnancy. In: Skinner JS, ed. Exercise testing and exercise prescription for special cases: Theoretical basis and clinical application. 2nd Ed. Philadelphia: Lea & Febiger, 1993.

Wolfe LA, Brenner IKM, Mottola MF. Maternal exercise, fetal well-being and pregnancy outcome. Exerc Sport Sci Rev 1994; 22(in press).

Wolfe LA, Hall P, Goodman LS, et al. Prescription of aerobic exercise during pregnancy. Sports Medicine 1989; 8:273–301.

Wolfe LA, Mottola MF. Aerobic exercise in pregnancy: an update. Can J Appl Physiol 1993; 18:119–147.

Wolfe LA, Ohtake PJ, Mottola MF, McGrath MJ. Physiological interactions between pregnancy and aerobic exercise. Exerc Sport Sci Rev 1989; 17:295–351.

Wolfe LA, Walker RMC, Bonen A, McGrath MJ. Effects of pregnancy and chronic exercise on respiratory responses to graded exercise. J Appl Physiol 1994; 76:1928.

EXERCISE AND THE QUALITY OF LIFE

ROY J. SHEPHARD, M.D., Ph.D., D.P.E., F.A.C.S.M.

Physicians have traditionally evaluated the outcome of any treatment, exercise included, in terms of an extension of lifespan. This approach has the advantage that statisticians can analyze precise numbers of deaths in the groups receiving active and placebo treatments. However, it may give an inappropriate estimate of the value of a particular treatment if the quality of the remaining years of life are either enhanced or worsened by the treatment.

This criticism is particularly valid when looking at the influence of exercise on older individuals. Even a vigorous program of regular physical activity may extend lifespan by no more than a few months, but it can reduce biologic age by as much as 10 to 20 years, thus minimizing terminal disability and deferring institutionalization.

This chapter looks at the issue of determining "quality of life" and its place in practice, particularly the assessment of responses to exercise programs that extend human longevity.

DEFINING QUALITY OF LIFE

The concept of quality of life was advanced as long ago as 1920, in the context of the work environment. Social scientists have continued to view the concept broadly, in terms of satisfaction with employment, income, family life, use of spare time, housing, and general environment, in addition to more specific aspects of health. The person with a good quality of life has both physical and material well-being, with an optimization of interpersonal relationships, social and recreational opportunities, and personal fulfillment. In part, there is movement toward the World Health Organization definition of health: "not the mere absence of illness, but the optimization of physical, emotional and social well-being." Some authors have suggested that certain of these issues fall outside the concerns of the physician, and they have thus proposed focusing on a narrower concept of "Health-related quality of life" or "Health status." However, many current instruments for the measurement of quality of life evaluate the full list of variables shown in Table 1.

Table 1 Suggested Elements for Inclusion in Assessment of the Quality of Life

Physical well-being: No restrictions on mobility or self-care
Psychologic well-being: Freedom from anxiety and depression
Social well-being: Good social contacts and support, intimate relationships
Good role performance: Able to earn living, perform household chores and other activities of daily living
Freedom from symptoms: Freedom from pain, fatigue, nausea, and disease specific symptoms

POTENTIAL VALUE OF QUALITY OF LIFE MEASUREMENTS

Assessments of the quality of life can be used to demonstrate the health importance of exercise programs in general or to compare the value of different exercise and rehabilitation programs. Scores are also useful in monitoring the progress of individual patients, in identifying psychosocial problems (when there is a large disparity between the physiologic data and the reported quality of life), in estimating the prognosis for individual patients, and in identifying regional disparities in population health. Health economists are also using quality of life increasingly as a method of assessing the cost-effectiveness of various types of treatment.

MEASURING INSTRUMENTS

Measuring instruments may be self-administered, based on an interview, or based on detailed functional assessment. The approach may be generic (a uniform procedure for all patients) or (if the person already has some disease or disability) specifically adapted to reflect a particular condition. Patients with a specific disorder (for example, rheumatoid arthritis) may resent (and thus cooperate poorly in completing) a lengthy questionnaire with many items that are irrelevant to their condition.

Early devices attempted to get a very simple global indication of the quality of life: for example, patients were asked to make a gamble ("How many years of survival would you give up in order to be rid of your disability") or to rate their quality of life on a scale of 1 through 10. One problem with this approach was that a given treatment might improve some aspects of life quality but worsen others, and this was obscured by the analysis (for example, an exercise program might lead to some temporary tiredness, but would greatly improve overall function after rest from the immediate activity session). Alternatively, observers calculated single or multiple scores based on the performance of various functional tests.

More recently multidimensional subjective scales that examine the different elements listed in Table 1 have been proposed. British investigators have looked at two dimensions (disability and distress), and others have added a third dimension of physical discomfort. Researchers in Europe have proposed as many as six dimensions, each rated on only a scale of two or three levels. The Nottingham Health Profile and the Sickness Impact Profile (Table 2) are two more complex instruments that are currently popular in North America. One difficulty in using multiple scales is that when evaluating differences between rival treatments, the observer must make many comparisons; there is therefore a danger that spuriously significant differences will arise. Finally, individual components of health and well-being can be explored using such instruments as the "Profile of Mood States" questionnaire (Table 3).

It is easy to see intuitively that 5 years of survival in a wheelchair does not offer the same quality-adjusted life expectancy as 5 years of life with full normal mobility. However, it is more difficult to determine how overall survival prospects should be adjusted to reflect a deterioration in the quality of life from a restriction of ambulation, particularly as there is much variation in the environmental barriers that are encountered, the available level of social support, and the individual's adaptation to and acceptance of disability. The value of good health to the patient also varies with its immediacy; most people substantially discount the avoidance of disability that will develop 30 or 40 years in the future.

It would be ideal to obtain the individual patient's perceptions of each of the items in Table 1, but it is difficult to know just how such disparate items can be combined mathematically to give a global indication of quality of life.

Scores for instruments such as the Nottingham Health Profile vary by age, gender, and socioeconomic status. This problem is particularly acute in a multicultural country. How valid is the measuring instrument when applied across cultural barriers? How can concepts of pain, discomfort, and disability be translated uniformly from one language or culture into a very different culture or milieu?

Most people eventually reach an age when they begin to report some disability. One simple global option is therefore to report the average period to the onset of any disability. The main weakness in such analyses to date has been the difficulty in defining disability, although progress is being made in describing the overall and instrumental activities of daily living. The age of onset of disability can be used as a simple method of evaluating early preventive measures, adopted by people who are initially free of symptoms. With a little more sophistication, however, it is also possible to calculate the patient's total number of years without disability. A comparison of the differences between the two scores in treated and untreated individuals then gives an estimate

Table 2 Items Evaluated in the Sickness Impact Profile

Variable	No. of Responses
Freedom of ambulation	12
Mobility	10
Self-care ability	23
Ability to manage home	10
Social interactions	20
Ability to communicate	9
Emotional health	9
Alertness	10
Normality of eating habits	9
Employment	9
Normal sleep-rest patterns	7
Involvement in recreation	8

Data from Bergner M, Bobbitt RA, Carter WB, Gilson BS. The sickness impact profile: developments and final revision of a health status measurement. Med Care 1988;26:724–735.

Table 3 Assessment of Psychological Well-Being by Profile of Mood States Questionnaire

Variable	No. of Items
Anxiety	9
Depression	15
Fatigue	7
Vigor	8
Confusion	7
Hostility	12

*Patients are asked to indicate on a 0 to 4 scale their feelings over the previous week.

of the success of rehabilitative measures that have been undertaken after the onset of symptoms.

In Canada, men have a total disability-free life expectancy of 61.3 years out of a total lifespan of 73.0 years, and the corresponding figures for women are 64.9 and 79.8 years. It is possible to use these figures to estimate the number of years of disability-free life expectancy that would be gained by the control of various diseases. The three top items are locomotor disorders (5.1 years), circulatory diseases (4.2 years), and respiratory disorders (2.2 years).

A final possibility is to calculate the number of years to the onset of clinically significant mental deterioration, an important statistic given the contribution of mental competence to continued independence.

EXERCISE AND THE COMPRESSION OF MORBIDITY

Some pessimists have argued that current measures of preventive medicine extend life span but do not reduce morbidity or enhance the overall quality of life, so that society is accumulating an increasing burden of handicapped elderly people. Fries in contrast has suggested that there is a compression of morbidity, as measures such as exercise allow old people to remain in good health until they approach their "ceiling" of life expectancy. Still others have suggested there has been a reduction of severe disability, but that extended survival has increased the burden of patients with minor disability. Unfortunately, it is difficult to resolve this controversy until methods of measuring quality of life have been further refined; available statistics suggest that in the population as a whole, longevity is increasing, but disability-free lifespan is remaining relatively static.

Nevertheless, there remains grounds for hope that disability-free lifespan is being extended in that subsegment of the population who exercise regularly. In particular, an active life-style is helping to reduce the need for institutionalization of the elderly and those who have become weak and frail as a result of chronic illness. Institutionalization is often due to a sudden catastrophe such as the onset of blindness or a major stroke. Exercise may offer a little help to avoid such morbidity by reducing resting blood pressure. Another problem that forces many seniors who are living alone to enter a nursing home is the sudden loss of social support, through death of a spouse or removal of a younger caregiving relation. Exercise can again make a small contribution by increasing the patient's social contacts and countering the depression that follows bereavement. A third important reason for institutionalization is loss of memory and a deterioration of cerebral function. In this case, a major benefit from exercise is unlikely, although some experiments have suggested that the scores on a variety of tests of mental ability are enhanced by participation in a regular exercise program. The biggest benefit from regular physical activity is likely in situations where physiologic function has become inadequate to meet the demands of daily living—aerobic power is insufficient to walk up a mild incline, muscle

Table 4 Relationship Between Physical Activity at Age 50 Years (Measured in Arbitrary Units) and Disability as Seniors

Current Disability	Activity at Age 50 Years (units)
None	9.3
Minor	8.1
Severe	7.7
Institutionalized	4.1

Data from Shephard RJ, Montelpare W. Geriatric benefits of exercise as an adult. J Gerontol 1988; 43:M86–M90.

strength is insufficient to lift the body mass from a chair, and flexibility is insufficient to dress unaided. Where the person cannot undertake such activities without help, the quality of life becomes very low. Moreover, in such a situation, the quality of life can be greatly enhanced by even a small exercise-induced training response.

Inevitably, there remain many reasons for institutionalization, dependency, and poor life quality where regular exercise is unlikely to be of help. Nevertheless, our empirical observations have shown that those who have established a high level of habitual activity by the age of 50 years have a substantially reduced likelihood of being institutionalized when they are seniors (Table 4). Quality of life measurements are likely to find increasing future use, both in demonstrating the overall value of an active life-style and in comparing the impact of different types of physical activity program on the health of various clinical populations.

SUGGESTED READING

Bergner M, Bobbitt RA, Carter WB, Gilson BS. The sickness impact profile: developments and final revision of a health status measurement. Med Care 1988; 26:724–735.

Fletcher A, Gore S, Jones D, et al. Quality of life measures in health care: Design, analysis and interpretations. Br Med J 1992; 305: 1145–1148.

Fries JF. Aging, natural death and the compression of morbidity. N Engl J Med 1980; 303:130–135.

Gruenberg EM. The failure of success. Millbank Memorial Fund Quarterly 1977; 55:3–24.

Hunt SM, McEwen J, McKenna SP. Measuring health status. Beckenham, Kent: Croom Helm Publishing, 1986.

Lawton MP, Brody AM. Assessment of older people: self-maintaining and instrumental activities of daily living. Gerontologist 1969; 9:179–186.

Paffenbarger R. Contributions of epidemiology to exercise science and cardiovascular health. Med Sci Sports Exerc 1988; 20:426–438.

Robine JM, Ritchie K. Healthy life expectancy: evaluation of global indicator of change in population health. Br Med J 1991; 302: 457–460.

Shephard RJ. Are we asking the right questions? J Cardiac Rehab 1982; 2:21–26.

Shephard RJ. Physical activity and quality of life. Quality of Life and Cardiovascular Care 1985; 1:40–44.

Shephard RJ. Fitness and aging. In: Blais C, ed. Aging into the twenty first century. Downsview, Ontario: Captus University Publications, 1991:22.

Shephard RJ, Montelpare W. Geriatric benefits of exercise as an adult. J Gerontol 1988; 43:M86–M90.

Wood-Dauphinee S, Küchler T. Quality of life as a rehabilitation outcome: Are we missing the boat? Can J Rehab 1992; 6:3–12.

EXERCISE PRESCRIPTION FOR THE HEALTHY AGED

ROY J. SHEPHARD, M.D., Ph.D., D.P.E.,
F.A.C.S.M.

The elderly form a growing segment of the North American population. Nevertheless, the task of prescribing exercise for the elderly patient remains controversial, with vigorous discussion of appropriate test methods, a suitable intensity and duration of exercise, safety precautions, and the likely benefits of physical activity. Indeed, because of excessive fears regarding the safety of moderate physical activity, many physicians do little more than advise their older patients to "be careful."

DEFINITION OF ELDERLY PATIENTS

The elderly are not a homogeneous group, and it is therefore necessary to define several distinct age categories before considering suitable test methods and exercise programming. Convenient subcategories are the "young-old" (65 to 75 years), the "middle-old" (75 to 85 years) and "very old" (over 85 years), but there are sometimes substantial differences of biologic age between individuals of identical calendar age. I therefore prefer a functional classification; the "young-old" are those who can live independently, with little or no restriction of their physical activity, the "middle-old" have developed some chronic disability, and the "very-old" have become almost totally dependent.

The Canada Health Survey of 1978–1980 found that 26.5% of those over the age of 65 years suffered from some limitation of physical activity; 8.9% were unable to perform major activities, and 85.6% reported chronic health problems. On average, Canadian seniors live for 8 to 10 years in the middle-old category and a year in the very old category before they die. Women are generally disabled for longer than men. This chapter focuses on exercise programs for ostensibly healthy elderly patients. However, I recognize that as age advances they constitute a diminishing fraction of a practice, that the dividing line between health and illness becomes progressively blurred, and that the onset of chronic disease does not necessarily preclude an exercise prescription.

EXERCISE TESTING OF THE ELDERLY

A typical exercise test protocol for the elderly includes many of the same items as for a younger individual, including information on maximum oxygen transport, electrocardiographic and blood pressure responses to graded exercise, muscle function, body composition, and flexibility.

Maximum Oxygen Transport

The main determinant of endurance performance is the ability to pump oxygen from the atmosphere to the working muscles, the maximal oxygen intake ($\dot{V}O_2$ max). In the very old, this can become the main factor limiting independent living (Table 1). The critical level for performing daily activities is probably an oxygen transport of 12 to 14 ml/[kg · min].

The aerobic function of the young-old can generally be tested by treadmill walking, cycle ergometry, or stair-climbing, although an older patient may need a little more time for familiarization with the laboratory and test equipment. Because of unstable knees, a light hand-support may be needed for treadmill walking and for stepping, and this will change the oxygen cost of a standard exercise test.

A treadmill walk to maximal effort is tolerated surprisingly well by the middle-aged and young-old. The traditional sign of a central, cardiovascular limitation of oxygen transport, a "plateau" of oxygen consumption, can be demonstrated in as many as three-quarters of tests. But even if a patient fails to reach a plateau, the peak oxygen intake seems very reproducible, with a test/retest correlation of 0.90. In contrast, if maximal tests are conducted on a cycle ergometer, the efforts of an older patient are commonly halted by local weakness of the quadriceps muscle, rather than by cardiovascular function.

Because of fears about the safety of maximal tests, an attempt is sometimes made to predict maximal oxygen intake from submaximal data. Unfortunately, such predictions become progressively more unsatisfactory as the patient becomes older, since the maximal heart rate shows a large and variable decrease with age. Attempts to estimate oxygen consumption from the rate of working on a treadmill or cycle ergometer are also unsatisfactory in the elderly. Treadmill walking becomes mechanically inefficient because the patient is nervous and takes short, tentative steps. Likewise, stiff joints and lack of recent familiarity with cycling give a mechanical efficiency of less than the assumed value of 23% when operating a cycle ergometer. Medications such as beta-blockers further impair the heart-rate response to a given intensity of exercise. Alternative approaches to the setting of an appropriate exercise prescription are a determination of their anaerobic threshold (the oxygen

Table 1 Approximate Normal Values for Directly Measured $\dot{V}O_2$max of Elderly Patients (ml/kg · min)*

| | Level of Cardiovascular Fitness | | |
Age (yr)	High	Moderate	Low
65	31	27	23
70	28	24	20
75	25	21	17
80	22	18	14
85	19	15	11
90	16	12	8

Values per unit of body mass are similar in men and women.

consumption associated with a significant hyperventilation and the accumulation of lactic acid) or a rating of perceived exertion (Table 2) corresponding to moderately intense effort.

As patients move into middle-old age, physicians become increasingly reluctant to recommend vigorous test exercise. A large proportion of the middle-old show electrocardiographic (ECG) abnormalities that would contraindicate vigorous exercise in a younger person. During the Canada Fitness Survey, 19% of subjects in the 60 to 69 year age-category saw themselves as unable to perform a simple submaximal step test, and 55% of potential subjects were "screened out" by health professionals conducting the tests.

A safer alternative is to observe some normal function such as the extent of daily activities, the normal pace of walking, or the heart rate developed at a moderate walking pace such as 1.3 m/sec (Table 3). The correlation between walking speed and maximal oxygen intake is only about -0.25, showing that 94% of the variation in walking pace is due to some other factor. The walking pace is also influenced by calf muscle strength; in subjects over the age of 65 years, the correlation between strength and walking pace is about 0.4. Plainly, such correlations do not allow the doctor to use walking pace to estimate either maximal oxygen intake or leg

strength, but it is nevertheless useful to base an exercise recommendation on what the patient can actually accomplish.

The very old may be unable to stand. Such patients can perform a progressive exercise test while seated in a straight-backed chair (Table 4). More commonly, the exercise capacity of the very old is assessed in terms of their ability to perform specific activities of daily living (ADL) (Table 5).

Electrocardiographic Changes

As patients become older, an increasing proportion show exercise-induced ECG abnormalities, including ST depression and premature ventricular contractions. De-

Table 2 Adjustment of Exercise Prescription Based on Perception of Effort

Rating of Effort	Numerical Value	Corresponding Fraction of Peak Oxygen Intake
Very light	9	50
	10	55
Fairly light	11	60
	12	65
Somewhat hard	13	70
	14	75
Hard	15	80
	16	85
Very hard	17	90
	18	94
Very, very hard	19	98
	20	100

Based on the original psychometric scale of Gunnar Borg, and evaluated by Sidney and Shephard in adults aged 65–85 years.

Table 3 Estimate of Fitness Based on Pace and Cardiac Response to Selected Speeds of Ambulation*

Speed	Normal Pace (m/min)	Normal Heart Rate (beats/min)
Slow	63	91
Normal	80	98
Fast	96	110
Maximal	116	131

*Normal values for male patients aged 55–66 years, with measured maximal oxygen intake of 33 ml/kg · min.
  Data from Cunningham DA, Rechnitzer PA, Donner AP. Exercise training and the speed of self-selected walking pace in retirement. Canad J Aging 1986; 5:19–26.

Table 4 Simple Chair-Stepping Test for the Prediction of Maximal Oxygen Intake*

Step Height (cm)	Oxygen Cost (ml/kg · min)	METS (Ratios to resting metabolism)
15.2	8.0	2.3
30.4	10.0	2.9
45.7	12.3	3.5
45.7	13.7	3.9

*Subject sits in a straight back chair and raises alternate legs to the height specified once every second. For the final test stage, the hands are also rested lightly upon the knees.
  Data from Smith EL, Gilligan C. Physical activity prescription for the older adult. Phys Sportsmed 1983; 11:91–101.

Table 5 Relationship Between $\dot{V}O_2$max and Ability to Perform the Activities of Daily Living

Class One:	Patient able to carry 11 kg (24 lb) up 8 steps, or can carry 36 kg (80 lb) or can shovel snow or spade soil or jog or walk at 8 km/h or can perform such recreational activities as skiing, squash, basketball, touch football and handball. $\dot{V}O_2$ intake > 21 ml/kg · min
Class Two:	If no to above, but patient can carry something up 8 steps, or have sexual intercourse or garden, rake, and weed or roller skate or dance the fox-trot or walk at 6.4 km/h on the level $\dot{V}O_2$ > 16 ml/kg · min
Class Three	If no to the above, but patient can shower without stopping, or mop floors or clean windows or hang a wash-load of clothing or walk at 4 km/h on the level or bowl or play golf or push a power mower $\dot{V}O_2$max intake > 11.5 ml/kg · min
Class Four	If no to the above and patient is unable to get dressed without stopping, or has symptoms when eating, when standing, when sitting, or when lying relaxed $\dot{V}O_2$max 7–11.5 ml/kg · min

Adapted from the concept of Lee, et al, 1988.

spite many false positive responses, particularly in women, such changes often reflect significant myocardial ischemia. Questions that arise are (1) is it safe for such individuals to undertake regular physical exercise, (2) should continuous ECG monitoring be provided while they participate in an exercise program, and (3) can the threshold for the appearance of ECG abnormalities (as seen in a laboratory test) be used to set limits to an exercise prescription?

Safety

A worst-case scenario can be based on the experience of cardiac rehabilitation programs. In one survey of 167 such programs, Van Camp obtained data on 51,303 patients and 2,351,916 hours of exercise. Results were similar to the experience of the Toronto Rehabilitation Centre Cardiac Program, where some 5,000 postcoronary patients have exercised for up to 20 years. Van Camp noted 21 incidents of cardiac arrest and eight myocardial infarctions across the 167 programs, with one cardiac arrest in 111,996 patient-hours of exercise, one infarct in 293,990 patient-hours of exercise, and one fatality in 783,972 patient-hours of exercise. Results were independent of program size and the availability of continuous ECG monitoring.

Continuous Monitoring

ECG monitoring is probably an expensive and unnecessary luxury, even for older patients with a prior myocardial infarction. DeBusk and associates arranged home exercise programs for postcoronary patients up to the age of 70 years, using heart-rate monitors and twice weekly telephonic transmission of the ECG signal to a supervising clinic. No patient developed any cardiovascular complications over 26 weeks of vigorous exercise, despite the absence of continuous ECG monitors, although a number of patients with high-risk conditions were excluded from the trial.

Prescription Ceiling

One important function of exercise testing is to set a prudent exercise "ceiling" a little below the intensity of effort that provokes myocardial ischemia. ST segmental depression is associated statistically with a twofold increase in the risk of exercise-induced cardiac emer-

gencies, but 50% or more of apparently positive records are "false positive" findings. In the remaining 50%, ST depression is a valid marker of myocardial ischemia, but during normal, everyday activities the ceiling defined in the laboratory may be reduced by vigorous contraction of small muscles, recent illness, emotional stress, and extremes of hot and cold weather.

ECG appearances and vulnerability to abnormal heart rhythms can both be influenced by many of the medications prescribed for the elderly. A watch must be kept for a possible diuretic-induced potassium loss. Beta-blockers and calcium channel antagonists also modify ST depression by altering exercise heart rate and/or modifying myocardial contractility.

Blood Pressure Responses

Many of the drugs prescribed for the elderly modify the blood pressure (BP) during and after exercise. Systolic BP normally rises progressively during exercise. However, if the myocardium has been weakened by chronic fibrotic degeneration, or left ventricular contractility is impaired by ischemia, the patient may find difficulty in sustaining BP against the increased afterload of vigorous exercise. Failure of the systemic BP to show the anticipated rise during a bout of physical activity is a warning that exercise should be halted urgently.

An abnormally low exercise BP, or its homologue, a poor exercise capacity, indicates a poor prognosis. Postural hypotension is another common problem of the elderly patient. If there are reports of fainting immediately after exercise, with no rhythm disturbances to account for this phenomenon, it may be worth undertaking a tilt-tolerance test.

Muscle Function

Standard laboratory approaches, such as dynamometric or a tensiometric determination of maximum isometric force, determinations of isokinetic and/or isotonic strength and endurance (using a device such as the Cybex II or the Kin-Com isokinetic tester), and measurements of isotonic strength (using an isotonic lifting frame) can be applied to the young-old and the middle-old (Table 6), although more encouragement is needed to elicit maximal effort as a person becomes older. Pain may also limit effort about an arthritic joint,

Table 6 Approximate Influence of Age, Sex, and Fitness Level on Handgrip Force (Newtons) as Recorded by Simple Mechanical Dynamometer

Age (yr)	Men			Women		
	High	Medium	Low	High	Medium	Low
65	480	430	380	290	250	210
70	450	400	350	265	225	185
75	420	370	320	240	200	160
80	390	340	290	210	170	130
85	360	310	260	180	140	100
90	330	280	230	150	110	70

and instability of the knee joints or poor balance may preclude the use of field performance tests such as a jump and reach test. Rapid spinal movements such as timed sit-ups and push-ups are unwise in those with a history of chronic back problems. Care must also be taken not to provoke an excessive rise of BP by prolonged isometric, isokinetic, or heavy isotonic straining against a closed glottis. Finally, in the frail elderly, there is a risk that sudden and overvigorous muscular effort could fracture osteoporotic bones.

Functional capacity may provide some guide to muscle function in the middle-old and very old. As previously noted, triceps surae strength is somewhat related to habitual walking pace. Another simple indicator of muscle condition is the ability of the quadriceps to lift the body mass from a chair.

Body Composition

Actuarial Tables

There are three difficulties in applying actuarial norms to the elderly: (1) progressive muscle wasting and bone mineral loss may give the older patient a normal body mass despite a substantial accumulation of body fat; (2) height measurements are complicated by kyphosis and vertebral collapse; and (3) the actuarial optimum applies to survival from the age of insurance, commonly purchased as a young adult, rather than indicating the optimal body mass for survival during the retirement years.

The optimal body mass thus rises with age (Table 7).

Skinfold Measurements

There are problems when measuring skinfold thicknesses in middle-old and very old patients. Undressing

becomes time consuming. Measurement errors arise because the skin moves independently of subcutaneous fat. The overlying skin is thinner and more compressible than in a younger person, and the ratio of deep to superficial fat also increases with age, so that the extent of obesity may be underestimated from measurements of subcutaneous fat. Age-specific formulas are thus recommended in order to predict the percentage of body fat from skinfold readings (Table 8).

Underwater Weighing

Underwater weighing assumes two body compartments, fat and lean tissue, each with a known and constant density. Bone mineral loss invalidates this assumption in the elderly patient. Underwater weighing remains technically possible in the young-old, but middle-old and very old patients find practical difficulties with the mechanics of the procedure. They are nervous about total immersion in a hydrostatic weighing tank, they may suffer hypotension subsequent to submersion, and there is a danger that they may slip on the wet decks of the tank if their balance is impaired. Many older patients have developed some chronic chest disease; this slows the expulsion of air from the lungs while they are underwater and delays gas equilibration during the determination of residual volume. The

Table 8 Equations for the Prediction of Body Density (D) and thus Body Fat from the Sum of Four Skinfolds (S = biceps + triceps + subscapular + suprailiac)

$$D = 1.1715 - Log_{10} (0.0779) \quad \text{(men)}$$
$$D = 1.1339 - Log_{10} (0.0645) \quad \text{(women)}$$

Based on the work of Durnin and Womersley (1974) for normal men and women over the age of 50 years.

Table 7 Influence of Age on Ideal Body Mass

Height (cm)	Society of Actuaries		Metropolitan Life		Andres (M and F)	
	M	F	M	F	50-59 yr	60-69 yr
147.3		48.5		52.5	55.0	58.4
149.9		49.9		53.4	56.8	60.5
152.4		51.2		54.5	58.4	62.5
155.0		52.6	60.9	55.7	60.5	64.5
157.5	57.6	54.2	62.0	57.3	62.5	66.8
160.0	58.9	55.8	63.2	58.9	64.5	68.9
162.6	60.3	57.8	64.5	60.5	66.6	71.1
165.1	61.9	60.0	65.9	62.0	68.6	73.4
167.6	63.7	61.7	67.3	63.6	70.9	75.5
170.2	65.7	63.5	68.6	65.2	73.2	78.0
172.7	67.6	65.3	70.0	66.6	75.2	80.5
175.3	69.4	66.8	71.4	68.0	77.5	82.5
177.8	71.4	68.5	72.7	69.3	79.8	85.0
180.3	73.5		74.3	70.7	82.0	87.5
182.9	75.5		75.9		84.5	90.0
185.4	77.5		77.7		86.8	92.5
188.0	79.8		79.5		89.3	95.2
190.5	82.1		81.6		91.8	97.7
193.0	84.3				94.3	100.2

Based on the observation of the Society of Actuaries, 1959, for subjects wearing indoor clothing, and the Metropolitan Life Insurance Co., 1983, and R. Andres, 1985 for unclothed subjects.

closed-circuit rebreathing procedure used during underwater weighing may also be complicated by poorly fitting dentures, and thus mouthpiece leakage. Because of the likelihood of chronic chest disease, it is essential to measure rather than to predict the residual gas volume, although one possible option is to make the measurement with the head out of the water.

Determinations of Lean Tissue

The loss of lean tissue provides an objective index of deteriorating physical condition, but measurements are quite difficult to make even in a well-equipped laboratory. Body potassium determinations require costly whole-body counting equipment, only available in large hospitals. Difficulties of data interpretation arise in seniors because the potassium–lean tissue ratio is reduced, and the ^{40}K radiation may also be screened from the counter by an increasing thickness of subcutaneous fat.

Estimates of body composition based on the dilution of deuterated or tritiated water again require sophisticated biochemical analyses, and are complicated by age-related changes in the water content of the fat-free compartment.

The measurement of whole body impedance is a simple office technique, and the equipment has been extensively promoted by the manufacturers, but major assumptions are needed about the electrical conductivity of lean tissue, which again depends on the water content of the body.

Flexibility

Flexibility becomes an increasingly important determinant of function as age increases. It is relatively specific to a given articulation, particularly in older people, where the impact of local anatomic peculiarities is compounded by the effects of arthritic change.

For those patients able to sit on the floor, the standard sit-and-reach test provides a reproducible measure of spinal flexibility (Table 9). Other joints can be assessed by a simple goniometer, but the quality of results is limited by the observer's success in aligning the goniometer with the axis of the joint.

Table 9 Approximate Flexibility, as Assessed by Sit and Reach Test*

Age (yr)	Men	Women
55	24	29
60	23	28
65	22	27
70	21	26
75	20	25
80	19	24
85	18	23
90	17	22

*A score of 25 cm is equivalent to the ability to touch the floor with the tips of the fingers.

EXERCISE PROGRAMS FOR THE ELDERLY

Principles of Exercise Prescription

The average physician may encounter the occasional masters-class athlete who is proposing to begin a fairly strenuous training program. But most older patients are merely seeking a prescription that will maintain reasonable physical condition and optimize their general health.

The health and performance of older patients can often be improved even by modest increases of physical activity. As conditioning begins, there is sometimes a considerable discrepancy between increases of score on formal fitness tests such as $\dot{V}O_2$max and improvements in tolerance of daily activities, perhaps because the main gains are made at the submaximal rather than the maximal level of performance.

Intensity

The traditionally recommended intensity of exercise for cardiorespiratory conditioning, 60% to 70% of $\dot{V}O_2$ max, was based on responses observed in young university students. Quite low intensities of effort can provide an effective basis of conditioning in elderly patients who have been sedentary for many years. Sidney and I compared various self-selected patterns of training in the young-old. A 33% gain of $\dot{V}O_2$max was seen over 7 weeks in subjects that averaged 3.3 training sessions/per week at 60% to 80% of their personal $\dot{V}O_2$max. However, a slower increment (10% over 14 weeks) was also seen in subjects who had exercised frequently, but who had failed to progress beyond 60% of their $\dot{V}O_2$max. Some subsequent authors have found gains of $\dot{V}O_2$max with training at only 30% to 45% of the maximal heart rate reserve.

There are several sound reasons for commending a relatively low intensity of effort to the elderly patient. Low intensity training reduces the likelihood of physical injury. The impact stress on the knee joint is some three times less during walking than during jogging. Further, the chances of provoking a cardiovascular emergency are reduced if training is restricted to moderate exercise. Finally, the consumption of fat is greater with prolonged bouts of moderate exercise than with shorter periods of more intensive effort.

Frequency and Duration of Effort

One hope of the exerciser is that life span will be increased. The extension of life span seems less if exercise is begun in old age (Table 10). Nevertheless, benefit is realized if the patient undertakes a critical volume of training. Studies of Harvard alumni showed that life expectancy was increased with an expenditure of 2.2 megajoules per week, and that benefit was maximized at 8.8 megajoules per week. Likewise, optimization of serum lipids required a weekly walking distance of at least 18 to 20 km. On the other hand, relatively brief

Table 10 Influence of Regular Physical Activity on Longevity

Age of Commencing Exercise	Years Gained
50–59	2.02
60–64	1.75
65–69	1.35
70–74	0.72
75–79	0.42

Based on data of Paffenbarger et al (1986) for added life to age 80 years as estimated from mortality rates.

periods of activity induce gains of muscle strength or flexibility, and some objectives (such as increased social contacts) are satisfied by program attendance alone.

In the frail elderly, prolonged exercise sessions are plainly impractical, at least when conditioning is first initiated. Thus, if a substantial volume of training is prescribed, such activity must be split into several sessions per day.

Safety of Exercise

In general, exercise programs for the elderly seem very safe, particularly if emphasis is placed upon doing only a little more than was accomplished in the preceding week.

Injury

There are few statistics on the likelihood of exercise-induced injuries in the elderly. Leg, ankle, and back lesions apparently occur with some frequency, and the Canada Fitness Survey suggested that injury was the second most common barrier to exercise in the elderly. One Canadian survey noted that 85% of diagnoses were of overuse, and only 4% of patients required surgical treatment. Surprisingly, stress fractures were less frequent than in younger age groups.

Injuries rise sharply even in a young adult once a critical weekly distance—40 to 50 km/week—is exceeded. Old people generally recognize their limitations, and are thus unlikely to engage in excessive competition. The incidence of some types of injury may even decline with age, due to a general decrease in the intensity of physical activity and adoption of safer pursuits. Safety can nevertheless be further enhanced by the development of age-specific sports leagues, along with rule modifications and skillful "officiating" to slow the pace of play. Violent muscular efforts and sudden twisting movements are undesirable. Straight leg lifts, traditional knee-bends, and hyperextension of the back have also been criticized by those with experience in programming for seniors.

The risks of collisions and falls are increased in the elderly patient, due to poor vision and hearing, disturbed balance, unstable knee and hip joints, reduced foot-lift, postural hypotension, and "drop-attacks." Osteoporosis also increases the likelihood that an impact will cause a fracture. Specific precautions in a seniors' program include the use of nonslip flooring and the choice of an environment that has been cleared of all obstacles. Impairments of balance, attacks of unconsciousness, and hypotension on leaving the water all increase the risks of swimming, and elderly patients should avoid swimming alone. However, rhythmic exercises in the water are well-suited to the needs of an older person.

Environmental Hazards

Aging compromises adaptations to extremes of both heat and cold. In the heat, problems due to a lack of fitness and poor cardiovascular function are compounded by greater body heat production (due to a poor mechanical inefficiency), a decreased secretion of sweat, an increased thickness of subcutaneous fat and poorer vascular regulation. Even moderate activity can cause fatalities in the frail elderly during bouts of unusually hot weather.

Exposure to cold and dry air is liable to provoke both bronchospasm and angina. Vulnerability to chilblains, frostbite, and hypothermia are all increased in the older patient. An inappropriate setting of the body's thermostat with a lesser capacity for vasoconstriction, is often compounded by treatment with drugs that increase heat loss and in some instances there may also be a lack of money to purchase adequate winter clothing.

Infections

Very strenuous activity can impair the immune function of a competitive athlete, but most seniors do not exercise to this intensity. Insipient diabetes and a poor blood supply to the skin can increase the likelihood of staphylococcal infections, ulcers, and slow-healing abrasions.

Death and Quality-Adjusted Life-Expectancy

When a middle-old or very old patient asks for advice about exercise, the common response of a cautious physician is "to be careful." However, if the prognosis of the "careful" individual is 9 years of partial dependency and a year of total dependency, there is much to commend a more carefree attitude towards pleasurable forms of exercise. On occasion, exercise may provoke an impending death, but it also improves overall prognosis and enhances life-quality, particularly by maintaining the individual's independence. Cross-sectional data suggest that the relative risk of provoking sudden death by exercise is actually lower in the elderly than in younger individuals, presumably because the older person exercises in a more prudent and less competitive manner.

Benefits of Exercise

Many of the accepted risks of a sedentary life-style have a differing magnitude in an elderly population. For example, the actuarial risk associated with a 20% excess of body mass drops from 225% in men aged 40 to 49 years to 119% at an age of 70 to 79 years. On the other hand, the actuarial risk of physical inactivity increases from 180% of standard in men aged 40 to 49 years to 285% in men aged 70 to 79 years. Particular benefits of exercise in the elderly include (1) the maintenance of independence, (2) the halting of osteoporotic changes, (3) social gains, and (4) relief of depression.

Independence

An active life-style does not materially inhibit the rate of loss of oxygen transport with aging (the average loss is still 0.4 to 0.5 ml/[kg · min] per year), but the exercise program moves the patient from a sedentary to an active aging curve. The training-induced increase in $\dot{V}o_2$max, about 10 ml/[kg · min] at any given age, is equivalent to as much as a 20 year reversal of aging. The $\dot{V}o_2$max of an active patient thus does not drop to the critical threshold needed for independent living (12 to 14 ml/[kg · min]) until the person has reached an age of 90 or 100 rather than 80 years.

Equally, training restores lean tissue, so that at any given calendar age the active patient is much further from the critical limit of muscle strength needed for independence. Conditioning is unlikely to reverse damage to articular surfaces, but greater strength can improve the stability of injured joints. Regular movement of joints through their full range of motion is particularly helpful in checking the slow loss of flexibility with aging.

Loss of independence sometimes reflects a deterioration of mental rather than physical function, and there are claims that mental function is enhanced by regular physical activity. It is unclear how far benefits reflect an exercise-induced increase of cerebral blood flow, and how far other less specific factors are involved, such as a general increase of arousal or greater interest in life.

Osteoporosis

Senescence is associated with a progressive loss of both mineral content and matrix from the bones, with a corresponding increase in the risk of fractures. Weight-bearing activity checks but does not entirely reverse this process.

Social Gains

The social world of the frail elderly becomes increasingly circumscribed, and an exercise class may provide a valuable occasion for friendly contact with other people.

Relief of Depression

Many patients exercise "to feel better." Exercise is helpful in lessening anxiety and relieving depression, particularly if patients are initially anxious or depressed.

Optimum Exercise Recommendation for the Elderly Patient

Safety

Most old people err on the side of caution. The physician should thus encourage activity rather than utter dire warnings. The ideal prescription leaves no more than a pleasant degree of tiredness on the following day. Prolonged muscular straining against a closed glottis must be avoided, and walking is preferred to jogging. The intensity should not provoke ECG abnormalities, chest pain, or a decline in BP. Moderation of the prescription is advisable during extremes of weather, unless the class can move to a swimming pool or an air-conditioned facility.

Effectiveness

Cardiovascular Function. Cardiovascular function is improved by any exercise that involves a substantial fraction of the body musculature. If the patient cannot stand, considerable conditioning is still possible through exercises involving the arms and shoulder girdle.

The elderly person gains some cardiovascular stimulation from heart rates in the range 110 to 120 beats/minute, but physical condition soon plateaus unless intensity is increased as fitness improves. Many patients have difficulty in palpating their heart rates. Other guidelines to an appropriate intensity include activity that allows continued conversation, that seems "somewhat hard," and that induces some sweating. Initially, bouts of activity may be limited to 10 to 15 minutes, but as condition improves the duration can be increased to 30 to 60 minutes per session.

Muscle Function. If an exercise program has an exclusive cardiovascular focus, this leads to an undesirable weakening of the arm muscles. However, the young-old can supplement cardiovascular training with a full range of isotonic, isometric, and circuit exercises, provided that individual contractions are held for only a few seconds, and an adequate recovery interval is allowed between contractions. The frail elderly can improve muscle condition by tensing one muscle group against another, or pressing periodically against the back of a chair or a bed-board. Weights such as books can also be secured to a short plank that is balanced on the ankles when lying in bed, in order to stimulate the leg muscles.

Flexibility. Major joints should be exercised regularly. If the joints are painful or unstable, suggest weight-supported activities in a heated pool. Flexibility can be improved by gentle stretching at the extremes of motion, using either the mass of the body or that of a partner as the driving force.

Osteoporosis. Exercise against an external force such as gravity seems necessary to conserve bone mineral. Walking provides a good stimulus to the lower limbs, hips, and spine, but weights must be held in the hands in order to strengthen the arm bones. Swimming and water-supported gymnastics probably do not correct osteoporosis.

Mood Elevation. Mental arousal is associated with

the proprioceptive stimulation of vigorous movements, even if the patient is confined to bed. Mood may also be enhanced by new social contacts, and the pleasant aesthetic experience of, for example, a brisk walk in the country.

Motivation

Up to 50% of patients drop out of formal exercise programs within 6 months of recruitment. Retention is favored by a matching of programs to the goals, aptitudes, interests, and skill levels of individual patients.

Goals. The primary goals of the older exerciser are usually an improvement of health and an increase of social contacts. Physicians should thus emphasize linkages between class participation, health, and independence, providing periodic feedback of gains in health-related fitness. It is also wise to choose programs that allow time for social interaction.

Aptitudes. It is often helpful to build on past aptitudes, suggesting the use of sporting equipment hidden in the corner of an attic. However, the success of this tactic depends on personality; in a very competitive individual, the poor performance of a previously mastered skill can have a negative impact on motivation.

Interests. Prescribed activities must be matched to the patient's interests and personality. An introverted person may react negatively to the enthusiastic locker-room atmosphere of some exercise classes, but respond positively to a graded walking prescription that allows enjoyment of the quiet of the countryside.

Skill and Fitness Levels. The expectations of the instructor should be matched to the patient's fitness level. It is sometimes very helpful to choose a class with an older leader. Specific classes for the obese and the setting of readily attainable goals reduce embarassment in the new recruit. Unsuccessful participation has a negative impact on both body image and motivation. The typical program drop-out is obese and a heavy smoker. This reflects a low overall interest of such individuals in health-related programs.

Other Motivational Tools. Positive feedback is vital. The exerciser can receive various types of feedback, physiologic (test scores), psychological (words of encouragement), and symbolic (T-shirts or pins to mark minor achievements). Compliance may be improved by a decision balance-sheet or contracts to attain specific fitness goals. Barriers to exercise should also be minimized—failing memory should be countered by telephone reminders and/or provision of transport to classes, and the costs of clothing and equipment should be kept to a minimum. Finally, as much as possible of the prescription should be built into normal daily living, walking rather than driving, and using hand rather than power tools in the home and garden.

SUGGESTED READING

American College of Sports Medicine. Guidelines for graded exercise testing and prescription. Philadelphia: Lea & Febiger, 1991.
Bortz WM. Disuse and aging. JAMA 1982; 248:1203–1208.
Cunningham DA, Rechnitzer PA, Donner AP. Exercise training and the speed of self-selected walking pace in retirement. Canad J Aging 1986; 5:19–26.
DeBusk RF, Houston N, Haskell WL, et al. Exercise training soon after myocardial infarction. Am J Cardiol 1979; 44:1223–1229.
Dishman R. Exercise adherence: Its impact on public health. Champaign, Ill: Human Kinetics Publishers, 1987.
Lawrence G. Aquafitness for women. Toronto: Personal Library Publishers, 1981.
Shephard RJ. Ischemic heart disease and exercise. London: Croom Helm, 1981.
Shephard RJ. Physical activity and aging. 2nd ed. London: Croom Helm, 1987.
Smith EL, Gilligan C. Physical activity prescription for the older adult. Phys Sportsmed 1983; 11:91–101.

INJURIES IN ATHLETES USING WHEELCHAIRS

DAVID C. REID, M.D., M.Ch.(Orth), F.R.C.S.(C)
R.S. BURNHAM, M.D., M.Sc., F.R.C.P.(C)

In 1948, Sir Ludwig Guttmann pioneered sports competition for spinal cord injured war veterans as an adjunct to their therapeutic exercise. Initially 16 disabled men and women competed at archery. Since that time wheelchair sport has grown rapidly in popularity and competitiveness, and in the 1992 Summer Paralympic Games, there were 3,032 competitors from 96 countries around the world. Concurrent with the increase in participation came a greater opportunity for competition and athletic excellence. Previously held records are regularly broken by large margins. This reflects the increased intensity and sophistication of training, the availability of adapted training facilities, improved coaching, and advances in sport equipment design. For instance, George Murray beat all able-bodied runners in the 1978 Boston Marathon with a time of 2:26:52. This record decreased to 1:47:10 by 1985, and is currently 1:17.

There is ample health justification for promoting the involvement of individuals with physical disabilities in such activities. Long-term morbidity and mortality figures for paraplegics are still poorer than for able-bodied individuals. As survival curves improve, however, cardiovascular disease is becoming as prevalent as traditional causes of death such as renal failure, respiratory infections, and gastrointestinal complications. Physical inactivity, smoking, obesity, atherosclerosis, and hypertension, along with some of the emotional distress, are all potentially modified by regular exercise and sport. Thus, wheelchair athletes no longer consider sport as simply a component of their rehabilitation. For many, it has become an important and healthy part of their recreational life-style. For others, preparing for, and participating in, national and international competitions is a full-time occupation, and considerable financial rewards and sponsorships may depend upon their performance. Wheelchair athletes are thus looking more and more to sport scientists for better ways to train, and to sport medicine professionals for improved techniques of injury prevention and treatment.

Unfortunately, sports medicine for athletes using wheelchairs is still in its infancy. Most of the research to date has consisted of case reports, case series, and cross-sectional surveys. These have been useful to profile injury prevalence and to identify which injuries are the most troublesome, in terms of the time lost from sport, as well as to single out those injuries requiring professional medical treatment. Randomized, well-controlled studies, investigating injury cause, prevention, and treatment are scarce. Therefore, the principles and techniques applied to able-bodied athletes are usually adopted for management of the injuries sustained by athletes using wheelchairs, despite the fact that their sport, equipment, injury profiles, and physiology are unique.

Epidemiologic research to date shows that injuries occur in association with wheelchair sport, and that the prevalence/incidence of this occurrence depends on the definition of injury. The most common injury site, although less troublesome in terms of time lost and professional treatment required, is the hand (Fig. 1). These are largely injuries to the skin. The next site in frequency, and by far the most troublesome, is the shoulder, followed by the elbow and wrist. Rotator cuff impingement syndrome and myofascial pain appear to be common diagnostic labels given to shoulder pain when wheelchair athletes are evaluated clinically. Musculoskeletal injuries can be of both acute onset and overuse types. Their occurrence seems correlated with the frequency and intensity of wheelchair sport and weight training, and with multiple sports involvement.

This chapter focuses on traumatic injury and thus does not dwell on the medical problems of competition. In general, physicians and therapists covering these events are faced with much the same issues as with able-bodied athletes. The wheelchair athlete must cope with jet lag, precompetitive anxiety, heat exhaustion, dehydration, respiratory infections, and gastrointestinal illness. However, intercurrent bladder infections and problems of distention, pressure sores, thrombosis, and increased heat dissipation problems are specific concerns. Pre-event site planning and inspection, including access for adapted vehicles and wheelchairs and appropriate toilet and shower design, are of great importance. Furthermore, the experience and mix of the medical team will differ from that selected to accompany an able-bodied team.

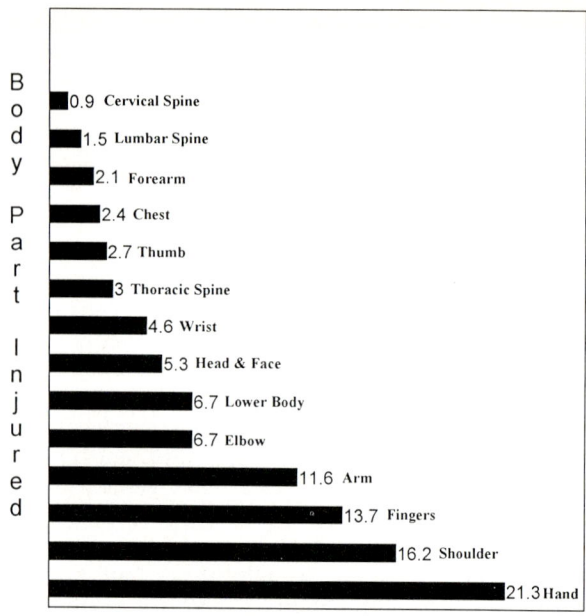

Percent of Total Injury (n=328)

Figure 1 Body parts injured by wheelchair competitors (percent of lesions). Hand and shoulder problems form the bulk of the "time loss" injuries.

INJURY CAUSES AND TREATMENT

An appreciation of the special conditions leading to major injuries provides some insight into methods of prevention and treatment.

Shoulder Pain

The vulnerability of the shoulder girdle in all wheelchair athletes is not surprising, since this area is stressed in day-to-day activities, training, and competition. Gellman et al. confirmed that the prevalence of shoulder pain increased with time since injury, such that 52% had problems within the first 5 years, and shoulder pain was universal by 20 years postinjury. Sie et al, reviewing 239 patients with spinal cord injury, found that 33% had shoulder pain severe enough to require medication or limit their functional activity. Alarmingly, there was a 92% prevalence in the group who had sustained these injuries 15 to 19 years previously.

Shoulder pain in wheelchair athletes may actually be referred from the neck or thoracic spine. However, most of the literature supports the concept that rotator cuff impingement (bursitis/tendinitis) is the most common cause of pain, followed by myofascial pain. There are multiple causes of shoulder rotator cuff syndrome in these athletes, but repetitive strain and overuse are likely causes. The shoulders of wheelchair competitors rarely get rest and recovery time, simply because of the demands of wheelchair propulsion during daily living. Superimposed on the basic demand is an intensive training schedule, as many wheelchair athletes are involved in several different sports concurrently and throughout the year. Careful attention to the structuring of training schedules, allowing adequate recovery time, is particularly important for the wheelchair athlete. Recurrent positioning of the shoulder in extreme forward flexion or flexion and internal rotation puts the rotator cuff in jeopardy of impingement under the coracoacromial arch. This impingement positioning is commonly assumed during everyday activities, as wheelchair competitors reach above their heads to obtain items that are high in relation to the wheelchair seat. Additionally, an overhead arm position is common, particularly in sports such as basketball. Weight training adds an extra load through the shoulder and it is often performed in an impingement position. Avoiding such positions by altering technique, such as using a decline bench instead of an incline bench for bench presses and shorter arch latissimus pull-downs, could alleviate some impingement stresses.

Recent research has suggested the possibility of a shoulder girdle muscle imbalance in wheelchair athletes. Shoulder rotator and adductor muscles are relatively weak in relation to the shoulder abductor muscles among wheelchair athletes compared to able-bodied controls. This imbalance is particularly exaggerated in shoulders that are clinically affected by rotator cuff impingement syndrome. Biomechanically, it is the downward pull of the shoulder rotator and adductor muscles that controls the upward humeral head pull provided by the deltoid (abductor) muscle and the upward push transmitted from the wheelchair tire to the arm. It is theorized that shoulder adductor and rotator insufficiency may allow a recurrent impingement of the rotator cuff muscles within the coracohumeral space by the upward migration of the humeral head, and subsequent encroachment on the acromiohumeral space. It is therefore recommended that strengthening programs around the shoulder include shoulder internal and external rotation, as well as adduction exercises, all of which can be performed easily using tubing or dental dam. Strengthening of the shoulder rotator muscles requires a well-stabilized scapula. Anecdotally, wheelchair competitors often assume a position of scapular protraction, both during sport and at rest. If the scapular retractor muscles (rhomboids and mid-trapezii) are insufficient to control scapular protraction, efforts to strengthen the shoulder rotator muscles will be impaired. Recent EMG research has identified rowing as an effective, easily performed exercise for scapular retractor strengthening by wheelchair athletes. Scapular retraction rowing exercises can conveniently be performed from a wheelchair, using surgical tubing.

Shoulder inflexibility may contribute to shoulder pain. Curtis et al found that spinal cord injured wheelchair athletes with shoulder symptoms had less shoulder extension and tendencies to less shoulder range of motion than those without shoulder pain. These tight muscle groups are predominantly of the anterior shoulder, in keeping with the observation of chronic scapula protraction posturing. Therefore, stretching of the anterior shoulder muscles, including shoulder extension, external rotation and scapular retraction, in addition to scapular retraction strengthening exercises, are recommended for wheelchair athletes. This routine may help to diminish the occurrence of upper and mid-trapezius myofascial pain frequently seen in wheelchair athletes.

Allowing adequate shoulder recovery time, minimizing impingement positioning, stretching anterior shoulder musculature, and strengthening the shoulder adductor, rotator, and scapular retractor muscles, should prevent some of the chronic shoulder disability and pain experienced by wheelchair athletes. When acute pain does occur, early assessment, diagnosis, and appropriate treatment is mandatory to avoid chronic problems. Measures to reduce acute inflammation, such as ice, anti-inflammatory drugs, and physiotherapy are often instituted early. If clinically warranted, diagnostic investigation may include x-rays (to rule out conditions like avascular necrosis of the humeral head) and arthrography/MRI (to rule out rotator cuff tears). Indeed, Bayley et al demonstrated a high incidence of rotator cuff tears in paraplegics complaining of chronic anterior impingement. Unfortunately, even when identified, the need for and role of surgical repair is still ill defined. This further emphasizes the need for early treatment and prevention of problems before irreversible tissue changes occur.

Hand Injury

The wheelchair athlete commonly sustains hand injuries, some of which are characterized by hand numbness and pain. Recent investigations that combined clinical and electrophysiologic assessments of the hands of wheelchair athletes found the most common site of entrapment was the median nerve at the carpal tunnel (carpal tunnel syndrome), followed by ulnar nerve entrapment at the wrist (Guyon's canal). The median nerve was most impaired at the proximal portion of the carpal tunnel, corresponding to the interface between the hand and wheelchair tire/rim during wheelchair propulsion. It was therefore hypothesized that recurrent trauma over the carpal tunnel contributed to the high prevalence of carpal tunnel syndrome in wheelchair athletes. Accordingly, an investigation was conducted to determine whether hand protection utilizing a glove padded with foam in the region of the carpal tunnel would minimize the median nerve dysfunction resultant from wheeling. It was found that measurable median nerve dysfunction did occur across the carpal tunnel with wheelchair propulsion, but that this was not minimized by utilizing the padded glove.

In our series, nearly one-half of all basketball injuries (25%) and abrasions (21.0%) involved the hand and wrist. Similarly in track, blisters (32%) and abrasions (30%) were the worst common injuries.

The major sources of these injuries include friction injuries incurred during acceleration and deceleration, debris on the wheel, inappropriate wheelchair design, and inadequate use of protective equipment. Gloves are the most commonly used protective equipment, but little thought has gone into the production and manufacturing of protective gloves for people using wheelchairs. Even if they are adequate when new, most athletes wear their gloves long past the point when they give useful protection. Theoretically, these common injuries could be greatly reduced by appropriate use of protective gear. When blisters do occur, meticulous attention is needed in order to allow rapid resolution. Careful scrutiny and follow up is needed to ensure that secondary infection does not complicate the recovery.

Tendinitis

Tendinitis comprises about 10.7% of injuries and a large proportion of the wrist problems. Unlike the common DeQuervain's tenosynovitis of the thumb tendons seen in the able-bodied athlete, the extensor and flexor tendons of the wrist are more commonly involved in the wheelchair athletes. One of the serious implications of this is the previously mentioned association with carpal tunnel syndrome. Early detection helps to alleviate chronicity.

Pressure Sores

Up to 10% of athletes report the development of or aggravation of existing pressure sores directly related to their physical activity. This is particularly seen in road racing, but is also noted in track and basketball players. Indeed, it has been reported that some competitive quadriplegic road racers induce or aggravate a pressure sore in order to cause a nociceptive source, increasing catecholamine output with the intent of improving race performance (autonomic dysreflexia or "boosting"). In view of the difficulty of healing these sores, and the debilitating effect of secondary infection, this is a significant problem. Careful attention to seat design, training techniques, and the duration of training sessions; awareness of previous devitalized areas of skin; prompt aggressive attention to "hot spots" on newly damaged areas, and education regarding the health risks of "boosting" can save months of treatment time. Good communication and confidence in the medical and therapeutic staff will allow early aggressive attention to these lesions.

Osteoporosis and Fractures

There is a generalized calcium loss and tendency for osteoporosis immediately following spinal trauma. As the individual becomes more active, this negative calcium balance is gradually corrected or the process slows down, probably influenced by increasing levels of glycosaminoglycans in the ground substance of the bones. Unfortunately lack of muscle contraction and decreased impact loading stresses through the paralyzed or weakened limbs results in progressive bone catabolism. Leg bone mineral density progressively decreases over at least 2 years postinjury, resulting in values of 40% and 60% of normal at the proximal tibia and femoral neck, respectively. Thus, the lower extremity bones are in a weakened state. In addition the limbs lack normal protective sensations, as well as the rapid muscle contraction and movement that normally reduces significant impacts and torques. Although one might anticipate a large incidence of fractures, overall they are relatively uncommon in the wheelchair athlete. In our review, we saw only seven fractures and two dislocations, comprising 2.6% of all injuries. Nevertheless, when osteoporotic fractures do occur, such injuries are serious problems. There are special points of recognition, treatment, and steps to avoid the complication of fractures in the wheelchair athlete.

Minimally displaced or small bone fractures may be overlooked by an athlete because protective sensation is lacking. Crepitus, a sudden increase in the range of motion of joints such as the hip, and a rapidly accumulated swelling of bruising should raise the suspicion of a fracture. Furthermore, dislocated or fractured major bones or joints may precipitate unusually forceful and frequent muscle spasms, or symptoms of autonomic dysreflexia (headache, blurred vision, facial flushing, goose bumps, and hypertension).

Unrecognized fractures may jeopardize the integrity of the overlying skin if they are not diagnosed or managed correctly. A simple closed injury can easily be converted into a potentially complicated open fracture. In addition, significant hemorrhage and sympathetic stimulation can give very rapid changes in blood pressure. Lastly, failure to manage a fracture adequately may lead to excessive tissue swelling, an increased tissue pressure, and potential compartment syndromes, which could jeopardize the viability of the limb.

The treatment of fractures requires special consideration. The choice is between open reduction, splinting, or treatment by limb care without splinting. An appropriate decision requires experience and a thorough knowledge of the potential benefits and complications of each fracture in each segment of the limb. Treatment should thus be determined in consultation with an orthopedic surgeon who has a special interest in the paraplegic individual.

Compartment Syndrome

Some of the complications usually seen with compartment syndromes (CS) may not be significant in the paralyzed limb, but muscle necrosis or skin slough, can lead to infection and electrolyte imbalance. Severe myonecrosis can precipitate renal failure and even death. It is not always easy to recognize impending acute CS, because dependent edema is almost a normal condition in some of these individuals. However, education of the athlete and awareness of coaches and medical staff can lead to early suspicion of an impending CS. Inasmuch as elevated commpartment pressures occur just as easily with contusions and crushing from falls or wheelchair collision, a routine clinical check of the tension in respective compartments and diminished pulses, can and should be carried out after each competition. The main point is to make the athlete aware of the potential for this syndrome.

Concussion (Closed Head Injury)

Concussion accounts for about 2% of all injuries. Most concussions are sustained by quadriplegic rugby players, probably a direct consequence of their poor balance and significant involvement of the musculature. In addition, many athletes strap their legs to their wheelchairs in order to assist in controlling involuntary leg spasms. Thus, the athlete and the wheelchair tend to act as a unit that moves and falls together, making the head a frequent and vulnerable point of contact. This is particularly true if the wheelchair tips over backwards. Although an unpopular suggestion, the use of helmets in wheelchair rugby should be considered.

COMMENTS

Over 40% of spinal injuries are sustained through motor vehicle accidents and sports such as football, diving, and gymnastics. Many of these individuals are relatively young. It is thus not surprising that a substantial proportion are attracted to the thrills and challenges of fast moving wheelchair competition.

In addition to the biomechanics of wheelchair propulsion, and individual pattern of muscle stress, imbalance, and flexibility, many mechanisms of injury in wheelchair athletes are sport specific. Causes include collisions, damage inflicted by wheelchair parts, mechanical failure of the wheelchair, spills, sports equipment and balls acting as missiles, difficult surfaces and terrains, poor techniques of wheeling, and lack of or poor protective equipment. It is particularly unfortunate that the injuries sustained during sports activities have serious ramifications for the every day life of these individuals.

Early detection of many injuries depends on the recognition of subtle clinical signs, because of the absence of normal protective sensation and a lack of subjective complaints. In some instances, the appropriate treatment of these injuries is at variance to what is presented for the able-bodied athlete, and hence special knowledge is required by those supervising their care.

Specialized seating and other chair modifications have decreased risks dramatically, but protective equipment such as gloves, helmets, and splints is still underused and inadequately researched.

SUGGESTED READING

Bayley JC, Cochran TP, Sledge CG. The weight-bearing shoulder: The impingement syndrome in paraplegics. J Bone Joint Surg 1987; 69A:676–678.

Biering-Sorensen F, Bohr HH, Schaadt OP: Longitudinal study of bone mineral content in the lumbar spine, the forearm and the lower extremities after spinal cord injury. Eur J Clin Invest 1990; 20:330–335.

Burnham R, May L, Nelson E, et al. Shoulder pain in wheelchair athletes – The role of muscle imbalance. Am J Sports Med 1993; 21: 238–242.

Burnham R, Newell E, Steadward R: Sports medicine for the physically disabled: The Canadian team experience at the 1988 Seoul Paralympic Games. Clin J Sport Med 1991; 1:193–196.

Curtis KA, Dillon DA. Survey of wheelchair athletic injuries: Common patterns and prevention. Paraplegia 1985; 23:170–175.

Ferrara MS, Buckley WE, McCann BC, et al. The injury experience of the competitive athlete with a disability: Prevention implications. Med Sci Sports Exerc 1992; 24:184–188.

Gellman H, Sie I, Waters RL. Late complications of the weight-bearing upper extremity in the paraplegic patient. Clin Orthop 1988; 233:132–135.

Givre S, Freed HA: Autonomic dysreflexia: A potentially fatal complication of somatic stress in quadriplegics. J Emerg Med 1989; 7:461–463.

Hoeberigs JH, Debets-Eggen HBL, Debets PML: Sports medical experiences from the International Flower Marathon for disabled wheelers. Am J Sports Med 1990; 18:418–421.

Jackson RW, Fredrickson A: Sports for the physically disabled — The 1976 Olympiad (Toronto). Am J Sports Med 1979; 7:293–296.

Martinez SF: Medical concerns among wheelchair road racers. Phys Sport Med 1989; 17:63–68.

McCormack DAR, Reid DC, Steadward RD, Syrotiuk DG. Injury profiles in wheelchair athletes: Results of a retrospective survey. Clin J Sport Med 1991; 1:35–40.

Nichols PJR, Norman PA, Ennis JR: Wheelchair users' shoulder? Scand J Rehabil Med 1979; 11:29–32.

Reid DC, Saboe L. Spinal trauma in sports and recreation. Clin J Sport Med 1991; 1:75–80.

Shephard RJ: Sports medicine and the wheelchair athlete. Sports Med 1988; 4:226–247.

Sherrill C, Adams-Mushett C, Jones JA. Classification and other injuries in sport for blind, cerebral palsied, les autres and amputee athletes. In: Sherril C, ed. Sport and disabled athletes. Champaign, Ill: Human Kinetics Publication, 1986:113.

Sie I, Waters RL, Adkins RH, Gellman H. Upper extremity pain in the post rehabilitation spinal cord injured patient. Arch Phys Med Rehab 1992; 73:44–48.

EXERCISE AND SPECIAL POPULATIONS

BO FERNHALL, Ph.D., F.A.C.S.M., F.A.A.C.V.P.R.

Mental retardation (MR) is the most common form of developmental disability in the western world, with an estimated prevalence of 3% in the United States. Approximately 7 to 8 million people are classified as having MR, and close to 1.5 million of these individuals are 55 years of age or older. This population has a two to four times higher risk of early mortality and morbidity than the general population. Persons with MR also have a much higher rate of institutionalization. Fifty to 60% of elderly persons with MR are institutionalized, compared to 5% to 8% of the general population. The most common medical problem in populations with MR is cardiovascular disease, and the prevalence rates of cardiovascular disorders in these persons residing in the community is considerably higher than for their peers without MR. Morbidity is further complicated by high rates of obesity; 40% to 60% of the population being classified as obese based on standard criteria.

It is now well established that exercise and physical fitness are important for health and well-being, particularly as they relate to the prevention of cardiovascular disease. However, persons with MR are generally not active individuals and the fitness levels of the average young adult with MR has been equated to that of a 60-year-old individual with coronary heart disease. Opportunities for special exercise programs for persons with MR are rare. The Special Olympics is the largest available program. However, while the Special Olympics may develop better socialization and physical skills, it does not generally improve the cardiovascular fitness of participants, nor does it impact on obesity. Thus, the preventive benefits of exercise are not often realized by persons with MR. Yet, since work performance has been related to cardiovascular fitness, achieving and maintaining some level of physical fitness is desirable because the jobs available to this population often require light to moderate activity.

Social policies in the past 25 years have emphasized deinstitutionalization and relocating persons with MR into community-based residences. Private practice physicians today are more likely to see and treat persons with MR than in the past. Thus, there is a need for medical professionals to be familiar with some of the specialized circumstances and problems associated with exercise in individuals with MR. An increase of physical activity and fitness levels, and a decrease in the incidence of obesity in this population may have important implications for both their mortality and morbidity.

DEFINITION AND ETIOLOGY

Mental retardation is defined by the American Association on Mental Retardation and the American Psychiatric Association as referring to "significantly subaverage general intellectual functioning existing concurrently with deficits in adaptive behavior and manifested during the developmental period." Table 1 displays the different categories of MR. All categories must be accompanied by maladaptive behavior, such as problems with communication, social skills, self care, or self direction. Furthermore, MR must be diagnosed before the individual reaches the age of 18 years. A diagnosis of substandard intelligence that is reached after the age of 18 is described as neurologic damage.

There are many potential causes of MR. Some are organic, including genetic disorders (e.g., Down syndrome, fragile X syndrome, phenylketonuria), maternal disorders (e.g., rubella, syphilis, fetal alcohol syndrome), birth trauma (e.g., anoxia), and diseases such as meningitis. Severe stimulus deprivation, malnutrition, and poverty can also contribute to MR. Individuals with MR usually have sensory, motor, and physical handicaps that make general exercise participation more difficult than for a person without MR. In addition to having multiple handicaps, many persons with MR have underlying congenital heart defects that limit their physical capabilities. Furthermore, MR is often accompanied by

Table 1 Categories of Mental Retardation

Category	IQ Range	Characteristics
Mild MR	50–70 Prevalence 60%–90% of subjects with MR	Live independently; work independently; marry, rear children; socially isolated; live near or in poverty
Moderate MR	35–55 Prevalence 7%–32% of subjects with MR	Significant adaptive behavior deficits; often work in sheltered workshops; most do not marry; have self care skills; problems with speech, socialization, and gait
Severe and profound MR	Below 40 Prevalence 4%–8% of subjects with MR	High incidence of motor, sensory, and physical handicaps; problems with activities of daily living and self care; often institutionalized

attentional deficit disorders that cause problems in the motivation of exercise participation.

EXERCISE AND FITNESS STATUS OF PERSONS WITH MR

Persons with MR have very low levels of cardiovascular fitness. Young adults with mild or moderate MR, without any limiting medical conditions, have mean $\dot{V}O_2$max values of 22 to 30 ml/kg/min (6 to 8.5 METS). Individuals with Down syndrome appear to have 10% to 20% lower $\dot{V}O_2$max values than their peers without Down syndrome. It is unclear why values are lower in individuals with Down syndrome, although this syndrome is associated with a greater incidence of congenital heart defects, which can have a negative influence on cardiovascular fitness. However, almost all published studies have described subjects without clinical evidence of limiting disease. All persons studied with MR have had lower than expected maximal heart rates (HR) (8% to 20%), a feature that is further exacerbated by Down syndrome. Individuals with Down syndrome typically have 10% lower maximal HR than persons having MR without Down syndrome. Low maximal HR limit peak cardiac output, which could explain the low $\dot{V}O_2$max values. It has also been suggested that motivation to perform is low in this population, although laboratory data suggest that the maximal testing of adults with MR produces both valid and reliable results.

The most commonly accepted reason for the low cardiovascular fitness levels observed is the sedentary life-style of persons with MR. However, this view is based on subjective observations rather than scientific data. There have been no studies on the physical activity patterns of populations with MR. The bigger problem arising from the low fitness levels may be the secondary effects of aging upon these individuals. If the rate of decrease in $\dot{V}O_2$max with age is the same in populations with MR as in those without MR, then by 50 years of age most persons with MR would be so severely limited that they could not perform even light physical work for a normal work day. The risk is greater for females than for males, since they generally begin adult life with lower cardiovascular work capacities than men.

Many persons with MR are obese, whether defined by BMI or by percent body fat. Their obesity has been linked not only to poor activity patterns, but also to diets high in fat and food energy. Overeating is a major problem for persons with mild and moderate MR, since food is often used as a reward by parents and/or center personnel. The average body fat reported for young adults with MR is 21% for men and 31% for women, with 42% of men and 61% of women falling into the obese categories (>20% body fat for men and >30% for women). Although persons with Down syndrome give the appearance of being fatter than those without Down syndrome, the percent of body fat tends to be similar in the two groups. A "fatter" appearance is more likely linked to shorter stature, shorter limbs, and skeletal muscle hypotonia, these features often being present in individuals with Down syndrome.

Low muscular strength and endurance have also been identified in this population. Average sit-up and push-up scores ranked in the first to second percentile for males with MR and in the fourth percentile for females with MR, when compared to their peers without MR. Young adults with MR also have only 78% of the expected upper body and 71% of the expected lower body isometric strength. Similar results have been shown for isokinetically measured strength. Again, individuals with Down syndrome had lower strength values than their peers without Down syndrome. It is generally hypothesized that the low values for muscular strength and endurance of populations with MR is due to inactivity and disuse, but this may not explain why persons with Down syndrome have even lower values.

EXERCISE AND FITNESS TESTING OF PERSONS WITH MR

Maximal exercise testing of individuals with MR can be both valid and reliable. In most such subjects, walking treadmill protocols have produced plateaus of $\dot{V}O_2$ as work rate is increased. Such plateauing is considered an objective criterion that $\dot{V}O_2$max has been achieved. Allowing subjects to stop exercising due to volitional fatigue before attaining a plateau of $\dot{V}O_2$ does not appear to change either $\dot{V}O_2$max or peak $\dot{V}O_2$ appreciably. Reliability coefficients are slightly lower than for populations without MR, but still in an acceptable range (0.92 to 0.94). Similar results have been shown using the Schwinn Air Dyne ergometer, but standard cycle ergometers have not yielded reliable and valid test results. Several investigators have reported problems with maintenance of the required pedal cadence and difficulties in achieving good efforts. Thus, if cycle ergometer testing is desired, I recommend using the Schwinn Air Dyne, which combines leg and arm work.

The sensitivity, specificity, and predictive accuracy of exercise testing for the detection of cardiovascular disease are unknown for populations with MR, as there are no data on groups of older persons with MR (>40 years of age). However, there is no reason to believe that exercise testing could not be used for this purpose, since individuals with MR can achieve good maximal test results. Even young persons with MR may present with significantly abnormal exercise electrocardiograms (ECG), presumably due to previously undetected congenital heart problems, or the early development of atherosclerotic heart disease. Table 2 gives recommendations for exercise test protocols that have been shown to yield valid and reliable results.

Maximal exercise testing is more difficult in persons with MR than in those without MR, because of attentional deficits and problems with task understanding, motivation, and communication. To increase the probability of obtaining accurate results it is important to: (1) familiarize subjects with both the laboratory and the tester; (2) provide ample task training; (3) provide

Table 2 Recommended Exercise Test Protocols

Treadmill		
Speed	*Grade*	*Time Interval*
3–5 km/h based on individual capability	2.5%–4.0% per stage start at 0%	2–3 minutes per stage

Familiarization with treadmill walking is essential!

Schwinn Air Dyne	
Work Rate Increments	*Time Interval*
Start at 25 watts 25 watt increments per stage	2–3 minutes per stage

Measurements: For either protocol, clinical measures such as blood pressure and ECG are obtained in standard manner. Oxygen uptake measures are also obtained in a normal manner, but may require substantial subject practice for valid results.

some safety features to ensure that subjects do not fall or fear falling; (4) tailor the protocol to the individual; and (5) provide an environment in which the participant feels like a contributing member.

If maximal testing cannot be conducted, submaximal field tests can be used to estimate cardiovascular fitness. However, submaximal tests are not as accurate for individuals with MR as for persons without MR. The 2.4 km walk-run, the Rockport walking test, and the modified Léger and Lambert shuttle run have all been validated for use in adults with MR. Popular submaximal cycle ergometer protocols such as the YMCA and Åstrand protocols are not valid for use with this population, because of errors in predicting the maximal HR (values are lower in persons with MR). The validated tests all have prediction errors of 15% to 20%, which is considerably greater than would be anticipated for persons without MR. Thus, caution should be used when interpreting the results of submaximal field tests with this population.

Strength and muscular endurance can be tested in much the same manner as in persons without MR. However, the test-retest reliability of many of the tests is much lower than for individuals without MR, suggesting that several trials should be used. When persons with MR are tested on isokinetic equipment, as many as four test sessions with three trials each are needed. Since a subject cannot be retested twice in any one day, the logistics of completing four clinical test sessions make it difficult to gather acceptable data. Test-retest reliability coefficients vary from 0.76 to 0.92 in populations with MR. The actual test-retest difference in the force produced may be as large as 10% to 19%, and such variance may not be acceptable. However, strength-based measures derived from testing on weight machines are easily obtained and reliable. Using standard techniques for 1 RM performance, test-retest reliability was 0.95 to 0.99, a range similar to data obtained from populations without MR.

Body composition can be evaluated by hydrostatic weighing in persons with MR, but obtaining reliable measures of residual volume may be difficult. Equally accurate results are obtained by using predicted residual volumes in this population. Skinfolds can be measured as accurately as in populations without MR. Generalized formulas for the prediction of body fat, based on three skinfold sites and corrected for age and sex, correlate well with the results obtained by hydrostatic weighing in persons with MR ($r = 0.84$ to 0.92). Similar correlations have also been found for predictions of body fat based on measurements of circumference, height, and body mass in individuals with MR (%fat = $13.5 + 0.487$ [waist circumference in cm] $- 0.527$ [forearm circumference in cm] $- 0.155$ [height in cm] $+ 0.077$ [body mass in kg]).

EXERCISE TRAINING IN PERSONS WITH MR

Many studies have found that persons with MR respond normally, or even better than expected, to traditional cardiovascular training programs. However, most of these studies have measured cardiovascular fitness using nonvalidated field tests. Data generated from studies that actually measured $\dot{V}O_2$max are less consistent. Several small studies without control groups have shown improvements in $\dot{V}O_2$max, ranging from 10% to 43%. There are also some investigations that show no improvement in $\dot{V}O_2$max with training, and yet others have shown that a 2.4 km run or treadmill performance was increased without a concomitant increase in $\dot{V}O_2$max.

Although it is clear that persons with MR do not necessarily respond to cardiovascular exercise training in an expected fashion, some distinguishing characteristics can be identified. It appears that persons with Down syndrome may not improve $\dot{V}O_2$max with training, or at least not in response to a standard program. Furthermore, most of the exercise programs that were shown to be effective continued for longer than the standard 10 to 12 week program. It seems that individuals with MR do not adapt to training as rapidly as persons without MR, and that programs continuing for 16 to 35 weeks can produce substantial improvements in $\dot{V}O_2$max.

Exercise intensity needs to be tightly controlled if training gains are to be realized. Most studies that found no increase in $\dot{V}O_2$max do not report what exercise intensity was used, whereas those that did find an increase used exercise intensities between 60% and 80% of the invididual's $\dot{V}O_2$max. Motivation is often a problem, and rewards have been used to increase motivation and adherence to prescribed exercise guidelines. It is difficult to improve cardiovascular fitness in this population without close exercise supervision and employment of appropriate motivational techniques. Guidelines for cardiovascular exercise prescription are presented in Table 3.

Although persons with MR have low levels of muscular strength and endurance, almost all research has shown improvements in response to training. The

Table 3   Guidelines for Exercise Prescription

Cardiovascular

Intensity	65%–85% of maximal HR. Maximal HR must be measured—cannot be estimated based on standard formulas.
Duration	15–60 minutes of aerobic activity. The activity may need to be varied and discontinuous in nature to keep interest and motivation.
Frequency	3–5 exercise sessions per week.
Program length	15 weeks or longer. The longer lasting programs produce better results, and may be needed to show improvements in $\dot{V}O_2$max.
Exercise mode	Any activity that uses large muscle groups. Running, jogging, treadmill walking, and Air-Dyne exercise are all effective.

Muscular Strength

Intensity	60%–80% of 1 RM, or 8–10 RM. May need to start at 30%–40% of 1 RM and progressively increase intensity to the desired level over a 3 week period.
Repetitions	8–10 per set. Standard Delorme type progressive program may also be used.
Sets	2–3 sets for each muscle group.
Rest interval	2–4 minutes between each set.
Frequency	3 times per week.
Program length	8–9 weeks before substantial improvements will be seen.
Exercise mode	Resistance training, preferably on weight machines, for safety reasons.

amount of improvement is related to the type of training employed, with more intense and longer duration programs eliciting the greatest response. Sit-up and pull-up performance can improve 30% to 200%. Training programs using weight machines can be expected to improve 1 RM strength measures by 25% to 100% over 8 to 10 weeks of training. It appears that individuals with MR respond to resistance training in an expected manner, developing gains similar to their peers without MR. Guidelines for muscular strength exercise prescriptions are presented in Table 3.

In persons with MR, it is difficult to decrease body fat and to have a significant impact on obesity through exercise training alone, without dietary intervention. Nevertheless, some individuals lose substantial amounts of body fat with training. Reductions in body fat through training programs have been most successful in obese women with MR, but long-term jogging programs have also produced substantial reductions of body fat in men. The probability of success in this population increases if the subject is obese at the start of the program, and/or if the program is continued for longer than 15 weeks. However, treatment of obesity through exercise training alone, without dietary intervention, cannot be recommended in persons with MR.

OTHER CONSIDERATIONS

The above discussion of exercise in populations with MR applies only to persons with mild or moderate MR. There is not enough information available to make general recommendations for individuals with severe or profound MR. Furthermore, since persons with mild and moderate MR are most likely to live and work independently, or semiindependently, the practical impact of exercise testing and training is greatest for them. The overall goal of any exercise program for individuals with MR should be to increase their overall work capacity, to

improve their general health, and to contribute to an overall sense of well-being. The success of such programs can have a significant impact on work productivity and the ability of persons with MR to live and function independently as contributing members of society.

SUGGESTED READING

Fernhall B. Physical fitness and exercise training of individuals with mental retardation. Med Sci Sports Exerc 1993; 25:442–450.

Fernhall B, Millar L, Burkett L. Maximal exercise testing of mentally retarded adolescents and adults: Reliability study. Arch Phys Med Rehabil 1990; 71:1065–1068.

Fernhall B, Tymeson G. Validation of cardiovascular fitness field tests for adults with mental retardation. Adapt Phys Activ Quart 1988; 5:49–59.

Fernhall B, Tymeson G. Graded exercise testing of mentally retarded adults: A study of feasibility. Arch Phys Med Rehabil 1993; 68:363–365.

Fernhall B, Tymeson G, Webster G. Cardiovascular fitness of mentally retarded individuals. Adapt Phys Activ Quart 1988; 5:12–28.

Pitetti K. A reliable isokinetic strength test for arm and leg musculature for mildly mentally retarded adults. Arch Phys Med Rehabil 1990; 71:669–672.

Pitetti K, Campbell K. Mentally retarded individuals: A population at risk? Med Sci Sports Exerc 1991; 23:586–593.

Pitetti K, Rimmer J, Fernhall B. Physical fitness and adults with mental retardation. Sports Med 1993; 16:23–56.

Pitetti K, Tan D. Cardiorespiratory responses of mentally retarded adults to air brake ergometry and treadmill exercise. Arch Phys Med Rehabil 1990; 71:318–321.

Pitetti K, Tan D. Effects of a minimally supervised exercise program for mentally retarded adults. Med Sci Sports Exerc 1991; 23: 594–601.

Rimmer J, Braddock D, Fujiura G. Prevalence of obesity in adults with mental retardation: Implications for health promotion and disease prevention. Mental Retardation 1993; 31:105–110.

Seidl C, Reid G, Montgomery D. A critique of cardiovascular fitness testing with mentally retarded persons. Adapt Phys Activ Quart 1987; 4:106–116.

Winnick JP, ed. Adapted physical education and sport. Champaign, Ill: Human Kinetics Books, 1990.

EXERCISE AND AIR POLLUTION

LAWRENCE J. FOLINSBEE, Ph.D.

Our environment contains a number of trace gaseous pollutants, including ozone (O_3), sulfur dioxide (SO_2), carbon monoxide (CO), nitrogen oxides, hydrocarbons, and many others. Community air pollution is an ancient problem, but real progress in understanding the health effects of air pollutants and the benefits from an improvement of air quality has occurred primarily over the past 40 years. The health effects of various air pollutants have been reviewed extensively, especially in the Air Quality Criteria Documents published by the U.S. Environmental Protection Agency. With regard to effects on exercise performance, three air pollutants merit particular concern: ozone, sulfur dioxide, and carbon monoxide. Both O_3 and SO_2 can have important effects on the respiratory tract and may cause ventilatory limitations to exercise, whereas CO has a direct effect on oxygen transport by hemoglobin. Three important variables determine exposure and, hence, our response to air pollutants: the ambient concentration of the gas; the duration of exposure; and the respiratory minute volume of the exposed individual. People who exercise heavily in polluted environments inhale a much greater quantity of air pollutants than their sedentary counterparts. Other factors may modify the actual quantity of gas that reaches the particular target site within the respiratory tract, such as the solubility of the gas and the route of inhalation (i.e., nose versus mouth). The presence of respiratory or cardiovascular disease can modify responses considerably, as will be seen in the cases of SO_2 and CO.

SULFUR DIOXIDE

SO_2 is a byproduct of many industrial processes, including cement manufacturing, ore smelting, pulp and paper manufacturing, sulfuric acid production, and processes that require the combustion of high sulfur fuels. Although SO_2 is a pervasive, widely transported pollutant usually present at low concentrations in the atmosphere, the higher concentrations in the vicinity of point sources are of the greatest concern.

Even at SO_2 levels in the vicinity of point sources, there is little effect on the respiratory tract of healthy individuals. However, individuals with asthma are nearly 10 times more sensitive to SO_2 than nonasthmatics. Nevertheless, most asthmatics respond to SO_2 only when the exposure is accompanied by exercise. Thus, the

major concern is with asthmatics who may be exposed to high concentrations of SO_2 while exercising near a point source. Respiratory symptom responses in asthmatics include chest discomfort, wheezing, and shortness of breath. Increased airway resistance and a decreased forced expiratory flow are seen immediately following SO_2 exposure. Responses range from almost none to as much as a ten-fold increase in airway resistance, or as much as a 60% decrease in FEV_1. Asthmatics with the most severe symptoms may find it necessary to use a bronchodilator, reduce their exercise level, or withdraw from the exposure. These observations strongly suggest that the performance of asthmatic athletes could be impaired by SO_2 exposure.

Responses to SO_2 have a rapid onset; marked changes can occur within 2 to 3 minutes. Although increased responses may be seen with longer exposures, responses are relatively insensitive to increases of exposure duration beyond about 10 minutes. Recovery from SO_2-induced bronchoconstriction is also rapid, seldom lasting longer than about an hour. There is then a "refractory period" lasting for about 3 to 4 hours, during which time the individual is less responsive to further SO_2 exposure. This refractory period is not associated with diminished airway responsiveness. Indeed, SO_2 is not thought to cause a change in airway responsiveness with either acute or prolonged exposure. There is no evidence of a late phase response (i.e., 4 to 8 hours after the initial exposure), nor is there any evidence of altered asthma status resulting from acute or chronic SO_2 exposure. Asthma severity seems to have only a minor effect on SO_2 response. Mild asthmatics, who are more likely to participate in outdoor exercise or competitive athletics, have similar SO_2 responses to individuals with moderate or severe asthma.

SO_2 is highly soluble and is efficiently removed in the moist upper airway, especially the nose. Responses to SO_2 exposure can be exacerbated by increased oral breathing or breathing air with a reduced water content (either cold or dry). It might thus be anticipated that responses to a given SO_2 exposure would be increased in dry winter weather compared to humid summer weather. The exacerbation of responses by cold-dry air or mouth breathing may be due, in part, to a diminished SO_2 removal in the upper airway.

Commonly used asthma medications can modify the effects of SO_2 on asthmatics. Bronchodilators such as albuterol (Proventil, Ventolin) or metaproterenol (Alupent, Metaprel) can markedly reduce or reverse the effects of SO_2. Cromolyn sodium (Intal) taken prior to exposure can partially inhibit the response to SO_2, but in the usual therapeutic dose, it is minimally effective. Theophylline (Uniphyl, Elixophyllin, Theobid, and others) and inhaled corticosteroids appear to have minimal, if any, prophylactic effect in modifying responses to SO_2 exposure. If regular medication is withheld, the SO_2 response of moderate asthmatics is about the same as when they are regularly medicated, even though their baseline pulmonary function deteriorates when medication is withheld. However, many mild asthmatics use a bronchodilator infrequently, on an "as-needed" basis,

This document has been reviewed in accordance with U.S. Environmental Protection Agency policy and approved for publication. It does not necessarily reflect the views of the agency and no official endorsement should be inferred. Mention of trade names does not constitute endorsement or recommendation for use.

often less than once a week. Such individuals may not carry medication during outdoor exercise, the primary activity during which the two events of exercise and inhalation of SO_2 from a stationary source plume may coincide. Thus it is inappropriate to assume that asthmatics, even those on a regular regimen of medication, will be "protected" from SO_2 exposure because of their use of medication. Asthmatic athletes or asthmatics who engage in regular outdoor exercise may wish to consider the prophylactic use of a beta-agonist prior to exercise, especially if this activity will occur in the vicinity of an SO_2 source.

OZONE

O_3 exists in the stratosphere, where it shields the earth's surface from ultraviolet light, and it is also formed in the troposphere by a complex photochemical reaction involving sunlight, oxygen, hydrocarbons, and nitrogen oxides, the latter two derived primarily from automobile emissions. Ozone is a highly reactive gas and if breathed at concentrations of several parts per million (ppm) it can induce potentially fatal pulmonary edema. Major metropolitan areas throughout the world have periodic elevations of ozone concentration, exposing millions of people to potentially harmful levels of O_3. Notable examples are Los Angeles and Mexico City, where levels often exceed 0.20 ppm for several consecutive hours.

O_3 exposure induces a number of symptoms, including cough, chest discomfort, and pain on deep inspiration, but not eye irritation. Many of these symptoms are thought to result from airway irritation and stimulation of the airway pain and cough receptors. Physiologic responses to O_3 include decreased lung volumes (i.e., FVC, IC, TLC) and expiratory flow rates (Fig. 1), increased airway resistance, a decreased tidal volume and increased breathing frequency during exercise, and increased airway responsiveness. Based on studies in which humans have undergone bronchoalveolar lavage after O_3 exposure, O_3 also induces airway inflammation, with erythema of the larger air passages, recruitment of neutrophils, and release of prostaglandins and other arachidonic acid metabolites. It is known from animal studies that O_3 damages pulmonary epithelia and it also appears to increase the permeability of the lung. There are clear indications from controlled human exposure studies that epithelial damage has occurred and that pulmonary repair processes are up-regulated.

Physiologic and symptomatic responses to O_3 are probably responsible for the observed effects on exercise performance. Several investigators have observed a decrease in peak $\dot{V}O_2$ both in healthy individuals and in trained athletes who are exposed to O_3 while exercising. These reductions in peak $\dot{V}O_2$ have been accompanied by reductions in maximal ventilation, maximal tidal volume (but not breathing frequency), and maximum power output. Marked symptoms of breathing discomfort and cough and sharp reductions in pulmonary function typically accompany the decrements of perfor-

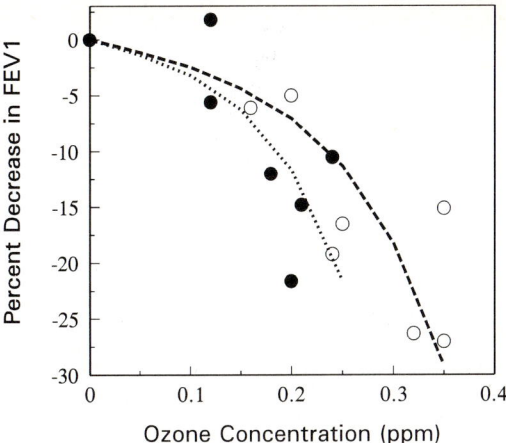

Figure 1 Percent decrease in lung function (forced expired volume in 1 second) after 1 hour continuous exercise exposures to O_3 concentrations of 0.12 to 0.35 ppm. Response curves have been estimated for two exercise intensities, based on respiratory minute volumes of 60 to 70 L/min (○ ○ ○) and 80 to 100 L/min (●●●). (From Folinsbee LJ. Ambient-air pollution and endurance performance. In: RJ Shephard, P-O Åstrand, eds. Endurance in sport [The encyclopedia of sports medicine 2]. Oxford: Blackwell Scientific, Human Kinetics, 1992:479–486; with permission.)

mance. Trained competitive athletes (cyclists and runners) who have been exposed to O_3 during heavy exercise indicate that they could not have performed maximally under those conditions and, in some cases, they were unable to complete a prescribed training or competitive simulation while exposed to O_3. The endurance time at a given rate of working during O_3 exposure was less than under control conditions. Such responses have been observed at O_3 concentrations as low as 0.18 ppm.

Although the breathing pattern is altered and airway resistance is increased slightly, the overall ventilation at submaximal work rates typically is unaffected. The rapid shallow breathing leads to a slight but negligible decline in alveolar ventilation. These exercise performance decrements do not appear to be due to interference with pulmonary diffusion of oxygen; O_3 exposure did not exacerbate a slight depression of arterial oxygen saturation that accompanied sustained heavy exercise (75% to 80% $\dot{V}O_2$max). There are no known effects of O_3 on cardiac output in humans. Decrements in $\dot{V}O_2$max and exercise performance are probably associated with the respiratory symptoms of cough and breathing discomfort that are caused by O_3 exposure. There is considerable intersubject variability in response to O_3; some individuals show few symptoms and have minimal physiologic responses, whereas others may be nearly incapacitated.

With continued or repeated exposure to O_3, responses become attenuated over a period of 3 to 5 days. Furthermore, residents of areas with high levels of oxidant air pollution such as Los Angeles tend to have milder responses to O_3 exposure than those who normally reside in an area with low levels of oxidants. The attenuated response in Los Angeles residents appears to be seasonal and is present primarily during and briefly after the summer/fall "smog season." Anecdotally, this is supported by reports from runners who experience the most symptoms from O_3 exposure in the late spring, at the beginning of the "smog season." However, the absence of symptoms does not indicate an absence of effect of O_3 on the respiratory tract. Both animal and human exposure studies have confirmed that, with repeated O_3 exposure, damage to the lung continues to occur even in the absence of respiratory symptoms and changes in pulmonary function. Thus, there is a continuing concern that individuals who are chronically exposed to O_3, especially those who are outdoors performing work or regular exercise, may have an increased risk of respiratory disease or an accelerated decline in lung function with aging. High ambient O_3 levels are best avoided by not exercising during the late morning or early afternoon hours, when O_3 levels tend to be at their peak.

Asthmatics who are exposed to O_3 experience slightly greater pulmonary function and airway resistance changes than healthy subjects. Both healthy and asthmatic individuals experience similar relative changes in airway responsiveness. However, this effect may be more problematic for asthmatics than for nonasthmatics, as it could result in increased responses to aeroallergens. Asthmatics experience increased numbers of asthma attacks during O_3 episodes and this problem is generally worse in children or adults who spend more time active outdoors on high-O_3 days.

In healthy adults, bronchodilators have little if any effect on O_3-induced responses. However, in asthmatics who have been exposed to O_3, these medications temporarily relieve an increase in airway resistance that tends to be greater in asthmatics than in healthy subjects. Nonsteroidal anti-inflammatory drugs such as indomethacin (Indocin) or ibuprofen (Advil, Motrin, Nuprin) inhibit the symptomatic and pulmonary function changes as well as some of the inflammatory responses. Antioxidants, such as vitamin C or E, may also prove beneficial, although evidence for their effects in humans is limited.

CARBON MONOXIDE

CO, a colorless and odorless gas, is a commonly occurring air pollutant that is a byproduct of incomplete combustion. Substantial CO exposure can occur in the interior of automobiles, parking garages, traffic tunnels, near busy streets, or in indoor environments contaminated by tobacco smoke or improperly ventilated combustion sources, particularly oil combustion space heaters and wood stoves. CO has a high affinity for hemoglobin and exposure to high levels of CO with resulting high concentrations of carboxyhemoglobin (COHb) can lead to death. At lower COHb levels, there is a reduction in exercise performance in healthy individuals and an increased risk of myocardial hypoxia in patients with a compromised coronary circulation.

The CO affinity of hemoglobin is about 240 times that of oxygen. The reversible binding of CO to hemoglobin not only reduces its ability to transport oxygen, but because of the leftward shift of the oxygen-hemoglobin dissociation curve, unloading of oxygen at the tissue level is impeded. CO can also bind to other proteins that have intracellular oxygen transport functions, such as myoglobin, although the effect that this may have on exercise performance is uncertain, especially at low levels of exposure. Because of its high affinity for hemoglobin, CO is cleared quite slowly from the blood, with a half time of 3 to 5 hours. COHb can be increased as a result of a brief exposure to a high concentration of CO (e.g., >100 ppm) or a longer exposure to a low concentration (<30 ppm). An hour of exercise in heavy traffic could raise blood levels of COHb to 3% to 5%. Further, once COHb is elevated, continued exposure to a relatively low concentration slows the pulmonary clearance of CO from the blood.

An increased COHb level impairs maximum exercise performance by reducing both $\dot{V}O_2max$ and the duration of short-term maximal exercise. These responses are thought to reflect reduced oxygen transport, due to the decreased number of available oxygen binding sites on the hemoglobin molecule and also an impaired tissue oxygenation due to the leftward shift of the oxygen-hemoglobin dissociation curve. The background level of COHb in healthy nonsmokers is about 0.7%, primarily derived from endogenous CO released as a result of hemoglobin degradation. There is a linear relationship between COHb levels and the decline in $\dot{V}O_2max$, with a 10% increase in COHb causing about a 10% decrease in $\dot{V}O_2max$ in healthy sea-level nonsmokers (Fig. 2). Although the lowest COHb levels shown to produce a statistically significant decrease in $\dot{V}O_2max$ is about 4%, even lower levels may have a small effect on maximum oxygen transport. Exposure to CO before endurance exercise could impair maximum performance. Although the $\dot{V}O_2max$ is depressed by relatively low levels of COHb, the $\dot{V}O_2$ during moderate submaximal exercise is unaffected by COHb levels below 15%. Compensatory responses such as increased cardiac output and increased blood flow permit maintenance of oxygen delivery in healthy individuals. Nevertheless, at the exercise levels that are maintained by highly trained athletes during competitive endurance events, the cardiovascular system is no longer able to compensate for the reduction in oxygen transport and reduced tissue oxygen delivery. The effects of CO may also be important to mountaineers, who perform heavy exercise at high altitude and, in addition, may be exposed to CO while cooking in their tents. Although the mechanisms responsible for hypoxia in altitude-exposed individuals and those exposed to CO are different, the effects of the two factors appear to be additive.

Patients with cardiovascular disease are at increased risk of angina pectoris, cardiac arrhythmia, and decreased ventricular performance when exercising during or after CO exposure. Individuals with healthy coronary circulations compensate for the decreased tissue oxygen delivery due to CO exposure by increasing coronary blood flow. Because many cardiac patients are unable to augment coronary flow, increased COHb levels increase

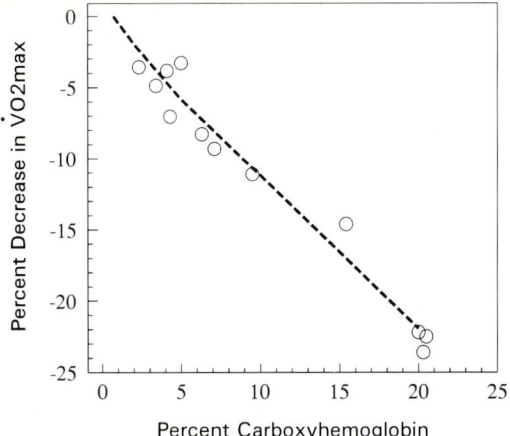

Figure 2 Effect of increased carboxyhemoglobin level on $\dot{V}O_2max$ in healthy men. The dashed line shows the linear regression from 5% to 20% COHb; the line was adjusted below 5% COHb to intersect the abscissa at 0.7% COHb, the mean resting level anticipated in unexposed subjects. (From Folinsbee LJ. Ambient-air pollution and endurance performance. In: RJ Shephard, P-O Åstrand, eds. Endurance in sport [The encyclopedia of sports medicine 2]. Oxford: Blackwell Scientific, Human Kinetics, 1992:479-486; with permission.)

the risk of myocardial hypoxia. Recent studies in patients with coronary artery disease have demonstrated that for each 1% increase in COHb above a nominal background level of 1%, there is a 4% decrease in the time to onset of ischemic electrocardiographic responses and a 2% decrease in the time to onset of angina. With increased COHb levels ($\geq 6\%$), the frequency of premature ventricular depolarization is also increased. Thus CO exposure presents a unique risk to patients with coronary artery disease who may be participating in cardiac rehabilitation programs; such individuals should be cautioned to avoid excess exposure to carbon monoxide. Patients with peripheral vascular disease can also be affected adversely by CO exposure. The time to the onset of ischemic leg pain is decreased in patients with intermittent claudication, even with slight elevations of COHb.

SUGGESTED READING

Adams WC. Effects of ozone exposure at ambient air pollution episode levels on exercise performance. Sports Med 1987; 4:395–424.

Folinsbee LJ. Ambient air pollution and endurance performance. In: RJ Shephard, P-O Åstrand, eds. Endurance in sport [The encyclopedia of sports medicine 2]. Oxford: Blackwell Scientific, Human Kinetics, 1992:479–486.

Folinsbee LJ. Human health effects of air pollution. Environ Health Perspect 1992; 100:45–56.

Folinsbee LJ, McDonnell WF, Horstman DH. Pulmonary function and symptom responses after 6.6 hour exposure to 0.12 ppm ozone with moderate exercise. JAPCA 1988; 38:28–35.

Folinsbee, LJ, Raven PB. Exercise and air pollution. J Sports Sci 1984; 2:57–75.

Gong H, Bradley PW, Simmons MS, Tashkin DP. Impaired exercise performance and pulmonary function in elite cyclists during low-level ozone exposure in a hot environment. Am Rev Respir Dis 1986; 134:726–733.

Horstman DH, Folinsbee LJ. Sulfur dioxide-induced bronchoconstriction in asthmatics exposed for short durations under controlled conditions: A selected review. In: Utell MJ, Frank R, eds. Susceptibility to inhaled pollutants, ASTM STP 1024, Philadelphia: American Society for Testing and Materials, 1989:195-206.

Linn W, Avol E, Shamoo D, et al. Repeated laboratory ozone exposures of volunteer Los Angeles residents: An apparent seasonal variation in response. Toxicol Indust Health 1988; 4:505–520.

United States Environmental Protection Agency. Air quality criteria for particulate matter and sulfur oxides. Research Triangle Park, NC: Environmental Criteria and Assessment Office. EPA Report No. EPA-600/8-82-029, 3 vol., 1982 (includes a second addendum in 1986).

United States Environmental Protection Agency. Air quality criteria for ozone and other photochemical oxidants. Research Triangle Park, NC: Environmental Criteria and Assessment Office. EPA Report No. EPA-600/8-84-020, 5 vol, 1986. (A new edition is available, but only in draft form).

United States Environmental Protection Agency. Air quality criteria for carbon monoxide. Research Triangle Park, NC: Environmental Criteria and Assessment Office. EPA Report No. EPA-600/8-90-045F, 1991.

AVOIDING HEAT ILLNESS DURING EXERCISE

KENT B. PANDOLF, Ph.D., M.P.H.

Exposure to heat stress while exercising can result in a number of heat illnesses. These illnesses include heat rash, heat cramps, heat syncope, exercise-induced heat exhaustion, water-depletion heat exhaustion, salt-depletion heat exhaustion, heat hyperpyrexia, and exertional heat stroke. Some heat illnesses are relatively minor and benign, such as heat rash and heat cramps, whereas others such as heat exhaustion and particularly exertional heat stroke can be potentially fatal.

This chapter presents guidelines for emergency medical technicians and physicians concerning the differential diagnosis of the various clinical syndromes resulting from overexposure to heat while exercising. Since prevention of heat illnesses is the ultimate goal, appropriate strategies are discussed from a practical standpoint. Avoidance of excessive heat stress during exercise is also discussed from the standpoint of proper assessment of the thermal environment utilizing available heat stress indexes. Adherence to these guidelines and preventive strategies should help to avoid the heat illnesses.

CHARACTERIZING HEAT ILLNESSES

Metabolic (exercise-induced) and environmental heat stress can result in a variety of heat illnesses (Fig. 1). The primary purpose of this section is not to detail the pathophysiologic manifestations of excessive heat exposure, but rather to present information that can be used for differential diagnosis of the various clinical syndromes resulting from overexposure to heat with particular emphasis on those syndromes that are more prevalent during exercise.

The information used in differential diagnosis was compiled from a variety of sources with greater detail available to the interested reader in the Suggested Reading. Since this chapter emphasizes prevention of these disorders, suggested readings are included that focus on medical treatment.

Heat rash (lichen tropicus; miliaria profunda; miliaria rubra; prickly heat) is a benign condition associated with an erythematous papulovesicular rash accompanied by sensations of prickling and/or tingling in the skin during sweating. It is most prevalent in hot environments with elevated humidity and slow air movement where the skin is continuously wetted by unevaporated sweat. The rash is generally localized to body areas that are covered with clothing and susceptible to sweat collection.

Heat cramps (mill cramps; miner's, stoker's, cane cutter's, or firefighter's cramps) are characterized by painful contraction or spasm of voluntary muscles in the abdominal wall and the extremities after strenuous physical exercise, extended thermal sweating, low salt intake (use of drinking water in fluid replenishment), and possibly development of a potassium deficit. The etiology of heat cramps is unknown, but they are observed mostly in individuals who are not acclimated to heat.

Heat syncope (heat collapse) is associated with sensations of giddiness or rapid physical fatigue during overexposure to heat. Sudden postural changes, unaccustomed physical exercise, or prolonged standing may result in fainting from peripheral vasodilation, collapse of vasomotor tone, venous pooling, hypotension, and/or cerebral anoxia. This disorder is sometimes associated with dizziness or light-headedness, nausea, epigastric discomfort, and occasionally with a desire to defecate.

Heat exhaustion (heat prostration) is of three types: exercise-induced heat exhaustion, water-depletion heat exhaustion, and salt-depletion heat exhaustion. The latter two disorders are thought to involve peripheral vascular collapse; however, pure types of heat exhaustion are rare. Deep body temperature is elevated, but is usually less than 40°C (104°F), and sweating generally remains profuse.

- *Exercise-induced heat exhaustion* is distinguished from the other two types of heat exhaustion by the absence of primary salt or water depletion. It occurs with intense physical exercise. The onset of symptoms is acute and associated with tetany, carpopedal spasms, abdominal cramps, syncope, and respiratory alkalosis.

- *Water-depletion heat exhaustion* can occur immediately following any period of heavy prolonged sweating. Inadequate replacement of water losses results in progressive water depletion. This disorder is characterized by intense thirst, vague discomfort, tingling sensations, lack of appetite, dizziness, fatigue, oliguria, rapid pulse, fever, and, in advanced stages, delirium and death. The advanced stages are rare when water is available. Skin, lips, mouth, and tongue are dry, and speaking may be difficult.

- *Salt-depletion heat exhaustion* is associated with inadequate replacement of salt losses during prolonged heavy sweating; the result is a progressive salt depletion. The characteristics are pallor, nausea and/or vomiting, fatigue, giddiness, muscle cramps and, in advanced stages, circulatory failure. Plasma sodium and chloride levels are low, and the sodium chloride content of the urine is negligible.

Exertional heat stroke and heat hyperpyrexia are illnesses distinguished by the degree of impairment in body temperature regulation. Heat hyperpyrexia is generally associated with a deep body temperature of 40.6° to 41.1°C (105° to 106°F) in an individual who is conscious, rational, and possibly still sweating. Hyperpyrexia is especially dangerous, because some individuals initially feel a state of well-being as body temperature

The views, opinions, and/or findings contained in this chapter are those of the author and should not be construed as an official Department of the Army position, policy, or decision, unless so designated by other official documentation.

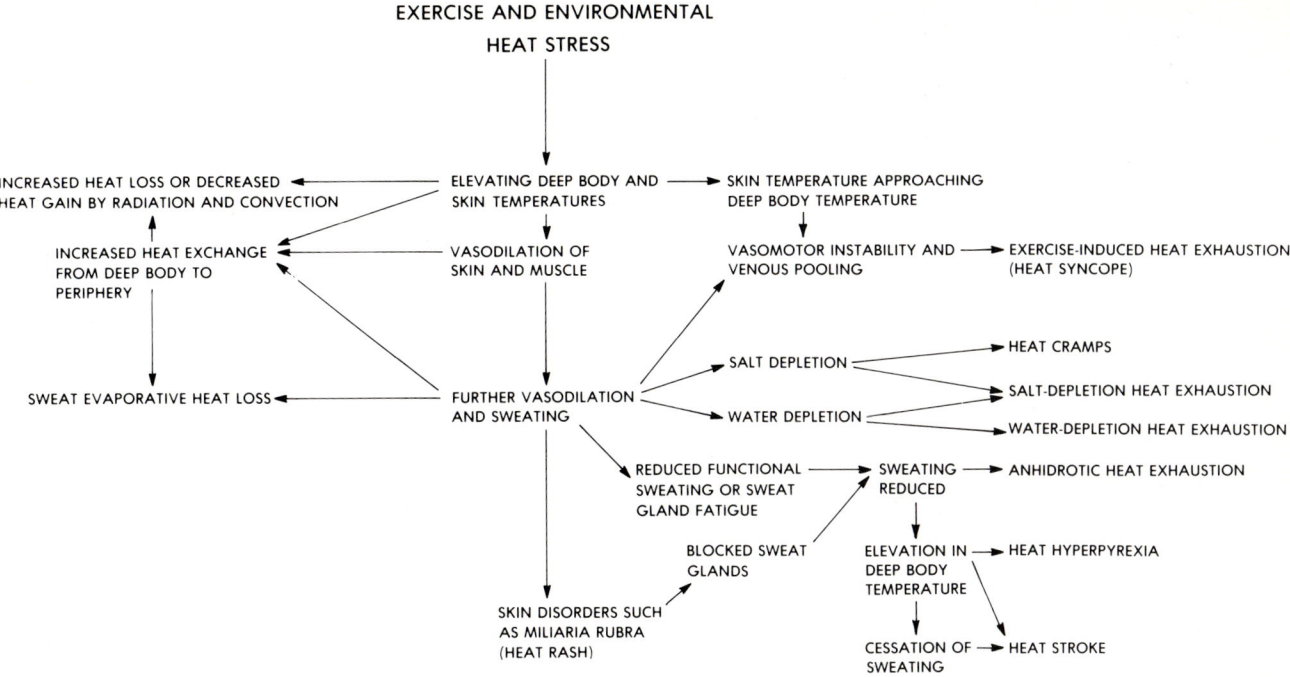

Figure 1 Mechanisms of thermoregulation during exercise-heat stress and causes of the various heat illnesses. (From Pandolf KB. Importance of environmental factors for exercise testing and exercise prescription. In: Skinner JS, ed. Exercise testing and exercise prescription for special cases. Philadelphia: Lea & Febiger, 1993:87–109; with permission.)

rises. If left untreated medically, heat hyperpyrexia and certain types of heat exhaustion can develop into heat stroke. Heat stroke is the most dangerous of the heat illnesses, and a true medical emergency. Heat stroke is frequently fatal. It is distinguished from heat exhaustion by clinically significant tissue injury. Exertional heat stroke differs from classical heat stroke in that it occurs primarily in physically active and healthy individuals rather than the elderly. Further, it is associated with rhabdomyolysis and acute renal failure. Exertional heat stroke presents as a failure in thermoregulation. It is usually of sudden onset with deep body temperature generally rising above 41.1°C (106°F), and associated with marked cerebral dysfunction and generalized anhidrosis. Other symptoms and signs include hypotension, diarrhea, vomiting, elevated serum enzyme levels, convulsions, and coma. It may result from overexposure to extremely high ambient temperatures, or from strenuous physical exercise in less severe heat.

PREVENTIVE STRATEGIES

Exercise-induced heat exhaustion and heat syncope can be minimized by ensuring prior heat acclimation, by grading the physical exercise to the degree of heat stress, and by avoiding sudden postural changes or sustained upright static exercise. Heat cramps and salt-depletion heat exhaustion can be prevented by adequate salt (10 to 15 g/day) and water intake; the latter is of great importance in avoiding water-depletion heat exhaustion. The two former disorders appear to be particularly prevalent in chronically hot climates, where salt and water needs are enhanced; therefore, caution should be used when advocating a moderation of salt intake in such climates. Heat rash and other skin disorders such as sunburn are associated with exercise-heat intolerance through reduced functional sweating. Heat rash is prevented by keeping the skin as dry as possible and by wearing clean, dry clothing that allows unimpeded sweat evaporation. The risk of sunburn can be decreased by clothing that provides solar protection and through the use of sunscreens. Heat hyperpyrexia and exertional heat stroke usually present as pronounced elevations of deep body temperature (in the range of 41° to 42°C). Some authors characterize heat hyperpyrexia by the lower deep body temperatures in this range with the athlete still able to sweat. Exertional heat stroke is associated with higher deep body temperatures and generally by a cessation of sweating. However, elevations in deep body temperature do not seem causally related to these illnesses, as both marathon runners and patients with passively-induced hyperthermia can sometimes tolerate deep body temperatures of 41.8° to 42°C while displaying minimal side effects. Heat hyperpyrexia and exertional heat stroke can be avoided by adapting the exercise to the anticipated climate, through proper prior heat acclimation, and by screening for athletes with a past history of heat illness.

Exercise–Heat Acclimation

The physiologic benefits of exercise-heat acclimation are a heightened sweating response, reduced heart rate, and lowered skin and deep body temperatures. Consequently, the exercise-heat tolerance is greatly improved. Figure 2 shows the improvement in exercise-heat tolerance of 24 young men who attempted 100 minutes of exercise at 49°C (120°F), 20% relative humidity for 7 consecutive days. These observations illustrate that no subject completed the 100 minute walk on day 1, 40% were capable by day 3, 80% by day 5, and all but one subject could complete the 100 minute walk by the seventh day of acclimation. Complete exercise-heat acclimation takes place after 10 to 14 days of exposure with about 75% of the physiologic adjustments occurring by the end of the first week.

Habitual physical exercise in the heat is the best method for developing heat acclimation. Daily 100 minute exposures represent the optimal time to induce exercise-heat acclimation. Athletes who expect to participate in events involving heat stress should train in the heat for at least 1 week before the event to help maximize their performance.

Aerobic Fitness

Scientists generally agree that high levels of aerobic fitness gained by endurance training reduce the physiologic strain during exercise in the heat. Figure 3 illustrates the findings from two authors in different hot climates (dry and wet, respectively) who independently report that maximal oxygen uptake accounts for between 42% and 46% of the variability in deep body temperature after 3 hours of exercise in the heat, or the number of days of exercise-heat acclimation needed to establish a plateau in deep body temperature. However, endurance training must induce significant elevations in deep body temperature during the training process in order to increase exercise-heat tolerance. Some hypothesize that a high level of aerobic fitness is a major factor in the small loss and rapid reacclimation of individuals after they stop exercising in the heat. Middle-aged and elderly men and women who are aerobically fit particularly gain in improved exercise-heat tolerance. Endurance athletes should be at peak levels of aerobic fitness in order to maximize these benefits related to improved exercise-heat tolerance, and possibly to minimize the risk of heat disorders.

Hydration State

Dehydration generally lowers endurance exercise performance and it also predisposes individuals to many of the heat illnesses. In addition, humans do not seem to adapt to chronic dehydration. Figure 4 shows that the sweating rate at a given deep body temperature is systematically reduced with increased dehydration levels

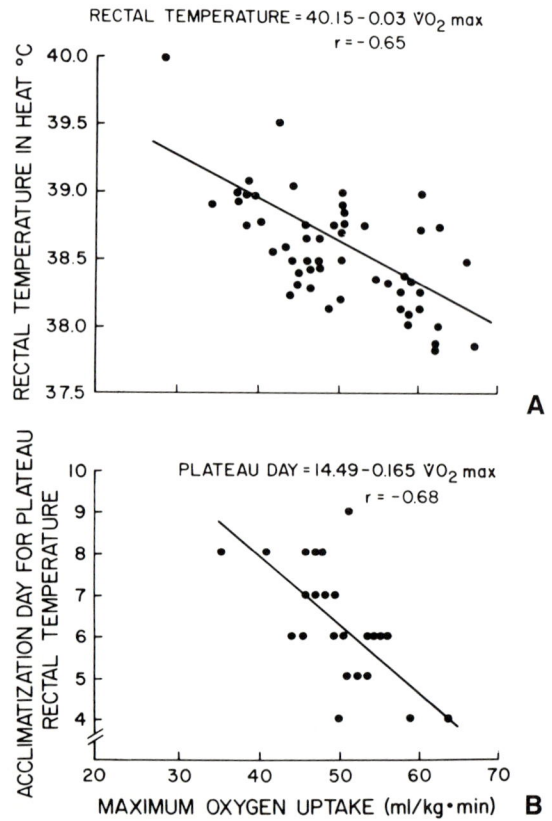

Figure 3 Relationship between maximal oxygen uptake and (*A*) final rectal temperature in a hot-humid environment or (*B*) the acclimatization day for a plateau in rectal temperature in a hot-dry environment. (From Armstrong LE, Pandolf KB. Physical training, cardiorespiratory physical fitness and exercise-heat tolerance. In: Pandolf KB, Sawka MN, Gonzalez RR, eds. Human performance physiology and environmental medicine at terrestrial extremes. Dubuque, IA: Brown & Benchmark, 1988:199–226; with permission.)

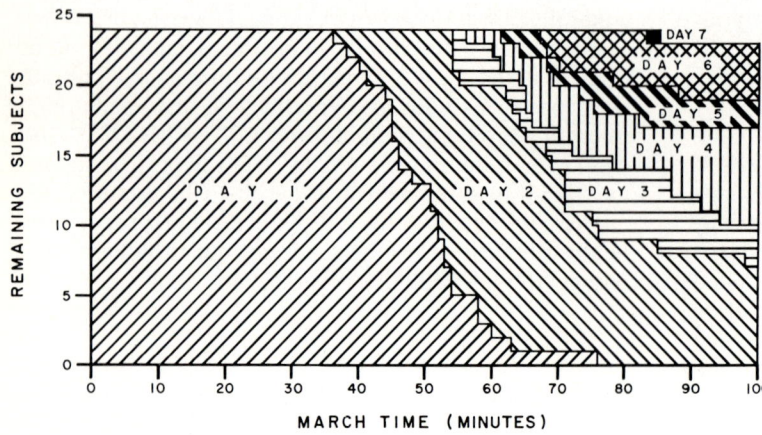

Figure 2 Relationship between improvement in exercise-heat tolerance (march time, min) and the number of remaining subjects (24 men) attempting 100 minutes of exercise (1.56 m · s⁻¹) at 49°C (120°F), 20% relative humidity over 7 consecutive days. (From Pandolf KB, Young AJ. Environmental extremes and endurance performance. In: Shephard RJ, Astrand PO, eds. Endurance in sport. Oxford: Blackwell, 1992:270–282; with permission.)

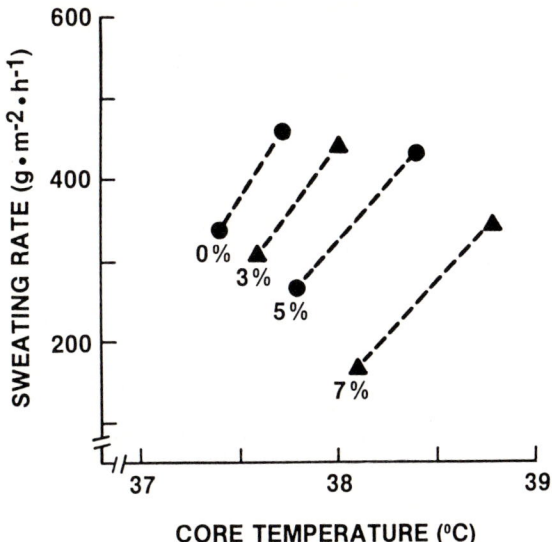

Figure 4 Relationship between mean whole-body sweating rate and final exercising core temperature when euhydrated (0%) and dehydrated by 3%, 5%, and 7% of body weight. (From Sawka MN, Pandolf KB. Effects of body water loss on physiological functions and exercise performance. In Gisolfi CV, Lamb DR, eds. Perspectives in exercise science and sports medicine. Vol 3. Fluid homeostasis during exercise. Carmel, IN: Benchmark, 1990:3–38; with permission.)

during exercise in the heat. The potential for heat dissipation through sweat evaporation is reduced, and susceptibility to many of the heat illnesses is increased. Ability to perform high-intensity physical exercise is decreased even at marginal levels of dehydration (1% to 2%). Greater dehydration levels are related to progressively larger reductions in exercise performance. Further, dehydration results in much larger reductions in exercise performance in hot compared to thermally-neutral environments. Dehydration is more likely to have a negative effect on prolonged endurance exercise than on short-term exercise. Thus, individuals should be strongly encouraged to avoid becoming dehydrated during exercise in the heat, and they should target a body weight loss of less than 2% in order to help avoid the heat illnesses.

Skin Disorders

Skin disorders such as heat rash and sunburn result in impaired sweating. They reduce exercise-heat tolerance, and may predispose an individual to heat illness. Heat rash over as little as 20% of the body surface causes an exercise-heat intolerance that persists for up to 3 weeks after the clinical rash has resolved. The heat intolerance associated with heat rash appears to depend on the specific region of the body that is affected and the contribution of that region to normal sweating responses. For instance, small areas of rash over the trunk may affect physiologic responses to heat stress as much as larger areas of rash on the limbs because of the greater sweating capacity of normal trunk skin. Mild whole-body

sunburn, induced at two times the minimal erythemal dose (MED), also impairs sweat gland activity during exercise in the heat. Sunburn appears to have a locally-mediated effect on both the responsiveness of the sweat glands and their capability to deliver sweat to the skin surface. More pronounced levels of sunburn, such as three or four MEDs, may have more profound thermoregulatory consequences during exercise-heat stress. These skin disorders deserve the same attention as lack of exercise-heat acclimation, low aerobic fitness, dehydration, and improper clothing as predisposing factors for heat illness.

Clothing

The proper choice of clothing for exercise in the heat helps to optimize endurance exercise performance and further reduces the risk of heat disorders. For hot environments, the solar protection of light-colored clothing is preferred during endurance exercise. Proper clothing should be relatively tight-fitting to allow for optimal evaporative heat transfer and to minimize wind resistance. Lightweight clothing prevents added metabolic heat production. A blend of synthetic and natural fibers offer thermal advantages and is more durable than clothing made from natural fibers. Endurance athletes should select clothing for performance in hot environments with a view to compensating for the air temperature, relative humidity, and solar load.

Heat Stress Indexes

Assessment of the thermal environment should consider the ambient temperature, humidity, wind velocity, and solar load in order to characterize the level of environmental heat stress imposed on the individual. One index of environmental heat stress applicable to athletic endurance performance is the wet bulb globe temperature (WBGT). The American College of Sports Medicine (ACSM) publishes a position stand concerning the prevention of thermal injuries during distance running, predicated in part on the WBGT index. For example, when the WBGT is greater than 28°C (82°F), ACSM recommends that athletic events should be curtailed or rescheduled until a lower WBGT is available. When the WBGT is at or below 28°C, ACSM suggests using color-coded flags to alert competitors and officials of the risk for heat stress. A red flag signals high risk and is related to a WBGT of 23° to 28°C (73° to 82°F), an amber flag denotes moderate risk with a WBGT of 18° to 23°C (65° to 73°F), and a green flag represents low risk with a WBGT below 18°C (65°F). These WBGT values are appropriate for individuals exercising in running shorts, athletic shoes, and a T-shirt. A different choice of clothing would require further adjustments in the WBGT values related to each risk category. ACSM also recommends that events where there is a likelihood of environmental heat stress should begin in the morning (before 8:00 AM), or in the evening (after 6:00 PM) to minimize the effects of the solar load.

Acknowledgment. The author wishes to thank Ms. Edna R. Safran for her editorial assistance in preparing this manuscript.

SUGGESTED READING

Armstrong LE, Pandolf KB. Physical training, cardiorespiratory physical fitness and exercise-heat tolerance. In: Pandolf KB, Sawka MN, Gonzalez RR, eds. Human performance physiology and environmental medicine at terrestrial extremes. Dubuque, IA: Brown & Benchmark, 1988:199.

Gonzalez RR. Biophysical and physiological integration of proper clothing for exercise. In: Pandolf KB, ed. Exercise and sport sciences reviews. Vol. 15. New York: Macmillan, 1987:261.

Hubbard RW, Armstrong LE. Hyperthermia: new thoughts on an old problem. Physician Sportsmed 1989; 17:97–113.

Leithead CS, Lind AR. Heat stress and heat disorders. Philadelphia: FA Davis, 1964.

Pandolf KB. Importance of environmental factors for exercise testing and exercise prescription. In: Skinner JS, ed. Exercise testing and exercise prescription for special cases. Philadelphia: Lea & Febiger, 1993:87.

Pandolf KB, Young AJ. Environmental extremes and endurance performance. In: Shephard RJ, Astrand PO, eds. Endurance in sport. Oxford: Blackwell, 1992:270.

Sawka MN, Pandolf KB. Effects of body water loss on physiological functions and exercise performance. In: Gisolfi CV, Lamb DR, eds. Perspectives in exercise science and sports medicine. Vol. 3. Fluid homeostasis during exercise. Carmel, IN: Benchmark, 1990:3.

Sawka MN, Wenger CB, Pandolf KB. Thermoregulatory responses to acute exercise-heat stress and heat acclimation. In: Fregly MJ, Blatteis CM, eds. Handbook of physiology. Section 4: Adaptation to the environment. New York: Oxford University Press, 1994; in press.

Wenger CB. Human heat acclimatization. In: Pandolf KB, Sawka MN, Gonzalez RR, eds. Human performance physiology and environmental medicine at terrestrial extremes. Dubuque, IA: Brown & Benchmark, 1988:153.

Yarbrough BE, Hubbard RW. Heat-related illnesses. In: Auerbach PS, Geehr EC, eds. Management of wilderness and environmental emergencies. St. Louis: Mosby, 1989:119.

EXERCISE IN THE COLD

ANDRÉ L. VALLERAND, Ph.D.

Humans have developed the technical capability to protect themselves, from a thermoregulation point of view, against almost any terrestrial extreme. With respect to the extreme cold, it is understood that the best technique to ensure survival resides in enhancing one's insulation, or reducing heat losses, by using a wide variety of new high-tech clothing and equipment. Excellent examples of the use of such technologies are displayed by winter Olympians, skiers, trekkers, joggers, and, in particular, polar adventurers. However, there are situations where technologic and behavioral strategies to increase insulation are simply not available, not appropriate, have lost their effectiveness, or have already been maximized. Faced with high rates of heat losses, survival would then reside in one's physiologic ability to maintain body temperatures via vasoconstriction and an enhanced metabolic heat production. This chapter focuses on thermogenesis during cold exposure, key factors that influence one's resistance to cold, hypothermia and its treatment, and finally implications for the winter athlete.

THERMOGENESIS TO SUSTAIN HOMEOTHERMY

Components of Thermogenesis

Although no one debates the importance of thermogenesis, or production of heat, in the cold, the various components and mechanisms involved in daily thermogenesis are rarely highlighted and often misconstrued.

Resting metabolic rate (RMR) accounts for the major portion of the daily energy expenditure while resting at thermal neutrality (TN) (Table 1). The thermic effect of food, exercise-induced thermogenesis, and thermoregulatory thermogenesis (TT) are the other three components of daily thermogenesis. Briefly, the thermic effect of food is made up of obligatory thermogenesis (a phase formerly known as the specific dynamic action, related to the absorption, breakdown, and storing of ingested nutrients) and facultative thermogenesis (a phase related to sympathetic nervous system activity). Exercise-induced thermogenesis represents the additional energy expenditure associated with standing, walking, and exercising. This component can vary from a negligible portion of the daily energy expenditure of a bed-ridden patient, to its highest in a marathoner, where such activity can burn as many as 8,400 kilojoules (2,000 kcal). The last component is TT. At thermal neutrality, TT is negligible. But in emergency situations where cold exposure is lengthy, energy expenditure can be as high as that of the marathoner mentioned. This is explained by the fact that although the cold-induced increase in metabolic rate can be relatively small compared to that of exercise, TT is increased *continuously,* in contrast to the *intermittent* nature of exercise.

Table 1 Components of Thermogenesis

Resting metabolic rate (RMR)

Thermic effect of food (TEF):
  Obligatory thermogenesis
  Facultative thermogenesis

Exercise-induced thermogenesis

Thermoregulatory thermogenesis:
  Shivering
  Nonshivering

TT can originate from shivering and/or nonshivering thermogenesis. Shivering is a form of involuntary rhythmic muscular contraction where no useful work is done. It is triggered by acetylcholine, and involves cellular processes similar to those occurring in other forms of skeletal muscle contraction. It is important to point out here that the conversion of chemical energy to mechanical work, which includes shivering, is not an efficient process, since about 75% of its energy is released as heat and only 25% is converted to high-energy compounds. So many muscle groups are recruited even during low intensity shivering that increased energy is demanded to fuel this muscular activity. Metabolic rate can be increased by up to five times RMR during shivering. Whether nonshivering mechanisms make a significant contribution to TT in humans and in which particular tissues, is unclear. Mechanisms unrelated to shivering can include ion pumping (i.e., Na/K pump) and futile metabolic cycles.

Fuel Utilization

Exercise and cold exposure are two distinct physiologic conditions where energy expenditure is enhanced: they have many similarities, in particular with respect to metabolic fuel utilization. In rats, cold exposure greatly enhances turnover, tolerance, oxidation, and uptake of plasma glucose. It has even been suggested that cold exposure stimulates peripheral tissue glucose uptake primarily via insulin-independent pathways, possibly similar to the well-known "insulin-like" effect of exercise. Increments in lipid metabolism and, in particular, FFA turnover have also been documented. In contrast, aside from changes in circulating substrates, very little was known about fuel metabolism in cold-exposed humans until very recently.

Using the well-known indirect calorimetry and nonprotein respiratory exchange ratio technique, it has been demonstrated recently that the cold-induced increase in heat production (fasting seminude subjects at rest for 2 hours at 10°C, 1 m · s⁻¹ wind) is associated with 588% and 63% increases in carbohydrate (CHO) and lipid oxidation, respectively, and an unchanged rate of protein oxidation. The proportion of substrate utilization is also dramatically altered. At TN, the greatest proportion of energy expenditure is derived from lipids (59%), but in the cold, there is a marked shift to CHO (51% of total energy expenditure). Entirely similar results have been observed with respect to CHO oxidation during cold water immersion. Attempts to determine the source of the substrates oxidized in the cold have been particularly revealing.

In humans, the utilization of circulating CHO is accelerated in the cold even in the presence of reduced blood insulin levels, suggesting a greater sensitivity of peripheral tissues to insulin. In addition, cold exposure increases the utilization of intramuscular glycogen (Fig. 1). This can be a factor limiting cold tolerance since low glycogen levels prior to cold water immersion (90 minutes in stirred 18°C water) significantly accelerate body cooling. Faster body cooling has also been observed

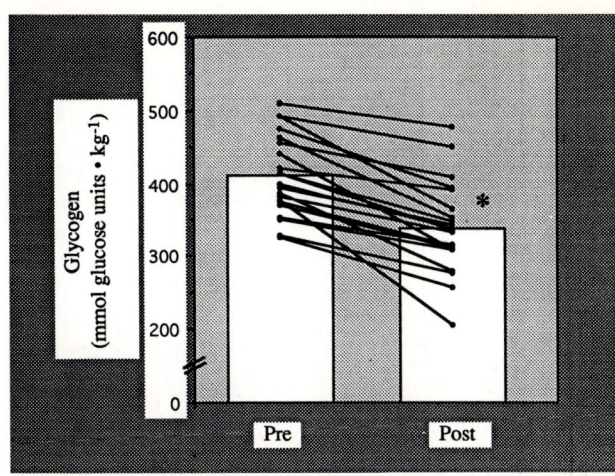

Figure 1 Muscle glycogen levels before and after cold water immersion (90 minutes at 18°C seminude). (From Martineau L, Jacobs I. Muscle glycogen utilization during shivering thermogenesis in humans. J Appl Physiol 1988; 65:2046–2050; with permission.)

when hypoglycemia is induced in cold-exposed individuals, suggesting that both low blood glucose and low muscle glycogen reserves should be avoided in the cold. It certainly appears as though there is a CHO dependence during TT, although the exact reasons remain to be elucidated.

What is the origin of the fatty acids oxidized in the cold? Recent cold exposure experiments have shown that blocking fatty acid release from white adipose tissue did not alter metabolic rate, lipid oxidation, or the rate of body cooling, suggesting that fatty acids from another source were being oxidized. Since plasma triglycerides (TG) were already known to represent another important source of fatty acids for oxidation during prolonged exercise, it was hypothesized that the same concept could apply to cold exposure. Unfortunately, plasma TG clearance was not found to be affected by the cold. It remains to be determined whether intramuscular TG (the only other potential source of fatty acids) represents a key source of readily available fatty acids for oxidation in the shivering muscles.

FACTORS THAT INFLUENCE RESISTANCE TO COLD

Heat Balance

It has been mentioned earlier that to prevent hypothermia, or at least delay its onset, it is essential that heat production be increased and/or heat losses be reduced. How do these *heat*-related concepts fit together and what is the link between body *heat* and body *temperatures*? The concept of whole body heat exchange is detailed in the heat balance equation below, which incorporates all routes for the gain and loss of heat [all terms are in W · m⁻² of body surface area (1 W = 1 J · s⁻¹)]:

$$\dot{S} = \dot{M} - (\dot{R} + \dot{C}) - \dot{E}_{persp} - \dot{C}_{resp} - \dot{E}_{resp}$$

where $\dot{M}$ is the metabolic rate, $\dot{R} + \dot{C}$ is the rate of dry heat exchange by radiation and convection, $\dot{E}_{persp}$ is the rate of evaporative heat loss from the skin, $\dot{C}_{resp}$ and $\dot{E}_{resp}$ are respectively the rates of convective and evaporative heat loss by the respiratory tract and $\dot{S}$ is the rate of heat debt (determined as the minute by minute balance of heat gains and heat losses). A negative $\dot{S}$ signifies a negative heat storage or a positive heat debt. Integrated over time, a total S (sum of instantaneous $\dot{S}$ in $W \cdot m^{-2}$, converted to kcal or kilojoules) will eventually correspond to a change in core temperature (T_{core}). Both the total S and the change in T_{core} have been used as indices of cold tolerance or resistance, although S is inherently a more robust measure, since it is based on more parameters than T_{core} alone.

As knowledge of the utilization of metabolic fuels during cold exposure expanded, it became increasingly evident that an enhancement of metabolic heat production could ensure warmer body temperatures by reducing the cumulative heat debt, therefore enhancing the individual's resistance to cold. Three types of interventions may be considered: the use of pharmacologic agents, dietary supplements, and exercise.

Pharmacologic Agents

The use of pharmacologic agents to enhance cold resistance is not a new idea. As early as 1942, it was reported that the ingestion of caffeine reduced the drop of mean skin temperatures (T_{sk}) in men who were exposed to cool ambient temperatures. Relatively similar results were found with the use of thermogenic mixtures of ephedrine and xanthines. Recent studies have established that β-adrenergic drugs (such as ephedrine) and xanthines (such as caffeine and theophylline) are effective thermogenic antiobesity agents. Studies involving mixtures of ephedrine/caffeine and ephedrine/caffeine/theophylline have documented a similar slowing of the drop of T_{sk} in the cold, accompanied by a warmer T_{core} and a reduced heat debt, these changes being consequent to a greater substrate oxidation and metabolic rate (Figs. 2 and 3). Although ephedrine/xanthine mixtures increase cold resistance, further work is required to determine their effectiveness during longer exposures and at deeper levels of hypothermia.

Dietary Supplements

The influence of dietary supplements in the cold has received a fair amount of attention, probably due to an abundance of literature about their usefulness during exercise. Moreover, energy substrate mobilization has been postulated as one factor limiting for TT. It was thus thought that enhancing energy substrate mobilization by feeding could enhance cold resistance. Although this theory seems in accord with the known facts in experimental animals, the corresponding metabolic data in humans is surprisingly unconvincing. We carefully rein-

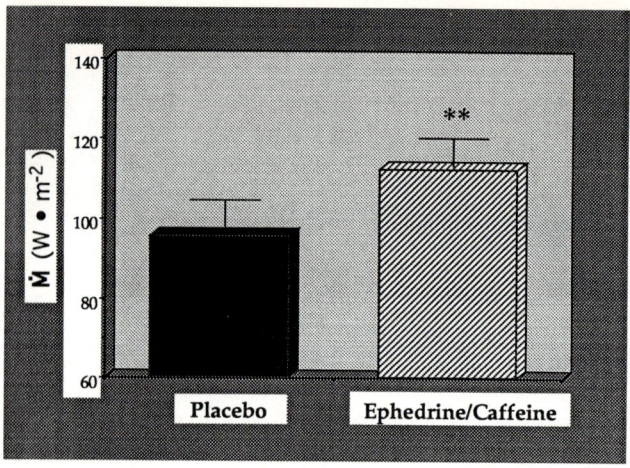

Figure 2 Average energy expenditure in cold air (3 hours at 10°C, 1 m·s⁻¹ wind, seminude) following the double-blind ingestion of either a placebo or an ephedrine/caffeine capsule (From Vallerand AL, et al., J Appl Physiol 1989; 67:438–444; with permission.)

vestigated the links between energy substrate mobilization, TT, and cold tolerance. Ingestion of various dietary supplements (1,400 kJ or ∼ 340 kcal of high-CHO or pure CHO) during either mild or more severe cold significantly enhanced energy substrate mobilization, exactly as expected. However, there were no associated changes in T_{core}, T_{sk}, M, or heat debt. We were unsure whether the above dosage of substrates was optimal, and a higher dose was tested in another study where cold-exposed men ingested as much as 3,000 kJ (710 kcal) of a high-CHO supplement in an effort to optimize substrate mobilization and thermogenesis. This high-energy supplement again had no beneficial effect on any thermal parameter, though it did increase CHO mobilization and oxidation at the expense of lipid mobilization and oxidation.

We hypothesized that dietary supplements might still have a beneficial effect at the higher metabolic rate associated with exercise in the cold. Results showed that ingesting a high-CHO supplement during intermittent exercise in the cold produced no beneficial effect on body temperatures or heat debt; it only increased CHO mobilization and oxidation at the expense of lipid mobilization and oxidation, without altering thermogenesis. Therefore it seems that dietary supplements alone are not as effective as originally thought in enhancing TT and cold resistance. Although energy substrate utilization is required to fuel thermogenesis in the cold, energy substrate mobilization does not appear to be a limiting factor for humans under normal conditions. Whether similar conclusions would be reached during conditions of energy deficiency in the cold, remains to be demonstrated.

Exercise

Although significant metabolic heat is produced through shivering alone, exercise-induced thermogen-

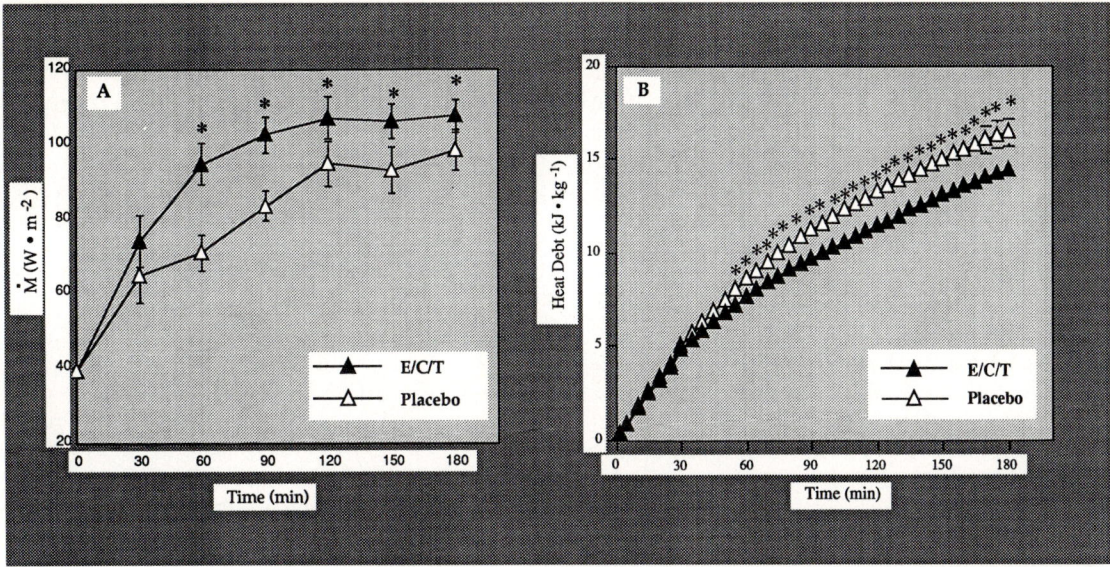

Figure 3 Average energy expenditure in cold air (3 hours at 10°C, 1 m · s⁻¹ wind, seminude) following the double-blind ingestion of either a placebo or an ephedrine/caffeine/theophylline capsule (ECT). (From Vallerand AL. Effects of ephedrine/xanthines on thermogenesis and cold tolerance. Int J Obes 1992; 17:S53–S56; with permission.)

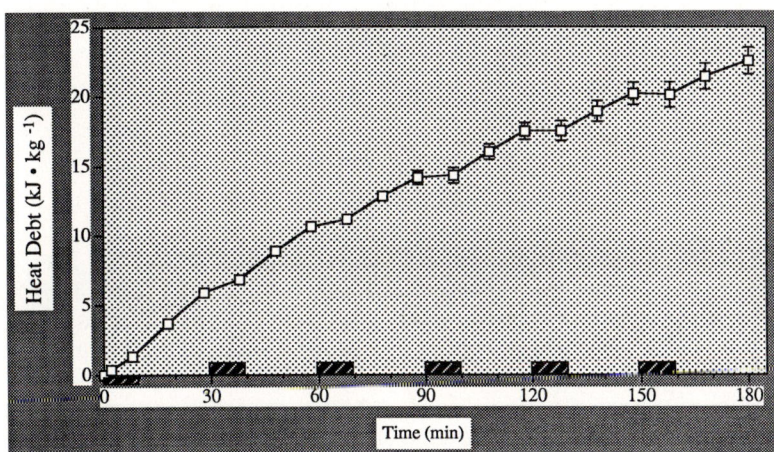

Figure 4 Cumulative heat debt in the cold air (3 hours at 0°C, 1 m · s⁻¹ wind) where intermittent exercise was performed (alternating 10 minutes treadmill walking, 20 minutes resting). Dark shaded areas on the x-axis represent the exercise periods.

esis can also become quite effective in defending the body against cold. Good examples are found in the swimmers who have crossed the English Channel (~ 18 hours at 16°C), the North American Great Lakes (~ >20 hours at 15° to 18°C), or even Glacier Bay, Alaska (~ 0.5 hours at 2° to 3°C). What is remarkable is that these feats have usually been performed while wearing minimum insulation! It is in our interest to try to explain these remarkable thermal performances, because there are unfortunately more unsuccessful immersions in cold water than the above hand-picked examples. First, it is likely that these participants, experienced and highly-trained swimmers, were somewhat habituated to cold water. Secondly, they probably had a substantial amount of insulative body fat. And thirdly, they probably knew exactly what their optimal swimming speed was in order to maintain body heat balance under the prevailing environmental conditions. The latter is not easily ac-

complished because water has a specific heat about 4,000 times that of air and a thermal conductivity about 25 times greater. When body heat travels from the core to the skin surface, heat is rapidly transferred to the water, quickly bringing the skin very close to water temperature. Any exercise intensity that inappropriately increases heat losses, particularly in cold water, accelerates body cooling.

In direct contrast to exercise in cold water, exercise in cold air consistently provides an optimal means of maintaining thermal balance. A good example is depicted in the experiment of Figure 4, where each intermittent bout of exercise almost flattened the heat debt profile in the cold (3 hours at 0°C), whereas the heat debt increased during each resting period. Nude men can maintain an elevated T_{core} when exercising at 10°C and can maintain thermal balance down to an air temperature of -10°C when the thermogenesis of moderate exercise exceeds heat losses. In air as cool as -30°C, exercise-induced thermogenesis can sustain a stable T_{core} when wearing heavy protective clothing. The problem with such clothing is the possible accumulation of sweat in the garment, the consequent high evaporative cooling and loss of insulating properties. Exercise in the cold can either accelerate or reduce the drop in T_{core}, depending on the balance between the increments in heat production versus the corresponding increments in heat losses. Another important aspect of thermal protection by exercising in the cold is simply how long the exercise can be maintained.

Interactions between exercise and cold stress depend greatly on the intensity of the cold exposure. Some situations result in combined shivering and exercise-induced thermogenesis. If the cold stimuli are strong enough and the exercise-induced thermogenesis is insufficient, additional thermogenesis from shivering helps to maintain T_{core}. For this reason, exercise in the cold delays the onset of any increase in plasma lactate, reduces plasma lactate levels during submaximal exercise, and increases plasma norepinephrine levels, in contrast to the values observed during exercise at TN. Further, the rate of oxygen consumption is higher during light exercise in the cold and part of the extra work is fueled by a greater glycogen utilization.

HYPOTHERMIA

Accidental hypothermia can be classified according to its severity and duration. Experts usually recognize mild hypothermia as starting at a T_{core} of about 35°C, moderate hypothermia between 30° and 34°C and severe hypothermia at <30°C. In the same fashion, the description of acute hypothermia is reserved for a duration of <6 hours, subacute hypothermia persists for 6 to 24 hours and chronic hypothermia for >24 hours. T_{core} is best determined with a rectal, oesophageal, or tympanic probe. Under field conditions, however, one may have to rely on oral readings. Nevertheless, efforts should be made to avoid being the author of an important case report where the victim's T_{core} could not be determined properly for lack of a suitable T_{core} probe. Although most electronic hand-held temperature indicators work very well and seem indestructible, they may become inaccurate or fail to function if left in the cold.

If T_{core} cannot be assessed, you can suspect mild hypothermia if your patient shivers vigorously and is still alert. However, if shivering is weak, if they make little attempt to protect themselves from the cold, and if they show profound mental confusion, you can suspect moderate to severe hypothermia; such patients must be treated as a medical emergency. There is much interindividual difference in response. One individual with 32°C of T_{core} may be conversant, whereas another will already be somnolent at 35°C. There are further differences in T_{core} according to the site chosen for measurement. Knowing these limitations, experts generally agree that hypothermia victims are likely to demonstrate the following symptoms, at a T_{core} of:

- <35°C: conscious and alert, with greatly increased shivering and vasoconstriction
- 32° to 34°C: conscious with mild/moderate clouding of mental capacities, but a very good chance of recovery.
- 30° to 32°C: a matter of serious concern due to severe clouding or loss of consciousness, and a slow but progressive reduction in shivering intensity.
- 30°C: unconscious, with acidosis, slow respiration, and limited heat production; the heart muscle does not respond either to medication or to electrical stimulation; remember that a 2°C afterdrop induced by rapid rewarming attempts can bring T_{core} to a dangerously low 28°C.
- 28°C: ventricular fibrillation is so common that it represents the main cause of death during the rewarming of such victims.
- 25°C: the patient slowly changes from homeotherm to poikilotherm, due to a marked depression in both heat production and heat conservation mechanisms: the victim is now at the mercy of the environment.

Note that low body temperatures do not themselves cause death, since therapeutic hypothermia to about 18° to 20°C has been used in surgery. It is therefore essential to re-warm and resuscitate any hypothermic victim before they are legally pronounced dead.

Treatment

Experts still debate the optimal method of rewarming following hypothermia. Although the list of possible methods is rather long, they can be divided into three general classes: passive rewarming, active external rewarming, and active internal rewarming. Passive rewarming consists of insulating the patient and letting shivering thermogenesis slowly rewarm a mildly hypothermic victim. Active external rewarming includes such methods as hot baths, radiant heat, hot water bottles, plumbed garments, electric blankets, warm water, and air mattress held at various temperatures and for varying periods of time. Methods of active internal rewarming comprise inhalation rewarming (breathing warm humidified air), warming by IV fluids, irrigation (nasogastric, bladder, pleural, colonic), microwave rewarming (in various volumes and/or temperatures and in varying combinations), and finally, for severe cases, extracorporeal circulation (use of a heat exchanger). In young, healthy and well-motivated experimental subjects, exercise-induced thermogenesis has been employed successfully as a rewarming technique following hypothermia as low as 31.2°C (inclusive of afterdrop). Even though exercise tends to exaggerate the extent of the afterdrop, this is compensated by a faster rate of rewarming thereafter. This is a bold and challenging new approach, since until now it was commonly believed that muscular activity could not be used as a method of rewarming below a T_{core} of 33°C.

RECOMMENDATIONS FOR THE WINTER ATHLETE

The interaction of exercise and cold produces significant physiologic changes that affect the winter athlete. Some recommendations follow:

- Cold weather competitions should be well marshalled so that hypothermic victims can be identified quickly and treated accordingly.
- Individual winter athletes should check weather conditions and dress appropriately to prevent hypothermia. A longer warm-up (15 minutes) can be valuable.
- It is advisable to run with a friend, or at least to inform others about your route or your expected time of arrival.
- The increased glycogen utilization associated with cold exposure could affect the endurance athlete. Further, the continuing demand for CHO in the face of glycogen depletion could lead to hypoglycemia. This will affect significantly not only muscle fatigue, temperature regulation, skilled performance, but also cerebral metabolism. It can also leave the winter athlete vulnerable to injuries.
- The winter athlete must pay attention to the body's warning signals about local cooling. Disregarding pain, numbness, and fatigue can be deadly. The same can be said about sweating in the cold: sweat destroys clothing insulation and is likely to increase evaporative cooling greatly. Persistent shivering after competition or exercise should be interpreted as indicating more extensive core cooling than was thought and should be a reason for concern.
- Since cold-induced diuresis affects blood volume, stroke volume, and heart rate at submaximal work intensities, it is important to stay well hydrated. It is also wise to avoid a negative energy and CHO balance: both have been associated with lessened resistance to cold.
- Both whole body and local cold acclimation are clearly of benefit; beneficial responses develop more readily at rest in the cold than during exercise. Note that the body has to be readapted to the cold every winter, though the extent of such readaptation may vary according to geographic location.
- Finally, hypothermic victims in isolated areas typically struggle until exhaustion in the mistaken belief that their only hope lies in reaching their destination. It is crucial to remember that an emergency bivouac offers a much better chance of survival, preventing exhaustion and further degradation of clothing insulation.

Acknowledgment. The assistance of Ms. I. Schmegner in the preparation of this manuscript is gratefully acknowledged.

SUGGESTED READING

Burton AC, Edholm OC. Man in a cold environment. New York: Hafner, 1955.

Doubt T. Physiology of exercise in the cold. Sports Med 1991; 11:367–381.

Jacobs I, Romet T, Kerrigan-Brown D. Muscle glycogen depletion during exercise at 9°C and 21°C. Eur J Appl Physiol 1985; 54:35–39.

Martineau L, Jacobs I. Muscle glycogen utilization during shivering thermogenesis in humans. J Appl Physiol 1988; 65:2046–2050.

Pandolf KB, Sawka MN, Gonzalez RR, eds. Human performance physiology and environmental medicine at terrestrial extremes. Indianapolis: Benchmark Press, 1988.

Shephard RJ. Metabolic adaptations to exercise in the cold. Sport Med 1993; 16:266–289.

Therminarias A. Acute exposure to cold air and metabolic responses to exercise. Int J Sports Med 1992; 13:S187–S190.

Vallerand AL. Effects of ephedrine/xanthines on thermogenesis and cold tolerance. Int J Obes 1993; 17:S53–S56.

Vallerand AL, Jacobs I. Energy metabolism during cold exposure. Int J Sports Med 1992; 13:S191–S193.

Vallerand AL, Tikuisis P, Ducharme MB, Jacobs I. Is energy substrate mobilization a limiting factor for cold thermogenesis? Eur J Appl Physiol 1993; 67:239–244.

EXERCISE AT HIGH ALTITUDES

BENJAMIN D. LEVINE, M.D.
JAMES STRAY-GUNDERSEN, M.D.

High altitude presents a unique challenge to athletic competition. Athletes must cope with hypoxia, cold, and dehydration, yet still maintain maximal performance. The timing of altitude exposure and the degree of acclimatization are also critical to a successful outcome. Physiological adaptation to high altitude may in fact be beneficial, and altitude training is frequently used by elite athletes to improve sea level performance. However, the objective benefits of altitude training and the optimal strategy of how high to live or train are controversial. On the one hand, acclimatization to high altitude results in central and peripheral adaptations that improve oxygen delivery and utilization. Moreover, hypoxic exercise may increase the training stimulus, thus magnifying the effects of endurance training. Conversely, hypoxia at altitude limits training intensity, which in elite athletes may result in relative deconditioning. We have therefore proposed that *living at altitude* but *training near sea level* will result in acclimatization without detraining, thereby improving sea level performance.

PHYSICAL FEATURES OF A HIGH ALTITUDE ENVIRONMENT

At high altitude, the barometric pressure is reduced, with a parallel decrease in the inspired partial pressure of oxygen (PIo_2); by 5,500 m (18,000 ft), the atmospheric pressure is reduced to one-half its sea level value and the PIo_2 is only 75 mm Hg (Fig. 1). *Hypoxia is thus the most prominent physiological manifestation of high altitude.* Temperature also decreases with altitude, at a rate of approximately 6.5°C/1,000 m. Other features include dry air (increasing the risk of dehydration), a decrease in air density and therefore air resistance, and an increase in the amount of ultraviolet light (4%/300 m), which increases the risk of sunburn.

EFFECT OF HIGH ALTITUDE ON EXERCISE AT ALTITUDE

Altitude induced hypoxia reduces the amount of oxygen available to perform physical work. Maximal aerobic power ($\dot{V}o_2$max) is reduced by approximately 1% for every 100 m above 1,500 m in normal individuals. For well-trained athletes, this effect is even greater, and reductions in $\dot{V}o_2$max and performance can be identified at altitudes as low as 500 m. Moreover, during exercise

---

This chapter was adapted with permission from Levine BD, Schecter MG. Exercise at high altitudes. In M Mellion, ed. Sports medicine secrets. Philadelphia: Hanley and Belfus, 1993.

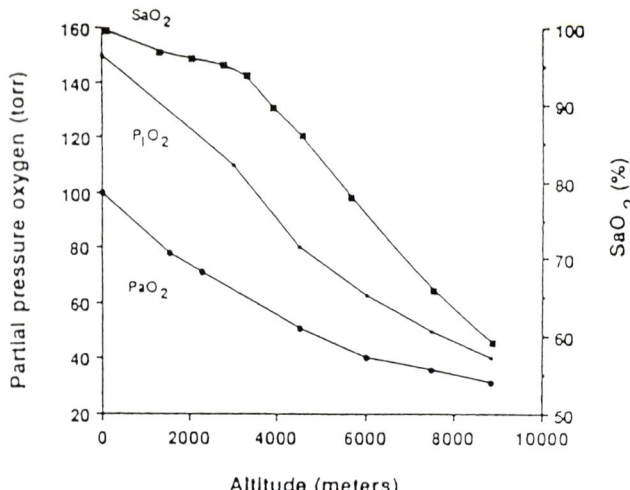

Figure 1 The relationship between altitude and inspired partial pressure of oxygen (PIo_2), with its associated effect on the arterial partial pressure of oxygen (Pao_2) and oxyhemoglobin saturation (Sao_2). Note the progressive fall in inspired-arterial gradient for oxygen with increasing altitude, presumably due to hyperventilation and decreases in the atmospheric-alveolar gradient for oxygen. Arterial oxygen saturation is well maintained at rest up to an altitude of 3,000 m, but falls acutely during exercise because of diffusion limitation in the lung (not shown). (Adapted from Hackett PH, Roach RC, Sutton JR. High altitude medicine. In: Auerbach PS, Gehr EC, eds. Management of wilderness and environmental emergencies. St. Louis: CV Mosby, 1989:1-34; with permission.)

at high altitude, ventilation is greater for any given submaximal workrate, as is blood lactate concentration, which increases the sensation of dyspnea and fatigue. However, *peak* blood lactate concentration is *lower* in individuals acclimatized to high altitude, a condition that has been termed "the lactate paradox."

In order to help understand the effect of altitude on exercise performance, it is useful to consider the "oxygen cascade," which describes the steps through which oxygen must pass: from the **environment** (determined by altitude achieved), into the **alveoli** (a function of ventilation and therefore the hypoxic ventilatory response), across the **pulmonary capillary** (limited by diffusion), to be transported by the **cardiovascular system** (a function of cardiac output and hemoglobin concentration) and eventually diffused into **skeletal muscle** (dependent on muscle capillarity and biochemical state) to be used by muscle **mitochondria** (influenced by oxidative enzyme activity) for aerobic respiration and ATP production (Fig. 2). The reduction in $\dot{V}o_2$max at altitude likely occurs because of diffusion limitation in the lung during exercise, which is exacerbated by the high pulmonary blood flow (cardiac output) of endurance athletes (Fig. 3).

Altitude affects endurance athletes and sprinters in different ways. For endurance events lasting longer than about 1 to 2 minutes, performance is significantly impaired at altitude, because of the hypoxia induced reduction in aerobic power. However, for short sprint events (400 m or less), most of the ATP required for muscular contraction of fast twitch fibers comes from

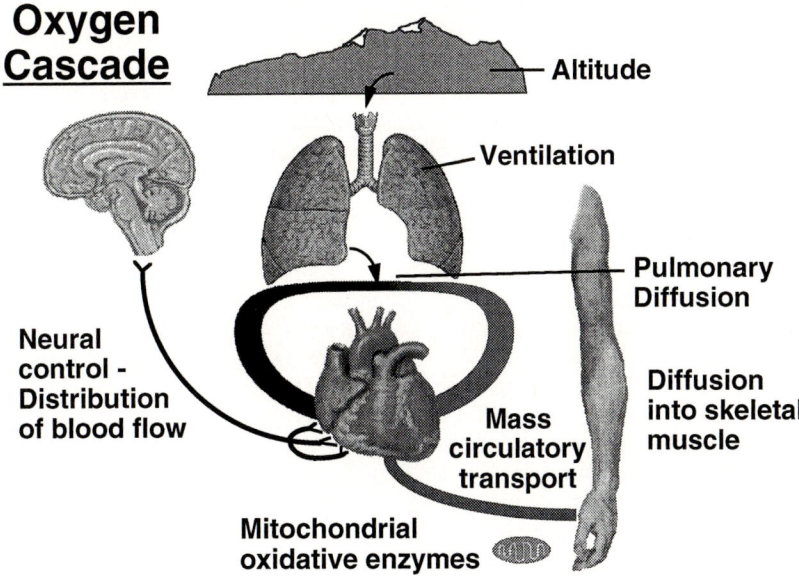

Figure 2 The "oxygen cascade," depicting the pathway of oxygen transfer from the environment to the skeletal muscle mitochondria.

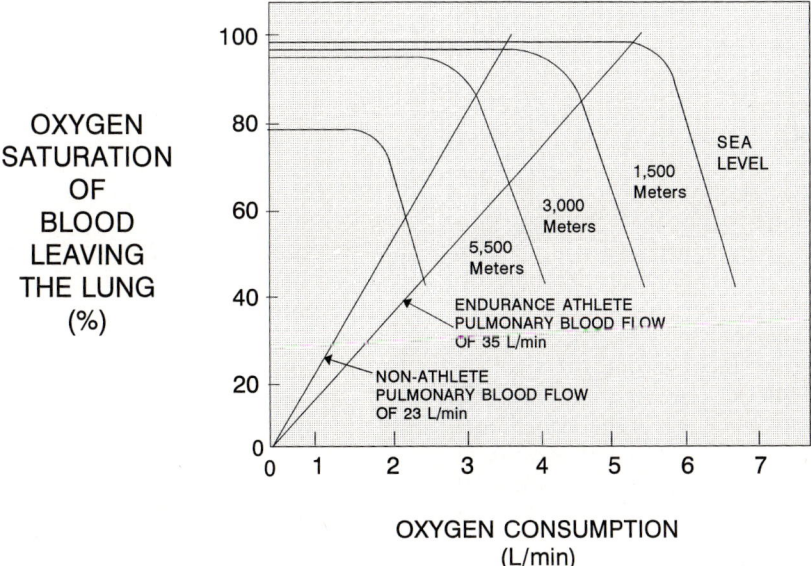

Figure 3 The effect of oxygen uptake and the requisite pulmonary blood flow (cardiac output) on the oxygen saturation of blood leaving the lungs at different altitudes. For an untrained individual with a $\dot{V}o_2$max of 3.5 L/min and a peak pulmonary blood flow of 23 L/min, the blood is well saturated at sea level and altitudes up to 1,500 m (5,000 ft) at peak exercise; but becomes progressively less saturated with exercise at increasing altitude. For an endurance athlete, however, who may have a $\dot{V}o_2$max of 5 L/min and a peak pulmonary blood flow of 35 L/min, diffusing capacity is closely matched to oxygen uptake and there is diffusion limitation even at altitudes between sea level and 1,500 m. This phenomenon likely occurs because there is much more plasticity in the capacity of the cardiovascular system to respond to training, compared to the lung where diffusing capacity is relatively constant. (Adapted and modified from RL Johnson. Pulmonary diffusion as a limiting factor in exercise. Circ Res 1967; 20(Suppl 1):I154-I160; with permission.)

glycolytic metabolism, which is not dependent on oxygen availability. The reduced air resistance at altitude thus actually improves sprint performance. That is why, for example, all the times in events shorter than 400 m in the Mexico City Olympics (2,100 m altitude) in 1968 were very fast and many world records were set. However, all events longer than 1,500 m were substantially slower than sea level times.

ACCLIMATIZATION

Chronic exposure to altitude stimulates the process of acclimatization, which includes a number of physiologic adaptations that improve *submaximal* work performance at altitude. These adaptations may affect oxygen transport along each step of the oxygen cascade. Increases in alveolar ventilation and reductions in mixed venous oxygen content are critical adaptations for maximizing exercise capacity at altitude. During exercise at extreme altitude (e.g., Himalayan mountaineers), chemoreceptor sensitivity, manifested as the hypoxic ventilatory response, may be one of the most important characteristics allowing work under conditions of severe hypoxia. The oxygen carrying capacity of the blood also increases, due to an increase in hemoglobin and hematocrit, thereby improving aerobic power. Moreover, the peripheral uptake of oxygen by skeletal muscle may be facilitated by increased capillary density, mitochondrial number, and tissue myoglobin concentration, as well as by increased concentrations of 2,3-diphosphoglycerate. Buffer capacity of skeletal muscle is also increased, which may improve anaerobic capacity and endurance. Finally, substrate utilization is enhanced by an increasing mobilization of free fatty acids and an increasing dependence on blood glucose, thus sparing muscle glycogen. This results in a decreased accumulation of metabolites such as lactate or ammonia during submaximal exercise. Although submaximal exercise capacity increases markedly with acclimatization, this effect is less dramatic with maximal exercise. At higher altitudes ($\geq$ 4,000 m), $\dot{V}O_2$max never returns to sea level values, despite prolonged acclimatization. However, at altitudes below 2,500 m, maximal oxygen uptake may approach sea level values after 1 to 2 weeks of acclimatization, at least in nonathletic populations.

The ventilatory changes begin immediately upon exposure to the hypoxic environment and continue to increase over the first few days at altitude. Hyperventilation causes a respiratory alkalosis, which stimulates renal excretion of bicarbonate over the first week in order to normalize acid-base balance. The sympathetic nervous system is activated acutely, with increases in both sympathetic nerve activity and arterial concentrations of epinephrine. This results in an increase in heart rate and cardiac output, so that tissue oxygen delivery remains near sea level values. By 2 to 3 weeks, systemic and regional blood flow have returned towards sea level values as oxygenation improves.

Hematocrit and hemoglobin concentration increase within 24 to 48 hours, because of a reduction in plasma volume rather than an increase in red cell mass. Erythropoietin begins to increase within the first few hours of hypoxia, and peaks by approximately 48 hours. Erythropoietin levels remain elevated for only 7 to 8 days at altitude, despite continued exposure, and red cell mass increases slowly in a time-dependent fashion. It may take as long as 1 to 2 years of continued altitude exposure for sea level natives to acquire the same red blood cell mass as high altitude natives who are exposed to the same altitude. Most of the metabolic changes appear to be complete by 3 to 4 weeks of altitude exposure. The ultrastructural changes in capillary density, mitochondrial number, and muscle fiber size probably take weeks to months to become complete.

There is abundant evidence that for competitions at altitude, this acclimatization process is critical and clearly improves performance *at altitude*. Therefore, if possible, adequate time for acclimatization should be allowed to maximize performance at altitude. Most of the short-term benefits of acclimatization are obtained after 2 to 3 weeks, which for a competition at altitude should allow maximal acclimatization while minimizing the detraining that may occur because of reduced training at altitude. Some athletes and coaches believe that if adequate time for acclimatization is not possible, then competing immediately upon arrival at altitude may be best. However, this hypothesis has not been rigorously tested.

Recreational athletes who hike, climb, or mountain bike but are not interested in athletic competition are also affected by the hypoxia of altitude. However, for nonendurance-trained individuals who plan to perform exercise at altitude, exercise training at sea level provides important advantages. In fact, the endurance and $\dot{V}O_2$max of such individuals when at altitude will improve to the same extent as the endurance and $\dot{V}O_2$max at sea level as the result of a training program pursued at sea level.

FAILURE OF ACCLIMATIZATION: HIGH ALTITUDE ILLNESS

With exposure to higher altitudes (> 2,500 m) and rapid ascent rates (> 300 m sleeping altitude/day above 3,000 m), a maladaptive state called acute mountain sickness (AMS) may develop. This is characterized by headache, nausea, anorexia, fatigue, and difficulty in sleeping. Fortunately, the process is usually mild and self-limited; in such cases, rest and analgesics are sufficient treatment. There is no evidence that competitive athletes are at any greater risk of developing AMS than are nonathletes, though exercise may exacerbate the development of AMS and should be reduced appropriately in symptomatic individuals. For patients who do not improve with rest, oxygen or descent to a lower altitude virtually always results in prompt symptom relief. Other effective treatments include acetazolamide, dexamethasone, and simulated descent using a portable hyperbaric bag. The problem is best prevented by limiting the rate of ascent, allowing for rest or acclimatization days, maintaining adequate hydration, avoiding alcohol or sedatives during the early acclimatization phase, and particularly limiting training volume and intensity during the first few days at altitude. The use of drugs to prevent AMS is discouraged in endurance athletes who are going to moderate altitude (below 3,000 m), unless a clear history of recurrent AMS is obtained.

In some individuals AMS may progress to a more severe and life-threatening form, including high altitude pulmonary (HAPE) or cerebral (HACE) edema. HAPE is characterized by dyspnea at rest, cyanosis, severe hypoxemia, and noncardiogenic pulmonary edema. The signs and symptoms of HACE include vomiting, ataxia, a reduction in the level of consciousness, and, in some cases, frank coma. Both of these syndromes can quickly result in death unless immediate descent occurs. Fortunately, both HAPE and HACE are very rare at the relatively low altitudes to which most athletes are exposed.

EFFECT OF HIGH ALTITUDE ON EXERCISE PERFORMANCE AT SEA LEVEL

The physiologic benefits of altitude training for endurance exercise must derive either from the development of acclimatization, an enhancement of the training effect by hypoxic exercise, or both. Athletes train faster and at greater aerobic power near sea level than at altitude (Table 1). During high intensity, interval type workouts, running speed, oxygen uptake, heart rate, and lactate are all lower at altitude, suggesting that interval workouts are best performed as close to sea level as possible. During base training, running speed and oxygen uptake are lower at altitude, but heart rate is the same as at sea level, and submaximal lactate is slightly higher. *The net balance between acclimatization and reduction in training intensity by hypoxia is the ultimate determinant of the outcome of altitude training in endurance athletes.*

Whether hypoxic exercise itself provides an enhancement of the training effect during altitude training is controversial, and probably depends on both the mode and the intensity of training. When a small enough muscle mass is used (i.e., one leg) so that the same absolute workrates can be performed under hypoxic and normoxic conditions, hypobaric hypoxic exercise results in greater increases in endurance, accompanied by greater increases in oxidative enzyme capacity than normoxic exercise training. Although one animal study using swimming rats suggested that the same synergistic effect can be observed in whole body exercise, this has been difficult to prove in humans. In general, controlled studies employing trained athletes have not been able to confirm a benefit of hypoxic exercise without concomitant acclimatization.

Many scientists, athletes, and coaches have been intrigued by the similarities between altitude acclimatization and endurance training. Numerous anecdotal reports since the 1940s have suggested that endurance athletes may achieve some benefit from altitude training for sea level performance. The ultimate result has depended on the type of athlete studied, the altitude achieved, and the methods of testing and training, with runners improving more than swimmers, and athletes training at lower altitudes improving more than those training at higher altitudes (> 4,000 m). Rarely considered in these studies, however, is the effect of supervised training per se. A training camp has the advantage of carefully supervised training and nutrition, quick and appropriate treatment of any injuries, and removal of the athlete from the stresses of every day life that may otherwise distract from training. Particularly in western societies without state-supported athletic programs, this factor may be very important to the improvement seen in uncontrolled studies. When appropriate control groups have been

Table 1 Training Workloads and Intensity Associated with Base and Interval Training at Altitudes of 2,700 and 1,200 m*

	Base training		Interval training	
	2,700 m	*1,200 m*	*2,700 m*	*1,200 m*
Percent of sea level 5 km speed	70.2 ± 2.0	80.9 ± 1.6†	98.1 ± 2.3	103.1 ± 1.1‡
Percent of sea level $\dot{V}O_2$max	62.5 ± 2.5	70.7 ± 2.4	82.5 ± 1.8	88.5 ± 0.8†
Heart rate (beats/min)	160 ± 4	163 ± 2	171 ± 2	181 ± 2†
Lactate (mmol/L)	4.1 ± 0.5	2.0 ± 0.3†	9.3 ± 0.8	11.9 ± 0.8†

*$\dot{V}O_2$max was measured in the laboratory at sea level (SL, 150 m) in 19 competitive distance runners. Average sea level velocity over a 5 km distance was derived from a time trial on the track. In the field at high altitude (2,700 m, n = 9) or near sea level (1,200 m, n = 10), a lightweight (800 g) device was used that contains a turbine flow meter and polarographic electrode to measure $\dot{V}O_2$, and that does not impede running performance (Cosmed K2). Heart rate (telemetry), capillary blood lactate concentration (membrane diffusion), and running speed were also measured during base and interval training; means ± SE.

†$p < 0.05$ compared to 2,700 m.

‡$p < 0.06$ compared to 2,800 m.

Data from Levine BD, Stray-Gundersen J. A practical approach to altitude training: where to live and train for optimal performance enhancement. Int J Sports Med 1992; 13(suppl 1):S209–S212.

included, living and training at altitude has not proven superior to similar training at sea level.

ALTERNATIVE STRATEGIES: "LIVING HIGH, TRAINING LOW"

We have proposed that living at altitude but training near sea level will result in acclimatization without detraining, thereby improving sea level performance. Preliminary data support this hypothesis, suggesting that blood volume can be expanded and maximal aerobic power, anaerobic capacity, and 5,000 m time can be improved by this practice. However, we lack final proof that this approach is better than sea level or altitude training, despite the fact that it has been used successfully by a number of international teams.

From a practical perspective, the critical question to answer for athletes and coaches is what is the appropriate "dose" of altitude and training? Specific issues include: (1) how high to live and how long to reside at altitude; (2) how high to train, and what kind of training is best; and (3) when to compete upon return to sea level? Adaptation to altitude depends on oxygen delivery to peripheral tissues, which decreases linearly with oxyhemoglobin saturation. Thus, red cell mass does not appear to increase until Pao_2 decreases below approximately 65 mm Hg, when arterial oxygen saturation begins to fall. For most individuals, this "threshold altitude" is approximately 2,200 to 2,500 m, though some small changes have been reported in endurance athletes living at altitudes as low as 1,250 m. Above 2,500 m such adaptations are likely to be greater with increasing altitude, unless AMS intervenes, or marked hypoxia (> 4,000 m) results in a catabolic state characterized by weight loss and reduction in muscle mass. Residence at an altitude of 2,500 to 2,800 m thus appears optimal to maximize acclimatization and minimize complications.

As far as training is concerned, high intensity, interval workouts should be conducted as close to sea level as possible, preferably below 1,500 m, in order to maximize running speed and training intensity. The appropriate altitude at which to conduct base training is less clear. Base training near sea level will allow a relatively normal training intensity and may prevent the loss of plasma volume that often accompanies altitude acclimatization. In contrast, base training at altitude, as long as it occurs at a low enough altitude to maintain similar running speeds and absolute workrates as at sea level, may facilitate an increase in mitochondrial oxidative enzyme activities and maximize peripheral oxygen utilization. It is important to emphasize, however, that altitude training is not a substitute for a focused, well-designed training program with appropriate rest and nutrition. A sample altitude training schedule is provided in Table 2.

Nutritional factors, particularly iron stores, play a critical role in the ability to respond to altitude training. In a series of studies we performed, involving competitive distance runners training at altitude, 12 of 41 participants (seven females, five males) had reduced iron stores as gauged from a low serum ferritin level. The athletes with low ferritin levels prior to altitude exposure (male and female) were unable to increase their volume of red cell mass (blood volume minus plasma volume) and did not increase their $\dot{V}o_2max$. Since iron is also a critical moiety in the synthesis of myoglobin, as well as mitochondrial cytochromes, iron deficiency may not only compromise oxygen carrying capacity, but may also inhibit oxygen extraction (a-v O_2 difference) and reduce O_2 flux, thereby limiting $\dot{V}o_2max$ and performance even in nonanemic athletes. Thus, iron stores must be normalized before undertaking a period of altitude training. This may require high doses of oral iron (200 to 250 mg of elemental iron/day in divided doses), which is usually best tolerated in liquid, pediatric preparation (Feosol, 1 to 2 teaspoons, t.i.d.).

Table 2 Sample Schedule of Altitude Training Based on 4 week "Mesocycle"*

Week 1 (Acclimatization Week—2,200 m–2,500 m)	
Mon.	Base training
Tues.	Base training
	PM base training
Wed.	Base training
Thurs.	Base training
Fri.	Base training
Sat.	Base training (or off)
Sun.	Long run
0/1/8 (# hard/ # long/ # total workouts)	
Week 2 (Medium Week)	
Mon.	Base training
Tues.	8 × 600 m, 105% 5 K race pace
	PM recovery run
Wed.	Base training
Thurs.	Base training
Fri.	Easy run
Sat.	5 K road race
	PM recovery run
Sun	Base training
2/0/9	
Week 3 (Hard Week)	
Mon.	Long run
	PM recovery run
Tues.	Base training
Wed.	5 × 1,000 m, 105% 5 K race pace
	PM recovery run, diet log
Thurs.	Base training
	PM base training
Fri.	Base training
	PM 10 × 200 m, 110% 5 K race pace
Sat.	Base training
Sun.	Long run
2/2/11	
Week 4 (Easy Week)	
Mon.	8/8/94 Easy run
Tues.	8/9/94 8 × 600 m, 105% 5 K race pace
	PM recover run
Wed.	8/10/94 Base training
Thurs.	8/11/94 Base training
Fri.	8/12/94 Base training
Sat.	8/13/94 Off
Sun.	8/14/94 Long run

*This schedule presumes that athletes begin a period of altitude training with substantial base training that includes regular interval workouts. They must also have normal iron stores. Many other strategies for altitude training exist that include shorter but repetitive cycles (see Dick 1992).

A final critical question is what is the appropriate timing for competition after a period of altitude training? Most athletes and coaches believe that the best performances are delivered 2 to 3 weeks after returning from altitude. This observation may be related to alterations in skeletal muscle acid-base balance that are changing rapidly after return from altitude. Alternatively, it may be necessary to have a period of normoxic training to maximize neuromotor coordination, particularly if all interval workouts have been performed under the slower training conditions of high altitude. When living and training occur at altitude, this empiric observation may well be true. However, when sufficient high intensity workouts are performed at low altitude to maintain foot speed and therefore neuromuscular coordination, the best time for a competition may well be immediately upon return from altitude, when the acclimatization is maximal. In fact, we have observed that for athletes who "live-high and train-low," 5,000 m time, anaerobic capacity, and maximal aerobic power are greatest in the first few days after return to sea level.

SUGGESTED READING

Adams WC, Bernauer EM, Dill DB, Bomar JB. Effects of equivalent sea-level and altitude training on $\dot{V}O_2$max and running performance. J Appl Physiol 1975; 39:262–265.

Dick FW. Training at altitude in practice. Int J Sports Med 1992: 13(suppl 1):S203–206.

Hackett PH, Roach RC, Sutton JR. High altitude medicine. In Auerbach PS, Gehr EC, eds. Management of wilderness and environmental emergencies. St. Louis: CV Mosby, 1989:1.

Hansen JR, Vogel JA, Stelter GP, Consolazio CF. Oxygen uptake in man during exhaustive work at sea level and high altitude. J Appl Physiol 1967; 26:511–522.

Levine BD, Roach RC, Houston CS. Work and training at altitude. In Sutton JR, Coates G, Houston CS, eds. Hypoxia: mountain medicine. Burlington, Vt: Queen City Publishers, 1992:192.

Levine BD, Stray-Gundersen J. A practical approach to altitude training: where to live and train for optimal performance enhancement. Int J Sports Med 1992; 13(suppl 1):S209–S212.

Maher JT, Jones LG, Hartley LH. Effects of high altitude exposure on submaximal endurance capacity of men. J Appl Physiol 1974; 37:895–898.

Mizuno M, Juel C, Bro-Rasmussen T, et al. Limb skeletal muscle adaptation in athletes after training at altitude. J Appl Physiol 1990; 68:496–502.

Peronnet F, Thibault G, Cousineau DL. A theoretical analysis of the effect of altitude on running performance. J Appl Physiol 1991; 70:399–404.

Reeves JT, Wolfel EE, Green HJ, et al. Oxygen transport during exercise at altitude and the lactate paradox: lessons from Operation Everest II and Pikes Peak. Exerc Sports Sci Rev 1992; 20:275–296.

Sutton JR, Reeves JT, Wagner PD, et al. Operation Everest II: oxygen transport during exercise at extreme simulated altitude. J Appl Physiol 1988; 64:1309–1321.

Terrados N, Jansson E, Sylven C, Kaijser L. Is hypoxia a stimulus for synthesis of oxidative enzymes and myoglobin? J Appl Physiol 1990; 68:2369–2372.

HAZARDS OF THE UNDERWATER ENVIRONMENT

ROBERT C. GOODE, D.Phil. (Oxon)

Five conditions related to the underwater environment that can lead to death are (1) hyperventilation and underwater swimming; (2) hyperventilation and sudden emersion from depth; (3) swimming position and unconsciousness; (4) hot tub immersion; and (5) acute exposure to cold water.

HYPERVENTILATION AND UNDERWATER SWIMMING

This activity is often practiced among young people and occasionally by skin diving classes. In an attempt to swim farther, the victim hyperventilates (overbreathes) for about eight to 15 breathes, dives into the water, and commences swimming underwater. In one instance, the subject remembered "making the turn" at the end of the pool and was later observed lying on the bottom at the "drop off" region. He had swum underwater for approximately 20 m in an apparently unconscious state before stopping all activity. One explanation for the unconscious state is based on the relation of oxygen and carbon dioxide content in the arterial blood to pressure of oxygen (PO_2) and carbon dioxide (PCO_2). With normal breathing, the arterial blood is almost fully saturated with oxygen. Hyperventilation can increase the amount of oxygen in simple solution, for as ventilation increases, the inspired oxygen/alveolar (arterial) pressure difference diminishes, with a resulting rise in arterial PO_2. The increase in O_2 content is not significant from a medical viewpoint. However, overbreathing also decreases the inspired alveolar (arterial) difference for CO_2, resulting in a lowered arterial PCO_2, and because the relationship between the CO_2 content of the blood and PCO_2 is curvilinear (as contrasted with the O_2 content of blood and PO_2 (which is sigmoid), the PCO_2 and CO_2 content of the blood drop significantly. A rising PCO_2 is a most potent stimulus to breathe. Lowering the arterial PCO_2 by overbreathing reduces this drive, so that it becomes easier to hold one's breath. During breathholding, metabolic activity results in a decrease and an increase in the blood content and pressure of O_2 and CO_2, respectively.

The subject who has hyperventilated dives in and

begins to swim underwater. This results in a continued consumption of O_2 and production of CO_2. In some subjects, the arterial Po_2 content and pressure drop to a point where brain O_2 requirements cannot be maintained and the subject becomes unconscious underwater. During this period, the CO_2 content and pressure continue to rise. Unfortunately, the pressure gradient does not increase sufficiently to stimulate the diver to surface and breathe (which would reoxygenate the blood and prevent unconsciousness).

As O_2 pressure declines, there is synergism between Po_2 and Pco_2 such that the drive to breathe is greater than that attributed to Pco_2 alone. Despite this increased drive, it is not sufficient to cause the subject to surface.

Treatment

In the incident described here, the subject was rescued by the author—the diver was not breathing, but after about four breaths of mouth-to-mouth resuscitation respiration re-commenced, and he was successfully resuscitated.

Prevention

It is not wise to hyperventilate before swimming underwater. If a breath-holding swimmer avoids respiratory gymnastics before diving, he or she will notice an increase in Pco_2 and a decrease in Po_2 while moving. These stimuli will interact and will result in a drive to breathing that is not likely to be denied—the subject will surface before becoming unconscious.

Swallowing type movements underwater are believed to move the diaphragm and rib cage sufficiently that the respiratory control system registers that a breath has been taken. This allows lower Po_2 values to develop and increases the possibility of unconsciousness due to oxygen lack (P. Dejours, personal communication).

HYPERVENTILATION AND SUDDEN EMERSION FROM DEPTH

Professor Herman Rahn of the Department of Physiology, SUNY, Buffalo (1963), was responsible for an explanation of a number of drownings that occurred when skin divers were coming up from deep water. In this scenario, a subject hyperventilates (see preceding section), dives down into the water, perhaps observes and/or performs some task, starts to resurface, and is found unconscious, close to the surface.

As the victim hyperventilates, the drive to breathe due to Pco_2 is reduced, and it does not rise sufficiently in time to cause the subject to resurface. The subject has increased the blood O_2 content slightly due to O_2 dissolved in simple physical solution. On reaching a depth of 10 m, the pressure of the water is such that it is equivalent to two atmospheres and as a result of pressure on the abdomen and rib cage, the volume of the lungs is reduced to approximately a half of the surface

value. If the time to reach the bottom was brief, the lung Po_2 would almost double, but there would be no increase in the O_2 content in the lung. Because of the increased Po_2, a small amount of oxygen would move into simple solution in the plasma. However, there would be no substantial increase in arterial content (at most, the Po_2 would approach 200 torr). When the arterial Po_2 falls to about 50 torr, most subjects experience a desire to breathe. The number of O_2 molecules required to generate a pressure of 50 torr in the diver would be approximately halved because of the reduced lung volume. If the subject, reacting to the low Po_2 stimulus, began to swim upwards, oxygen would continue to diffuse from the lung to the arterial blood and on to the cells. The ambient pressure would decrease with resurfacing. Near the surface, the water pressure is little more than one atmosphere. As a result, the pressure on the rib cage and diaphragm would be reduced by a half and the lung volume would increase. With the sudden increase in volume and a steadily decreasing number of O_2 molecules, the Po_2 would plunge in the lungs and arterial blood, resulting in an insufficient oxygen supply to the brain and subsequent unconsciousness.

Treatment

Treatment is as described for hyperventilation and underwater swimming.

Prevention

Do not hyperventilate. This limits the depth of your dive. The arterial Pco_2 rises quickly, causing you to surface well before your Po_2 falls to a point where unconsciousness results.

BODY POSITION AND UNCONSCIOUSNESS

On occasion, competitive swimmers have completed a race such as a 100 meter free style, touched the end of the pool for the finish, stood up (in the shallow end or shallow pool) so that the upper part of their body was out of the water, and fainted.

The muscular effort of the swimmer has resulted in the diversion of much blood flow to active muscles. The act of suddenly standing up results in some blood moving from the head toward the thorax, due to the effects of gravity. The sudden loss of water pressure on the thorax also causes thoracic pressure to decrease. As a consequence of gravity and the decreased pressure in the thorax, the blood flow to the brain is reduced and unconsciousness results. At times, competitive swimmers will hyperventilate, reducing their arterial CO_2 pressure. A lowered arterial Pco_2 can result in a vasoconstriction of the cerebral blood vessels. The reduced Pco_2 also inhibits the release of oxygen from hemoglobin. The combination of sudden change in posture and hyperventilation can easily lead to a sufficient reduction in O_2 supply to the brain to cause unconsciousness.

Prevention

Swimmers should not stand up suddenly when they finish a race, but remain in the water (no more than the head out) where the water envelope can help to maintain both venous return and an adequate cerebral blood pressure. Floating in a horizontal position, head out, is a preferred body position at the end of a race. This ensures a more uniform arterial blood pressure and helps to maintain cerebral blood flow and O_2 supply. In addition, finish line judges should be ready to act in an emergency.

HOT TUB IMMERSION

The fourth hazard associated with immersion is that of putting oneself into very warm water. Fatalities have been associated with exercise, older age, and alcohol. One scenario involved an active teenage boy who was found drowned in a hot tub. There was no sign of foul play, drugs, alcohol, or heart failure.

The victim had been weight training before immersing himself in the tub. One explanation for this death is related to the fainting episode of the swimmer described earlier. The subject's body temperature and skin temperature were likely elevated as a result of the exercise, since he was an enthusiast. Immersion in hot water would assist in a further diversion of blood from the core to the skin, in addition to that that had been redistributed to the skeletal muscles as a consequence of the exercise. It is possible the subject fainted as a consequence of inadequate flow to the brain while he was in the hot water. An additional adverse factor could have been introduced as the subject stood to step out of the tub. At this point, some of the compression effect of the water would have been lost. In addition, the sudden upward movement with gravitation effects could have contributed to the failure to provide an adequate blood flow to the brain. The lack of blood flow and thus lack of oxygen could have led to unconsciousness and finally drowning and/or asphyxiation.

An elderly man was found at the bottom of a hot tub. His death was not attributed to heart failure. It is possible the overall peripheral vasodilation could have reduced venous return such that he became unconscious, or as above, on exiting, the effect of gravity, and loss of compression could have contributed to his death.

Alcohol has been associated with death in hot tubs. Many victims who have died in hot tubs have had high levels of blood alcohol. Alcohol is a peripheral vasodilator and could act along with the heat of the water to divert blood flow from the core of the body to the skin. Fainting could occur while the victim was immersed or on climbing out of the tub (see above).

Prevention

If one has a tendency toward fainting, it is unwise to use hot tubs, especially after vigorous exercise. It is often desirable to climb immediately into a hot tub after exercise, but such individuals should not do it alone.

Similarly, seniors and persons who have consumed alcohol should not go into hot tubs alone. Water conducts heat to and from the skin some 20 times more efficiently than air—a temperature of 38°C in water can have far more physiologic effect than a similar temperature in air. Moderation is recommended in water temperature, in the time immersed, and in the amount of alcohol consumed.

SUDDEN COLD WATER IMMERSION

Long-term hypothermia (>30 minutes, water $\sim 5°C$) is known to cause death. It is generally agreed that this event is a consequence of a loss of core temperature and gradual cooling of the brain. Short-term immersion deaths (within a few minutes) may result from one or many factors (Goode et al, 1975). During the initial immersion phase, cold water can stimulate an increase in ventilation, equivalent to that reported for vigorous exercise (~ 90 L/min). The rate of change in temperature as well as the absolute value is believed to be the major drive to increased breathing. The increased ventilation results in a sudden fall in arterial CO_2. Sudden changes in Pa_{CO_2} have been associated with arrhythmias. It is possible that death may be a result of heart failure.

A second proposed mechanism is that of a vagal arrest of heart action, due to cold water coming in contact with the back of the throat. The increased drive to breathe due to the cold stimulation could lead to inhalation of water and provoke such a response.

If the subject is wholly immersed, in addition to the drive to breathe due to the cold stimulus, there is often an increasing Pa_{CO_2} and a falling Pa_{O_2}, as well as a neurogenic drive to breathing from active muscles and higher centers. The subject is likely to inhale water, leading to drowning, and/or vagal arrest or heart failure.

A further complication is an apparent loss of strength and coordination (within 3 minutes, at a water temperature of 8°C). This could hinder one's ability to climb out of a pool or hold on to a ladder.

Treatment

For hypothermia, a warm bath (at a temperature that the rescuer's elbow can just tolerate) is given, with the whole body (including the arms and legs, but not the head) immersed until a normal body temperature is restored (Hoskin et al, 1986).

For sudden immersion, a hot bath is given, and if inhalation of water has occurred or might have occurred, the victim should immediately be transported to hospital.

In both cases, long- and short-term hypothermia, the victim should also be treated for shock.

Prevention

Flotation suits that prevent heat loss from areas such as the groin, under the arms, and head are a must for people who work or play on or near cold water (snow-mobilers, sailors, fishers, police, and coast guards).

Subjects can learn not to overbreathe when they are suddenly immersed, which will prevent the abrupt decrease in $Paco_2$ as well as the inhalation of water.

SUGGESTED READING

Goode RC, Miller R, Duffin J, et al. Sudden cold water immersion. Respir Physiol 1975; 23:301–310.

Hoskin RW, Melinyshyn MJ, Romet TT, Goode RC. Bath rewarming from immersion hypothermia. J Appl Physiol 1986; 61: 1518–1522.

Rahn H. Oxygen stores of man. In: Neil E, Joels N, eds. Oxygen in the animal organism. Oxford: Pergamon Press, 1963:609–619.

CIRCADIAN RHYTHMS, JET LAG, AND THE ATHLETE

JONATHAN FRENCH, Ph.D.

This chapter focuses on the implications of circadian rhythmicity for the international athlete. Simple techniques are described that can minimize the effect of the circadian dysrhythmia or "jet lag" faced by the athlete who must travel across multiple time zones to compete. Controlled light exposure is a new and powerful technique that also is described since it has become refined enough for practical use. The information is presented in the hope that the effects of circadian dysrhythmia will not prevent the athlete from performing at peak levels in international events.

CIRCADIAN RHYTHMS

There is a profound cyclicity in nature recognized since antiquity. The length of available sunlight, the tides, and the weather all have regular cycles. The life that developed on Earth makes use of these geophysical cues to guide the expression of important biological events. Seasonal cues, for example, trigger mating, migration, and hibernation behaviors. Cycles that occur within a 24 hour period, like the length of day, are used to cue important physiologic events such as arousal, hormonal, enzymatic, and body temperature patterns. This discussion focuses on those cyclic events that occur within a 24 hour period, called circadian rhythms (circa-meaning "about" and -dian meaning "daily"); their disruption can have immediate impact on an athlete's performance.

Athletes know that they perform better at certain times of day than at others. For example, competing at 3:00 AM is extremely difficult, because at that time the body is used to sleeping. Yet, an athlete who travels to an event that is several time zones removed from normal, without preparation, may be entering an event at a time when their body will respond as if it was 3 AM, competing against other athletes who are at their performance peak. Even a single time zone change can make a difference to the outcome of an athletic competition. For example, there is evidence that west coast professional football teams perform poorly when visiting east coast teams during the day and better when they play east coast teams at night. Proper management of circadian rhythms is important to sharpening the competitive edge for individuals and teams. Other studies suggest that between 1 and 5 PM is the best time of day to perform many types of exercise.

Circadian cycles are regulated by what has been called a central biological "clock"; a more realistic description would refer to a series of neurohormonal oscillators, functioning in synchrony. The predominant oscillator is located in the suprachiasmatic nucleus (SCN) of the hypothalamus. The rising and setting of the sun are the primary cues used by the SCN to regulate circadian cycles (a process called entrainment). The SCN receives information about ambient illumination from the retina by way of the retinohypothalamic tract. In the absence of environmental cues, circadian cycles are considered to be free running and revert to an endogenous 25 hour rhythm.

The pineal, an endocrine gland that overlies the tectum of the midbrain, also is important to circadian cyclicity. It receives nerve fibers from postganglionic sympathetic neurons that arise in the superior cervical ganglion. Pinealocytes secrete the hormone melatonin in response to information about environmental light that is received from the SCN. Plasma levels of melatonin increase precipitously about dusk and decrease about dawn. Elevated plasma melatonin induces sleepiness, suggesting that it may be an endogenous fatiguing agent. Melatonin also communicates systemically information about ambient darkness cyclicity to various organ systems of the body (for a more detailed description, see Reiter, 1991).

The area of research known as chronobiology, which studies the influence of light and dark cycles on biological systems, has experienced tremendous growth in the past few years as the functioning of the SCN, the pineal gland, and physiologic cycles have become better understood. The administration of medicines (e.g., anti-cancer drugs or anesthetics) might be better timed to target the peak activity of the processes they are designed to inhibit. Circadian cyclicity of heart rate, blood pressure, and body temperature have important implications for diagnosis. Similarly, timed exposure to light and exogenously administered melatonin are recent techniques that provide a means to attenuate the physiologic effects of transmeridian travel.

JET LAG

Jet lag is a popular term for circadian dysrhythmia. It is caused by rapid travel to another time zone where light, dark, and other cues are quite different from the established cues. In fact, jet lag is often conceived as a mismatch between established internal cycles and new environmental cues, primarily light and darkness. Specific rhythms re-entrain at different rates. For example, body temperature recovers from a time zone shift later than physical strength and, for a while, the disharmony between internal circadian cycles can further aggravate the jet lag.

In general, it is easier and faster for circadian cycles to recover from westward than from eastward travel.

Table 1 Simple Strategies to Adjust to Jet Lag

Avoid the sun as much as possible before you travel.
Once there, get as much sunlight as possible, indoors and out.
Eat meals consistent with the time zone (e.g., lunch at lunch time).
Avoid alcohol.
Set your watch to the new time zone before travelling. Get used to thinking about the time at your destination.
Sleep at a time consistent with your new time zone. Avoid long naps.

(Westward travel is thought to delay the sleep cycle, providing more time to sleep, and is a forward adjustment of the cycle, which is generally regarded as easier to accomplish.) Physically fit individuals can recover more quickly from the effects of transmeridian travel than less active persons. To ensure adequate recovery, normal individuals require about 1 day for each time zone that has been crossed. However, in one study of the U.S. women's soccer team, mood, anaerobic power, peak strength, and work capacity were disrupted for only 2 days after jet travel across six to nine time zones (Hill et al, 1993). Most other symptoms were absent after 4 days.

To prepare minimally against circadian dysrhythmia the international athlete should follow the simple guidelines recommended in Table 1. To prepare more fully, the controlled light exposure guidelines in Figures 1 and 2 should also be followed.

STRATEGIES FOR THE ATHLETE

The best option for an athlete would be to travel to the meet site a week or two ahead of time and begin to work out in the new conditions. In many ways, travel by boat would be the best strategy since gradual and steady adjustment would be possible. For a journey across six time zones, the normal traveler should arrive about 6 or 7 days before. For many athletes this is just not feasible. In order to perform at peak in a distant time zone and get there more quickly, an athlete must artificially resynchronize circadian cyclicity. It is for these people that the recommendations in this chapter are made.

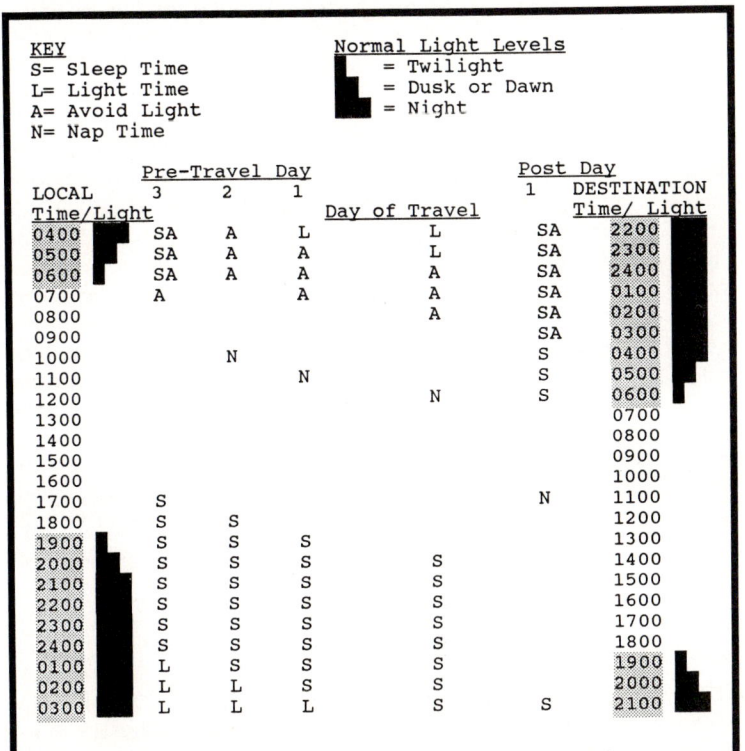

Figure 1 Recommended light management for a traveler crossing six time zones eastward (phase advance).

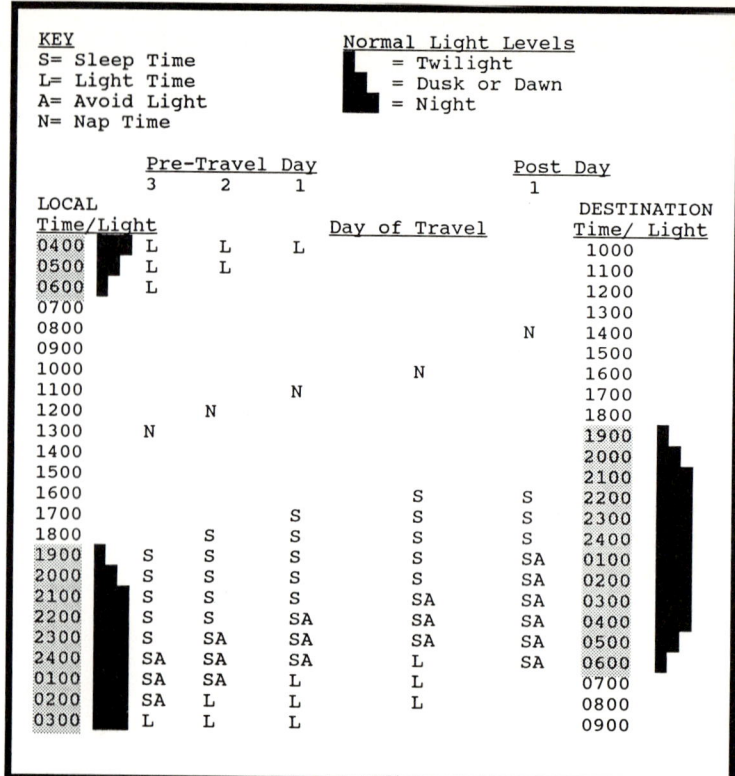

Figure 2 Recommended light management for a traveler crossing six time zones westward (phase delay).

Food

There is little evidence that any special diet can effectively counter jet lag. However, some general food guidelines might be useful to the international athlete. For example, carbohydrate rich meals can increase the serum levels of tryptophan and thus induce the behavioral changes typical of increased brain serotonin and possibly melatonin levels (since serotonin is a substrate for melatonin). Foods high in carbohydrates or in tryptophan (legumes, grains, nuts) may promote sleepiness (hence night-time adaptation). Conversely, high-protein breakfasts and lunch may enhance catecholamine activity and promote wakefulness (hence day-time adaptation to a new location). Most athletes are extremely familiar with the effects of diet on their performance; they are not likely to alter their food regimens, nor should they grossly alter their typical food intake.

Sleep Hygiene

Sleep is best taken in a dark, quiet environment. The traveler should be encouraged to carry ear-plugs and cloth protectors to wear over the eyes in case the environment is not conducive to restful sleep. Sleep is best after a light meal of easily digestible foods (e.g., pasta rather than steak). Sleeping on the flight to the competition should be strongly encouraged. Naps are a good idea to counter the fatiguing effects of jet lag but they should not last for more than an hour or two. Also, naps should not be too close to the new sleep time, since

they could interfere with getting a good rest at the right (entraining) time of night. Techniques of stress control, particularly the stresses that accompany competition and travel to foreign lands, promote sleep and should be considered an important part of team management.

Drugs

In general, sleep promoting drugs are avoided by athletes, particularly since they must submit to doping controls. Still, some evidence suggests that benzodiazepines may reduce jet lag. Sleep promoting medications are certainly helpful for the athlete, coaches, and trainers who wish to sleep on the airplane.

If the traveler is having trouble staying awake after a nap or during the day, caffeine can help. Caffeine is very effective in increasing vigilance, mood, and reaction time in a dose-dependent manner. People who are not used to caffeine should be careful as the effects can be powerful. Caffeine should not be taken for at least 6 hours prior to the desired sleep period. Various sources include coffee (5 oz cup has 64 to 124 mg), tea (5 oz cup has 9 to 50 mg) and chocolate (1 oz has 1 to 35 mg). Various 12 oz cans of cola beverages may have between 35 and 54 mg of caffeine.

Controlled Light Exposure

The trainer/physician should consider whether it is in the athlete's best interest to avoid a circadian phase shift. For example, it may be that the athlete will be competing at 10 AM at the destination. If that is a 6 hour westward time zone difference, it would correspond to 4 PM (see Fig. 2), which could be the athlete's peak physical performance time. Strategies for not shifting circadian rhythms include doing everything at the same time at the new destination as at home. Watches should be kept to home time, meals and sleep should be scheduled as at home, and light exposure should be the same as at home as much as possible.

If a circadian shift is a reasonable option, controlled exposure to light is a simple technique that has reportedly met with growing success. The ability of light to shift circadian rhythms in humans is an area of great interest to chronobiologists. The first human phase response curve for light was recently demonstrated by Minors et al, 1991. They showed that a 3 hour pulse of about 9,000 lux of light (equivalent to a partly cloudy day) slightly after the circadian temperature minimum could advance the rhythm by over an hour. Three such light exposures advanced the rhythm by almost 6 hours. This would be the equivalent of sending someone eastward across 6 time zones with just a few hours of light preparation over 3 days. Conversely, light given about 3 hours before the temperature minimum caused a phase delay, or sent the body clock in a westward direction.

The circadian temperature curve peaks about 4 PM while the nadir occurs about 4 AM in normally entrained individuals. Since the phase response curve for light is based on temperature minimums, an oral digital thermometer is useful to refine this technique. About a week prior to travel, an athlete should record oral temperature while awake every 2 hours for 2 days. Between 1 PM and 6 PM, temperatures should be recorded every hour to determine when the temperature normally peaks. The minimum temperature should be about 12 hours after the maximum temperature.

The first light schedule (Fig. 1) details light exposure and avoidance periods for a traveler going 6 hours eastward. The second schedule (Fig. 2) is for a person going 6 hours westward. Based on the information presented in this chapter, it should be possible to recreate the schedules for trips of longer or shorter distances. The thermometer is also helpful to ensure that when the traveler rises 4 AM on the first day of travel (Day 3 Pre-travel in Fig. 1), oral temperature is rising. Similarly, oral temperature should be decreasing when the traveler rises at 1 AM on the first day of travel going west (see Fig. 2). This can easily be accomplished by sampling temperature every 10 minutes before light exposure begins. The only essential times on either schedule are the times to get as much light as possible (L) and the times to avoid light (A). All other times indicated for sleep (S) or naps (N) are recommended times.

Light exposure should be from a source at least as intense as a bright make-up mirror of the type used by actors (about 3,000 lux). Two or three 150 watt lamps brought into the bathroom and placed very near the mirror without a lamp shade may be sufficient if the athlete sits about arms length from the mirror and turns on all the lights available in the bathroom. Intensity of light is more important than whether the light is fluorescent or incandescent. A standard four bulb fluorescent light fixture can also generate almost 3,000 lux at a distance of 5 to 10 cm. Commercial light sources are available that have a much better illuminance and since they can be worn in a visor, they allow mobility. The devices usually include more sophisticated schedules for light exposure.

Both figures show the local time on the left and the new time zone (6 hours displaced) on the right. Shaded portions of the figures indicate the likely outdoor light levels at each location, both at home and at the destination. The times indicate when an event starts and each event on the schedule lasts 60 minutes. For example, the last 'L' on the first day (Day 3 Pre-Travel) in schedule II starts at 0600 and ends at 0700. The schedules require that the athlete sit rather quietly in front of the light to avoid raising oral temperature by physical activity. This would be a good time to accomplish tasks for which it is otherwise hard to find time such as paying bills or reading a book or magazine. Advise the athlete to prepare carefully the things they have decided to do during the light exposure time the night before so as to maximize the actual light exposure time. The athlete should be cautioned not to go more than a few meters (1 to 2) from the light source if possible. It is a good idea to advise the athlete to retire early (although not too early) on the night before the first night on the new schedule. Times on the schedule where no letter appears requires only that the traveler be awake and active. Exercise should be taken at normal times.

The scheduled light exposure times (L) and avoidance times (A) are based on the supposition that the light will be effective in shifting the biological clock by about an hour with each day of exposure to the 3 hour regimen. Therefore, the times to seek light and to avoid light are shifted appropriately on the schedules. Nap times (N) are selected to somewhat correspond with when most individuals experience a (local) late morning/early afternoon drowsiness, shifted by about 1 hour daily. The circadian phase advance schedule (Fig. 1) for eastward travel should cause the oral temperature minimum to occur earlier by over an hour every day of exposure. All other events were adjusted accordingly. The phase delay schedule (Fig. 2) for westward travel should cause the temperature minimum to occur later and all other adjustments were made accordingly. The amount of sleep time available to the athlete is much greater in Figure 2, so it would be useful to have the athlete try to sleep around the normal sleep times at the destination. As mentioned earlier, it is less stressful for most to travel westward (phase delay). It might be easier on the athlete to avoid attempts to pre-shift prior to travel and save the effort for the trip back. Otherwise, for both schedules, the athlete should be using time at the destination before the plane takes off. For example, set watches and clocks at the new time and start planning meals and naps in accordance with the new time. The post arrival (Post-day 1) events on the schedules should begin as soon as the plane lands.

As much sleep as possible should be taken on the

airplane since it could be as much as 34 hours before the traveler will get a good bedrest again. The dark glasses and ear plugs facilitate airplane rest, as will a blanket placed on the lower back. There are often empty rows on airplanes and, with the flight attendant's permission, the traveler can occupy one for an even better sleep than in the chair. The athlete should be cautioned not to nap for more than a few hours after landing in order to promote sleep at the appropriate time later in the day.

THE FUTURE

A phase response curve for melatonin has recently been described (Lewy et al, 1992), which predicts schedules like those for light except for melatonin administration. Although the melatonin technique may be avoided by athletes wary of any chemical compound, it seems to be a powerful new way to reset the circadian clock. It is easier than controlled light exposure, as well, since long hours in front of a bright light are not necessary. A 2 to 10 mg dose of melatonin between 4 and 5 PM on the day before and the day of travel provides about 6 to 8 hours of phase advance (eastward preparation). Conversely, the same dose between 4 and 5 AM 2 days before travel may induce a westward shift in circadian cycles. However, it is difficult to obtain medical quality melatonin. Travelers might utilize foods high in carbohydrates or tryptophan to elevate melatonin at the appropriate times. In the future, melatonin may be available as an anti-jet lag compound. Further developments must await more empirical data.

It is ambitious to recommend light exposure schedules to a large number of individuals. I hope that these suggested techniques are robust enough to be of some help. Any responses regarding the usefulness of these techniques, after they have been tried, will be greatly appreciated by the author and incorporated into future versions of this material. However, there is enough evidence now to indicate that controlled light exposure can blunt the effects of transmeridian travel and help an athlete give the best possible performance at the event, wherever it may be.

SUGGESTED READING

Coleman RM. Wide awake at 3:00 am. New York: W.H. Freeman, 1986.

Hill DW, Hill CM, Fields KL, Smith JC. Effects of jet lag on factors related to sport performance. Can J Appl Physiol 1993; 18:91–103.

Lewy AJ, Saeeduddin A, Latham Jackson JM, Sack RL. Melatonin shifts human circadian rhythms according to a phase response curve. Chronobiol Int 1992; 9:380–392.

Minors DS, Waterhouse JM, Wirz-Justice A. A human phase response curve. Neurosci Lett 1991; 133:36–40.

Moore-Ede MC. The twenty-four hour society. Reading, Ma: Addison Wesley, 1993.

Reiter RJ. Melatonin: the chemical expression of darkness. Mol Cell Endocrinol 1991; 79:153–158.

BLOOD DOPING AND PERFORMANCE

E. RANDY EICHNER, M.D., F.A.C.S.M.

Blood has long fascinated athletes. It is said that ancient gladiators drank the blood of vanquished foes for courage, and it is known that modern Olympians (American cyclists in 1984) infused the blood of valued friends for endurance. Besides their fascination with blood, modern athletes cleave to the ancient credo that "more is better." When it comes to blood doping, alas, this credo can be deadly.

Blood doping, more precisely termed *blood boosting, blood packing,* or *induced erythrocythemia,* is the artificial raising of hematocrit (hemoglobin concentration) by transfusing red blood cells or by injecting recombinant human erythropoietin (rhEPO). The underlying rationale is that, by raising hematocrit without unduly raising blood viscosity, one can enhance aerobic endurance — and thus athletic performance — by enhancing oxygen delivery to the working muscles.

METHODS OF BLOOD DOPING

The methods for blood doping vary. Probably the most common method is removing 1 to 1.5 liters of blood from the athlete and freezing the red blood cells for 8 to 12 weeks (or longer), while the athlete retrains from the enervating effects of the acute anemia and regenerates red cells to return to his or her baseline hematocrit and aerobic power. Then, a few days (or weeks) before the key race or event, the red cells are thawed and infused into the athlete, boosting the hematocrit to 50% or so.

There is reason to believe that, in certain countries, the use of rhEPO may now have superseded blood transfusion as the preferred means of blood doping. This method is especially dangerous, because the more rhEPO given, the higher the hematocrit will rise. In theory, and based on analogy with patients who develop erythropoietin-secreting tumors (cerebellum; liver), in a few weeks (or months) the hematocrit could increase to

70% or higher in an athlete foolish enough to overdose steadily with rhEPO.

FIRST USE OF BLOOD DOPING

Research on blood doping began during World War II, when Allied bomber planes began flying higher over Germany to avoid antiaircraft guns. The U.S. Naval Medical Research Institute explored whether the blood doping of pilots would prevent adverse physiologic and behavioral symptoms from hypoxia at high altitude. By transfusing a liter of homologous blood, hematocrits in five healthy young men were raised from normal to the range of 55% to 58% over 4 days. No adverse effects followed the blood doping.

A key finding with implications for athletic performance was that, compared with a control group, the blood-doped men had lower heart rate responses when they exercised on a treadmill, both at simulated altitude and at sea level.

RATIONALE

The rationale for blood doping is firm; in theory, it should work. In elite endurance athletes, the blood adapts in ways that enhance performance. A cardinal adaptation is an increase in baseline plasma volume, in the range of 10% to 20%, depending on volume and intensity of aerobic training. This adaptation tends to dilute the hematocrit, giving rise to the common condition known as "sports anemia."

"Sports anemia" is a misnomer. The expansion of plasma volume, acting in concert with the adaptations of an "athlete's heart," is not a detriment, but is rather a benefit to function. The expansion in plasma volume increases the cardiac stroke volume enough to outstrip the fall in hematocrit, so that the net effect, based on the Fick equation, is an increase in oxygen delivery to working muscles. In other words, the expansion of plasma volume from aerobic training makes for a better athlete.

It also seems likely, based mainly on cross-sectional data but also on sparse longitudinal data, that the red cell mass increases in elite aerobic athletes such as marathoners. In other words, intense, long-term aerobic training may expand both plasma volume and red cell mass, producing, in essence, more blood. In athletes who are not training at altitude, the gain in plasma volume outstrips the gain in red cell mass, keeping the hematocrit low. The elite marathoner, for example, has *more* blood, but *thinner* blood, easy to pump to the working muscles and thus prone to increase endurance performance.

The rationale of blood doping, then, is to augment the red cell mass slightly further: enough to ferry more oxygen to the muscles, yet not so much as to increase blood viscosity meaningfully. It is assumed that the "ideal" hematocrit for world-class endurance performance is approximately 50%, a level below that linked to ominous rises in blood viscosity. At such a hematocrit, it is thought that "ideal" amounts of oxygen will be carried from the lungs: enough to saturate the maximal oxidative capacity of working muscles, thus fostering the athlete's supreme oxygen consumption and peak endurance performance.

OBSERVATIONS AND RESEARCH

The concept that the ideal hematocrit for peak endurance performance is approximately 50% is only a hypothesis, based partly on anecdotal observations and partly on emerging results of laboratory and field research on blood doping in athletes.

Key anecdotal observations occurred at the 1968 Olympic Games, held in Mexico City, 2,225 meters above sea level. At this altitude, nearly all the men's distance races were dominated by Kenyans or Ethiopians, athletes born, bred, and trained in the highlands. It was assumed that these men had high hematocrits that gave them a competitive edge at low ambient pressures. The hematocrits of the 1968 African winners are not known, but the Tarahumara Indians, also good distance runners, who live in Mexico's Sierra Madre at altitudes similar to those of the Kenyan highlands, have hematocrits in the 50% range.

After the 1968 Olympic Games, research on blood doping and athletic performance accelerated. By 1972, the pioneering but uncontrolled research of Ekblom et al showed that the reinfusion of autologous red cells increased both maximal oxygen uptake and running time to exhaustion, the former by 9% and the latter, tested by brief all-out treadmill runs, by as much as 23%.

This investigation seemed to trigger more anecdotal observations suggesting that blood doping can help athletes win distance races. Blood doping was used by at least a few endurance athletes in the 1972, 1980, and 1984 Olympic Games, and by a U.S. Nordic skier in 1987. Besides the few athletes who have admitted to blood doping, other winners have been accused of it, including East German and Italian distance runners, and Soviet cross-country skiers.

Among a host of studies of blood doping conducted since 1972, three of the best-designed and controlled investigations, all using freeze-preserved, autologous red cells, agree that blood doping enhances endurance performance. The first was a double-blind, sham-control, crossover study of 11 elite male track athletes. The transfusion of 2 units of autologous red cells increased maximal oxygen uptake by 5% and brief, all-out running time to exhaustion by 35%. The second was a double-blind, sham-control study of 12 experienced male distance runners. After they had received 2 units of autologous blood, their mean time for an 8 km treadmill run was 45 seconds faster than when they received an equal volume of saline. The third was a sham-control study of six highly-trained male distance runners in Albuquerque, New Mexico; the performance was gauged from the time it took to race 10,000 meters on an outdoor track. Blood boosting cut the mean race time by 69 seconds. Another recent study, perhaps less well controlled than the previous three, suggests that blood doping also speeds the race time of cross-country skiers.

No study is perfect, but when all studies are viewed together, blood doping seems to enhance performance. A 10,000-meter runner from sea level, for example, stands to gain at least a few seconds from blood doping, especially if the race is run at altitude, but also, it seems, if the race is at sea-level. In the Olympic Games, a few seconds may be the margin of victory over this distance.

EXPERIENCE WITH RHEPO

If doping with autologous blood enhances performance, doping via rhEPO would certainly be expected to do the same. One study of the effect of rhEPO on performance has already appeared. For 6 weeks, 15 trained, male physical education students took rhEPO injections three times a week. Their mean hematocrit rose from 45% to 50%. On treadmill tests, their mean maximal oxygen uptake increased 8%; brief, all-out running time to exhaustion also improved by 17%. The increase in maximal oxygen uptake declined toward baseline a few weeks after stopping the rhEPO. This study lacked a placebo control group and was poorly controlled for possible training effects over the 6 weeks, but nevertheless it suggests that the performance benefits of blood doping via rhEPO are similar to those via blood transfusion.

This study also suggests the existence of an "erythropoietin-induced exercising hypertension." In other words, rhEPO seems to accentuate the normal, exercise-induced rise in systolic blood pressure. During submaximal exercise (cycling at a workrate of 200 W), systolic blood pressure increased from a mean peak of 177 mm Hg *before* taking rhEPO to a mean peak of 191 mm Hg (highest value, 245 mm Hg) *while* taking rhEPO. This troubling accentuation of blood pressure occurred during exercise that was judged as moderate by heart rate (140 beats/minute) and perceived exertion (12 to 13 points on the Borg scale). Resting blood pressures did not increase significantly on rhEPO, although the resting diastolic pressure tended to rise. In a recent study where rhEPO was used to treat chronic orthostatic hypotension, however, three of eight patients (most of whom were mildly anemic before they took rhEPO) developed hypertension at rest. Apparently rhEPO may increase blood pressure, both by increasing hematocrit (because hemoglobin binds and inhibits nitric oxide, an endogenous vasodilator) and (based on a rodent model) by directly constricting renal and other arterioles. For athletes abusing rhEPO, a concomitant, sharp rise in both hematocrit and exercising blood pressure could have dire implications.

DANGERS OF ABUSING RHEPO

Some athletes are abusing rhEPO. The prevalence of abuse at present seems small, but for some individuals the consequences may be grave. Evidence of abuse is as yet circumstantial. A few athletes in Europe and the United States have admitted their abuse of rhEPO to a few doctors and journalists. A 1989 poll of 1,015 Italian athletes revealed widespread knowledge of doping methods and suggested that at least 7% of top-ranking athletes used autologous red cells in blood doping. Informed physicians have told journalists that some European cyclists also abuse rhEPO.

What befell some of these cyclists raises alarm about rhEPO abuse. Beginning in 1987, when rhEPO arrived in Europe, and continuing into 1990, at least 18 competitive Dutch or Belgian cyclists have died, most of them suddenly and unexpectedly. Some of them cycled for a professional team that was notorious over the years for abusing drugs. Most experts agree that such a spate of deaths among elite cyclists is atypical. The modes of death are also atypical in some cases. Details are sparse, and it is unlikely that all 18 deaths are from the same cause. Officials deny that rhEPO was involved in any death, claiming that most were from heart problems, congenital or acquired, including four "ischemic cases" (presumably coronary artery disease) and six "post-viral cases" (presumably myocarditis). Yet press accounts suggest that some of the deaths occurred not during racing, as might be expected from cardiac deaths in elite athletes, but in the days after racing, while the competitors were sleeping in bed or resting on a beach.

Plausibly, a cyclist abusing rhEPO might start a race with a hematocrit of 55% to 60%, and—because of sweating and dehydration—end the race with a hematocrit of over 60%. If the last dose of rhEPO were taken just before the race, it would continue to act over the next few days, keeping the hematocrit higher than it otherwise would be. A high hematocrit, elevated blood viscosity, and dehydration—along with hours on the saddle—would increase the risk of postrace thrombosis in pelvic or leg veins, predisposing the individual to pulmonary embolus. A Dutch-sponsored cycling team withdrew from the 1991 Tour de France when they became ill from Intralipid that they had infused (to promote recovery). The preparation apparently turned rancid after storage in a hot car trunk. Intravenous infusions of such lipid solutions may well increase the risk of thrombosis.

These same factors, plus a sharp rhEPO-evoked rise in exercising blood pressure, might predispose to stroke or, depending on the status of the individual's coronary arteries and possible abuse of other drugs (anabolic steroids; amphetamine), myocardial infarction or arrhythmia.

Another spate of mysterious sudden deaths in elite endurance athletes has been reported from Sweden. In the 3 years leading up to June, 1992, six orienteers, who comprised 3% of world-class orienteers and who occasionally trained together, died during racing or training. The putative cause of the deaths was myocarditis, perhaps from *Chlamydia pneumoniae,* but one wonders whether drug or rhEPO abuse was also involved.

WHAT CAN BE DONE?

Abuse of rhEPO cannot be detected by urine testing, and the International Olympics Committee does not yet allow blood testing. Even when blood testing becomes routine, rhEPO abuse will be difficult to prove, because rhEPO is identical to native or endogenous EPO. Any injected rhEPO would mix with native EPO, and the half-life of rhEPO is short, so that any increase of EPO level (from injection of rhEPO) would disappear within a day or two.

The use of rhEPO in sports is thus illegal, but it cannot presently be detected. Among possible remedies, three are commonly debated: (1) mark the drug so that it can be distinguished from native EPO; (2) control the distribution of the drug, as we currently do for narcotics; and (3) sanction the drug, but monitor athletes and bar from competition anyone with a high hematocrit and/or with a hematologic profile diagnostic of rhEPO use. We should also educate athletes and coaches about the dangers of abusing rhEPO.

None of these remedies seems likely to be very effective. Those who make rhEPO do not want to mark it, arguing that it may then become antigenic. Controlling the dispensation of rhEPO may tarnish its reputation and will encourage an underground market. Sanctioning the drug will encourage some athletes to "dope up to the line" to gain an edge or to "keep up with my competitors."

Barring athletes with a "high hematocrit" raises questions and may prompt lawsuits. How high is too high? Is 55% too high for a male distance racer? Is 50% too high for a woman? By and large, this is probably true. But could a dishonest athlete who was abusing rhEPO claim he or she had inherited a high hematocrit, trained in the mountains, or become dehydrated from a gastrointestinal illness, thus showing a spuriously high hematocrit?

Rarely, an athlete can excel because of inheriting a high hematocrit, as in the 1991 report concerning a Finnish distance athlete who had an autosomal dominant erythrocytosis caused by increased sensitivity to native EPO. At the time of the report, his age was 53, his hematocrit was 68%, and in his athletic prime he had won several Olympic gold medals in cross-country skiing.

We need more research on natural hematocrit levels among elite distance racers, such as the Kenyans, born and bred at altitude. Presumably, because of the gain in plasma volume with endurance training, the hematocrit even here will rarely exceed 55% in a man, or 50% in a woman.

Finally, we need better hematologic profiles to detect blood doping. As already shown in cross-country skiers, recent autologous blood transfusion (within a week) can be detected in about half the recipients by a single blood sampling, if the profile reveals a high hematocrit (hemoglobin concentration) and a low serum EPO level.

As for recent abuse of rhEPO, promising blood profiles would include markers for "newborn" red cells, such as subtle elevations in reticulocyte count or red cell creatine content, or an increase in the percentage of large red cells, or macrocytes. Other promising tests include the serum level of soluble transferrin receptor, which should increase from rhEPO-induced erythropoiesis, or the detection of macrocytes, which are also hypochromic, suggesting response to rhEPO and an early, functional iron deficiency.

A 1993 report compared red cell indices (as determined by an automated cytoanalyzer) in 20 athletes who took rhEPO for 30 to 45 days, versus 240 elite athletes not taking rhEPO. Most of those taking rhEPO had greater blood percentages of macrocytes, and a cut-off value for the percentage of hypochromic macrocytes was surpassed by 50% of those taking rhEPO, but by none of the control athletes.

The International Ski Federation now mandates blood sampling of athletes to detect such doping, and a similar proposal is under study by the International Olympic Committee. We should soon be able to detect and deter blood doping, be it from autologous transfusion or rhEPO, once we can sample blood from athletes, unannounced and year-round, both in training and randomly in competition.

SUGGESTED READING

Berglund B, Birgegard G, Wide L, Pihlstedt P. Effects of blood transfusions on some hematological variables in endurance athletes. Med Sci Sports Exerc 1989; 21:637–642.

Brien AJ, Simon TL. The effects of red blood cell infusion on 10-km race time. JAMA 1987; 257:2761–2765.

Casoni I, Ricci G, Ballarin E, et al. Hematological indices of erythropoietin administration in athletes. Int J Sports Med 1993; 14:307–311.

Eichner ER. Sports anemia, iron supplements, and blood doping. Med Sci Sports Exerc 1992; 24:S315–S318.

Ekblom B, Berglund B. Effect of erythropoietin administration on maximal aerobic power. Scand J Med Sci Sports 1991; 1:88–93.

Hoeldtke RD, Streeten DHP. Treatment of orthostatic hypotension with erythropoietin. N Engl J Med 1993; 329:611–615.

Klein HG. Blood transfusion and athletics: Games people play. N Engl J Med 1985; 312:854–856.

Scarpino V, Arrigo A, Benzi G, et al. Evaluation of prevalence of "doping" among Italian athletes. Lancet 1990; 336:1048–1050.

CONTROL OF DRUG ABUSE IN SPORT

NORMAN GLEDHILL, Ph.D.

The analysis of competitors' urine was introduced during the 1968 Olympics. Earlier attempts at doping control had involved clumsy luggage and dormitory searches. Since that time, the sophistication of the doping control program has been enhanced substantially and modifications are incorporated frequently. Such modifications often involve the addition to the banned list of previously permitted drugs or the removal from the banned list of previously prohibited drugs. Hence, it is essential for physicians who treat athletes to update their knowledge of doping control on a regular basis. This chapter provides an overview of the current doping control program along with details on banned drugs and banned manipulations, highlighting recent modifications.

THE DOPING CONTROL PROGRAM

Doping control was introduced into various sports in the 1960s, including those controlled by the International Olympic Committee (IOC). In 1988 the IOC defined doping as "the administration of or use by a competing athlete of any substance foreign to the body or of any physiological substance taken in an abnormal quantity or taken by an abnormal route of entry into the body with the sole intention of increasing in an artificial manner his/her performance in competition." International Sports Federations (ISFs) and National Sport Organizations (NSOs) generally employ the following working definition of doping; "the use of any substances contained in the current IOC banned drug list by a competitor, or the administration or supply of these substances to a competitor by another person such as a physician, physiotherapist, team leader, coach, parent or other person." The Medical Commission of the IOC established a list of banned drugs, which is updated regularly. Also, since the accurate analysis of drugs in urine necessitates very sophisticated analytical techniques plus an extensive knowledge of the body's metabolism of the drugs in question, the IOC accredits select laboratories around the world to conduct the testing.

The IOC conducts doping control at all Olympic events. ISFs and NSOs conduct doping control at major competitions, at training camps, and year-round, out of competition. The IOC's banned drug list is utilized whenever doping control takes place and the analysis of urine samples is conducted only in IOC accredited laboratories. However, ISFs and NSOs occasionally supplement the IOC's banned drug list with additional drugs or manipulations that have not yet been banned by the IOC. Such additions are communicated widely to the athletes and other personnel involved. The IOC Medical Commission also has established detailed procedures for the conduct of doping control, and they have become the standard internationally. Whether doping control is carried out at a competition or during training, the procedures involve several crucial steps that must be adhered to fastidiously. These procedures comprise:

1. Selection of the athlete to be tested.
2. Collection and coding of A and B urine samples.
3. Secure storage and transport of the samples to an IOC accredited laboratory.
4. Analysis of the A sample.
5. Reporting of any positive tests to the appropriate authorities.
6. Analysis of the B confirmation sample.
7. Imposition of sanctions.

At competitions, the selection of the athletes for testing can be entirely random or by virtue of the athlete's placing in an event. A doping control marshall notifies the athletes that they have been selected for testing and accompanies the competitors thus identified at all times following notification. Notification of selection acknowledgments are signed by the athletes and they have the option of being accompanied throughout the doping control procedure by an advisor of their choosing. Failure by an athlete to comply with doping control is generally treated as a doping infraction. From the time of notification until the urine samples have been collected, athletes are allowed to consume only sealed drinks that are provided by the doping control authority. The accompanying marshalls are responsible for ensuring that the athletes do not smuggle samples of blank urine into the doping control area (in containers or bags strapped to the body), or empty their bladders and replace the urine with blank urine via a catheter. Upon arrival at the doping control area, each athlete's identity is verified by the doping control officer, and once inside the area the athlete is accompanied constantly by a chaperon until the urine sample has been provided.

The athletes are extensively involved in the sample handling process. They choose a sterilized collection vessel that is sealed in a plastic bag from a selection of such vessels. They then void into the container under the unobstructed view of a same gender chaperon. The athletes then select (from a number of options) a sealed transport pack containing the coded A and B sample containers. They also select a uniquely coded label, plus the related transport pack seals, and then observe the label being attached to the bottles plus the documentation forms. The unique identification code is sometimes also etched onto the glass bottle. The athletes divide the urine sample between the A and B containers, and the bottles are then sealed, generally by crimping. The lids of the bottles may also be sealed with a coating of wax, which cannot be violated without leaving evidence. The athletes next package the A and B containers into their respective transport packs along with the completed documents, and then seal the transport packs with tamper proof, uniquely coded tabs.

On the completion of the sample collection procedure, the chaperons and doping control officers sign a copy of the documentation and give it to the athletes. The samples are then stored securely under refrigeration until they are sent to the laboratory. To deliver samples to the laboratory, the transport packs are put in containers that are sealed with tamper proof tabs. The entire chain of custody in the handling of the samples, from the doping control officer to the laboratory, is carefully documented.

IOC ACCREDITED DRUG-TESTING LABORATORIES

The detection of banned substances or their metabolites in urine can be very difficult; when analyses are undertaken during a major competition such as the Olympic Games, the volume of tests is also large and the results must be available in 24 to 48 hours. To become accredited, a laboratory must meet a number of administrative requirements and must identify correctly the drugs presented in 10 unknown urine samples. All IOC accredited laboratories must be re-accredited annually by correctly analyzing 10 unknown urine samples. The laboratory must supply documentation regarding the methods of analysis employed, the expertise of laboratory personnel, and the laboratory's research program, also documenting the procedures followed in receiving, storing, and handling the samples. If a laboratory fails to meet the re-accreditation standards, it is suspended at the Phase 1 or Phase 2 level (Table 1). A list of the laboratories currently accredited by the IOC is provided in Table 1.

DOPING CLASSES, DOPING METHODS, AND EXAMPLES OF BANNED DRUGS

The IOC list of doping classes, doping methods, and restricted drugs is contained in Table 2. Category I in this table contains a list of the pharmacological classes of banned substances. A list of representative samples from each of the five doping classes in Category I is contained in Table 3. No substances in the banned classes can be used for the medical treatment of competitors, even if the substance is not listed specifically. The term "and related substances" (which means drugs that are related to that class by their pharmacologic action and/or chemical structure) is appended to the end of the example drug list in each category. Thus, new but related drugs that may be developed prior to any subsequent revision of the list are also banned. Caffeine is a special case, in that a urine specimen is not considered positive until the concentration of caffeine exceeds 12 μg/ml. The normal ingestion of coffee, tea, or other drinks containing caffeine will not cause this limit to be exceeded or even remotely approached. However, the ingestion of caffeine tablets or the use of caffeine suppositories or injections may result in a positive doping test.

Category II lists the doping methods banned by the IOC. Blood doping via the transfusion or reinfusion of blood or the use of erythropoietin, all of which increase red cell mass, are banned. As well, the use of substances or methods that alter the integrity and validity of urine samples is prohibited. Examples of these banned manipulations are catheterization, urine substitution, inhibition of renal excretion (by probenecid and related compounds), and urine tampering (by epitestosterone application).

Category III contains classes of drugs that are subject to certain restrictions. Alcohol and marijuana are not prohibited by the IOC. However, an athlete's blood or breath alcohol level or the presence of marijuana in urine may be determined at the request of an ISF or NSO. Injectable and oral anaesthetics are permitted with certain restrictions: agents such as procaine (Novocain) and lidocaine (Xylocaine) can be used, but cocaine cannot; local or intra-articular injections are permitted, but intravenous injections are not; vasoconstrictors must not be present, and any use of permitted anaesthetics must be medically justified and documented.

The use of corticosteroids is banned except for topical use (ear, eye, and skin), inhalation therapy (asthma, allergic rhinitis), and local or intra-articular

Table 1 Current IOC Accredited Laboratories (March, 1993)

Athens*	Indianapolis	Oslo
Barcelona	Lausanne	Paris
Beijing	Lisbon	Prague†
Cologne	London	Rome
Copenhagen†	Los Angeles	Seoul†
Ghent	Madrid	Sydney
Helsinki	Moscow	Tokyo
Huddinge		

*Phase 1: The laboratory is temporarily suspended from international testing. At the national level, the laboratory may perform screening procedures but positive A samples must be confirmed by a fully accredited IOC laboratory and the corresponding B sample must be analyzed by a fully accredited IOC laboratory.

†Phase 2: The laboratory can perform international testing, but it is temporarily suspended from confirmation of positive A samples and analysis of B samples. Confirmation of the A samples and analysis of the B samples must be performed in a fully accredited IOC laboratory.

Table 2 IOC Categories of Doping Classes and Methods

I Doping classes
  A. Stimulants
  B. Narcotics
  C. Anabolic agents
  D. Diuretics
  E. Peptide hormones and their analogues
II Doping methods
  A. Blood doping
  B. Pharmacologic, chemical, and physical manipulations
III Classes of drugs subject to certain restrictions
  A. Alcohol
  B. Marijuana
  C. Local anaesthetics
  D. Corticosteroids
  E. Beta-blockers

Table 3   Representative Examples from the Doping Classes in Category I

A. Stimulants

Amfepramone	Crothetamide (component of "micoren")	Methylephedrine
Amfetaminil	Dimetamfetamine	Methylphenidate
Amineptine	Ephedrine	Morazone
Amiphenazole	Etafedrine	Nikethamide
Amphetamine	Ethamivan	Pemoline
Benzphetamine	Etilamfetamine	Pentetrazol
Caffeine*	Fencamfamin	Phendimetrazine
Cathine	Fenetylline	Phenmetrazine
Chlorphentermine	Fenproporex	Phentermine
Clobenzorex	Furfenorex	Phenylpropanolamine
Clorprenaline	Mefenorex	Pipradol
Cocaine	Mesocarbe	Prolintane
Cropropamide (component of "micoren")	Methamphetamine	Propylhexedrine
	Methoxyphenamine	Pyrovalerone
		Strychnine

and related compounds

B. Narcotic Analgesics

Alphaprodine	Dihydrocodeine	Morphine
Anileridine	Dipipanone	Nalbuphine
Buprenorphine	Ethoheptazine	Pentazocine
Dextromoramide	Ethylmorphine	Pethidine
Dextropropoxyphen	Levorphanol	Phenazocine
Diamorphine (heroin)	Methadone	Trimeperidine

and related compounds

C. Anabolic Agents

i) Androgenic Anabolic Steroids

Bolasterone	Mesterolone	Oxandrolone
Boldenone	Metandienone	Oxymesterone
Clostebol	Metenolone	Oxymetholone
Dehydrochlormethyl-testosterone	Methyltestosterone	Stanozolol
Fluoxymesterone	Nandrolone	Testosterone**
	Norethandrolone	

and related substances

ii) Other Anabolic Agents

Beta-2 agonists (e.g., clenbuterol, bitolterol, orciprenaline, rimiterol)

D. Diuretics

Acetazolamide	Canrenone	Furosemide
Amiloride	Chlormerodrin	Hydrochlorothiazide
Bendroflumethiazide	Chlortalidone	Mersalyl
Benzthiazide	Diclofenamide	Spironolactone
Bumetanide	Ethacrynic acid	Triamterene

and related compounds

E. Peptide Hormones and Their Analogues

Chorionic Gonadotrophin (HCG-Human Chorionic Gonadotrophin) — The administration to males of HCG and other compounds with related activity leads to an increased rate of production of endogenous androgenic steroids and is considered equivalent to the exogenous administration of testosterone.

Corticotrophin (ACTH) — Corticotrophin has been misused to increase the blood levels of endogenous corticosteroids to obtain the euphoric effect of corticosteroids. The application of Corticotrophin is considered to be equivalent to the oral, intramuscular, or intravenous application of corticosteroids.

Growth hormone (HGH, somatotropin) — The misuse of HGH in sport is unethical and dangerous due to the various adverse side effects (e.g., allergic reactions, diabetogenic effects, and acromegaly) when applied in high doses.

All the respective releasing factors of the above hormones or their analogues are also banned.

Erythropoietin (EPO) is the glucoprotein hormone produced in human kidney which regulates the rate of synthesis of erythrocytes.

---

*A urine specimen will be considered positive if the concentration of caffeine exceeds 12 µg/ml.

**The presence of a testosterone to epitestosterone ratio greater than six to one in the urine of a competitor constitutes an offense unless there is evidence that this ratio is due to a physiological or pathological condition. Ratios between six to one and ten to one will be reviewed further before considering the results as positive or negative.

injections (with written medical notification). The oral, intramuscular or intravenous injection of corticosteroids is not permitted. The IOC Medical Commission has noted that there is a wide range of effective alternative preparations available to control hypertension, cardiac arrhythmias, angina pectoris, and migraine. Hence, due to the continued misuse of beta-blockers in some sports in which physical activity is of minor importance, the IOC Medical Commission reserves the right to test athletes from such sports whenever it deems appropriate. These sports are unlikely to include endurance events, in which beta-blockers would impair performance capacity. Tests for beta-blockers are performed at the request of an ISF or NSO (for example, in archery, shooting, biathlon, modern pentathlon, bobsleigh, diving, luge, and ski jumping), and at the discretion of the IOC Medical Commission. Examples of beta-blockers include acebutolol (Sectral), alprenolol, atenolol (Tenoretic, Tenormin), labetalol (Normodyne, Trandate), metoprolol (Lopressor), nadolol (Corgard), oxprenolol, propranolol (Inderal, Inderide), sotalol, and related substances.

NONDETECTABLE DOPING

The policy of the IOC's Medical Commission is to "ban only those drugs or methods for which suitable analytical procedures can be derived, which unequivocally detect compounds in urine samples." However, there are some notable exceptions to this policy. Blood doping is banned, but no reliable analytic technique is yet available to detect its use. The current state of the art in detecting blood doping requires blood rather than urine sampling; two samples are taken 1 to 2 weeks apart, and the levels of hemoglobin plus erythropoietin are compared. However, only 50% of athletes who have been involved in blood doping can be detected by use of this procedure.

Human Growth Hormone (HGH) is an endogenous substance; detection of its misuse is extremely difficult, because urine levels do not directly reflect plasma levels, and HGH disappears rapidly from the system. The recent development of synthetic HGH and its reported availability to athletes has further exacerbated this problem. Erythropoietin (EPO) is an endogenous hormone that stimulates red blood cell production. The recent availability of synthetic EPO has resulted in some athletes utilizing this drug instead of blood doping. Since an elevated body EPO is rapidly reduced to normal, the administration of this hormone cannot presently be detected. Bicarbonate doping (soda loading) refers to the oral ingestion of sodium bicarbonate to increase the body's bicarbonate buffering system, thereby enhancing anaerobic performance by delaying the fall in intramuscular pH. The IOC has not yet identified bicarbonate

doping as a banned method, but some NSOs have prohibited this manipulation.

RECENT MODIFICATIONS TO THE IOC LIST OF DOPING CLASSES AND METHODS

Beta-2 agonists such as bitolterol (Tornalate), orciprenaline, and rimiterol are now banned. Salbutamol and terbutalin (Brethine, Bricanyl) remain as permitted beta-2 agonists, but only if administered by inhalation. Physicians wishing to prescribe these permitted drugs for a competitor must provide written notification to the IOC Medical Commission. Codeine has been taken off the list of banned substances, and its use is now permitted for medical purposes. However, the use of codeine by an athlete must still be declared. The name of the banned group androgenic anabolic steroids was changed to anabolic agents, with identification of two sub-groups: (1) androgenic anabolic steroids and (2) other anabolic agents (beta-2 agonists, such as the recently added clenbuterol). Beta-blockers have been reclassified as drugs subject to certain restrictions, indicating that tests for their administration should be undertaken on request and only in those sports in which beta-blockers are likely to enhance performance. The expression "by inhalation" was added to the section dealing with corticosteroids. It now reads: "Any team doctor wishing to administer corticosteroids by local or intra-articular injection, or by inhalation, to a competitor must give written notification to the IOC Medical Commission." The presence in a competitor's urine of a testosterone (T) to epitestosterone (E) ratio greater than six to one will be reviewed further before it is considered to be positive or negative. T/E ratios beyond ten to one are considered as positive.

SUGGESTED READING

American College of Sports Medicine. Position stand on blood doping as an ergogenic aid. Med Sci Sports Exerc 1987; 19:540–543.

American College of Sports Medicine. Position stand on the use of anabolic-androgenic steroids in sports. Med Sci Sports Exerc 1984; 16:13–18.

Cowart VS. Human growth hormone, the latest ergogenic aid? Physician Sportsmed 1988; 16:175–185.

Dodd SL, Herb RA, Powers SK. Caffeine and exercise performance; an update. Sports Med 1993; 15:14–23.

Lamb DR. Anabolic steroids in athletics: how well do they work and how dangerous are they? Am J Sports Med 1984; 12:31–38.

Laties VG, Weiss B. The amphetamine margin in sports. Federation Proceedings 1981; 40:2689–2692.

Leith W. EPO and cycling. A look at the recent mysterious deaths of eighteen healthy Dutch and Belgian cyclists. Athletics 1992; July:24–26.

Macintyre JG. Growth hormone and athletes. Sports Med 1987; 129–142.

Wagner JC. Enhancement of athletic performance with drugs; an overview. Sports Med 1991; 12:250–265.

PSYCHOLOGICAL ASPECTS OF SPORTS MEDICINE

IMPROVING COMPLIANCE WITH EXERCISE PROGRAMS

ROBERT J. SONSTROEM, Ph.D.

Adherence to exercise programs remains a critical problem in sports medicine. A variety of theories, variables, and methods have been applied to predicting and promoting exercise participation, with less than consensual success. This chapter presents a different approach, which emphasizes influencing participants directly on the gymnasium floor or playing field. Self-esteem enhancement techniques are being used successfully in contemporary educational programs, assertiveness training, psychotherapy, and drug and alcohol rehabilitation programs. These techniques feature interactions between people and personal achievements and are already inherent in exercise settings. Planning to emphasize these techniques within activity sessions promises that more people will be reached and that they will be reached more vitally. The self-enhancement mechanisms discussed here have been selected both from self-esteem theory and from practical educational and clinical programs attempting to change self-esteem.

The validity of this approach involves at least three postulates. First, self-esteem guides future behavior. People's feelings about themselves and their abilities strongly influence their behavior within a given environment. Developing positive self-regard about one's abilities to exercise is seen as a basis for promoting physical activity participation and adherence. A second payoff from utilizing these techniques is that they are founded on important learning and performance reinforcement principles. Finally, many group exercise programs incorporate an ultimate goal of leading participants to internalize the exercise process so that they can continue their own regimens independently. Psychologically, this is believed to involve the development of an intrinsic motivation to exercise. Many of the techniques used to enhance self-esteem also foster intrinsic motivation.

For present purposes, the application of self-enhancement techniques is assumed to occur in group exercise programs conducted under the direction of one or more exercise leaders. These individuals serve a vital function as facilitators of the self-enhancement processes. Successful internalization of these processes will produce fulfilled participants who are capable of continuing individual programs without detailed supervision.

BACKGROUND

Positive self-esteem is regarded by clinicians as the premier indicator of favorable life adjustment. However, self-esteem is resistant to change after adolescence. When changes do occur, they are generally in response to intensive and extensive participation in activities of high importance to the individual. Self-esteem is multidimensional. People tend to have discrete evaluations of themselves as social persons, as professionals, as comics, as physically competent people, and as family members. Presumably, the contribution of each of these to global self-esteem is directly proportional to its importance to the individual. Increasing competence in an important domain is believed to affect self-regard favorably. Exercise participation and physical fitness are viewed as socially desirable attributes in today's society. This fact, coupled with the high intrinsic regard most people hold for their bodies, should enhance the importance of physical competence and fitness for all members of an exercise class. The challenge for the exercise leader(s) is to ensure success experiences for participants. Thus, self-esteem is positively affected by increased competence in an important domain, simultaneously increasing the importance of that domain to the individual.

Feelings of personal competence derived from experiences of success are thought to be an important dimension of self-esteem. Self-acceptance, or self-love, is generally considered an important second dimension. Self-accepting people see themselves accurately, admit to their weaknesses, and, while seeking to correct their shortcomings, live happily and creatively with this awareness. Mechanisms to enhance personal competence and self-acceptance must be linked with exercise program activities in planning for a growth in self-esteem.

AGENTS OF CHANGE

Self-esteem will not change in a mental vacuum. The development of physical fitness does not automatically

608

Table 1 Mechanisms of Self-Esteem Change (Principles of Operation to be Emphasized by the Exercise Leader)

Self-evaluation
    Promote self-awareness
    Provide constructive feedback
    Recognize strong points
    Discuss weaknesses positively
    Accept the individual as he/she is
Success experiences
    Instil a standard of individual improvement
    Assess goal importance for the individual
    Assist in setting realistic goals
    Positive reinforcement
Social reinforcement
    Publicly identify progress
    Teach others to praise
    Arrange for group discussions
    Find an appreciative ear
Process internalization
    Lead in cognitive restructuring
    Inculcate personal responsibility for exercise behavior
    Teach self-monitoring/instructional techniques
    Teach self-talk and self-praise

enhance self-perceptions. Rather, the person must be psychologically involved in the process, cognitively monitoring and emotionally appreciating changes to the physical self. For present purposes, the selected mechanisms of change (agents) have been organized under four rubrics: Self-Evaluation, Success Experiences, Social Reinforcement, and Process Internalization (Table 1). The content and order of these four categories is somewhat arbitrary, as change agents are used in an interactive fashion throughout a program.

SELF-EVALUATION

Self-awareness must be present for change to occur. The theory of "objective self-awareness" stipulates that an individual's attention must be directed inwardly for change to occur. Heightened physical and emotional activation serve to direct a person's attention inwardly. It is difficult to be unaware of oneself in a process that involves perspiration, increased heart rate, and shortness of breath. Self-awareness is fostered further by pre- and post-exercise stretching, by self-monitoring of heart rate, and by regulation of exercise pace. Maintenance of a logbook throughout an exercise program keeps such experiences at the front of personal awareness.

Self-evaluation is also promoted by feedback, based upon tests administered at program entry. Theory suggests that accurate self-perceptions are fundamental to well-adjusted people. A knowledge of one's abilities should also increase sensitivity to change. Ewart and colleagues found that patients perceived their personal fitness more accurately after receiving their entry test performance evaluations. The impact of objective feedback can be both magnified and tempered by feedback from the instructor, who seeks to reconcile strong points, weaknesses, and self-acceptance with the development of realistic goals for the individual participant. Exercise leaders should emphasize the extent of individual differences in genetic endowment and previous training. Participants should realize that endo-mesomorphs as compared to ectomorphs may experience greater difficulty in learning to jog several kilometers.

Self-recognition of strong points and an ability to discuss weaknesses positively can be facilitated if an appropriate atmosphere is created by the class leader. Exercise leaders become "important others" in the lives of participants and are essential facilitators for self-esteem enhancement. Leaders who project an acceptance of people as they are, will help participants to realize that a physical weakness is not a reason to think poorly of one's self. Individuals must come to accept certain weaknesses, rather than ignore them, as they attempt to minimize their shortcomings. Good leaders understand the "Looking Glass" principle, "we are what we think others think we are." Private discussion with the leader will often personalize feedback for the individual and serve to establish its salience.

SUCCESS EXPERIENCES

Exercise leaders must instil a standard of individual improvement in their classes. If the processes discussed under Self-Evaluation are being implemented, this should not be difficult. In their early stages, adult exercise programs rely on preset standards, controlling exercise intensity and duration at a uniform level commensurate with individual ability. After a short time, however, individual differences in fitness gains encourage a greater emphasis on individualized programs. At this point, the leader should assist the participant in planning new personal goals. The instructor can assess various goals and their importance to the individual. How high are the person's cardiorespiratory goals? How important are these goals? Does the person desire stronger shoulders, sturdier legs, or greater flexibility? As the program progresses, the participant must assume ever greater responsibility for realizing these goals; the role of the leader becomes to assist in setting realistic goals. The leader who is interested in creating a positive atmosphere for change *will expect* change. All of the leader's expressions and gestures must indicate acceptance of the idea that a person will change. Genuine interest in the participants will prime a recognition of such change, small though it may be. Procedures to this point have been dedicated to making exercise achievement more personal and more important to the individual. If the leader now conscientiously reinforces progress, the personal importance of exercise achievement will continue to grow in the person.

SOCIAL REINFORCEMENT

Creation of an atmosphere promoting growth is facilitated if the class leader publicly identifies progress. Besides the obvious advantages of providing powerful reinforcement and sanctioning change, such a practice nullifies current societal structures banning personal praise. When is the last time someone said to you, "Nice job, Mary! You're certainly an outstanding teacher/physician/coach." We don't receive this type of reinforcement and we don't expect to give it. Therefore, our self-concepts remain static, clinging to self-perceptions developed years ago. On the other hand, when we either give praise or receive it, we endorse the principle of change. By giving and receiving praise we also recognize personal worth and acceptance. The leader interested in creating an environment that fosters personal growth, teaches others to praise. Personal praise for others is more apt to come from people who are themselves self-confident. Self-esteem therapies reverse this process, using the praise of others as a means of enhancing personal self-esteem. This has the net effect of increasing the personalized feedback received in the process of internalizing experiences of success. Social support can be increased through group discussions. These emphasize goals and progress toward goals, and provide personalized feedback additional to that provided by program leaders. Activities that can give direction to such discussions include: "My Goals in this Program," "Pride Line" (recent accomplishments), and "Joe's Day" (group reactions to the perceptions of a single individual regarding his or her goal, progress, and obstacles). Participants are also encouraged to find an appreciative ear outside of the program; someone in their private world who is interested in them, their exercise, and their progress toward fitness goals. This person may be a spouse, a relative, a friend, or a business acquaintance. Having someone who asks questions about the program and reinforces progress, has the effect of keeping exercise experiences in the participant's mind throughout the week. Discussants are ideally "important others" for the individual.

PROCESS INTERNALIZATION

Additional techniques may be needed to internalize personal successes. Some people need to restructure their thinking about themselves in relation to exercise. Cognitive misconceptions about reality are stressed by clinicians such as Albert Ellis. Such cognitive distortions are particularly prevalent in people with low self-esteem and they are apt to preclude personal growth. Several of the distortions likely to be found in physical activity programs are listed below:

1. *Past history determines present behavior.* This distortion is particularly relevant for people who felt inadequate at games and sports during their youth. It may also be applicable to those who have dropped out of other programs.
2. *Complete competence is required for worthiness (all-or-none thinking).* Unreasonably lofty goals invite subsequent defeat. Sometimes, people enter exercise programs with the idea that in 4 months they will run marathons or be able to best the neighbor who logs 50 km weekly. The associated lack of self-acceptance must be altered by knowledge, activity experiences, and discussion. The ubiquity of unrealistic, lofty goals compels leader attention, particularly in the early stages of a program.
3. *Human unhappiness is externally caused.* A converse of this irrational belief is that human happiness is externally caused. Certain program participants are so prone to praise a program for the benefits they receive that they fail to appreciate their own involvement in the process. The personal achievements of exercise participants should be reinforced. Exercisers must feel personally responsible for their successes, for their fitness progress, and for their health.
4. *Conclusions based on a single incident (overgeneralization).* People with a low self-esteem are particularly prone to this type of irrational belief. For example, a single overuse injury can lead such people to assume that they lack the body build or the constitution for exercise.
5. *Overestimating negative and underestimating positive events (magnification and minimization).* These processes come naturally to people with low self-esteem. Instructor interpretation of performance and norms is very important.

Such common misconceptions can be corrected by the proper interpretation of fitness gains realized within a program.

After the first weeks in an exercise class, leaders should begin the slow process of inculcating a sense of personal responsibility for exercise behavior. This involves early participation in the formulation of goals. Always, the instructor *teaches self-monitoring/instructional techniques.* These begin with program-imposed procedures: warm-up/stretching, heart rate and perceived exertion monitoring, and attention to cooldown. Later, individuals are encouraged to alter warm-up and cool-down routines, based on perceived needs. Free choice, based on personal interests, is emphasized in the recreational segments of a workout. Participants are taught to monitor breath control, tenseness, and pace as they jog. The middle and later stages of a training program should include options for selecting training modalities and for flexible daily workloads, based on personal monitoring within limits imposed by safety concerns. Most importantly, participants should be impressed with the idea that they, personally, are responsible for their own attendance at class sessions. Good attendance is fostered if goals are set for long time periods. Attendance lapses are apt to occur, and relapse training should be included within a program.

Self-talk is used to make achievement and self-direction more meaningful to the participant. If an exercise class incorporates praise, it becomes easier for people to praise themselves. Self-direction may include monitoring the body during exercise and motivational directives. Some examples are:

"Next week I'll try to maintain the increased output I've achieved this week across all three sessions. The following week I'll add half a kilometer to my jogging."

"I must slow up if I'm going to cover three kilometers."

"My back is tender today. It's best if I stop at 20 situps."

Types of praise might include:

"Wow, what a job I've done. I was tired after two laps but I slowed my pace as I've been taught to do."

or:

"The last three kilometers were a breeze. What a body I've got."

It may be suspected that exercise participants engage in these thoughts anyway. Some probably do. But it is also true that some dwell on the unpleasant aspects of exercise and many are active without exercising their minds and emotions properly. In learning self-talk, participants are strongly encouraged to speak aloud. With time, self-consciousness diminishes and the process develops authenticity as a means of uniting mind, emotion, and physical capabilities.

COMMENTS

Many of the mechanisms of enhancing self-esteem identified here are already used in exercise programs for purposes other than enhancement of self-esteem. However, such mechanisms must be consciously operationalized and applied before an optimal enhancement of self-esteem can be achieved. Participants must be cognitively and emotionally impressed with the importance of the gains that they achieve. Rather than advocating a permissive philosophy that extols the worth of the individual in all contexts, these self-enhancement procedures emphasize competence.

The processes presented place a heavy reliance on floor leadership. Instructors need not be clinical psychologists, but they need background knowledge and orientation in terms of the structure of self-esteem and the manner in which self-esteem can be changed. They should have the skills to teach mechanisms of change to participants. Finally, they should have a conscientious concern for people; this will lead to accurate evaluation and positive monitoring of participant progress.

SUGGESTED READING

American College of Sports Medicine. Resource manual for guidelines for exercise testing and prescription. Vol. 2. Philadelphia: Lea & Febiger, 1992.

Baumeister RF, ed. Self-esteem: The puzzle of low self-regard. New York: Plenum Press, 1993.

Canfield J, Wells HC. 100 Ways to enhance self-concept in the class-rooms: A handbook for teachers and parents. Englewood Cliffs, NJ: Prentice-Hall, 1976.

Dryden W. Counseling individuals: The rational-emotive approach. New York: Taylor & Francis, 1987.

Fox KR, Corbin CB. The physical self-perception profile: Development and preliminary validation. J Sport Exerc Psychol 1989; 11:408–430.

Pope AW, McHale SM, Craighead WE. Self-esteem enhancement with children and adolescents. New York: Pergamon Press, 1988.

Rosenberg M. Conceiving the self. New York: Basic Books, 1979.

Sonstroem RJ. Exercise and self-esteem. Exerc Sport Sci Rev 1984; 12:123–155.

Sonstroem RJ, Harlow LL, Josephs L. Exercise and self-esteem: Validity of model expansion and exercise associations. J Sport Exerc Psychol (in press).

Sonstroem RJ, Morgan WP. Exercise and self-esteem: Rationale and model. Med Sci Sports Exerc 1989; 21:329–337.

Wylie RC. The self-concept: Theory and research on selected topics. Vol 2. Lincoln, NB: University of Nebraska Press, 1979.

EXERCISE FOR MOOD ENHANCEMENT

LARRY M. LEITH, Ph.D.

Traditionally, mood is defined as a conscious state of mind or predominant emotion. Mood has also been described as transient, fluctuating affective states. It is normal to experience temporary mood swings as a part of everyday living. Our mood is affected by a variety of factors. A reprimand from our boss, a snub from a significant other, a flat tire, or losing our wallet can all put us into a vile mood. Similarly, a pat on the back, an enjoyable date, or a lottery ticket win can immediately put us in an excellent frame of mind. Another activity that has excellent potential for affecting our mood is exercise. The relationship between exercise and mood is the primary focus of this chapter.

DIAGNOSIS AND TRADITIONAL TREATMENTS

Mood aberrations were traditionally diagnosed only when the individual's problems were severe enough to require professional intervention. Serious depression, anxiety, or a bipolar affective disorder invariably culminated in a *DSM-III* diagnosis by a trained professional. Once the diagnosis was established, the immediate treatment for these disorders involved the use of psychoactive drugs.

Depressive episodes were most often treated with tricyclic antidepressants, and in some cases with monoamine oxidase inhibitors. Drug therapy for anxiety typically involved the use of minor tranquilizers, especially the benzodiazepines. And finally, bipolar affective disorder, which represents the most drastic form of mood swing, was most often treated with lithium carbonate. Although these drugs have been proven necessary and effective in the handling of serious mood disturbances, their use is often associated with serious side effects.

In most cases, disturbances of mood are not severe enough to justify this type of intervention. Clearly, alternative modes of diagnosis and treatment are required for these instances of nonclinical mood change.

Over the past 20 years, researchers have attempted to chart day-to-day changes in mood by psychometric assessment. The most common measurement technique involves use of the Profile of Mood States (POMS), an instrument consisting of 65 five-point adjective rating scales factored into six mood scores: (1) tension-anxiety, (2) depression-dejection, (3) anger-hostility, (4) vigor-activity, (5) fatigue-inertia, and (6) confusion-bewilderment. The POMS was originally developed as a means of measuring current mood states in individuals undergoing counseling or psychotherapy. Although other psychometric instruments such as the Mood Adjective Checklist, the Affectometer, and the Positive Affect and Negative Affect Schedule (PANAS), are being utilized more frequently, the POMS remains the most popular method for the psychometric assessment of individual mood states.

EXERCISE: AN ALTERNATIVE APPROACH TO MOOD ENHANCEMENT

It is tempting to speculate that interest in the exercise-mood relationship developed as a result of the frequently quoted "feel better" phenomenon; those who involve themselves in regular physical exercise commonly report that exercising makes them feel good. Although pervasive in the exercise literature, it is only recently that this relationship has been assessed using objective test scores. In a comprehensive literature review, I located 28 empirical studies that investigated the exercise-mood relationship. A capsule summary reveals that 21 of these studies were associated with significant improvements in mood scores, five studies reported no changes, and two studies experienced a worsened mood following exercise. Although these results are by no means unequivocal, they provide grounds for cautious optimism concerning the exercise-mood relationship. The remainder of this chapter offers the sports medicine practitioner a working knowledge of how exercise affects participant mood.

Elements of Mood Influenced by Exercise

Because mood is a multidimensional concept, it is not sufficient merely to report improvement or lack of improvement in mood after involvement in an exercise program. Although this technique has been utilized in several recent literature reviews, a more appropriate analysis involves looking at the specific elements of mood that are affected by exercise. The latter approach provides the practitioner with a better understanding of when exercise may be appropriate as a method of mood enhancement.

In empirical studies conducted to date, the elements of mood most often affected by exercise are, in descending order, tension-anxiety, confusion-bewilderment, depression-dejection, anger-hostility, vigor-activity, and fatigue-inertia. The first three subscales are improved approximately 50% more often than the last three subscales, suggesting that exercise may be most appropriate for dealing with the mood states of tension-anxiety, depression-dejection, and confusion-bewilderment.

Qualitative Aspects of Exercise for Mood Enhancement

Having established that exercise can indeed result in mood enhancement, the next logical step is to determine the specific characteristics of an exercise program most conducive to positive change. The mode of physical activity, the length of the exercise program, and the frequency, intensity, and duration of activity all must be considered when utilizing exercise for mood enchancement. Finally, it is necessary to determine whether fitness gains are necessary for the participant to experience positive changes of mood.

Exercise Mode

Most studies investigating the exercise-mood relationship have utilized running and/or walking as the mode of physical activity. However, a wide variety of other types of exercise have been associated with improvements in mood, including swimming, cycling, yoga, Tai Chi, basic training in an army camp, rowing, weight lifting, aerobic dance, and "unspecified" aerobic exercise programs. Several researchers have attempted to compare different exercise modes in terms of their potential to enhance mood, but no one exercise mode has emerged as superior to its alternatives. It would appear, however, that all of these activities involve the use of large muscle masses, and most are aerobic in nature.

Length of Exercise Program

Significant improvements in mood have been reported following exercise programs lasting 5 months or more, 12 to 15 weeks, and 6 to 10 weeks. Such findings suggest that the length of the exercise program is not critical for improvements in mood to be experienced. This viewpoint is reinforced by an increasing number of experiments documenting improvements of mood after a single bout of exercise. This observation should come as no surprise since the mood score reflects immediate mood states. Exercise may, therefore, be used as a single treatment intervention. Of special significance to the sports medicine practitioner, however, is the implication that chronic exercise may serve an important preventive function. By inducing positive mood changes on a day-to-day basis, exercise may prevent the build-up of negative mood states. For this reason, chronic involvement in an exercise program is recommended as a means of optimizing mood.

Exercise Frequency

Most studies reviewed have required exercise to be performed three times per week. Exercise frequencies of once, twice, and seven times per week have also been associated with improved mood in the participants. In accordance with the "preventive" notion suggested above, it seems reasonable to suggest a minimum exercise frequency of three times per week as an approach to mood enhancement. More exercise sessions per week could provide even more benefit, but only if the participant does not view the added workload as a chore. If the frequency of the exercise program is perceived as tedious, the benefits may be lost, and too frequent involvement in an exercise program may actually worsen mood. For this reason, except in the case of elite athletes, exercising 7 days per week is not recommended if the primary goal is mood enhancement. A maximum of 5 days per week is a reasonable guideline.

Exercise Intensity

Many studies examining the exercise-mood relationship do not report exercise intensities. Of those that do, exercise intensities of 60% to 85% maximal heart rate were commonly utilized. Because most of these studies report exercise intensities covering a substantial range, such as 70% to 85%, 65% to 85%, or 60% to 80% of maximal heart rates, it becomes very difficult to compare individual exercise intensities in terms of their mood elevating effects. The most recent research suggests that as exercise becomes more strenuous, mood appears to worsen. In addition, some evidence suggests that as exercise intensity increases, there are increases in not only the participant's rating of perceived exertion (RPE), but also negative feeling states. This suggests a possible moderate correlation between RPEs and negative affect; when we feel we are exercising too hard, our mood worsens. This observation has a good deal of intuitive merit. The implication for the sports medicine practitioner is that if exercise is to be used for mood enhancement, it should be of mild to moderate intensity.

Exercise Duration

Most of the studies reviewed involved exercise sessions of 20 or more minutes duration with the majority of studies employing 40 to 60 minute sessions. Exercise duration apparently had no impact on the extent of mood changes in the participants. Mood improvements have been reported after exercise sessions of 20 minutes, but no data are available utilizing shorter exercise durations. This is unfortunate, since we do not yet know whether exercise-induced mood changes develop within the first 5 or 10 minutes of exercise and then plateau for the duration of the activity, or whether they appear progressively throughout the entirety of a longer session. Information of this nature would be of practical significance to the exercise practitioner. In the meantime, a minimum-maximum exercise duration range of 20 to 60 minutes is recommended. I firmly believe that even shorter periods of exercise will prove an effective method of mood enhancement as research continues to accumulate.

Importance of Fitness Gains

Most studies examining the exercise-mood relationship have neither measured nor reported fitness changes in the participant. In studies that have documented fitness gains, significant improvements in mood have been reported. However, an even larger number of studies not documenting or experiencing fitness gains have also been associated with mood enhancement. These findings taken cumulatively suggest that improvements in fitness are not necessary in order for the participant to experience beneficial mood effects. This observation appears reasonable in view of the fact that mood represents immediate feeling states. We have already commented that mood improvements have been documented after single

Table 1 Prescribing Exercise for Mood Enhancement

When indicated?	Complaints from athlete concerning mood
	Behavioral observation by the coach or therapist (i.e., the athlete appears depressed, anxious, or lethargic)
	As a preventative technique
How measured?*	The Profile of Mood States (POMS)
	The Mood Adjective Checklist
	The Affectometer
	The Positive Affect and Negative Affect Schedule (PANAS)
Aspects of mood most affected?	Anxiety, depression, and confusion
	Some benefit for vigor, fatigue, and hostility
Mode of exercise?	Any aerobic exercise involving the large muscle groups; jogging and walking have been used most frequently
Length of exercise program?	Not critical, but 6–15 week programs have been used most frequently
Frequency?	3–5 times per week
Intensity?	Mild to moderate
Duration?	Minimum/maximum of 20–50 minutes per session
Fitness changes?	Not necessary

*References for measurement instruments are provided in the Suggested Reading section.

bouts of exercise. Therefore, prolonged exercise programs resulting in fitness gains are not necessary prerequisites of mood enhancement. Indirectly, however, the time required to experience fitness gains should serve a positive function by providing a cumulative mood enhancing effect.

PRACTICAL APPLICATIONS FOR THE PRACTITIONER

Exercise appears to provide a valuable alternative treatment for nonclinical forms of mood disorder. There is every reason to believe that it is also effective in preventing major disturbances of mood state. A summary of the major recommendations is provided in Table 1.

SUGGESTED READING

Dyer JB, Crouch JG. Effects of running on moods: A time series study. Percep Mot Skill 1988; 67:43–50.

Kamman R, Flett R. Measure of current level of general happiness. Austral J Psychiat 1983; 35:259–265.

LeUnes A, Hayward SA. Annotated bibliography on the Profile of Mood States in sport. J Sport Behav 1988; 11:213–239.

McIntyre CW, Watson D, Cunningham AC. The effects of social interaction, exercise, and test stress on positive and negative affect. Bull Psychonomic Society 1990; 28:141–143.

McNair DM, Lorr N, Droppleman LF. Manual for the Profile of Mood States. San Diego: Education and Industrial Testing Service, 1971.

Nowlis V. Research with the mood adjective checklist. In: Tomkins SS, Izare CE, eds. Affect, cognition, and personality. New York: Springer, 1965:125.

Watson D, Clark LA, Tellegen A. Development and validation of brief measures of positive and negative affect: The PANAS scales. J Pers Soc Psychol 1988; 54:1063–1070.

EXERCISE FOR CONTROL OF ANXIETY

STEVEN J. PETRUZZELLO, Ph.D.

Anxiety has become a tremendous mental health problem in the United States. Estimates from the late 1970s and mid-1980s have indicated that approximately 20% of the U.S. adult population experiences some type of mental disturbance, with anxiety (including panic attacks, phobic disorders, and obsessive-compulsive disorders) being most prevalent (affecting some 13 million people). From such prevalence rates, it has been estimated that 29% to 38% of U.S. adults are likely to experience a significant mental health problem at some point during their lifetime.

Anxiety results from a failure to deal effectively with mental stress. It can be characterized as a negative cognitive appraisal, typified by worry, self-doubt, and apprehension. This negative appraisal develops out of a perceived degree of uncertainty, or lack of control, over situational demands, perceived lack of resources for dealing with such demands, and negative interpretations of arousal symptoms (e.g., increases in heart rate). Anxiety is commonly distinguished as being of a trait or state nature. The level of trait anxiety reflects a general predisposition, or relatively stable component of personality, causing the individual to respond across a variety of situations with consistently high or low levels of anxiety. State anxiety, on the other hand, fluctuates as a consequence of a particular situation. State anxiety is often caused by dwelling on negative outcomes, negative self-talk (e.g., self-doubt, self-reproach), or through misinterpretation of physiologic signals. Behavioral manifestations of anxiety include increased avoidance behaviors, muscle tension, trembling, sweating, labored breathing, an inability to concentrate, restlessness, and irritability.

A number of treatment options can help individuals suffering from anxiety. Primary care providers often choose pharmacologic treatments for such disorders. Some estimates have suggested that more than 60% of currently used antianxiety drugs are prescribed by general practitioners and internists. Although effective in correcting anxiety, such psychotropic treatments can have undesirable side effects and cannot be tolerated by some patients. Fortunately, other options are available and are being used. Exercise has been suggested as a potential treatment for anxiety disorders. A 1983 survey of over 1,700 primary care physicians (published in *Physician & Sportsmedicine*) indicated that 60% prescribed exercise (walking, swimming, bicycling, or running) for patients who were suffering from anxiety. In 1984, the Office of Prevention of the National Institute of Mental Health convened a workshop to examine the role of exercise as a strategy for coping with stress. This workshop concluded that anxiety, as well as other problems associated with mental stress, needed to become a topic of immediate concern, with a particular focus on the effectiveness of exercise as a means of treatment.

Establishment of the extent to which exercise is an effective treatment for mental disorders like anxiety would be helpful on a number of fronts. First, it would remove or reduce the need for reliance on drug therapies. Further, demonstration of the efficacy of exercise in dealing with psychological problems like anxiety would encourage less reliance on health care providers and allow an increase in self-regulatory strategies. It would also shift the emphasis away from treatment and toward prevention. Exercise may finally prove to be a more cost-effective means of both treatment and prevention, whether prescribed as a treatment in and of itself or in conjunction with more "traditional" therapies (e.g., drugs, psychotherapy).

PREVENTION AND TREATMENT

The current consensus regarding exercise and anxiety reduction was developed at the 1992 International Conference on Physical Activity, Fitness, and Health. A number of specific conclusions were reached about exercise as a technique for anxiety reduction. Although alternative strategies are available for ameliorating the effects of anxiety (e.g., relaxation, meditation, cognitive restructuring), exercise not only corrects anxiety, but seems to offer many other benefits as well.

One way to prevent the development of clinical manifestations of anxiety is through a lifestyle that includes regular aerobic exercise. There is consistent evidence that physically fit individuals are less trait anxious than those who are unfit. Furthermore, fit individuals are able to deal with acute stressors more effectively than their unfit counterparts. Such stressors are cognitively appraised as less threatening and any physiologic reactions (e.g., an increased output of norepinephrine and cortisol) occur more quickly to stressor onset and dissipate more quickly once the stress has ended. In essence, the fit patient spends less time dealing with the stressor, both psychologically and physiologically.

Once anxiety has manifested itself, aerobic exercise is effective in alleviating its effects. This has been shown for both acute and chronic exercise.

Acute Exercise

Acute exercise has been associated with reductions in state anxiety, regardless of whether the anxiety is assessed via self-report, physiologic reactions, or behavioral means. Such findings clearly do not support antiexercise notions that have survived in parts of the literature for years. For example, the Pitts-McClure hypothesis that lactate, a metabolite from exercise, causes anxiety attacks has been consistently and convincingly refuted, yet it is still sometimes offered as a rationale against the use of exercise for treating anxiety disorders. In general, exercise is no more effective than other known anxiety-reducing treatments. This statement must be qualified, however, given that significant studies have shown exercise to be more effective in reducing muscular tension than treatments like quiet rest or even some antianxiety drugs (e.g., meprobamate [Deprol, Equanil, Miltown]). The anxiolytic effects also persist for a longer time after exercise than for other treatments.

Anxiolytic effects seem more consistent after exercise that is rhythmic and aerobic in nature (e.g., walking, swimming, running; cardiorespiratory/aerobic endurance) rather than intermittent (e.g., weight training; muscular strength/endurance). Unfortunately, there has been little examination of the latter as a method of anxiety reduction. Given that intermittent exercise is a reliable method of reducing depression, it is possible that with more systematic study the same will be found for anxiety reduction.

In terms of "prescription," the "dose" of exercise (intensity, duration, and frequency) necessary to achieve anxiolytic effects remains unknown. It has been suggested that patients must exercise at more than 70% of maximal heart rate for *at least* 20 minutes in order to reduce anxiety, but this has not been confirmed. Some studies have shown that exercise intensities as low as 40% of predicted maximal heart rate still reduce anxiety. With respect to exercise duration, my colleagues and I have found that exercise durations of as little as 5 minutes reliably reduce anxiety. Although the minimal "dose" is as yet unknown, it does appear that a patient who follows the American College of Sports Medicine's guidelines for improving cardiorespiratory fitness will also experience psychological improvements, but for a variety of reasons it is probably not wise to *begin* an exercise program at these levels. Fortunately, it appears that some benefit can be gained from shorter duration and less intense bouts of physical activity.

As previously noted, the anxiolytic effects generally begin 5 to 10 minutes after exercise and last for at least 2 hours. Such effects do not last indefinitely, but acute bouts of exercise can be used to reduce state anxiety and in this way may prevent chronic anxiety. It is also possible that the intensity and duration of an exercise bout will influence the duration of the anxiolytic effects, but this remains to be demonstrated.

Finally, with regard to acute effects, subject characteristics do not seem to affect the anxiety-reducing impact of exercise differentially. Young or old, male or female, and "normal" or clinical samples have all exhibited decreases in state anxiety after exercise. Some studies have shown larger decreases in anxiety in those individuals with initially higher levels of anxiety, but just as many have shown reductions when initial anxiety levels were "normal" or low.

Chronic Exercise

As noted, there is a small to moderate relationship between the degree of physical fitness and trait anxiety. Physically fit patients (usually assessed in terms of aerobic power) have less trait anxiety and are less neurotic than unfit individuals. This relationship does not, however, demonstrate that fitness *caused* the differences in anxiety. Although regular physical activity may indeed be the cause, it may also be that individuals engaged in regular physical activity live life-styles conducive to better health (e.g., better nutrition, less substance abuse).

More telling are those studies that have examined the effects of exercise training programs on subsequent trait anxiety. Training programs ranging from as little as 4 weeks to more than 15 weeks in length have been examined. The largest effects, in terms of reduced anxiety, were found for programs that exceeded 15 weeks in duration. As with state anxiety, no systematic relationships were uncovered relating response to the intensity and duration of the exercise stimulus. Again, there has been very little work examining the mode of exercise, but some preliminary studies with clinically anxious patients have shown similar reductions for both aerobic (i.e., cardiorespiratory endurance) and nonaerobic (i.e., muscular strength/endurance) forms of exercise.

A couple of issues are worth noting. First, given the relationship between fitness and anxiety and the reduction of trait anxiety with exercise programs of sufficient length, it appears that a certain amount of physical activity may be required to maintain anxiety at "normal" levels. Physical activity below such levels seems associated with numerous problems, including a decreased ability to deal with stress. Based on the notion of a minimal level of physical activity for effective functioning, some authors have discussed the idea that a sedentary life-style is a violation of our genetic heritage. We essentially have a biopsychological system that functions best with at least moderate and regular physical activity. A second point derives from clinical studies where exercise training has been used as an alternative or adjuvant to traditional treatment. Subjects in these studies invariably have noted that exercise was *more* important than medication or psychotherapy in bringing about their improvement. Whether because of enhanced physical functioning, development of a sense of personal mastery, or a feeling or self-control, such accounts highlight the potential importance of including exercise in treatment protocols.

RECOMMENDATIONS

It is truly unfortunate that so little is known about how an exercise program should be structured to reduce anxiety. Indeed, we still do not know how to keep people engaged in regular programs of physical activity for the derivation of either physiologic *or* psychological benefits. Based on previous investigations, however, a number of recommendations can be made.

The first, and perhaps most important, step in getting an individual involved in an exercise program, is to evaluate the goals and needs of that individual. Ideally, the individual should be involved in such evaluations and decision making, in order to enhance feelings of control and to give a sense of commitment to the exercise program that develops out of such discussion. This should help the health care provider (whether physician, therapist, or counselor) to assist in developing an exercise program that is neither too difficult nor too restrictive. This should also ensure that unrealistic expectations are eliminated at the outset, since filling out the exercise prescription should not itself become another source of anxiety.

As we do not yet know the minimal levels of either intensity or duration needed to achieve anxiolytic effects, or the optimal levels for maximizing such benefits, it seems prudent to begin a program with light, self-selected exercise lasting at least 10 to 30 minutes per bout. It is important that the activity be chosen by the individual rather than by the health care professional. This will help to instill a sense of control and will diminish the possibility of dislike for the activity. It may be necessary to provide the person with a menu of activity options, from which she or he can choose one or more activities. Based on what is currently known, rhythmic, cardiorespiratory/aerobic endurance activities should be suggested as the primary options. Sample activities would include walking, easy jogging, hiking, swimming, and cycling. Walking is perhaps one of the most underrated forms of beneficial physical activity. It is a low-impact, easy-to-do form of exercise that does not require special equipment or clothing and can be done nearly anywhere. In the early stages of exercise adoption, especially for individuals who have been sedentary for extended periods, such activity would (1) be a useful starting point, (2) provide adequate fitness benefits, (3) maintain compliance and/or minimize drop-outs, and (4) provide a basis for a graded program to be instituted as adaptation occurs.

Beginning an exercise program at an easy or light pace is important, especially for those suffering from an anxiety disorder. Physical inactivity is often associated with such disorders. Exercise for individuals who are suffering from such problems is likely to be beneficial, but nevertheless initial efforts may be difficult, due to prolonged inactivity. Such individuals should be closely supervised by qualified health care professionals who can provide encouragement, reassurance, and assistance as necessary. In the early stages of an exercise program, individuals need to learn, both from the health care professional and experientially, that the sensations of muscular exertion are normal with exercise. Starting with an easy pace will minimize such sensations and allow a gradual adaptation to them; increases in intensity and duration can be made more easily with time. Minimization of unpleasant feelings and perhaps even increasing positive feelings during the activity enhance enjoyment, and thus help to maintain patient compliance.

Until the person has developed sufficient confidence to exercise alone or unsupervised, the intensity of effort should be closely monitored. Although the pulse rate is often used as a measure of intensity, the individual *perception* of effort may be more important. Familiarization with an effort rating like the Borg Rating of Perceived Exertion scale is useful. Intensity can still be revised upward, as responses to exercise change over time. It is useful, in those instances where it does not create more anxiety, to have the patient record in an exercise log or diary the type, duration, and intensity of exercise each time it is performed. This allows regular evaluation by the health care professional and the individual can monitor his or her own progress, thereby enhancing feelings of well-being.

The available evidence points to the fact that maintenance of a physically active life-style can prevent the development, or lessen the impact, of clinical affective disorders. In those instances where treatment is necessary, a graded program of rhythmic, aerobic exercise can be useful adjuvant therapy. In addition to the physiologic benefits that can accrue, such treatment has been demonstrated to decrease chronic anxiety and general neurotic symptoms.

SUGGESTED READING

Johnsgard KW. The exercise prescription for depression and anxiety. New York: Plenum, 1989.

Landers DM, Petruzzello SJ. Physical activity, fitness, and anxiety. In: Bouchard C, Shephard RJ, Stephens T, eds. Physical activity, fitness and health. Champaign, IL: Human Kinetics, 1994, pp. 868–882.

Landers DM, Petruzzello SJ. The effectiveness of exercise and physical activity in reducing anxiety and reactivity to psychosocial stressors.

In: Quinney HA, Wall AE, Gauvin L, eds. Active living proceedings. Champaign, IL: Human Kinetics, 1994, pp. 77-82.

Martinsen EW, Hoffart A, Solberg OY. Aerobic and non-aerobic forms of exercise in the treatment of anxiety disorders. Stress Med 1989; 5:115–120.

Morgan WP, Goldston SE, eds. Exercise and mental health. Washington, DC: Hemisphere, 1987.

Orwin A. The running treatment: A preliminary communication on a new use for an old therapy (physical activity) in the agoraphobic syndrome. Br J Psychiatry 1973; 122:175–179.

Petruzzello SJ, Landers DM. A meta-analysis on the anxiety-reducing effects of acute and chronic exercise: Outcomes and mechanisms. Sports Med 1991; 11:143–182.

Sexton H, Maere A, Dahl NH. Exercise intensity and reduction in neurotic symptoms: A controlled follow-up study. Acta Psychiatr Scand 1989; 80:231–235.

EXERCISE AND A HEALTHY LIFESTYLE

RICHARD S. CROW, M.D.
DAVID R. JACOBS, Jr., Ph.D.

There is much evidence that regular physical activity is beneficial for physiologic function and has positive effects on other health behaviors. In addition, physical activity is believed to have a direct effect on health. Observational studies and clinical trials reveal that physical inactivity is significantly associated with major cardiovascular disease risk factors, hypertension, diabetes mellitus, coronary heart disease, and osteoporosis. However, the most compelling reason for recommending lifelong physical activity is its influence on the individual's quality of life. Maintenance of physical fitness for less than maximal effort enhances a person's ability to perform the activities of daily living (ADL) without restriction. Physical independence and the ability to participate in diverse activities of life—from active work/play, to child rearing and self-care—is the essence of a high quality of life. Therefore, physical activity is important to the quality of life, through its effects on physiologic function and disease prevention.

A primary concern of the practitioner is "to do no harm" when recommending any intervention. The fact that habitual activity may protect against coronary disease does not preclude some excess risk of sudden death during exercise, particularly in untrained individuals. Similarly, musculoskeletal and other injuries resulting from vigorous activity are a legitimate issue in assessing the risks versus the benefits of regular physical activity. Health professionals should therefore be knowledgeable about any special medical condition in the counseled individual when recommending the type, frequency, and intensity of physical activity.

REDUCED PHYSICAL ACTIVITY IN INDUSTRIAL CULTURES

Until recently, on an evolutionary time scale, all humans lived a hunter-gatherer existence. During human evolution, many of the survival adaptations of subsistence cultures were linked with the need for regular physical activity. Profound changes have occurred in the level and regularity of physical activity over the last 1 or 2 centuries, largely as a result of technologic advances. We postulate that these departures from our evolutionary legacy are likely related to the widespread expression of chronic disease risk factors (hypercholesterolemia, obesity, hyperinsulinemia, hypertension, hypercoagulability, hyperglycemia, and reduced bone mineral density) in the physically inactive. At the same time, better medical care and nutrition protect modern individuals from early death by starvation, trauma, and infection, allowing a longer lifetime and the exposure of most people to the risk of chronic diseases. Though it is likely that physical inactivity plays a role in the development of these chronic diseases, their prevention should not be the sole reason for people to increase their physical activity levels.

Research should be focused on preserving the quality of life as well as its prolongation. Although physical activity is recommended for its positive effects on risk factors and as a means of reducing morbidity and mortality, we maintain here that the quintessential benefit of regular physical activity is in the enhancement of physical fitness and the quality of life. In contrast with physical activity or skeletal and muscular movement, physical fitness relates to efficiency in performing work. Components of fitness include aerobic fitness, muscular strength and endurance, body composition, and flexibility. These attributes of fitness are important to efficient performance of a full range of ADL. We recommend, therefore, that practitioners shift toward physical activity advice for its advantageous effects on physiologic function and the quality of life of their patients.

PHYSICAL ACTIVITY AND OTHER HEALTH BEHAVIORS

Circumstantial evidence suggests that other health behaviors are positively influenced by regular physical activity. Unhealthy behavior, however (e.g., smoking, food and substance abuse), is influenced by many factors in life, of which physical activity is only one. Thus, correction of sedentary habits may not be sufficient to alter other adverse behaviors.

Physical activity is well documented to influence body weight and reduce obesity, to increase energy intake, and to improve exercise tolerance. Associations with other health behaviors (smoking, substance abuse, risk taking, stress management) are small, statistically insignificant, or have not been adequately studied. These comments thus represent our view of the current state of knowledge. Perhaps expectations about the positive influences of physical activity are too high in some health professions. Or perhaps physical activity assessment tools are too crude. It remains possible that a program of physical activity would be a useful alternative behavior when efforts are being made to stop smoking or to improve other health behaviors, but this has not been consistently demonstrated.

IMPROVING SUBMAXIMAL EXERCISE PERFORMANCE

In our view, habitual physical activity is to physiologic function what vitamins and minerals are to good nutrition. The lack is often not perceived until symptoms are manifest, or a "difference" is noticed after beginning supplementation or an exercise program. Adaptation to reduced muscle activity is rapid, with an accelerated rate of functional impairment and consequent lack of fitness the consequence. Typical effects of habitual exercise (the training response) include adaptive responses to the functional stresses imposed by the increased metabolic, physical, or mechanical demands of exercise. If the appropriate type of exercise is performed, at the proper intensity, duration, and frequency, sedentary persons of all ages can achieve significant improvement in physical fitness and health. For exercise to produce a training response, it must impose an added demand on function; and for improvement to continue, this demand must increase slowly but progressively over days, weeks, or months. For extremely inactive individuals, a small increase in leisure time physical activity can cause a dramatic increase in exercise tolerance, whether or not maximal exercise capacity is increased. If individuals are enabled to work harder and longer at a task before becoming fatigued, or if they perceive their appearance has improved, then their self-image or feelings of well-being may be enhanced. Gains in submaximal fitness are therefore a key element in understanding the potential influence of physical activity on the quality of life.

When recommending physical activity, the health professional needs to consider specific health goals for the individual, including exercise tolerance, recent exercise experience, age, clinical status, interests, skills, and opportunities. We make recommendations according to the person's stage of life.

Children and Young Adults (1 to 24 Years)

Physical activity and life-style behaviors begin in childhood, with introduction to structured sports, play, and fitness building. In this age group, the focus of physical activity should be on the development of exercise skills through individual and team sports as a foundation for an active life-style as an adult. Emphasis on large muscle groups, dynamic exercise, strengthening, and flexibility are the goals. Physical activity as "play" should be emphasized. The outcome sought is enhanced body awareness and enjoyment of movement, with the development of personal exercise skills, self-confidence, and a lifelong interest in regular and vigorous physical activity.

Adults (25 to 64)

The goal of physical activity in this age group is to maintain muscle mass, enhance cardiovascular fitness and psychological well-being, and maintain optimal body weight and composition. During these years individuals typically become less physically active (for instance, after marriage or on entering a profession). The reduction of habitual activity is paralleled by a progressive decline in physical work capacity and in resting metabolism. Appetite, however, fails to adjust in the same direction and weight gain is almost universal.

A physical activity strategy for the mid-years of adult life should consist predominantly (more than 75% of time) of endurance activities performed frequently (≥ 3 times per week) at a moderate intensity ($\geq 50\%$ of aerobic capacity). Activities should be selected that are convenient and enjoyable and cause up to 1,200 or more kilojoules (300 or more kcal) to be expended per session. Maintenance of work capacity, muscle mass, and flexibility is the most desired physiologic outcome. A regular program of more moderate intensity activities, such as gardening, house cleaning and repair, child care, and other tasks of daily living, is also an effective alternative. Although improvement in chronic disease risk factors will likely occur, this is not the primary focus. The potential benefits in quality of life include better weight management, a positive self image, self-sufficiency in tasks around the house and in the garden, and renewed pleasure at sport or in play with children and peers.

Older Adults (65 and Older)

Physical activity is particularly beneficial in older adults. Between 1985 and the end of this century we can expect a 50% increase in the proportion of the population aged 65 and older in the developed countries. There is an inevitable decline in function and structure with aging. A distinction can be made between "usual aging," in which extrinsic factors (gain of fat weight and poor exercise tolerance) accelerate the intrinsic effects of aging on function, and "successful aging," in which extrinsic factors can play a positive rather than a negative role.

The major goals of physical activity in older adults are retention of musculoskeletal function and lean body mass, muscle strength and mass, bone mineral content, connective tissue strength, range of motion, and the ability to maintain self care and enjoy leisure-time pursuits. These are also goals in middle age, but may be more easily attainable in younger people. In the elderly, however, the routine ADL eventually become impossible unless function has been maintained by ongoing regular physical activity. The obligatory effects of aging, including reduced maximal aerobic power and muscle strength, result in reduced physical fitness. A gradual reduction in the basal metabolic rate occurs with age, without a proportional reduction of the demand for essential nutrients. Happily, a person who is physically more active can have a higher food intake and a more adequate intake of essential nutrients without developing obesity. Excess body weight and a marginal intake of essential nutrients make walking, stair climbing, getting up from a bed or a chair, entering a bus or train, and self-care activities more difficult, fatiguing, and eventually impossible. As exercise tolerance diminishes, a large and increasing proportion of older citizens live below or near "thresholds" of physical capacity, a short step from dependence. Physical activity training can readily produce a profound improvement of functions in old age and can effectively postpone physical deterioration for many years.

By way of example, consider an 80-year-old sedentary male with a maximal exercise capacity of 4.5 mets. In such an individual activities such as slow walking (3.2 km/h; 2 mph), billiards, horseback riding (walking pace), and slow ball room dancing are performed at 50% of maximal exercise capacity. Calisthenics, gardening, walking (4.8 km/h; 3 mph), and slow swimming require over 75% of maximal capacity. Thus, minor intercurrent illness, weight gain, or extended periods of inactivity bring such an individual's exercise capacity below the minimum necessary for independent function. A regular physical activity program targeting cardiovascular fitness, psychological well-being, maintenance of optimal body weight and composition, muscular endurance, muscular strength, and flexibility for leg, thigh, back and shoulders, can result in major gains in submaximal

exercise tolerance. Simple activities that use familiar skills should be recommended. Walking, games, stretching, flexibility, and muscular toning activities should be encouraged. The use of short, intermittent, tonic skeletal muscle contractions rather than prolonged static exercise should be recommended for increasing muscle strength. Such activities should be easy to perform, with slow progression. Exercise that increases heart rate to 30% to 45% of maximal estimated heart rate reserve for age can be as effective, and safer, for increasing exercise tolerance in seniors than more intense exercise requiring 60% to 75% of heart rate reserve. Gains of 10% to 15% in submaximal exercise capacity can be anticipated, with resultant enormous improvements in daily function, self confidence, and quality of life. Positive changes in other health behaviors and in cardiovascular disease risk factor levels, if they occur, should be considered an added bonus.

Acknowledgment. The authors thank Henry Blackburn, M.D. for his helpful editorial comments.

SUGGESTED READING

Astrand PO, Rodahl K. Textbook of work physiology. New York: McGraw-Hill, 1986:574.

Badenhop DT, Cleary PA, Schaal SF, et al. Physiologic adjustments to higher- or lower-intensity exercise in elders. Med Sci Sports Exerc 1983; 15:496–502.

Blackburn H. Physical activity and coronary heart disease: A brief update and population view. J Cardiac Rehab 1983; 3:101–111.

Blair SN. Exercise and health. Sports Science Exchange 1990; 3(29):

Blair SN, Ellsworth NM, Haskell WL, et al. Comparison of nutrient intake in middle-aged men and women runners and control. Med Sci Sports Exerc 1981; 13:310–315.

Blair SN, Jacobs DR, Powell KE. Relationships between exercise or physical activity and other health behaviors. Public Health Rep 1985; 100:172–180.

Epstein LH, Wing RR. Aerobic exercise and weight. Addict Behav 1980; 5(4):371–388.

Powell KE, Thompson PD, Caspersen CJ, Kendrick JS. Physical activity and the incidence of coronary heart disease. Ann Rev Public Health 1987; 8:253–287.

Rowe JW, Kahn RL. Human aging: Usual and successful. Science 1987; 237:143–149.

Siscovick S, Laporte R, Newman JR. The disease specific benefits and risks of physical activity and exercise. Public Health Rep 1985; 100:180–188.

Siscovick DS, Weiss NS, Fletcher RH, Lasky T. The incidence of primary cardiac arrest during vigorous exercise. N Engl J Med 1984; 311:874–877.

MEDICAL ASPECTS OF SPORTS MEDICINE

EXERCISE AND PREVENTIVE MEDICINE

STEVEN N. BLAIR, P.E.D.
BEVERLY F. TREMAIN, M.Sc.

BACKGROUND

Numerous studies over the past 40 years clearly illustrate that regular participation in physical activity makes important contributions to the promotion and maintenance of health and function. Evidence supporting the healthful aspects of exercise comes from studies in epidemiology, pathology, clinical medicine, and laboratory experiments with humans and animal models. In addition to scientific evidence on the relation of physical activity to health, it is also logical that a physically active life-style is an inherent characteristic of our species. *Homo sapiens* have evolved from our early human ancestors over the past 4 million years, and for most of that time we have existed as scavengers or hunter/gatherers, ways of life that required relatively high energy expenditures. With the development of cities, industrialization, and use of fossil fuels for energy, the physical activity demanded of residents in highly industrialized societies has dropped to low levels. Indeed, in present day North America, many of us can get through the day without taking any strenuous activity and engaging in very little moderate intensity activity. Labor-saving devices are ubiquitous at home, at work, and during our leisure time, helping to maintain extremely sedentary life-styles.

Public health, scientific, and medical organizations are now recognizing the importance of adequate physical activity to health. In 1992, the American Heart Association recognized physical inactivity as a major risk factor for coronary artery disease, giving it the same status as smoking, high blood pressure, and high cholesterol. A joint statement by the American College of Sports Medicine (ACSM) and the U.S. Centers for Disease Control and Prevention (CDC) identified physical inactivity as a major public health problem, with approximately 24% of adult U.S. residents currently classed as sedentary.

Major objectives of the U.S. Public Health Service Healthy People 2000 project are to increase participation in moderate daily physical activity to "at least 30% of people" and to reduce the proportion of those with sedentary life-styles to "no more than 15% of people." Additional objectives target schools, worksites, and communities as appropriate settings to promote lifetime physical activity. The project also seeks "a stronger focus by primary care providers on the physical activity patterns of their patients."

PHYSICAL ACTIVITY, FITNESS, AND HEALTH

Sedentary and unfit individuals are at substantially increased risk for several chronic diseases. Several recent prospective studies have shown much higher death rates in men and women who were either inactive or physically unfit. Data from our studies of patients examined at the Cooper Clinic show a steep inverse gradient for all-cause, cardiovascular disease, and cancer mortality across physical fitness groups. The respective age-adjusted all-cause death rates per 10,000 person-years of follow-up across low, moderate, and high levels of physical fitness are 64, 26, and 20 in men and 40, 16, and 7 in women. The gradient for cardiovascular disease mortality across fitness groups is even steeper.

The Harvard Alumni Study conducted by Paffenbarger and colleagues has contributed greatly to our understanding of the relation between physical activity and health. Their recent report on the impact of changes in the habitual physical activity of alumni is one of the most important physical activity epidemiology studies of the past 25 years. The investigators followed 10,269 men for up to 19 years, having made an initial assessment of their physical activity habits in 1962 or 1966. The participants' activity patterns were re-evaluated in 1977, and deaths in the cohort were recorded from 1977 to 1985. Men who were sedentary at both assessments had significantly higher death rates than men who had been sedentary initially, but became active by the 1977 evaluation. Men who were active at both evaluations had the lowest death rates. Perhaps the most striking feature of this research was the comparable reduction of risk for several beneficial changes in risk factors. The respective reductions in risk of coronary heart disease mortality for stopping smoking, starting to exercise, and remaining free of hypertension and obesity are presented in Figure 1. This study supports the hypothesis that starting to exercise is as important a means of reducing coronary heart disease risk as is stopping smoking.

Our research group has also evaluated the impact of changing physical activity on the risk of all-cause mortality. We followed 10,288 men who had received two ex-

aminations at the Cooper Clinic. There were 275 deaths during the 52,069 man-years of follow-up after the second examination. Men who had converted from a sedentary to an active way of life from the first to the second examination had a reduction in risk of death of approximately 50% when compared with men who had remained inactive (Fig. 2). The reduction in risk in the men

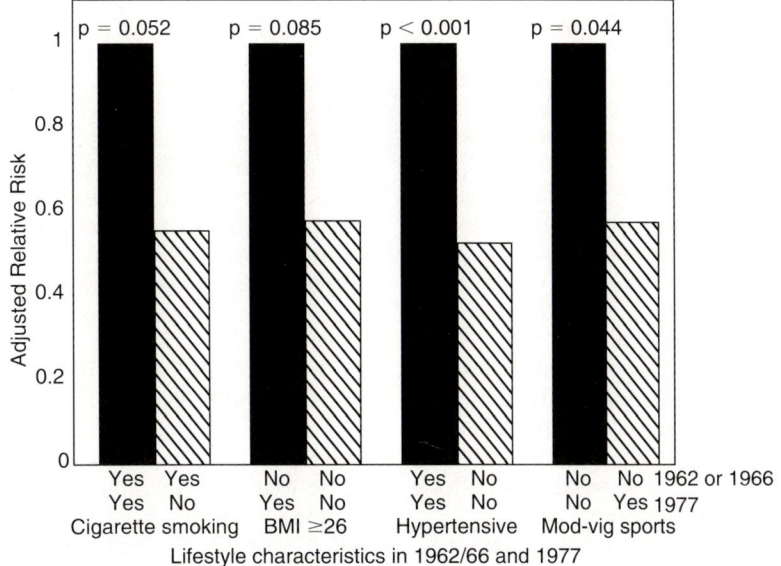

Figure 1 Adjusted relative risks (each relative risk is adjusted for age and all other variables in the figure) for coronary heart disease mortality by changes in life-style characteristics. The solid bars represent men who had unfavorable characteristics at baseline (in 1962 or 1966) and at follow-up (in 1977). The striped bars show the adjusted relative risks for men who made favorable changes on the variable of interest between baseline and follow-up. There were 10,269 men in the cohort, with 130 deaths from coronary heart disease. (Data from Paffenbarger et al, 1993. Figure from Blair SN. Research Quarterly for Exercise and Sport, 1993: 64:365-376; with permission.)

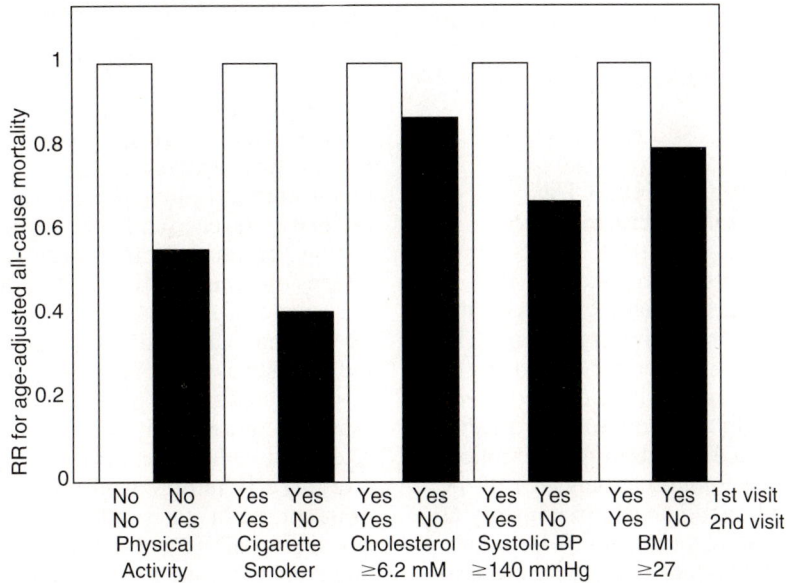

Figure 2 Relative risks (RR) for age-adjusted all-cause mortality are shown for changes in life-style characteristics in 10,288 men with two examinations at the Cooper Clinic during 1970 to 1989. There were 275 deaths during 52,069 man-years of follow-up. The white bars represent men who were at risk on the variable at both examinations and the black bars represent men who made favorable changes in risk factors from the first to the second examination. (From Blair SN. Research Quarterly for Exercise and Sport, 1993; 64:365-376; with permission.)

who became active was comparable to the benefit gained by stopping smoking, as in the Paffenbarger study. Furthermore, starting to exercise was associated with a greater reduction in risk than that realized by lowering blood pressure or cholesterol, or losing weight. The data from these two studies on change in activity and risk reduction provide important additional support for the causal hypothesis regarding physical activity and health.

The strongest evidence of health benefits from physical activity is for cardiovascular disease, but data are also accumulating that show an impact of habitual physical activity on other diseases. It is now reasonable to assume that sedentary habits increase the risk for colon cancer, and perhaps for prostate, breast, and lung cancer as well. Non-insulin-dependent diabetes mellitus appears to be delayed or prevented by regular physical activity, and a lifetime of active living may reduce loss of bone mineral density and subsequent osteoporosis.

We know for certain that physical activity improves physical fitness. The importance of physical fitness, both cardiorespiratory and musculoskeletal, to function is increasingly recognized. Higher levels of physical fitness are especially beneficial to older individuals. Elderly persons with adequate amounts of muscular strength are less likely to fall. Fit individuals also have a higher level of function in daily activities and are less likely to suffer from functional limitations or disabilities.

In summary, we can now be assured that physical activity is an important health habit, and increasing attention to this issue is needed by medical practitioners. Typically, exercise promotion in the medical setting occurs after the onset of disease rather than as a means of primary prevention. Exercise rehabilitation is valuable, but additional emphasis needs to be placed on the role of physical activity in primary prevention. Helping patients establish a regular pattern of physical activity will reduce their risks of cardiovascular disease, colon cancer, non-insulin-dependent diabetes mellitus, and obesity, and will improve their functional capability and overall sense of well being.

CURRENT STATUS OF PHYSICIAN COUNSELING ON EXERCISE

Although many physicians appreciate the role of exercise in health promotion, few make exercise counseling a priority in primary preventive treatment. The concept of exercise as preventive medicine needs to be incorporated into medical practice. Patients should be encouraged to take more responsibility for their health, and physical activity is a valuable step in that direction.

Williford and colleagues found that only 48% of the physicians they surveyed obtained an exercise history as part of a routine physical examination, and 70% did not develop exercise prescriptions. Only 23% of the physicians were familiar with the ACSM guidelines for exercise prescription. Similarly, Valente and colleagues researched physicians' beliefs on the importance of several risk factors in preventing disease, looking at their information gathering practices, and their abilities in the

practice of health promotion. The promotion of aerobic exercise was thought to be very important by 72% of practicing physicians, but paradoxically only 53% of physicians reported gathering any information about exercise history and only 30% reported that they were prepared to counsel patients on exercise. The physicians were also asked about their potential success at counseling patients if they were given proper educational resources. About 5% of the physicians revealed that they experienced success with exercise promotion.

One of the objectives in the Healthy People 2000 program is to "increase to at least 50% the proportion of primary care providers who routinely assess and counsel their patients regarding the frequency, duration, type, and intensity of each patient's physical activity practices." However, a baseline measurement in the Healthy People 2000 document indicates that currently only 30% of primary care physicians counsel sedentary patients on the benefits of regular activity.

STRATEGIES FOR INTEGRATING EXERCISE COUNSELING INTO MEDICAL PRACTICE

Barriers to the promotion of physical activity include getting individuals to start exercising and also in keeping them involved in a physical activity program. All too often, clinicians have assumed that their patients are ready for a strenuous exercise program and that they will follow a regimented exercise prescription. However, data show that a relatively small percentage of the population finds activity enjoyable and is ready to make major changes in their personal exercise habits. New approaches must be developed and implemented to help more patients become more active more of the time.

Life-style Exercise

We believe that the single most important component of the exercise program is the total energy expenditure demanded by the increased activity. Too much emphasis in the past has been placed on high intensity exercise and on continuous exercise sessions lasting 30 minutes or more. Life-style modifications, with a focus on accumulating additional physical activity over the course of the day, may be more acceptable to more people than the traditional exercise prescription. With the life-style approach, the individual incorporates several bouts of physical activity into a typical day. For example, rather than undertaking a specific 30 minute session of walking or running, a person could incorporate three 10 minute walks into their normal day. More frequent use of stairs rather than elevators or escalators, developing active hobbies such as gardening, and participating in active recreational pursuits are all ways to build increased energy expenditure into the normal daily routine. If the energy expenditure accumulated in several short bouts of activity equals that of a single session in the traditional exercise program, we postulate that comparable health benefits will be realized. These two methods of increasing overall energy expenditure are illustrated in Figure 3.

Readiness for a Change of Health Behavior

The traditional approach to exercise counseling is to assume that an individual is ready to begin exercising, so that all the physician has to do is to write an exercise prescription. In fact, many patients have an extreme dislike of exercise and are unlikely to make major changes in their exercise behavior without a careful consideration of several psychosocial characteristics and principles of behavioral change. Health professionals who adopt directive and regimented exercise intervention tactics may only encourage failure of the patient to make the desired changes. Prochaska and colleagues developed the Transtheoretical Model of Behavioral Change, which emphasizes the individual's stage of readiness for behavioral change. The six stages of this model are precontemplation, contemplation, preparation, action, maintenance, and termination.

The precontemplation stage includes individuals who have no serious intentions of changing their health behavior. These individuals have not yet evaluated the pros and cons of making a change, and are not ready to make an attempt to start exercising. Individuals who are at this stage should be informed about the health risks of sedentary living; they should also be helped to understand that they are currently quite inactive and should consider augmenting their habitual activity.

Contemplators are individuals who are seriously considering a change in life-style behavior, but they are not sure of how to proceed and have not yet initiated any changes. The physician should encourage such individuals to evaluate the benefits of becoming more physically active, and should provide appropriate support and advice to help them get ready to implement a more active life-style.

The preparation stage involves seeking advice, gaining knowledge, or taking other action in order to change personal behavior. The individual should begin to develop specific plans on how she or he can increase daily activity.

Individuals in the action stage begin to make changes. Techniques that offer appropriate help at this stage include contingency management and problem solving. Physicians should be prepared to help their patients evaluate progress, develop ways of overcoming barriers to activity, and use stimulus control techniques. One common problem at this stage is that people are unprepared for the sacrifices that will be needed and the negative consequences that may arise as behavioral change is initiated.

The maintenance stage involves keeping the behavior as consistent as possible. The individual needs to develop skills to facilitate a return to regular physical activity after unavoidable breaks in the routine. Identification of sources of social support from family, friends, and co-workers can be helpful in maintaining a more active way of life.

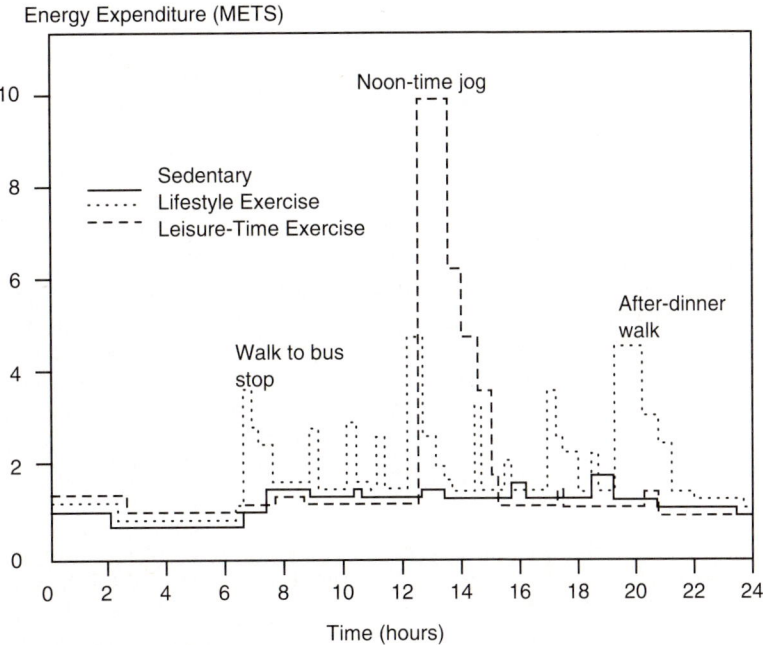

Figure 3 Theoretical patterns of physical activity over 24 hours. The solid line indicates the energy expenditure over the course of a day for a sedentary person. The dashed line represents the energy expenditure of an individual who engages in planned, vigorous exercise during leisure time, but is otherwise sedentary. The dotted line illustrates energy expenditure for an individual with a sedentary job who seeks opportunities to integrate short bouts of physical activity into the daily routine. Comparable health effects are expected for leisure-time exercise and life-style exercise if the total daily expenditure is the same. (From Blair SN, Kohl HW, Gordon NF. Physical activity and health: A lifestyle approach, Med Exerc Nutr Health 1992: 1(1), 54-57; reprinted by permission of Blackwell Scientific Publications, Inc.)

What is Your PACE Score?

This form will help your doctor understand your level of physical activity. Please read the entire form and then choose the number that best describes your *current* level of physical activity or your interest in physical activity. Do not include activities that you do as part of your job.

"**Vigorous**" exercise includes activities like jogging, running, fast cycling, aerobics classes, swimming laps, singles tennis, and racketball. Any activity that makes you work *as hard as jogging* and that lasts *20 minutes* at a time should be counted. These types of activities usually make you sweat, get out of breath, and your heart beats hard. (Do not count weight lifting.)

"**Moderate**" exercise includes activities like brisk walking, gardening, slow cycling, dancing, doubles tennis, or hard work around the house. Any activity that makes you work *as hard as brisk walking* and that lasts at least *30 minutes* at a time should be counted.

| Circle One Number Only | Current Physical Activity Status |

1. I do not exercise or walk regularly now, and I do not intend to start in the near future.
2. I do not exercise or walk regularly, but I have been thinking of starting.
3. I am trying to start to exercise or walk. (or) During the last month I have started to exercise or walk on occasion (or on weekends only).
4. I have exercised or walked infrequently (or on weekends only) for over 1 month.
5. I am doing vigorous or moderate exercise less than 3 times per week (or moderate exercise less than 2 hours per week).
6. I have been doing moderate exercise 3 or more times per week (or more than 2 hours per week) for the last 1-6 months.
7. I have been doing moderate exercise 3 or more times per week (or more than 2 hours per week) for 7 months or more.
8. I have been doing vigorous exercise 3-5 times per week for 1-6 months.
9. I have been doing vigorous exercise 3-5 times per week for 7-12 months.
10. I have been doing vigorous exercise 3-5 times per week for over 12 months.
11. I do vigorous exercise 6 or more times per week.

Figure 4 Method for self-assessment of physical activity leading to assignment of a PACE score.

The final stage of the model is termination. When applied to physical activity, it does not mean that the activity has been terminated, but rather that the sedentary life-style has been terminated. Those at the termination stage have clearly adopted the behavior and have incorporated it into their life-style to the point that there is no danger they will slip back into their old habits. One characteristic of this stage is an increased sense of self-efficacy.

Physician-Based Assessment and Counseling for Exercise (PACE)

PACE is a resource for physicians that use the stages of change model. It was developed by clinicians and scientists at San Diego State University in a project supported by the CDC. The PACE program is designed to make the physicians' role in exercise promotion effective. The program offers tactics that can be incorporated into a normal office routine. Recognizing that time is limited, PACE seeks the most efficient use of brief doctor-patient encounters. It provides an effective method of modifying exercise habits, with attention given to understanding the sociological, psychological, and emotional factors that may hinder an appropriate change of behavior.

The PACE program is divided into several sections, which include the physician's role in health promotion, reasons for exercise promotion, and the risks of promoting exercise. The program outlines specific tactics for the physician and provides specific guidance for effective health counseling methods. The counseling program begins by determining each patient's PACE score (Fig. 4), which is used to identify the patient's stage of readiness for an increase of physical activity. This part of the PACE program can be administered by the office receptionist or other designated staff members. Interpretation of the PACE score is simple and straightforward. Individuals with a score of 1 (about 10% of the North American population) are precontemplators. Contemplators are those with a score of 2 to 5; this group comprises about 50% of the population. A score of 6 to 10 places an individual in the active stage, and almost 40% fall into this group.

Different intervention and counseling tactics are proposed for patients in the various stages. For the

Table 1 Guidelines for Exercise Testing and Participation

	Apparently Healthy		Higher Risk*		
	Younger ≤40 Years (Men) ≤50 Years (Women)	Older	No Symptoms	Symptoms	With Disease†
Medical exam and diagnostic exercise recommended prior to:					
Moderate exercise‡	No‖	No	No	Yes	Yes
Vigorous exercise§	No	Yes¶	Yes	Yes	Yes
Physician supervision recommended during exercise test:					
Sub-maximal testing	No	No	No	Yes	Yes
Maximal testing	No	Yes	Yes	Yes	Yes

*Persons with two or more risk factors or symptoms.

†Persons with known cardiac, pulmonary, or metabolic disease.

‡Moderate exercise (exercise intensity 40% to 60% Vo_2max) — Exercise intensity well within the individual's current capacity and can be comfortably sustained for a prolonged period of time (i.e., 60 minutes, slow progression, and generally noncompetitive).

§Vigorous exercise (exercise intensity >60% Vo_2max) — Exercise intense enough to represent a substantial challenge and which would ordinarily result in fatigue within 20 minutes.

‖The "no" responses in this table mean that an item is "not necessary." The "no" response does **not** mean that an item should not be done.

¶A "yes" response means that an item is recommended.

From ACSM Guidelines for Exercise Testing and Prescription (4th ed). Lea & Febiger, 1991; with permission.

precontemplators, the benefits of physical activity, the hazards of inactivity, and road blocks to physical activity are discussed. The contemplators are given information on beginning a program, including a discussion of their preferred activity, means of identifying social support, and of recognizing barriers to physical activity. The physician also investigates the patient's self-efficacy for beginning an exercise program and discusses rewards and incentives. For those patients who are already active, the physician's primary concern is to provide the support that will help them to continue their active life-style. An elaboration of these tactics is beyond the scope of this chapter, but interested physicians are encouraged to obtain the PACE materials for review (see Suggested Reading). Simplicity, low cost, professional guidelines, and theoretically-based methods are advantages to using the PACE program.

EVALUATION PRIOR TO EXERCISE

The familiar adage of "see your doctor before beginning an exercise program" is often voiced more for liability avoidance than for protection of the patient. A substantial majority of the population can begin a moderate exercise program without seeing a doctor and without having extensive tests. The expense and time involved in completing elaborate testing protocols to clear patients for exercise participation can create a barrier to increased physical activity. One must consider the substantial risk associated with sedentary habits when evaluating the cost-benefit ratio of extensive pre-exercise medical evaluations. Much of the information needed to identify patients who might need a more

extensive pre-exercise evaluation is already available to the physician, such as a medical history, exercise history, family history, blood pressure, weight, and other clinical data. The ACSM guidelines for risk stratification, based on age, major cardiac risk factors, medical conditions, and sex, are given in Table 1.

Acknowledgment. We thank Melba Morrow for preparing the figures and tables, proofreading, and production of the final draft of the manuscript, and Dr. James Sallis for comments on the section about the PACE materials.

SUGGESTED READING

American College of Sports Medicine. Guidelines for exercise testing and prescription. 4th Ed. Philadelphia: Lea & Febiger, 1991.

American College of Sports Medicine. Exercise lite kit. Available from the College, P.O. Box 1440, Indianapolis, IN 46206-1440. Telephone (317) 637-9200.

American Heart Association Statement on Exercise. Benefits and recommendations for physical activity programs for all Americans. Circulation 1992; 86:340–344.

Blair SN. Living with exercise. Dallas: American Health Publishing Company, 1991.

Blair SN. 1993 C. H. McCloy research lecture: Physical activity, physical fitness, and health. Res Q Exerc Sports 1993; 64:365–376.

Blair SN, Kohl HW, Gordon NF, Paffenbarger RS Jr. How much physical activity is good for health? Ann Rev Publ Health 1992; 13:99–126.

Centers for Disease Control. Physician-based assessment and counseling for exercise manual. Atlanta: CDC, 1991.

Paffenbarger RS, Hyde RT, Wing AL, et al. The association of changes in physical-activity level and other lifestyle characteristics with mortality among men. N Engl J Med 1993; 328:538–545.

Patrick K, Sallis JF, Long B, et al. Physician-based assessment and counseling for exercise: Background and development. The Physician and Sportsmedicine, in press.

Pender NJ, Sallis JF, Long BJ, Calfas KJ. Health care provider counseling to promote physical activity. In: Dishman RK, ed. Advances in exercise adherence. Champaign, Il: Human Kinetics, in press.

Prochaska JO, DiClemente CC, Norcross JC. In search of how people change: Applications to addictive behaviors. Am Psychol 1992; 47:1102–1114.

U.S. Department of Health and Human Services. Promoting health/ preventing disease. Year 2000 health objectives for the nation. Washington, DC, Winter 1990.

Valente CM, Sobal J, Muncie HL, et al. Health promotion: physicians' beliefs, attitudes, and practices. Am J Prev Med 1986; 2:82–88.

Williford HN, Barfield BR, Lazenby RB, Olson MS. A survey of physicians' attitudes and practices related to exercise promotion. Prev Med 1992; 21:630–636.

MEDICAL MANAGEMENT OF MASS PARTICIPATION EVENTS

DAN TUNSTALL PEDOE, D.Phil., F.R.C.P.

Mass participation events attract thousands of variably trained and acclimatized participants to events that may be physically very demanding, cover difficult or even dangerous terrain, and may be held under stressful climatic conditions.

Participants may be young, middle-aged, or even elderly. Novices may have entered from "bravado" or for "fun," having seen some media coverage of the event and may be unaware of the best method to prepare for the event or safe strategies for completing it. Some participants may have entered as a form of "illness denial" after recovery from major medical or surgical events, and many enter having been sponsored to raise money for a particular charity. Their enthusiasm for the event may therefore be "indirect" and they may well persist in taking part against sensible medical advice. Particularly if the event has attracted media attention and has been expensive to enter they will expect a high level of medical support, before, during, and after the event.

Local hospitals and medical facilities will not take kindly to a mass influx of participants with "self-induced injuries" if things go badly on the day of the event. Sponsors have often made a major financial investment in the event; this has made it possible, and they will expect only favorable media coverage. Certainly, they will be unhappy if deficiencies in the medical coverage or organization are revealed by any dramatic adverse events.

Medical support for mass participation events is directed at minimizing the potential risks and avoiding the worst scenario where local medical emergency services and hospitals are flooded with casualties. Medical support for such events therefore requires considerable planning and cannot be recruited at the last moment. It should aim to deal with all but the most serious medical problems.

Medical support includes (1) medical input in pre-event planning; (2) education of the participants, organizers and medical support staff in possible hazards, their avoidance and treatment; (3) organization of medical and related support services for the event; (4) liaison with local medical services and hospitals; (5) liaison with the media to make sure they give accurate and helpful information; and (6) collecting and reporting the numbers and types of medical and first aid contacts and relating these to the specific conditions of the event so that arrangements can be constantly improved.

As medical director of the London Marathon, which now has >25,000 participants each year, I will be drawing examples from that event, and from other mass events in which I have participated. Nevertheless, the general principles apply to any major endurance event, which may include road races, triathlons, popular cycling events, and ultra-long distance cross-country ski and ice skating events. For simplicity's sake, I refer to runners, but the term can usually be used to cover other types of endurance event participants.

THE MEDICAL DIRECTOR

Mass participation events must have an identifiable medical advisor or director, who acts as the ultimate arbiter on questions of safety and medical organization and is the media contact for such questions. Ideally, this advisor is medically qualified and must be able to devote the necessary time to the task. If such a medical doctor is not available, a medical committee chaired by a health professional who has an appropriate background in the sport can bring together the necessary expertise. Most events will have a de facto subcommittee of health professionals who help with the recruitment and involvement of their own colleagues and interrelate with the event organizers through the medical director.

EVENT PLANNING

Most major events require several months of planning. The medical director should be involved in that process, to minimize risks to the participants.

The Course

In mass participation events, participants must be under observation at all times and be readily accessible for evacuation, as it is possible for someone to collapse at any point on the course, or wander off it in a confused state if they become hypothermic or hyperthermic. Evacuation by ambulance must be possible without disrupting the whole event.

The course must be safe for the numbers planned, with no sudden early pinch points. Multiple start points may be needed. Some road hazards are not obvious when running in a large pack of runners and a runner who trips and falls may be a major hazard.

Some degree of hazard may unwittingly be introduced by the organizers' wish to accommodate demands of the media or of the sponsors, without whom the event might not be possible. Where this occurs, compromise may be needed.

The Finish

The finish line must be protected from spectators and allow steady egress of the competitors, giving them ready access to their clothes, medical facilities, food and drink, their relatives and friends, and transport home.

Food and Drink

Food and drink must be appropriate for the requirements of participants in a given event and appropriately spaced around the course, in adequate amounts. Nutrients must also be readily available at the finish, when the participants will be fluid and carbohydrate depleted. Water should always be available but it must be potable and not carbonated. Sports drinks containing carbohydrate and weak salt solution ("glucose electrolyte drinks") become more necessary as the duration of the event increases (> 4 hours), and in ultra-endurance events food becomes necessary during the event as well as at the finish.

Local businesses may supply drinks such as champagne, orange juice, and beer. If these are available only at an occasional feeding station or at the finish, they will be much enjoyed by the "fun runners" and can be ignored by the serious participants. They pose no real hazard, but alcohol in significant amounts during or before an event could be hazardous in a cycle, skating, or ski race where levels of incoordination from fatigue might be increased, posing a threat to the safety of participants.

Free Drugs

Sponsor involvement in food and drinks has extended to "free drugs" in the pre-race goody bag given to all competitors, for at least one U.S. Marathon. Aspirin and a non-steroidal anti-inflammatory drug were distributed to all competitors. Both of these drugs may cause gastrointestinal hemorrhage, which is already more frequent in endurance running. They also may have other dramatic effects. Inclusion of even a widely used product in such a way implies the approval of the event organizers. I think such promotion is ill-advised and could lead to litigation.

General Care of Participants

Logistics for the care of participants, including access to toilets, the provision of prerace drinks and feeding stations, the refreshment available during and after the event, the mechanism and timing of when they have to get stripped off, and methods for reuniting them with their clothes and personal effects at the finish without undue delay, should all be planned well in advance. For events such as major road races, guidelines have been produced by various international and national running organizations. The medical director may not need to take a major role if the organizers are experienced, but she or he should know what is planned. Problems are more likely to arise with new events not conforming to previous well-established protocols (e.g., marathon aerobic sessions), or if the number of participants is dramatically increased.

Selection of Participants

Medical Certificates

Entry to mass participation events is usually *not* dependent on medical criteria, because of the onus this would place on the event organizers to screen aspiring participants. Medical certification of "fitness to compete" may be practicable for small events attracting local nationals only, where the credentials and signatures of the doctors signing the certificates could be checked, but it becomes quite impracticable for major events attracting large numbers, and for international entries (where the validity of documents would be almost impossible to check).

The value of certificates of fitness to compete is in any case debatable. Doctors "playing safe" may use any medical condition to prevent legitimate participation. Conversely, medical problems may be occult and can arise after the medical certificate has been issued.

Responsibility has to be shifted from the organizers to the participants, by a process of **early selection,** preferably several months before a major event such as a marathon, giving novices time to train properly, **education of the entrants,** and **incentives** for sick or injured participants to withdraw before the event. The best incentive for such withdrawal is a guaranteed entry for the following year. This idea has been copied by the London Marathon from New York, with the difference that New York does allow late entries to be replaced from a waiting list, whereas the London Marathon does not replace the "sick, lame and injured," but allows for the 25% who are expected to withdraw by overbooking (like an airline), accepting more entries than they really want in the race on the day.

In practice, although oversubscribed major events may reduce the numbers of entrants by means of a lottery system, they also optimize the flow along the course and through the finish by cutting the top off the normal distribution curve of finishing times. An entrant submitting a projected finish time of 4 hours for the London marathon, the modal time, is less likely to be accepted than one suggesting 3 hours or 5 hours.

Age Limitations

Depending on the event, the medical director may advise on age categories. These are fixed by some sports organizations. The International Marathon Medical Directors Association (IMMDA) has advised that it is potentially hazardous to allow runners of under 18 to participate in a full marathon run.

Whilst evidence for lasting musculoskeletal damage in children training or competing in long distance events is controversial, children are not "free agents"; they also have inferior thermoregulatory control, are relatively inefficient runners, are more prone to intercurrent infection, and would do better eventually as runners by training for shorter distances.

The London Marathon has a childrens' race associated with it—the Mini Marathon—which has stopped rather intemperate press attacks on the organizers for not allowing children to take part in the marathon itself. The pressure is usually from ambitious parents who hope to bask in the reflected glory of their childrens' success. The sight of ambitious parents screaming at exhausted children to egg them on should not be part of a "fun event." Other mass participation events, such as shorter runs or swimming events, may well be family affairs, where younger athletes can happily take part if not compete with adults.

Some prestige events, such as the Boston Marathon, have nonmedical entry qualifications; they require a certain time standard in a marathon within the year previous to entry, thus excluding novices. Some triathlons have similar entry criteria.

Prerace Education

Many events send participants prerace training advice. The London marathon, since its inception, has sent simple medical and training advice with the acceptance letter. The medical advice has been widely copied (Fig. 1). The advice sheet or mailing cautions runners with medical problems to consult their own doctor, and warns them of symptoms and medical conditions that should restrain them from running or competing. It also suggests that if they cannot run 24 km (15 miles) reasonably comfortably 1 month before the marathon (42 km) they should not be taking part!

Seminars for participants can be held at intervals before an event. Material can be produced for newspapers and magazines that participants are likely to read.

Education of first-aiders and medical staff involved with the event, including local accident and emergency staff may also be necessary. This must begin some time before the event. A meeting of medical and first aid staff or at least the senior members for a full briefing before the event is also desirable.

MEDICAL AID STATIONS AND STAFFING

Aid Stations

Medical support for an event covering a long course, or as in a triathlon a series of courses, requires a certain number of fixed stations, supplemented by mobile medical vehicles. The latter may just evacuate casualties, or may act as mobile medical aid posts, tracking the event. The precise requirements vary with the event. Mobile medical stations can cut across and serve as fixed stations early and late in the event. Some or all of the course may not be suitable for a mobile vehicle to follow the participants. Where there are no aid stations or patrol vehicles, a certain number of spotters or marshals with mobile phones or two-way radios are needed, so that participants in distress can be reported promptly to the event organizers, and rescued if necessary. Most aid stations are used as "pit stops" by runners requiring massage, a blister dressed, or some other minor treatment before they continue the event, but a few serious problems may present.

Medical Disqualification

Medical personnel may wish to restrain a participant from continuing, particularly if the individual is confused, aggressive, and poorly coordinated, showing signs of hypoglycemia or hyperthermia. Whether they have the authority to do so depends on the event. If runners are significantly confused and disoriented when questioned on personal details, every attempt should be made both to assess them fully (including the measurement of rectal temperature) and to treat them appropriately. Uncoordinated runners who are mentally clear may continue to run if periodic assessment can be organized.

Location and Visibility of Aid Stations

There are advantages in medical and feeding stations being adjacent to each other, for mutual support and better communications, as well as easier identification of medical aid posts for the participants. In events with many spectators, the runners may not see the first aiders hidden in the crowd, but will find them if they are always downstream of a water station. The London marathon has had over 1,000 runners seek aid at one post that followed a series of inconspicuous aid posts. The medical center at the finish also needs to be well signposted and obvious. Participants should be given a map of the finish facilities on which the medical center is conspicuously marked, as should the information tent or caravan.

Staffing

The vast majority of staff can be first-aiders. In Britain, we have St John (St Andrew in Scotland) and the Red Cross, who are highly organized and have their own doctors and nurses but are principally first-aiders. They can supply ambulances, first-aid buses, and even cardiac vehicles and they have their own communications systems that can link in with police and civic ambulance control. In the United States, medical support is often recruited from local hospitals, with nurses, doctors and medical students, supplemented by Radio Hams (for

should be cancelled. A red flag (WBGT 73 to 82 or 23 to 28) advises caution. Facilities for runners to weigh themselves at the start and put their weight on their running number so that they can be checked along the course for excessive fluid loss would seem a sensible precaution, but such a tactic depends on runner cooperation and the availability of accurate scales.

Unfortunately, if an event starts early and lasts for several hours, the conditions are not predictable; slower, fatter runners may remain on the course long after the leaner fitter runners have finished.

My only personal experience of hazard warnings was in New York in 1984. The race organizers had warned the assembled runners at the start of a heat hazard, with an expected hot day (in November) after a cool period. The temperature rose above 80° F, with near 100% humidity. I did not see a single runner drop out at the start, and they all seemed to start at their usual pace. I added 20 minutes to my previous worst time, ran that schedule, and drank copiously whenever I could, passing thousands of "runners" who were already walking at 14 km (one third of the distance). Hundreds had to be evacuated to hospital, despite the warnings by the organizers.

A really serious electrical storm, hurricane, tornado warning, black ice, or blizzard could make an event so hazardous that it would have to be cancelled. Practically, major events should be scheduled for a time of year and location where extreme climatic conditions are most unlikely.

Timing the Start of the Event

Where heat is a potential hazard, races may have to be started before dawn and frequent sponging and water spray stations as well as drink stations will be needed. Runners should be advised to run in the shade where they can.

Other factors such as oxidant air pollution (which often peaks in the afternoon) may also have to be taken into account. Too often where television coverage is involved, the media dictate the timing of the start, but should there be a sudden heat wave, moving an event forward in time (on the same day) is usually more practicable than postponing it, provided that the media are willing to broadcast the changes.

Entrant Identification

Runners are usually identified by a race number with a Bar code that can be read by a computer input device. Runners are listed in the program on that basis, and are logged on to the computer database by their running number. Unfortunately this is not an infallible form of identification, as runners may not be competing under their own number. An unconcious or dead runner is probably who he or she appears to be, but the individual has to be formally identified before any news of the identity can be released. The London marathon has the facility to block access to a runner's details on the computer database. This is necessary to stop press

diligence in releasing stories prematurely, before the facts have been verified and relatives have been located and acquainted with the facts.

Deaths or Major Casualties

The medical director of a major event needs to have delegated direct patient management, so that he or she can deal with the media should a tragedy occur. We have had three deaths from 275,000 marathons completed in London, and despite warning the press of the risks, the reaction of the some of the popular press to the first death was quite intemperate. As medical director, one should be prepared to counsel the relatives, attend the necropsy and the inquest, and help protect the relatives from excessive media attention. The press react better to being kept fully informed by the most senior person available, who should be honest with them as to what is known and what is conjecture.

Liaison with Local Hospitals

The medical director should inform local hospital emergency departments in advance of the details of the event and its possible impact on them and the type of casualty that they might receive (and even on how to manage them, if the problems are likely to be unusual for a duty casualty officer). The letter should contain information on how the medical director can be contacted on the day, and how hospital casualties can be transported to the finish, to their clothes and relatives, once they have been "patched up." Arrangements should also be made to collect details of hospital casualties, subsequent to the event. Press interference, chasing details of major casualties, can make hospitals uncooperative and this aspect of the medical director's work difficult.

TYPES OF CASUALTY

The London marathon classifies casualty contacts into:

(a) Social (ask for a drink or bandage and treat themselves).

(b) Musculoskeletal—mainly cramp, but some more serious injuries such as fatigue fractures, falls, etc. Diagnosis, often by first-aiders, can mean that runners who stagger on are misdiagnosed;

(c) Skin and topical—chafing of the groin and nipples, blisters, subungual hematomas, etc.

(d) Constitutional—collapse, hypo- and hyperthermia, fits, vomiting, cardiac problems, headaches, etc.

The first-aiders and medical staff must all be fully briefed on the symptoms and signs of more serious exercise-related problems, such as those resulting from thermal stress and hypothermia. Collapsed and disoriented runners *must* have a rectal temperature taken. Although aural temperatures are becoming more widely used, the rectal temperature is the basis for most systems of casualty classification; if readings stay high at the end of a race, this is an urgent indication for action.

Because of difficulties with the definition of thermal injury, which is based on nonexercising populations (e.g., When does "Heat Exhaustion" become "Heat Stroke"?), Roberts has produced a classification of exercise-related collapse, based on rectal temperatures, mental state, and ability to drink and walk. This gives useful guidelines for such cases.

The main priority is to give intravenous (IV) fluids to runners who cannot drink, particularly if they continue to lose fluid from vomiting or diarrhea, and to cool runners whose temperature remains high. In the London Marathon, for simplicity we define hypothermia as a rectal temperature lower than 35° C and hyperthermia as a persistent rectal temperature higher than 40° C 10 minutes after ceasing to run. Rectal temperatures of >42° C may be found; these patients must be treated enthusiastically, to prevent rhabdomyolysis and subsequent renal failure. Mental confusion, persistent cramps, vomiting, and diarrhea are all markers of a serious case, but usually these respond rapidly to IV fluids, fanning, sponging, and administration of 50% glucose.

A full description of the medical problems encountered in road races is beyond the scope of this chapter. It should be appreciated that even short runs can produce dramatic collapses and there may be more sick runners after a 10 km or half marathon, because these events attract more untrained individuals.

Triathlons have the potential for trauma from cycling accidents. One English triathlon championship, before the introduction of wet suits for these events, resulted in a serious incidence of hypothermia; even swimmers who did not have to be rescued became amnesic for the last part of the swim and several minutes afterwards, symptoms implying a serious drop in core temperature.

Hospital casualties from these events tend to be the more serious musculoskeletal problems, runners who collapse between aid stations and are evacuated by the routine ambulance service, and the more serious collapses and the cardiac events, passed on from the medical stations. Experience of the London Marathon is that very few casualties require admission, perhaps 1 in 10,000 runners.

SUGGESTED READING

American College of Sports Medicine. The prevention of thermal injuries during distance running. Med Sci Sports Exerc 1987; 19:529–533.

Roberts WO. Exercise related collapse. Phys Sports Med 1989; 17(5):49–59.

Tunstall Pedoe DS. Popular marathons, half marathons and other long distance runs: recommendations for medical support, Recommendations of a consensus conference. Br Med J 1984; 288:1355–1359.

CARDIOVASCULAR SYMPTOMS IN SPORTS MEDICINE

ROY J. SHEPHARD, M.D., Ph.D., D.P.E., F.A.C.S.M.

This chapter discusses common cardiovascular symptoms seen in sports medical practice, looking at etiology, differential diagnosis, and evaluation regarding the young, well-conditioned athlete and the middle-aged exerciser.

CHEST PAIN

Young Athlete

Differential Diagnosis

Angina is uncommon in the young athlete (Table 1). In the adolescent, potential causes of angina include a gross increase of myocardial oxygen demand associated with a congenital lesion (aortic or pulmonary valvular stenosis, aortic stenosis, bicuspid aortic valve with stenosis or regurgitation, Marfan's syndrome with aortic regurgitation), mitral regurgitation associated with mitral valve prolapse, a gross deficiency of coronary perfusion (particularly an anomalous coronary artery), a relative increase of cardiac work-rate due to idiopathic hypertension or rarely a pheochromocytoma, hypertrophic cardiomyopathy, or a low arterial oxygen content (nutritional anemia, sickling disease, or extreme altitudes). In the third decade of life, some patients may also develop sufficient coronary atheroma to cause angina and even myocardial infarction.

Chest pain during exercise sometimes accompanies ventricular premature beats, but often reflects noncardiac causes such as an anxiety state, a "stitch," tenderness of the chest muscles after very prolonged exercise, osteoarthritis of the upper spine or shoulder, pleurisy, or a persistent effect of thoracic surgery or trauma.

Evaluation

A simple history often serves to distinguish relatively benign causes of chest pain from true angina. An anxiety state usually has other prominent symptoms such as weakness, giddiness, breathlessness, and a choking sensation; often, there is also vaso-regulatory asthenia, with a poor blood pressure (BP) response to a change of posture. A "stitch" is an unpleasant, sharp, and rather severe pain associated with prolonged and vigorous effort. It appears to be related to spasm or ischemia of

Table 1 Differential Diagnosis of Angina
in Young Athlete

Increased myocardial oxygen demand
   Congenital lesions—Pulmonary stenosis
     Aortic stenosis
     Aortic regurgitation
     Marfan's syndrome
   Mitral prolapse/regurgitation
   Idiopathic hypertension
   Pheochromocytoma
   Hypertrophic cardiomyopathy

Impaired coronary flow
   Anomalous coronary artery
   Coronary atheroma

Reduced arterial oxygen content
   Nutritional anemia
   Sickle cell disease
   Extreme high altitudes

Nonanginal pains
   Ventricular premature beats
   Anxiety state
   "Stitch"
   Tenderness of chest muscles
   Osteoarthritis
   Pleurisy
   Thoracic surgery or trauma

the diaphragm and is diagnosed from its late onset and characteristic location (laterally, over the lower part of the chest wall).

Osteoarthritis of the shoulder joint or spine can occasionally be confused with angina, particularly if the pain radiates into the left arm. There may be a history of injury. Moreover, if there is such a lesion, the same sensation can usually be elicited by passive manipulation of the shoulder or spine. Crepitations may be felt over the joint and radiographs may reveal typical osteophytes, although the severity of pain is not always well matched to the extent of radiographic abnormalities.

Both pleurisy and the after-effects of thoracic surgery or trauma give rise to sharp pains distinguished by their relation to the breathing cycle. Comparable sensations can be elicited by deep breathing at rest.

A classic case of angina is fairly readily recognized. The pain is brought on by an increase of cardiac work-rate (vigorous exercise, such as hurrying up a hill, exposure to cold air, or anxiety) and it is quickly relieved by a reduction of cardiac work-rate (rest, warmth, lessening of emotional stress, or reduction of BP by administration of nitrites). The pain begins in the mid-line of the chest, but typically radiates along the inner aspect of the left arm, up into the root of the neck or behind the ear; when first diagnosed, the pain is only moderate in intensity and a given attack lasts for less than 2 minutes. If the origin is atheromatous, there is usually a history of cardiac risk factors, and an anginal attack can often be linked to the appearance of a typical horizontal or downsloping ST segmental depression on a stress electrocardiogram (ECG) (note that an anxiety state with hyperventilation can lead to junctional ST depression, while if the cause of myocardial ischemia is

pulmonary stenosis, the ST displacement will be most obvious in Leads V1-V2). A stenotic cause (often including a bicuspid aortic valve) can be diagnosed from the associated murmurs; with aortic stenosis, BP also tends to fall during exercise. A prolapse of the mitral valve can often be visualized on echocardiography; typically, it has little impact on ventricular function, but any regurgitant flow can be estimated by Doppler flow measurements. Idiopathic hypertension and a pheochromocytoma are signaled by a high and labile resting BP, with an unexpectedly large rise of BP during exercise. Hypertrophic cardiomyopathy is a somewhat controversial diagnosis, and it must be distinguished clearly from a normal, physiologic response to vigorous training by echocardiography and scintigraphy. Many athletes show a large ventricular cavity and a thick ventricular wall. However, a healthy hypertrophy is associated with a normal rate of diastolic filling and an absence of perfusion defects. A hemoglobin reading, determination of iron saturation, and if necessary a plasma volume determination should identify the various types of anemia. If all of these leads prove negative, coronary angiography should be considered to seek an anomalous cardiac vascular supply.

Myocardial infarction is differentiated from angina mainly in terms of the severity of the incident. The pain of an infarction is again felt in the mid-line, but it has a much more severe, vise-like quality. The patient is often pallid and shows signs of collapse. The symptoms usually persist for 20 minutes or longer, despite rest and sedative medications. A major infarction is fairly readily diagnosed, but smaller infarcts can be confused with acute gastritis, a grumbling appendicitis, or exacerbation of an ulcer. The diagnosis of infarction is confirmed by a characteristic evolution of the resting ECG and an increase of serum enzyme levels (CK, LDH, SGOT), although it should be noted that a prolonged bout of exercise such as a marathon run can in itself lead to a substantial increase of serum enzymes, including some increment of the supposedly cardiac specific isozymes of LDH.

Older Fitness Exerciser

Differential Diagnosis

In those over the age of 30 years, the most probable cause of an exercise-related chest pain is angina secondary to coronary atherosclerosis (Table 2). Cardiomyopathy is also possible. At this age, a congenital lesion is unlikely to have remained undiagnosed. Anemia and exposure to low oxygen pressures remain potential causes, as do various forms of hypertension and an acquired aortic valvular stenosis or a regurgitant lesion. If exercise is pursued to the point of congestive failure, hepatic congestion can also give rise to pain in the upper right quadrant of the abdomen.

Of noncardiac causes, there is an increased likelihood of anxiety about the heart in older subjects. A "stitch" remains a possibility if the person has exercised long and hard. Osteoarthritis of the shoulder or disc

Table 2 Differential Diagnosis of Angina
in Fitness Exerciser

Cardiac causes
  Coronary atherosclerosis
  Cardiomyopathy
  Poor oxygen supply (anemia, high altitudes)
  Increased work-rate (hypertension, aortic stenosis or regurgitation)

Noncardiac causes
  "Stitch"
  Anxiety state and/or ventricular premature contractions
  Osteoarthritis (shoulder or spine)
  Rotator cuff/hyperabduction syndrome
  Pleurisy
  Thoracic surgery or trauma
  Hepatic tenderness (secondary to congestive failure)
  Visceral disorders (hiatus hernia, peptic ulcer, gall-stone, colic)
  Malingering

degeneration is more likely in this age group, as are a rotator cuff/hyperabduction syndrome, pleurisy, and thoracic surgery or trauma. There is also a potential for confusion with visceral disorders (hiatus hernia, gastric and duodenal ulcer, passage of gall-stones, and colic). Finally, the occasional athlete who is highly paid and having difficulty meeting the demands of training may be suspected of malingering.

Evaluation

Many of the noncardiac causes of chest pain can be eliminated by history, particularly the absence of any relation of symptoms to exercise, with no evidence of rapid alleviation by rest. Orthopedic problems can be revealed by passive movement of the affected region, although there is sometimes a misleading history of precipitation by effort such as carrying a golf bag. Gall-stones and colic should give a history of waxing and waning rather than steadily increasing pain. A barium meal will help to distinguish a hiatus hernia, while a test meal may be useful in the differential diagnosis of a peptic ulcer.

If true angina is suspected, the patient should first be evaluated for cardiac risk factors (particularly cigarette smoking, obesity, a sedentary life-style, hypertension, an adverse lipid profile, glycosuria, and in women the use of oral contraceptives). Typically, ST segmental depression will be observed in a graded stress test, significance being attached to a horizontal or downward sloping depression of 1 mm or more. Even if testing is confined to a "high-risk" population there are a substantial proportion of "false-positive" findings. If symptoms are marked, a positive stress ECG should be followed by more sophisticated cardiac evaluation (echocardiography, scintigraphy). If there is evidence of a perfusion defect, coronary angiography should ultimately be carried out to determine if the lesion is suitable for angioplasty.

In a substantial proportion of older patients, myocardial ischemia appears to be clinically "silent." The merits of extensive evaluation of the symptom-free patient remain controversial. But patients with silent ischemia (particularly if associated with thickening of the ventricular septum or mitral valve prolapse) seem at particular risk of sudden death during exercise. In terms of the safety of exercise prescription, it is sometimes possible and certainly useful to encourage a coronary-prone patient to learn to recognize the sensations associated with more modest degrees of myocardial ischemia. The affected patient may sense a "fullness" or "tightness" in the chest or a constriction of the throat, which are useful indications to halt exercise briefly until the sensation passes.

The likelihood of a true infarct also increases progressively with age. The differentiation from angina is as described in the young athlete.

PALPITATIONS

Young Athlete

Differential Diagnosis

It is remarkable that whereas the average person is unconscious of the heart beating except during very vigorous exercise, abnormalities of heart rhythm are nevertheless readily sensed as palpitations. Factors predisposing to abnormalities of rhythm include vigorous vagal activity, an alteration of plasma composition (for example, hyperkalemia following rigorous dieting or prolonged exercise), anxiety and associated catecholamine release, abuse of stimulant drugs such as the amphetamines, the over-use of sympathomimetic amines (for example, in treating exercise-induced bronchospasm), an accumulation of nicotine or caffeine [including attempts at caffeine doping!], alcohol abuse, and an acute or chronic viral myocarditis. If ignored, such problems can predispose to syncope, cardiac arrest, and/or arrhythmic death.

The likely differential diagnosis in the young athlete (Table 3) includes various forms of heart block, abnormalities of conduction, and ventricular premature contractions.

In sinu-atrial block, the P-R interval of the ECG is progressively increased until one or more impulses fail to reach the ventricle (a Wenckebach-type block). Sometimes, there may also be a QRS complex without a preceding P wave ("ventricular escape"). More rarely, the P-R interval remains constant until there is a "pause," when an entire complex is missing (Mobitz-type block); this type of abnormality is more prone to progress to independent atrial and ventricular rhythms (third degree block). Sometimes, patients may alternate between a normal sinus rhythm and a nodal rhythm in a manner that simulates sinus arrhythmia. A high level of vagal tone is usually responsible, and many healthy endurance athletes show first degree block.

Partial right bundle block is another common finding in endurance athletes, and does not seem of

Table 3 Differential Diagnosis and Etiology
of Palpitations in Young Athlete

Differential diagnosis
  Sinu-atrial block
    Wenckebach type
    Mobitz type
  Premature ventricular contractions
  Wolff-Parkinson-White syndrome

Etiology
  Vagal hypertonia
    Nicotine, alcohol, or caffeine abuse
  Hyperkalemia (dieting, prolonged exercise)
  Anxiety-state
  Amphetamine abuse
  Overuse of bronchodilator amines
  Acute or chronic myocarditis

Table 4 Differential Diagnosis and Etiology
of Palpitations in Fitness Exerciser

Differential diagnosis
  As in young athlete, plus
    Atrial fibrillation
    Atrial flutter

Etiology
  Coronary atherosclerosis
  Nicotine or alcohol abuse
  Over-vigorous dieting
  Anxiety
  Rheumatic heart disease
  Acute myocarditis
  Gall bladder disease
  Heart failure

serious portent. However, left bundle block is usually associated with myocardial disease.

Premature ventricular contractions (PVCs) may arise in the sinus, atrium, atrioventricular (AV) node, or ventricle, and are probably the most common reason for sensing a sudden "thump" in the chest. Although sometimes called extrasystoles, they tend to replace a normal beat, rather than adding to the total number of beats. If the PVC is of supraventricular origin, there is a normal QRS complex, but if the contraction originates within the ventricle, the QRS complex is broadened and has an abnormal waveform.

The Wolff-Parkinson-White (WPW) syndrome presents a superficially similar picture. In the WPW disorder, an accessory conduction path bypasses the normal conduction delay imposed by the AV node. The P-R interval is thus less than 120 msec, and it is followed by an abnormal QRS complex, with a strong possibility of allowing a re-entrant rhythm and ventricular fibrillation.

Evaluation

Most of the above possibilities can be distinguished by a resting ECG. A history should look for smoking, alcohol abuse, administration of sympathomimetic amines, weight-loss by dieting, diuretics, or sauna, evidence of anxiety, and caffeine doping (the last, particularly in the endurance competitor). In doubtful cases, measurements of serum potassium and serum or urinary caffeine levels may be useful, and if manipulation of body weight is suspected the formula developed for the evaluation of body mass in wrestlers may be applied. Holter monitoring and a stress ECG may be helpful in distinguishing a vagal origin of aberrant rhythms. Vagal tone is decreased with exercise, so that the rhythm usually becomes more normal when exercise is begun. On the other hand, in the rare instances with an ischemic cause, symptoms become worse with physical effort. Other possible methods of evaluation that would rarely be used in a young exerciser include a reduction of vagal tone by atropine administration and atrial pacing.

Fitness Exerciser

Differential Diagnosis

Vagal hypertonia is unlikely as an explanation of arrhythmias in the middle-aged fitness exerciser (Table 4). The condition is often attributable to coronary atherosclerosis. Many of the other potential causes are as in a young athlete. Smoking, alcohol abuse, and over-vigorous dieting are more probable factors, while anxiety is more likely to be related to problems encountered at the office than to anxieties about athletic competition. Occasionally, a diseased gall bladder or heart failure may be a contributory cause. Atrial fibrillation or flutter may be an aftermath of rheumatic infection, while abnormalities of conduction and re-entrant rhythms are often attributable to ischemia of the conducting pathways.

Adverse features of PVCs include an increase in their frequency with an increasing intensity of exercise, runs of two or more premature contractions, a polyfocal origin (as shown by variations in the ECG format of the aberrant beats), and occurrence early in the repolarization cycle. If ignored, adverse types of PVC can progress to ventricular tachycardia and ventricular fibrillation. On the other hand, as in younger individuals, occasional unifocal PVCs have little influence on the likelihood of either myocardial infarction or sudden death.

Indications for a cautious approach to exercise prescription include sino-atrial block, marked AV block, left bundle branch block, and adverse forms of ventricular premature contraction.

Evaluation

The evaluation is generally as in a younger individual, with many of the decisions being based on history and a resting ECG. If ischemia is the underlying cause, a worsening of the ECG during a progressive stress test is a useful diagnostic sign, and there may also be ECG evidence of general myocardial ischemia during exercise. In such a situation, it is useful to determine the rate/pressure product at which abnormal rhythms become marked and to set an exercise prescription a little below this threshold. A sick sinus syndrome can be identified by an impaired response to manipulations of autonomic tone (infusions of atropine and isoproterenol). Infra-His conduction abnormalities can be brought out by atrial pacing.

SYNCOPE AND NEAR-SYNCOPE

Young Athlete

Syncope essentially reflects a failure of the cerebral circulation to satisfy the oxygen demands of the brain. Since a classic exercise test is pursued to maximal cardiac demand, there is inevitably a situation of near-syncope in maximal effort tests. Nevertheless, if collapse occurs during an endurance competition, the patient should be checked for hyperthermia. In a cool environment, the cutaneous vasodilatation associated with submaximal exercise becomes replaced by a marked cyanosis as the arterial flow to the skin is reduced, and this changes again to an ashen pallor as the veins constrict in a final attempt to sustain preloading of the heart in all-out effort. Under hot and humid conditions, the cutaneous vasodilatation persists to heavier intensities of exercise, speeding the onset of syncope. In both cool and hot conditions the declining cerebral flow is signaled by a loss of coordination, a staggering gait, and a confused response to questioning. If the person warms down by gentle exercise such as slow walking, a normal cerebral blood flow is quickly restored and no harm results. However, if the upright posture is maintained (particularly in a hot and humid environment, as in an outdoor stadium or a crowded shower area) there may be a dramatic fall of BP, sometimes progressing to a loss of consciousness, myocardial ischemia, and even brain damage.

Syncope should be distinguished from a vaso-vagal attack (Table 5), although the two conditions may be associated. A vaso-vagal attack is often induced by a profound emotional shock. There is a sudden slowing of the heart (as opposed to the tachycardia of syncope), the skin is cold and clammy (whereas it is often hot in syncope), and the muscle blood vessels are widely dilated.

Other possible causes of syncope to be considered include hypoxia (exercise at altitudes above 2,500 meters, breath-hold diving), hypoglycemia (particularly in a diabetic, and in those participating in events of 2 hours duration and longer), hypocapnia (anxiety hyperventilation), syncopal migraine, certain forms of epilepsy, pressure on the carotid sinus (for instance, in wrestling), hypovolemia (repeated heat exposure or deliberate fluid loss in attempts to make a given weight category), congenital heart abnormalities (particularly an exercise-induced reversal of shunt), aortic stenosis or regurgitation, hypertrophic cardiomyopathy (obstructive or non-obstructive), heart block associated with the various arrhythmias discussed above (a Stokes-Adams attack), and decompression sickness with collapse.

Many of these conditions will be distinguished by ancillary features of their history. A resting ECG and

Table 5 Differential Diagnosis of Syncope in Young Athlete

Vaso-vagal attack
Hypoxia (high altitude or breath-hold dive)
Hypoglycemic collapse (diabetics, other long-distance competitors)
Hypocapnia (anxiety states)
Syncopal migraine and epilepsy
Carotid sinus compression
Hypovolemia (heat or weight loss)
Congenital heart disease (reversed shunt)
Aortic stenosis or regurgitation
Hypertrophic cardiomyopathy
Heart block (Stokes-Adams attack)
Decompression sickness

Holter monitor are usually required, and echocardiography may be needed if a cardiac pathology is suspected. Aortic stenosis is indicated by a failure of BP to show the anticipated rise with an increase of work-rate during a laboratory stress test.

Fitness Exerciser

In older individuals, BP may fail to show the anticipated rise or even decrease as exercise continues. This reflects a relative insufficiency of oxygen supply to the myocardium, often due to aortic stenosis, and it is an urgent warning that syncope is approaching.

In addition to the causes of syncope listed for the young athlete, causes for the older adult (Table 6) include a large capacity of the leg veins (an unfit person with a tendency to varicosities who is exercising in a hot environment), over-vigorous palpation of the carotid pulse to monitor exercise heart rate, the use of hypotensive drugs, and (after cardiac surgery) dysfunction of a prosthetic valve. Abnormalities of heart rhythm may include bradycardia (particularly a sick sinus syndrome), supraventricular and ventricular tachycardia, and ventricular fibrillation. The abnormalities of rhythm often reflect myocardial ischemia, being brought to light by the increase of cardiac work-rate and increase of circulating catecholamines during exercise.

The main bases of evaluation are history, resting ECG, Holter monitoring, a laboratory stress test, manipulations of autonomic tone, and the response to atrial pacing.

DYSPNEA

Young Athlete

Dyspnea may be defined as an unpleasant shortness of breath. It commonly arises when the tidal volume exceeds 50 percent of the individual's vital capacity; athletes readily confirm that the breathlessness that they experience during maximal effort can be extremely unpleasant, although there is sometimes a 20 percent discrepancy between the dyspnea threshold in hypercapnia and in exercise, presumably because other aspects of competition distract the mind from respira-

Table 6 Differential Diagnosis of Syncope
in Fitness Exerciser

As in young athlete, plus:
    Poor venous tone (unfit, varicosities)
    Carotid palpation (exercise prescription)
    Hypotensive drugs
    Malfunction of prosthetic valve
    Sick sinus syndrome
    Supraventricular tachycardia
    Ventricular tachycardia
    Ventricular fibrillation

Table 7 Differential Diagnosis of Dyspnea
in Young Athlete

Exercise-induced bronchospasm
Air-pollutant exposure
Anxiety hyperventilation
Anaerobic activity
Decompression sickness (chokes)
Thoracic or mediastinal emphysema

Table 8 Differential Diagnosis of Dyspnea
in Fitness Exerciser

Chronic chest disease
Cigarette smoking
Exposure to industrial pollutants
Exercise-induced bronchospasm
Anxiety state
Pneumothorax
Cardiac failure

line test also reveals increased responsiveness of the airways. Other causes will be suggested by the history.

Fitness Exerciser

In older patients, chronic chest disease due to repeated infection, smoking, or exposure to industrial pollutants is a more common cause of dyspnea than exercise-induced bronchospasm (Table 8). A poor vital capacity and a tendency to expiratory collapse of the airways lead to an early and unpleasant breathlessness when attempts are made to engage in vigorous exercise. Frequently, this tendency is exacerbated by anxiety, hyperventilation relative to the metabolic demands of the task, and a muscle weakness that leads to early anaerobiosis.

Less common causes of dyspnea include a pneumothorax (provoked by hyperventilation, particularly in an emphysematous subject) and cardiac failure associated with myocardial ischemia.

Evaluation for chronic pulmonary disease will include routine tests of pulmonary function (spirometry, flow/volume loops, diffusing capacity) and methacholine sensitivity. If these tests prove negative, a careful stress test should be undertaken to exclude exercise-induced myocardial ischemia. An early and excessive dyspnea provides clinical warning of pulmonary congestion due to decompensation of a failing heart. There is usually an associated fall in systemic blood pressure.

The perception of breathlessness provides one simple way of regulating the intensity of an exercise prescription for the older fitness exerciser, since difficulty in talking and a feeling of respiratory discomfort are first sensed when the anaerobic threshold is passed, at about 70% of maximal oxygen intake for a large muscle task. This approach is particularly useful in situations where the pulse rate cannot be monitored (for instance, when administering beta-blocking drugs or after cardiac transplantation.

tory sensations. Dyspnea is often encountered when exercising underwater, as the increase of barometric pressure increases airflow resistance for a given respiratory minute volume. In such situations, the basic mechanical requirements of chest ventilation are supplemented by the work the chest must perform against the resistance of the surrounding water and an appreciable respiratory impedance associated with any breathing equipment that is worn.

The usual clinical source of chest discomfort in a young athlete is an exercise-induced bronchospasm (Table 7). The patient may report a history of allergies, and the dyspnea is typically seen after a few minutes of vigorous activity — particularly if the atmosphere is dry and cold. The predominant symptoms are cough, wheezing, and tightness in the chest and throat, and relief is usually obtained very quickly from a bronchodilator. Exposure to certain air pollutants, particularly the oxides of sulfur and ozone, increases the tendency to bronchospasm and thus dyspnea during exercise. Other sources of excessive breathlessness are anxiety hyperventilation, hypoxia (altitudes greater than 2500 m), anaerobic activity with a massive lactacidosis, respiratory manifestations of decompression sickness (the "chokes"), and thoracic or mediastinal emphysema (ascent from a dive with breath-holding).

Exercise-induced bronchospasm can be demonstrated as a decrease of forced expiratory volume $> 10\%$ during exercise in a cold, dry atmosphere. A methacho-

EXERCISE IN THE PATIENT WITH A CARDIOVASCULAR DISORDER

ROY J. SHEPHARD, M.D., Ph.D., D.P.E.,
F.A.C.S.M.

This chapter provides an overview of the response to exercise in various types of cardiovascular disorder and presents appropriate management plans for both the young athlete and the middle-aged fitness exerciser.

SYSTEMIC HYPERTENSION

Moderate exercise makes a useful contribution to treatment in many patients with mild systemic hypertension. Although the long-term reduction of blood pressure (BP) associated with regular endurance training is fairly small (5 to 10 mm Hg, averaged across a population sample), it compares favorably with the population response to many types of drug treatment, while the side-effects are generally less serious than for drug therapy. Initial examination should make sure that the patient is truly hypertensive rather than merely anxious in the doctor's examining room. The severity and the consistency of any hypertension should be established, and examination should exclude aortic stenosis, renal abnormality, or pheochromocytoma.

Young Athlete

If a young athlete shows a resting hypertension, and (as is likely) there is also an exaggerated BP response to exercise, the training plan should be modified. The duration of muscle contractions should be shortened and the recovery intervals lenthened. In very severe cases, it may be desirable to avoid weight-lifting, straining against a closed glottis, and prolonged bouts of endurance activity. However, there is no real agreement on a dangerous ceiling of BP, and the only potential dangers in most athletes with idiopathic hypertension are the rupture of a cerebral aneurysm and aortic dissection.

In most competitive athletes, the basis of treatment is salt restriction and diuretics. If the resultant fluid loss is excessive, this may impair endurance performance. If beta-blockers are used, there may be conflict with doping regulations, particularly in sports requiring a skilled performance (for example, pistol shooting). In such cases, alternative hypotensive agents should be used.

Fitness Exerciser

As in young athletes, there is an above-average rise of BP during physical effort, and this is an important argument against allowing over intensive bursts of activity. Prolonged straining against a closed glottis, the lifting of heavy weights, and the prolonged support of body weight are all best avoided if there is more than mild hypertension. Potential hazards of an excessive rise of BP in an older person include hypertrophic cardiomyopathy (evaluated by echocardiography), anginal pain (with possible progression to cardiac failure), myocardial infarction, ventricular fibrillation, and rupture of an atheromatous aorta.

Careful note must be taken of any medications that have been prescribed for hypertension. Diuretics reduce plasma volume, increasing the tendency to syncope, while beta-blocking agents greatly reduce the increase of heart rate (HR) with exercise, preventing a HR-based exercise prescription. Recommendations of an appropriate exercise intensity should be based rather on the ventilatory response, a rating of perceived exertion, or the distance to be covered in a given time. It is also desirable to test renal function in the patient with severe hypertension, since renal complications are exacerbated by exercise.

The mechanisms whereby the mildly hypertensive patient benefits from exercise have yet to be fully elucidated, but one factor is certainly a correction of any associated obesity. It is thus important that the increase of energy expenditure associated with therapeutic exercise be linked to a moderate restriction of food intake. When seeking an increase of fat metabolism, prolonged, moderate exercise (for example, an hour of brisk walking per day) is more effective than a shorter burst of more intensive exercise.

The optimal prescription for the active mild hypertensive is a restriction of salt intake, exercise, and possibly a mild diuretic. Beta-blocking agents should be reserved for severe and refractory cases.

PULMONARY HYPERTENSION

Resting pulmonary hypertension is sometimes observed with prolonged residence at high altitudes (>3500 m). It is also a consequence of an increased pulmonary flow (for instance, a large left to right intracardiac shunt). Other causes include sickle cell disease, schistosomiasis, generalized rheumatic disease, multiple pulmonary emboli, and various types of chronic chest disease.

The capacity of the pulmonary circulation is typically about three times the resting blood flow, so that pulmonary pressures inevitably rise during vigorous exercise. This trend is further exacerbated if exercise is performed at altitudes above 2,500 m, and is inevitably greater if the resting pressure is increased.

The ability to exercise is usually determined by the primary disorder. The patient must be monitored regularly for signs of right ventricular strain and abnormalities of heart rhythm, and the exercise prescription must be moderated if condition is deteriorating.

ARRHYTHMIAS

Regular exercise is unlikely, in itself, to correct abnormalities of resting heart rhythm. However, it may reduce dependency on nicotine and caffeine and thus help to remove a cause of dysrhythmia. If the activity is of a pleasant, relaxing type, it can also help to correct anxiety, and if the cause of the dysrhythmia is myocardial ischemia, the training-associated decrease of cardiac work-rate and improvement of coronary perfusion can have a positive influence on prognosis. It is particularly important that the symptom such as occasional palpitations or thumps in the chest not be allowed to develop into a debilitating phobia, with progressive invalidism.

Bradyarrhythmias

Sports that require skill and aerobic activities are permissible in such conditions as sinus node dysfunction, atrioventricular (AV) block, and AV dissociation, provided that the degree of dysrhythmia does not increase with exercise. If there is a complete congenital or acquired AV block, skill or aerobic activities at an amateur level are again acceptable, provided that a stress test demonstrates an adequate increase of HR and cardiac output during exercise. Power sports where there is a danger of collision should be avoided by those wearing pacemakers.

Premature Complexes

Atrial premature complexes and AV junctional complexes are typically benign, although patients should be evaluated for dilated cardiomyopathy and right ventricular dysplasia.

Premature ventricular contractions (PVCs) are of concern if they become more frequent during exercise, if they are polyfocal in origin, if they occur early during the repolarization cycle, or if there is evidence of associated myocardial ischemia. A laboratory stress test should establish the intensity of exercise where dysrhythmias become marked. The prescribed activity should then be held some 10% below the dysrhythmia threshold. The patient should further be advised to moderate exercise momentarily if the frequency of PVCs is increasing, if the climate is unusually hot or cold, or if there is anxiety from social or business worries. Care must be taken to sustain fluid and mineral balances in warm weather. Fiercely competitive activities such as ice-hockey or squash are probably best avoided, since these lead to higher serum catecholamine levels for a given intensity of exercise. Swimming should not be undertaken alone, particularly if there is a suspicion of the Stokes-Adams syndrome. Underwater exploration should also be forbidden.

Supraventricular and Junctional Tachyrhythmias

Atrial fibrillation is usually due to valvular disease, myocardial ischemia, or degenerative cardiomyopathies, although it can sometimes arise without cardiac pathology or in the Wolff-Parkinson-White syndrome. Aerobic and skill sports are acceptable in such patients, provided that the ventricular rate is slow or is well controlled by therapy. However, risky environments such as underwater exploration are to be avoided, and the intensity of effort is best kept below the anaerobic threshold. Beta-blocking agents such as propranolol (Inderal) are frequently administered to such patients. These agents cause a decrease of myocardial contractility and a greatly restricted rise of HR during exercise (so that HR is no longer a guide to exercise prescription), but the slower ventricular rate usually leads to a larger cardiac output in those with tachyrhythmias. Digitalis preparations increase myocardial contractility as well as slowing ventricular rate, but excessive doses may provoke arrhythmias. Excessive doses of quinidine may provoke a complete heart block; they also tend to cause hypotension and respiratory depression.

Control of ventricular rate is much less likely to be achieved in patients with atrial flutter, and in such individuals exercise must usually be limited to mild walking.

Ventricular tachyrhythmias

A slow ventricular tachycardia is sometimes seen in young athletes due to a high level of vagal tone. This is relatively benign, and is usually over-ridden by the increase of HR with exercise. In older individuals, ventricular tachyrhythmias are usually associated with organic disease such as myocardial ischemia or a cardiomyopathy. If the ventricular rate is moderate (130 to 150 beats/min) and a normal rhythm is established with exercise, patients who are receiving antiarrhythmic medication may undertake moderate aerobic exercise (below the anaerobic threshold). If the ventricular rate is higher, the cardiac output is low, and there is a grave danger of progression to ventricular fibrillation. In such individuals, all forms of vigorous exercise are contraindicated.

VALVULAR HEART DISEASE

Mitral Stenosis

Mitral stenosis is almost always a long-term consequence of rheumatic heart disease, and with better control of streptococcal infections in childhood, the incidence is falling. Often, there is an associated incompetence of the mitral valve and/or congestive failure.

In the patient who has a mild stenosis (New York Heart Association Classes I and II) there is no objection to participating in sports with a relatively low energy demand (for example, cricket, golf, rifle-shooting, and bowling). If the disease has progressed to cardiac failure (New York Heart Association Classes III and IV), both the peak cardiac output and the ejection fraction are low; only 25 to 30% of the ventricular contents may be ejected at rest, and this fraction falls further during exercise. There is a compensatory peripheral vasoconstriction that further reduces exercise tolerance. All forms of prolonged effort should be avoided by such patients. However, as in other forms of cardiac disease, one key to an improvement of condition is a reduction of cardiac work-rate. The reductions of HR and BP induced by gentle endurance exercise (moderate walking or swimming) can thus supplement such measures as a reduction of salt intake, the administration of diuretics, and the use of ACE inhibitors. The strengthening of the skeletal muscles may contribute to the improved performance of such patients.

Mitral Regurgitation

Mitral regurgitation may arise as a consequence of acute infectious myocarditis, rheumatic heart disease, or myxomatous degeneration of the bicuspid valve. Moderate regurgitation is better tolerated than a pure mitral stenosis; the regurgitant fraction determines the severity of overload placed upon the left atrium and ventricle.

Activities that require strong static efforts are liable to increase the regurgitant fraction, and are thus to be avoided. The severity of the lesion must be assessed by symptoms, the intensity of the murmur, the type of heart rhythm, any electrocardiogram (ECG) signs of left ventricular or left atrial strain, any enlargement of atrial or ventricular cavities at echocardiography, the extent of reflux seen on Doppler echocardiography, the normality of the exercise stress test, and the normality of the cardiac rhythm on Holter monitoring. Assuming an absence of symptoms and relatively normal cardiac function, the patient may be allowed to compete in all except prolonged sports such as distance running, cycling, and cross-country skiing. If there are symptoms and a moderate regurgitant fraction, the patient should be encouraged to concentrate on skill activities and team games, choosing the less demanding playing positions. Walking, swimming, and golf may still be helpful to the patient with moderate to severe mitral insufficiency, but the clinical condition must be monitored regularly, and the intensity of activity must be reduced if there is a temporary worsening of cardiac function.

Mitral Valve Prolapse

Mitral valve prolapse is often an isolated finding, although it may be associated with Marfan's syndrome, ischemic cardiopathy and weakness of the papillary muscles, hypertrophic cardiomyopathy, or a myxomatous degeneration of the mitral valves. Sometimes (in the floppy valve syndrome) there may be a prolapse of several intracardiac valves.

The investigation of mitral valve prolapse is the same as for mitral regurgitation. Primary prolapse is a common condition in athletes, and requires no more than an annual evaluation to ensure that the prolapse is not worsening or giving rise to arrhythmias. Competitive sports are generally to be avoided in secondary valve prolapse; the treatment is determined by the underlying condition, but exercise is normally to be held below the anaerobic threshold. If there is significant regurgitant flow, this is a further determinant of the intensity and duration of activity that is allowable.

Aortic Stenosis

Aortic stenosis may be congenital or a consequence of disease. It has a sinister prognosis. Attempts to exercise in such patients can be associated with syncope, left ventricular failure, and sudden death; in the long term, vigorous activity may also worsen any preexistent cardiopathy. The diagnosis of a valvular stenosis can usually be reached by auscultation, but arterial catheterization and measurement of the valvular pressure gradient is needed to ascertain its severity.

An adverse reaction to exercise is indicated by failure of BP to show the anticipated rise during a graded stress test. A strenuous exercise program is generally contraindicated, but some recent reports have shown that patients with mild lesions, a healthy myocardium, and a good coronary vasculature can undertake moderate endurance exercise successfully.

Caution is needed even after surgical correction of the stenosis; the capacity of the prosthetic valve is limited, it may cause hemolysis or hemorrhage, and a risk of sudden death persists—particularly if there are abnormal heart rhythms or myocardial ischemia.

Aortic Regurgitation

The most common cause of aortic regurgitation in an athlete is a deformed bicuspid aortic valve, but Marfan's syndrome is another possibility. In an older exerciser, possible etiologies include rheumatic heart disease, infective endocarditis, and myxomatous valve degeneration.

The extent of regurgitation must be judged from the intensity of the diastolic murmur, any ECG signs of left ventricular strain, the wall and cavity dimensions at echocardiography, the normality of the exercise stress test, and the absence of arrhythmias at Holter monitoring. Decisions about exercise participation follow the same guidelines noted for mitral regurgitation.

Other Valvular Diseases

Tricuspid stenosis can occasionally present as a congenital disorder, but is usually associated with other valvular lesions, particularly in rheumatic heart disease. The treatment is analogous to that of a person with severe left-sided stenosis. There is unlikely to be any desire for competitive sport, but with careful monitoring for right atrial strain, function may be improved by gentle walking.

Tricuspid regurgitation is commonly seen in rheumatic heart disease and is often secondary to severe left-sided heart failure. The exercise potential is very limited, as in an uncomplicated but severe case of left-sided failure.

Acquired pulmonary regurgitation is usually caused by severe pulmonary hypertension (see above).

CONGENITAL HEART DISEASE

Although there are a great range of forms of congenital heart disease, most are likely to be treated surgically at an early age, and if the operation has been successful, the great majority of such patients have an exercise tolerance that compares favorably with that of the average sedentary person.

Small septal defects may remain untreated. Normally, blood is shunted from the left to the right side of the heart, with no problem other than a slight pulmonary hypertension. However, there is a danger that in vigorous exercise a further increase of blood flow through an already overloaded pulmonary circulation can lead to a reversal of the intracardiac shunt, with intense, disabling cyanosis, or even a loss of consciousness. The septal lesions may also affect the conducting system, with abnormalities of heart rhythm, as previously discussed.

A mild pulmonary stenosis may have remained untreated. A characteristic systolic murmur is audible over the pulmonary valve, and the extent of the lesion can be verified by venous catheterization. The impact on right ventricular function can be gauged from the extent of hypertrophy on posteroanterior (PA) radiographs and/or echocardiography, and evidence of right heart strain on both the resting and the exercise ECG; provided that there is no evidence of such strain, there seems no reason to impose any restrictions upon exercise in such patients.

MYOCARDITIS

Acute viral myocarditis was once held to be a common cause of sudden death during exercise. The question is difficult to resolve, for if a person dies unexpectedly, there is often a tendency for relatives to recall some infection that might have passed unnoticed in the absence of the catastrophe. One of the 7,000 patients exercising in the Toronto Rehabilitation Centre postcoronary rehabilitation program died at the eighth kilometer of a distance run, and in retrospect it was suggested that he had developed but not reported an influenzal infection a few days before the event. However, systematic analyses of exercise-induced sudden deaths, including autopsy reports, suggest that viral infections make a very small contribution to the total number of incidents.

ECG evidence of myocarditis is minimal. The commonly suggested indicators of myocarditis are Q waves and ST elevation, but such findings are also observed sometimes in healthy athletes. The only effective preventive measure is thus to avoid strenuous exercise during and immediately after an illness that appears to have a viral origin. If there is indeed a residual myocarditis, an intelligent patient can usually sense a lack of full recovery.

CONGESTIVE HEART FAILURE

According to the Frank/Starling relationship, an increase of end-diastolic volume increases the stroke volume of the heart until a plateau is reached. Any further increase of ventricular size is then associated with a decreasing ejection fraction; this is the stage that a patient has reached with decompensation and pump insufficiency. The heart wall has become sufficiently distended that the normally inter-digitating actin and myosin filaments have become longitudinally separated from each other, and cannot interact properly to produce an effective contraction.

The overfilling of the ventricles can result from difficulty in ejecting blood (an aortic valvular stenosis, an aortic vascular stenosis, or a high peripheral impedance due to sclerosed arteries and weakened muscles), back-flow of blood through incompetent valves, a reduction of myocardial contractility (for example, an excessive use of calcium-channel blocking drugs, or exercise-induced myocardial ischemia), paradoxical movement of the ventricular wall, or an excessive blood volume.

There is little danger in pursuing exercise while the patient is operating on the ascending limb of the Frank/Starling curve; indeed, as previously discussed, such moderate activity will have beneficial long-term consequences for the person with congestive heart failure. However, exercise prescription should be preceded by an optimization of clinical condition, including a reduction of fluid and salt intake, the administration of diuretics, and the use of hypotensive medication if appropriate. On the other hand, it is dangerous for the patient to pass into the phase of decompensation. The patient will often comment on increasing breathlessness and a decrease of exercise tolerance if condition is worsening. Clinical signs such as basal rales, congested neck veins, and ankle edema will give further warning that re-evaluation is needed. Echocardiography and nuclear cardiology should be used to establish or to re-evaluate acceptable levels of exercise for such individuals.

CARDIAC TRANSPLANT PATIENTS

Most experience to date has been with orthotopic transplantation (the transplanting of a carefully matched donor heart, with excision of the diseased heart). Heterotopic transplantation (where the recipient's heart is left intact) generally seems less successful, particularly during exercise, where the recipient heart develops a tachycardia before the donor heart does.

The essential characteristic of the orthotope is that the heart has no nerve supply. Unlike the dog, there is little or no regeneration of either afferent or efferent nerves, even if the patient survives for as long as 10 years after the operation. The initial adjustment to exercise comes through an increase of venous return and a decrease of peripheral resistance, the combination of altered pre-load and after-load augmenting stroke volume. Over the course of several minutes of vigorous activity, there is an eventual tachycardia associated with an increase of circulating catecholamines, and these same hormones also induce an increase of myocardial contractility, with a further augmentation of stroke volume. However, the peak cardiac output and the peak oxygen transport tend to be lower than in a normal person of similar age.

A number of authors have now implemented training programs for periods of up to 1 year following cardiac transplantation, and they have noted a substantial improvement of peak performance, to the point that one patient has now successfully run a marathon distance after transplantation. Since exercise induces little immediate change of HR, exercise prescription must be based on perceived exertion, ventilatory or BP responses, and walking pace, as in the person who is being treated by beta-blocking agents. The observed effects of training seem larger than can be explained by spontaneous recovery of the transplanted heart, although controlled experiments of exercise have yet to be carried out. The basis for any training-induced improvement of condition remains unclear, but one well-documented response to conditioning is an increase of lean tissue mass. During the perioperative period, there is a substantial loss of lean tissue due to bed rest, and such protein loss is exacerbated by the steroid medications used to counter acute rejection episodes. Weak muscles therefore lead to heavy after-loading of the myocardium, and much of the benefit of regular exercise may arise from a restoration of muscle strength. If so, the recovery process might be speeded by the introduction of light isometric or isotonic activity.

As in myocardial infarction, the patient who has received a heart transplant initially tends to show an anxiety-depression reaction, and the training-induced recovery of function is associated with a reduction of such symptoms. Complications of the operation include periodic episodes of donor tissue rejection and an early development of atherosclerosis. Care should therefore be taken to avoid vigorous exercise if a rejection episode is developing. Particular caution is necessary if beta-blocking medication has been prescribed, since this cuts off the last remaining mechanisms for an increase of myocardial contractility and HR.

CORONARY ARTERY DISEASE

Role of Exercise in Prevention

There is now increasingly solid evidence that regular physical activity can play an important role in lessening the likelihood of ischemic heart disease, even after correcting data for possible confounding or intermediary factors such as an exercise-mediated decrease of cigarette smoking. Although emphasis was initially laid on the prevention of coronary atherosclerosis by exercise at or near the anaerobic threshold, more recent studies have suggested that benefit is also obtained from moderate pursuits such as rapid walking and regular stair climbing. The key factor in prevention seems an increase of leisure energy expenditure. Some benefit is observed with the deliberate usage of 2 MJ (500 kcal) per week, and a maximum response is seen when activity is increased by about 8 MJ (2000 kcal) per week. The favorable impact of regular exercise is most clearly documented for the prevention of sudden death and cardiovascular death. During middle-age (35 to 39 years), a person who has conserved the habit of regular physical activity has the expectation of living 2 years longer than someone who is sedentary. However, by the age of 75 to 79 years, this advantage has dropped to 0.3 to 0.4 years. Perhaps more significant from the viewpoint of the patient, there are even larger gains in the quality adjusted life span.

A number of exercise responses undoubtedly contribute to the prevention of ischemic heart disease. The added energy expenditure reduces obesity, augments the HDL/total cholesterol ratio, and may also have a favorable influence on the tendency of the blood to coagulate, thus lessening the progression of atherosclerotic lesions. At the same time, the decrease of HR and BP decrease the cardiac work-rate for a given external energy expenditure, while the slower HR gives more opportunity for ventricular perfusion; all three of these changes lessen the likelihood that a given exercise requirement will induce myocardial ischemia, ventricular fibrillation, and sudden death.

There has in the past been much controversy regarding the need for a medical examination and/or a stress ECG if an older, coronary-prone person is planning to initiate an exercise program. A consultation may be desirable if there is a wish to make a sudden return to a strenuous sport pursued 20 years earlier, but if the proposal is for a prudent and gradually progressive program of rapid walking, an exercise ECG is not particularly helpful. False positive tests are frequent, and the ECG report may therefore serve to create an unwarranted cardiac neurosis. Moreover, even if an observed ST segmental depression is a true positive result, the advice to the patient (a gentle progression of rapid walking) remains essentially unchanged by the findings from the stress test. Provided that the patient feels no more than pleasantly tired the next day, the amount of exercise that has been undertaken is appropriate. The main cause of cardiac problems is lack of compliance with an exercise regimen, rather than overexertion. Exercise should therefore be made as simple as possible, using a minimum of equipment and specialized clothing. The best arrangement is to incorporate the activity into the daily routine — for example, a gradual progression from walking one bus-stop to a 2 to 3 km rapid walk or bicycling to and from work each day. As condition improves, the basic activity can be supplemented by other large muscle tasks: use of a hand mower rather than a motorized lawn mower, other forms of gardening with hand tools, swimming in the summer, cross-country skiing in the winter, and the increasingly rapid ascent of stairs in the office block.

Exercise in Rehabilitation

Practical experience has now firmly established the value of exercise in rehabilitation following myocardial infarction, although attempts to demonstrate this point by controlled experiments have been hampered by (1) a crossover of patients between exercise and control groups, (2) difficulty in accumulating sufficient numbers of patients for randomization, and (3) failure to stratify patients in terms of the severity of their disease. Nevertheless, several investigators have combined individually inconclusive trials by the technique of meta-analysis, and in this way have shown that involvement in an exercise-centered rehabilitation program reduces the risk of a fatal recurrence by 20 to 30%. The risk of a nonfatal recurrence is essentially unchanged, but the severity of such recurrences may also be reduced. Finally, and perhaps most importantly, the quality of life is greatly upgraded as the patient changes from a cardiac cripple to a person able to enjoy all the pleasures of life that they may desire, including (with appropriate preparation) such grueling challenges as completion of a marathon run in a little over 3 hours.

Rehabilitation usually proceeds through at least three phases. The first phase begins in the hospital, with carefully graded and closely monitored activities beginning as soon as 24 hours following a mild infarction.

After discharge, the second phase proceeds for 2 to 3 months, with the patient attending exercise classes at an out-patient rehabilitation facility two to three times per week. Condition is assessed through a graded exercise test, and an initial exercise prescription is set at a level below that provoking deep ST depression or dysrhythmia. The patient is taught the technique of alternate rapid and slow walking, is shown how to count the pulse rate by light carotid palpation, and is taught to recognize any symptoms such as moderate angina and PVCs. Advice is also offered on the purchase of clothing, walking shoes, and watches suitable for pulse counting. Opportunity is taken before each exercise class begins to review any problems that have developed (on a group or an individual basis, as appropriate), and to make periodic recommendations about other changes of life-style (such as smoking cessation, reduction of body weight, and dietary modification). Parallel classes are arranged for spouses to provide additional support for the required exercise program, and to allow a joint discussion of any occupational, domestic, or sexual problems that may be limiting the response to treatment. If there are major overt or denied psychological problems, hypnotherapy may be a useful adjunct to the exercise regimen.

The exercise prescription is normally presented in terms of a walking distance, a time to cover the required distance, and a pulse rate ceiling. Progression to a faster pace and/or a longer distance is allowed if the patient is completing the current prescription without symptoms and consistently has a heart rate below the specified ceiling. Typical rates of progression for a small, uncomplicated infarction and for a larger infarction with persistent dysrhythmia or anginal pain are illustrated in Table 1. Some centers provide all patients with continu-

Table 1 Exercise Prescription After Myocardial Infarction*

| Time | Exercise Prescription | |
	Small infarct	Major infarct
Weeks 1–2	1.6 km/16 min	1.6 km/30 min
3–4	3.2 km/32 min	2.4 km/42 min
5–6	4.8 km/48 min	3.2 km/50 min

*Typical rate of progression of Toronto Rehabilitation Centre patients who enter stage III program after a small myocardial infarction (initial maximal oxygen intake 25 ml/kg · min) and after a more severe infarct with persistent VPBs (symptom-limited maximal oxygen intake 15 ml/kg · min).

Further progression is allowed when the heart rate is consistently below the target value (60% of the symptom limited maximal oxygen intake), the patient is reporting no more than pleasant tiredness on the day following an exercise session, and exercise provokes no increase of PVCs.

ous ECG monitoring during Phase II, but this seems an unnecessary expense. One potential compromise is to restrict this facility to patients who show complications at their initial exercise test. A second option, adopted at the Toronto Rehabilitation Centre, is to apply telemetry to patients who report symptoms while meeting their prescribed exercise. Since the prescription has been established to avoid symptoms, the number of patients requiring such monitoring is relatively small.

After 2 to 3 months of closely supervised activity, the extent of supervision can be progressively reduced, and in uncomplicated cases the site of exercise can become a community exercise facility. In Toronto, our practice is for the patients to attend the Rehabilitation Centre once a week for a further period of 1 year. The program at the Centre includes a general discussion of life-style and problems, a review of the home prescription as reported on an exercise log, a group warm-up with 10 minutes of stretching and light calisthenics, performance of the endurance prescription under close observation, a "fun" activity such as a gently-paced game of volleyball, and a careful cool-down. The prescription is also carried out away from the Centre four to five times per week. A laboratory stress test is performed at 6 month intervals, and other medical advice is available as needed. By the end of the year, a typical patient is covering 4.8 km in 42 min if under the age of 45 years, and in 45 minutes if over the age of 45 years.

The patient must be encouraged to sustain this level of exercise regularly for the rest of his or her life. In the US, the limitations of most medical insurance schemes preclude a longer period of supervised activity, but in Toronto we encourage patients to attend the Centre once per month for a further 3 years in order both to monitor progress and to increase compliance with the exercise prescription. While some centers report drop-out rates of 50% and more for a 4 year period, our approach has encouraged more than 80% of patients to sustain the minimum maintenance prescription of three exercise sessions per week. Some 50 of over 7000 patients have developed their condition to the point of completing a marathon run, and although the peak oxygen transport at entry to our program has been typical of the average postcoronary patient (25 to 30 ml/kg · min), some of the Marathon participants have increased their maximal oxygen intake to over 60 ml/kg · min. The program has nevertheless proven remarkably safe; the risk of exercise-related death has been about 1 incident per 100,000 hours of unsupervised exercise, while there is about 1 cardiovascular incident for 300,000 hours of supervised activity. The long-term overall death rate, about 0.8% per year, is much lower than in most centers, and the figure is particularly low (0.5% per year) for those who have elected to reach marathon standards. Plainly, the Toronto pattern of exercise-centered rehabilitation is a very effective therapy for the postcoronary patient.

RECOMMENDATIONS

With a few specific exceptions, moderate physical activity is beneficial for patients with cardiovascular disorders. The recommended intensity and duration of such activity varies with the diagnosis and must also be based upon a careful evaluation of cardiac function in the individual. In particular, regular endurance exercise

plays an important role in preventing the development of clinical manifestations of ischemic heart disease. Following infarction, a careful progression of physical activity greatly enhances the quality of life, and probably reduces the likelihood of a fatal (but not a nonfatal) recurrence.

SUGGESTED READING

Blair SN, Painter P, Pate RR, et al. Resource manual for guidelines for exercise testing and prescription. Philadelphia: Lea & Febiger, 1988.
Kavanagh T. The healthy heart program. Toronto: Van Nostrand Reinhold, 1980.
Lubich T, Venerando A. Sports cardiology. Bologna: Aulo Gaggi, 1979.
Plas F. Guide de cardiologie du sport. Paris: Laboratoires Besins-Iscovesco, 1976.
Roskamm H, Reindell H, Konig K. Körperliche activitat und herz- und krieslauferkrankungen. Munich: Johann Ambrosius Barth, 1966.
Rost R. Athletics and the heart. Chicago: Year Book Medical Publishers, 1986.
Shephard RJ. Ischemic heart disease and exercise. London: Croom Helm, 1981.
Shephard RJ, Miller HS. Exercise and the heart in health and disease. New York: Marcel Dekker, 1992.

EXERCISE IN THE TREATMENT OF POSTCORONARY AND BYPASS PATIENTS

BARRY A. FRANKLIN, Ph.D.

Coronary atherosclerosis involves a localized accumulation of lipid and fibrous tissue within the coronary artery, progressively narrowing the lumen of the vessel. Fatty streaks may progress to fibrous plaques and eventually to atheromata. Clinically significant lesions, producing myocardial ischemia and left ventricular (LV) dysfunction, often occur with obstructions that exceed 75% of the vessel's cross-sectional area (Fig. 1). Such lesions may become complicated by hemorrhage, ulceration, calcification, or thrombosis, leading to angina pectoris, myocardial infarction (MI), or sudden cardiac death. More than 1.5 million Americans have a MI each year, at an estimated cost of $88.2 billion annually.

Although the degree of LV dysfunction and residual myocardial ischemia largely determine the risk of future cardiac events, risk status can be influenced by numerous interventions and life-style habits (Fig. 2). Multicenter trials have confirmed that mortality from acute MI can be decreased by approximately 25% with early (within 3 hours) thrombolytic reperfusion. Patients at moderate risk may likely experience a reduction in mortality from

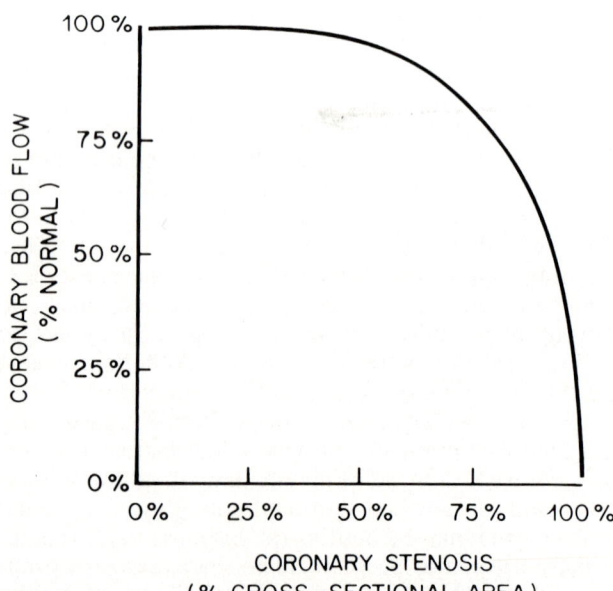

Figure 1 Relationship between coronary blood flow and coronary artery stenosis. Myocardial perfusion is not significantly reduced until the obstruction exceeds 75% of the vessel's cross-sectional area.

successful percutaneous transluminal coronary angioplasty (PTCA) or coronary artery bypass graft surgery (CABGS). Risk factor interventions aimed at smoking cessation and lipid/lipoprotein modification, and efficacious drugs, including beta-blockers and aspirin, have

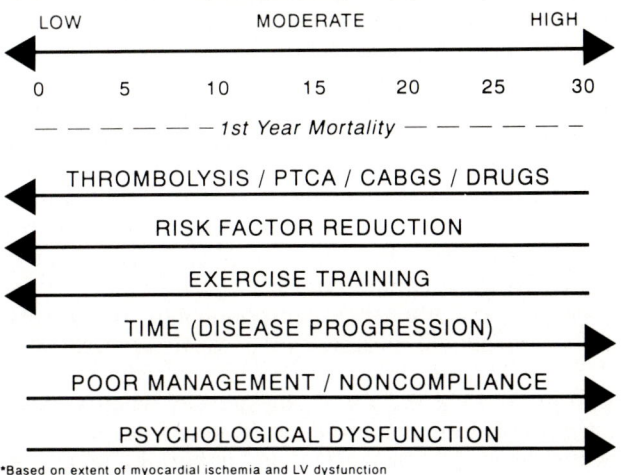

RISK STRATIFICATION CONTINUUM*

LOW   MODERATE   HIGH

0   5   10   15   20   25   30

— — — — 1st Year Mortality — — — —

THROMBOLYSIS / PTCA / CABGS / DRUGS

RISK FACTOR REDUCTION

EXERCISE TRAINING

TIME (DISEASE PROGRESSION)

POOR MANAGEMENT / NONCOMPLIANCE

PSYCHOLOGICAL DYSFUNCTION

*Based on extent of myocardial ischemia and LV dysfunction

Figure 2 Variables that may potentially influence the patient's risk status (PTCA = percutaneous transluminal coronary angioplasty; CABGS = coronary artery bypass graft surgery).

produced significant reductions in cardiovascular-related morbidity and mortality. Moreover, randomized trials of secondary prevention have demonstrated increased survival with regular dynamic exercise. In contrast, time (disease progression), poor patient management or compliance, and psychological dysfunction, manifested as hostility and/or social isolationism, can lead to increased risk and an adverse prognosis.

This chapter addresses the physiologic basis and rationale for exercise in the treatment of the post-MI and CABGS patient, with specific reference to patient evaluation and assessment, contraindications, exercise prescription, chronic adaptations to training, exercise trainability, and potential risks of exercise therapy.

PATIENT EVALUATION

Before beginning an exercise program, patients with coronary artery disease (CAD) should undergo a complete medical history, physical examination, and a graded exercise tolerance test. Other evaluations may include subcutaneous skinfold thickness measurements for assessment of relative body fatness and ideal weight; standard spirometry; flexibility testing (e.g., sit-and-reach test); hand grip dynamometry; and a 12 to 14 hour fasting serum lipid and lipoprotein profile. Some programs also administer objective inventories (e.g., Minnesota Multiphasic Personality Inventory, Jenkins Activity Survey) to screen for the psychosocial dysfunction that often follows an acute coronary event.

Exercise testing of the cardiac patient permits evaluation of the following variables: aerobic power of the body, that is, the peak or maximal oxygen uptake ($\dot{V}o_2max$); hemodynamics, assessed by the heart rate

(HR) and blood pressure (BP) responses; limiting clinical signs or symptoms (e.g., angina pectoris); and associated changes in electrical functions of the heart, especially supraventricular and ventricular arrhythmias and ST-segment displacement. Standard lower or upper extremity tests, employing either the treadmill, cycle ergometer, or arm-crank ergometer, have the advantage of reproducibility and quantitation of physiologic responses to known external work rates. Although the majority of physicians still prefer "low level" testing soon after MI or CABGS, terminating the test when a predetermined, submaximal HR, work rate, or perceived exertion is achieved, stable patients are generally taken, in the absence of adverse signs or symptoms, to peak effort or volitional fatigue.

Clinical variables that should be monitored during the test include BP (cuff method), HR, and multiple lead electrocardiograms (the use of multiple leads increases sensitivity but may reduce specificity in detecting myocardial ischemia). Although the monitoring of 12 or more leads is recommended by some clinicians, we have found that recording three leads is adequate for most clinical situations and favor the precordial leads V_1, V_5, and avF. Other informative variables include perceived exertion ratings and the direct measurement of expired gases for $\dot{V}o_2max$ that, in cardiac patients, may be markedly overestimated when it is predicted from exercise time or work rate.

Because the ST-segment abnormalities that may develop during exercise are uninterpretable in the presence of digitalis, substantial ST-segment depression at rest, left ventricular hypertrophy, left bundle-branch block, or the pre-excitation (Wolff-Parkinson-White [WPW]) syndrome, exercise testing with myocardial perfusion imaging (e.g., thallium-201 scintigraphy) is often recommended to screen for myocardial ischemia in patients with these conditions.

Exercise stress testing should be performed regularly on post-MI and CABGS patients, generally beginning 2 to 6 months after starting a physical conditioning program, and continuing at least yearly thereafter. It is important to assess the patients response to the exercise stimulus periodically as well as to exclude the possibility of a deterioration in clinical status.

CONTRAINDICATIONS

Absolute contraindications are those known or suspected medical conditions that preclude or delay entrance into or continuation of an exercise-based cardiac rehabilitation program. These include unstable angina pectoris, severe aortic stenosis, uncontrolled atrial or ventricular dysrhythmias, acute congestive heart failure, third degree heart block (without pacemaker), and other medical conditions that could be aggravated by exercise (e.g., active myocarditis, acute systemic illness or fever, or uncontrolled diabetes). In addition, certain pathophysiologic abnormalities, including left ventricular dysfunction, myocardial ischemia, and worrisome ventricular arrhythmias, may require medical and/or surgical interventions before initiating the exercise training program.

Recently, concerns have been raised regarding the potential deleterious effects of vigorous exercise training for patients with silent myocardial ischemia, that is, exertional ST-segment depression without symptoms, or those recovering from large anterior wall MI. Others, however, suggest that increased fibrosis, infarct expansion, and a deterioration in left ventricular function are unlikely outcomes of exercise training. Until these controversies are resolved, it seems prudent to recommend a more moderate training intensity for patients with these anomalies, compensating for the lower intensity by an increased exercise frequency, duration, or both.

EXERCISE PRESCRIPTION

In addition to sustained compliance, the effectiveness of an exercise program for post-MI and CABGS patients is, to a large extent, predicated on an appropriate exercise prescription. Three phases are included in the typical exercise session: warm-up, stimulus phase, and cool-down. The stimulus or endurance phase should be prescribed with respect to mode, intensity, frequency, and duration of exercise.

Mode

Simple exposure to orthostatic or gravitational stress (e.g., intermittent sitting or standing during the bed rest stage of hospital convalescence [Phase I]) and slow walking can obviate much of the deterioration in exercise performance that normally follows acute MI.

Large muscle group, continuous exercise, such as walking, jogging, stationary cycling, swimming, rowing, stepping on and off a bench, or stair climbing, is appropriate for outpatient (Phase II-IV) cardiovascular endurance conditioning. Because of the limited degree of transfer of training benefits from the legs to the arms, and vice versa, both sets of limbs should be exercised. Equipment suitable for upper-body training includes rowing machines, wall pulleys, simulated cross-country skiing devices, and arm or combined arm-leg ergometers. In our experience, work rates approximating 50% of those used for leg training are appropriate for arm training. Since the chronotropic reserve for arm exercise is slightly reduced relative to leg exercise, we decrease the prescribed heart rate for leg training by approximately 10 to 15 beats/min for arm training.

Mild-to-moderate resistance training can also provide a safe and effective method for improving muscular strength and endurance in selected cardiac patients. To prevent soreness and injury of the skeletal muscles, patients may perform 1 to 3 sets of each exercise, using a weight load that will allow the completion of 12 to 15 repetitions comfortably.

Intensity

The prescribed exercise intensity should be above a minimal level that promotes cardiorespiratory fitness and/or health benefits, yet below the metabolic load that evokes abnormal signs or symptoms. For most cardiac patients, the threshold intensity for aerobic conditioning probably lies between 40% and 60% of their personal $\dot{V}O_2max$; moreover, considerable evidence suggests that the threshold increases in direct proportion to the pretraining $\dot{V}O_2max$ (Fig. 3). Improvement in aerobic power with low-to-moderate training intensities suggests that the interrelation among the training intensity, frequency and duration may permit a decrease in the intensity, with partial or total compensation by increases in the exercise duration or frequency, or both.

An exercise intensity corresponding to 70% to 85% of the individual's maximal HR, which approximates 57% to 78% of their $\dot{V}O_2max$, is considered more appropriate than the threshold intensity when seeking cardiorespiratory conditioning. Ratings of perceived exertion may serve as a useful and important adjunct to HR as an intensity guide, with the goal of keeping the exercise at a moderate level. Ratings greater than 13 or 14 on the conventional Borg scale (6 to 20), corresponding to "somewhat hard" exertion, indicate an exercise training intensity that is too high, regardless of the individual's HR response. Finally, it should be emphasized that numerous health benefits can be derived at exercise intensities that are below those generally prescribed to improve the $\dot{V}O_2max$.

Frequency

Although deconditioned cardiac patients may improve their cardiorespiratory fitness with only twice-weekly exercise sessions, 3 or 4 evenly spaced workouts per week appear to represent the optimal training frequency. Additional benefits of 5 or more training sessions per week appear to be minimal, whereas the incidence of orthopedic injury increases abruptly with such a frequency.

Duration

The duration of exercise required to elicit a significant training effect varies inversely with the intensity; the greater the intensity, the shorter the duration of exercise necessary to achieve favorable adaptation and improvement in $\dot{V}O_2max$. Exercise for 10 to 15 minutes improves aerobic power, but 30 to 45 minute sessions are even more effective. Recent studies have shown similar training effects in subjects who completed three 10 minute bouts of moderate intensity exercise per day versus those who performed one "long" exercise bout of 30 minutes duration.

BENEFITS AND LIMITATIONS OF EXERCISE TRAINING

Common reasons for exercise training of patients with CAD include improvement in functional capacity, cardiac function, coronary risk factors, psychosocial well-being and reduced morbidity and mortality (Fig. 4).

THEORETICAL THRESHOLD INTENSITIES
FOR TRAINING CARDIAC PATIENTS

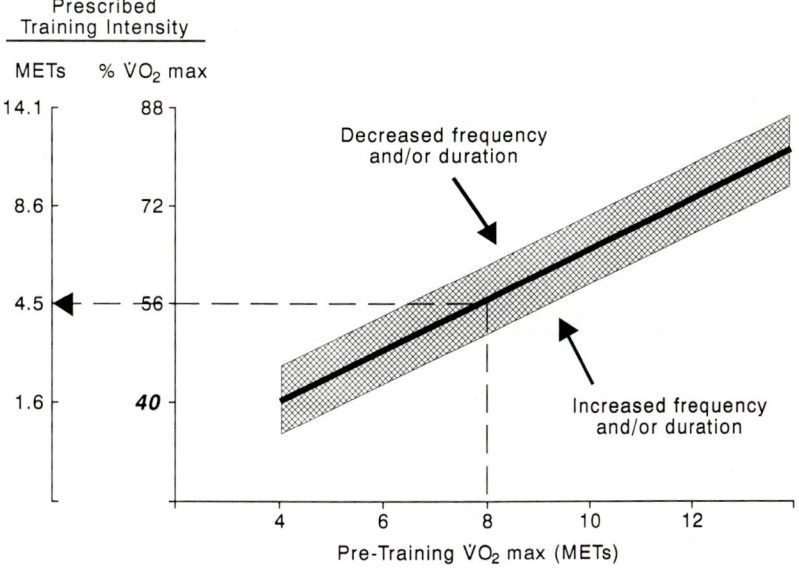

Figure 3 Theoretical relation between pretraining $\dot{V}O_2$max (METs) and the minimal intensity for exercise training, expressed as a percentage of the $\dot{V}O_2$max. The threshold intensity for training increases in direct proportion to $\dot{V}O_2$max before training; however, it can be modulated by altering the exercise frequency and/or duration. For example, a patient with a peak power output of 8 METs would exercise at approximately 56% of his $\dot{V}O_2$max, or 4.5 ± 0.5 METs, to further increase his functional capacity.

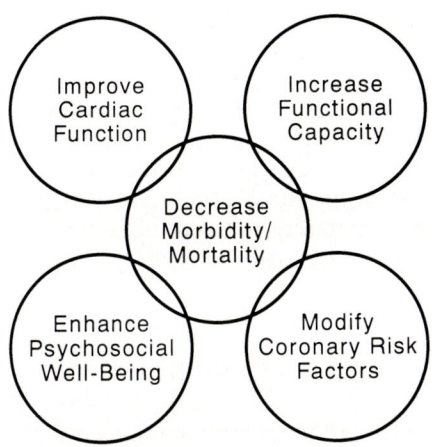

Figure 4 Common reasons for exercise training of patients with coronary artery disease.

Functional Capacity

Although a "spontaneous" increase in aerobic power generally occurs between 3 and 11 weeks after a clinically uncomplicated MI, even in patients who undergo no formalized exercise training, such training can further augment the gains in $\dot{V}O_2$max and relieve symptoms in a majority of patients with CAD. This is particularly important since most patients with clinically manifest CAD have a subnormal functional capacity (50% to 70% of age and gender-predicted norms), and some of these individuals may be limited by angina pectoris at relatively low levels of exertion. Because a given submaximal task requires a relatively fixed oxygen consumption (ml/[kg · min]), the cardiac patient finds that after a physical conditioning program, she or he is working at a lower percentage of capacity, with a greater reserve of power.

Cardiac Function

The effects of chronic exercise training on the autonomic nervous system appear to play a key role in reducing exertional angina. Vagal tone appears to be enhanced at rest, whereas sympathetic drive (and resulting circulating catecholamine levels, particularly norepinephrine) is attenuated during exercise. The consequence is a reduction in the HR and/or BP and myocardial O_2 demand at any given somatic O_2 uptake or submaximal power output. Reduced myocardial O_2 demands presumably allow the cardiac patient to perform at a higher "symptom-limited" work rate before reaching a reproducible rate-pressure product (ischemic threshold).

The effects of exercise training on myocardial perfusion and ejection fraction are less clearly understood. Attempts to use thallium-201 exercise scintigraphy and multiple-gated image acquisition scans before and after physical training have produced conflicting, and often unremarkable data, whereas angiographic studies in group trials attempting to demonstrate revascularization have, without exception, yielded disappointing results. Thus, we lack direct evidence that exercise increases human coronary collateralization or vessel diameter.

Any improvements in coronary blood flow may be related to the decreased HR response to submaximal

Table 1 Patient Characteristics Associated with Exercise-Related Cardiovascular Complications

Clinical Status

Multiple myocardial infarctions
Impaired left ventricular function
  (ejection fraction < 25%)
Rest or unstable angina pectoris
Serious dysrhythmias at rest
High-grade left anterior descending lesions and/or significant
  (≥ 75% occlusion) multi-vessel atherosclerosis on angiography
Low serum potassium

Exercise Test Data

Low or high exercise tolerance (power output ≤ 4 METs or
  ≥ 10 METs)
Chronotropic impairment off drugs (heart rate < 120
  beats/min)
Inotropic impairment (decrease in SBP with increasing work
  rates)
Myocardial ischemia (angina and/or ST-depression ≥ 0.2 mV)
Malignant cardiac dysrhythmias (especially in patients with
  impaired left ventricular function)

Exercise Training Participation

Disregard for appropriate warm-up and cool-down
Consistently exceeds prescribed training heart rate (intensity
  violators)

Other

Cigarette smoker
Male gender

SBP = systolic blood pressure; 1 MET (metabolic equivalent) = 3.5 ml O_2/kg/min

exercise. Because coronary blood flow occurs predominantly in diastole, the period of the cardiac cycle available to coronary perfusion is increased. Thus, a conditioning bradycardia appears to play a critical role in the prevention of ischemia in patients with CAD, by increasing coronary blood flow and reducing O_2 demands on the myocardium.

Coronary Risk Factors

Aerobic exercise training programs can result in modest decreases in body mass, fat stores, BP (particularly in hypertensives), total blood cholesterol, serum triglycerides, and low-density lipoprotein (LDL) cholesterol, with increases in the "antiatherogenic" high-density lipoprotein (HDL) cholesterol subfraction.

Psychosocial Well-Being

Exercise training may also improve well-being and self-efficacy in some patients with CAD. Several groups of investigators have reported an improved quality of life and reduced depression in clinically depressed post-MI patients following exercise-based cardiac rehabilitation programs. However, most randomized, controlled studies of exercise training have found little or no effect in modulating the psychosocial dysfunction complicating acute MI.

Morbidity/Mortality

Two meta-analyses have now shown that cardiac rehabilitation after MI provides a 20% to 25% reduction in total and cardiovascular-related mortality; however, neither study found a significant decrease in the incidence of nonfatal recurrent events. The exercise dosage adopted in these studies generally ranged from 50% to 75% $\dot{V}O_2$max for 20 to 60 minutes, two to four times per week. Such findings suggest that the reduction in fatal cardiac events after cardiac rehabilitation may be achieved with mild-to-moderate exercise intensities. Decreased vulnerability to dysrhythmias and

increased resistance to ventricular fibrillation have been postulated as mechanisms compatible with a specific, training-related protection against sudden coronary death. Recent studies have also shown that regular exercise provides protection against the triggering of MI by strenuous exertion (≥ 6 METs). Unfortunately, similar data on patients following CABGS or PTCA are lacking.

Limitations

There are, however, finite limits to the benefits that exercise training offers in the primary and secondary prevention of heart disease. Contrary to the speculation of a few overzealous enthusiasts, regular exercise training, regardless of the intensity, duration, or both, does not confer "immunity" to CAD or, for that matter, reinfarction. Even marathon running after MI will not necessarily prevent progression of the disease.

EXERCISE TRAINABILITY

Variables potentially affecting exercise trainability (that is, the cardiorespiratory response to physical conditioning) include medications (particularly the use of β-adrenergic blockers) and LV dysfunction. Although it has been suggested that β-blockade may alter or impair exercise training effects, cardiac patients derive considerable aerobic benefit from an exercise training program in the presence of either cardioselective or nonselective β-blocking agents, even if these are taken in therapeutic doses, with a resultant reduction of training HR. Moreover, endurance exercise training appears to be safe and effective in patients with impaired LV function, despite a lack of improvement in resting hemodynamics or ejection fraction. In contrast, post-MI patients who have **both** LV dysfunction and exercise-induced myocardial ischemia show little or no increase in $\dot{V}O_2$max after early outpatient (Phase II) cardiac rehabilitation.

Table 2 Recommendations to Reduce the Incidence of Cardiovascular Complications During Exercise

Ensure medical clearance and follow-up, including serial exercise testing.
Provide on-site medical supervision of moderate and high risk patients.
Establish an emergency plan.
Use continuous or intermittent electrocardiographic monitoring for selected patients.
Emphasize appropriate warm-up and cool-down procedures.
Promote patient education.
Emphasize strict adherence to prescribed training pulse rates.
Reduce exercise intensity in "high risk" patients.
Maintain supervision during the recovery period.
Modify recreational game rules and minimize competition.
Adapt the exercise intensity to the environment.

RISKS OF EXERCISE

The incidence of major cardiovascular complications in supervised cardiac rehabilitation programs is relatively low: one study estimated 1 cardiac arrest per 111,996 patient-hours, 1 MI per 293,990 patient-hours, and 1 fatality per 783,972 patient-hours of exercise. It should be emphasized, however, that this seemingly low morbidity and mortality rate applies only to medically supervised programs equipped with a defibrillator and appropriate emergency drugs. Recent reports indicate that over 80% of all patients with cardiac arrests occurring under such conditions are successfully resuscitated.

Although it is difficult to identify cardiac patients who may be predisposed to cardiovascular complications during exercise training, a profile of the "high risk" patient is beginning to emerge (Table 1). However, due to the vagaries of the atherosclerotic process, the accuracy in predicting which patients will have a cardiovascular complication during exercise remains imperfect. Recommendations to reduce the incidence of cardiovascular complications during exercise are shown in Table 2.

RECOMMENDATIONS

Exercise training remains a pivotal component of rehabilitative care for post-MI and CABGS patients.

Although exercise alone should not be expected to alter global coronary risk status, it may act as a facilitator, especially when combined with education and behavior modification. Incorporating more aggressive efforts at smoking cessation and diet-drug management for hypercholesterolemia should further enhance the efficacy of cardiac rehabilitation programs.

SUGGESTED READING

Arvan S. Exercise performance of the high risk acute myocardial infarction patient after cardiac rehabilitation. Am J Cardiol 1988; 62:197–201.

Blumenthal JA, Emery CF. Rehabilitation of patients following myocardial infarction. J Consult Clin Psychol 1988; 56:374–381.

DeBusk RF, Blomqvist CG, Kouchoukos NT, et al. Identification and treatment of low-risk patients after acute myocardial infarction and coronary-artery bypass graft surgery. N Engl J Med 1986; 314:161–166.

Fletcher GF, Froelicher VF, Hartley LH, et al. Exercise standards: A statement for health professionals from the American Heart Association. Circulation 1990; 82:2286–2322.

Franklin BA. Safety of outpatient cardiac exercise therapy: Reducing the incidence of complications. Phys Sportsmed 1986; 14:235–248.

Franklin BA. Aerobic exercise training programs for the upper body. Med Sci Sports Exerc 1989; 21:S141–S148.

Franklin BA. Exercise training and coronary collateral circulation. Med Sci Sports Exerc 1991; 23:648–653.

Franklin BA, Gordon S, Timmis GC. Amount of exercise necessary for the patient with coronary artery disease. Am J Cardiol 1992; 69:1426–1432.

Franklin BA, Hellerstein HK, Gordon S, Timmis GC. Cardiac patients. In: Franklin BA, Gordon S, Timmis GC, eds. Exercise in modern medicine. Baltimore: Williams & Wilkins, 1989:44.

Gattiker H, Goins P, Dennis C. Cardiac rehabilitation: Current status and future directions. West J Med 1992; 156:183–188.

Greenland P. Efficacy of supervised cardiac rehabilitation programs for coronary patients: Update 1986 to 1990. J Cardiopulmonary Rehabil 1991; 11:197–203.

Hammond HK. Exercise for coronary heart disease patients: Is it worth the effort? J Cardiopulmonary Rehabil 1985; 5:531–539.

Health and Public Policy Committee. American College of Physicians. Cardiac rehabilitation services. Ann Intern Med 1988; 109:671–675.

O'Connor GT, Buring JE, Yusuf S, et al. An overview of randomized trials of rehabilitation with exercise after myocardial infarction. Circulation 1989; 80:234–244.

Oldridge NB, Guyatt GH, Fisher ME, Rimm AA. Cardiac rehabilitation after myocardial infarction: Combined experience of randomized clinical trials. JAMA 1988; 260:945–950.

Shephard RJ. Exercise in secondary and tertiary rehabilitation: Costs and benefits. J Cardiopulmonary Rehabil 1989; 9:188–194.

Van Camp SP, Peterson RA. Cardiovascular complications of outpatient cardiac rehabilitation programs. JAMA 1986; 256:1160–1163.

EXERCISE AND HYPERTENSION

AARON R. FOLSOM, M.D., M.P.H.

Arterial hypertension (or high blood pressure [BP]: systolic BP ≥ 140 mm Hg or diastolic BP ≥ 90 mm Hg) is a major public health problem. Its prevalence in many industrialized countries approaches 25% among adults, in general, and over 50% among the elderly. It is one of the most important causes of renal and cardiovascular diseases, including myocardial infarction and stroke. The etiology of high BP is uncertain, but identified risk factors include a family history of hypertension, African ancestry, high sodium chloride intake, excessive body weight, excessive alcohol consumption, deficient intake of potassium, and insufficient physical activity.

Adequate detection and pharmacologic therapy of individuals with high BP clearly reduces the likelihood of the cardiovascular-renal complications of hypertension, and considerable medical resources have been directed towards this approach. However, long-term antihypertensive medication is costly, can cause important side effects, and requires good compliance to be fully effective. Recently, hypertension experts have encouraged nonpharmacologic, life-style approaches to help control and even to prevent the onset of hypertension. This chapter reviews the role that exercise may have in the prevention and treatment of hypertension.

EPIDEMIOLOGIC ASSOCIATION BETWEEN INSUFFICIENT EXERCISE AND HYPERTENSION

The most conclusive evidence on whether exercise might prevent high BP would come from a long-term clinical trial in which normotensive individuals would be randomized to either exercise or not, with follow-up to determine hypertension incidence rates in the two groups. Unfortunately, such a trial has not been conducted and does not seem feasible because of a large sample-size requirement, an anticipated high drop-out rate, low compliance by both the exercisers and sedentary controls, and the long duration required. Research on the independent relation between physical activity and hypertension is further complicated by exercise's strong influence on obesity, weight loss, and associated metabolic relationships that themselves affect BP level.

Longitudinal Studies

Longitudinal cohort studies, without randomization, offer the best available evidence on the role of habitual exercise in preventing hypertension. At least four such longitudinal studies exist. Paffenbarger et al (1983) studied nearly 15,000 Harvard male alumni, who reported their leisure-time physical activity 16 to 50 years after college entrance. During a 6 to 10 year follow-up, 681 participants reported having developed hypertension. The presence or absence of a background of collegiate sports did not influence the risk of hypertension, nor did stair-climbing, walking, or light sports played by alumni. However, alumni who did not engage in vigorous sports were at 35% greater risk of developing hypertension than those who did, and this relation held at all ages, 35 to 74 years. The risk associated with a lack of strenuous exercise was independent of parental history of hypertension, body mass index (BMI), and weight gain since college. After adjustment for these other characteristics, the relative risk of hypertension in the less active subjects was 1.52 (95% confidence interval; 1.18 to 1.86). The authors thus estimated that at least 25% of the hypertension in this study population was due to lack of vigorous exercise.

Using the same physical activity questionnaire, Paffenbarger et al (1991) also surveyed 5,463 University of Pennsylvania male alumni who were initially free of hypertension. A total of 739 developed hypertension over the subsequent 15 years. Adjusted for age, men who habitually engaged in vigorous sports had a 19% to 29% lower risk of developing hypertension than men who reported no participation in sports. However, when adjusted for other risk factors (obesity, weight gain, and parental hypertension), the relative risk of hypertension associated with no participation in vigorous sports was only 1.06 (95% confidence interval: 0.86 to 1.31). In addition, vigorous sports play did not reduce the risk of mortality among hypertensives, although freedom from obesity and cigarette smoking did.

Folsom et al studied the two year incidence of hypertension, based on self-reports, in a cohort of nearly 42,000 women aged 55 to 69 years. On follow-up, 218 women reported a new physician-diagnosis of hypertension. A low level of reported leisure physical activity, based on three questions, was associated with a 40% greater age-adjusted incidence of hypertension (95% confidence interval: 10% to 70%). However, after adjustment for BMI, waist-to-hip ratio, age, and cigarette smoking, the association of physical activity with hypertension was no longer statistically significant.

Blair et al examined over 6,000 adults aged 20 to 65 years who were initially free of cardiovascular disease and hypertension. On the basis of a maximal treadmill exercise test, participants were classified as "fit" or "not fit," defined by the 85th percentile of treadmill performance of the persons tested. A total of 240 cases of new hypertension, based on self-report of hypertension or use of antihypertensives, developed over an average of 4 years follow-up. After adjustment of data for sex, age, baseline BP, and BMI, the risk of hypertension in the low fitness group was 1.52 times the risk of persons in the high fitness group (95% confidence interval: 1.08 to 2.15).

Thus, these four longitudinal studies indicate exercisers have a 20% to 50% lower age-adjusted hypertension risk than do sedentary adults. Although the association is weakened with statistical adjustment for BMI and other risk factors, one could argue that such (over) adjustment distorts the full effect of exercise, because BMI, itself, is influenced by physical activity level. More longitudinal studies are clearly needed, especially those with validated assessments of physical activity level combined with longitudinally-repeated BP measurements to define the precise incidence of hypertension.

Other Studies

There have been numerous cross-sectional epidemiologic studies of exercise and hypertension. These have included studies of hypertension in relation to occupational activity, leisure time physical activity, performance on fitness tests, and in athletes versus nonathletes. Both within-population and between-population comparisons have been made. Such cross-sectional studies do not consistently demonstrate a relation between lack of exercise and hypertension, but they may suffer from several biases. The most important biases are that persons with hypertension may have chosen or been advised to reduce their exercise and that account may not have been taken of other factors related to both hypertension and sedentary life-style.

EXPERIMENTAL EFFECTS OF EXERCISE TRAINING

Dozens of trials have evaluated whether increased physical activity can lower BP level. Studies in humans have included both hypertensive and normotensive individuals. Most trials have lasted less than 6 months, and therefore relate less to the primary prevention of hypertension than to the control of high BP. At least three meta-analyses summarizing these exercise trials have been conducted since 1990. The most salient conclusions are summarized in Table 1.

Hagberg reported the outcome of a meta-analysis of 25 chronic exercise studies in persons with essential hypertension. Two-thirds of the studies individually showed some BP reduction by exercise. The pooled average reduction with training was 10.8 mm Hg for systolic BP and 8.2 mm Hg for diastolic BP. Additional interesting conclusions were that women may benefit more than men, nonobese more than the obese,

Table 1 Conclusions from Overviews of Trials of Exercise and Blood Pressure (BP)

- The net reduction in BP with exercise is approximately 7–9 mm Hg, somewhat higher for systolic than diastolic BP.
- Better-designed trials report smaller reductions than do poorer-designed studies.
- Both hypertensives and normotensives benefit.
- Women may benefit more than men.
- Efficacy appears to be independent of weight loss, and may be larger in nonobese than obese subjects.
- Moderate intensity (40%–50% of aerobic power) appears sufficient; in fact, moderate intensity may be more efficacious than heavy intensity.
- Training of ≥3 weeks duration is needed; longer training may or may not improve BP further.
- BP returns essentially to the pretreatment value if the patient stops exercising.

moderate-intensity exercisers more than heavy exercisers, and that resistance training, as well as aerobic exercise, seemed efficacious.

Arroll and Beaglehole summarized 22 experimental investigations of habitual activity in humans (hypertensive or normotensive), published since 1980. Only 13 of these 22 studies had a control group, and of these 13, only one study did not have an identifiable major flaw. The pooled analysis indicated that exercise reduced BP in both hypertensive and normotensive persons, independent of any concomitant weight loss. The average reduction in the better-designed studies was approximately 6 to 7 mm Hg for both systolic and diastolic BP. The better-designed trials reported smaller reductions than did poorer-designed studies. All types of activity, including circuit weight training, lowered BP. Activity performed daily produced a greater BP reduction than when performed three times per week.

Spataro et al reported, in abstract, the pooled results of 150 controlled and uncontrolled training studies published over the last 52 years. Overall, there was a reduction of systolic and diastolic BP, respectively, of 9 and 6 mm Hg in exercisers, versus 2 and 1 mm Hg for nonexercising controls.

In addition to human trials, Tipton has reviewed rat studies of exercise to lower BP. These studies include normotensive, surgically hypertensive, and genetically-hypertensive animals, who were typically subjected to running or swimming. Results of these trials are inconsistent, with decreases, increases, and no changes in BP having been reported. The most consistent improvement in BP was seen for swimming rats.

Thus, the human literature suggests strongly that a small to moderate reduction in BP can be achieved with habitual physical activity.

MECHANISMS BY WHICH EXERCISE MAY REDUCE OR PREVENT HIGH BLOOD PRESSURE

By Poiseuille's law, BP is the product of cardiac output and total peripheral resistance. Thus, mechanisms by which exercise may reduce BP must involve reductions of cardiac output and/or peripheral resistance.

Numerous mechanisms have been hypothesized (Table 2), but for none of them is evidence consistent or conclusive. Moreover, there are no longitudinal studies of mechanisms lasting for more than a few months. Improvements in sympathetic vascular tone and insulin resistance are the best documented theories.

RECOMMENDATIONS

Primary Prevention

The totality of epidemiologic evidence is scant but generally suggests that regular exercise can help to prevent hypertension. In addition, regular exercise can help to prevent adult weight gain, which is itself a major

Table 2 Hypothesized Mechanisms for Reduction of Blood
Pressure with Exercise Training

Reduced cardiac output and/or peripheral resistance due to:
- Decreased sympathetic tone, perhaps due to decreased
  catecholamine release and/or decreased beta-adrenergic
  receptor activity.
- Improved insulin sensitivity, resulting in an increase in renal
  sodium excretion and a decrease in adrenergic stimulation.
- Decreased plasma levels of renin/aldosterone, resulting in
  increased renal sodium excretion.
- Altered transport of intracellular sodium and other cations.
- Altered baroreceptor or neural control, perhaps through
  central opioid or seratonergic mechanisms.
- Decreased blood viscosity.
- Altered dietary habits (e.g., decreased intake of sodium and
  fat, increased intake of potassium).

risk factor for hypertension. As a result, numerous advisory groups have recommended regular exercise to prevent the onset of high BP. For example, the U.S. National High Blood Pressure Education Program Working Group on Primary Prevention of Hypertension recently advocated increased physical activity of low to moderate intensity, along with weight control, reduced sodium chloride intake, and reduced alcohol consumption, as important ways to prevent the development of high BP. All adults, and especially those with high "normal" BP ($\geq$ 130/85 mm Hg), should be encouraged to engage in regular exercise.

Hypertension Control

Evidence that exercise can reduce BP level is moderately strong. It is therefore recommended widely as a nonpharmacologic adjunct in the treatment of patients with hypertension. For many individuals with mildly elevated BP, good adherence to exercise, in conjunction with other nonpharmacologic measures, can reduce BP level below the treatment goal of 140/90 mm Hg, thus eliminating the need for antihypertensive drugs. Other hypertensive patients, including those with moderate or severe hypertension ($\geq$ 160/95 mm Hg), generally require pharmacologic control first. With the addition of exercise and other nonpharmacologic therapy, medication can often be reduced subsequently.

The safe prescription of exercise is discussed elsewhere in this book. Exercise in the hypertensive patient requires special consideration. Hypertensives are at increased risk of most cardiovascular diseases, including coronary disease and sudden death. Hypertensive patients greater than 35 years of age, therefore, require a thorough medical evaluation, including a physical examination and exercise testing. Antihypertensive drugs increase the rate of false positive exercise tests, so thallium exercise testing may be required as a confirmatory test.

Accepted guidelines recommend aerobic exercise three to four times per week for 20 to 60 minutes per session. This pattern of exercise is also recommended for hypertensive patients. Since clinical trials suggest that vigorous exercise offers no advantage over moderate

exercise, hypertensives generally should exercise at 40% to 50% of their maximal aerobic power (or a corresponding percentage of their maximal heart rate). Isometric exercise is not recommended. However, resistance weight training is acceptable, if it is closely monitored, and if heavy resistance and the performance of the Valsalva maneuver are avoided. Patients taking antihypertensive medications should be advised to cool down adequately after exercise to help prevent postexercise hypotension.

Most antihypertensive drugs, in particular calcium antagonists, angiotensin converting enzyme inhibitors, alpha-receptor blockers, and vasodilators, are well tolerated by hypertensive patients who exercise. Although not contraindicated, diuretics are less desirable; they increase the risk of dehydration, and may lead to hypokalemia unless a potassium-sparing diuretic is used. Beta-blockers are also less desirable in the hypertensive exerciser, because these agents decrease heart rate, cardiac output, muscle blood flow, and heat dissipation. Beta-blockers also may reduce exercise capacity. If beta-blockers are indicated for other reasons, selective beta$_1$-blockers are preferred.

Because many antihypertensive drugs induce bradycardia, patients placed on antihypertensive agents may require adjustment of their training heart rate. Exercise testing after drug therapy has been stabilized can help to identify an appropriate target heart rate. Since the timing of the antihypertensive dose may influence the exercise heart rate, the exercise test should be done at the same time of day that the patient plans to exercise.

SUGGESTED READING

Arroll B, Beaglehole R. Does physical activity lower blood pressure: A critical review of the clinical trials. J Clin Epidemiol 1992; 45:439–447.

Blair SN, Goodyear NN, Gibbons LW, Cooper KH. Physical fitness and incidence of hypertension in healthy normotensive men and women. JAMA 1984; 252:487–490.

Folsom AR, Prineas RJ, Kaye SA, Munger RG. Incidence of hypertension and stroke in relation to body fat distribution and other risk factors in older women. Stroke 1990; 21:701–706.

Franklin BA, Gordon S, Timmis GC. Exercise prescription for hypertensive patients. Ann Med 1991; 23:279–287.

Gordon NF, Scott CB, Wilkinson WJ, et al. Exercise and mild essential hypertension: Recommendations for adults. Sports Med 1990; 10:390–404.

Hagberg JM. Exercise, fitness, and hypertension. In: Bouchard C, Shephard RJ, Stephens T, Sutton JR, McPherson BD, eds. Exercise, fitness, and health: A consensus of current knowledge. Champaign, Ill: Human Kinetics, 1990:455.

National High Blood Pressure Education Program Working Group: Report on Primary Prevention of Hypertension. Arch Intern Med 1993; 153:186–208.

Paffenbarger RS Jr, Jung DL, Leung RW, Hyde RT: Physical activity and hypertension: An epidemiological view. Ann Med 1991; 23:319–327.

Paffenbarger RS Jr, Wing AL, Hyde RT, Jung DL: Physical activity and incidence of hypertension in college alumni. Am J Epidemiol 1983; 117:245–257.

Spataro JA, Martinez JGR, Tran ZV: The effects of exercise training on human hypertension: A meta-analysis of studies [Abstract]. Circulation 1992; 86 (Suppl 4):I–673.

Tipton CM: Exercise, training and hypertension: An update. Exerc Sports Sci Rev 1991; 19:447–504.

EXERCISE TESTING IN PEDIATRIC CARDIOLOGY

RICHARD ROST, M.D.

The evaluation of physical working capacity in children and adolescents is claiming increased attention for several reasons. Entry into top performance training and competition now occurs at a very young age. In many sports, childhood training is an unavoidable precondition for any athlete who wants to reach world class. The assessment of physical performance capacity in children is also important from the viewpoint of general health, including prevention, treatment, and rehabilitation. These more general aspects of exercise testing are of particular importance from the cardiologic point of view, and form the basis of this chapter.

Living conditions in industrialized regions increasingly prevent children and adolescents from realizing their natural impulse to exercise. The resulting sedentary life-style contributes greatly to the growing incidence of cardiovascular diseases in adults. Ergometric investigations thus provide the basis for general and individual preventive training programs in childhood.

The positive experience with exercise therapy in adult cardiac patients is increasingly translated into the management of cardiac conditions in children. Exercise therapy is even more important in children, given their natural desire for physical activity. Whereas in industrialized societies a sedentary life-style is considered normal in adults, in children it is seen as a symptom of disease and frequently brings about social alienation. Cardiac conditions in children are frequently a reason for prohibiting physical activity, thereby causing more harm than the cardiac condition. Most cardiac conditions in childhood are of congenital origin. Advances in cardiac surgery now allow very early correction of the more serious conditions. Therefore, ergometric assessment of physical performance capacity is needed even more, in order to provide exact data as a basis for training programs in the treatment and rehabilitation of young cardiac patients both before and after surgical interventions.

Ergometric investigation in children has been badly neglected. Sophisticated ergometric stress testing is now a basic method of adult cardiologic office practice, but (at least in Germany) ergometric investigations of children, even in university pediatric hospitals, frequently still consist of tests such as kneebendings or stair running, if they are done at all. Data on the normal performance capacity of children are extremely rare when compared to information about adults. Among reasons for these deficiencies, we may note that (1) coronary artery disease (CAD) gives an important impetus to ergometric investigations in adults, and (2) the equipment developed for investigation of adults does not fit the investigation of very young children.

TESTING METHODS

In Europe, ergometry in adults is performed nearly exclusively on a cycle ergometer (CE), whereas in the United States and other western countries, treadmill (TM) testing plays a major role. From a physiologic point of view, the TM may have some advantages, since it allows the recruitment of larger muscle groups and therefore a patient can develop a higher cardiac work load. From a cardiologic point of view, however, CE has to be favored, taking into account the better possibility of electrocardiogram (ECG) and arterial blood pressure (BP) recording. The subsequent discussion therefore refers only to CE.

Test Protocol

From a cardiologic point of view, the best schedule of stress testing is a ramp protocol (a stepwise increase of work rate); this experience of "adult" ergometry holds true in pediatric cardiologic stress testing. In our routine protocol we start at a work rate of 0.5 watts/kg body mass, and increase this loading by 0.5 watts/kg each second minute, until a preselected endpoint is reached. Such endpoints include subjective exhaustion or a predetermined heart rate (e.g., 170 beats per minute [bpm]) depending on the question to be answered. Classical clinical reasons for halting a test also must be observed, as in adults. The same holds true for emergency and technical equipment, which must meet the same standards as in "adult" ergometry.

INTERPRETATION OF RESULTS

During ergometry, many parameters can be measured. From a practical cardiologic point of view, the most important are physical performance capacity, ECG, and BP. These parameters are therefore discussed in detail.

Physical Working Capacity

The assessment of physical performance capacity in children is more difficult than in adults because of the dynamic processes of growth, maturation, and sexual differentiation. Since children are smaller and for biologic reasons need the protection of adults, the general belief is that their performance capacity is lower than in adults. This opinion is correct in absolute terms, but incorrect in relative units. The working capacity of children per unit of body mass surpasses adult values. Two reasons for this fact can be mentioned:

- Children are smaller and therefore have a larger ratio of body surface to body mass. Smaller creatures are relatively more efficient than larger ones.
- Children are generally better trained than grownups, since they are more active.

However, the statement that children are more efficient than adults deserves further discussion. The aerobic performance of children is greater, but their anaerobic capacity is less than in adults.

Maximal Working Capacity (MWC)

In order to assess MWC by stress testing, a maximal cardiovascular strain must be assured. This can be assumed if a maximal heart rate (HR) of at least 200 − years of age is achieved. Adults aged 20 to 30 years have an MWC of 3 watts/kg for male and 2.5 watts/kg for female subjects. Figure 1 demonstrates the results that we have found in children and adolescents between 6 and 18 years of age. Average boys up to 10 years of age have an MWC of 3.5 watts/kg, whereas the MWC in girls of similar age is slightly but significantly lower at 3.3 watts/kg. After the onset of puberty, girls develop the typical female fat distribution, with a relative decrease of lean body mass (LBM) and a decrease of MWC to the values mentioned above for women.

The findings of a lower relative performance capacity in girls before puberty is surprising, and contrasts with general beliefs. However, it can be seen in nearly all investigations of working capacity in children. Various hypothesis have been advanced to explain such differences, particularly socio-cultural reasons associated with the traditional gender roles of male and female subjects ("boys are playing soccer, whereas girls are playing with dolls"). A basically diminished power of female skeletal muscle has been proposed by Burmeister. However, if working capacity is expressed relative to LBM, such differences disappear. One reason is a larger fat compartment seen already in girls before puberty; this could be an effect of maternal hormones transported across the placenta during pregnancy.

Physical Working Capacity 170 (PWC 170)

A major problem of CE stress testing in young children is a fairly low muscle power. Children may find it difficult or even impossible to reach the above mentioned maximal HR criteria. One frequently used solution is to apply a submaximal test protocol and estimate the work rate achieved at HR of 170 bpm by interpolation between the results observed at work intensities below and above 170 bpm or if necessary making a slight extrapolation. A HR of 170 bpm is normally a submaximal load for children. The normal PWC 170 in adult males is about 2.5 watt/kg and in adult females is 2.0 watt/kg, independent of age. The value for men is also valid for boys (Fig. 2), whereas girls demonstrate slightly lower values (2.4), decreasing further during puberty to the values expected in adult women.

These results are in contrast to the findings of Mocellin and Rutenfranz, who demonstrated that age-dependent values of PWC 170 were lower in early childhood. However, if the PWC 170 shows no age-dependency in adult life, there is no fundamental reason why it should be age-dependent in childhood. The HR 170 is a small percentage of MWC in the young, but a large percentage in older adults—hence the age-dependence of MWC, but not PWC 170.

Aerobic Performance (AP)

Maximal oxygen uptake ($\dot{V}O_2max$) is generally considered to be the most important indicator of AP. According to a literature survey by Bar-Or, the statements made for MWC are also true of $\dot{V}O_2max$. In absolute terms, the AP of children is lower than in adults. However, when expressed relative to body mass, the $\dot{V}O_2max$ is about 50 ml/[kg · min] in boys and 45 ml/[kg · min] in girls, both values being larger than in norms grown-ups (men: 40 to 45 ml/[kg · min] and

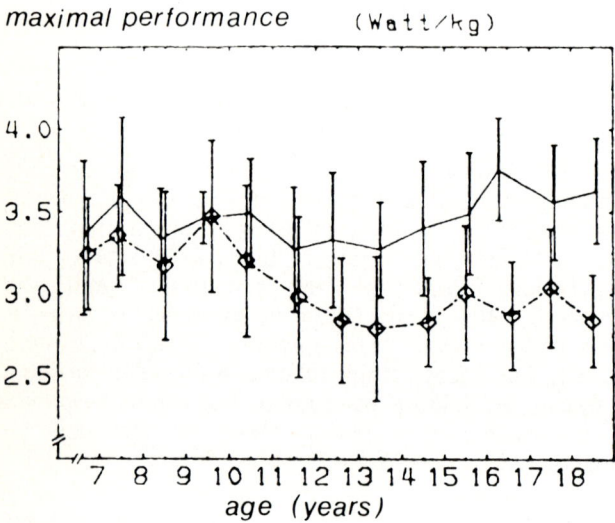

Figure 1 Maximal performance capacity in relation to body mass. Solid line: Boys, interrupted line: girls. (From Klemt U. Die kardiopulmonale leistungsfähigkeit im Kindes und Jungendalter. Sport und Buch. Köln: Strauss, 1988; with permission.)

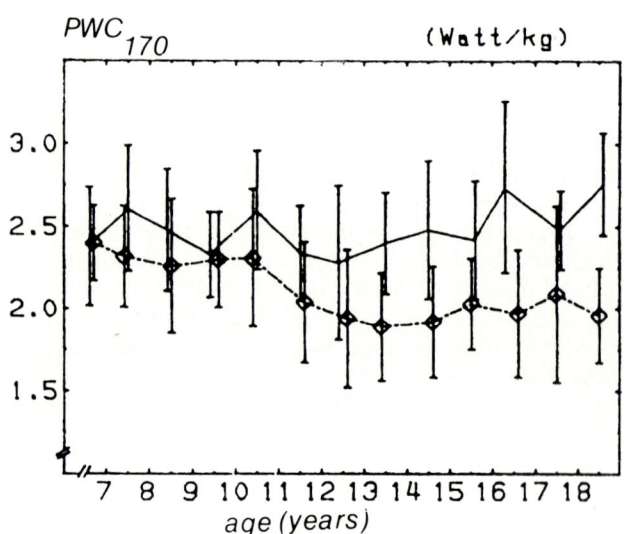

Figure 2 PWC 170 in relation to body mass (compare with Fig. 1).

women 32 to 35 ml/[kg · min]). The sex differences and the age-dependent development in boys and girls are the same as have been described for MWC. Our results (Fig. 3) agree with these statements.

Anaerobic Performance Capacity (AAPC)

Whereas the AP per unit of body mass is greater in children than in adults, the contrary is true for AAPC. The most important test of AAPC is the blood lactate concentration (LA). However, observations can also be based on ergospirometry, using ventilatory threshold instead of LA aerobic-anaerobic threshold (AAT) and maximal respiratory quotient instead of maximal LA. Figures 4 and 5 demonstrate an age-dependent increase of maximal LA. The younger the children, the lower are the maximal LA concentrations. Paradoxically, there is an opposite decrease of weight-related AAT, since a given LA concentration reflects a higher percentage if the maximum value is smaller. For this reason, the LA performance curve in children is shifted to the right (Fig. 6), as in very well-trained endurance athletes who are also unable to achieve high LA concentrations.

The question arises why children do not reach the same maximal LA concentrations as grown-ups. Various hypotheses are discussed in the literature. There may be a lower will to achieve peak effort in children. However, the same phenomenon can be seen in children who perform competitive athletics and who have much more

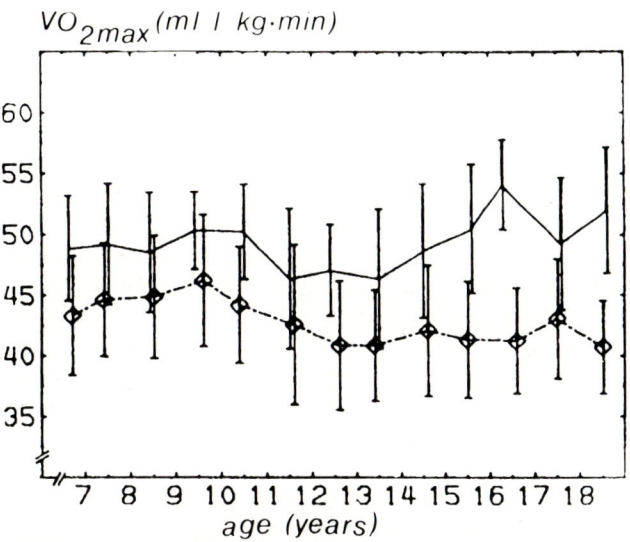

Figure 3 $\dot{V}O_2$max in relation to body mass (compare with Fig. 1).

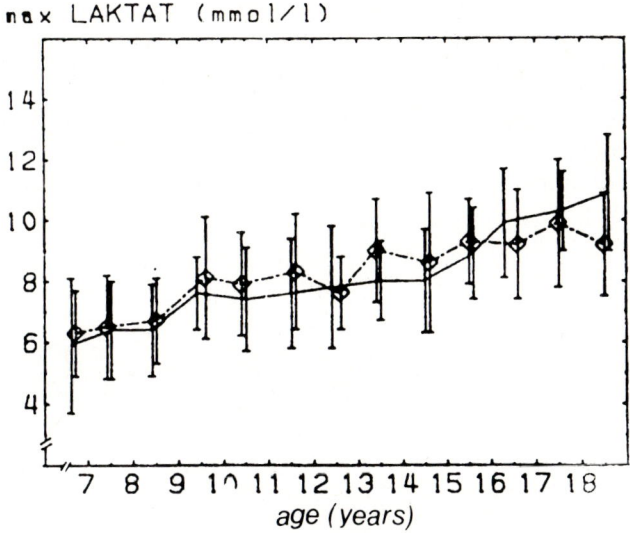

Figure 4 Maximal lactate concentration in stress testing (compare with Fig. 1).

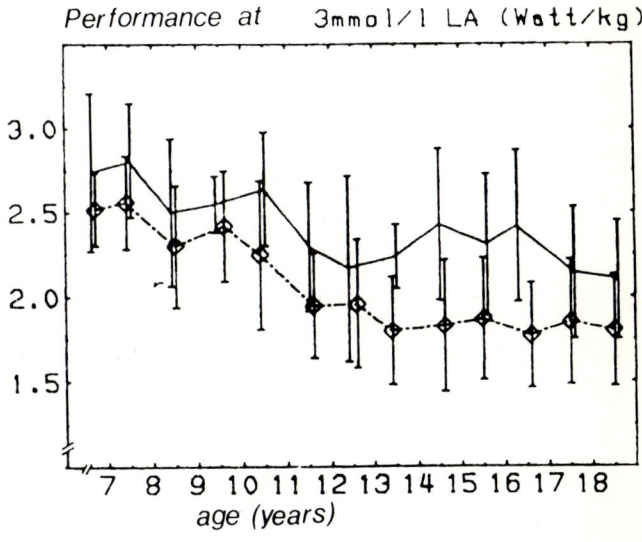

Figure 5 Power output per unit of body mass corresponding to a lactate concentration of 3 mmol/L (compare with Fig. 1).

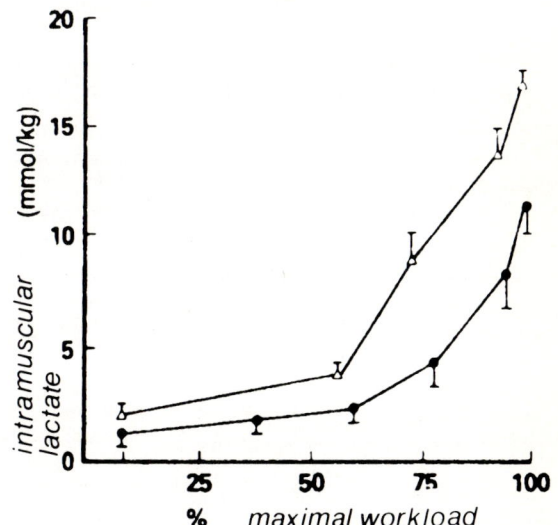

Figure 6 Intramuscular lactate concentration during stress testing in boys and in male adults. (From Erikson B, Karlson J, Saltin B. Muscle metabolites during exercise in pubertal boys. Acta Paediatr Scand (Suppl.) 1971; 217:154; with permission.)

ambition to perform strenuously than do most adults. Another explanation might be the relatively smaller skeletal muscle mass and therefore a comparatively larger distribution volume for LA as it leaves the active muscle. However, the intramuscular LA concentration is also lower in children (see Fig. 6). The most frequently accepted hypothesis is thus that anaerobic enzyme systems are less efficient in children. Erikson et al found lower concentrations of key anaerobic enzymes such as phosphofructokinase in muscle biopsies of children. It may not be easy to accept that the basic system of anaerobic metabolism in children is at a lower level of maturity than the more complicated aerobic system, but nevertheless this theory is widely accepted today.

Electrocardiogram

The stress ECG does not play the same role in children as in "adults" ergometry, since the detection of CAD is only a very rare indication for stress testing in children. However, congenital coronary abnormalities can occasionally cause myocardial ischemia and even sudden death during exercise. If there is any suspicion of such a condition, the stress ECG becomes of considerable importance, as in CAD. A "positive" stress ECG in terms of ST depression might generally be considered a "false positive" indication of ischemic conditions. However, it can signal nonischemic cardiac conditions that are typically seen in the young, such as myocarditis, mitral valve prolapse, or cardiomyopathy. Pseudoischemic repolarization abnormalities may be the consequence of myocardial hypertrophy (e.g., in aortic stenosis). Particular indications for recording a stress ECG in children and adolescents include:

- Striking findings in the resting ECG, such as substitutional rhythms or repolarization abnormalities (Figs. 7 and 8). Their disappearance during exercise generally confirms that they are insignificant. However, the disappearance of ST-depression during exercise can also be found in

cardiac conditions such as hypertrophic cardiomyopathy. If there is any suspicion of hypertrophic cardiomyopathy, it must be further elucidated, for example by echocardiography.
- Cardiac arrhythmias are frequently found during stress testing, even if the most important method of detecting arrhythmias in children is Holter monitoring, as in adults. In the case of exercise-induced arrhythmias, a careful investigation of the basic cardiac condition is important to minimize the potential risk of physical activity.
- Assessment of congenital conduction abnormalities, the most important being the WPW and the QT syndromes.

WPW syndrome. The Wolff-Parkinson-White (WPW) type of pre-excitation may be a potential risk during physical activity if paroxysmal tachycardias in the form of atrial fibrillation are conducted via the bundle of Kent to the ventricle, triggering fatal ventricular fibrillation (VF). If children or adolescents with WPW complain of tachycardias, this possibility must be excluded. A stress ECG can be helpful for this purpose. If the delta wave disappears during exercise, this means the electrical bypass cannot conduct high frequencies, excluding a risk of VF.

QT syndrome. The QT syndrome implies a risk of sudden death during physical activity. This syndrome is frequently not clearly seen in the resting ECG. If there is any clinical suspicion of this syndrome (for example, in the case of syncopes) a lengthening of the frequency-related QT-time may be helpful in reaching a correct diagnosis.

Arterial Blood Pressure

The objective of measuring BP during stress testing in "adult" ergometry is predominantly to assess hypertension and to a lesser degree to assess cardiac function. Regarding the first objective, the incidence of hypertension is low in childhood, so that the stress BP has a lower impact in pediatric ergometry. Nevertheless, the measurement of BP during stress testing may deliver some useful clinical hints even in children.

In order to evaluate the stress BP, reference values are needed. The increase of BP during exercise is smaller in children than in adults as a consequence of their lower

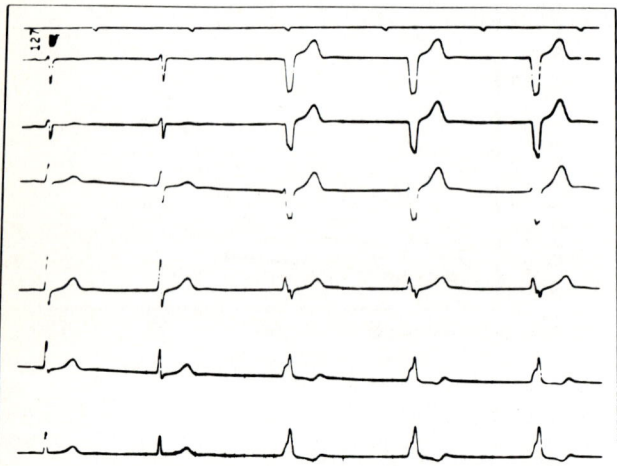

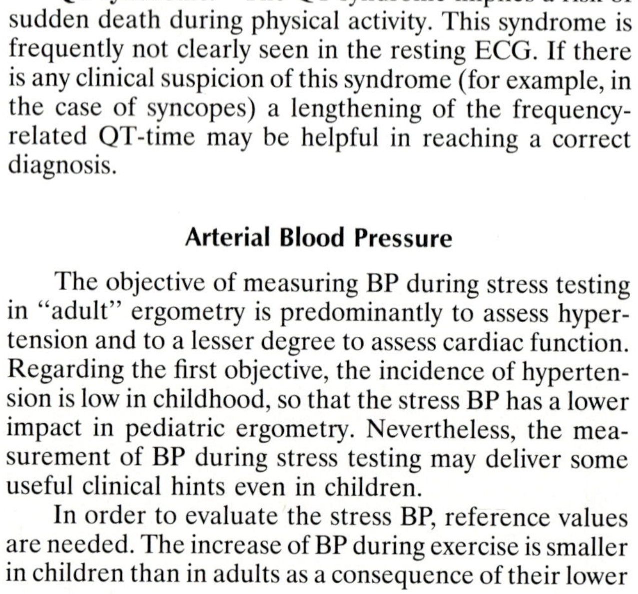

Figure 7 Healthy boy, showing ventricular substitutional rhythm that disappeared during exercise.

Figure 8 Typical pseudoischemic ST depression frequently seen in children. The abnormality disappears during exercise.

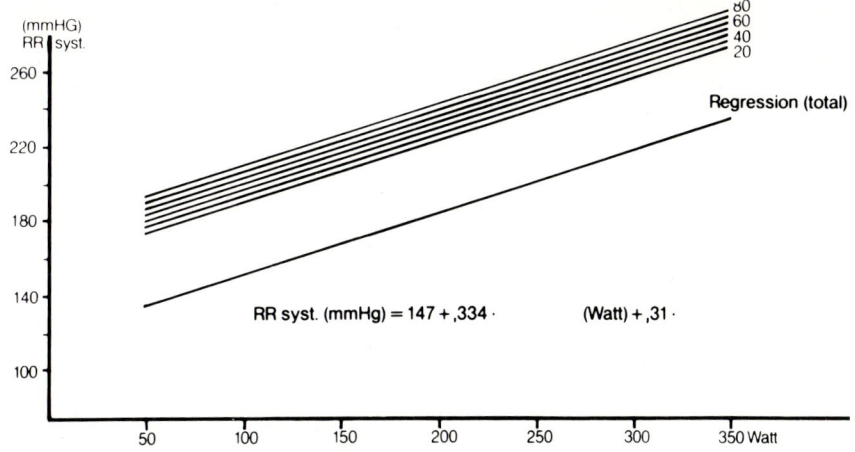

Figure 9 Schedule to assess arterial blood pressure during exercise depending on work rate and age. Regression line and age dependent standard deviation-lines. (From Heck H, Rost R, Hollmann W. Normal values for blood pressure in bicycle ergometry. In: Löllgen H, Mellerowicz H, eds. Progress in ergometry. Berlin: Springer, 1984:201; with permission.)

Figure 10 Arterial blood pressure during exercise as an indicator of subsequent hypertension. The diagram demonstrates the resting blood pressure an average of 5 years after the first investigation. The upper diagram summarizes the results of those subjects who have been classified as "exercise positive" (blood pressure too high according to the criteria given in Fig. 9). Exercise negatives (lower diagram) were normal at rest and during exercise. Open columns: normotensive, closed columns manifest hypertension, dotted area borderlines. The first columns (Y) depict younger subjects (less than 45 years), the second (O) subjects older than 45 years, and the last ones (T) the total sample. Of those who were exercise-negative at the first examination, occasional subjects developed borderline but none developed manifest hypertension (in contrast with those who were exercise-positive). In the young group, the percentage of manifest hypertension was much lower than in the elder sub-sample.

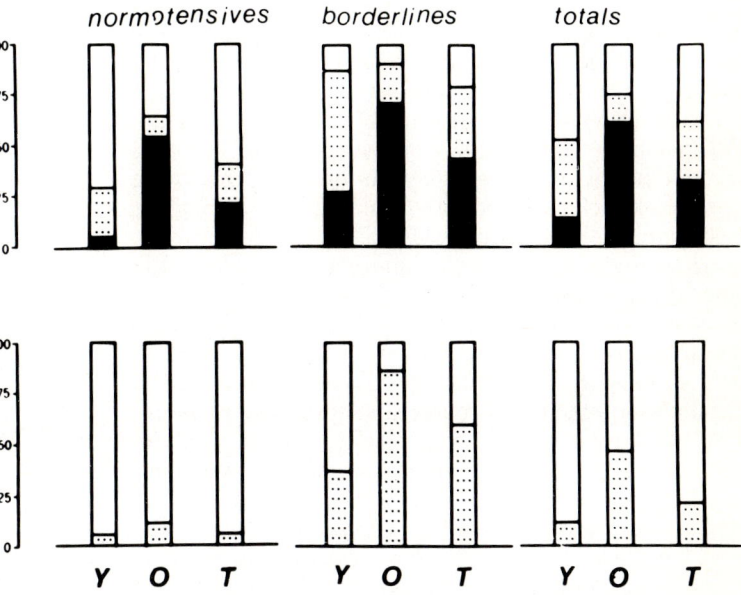

peripheral resistance. Heck has estimated regression lines for stress BP that can be used for children (Fig. 9). In adults, those who demonstrate an excessive increase of BP during exercise ("exercise hypertension") frequently develop a resting hypertension subsequently (Fig. 10). This also seems true of young people, although the percentage is lower than in older individuals. Bar-Or and co-workers found that 11% of children and adolescents who demonstrated an "exercise hypertension" developed a resting hypertension in the next 3 to 14 years, whereas this was not seen in any case of the control group. Measuring the stress BP can thus be considered a screening test for children and adolescents who are prospective hypertensives.

An abnormal stress BP may also be useful in the assessment of congenital cardiovascular conditions. According to Taylor, an excessive stress BP in coarctation of the aorta underlines a need for surgical correction.

The same may also be true in aortic stenosis if low or no increase of stress BP is seen.

SUGGESTED READING

Amecke F, Rost R. Prognostic significance of an overshooting exercise blood pressure as an indicator of subsequent manifestation of hypertension. In: Löllgen H, Mellerowicz H, eds. Progress in ergometry. Berlin: Springer, 1984:212.

Bar-Or O. Pediatric sports medicine for the practioner. New York: Springer Verlag, 1983.

Burmeister W, Rutenfranz J, Svresny W, Radny H. Body cell mass and physical performance capacity of school children. Int Z Angew Physiol 1972; 31:61.

Davies C, Barnes C, Godfrey S. Body composition and maximal exercise performance in children. Hum Biol 1972; 44:195.

Erikson B, Karlson J, Saltin B. Muscle metabolites during exercise in pubertal boys. Acta Paediatr Scand (Suppl) 1971; 217:154.

Heck H, Rost R, Hollmann W. Normal values for blood pressure in bicycle ergometry. In: Löllgen H, Mellerowicz H, eds. Progress in ergometry. Berlin: Springer, 1984:201.

Klemt U. Die kardiopulmonale leistungsfähigkeit im Kindes und Jugendalter. Sport und Buch. Köln: Straub, 1988.

Mocellin R, Rutenfranz J. Methodische untersuchungen zur bestimmung der körperlichen leistungsfähigkeit (W170) im kindesalter. Z Kinderheilk 1979; 108:61.

Rost R. Athletics and the heart. Chicago: Year Book, 1987.

Rost R, Hollmann W. Belastungsuntersuchungen in der praxis. Stuttgart: Thieme, 1982.

Taylor S, Donald K. Circulatory studies at rest and during exercise in coarctation of the aorta before and after operation. Br Heart J 1960; 22:117.

EXERCISE AND CONGESTIVE HEART FAILURE

JACK GOODMAN, Ph.D.

Congestive heart failure (CHF) occurs in approximately 1% of the population, and has a 5 year mortality rate of about 60% in men, and about 45% in women. The 3 year mortality rate for those with a class III to IV ventricle (NYHA) is approximately 75%. In addition, CHF remains the most common cause of hospital admissions for those over 65 years of age. Despite the significant decline in coronary artery disease during the past 20 years, the incidence of CHF has doubled over the same period, posing a continuing challenge for the clinical cardiologist.

Exercise tolerance is greatly reduced in CHF, with dyspnea upon effort being one of the hallmark features of this condition. The limitations to exercise appear to be a complex interaction of central and peripheral phenomena, the former being a manifestation of the primary disease process, and the latter a compensatory maladaptation exerted through neurohumoral pathways in an attempt to preserve tissue perfusion. Large scale trials have identified exercise intolerance (e.g., a poor maximal oxygen consumption, or $\dot{V}o_2$max) as a good predictor of early mortality in such patients, and the quantification of exercise performance is now a widely accepted method of monitoring clinical status, efficacy of treatment, and functional consequences of CHF.

PATHOPHYSIOLOGY OF CHRONIC HEART FAILURE

Ischemic and nonischemic cardiomyopathies are both characterized by a depressed slope of the ventricular function curve, the rate and extent of fiber shortening being profoundly reduced. This is manifest as a reduced cardiac output, ejection rate, and ejection fraction (EF). Most clinical laboratories define a "normal" EF as 45% or more, with an increase of 5% (EF units) during exercise. In patients with CHF, left ventricular (LV) EF typically remains unchanged or declines during exercise.

In compensated CHF, numerous mechanisms are employed in order to support the cardiac output response during exercise or to sustain systemic hemodynamics, including (1) use of the Frank-Starling mechanism (increased end-diastolic volume [EDV]), (2) LV hypertrophy or dilatation, (3) expansion of blood volume (via the renin-angiotensin system), (4) enhanced O_2 extraction (via increases in 2,3-DPG), (5) increased peripheral anaerobic metabolism, and (6) increased sympathetic discharge. As depicted in Figure 1, a number of these short- and long-term maladaptive responses directly affect exercise tolerance, through central or peripheral actions on the cardiovascular system.

LIMITATIONS TO EXERCISE PERFORMANCE IN CHF

Three broad explanations (Table 1) may provide a conceptual framework for establishing the functional limits to $\dot{V}o_2$max. Depressed LV function and/or an abnormal chronotropic response to exercise (through a diminished response to adrenergic/sympathetic stimulation) directly contribute to a centrally-limited $\dot{V}o_2$max. Myocardial damage limits tension development, and long-term ventricular remodeling leads to a thin-walled, dilated ventricle. Although this helps to maintain stroke volume, wall stress is greatly increased, and the end-diastolic reserve is quickly exhausted. Peripheral factors include an impaired vasodilatory response, secondary to both neurohumoral abnormalities and vascular smooth muscle remodeling. In addition, intrinsic skeletal muscle dysfunction is present, including a reduced oxidative capacity and altered energy metabolite production and/or recovery.

Central Limitations

Cardiac Function

The limited cardiac reserve in CHF is an obvious cause for limited exercise capacity. However, it does not explain either the poor relationship between most indices of cardiac function and $\dot{V}o_2$max, or the wide variation in exercise performance seen in patients with equally poor LVEFs. Resting LVEF correlates poorly with most measures of exercise capacity ($\dot{V}o_2$max, maximal work rates). Some studies have reported a weak correlation between right ventricular EF and exercise capacity, but in general the association is weak and inconsistent. A "down-regulation" of β-adrenergic re-

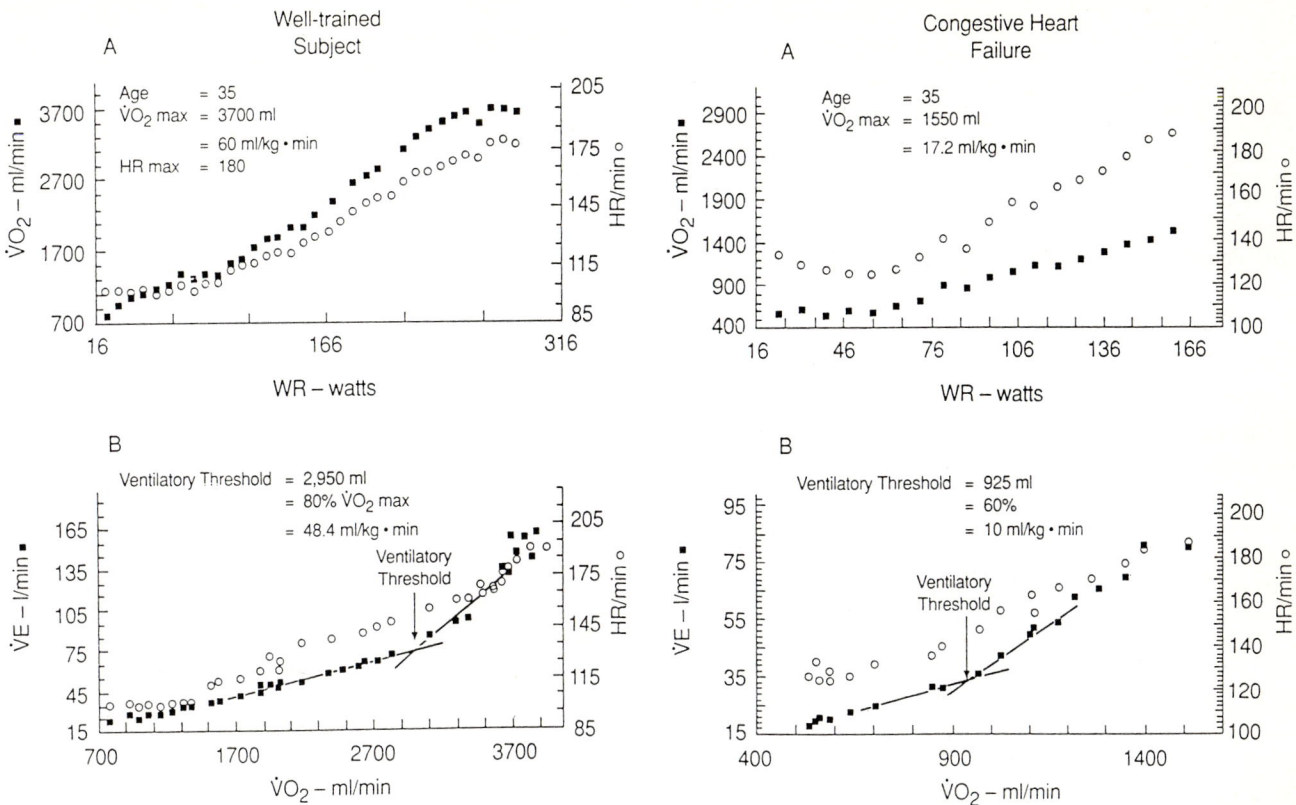

Figure 1 Actual data from graded exercise with measurement of heart rate, oxygen consumption, and ventilation in a well trained subject (*left*) and a patient with CHF (*right*). Both subjects demonstrated a well-defined plateau in oxygen consumption and heart rate (*A*), with a considerably lower peak work rate and $\dot{V}O_2$max seen in the CHF patient. Graph *B* for each subject illustrates the determination of the ventilatory (anaerobic) threshold using $\dot{V}E/\dot{V}O_2$ criteria.

Table 1 Limitations to Exercise in Chronic Heart Failure and Potential Effects of Exercise Training

Factors Affecting Exercise Response	Clinical/Experimental Evidence	Potential Effect of Exercise Training
Cardiac factors		
Depressed contractility	↓ dP/dT; depressed EF	↑ In some animal/human studies
Exhausted end-diastolic reserve	LV dilatation; ↑ diastolic function; ↑ ANP	?
Depressed adrenergic responsiveness	Chronotropic incompetence	?
Peripheral circulatory factors		
Reduced vasodilatory reserve	Impaired local ischemic blood flow response	↑ Vascular blood flow and conductance
Elevated peripheral resistance	↑ exercise pressor response/endothelial remodeling	↓ Peripheral resistance
Reduced skeletal muscle capillarity	Skeletal muscle biopsy data; ↓ capillary fiber ratio	↑ Capillarity
Neurohumoral factors		
Elevated catecholamines	↑ Systemic pressure; ↑ arrhythmias	↓ Catecholamine secretion with exercise
Renin-angiotensin-aldosterone activity elevated	↑ Renin; systemic blood pressure	↓ Systemic blood pressure
Increased antidiuretic and natriuretic hormones	↑ ANP	?
Intrinsic skeletal muscle factors		
Muscle atrophy	NMRS and biopsy data, especially slow-twitch fibers	↑ Muscle tone and strength
Decreased oxidative enzyme activity	Biopsy data; Krebs cycle enzyme activities ↓	↑ Marker oxidative enzyme activity
Altered metabolites	↓ ATP/ADP ratios; ↓ PCr and recovery during exercise	↑ Recovery rates, ↑ [intramuscular]
↑ Intramuscular acidosis	↓ pH (NMRS studies); ↑ lactate	↑ Buffering, ↓ anaerobic metabolism

ADP = ; ANP = ; ATP = ; dP = ; dT = ; LV = left ventricular; NMRS = nuclear magnetic resonance spectroscopy; PCr = phosphocreatine.

ceptors in CHF may explain the limited heart rate reserve during exercise, and a reduced inotropic response may produce an inadequate systemic pressure, resulting in hypoperfusion of the exercising muscles.

Diastolic dysfunction may contribute to a global LV failure, and may help to explain why measures of systolic function correlate poorly with exercise capacity. It is for this reason that some have classified CHF patients as having either systolic or diastolic failure.

Pulmonary Function

Dyspnea is a common clinical finding in CHF. Originally it was suggested as causing an early cessation of exercise, secondary to transient pulmonary edema. Increased LV end-diastolic pressure, and elevated pulmonary capillary wedge pressure (PCWP) can alter lung mechanics via increases in interstitial fluid, thereby reducing lung compliance. Theoretically, stimulation of so-called "J-receptors" in the lung may stimulate the "J-reflex," causing an increased breathing frequency and a sensation of breathlessness. However, despite the presence of an elevated PCWP in CHF, it is unlikely that the high wedge pressure contributes to exercise intolerance, as it correlates poorly with exercise capacity. Although most CHF patients do not develop arterial blood desaturation during exercise, abnormalities in the ventilation-perfusion relationship may contribute to a large minute ventilation. Recent data suggest that patients with CHF have enlarged dead space volumes and demonstrate a higher respiratory energy cost during exercise, which may contribute to the widely reported dyspnea during both graded exercise testing and vigorous exercise.

Peripheral Limitations

Neurohumoral Factors and Exercise Capacity

Neurohumoral activation is the hallmark compensatory response to CHF, contributing directly to peripheral vasoconstriction and a poor exercise capacity in these patients. Elevated plasma catecholamines are widely reported in CHF, regardless of the form of treatment received, and such increments are well correlated with early mortality. However, it is unclear if elevated catecholamine levels help to cause circulatory dysfunction (e.g., by actively increasing vasoconstrictor tone during exercise), or are simply a marker of the severity of CHF. An elevated activity of the renin-angiotensin-aldosterone system has been closely linked with an elevation of resting arterial resistance. Despite the observation that plasma renin activity (and norepinephrine) increases with exercise, the acute administration of angiotensin converting enzyme (ACE) inhibitors does *not* alter exercise tolerance in CHF. This has led some investigators to question the role of neurohumoral activation *during* exercise itself. Furthermore, the improvement in exercise performance after chronic ACE inhibition is modest, and is only evident after months of therapy.

Local Muscle Perfusion

Hypoperfusion of skeletal muscle may be the primary stimulus for dyspnea and the resultant limitation to exercise in CHF. A reduction in forearm blood flow in CHF during exercise was first reported some 30 years ago. Subsequently, others have demonstrated a diminished arterial and venous vasodilatory capacity in CHF. In addition, maximal vasodilatory function is impaired during exercise, despite the presence of a metabolic dilator influence. Preliminary data from our laboratory have demonstrated a positive linear relationship between vascular conductance and $\dot{V}o_2max$ in CHF, underscoring the critical dependence of $\dot{V}o_2max$ upon an adequate vasodilatory response to exercise. Furthermore, we have observed that CHF patients who demonstrate a superior exercise response relative to others with similar CHF do so because of a favorable response of their total peripheral resistance.

The exact cause of the impaired blood flow response is unclear. Aside from the neurohumoral factors summarized above, suspect neurohumoral agents include vasopressin (which is increased in CHF) and factors related to local regulation of vessel diameter, including endothelin (a vasoconstrictor) and altered endothelium dependent relaxing factor. Both of these latter factors have been implicated in an endothelium-related impairment of vasodilatation in CHF.

Muscle Energetics and Morphology

The use of nuclear magnetic resonance spectroscopy (NMRS) and needle biopsy sampling has revealed that patients with CHF have an intrinsic abnormality of the skeletal musculature. Histochemical and biochemical analysis of biopsy samples reveal an atrophy of slow-twitch (type 1) muscle fibers and a diminished oxidative enzyme activity, levels of oxidative enzymes being positively correlated with $\dot{V}o_2max$. In addition, increased connective tissue in the interstitial space has been reported. Studies using NMRS have demonstrated a lower intracellular pH at a given workrate, and abnormalities in high-energy phosphate and phosphocreatinine kinetics during handgrip exercise. These observations suggest a greater reliance on glycolytic pathways during exercise in CHF. Such findings are unexplained by the peripheral blood flow response.

Recent studies have also revealed that the muscle fatigue seen in CHF is not related to central motor drive or neural transmission, but is local in nature. It must therefore be due to alterations in the chemical or architectural milieu of the muscle. The mechanism responsible for the altered intrinsic state of the muscle is unclear; chronic deconditioning may contribute strongly, since training can reverse many of the deficits seen in CHF (see below), and a reduced nutritive flow to muscle may be matched by a "down-regulation" of energy metabolism.

Collectively, the alterations in neurohumoral, muscle, and vasodilatory function may explain a peripherally-mediated impairment of exercise that follows this sequence:

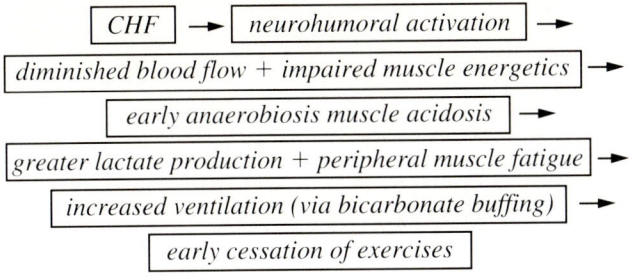

CHF → neurohumoral activation →

diminished blood flow + impaired muscle energetics →

early anaerobiosis muscle acidosis →

greater lactate production + peripheral muscle fatigue →

increased ventilation (via bicarbonate buffing) →

early cessation of exercises

EXERCISE TESTING IN CHF

Exercise testing in CHF has many purposes, including the objective quantification and grading of clinical status, documentation of functional capacity, and monitoring the efficacy of various interventions. In normal subjects, direct assessment of $\dot{V}O_2$max during graded exercise is both precise and reproducible (coefficient of reliability = 0.95), providing an objective means by which limitations to exercise can be identified. Repeated measures of $\dot{V}O_2$max vary by only 2% to 4%. However, "maximal" test data must be interpreted cautiously in CHF, particularly when "maximal" oxygen uptakes are less than 15 to 20 ml/(kg · min). Less than 50% of those tested reach a quantifiable "plateau" in oxygen consumption, despite a further increment of workrate. Consequently, many CHF patients demonstrate a "peak" oxygen consumption, which might increase considerably with further habituation to the test protocol. In addition, cycle ergometry often produces early fatigue local to the legs, significantly limiting peak $\dot{V}O_2$. Notwithstanding these limitations, graded exercise testing with measures of gas-exchange permits determination of various cardiorespiratory parameters that help to assess the clinical status of the patient (Table 2), and facilitate the differentiation of pulmonary versus cardiac limitation of effort.

Patients with CHF have a sharply reduced $\dot{V}O_2$max, most likely due to the interaction of factors that vary widely from patient to patient, including (1) tolerance of elevated PCWP without dyspnea, (2) adequacy of chronotropic response to exercise, (3) decrease of peripheral vascular resistance during exercise, (4) reduction of oxidative potential, and (5) ventricular dilatation and adequacy of systolic reserve.

An objective classification of CHF patients based upon direct measures of $\dot{V}O_2$max and the anaerobic threshold (discussed below) has been developed (Table 3). This approach may offer an advantage over the traditional functional classification using the NYHA criteria.

Anaerobic Threshold

Patients with CHF exhibit a substantially lower anaerobic threshold (AT) than normal subjects, which reflects an early transition to anaerobic metabolism for reasons already summarized. Exercise performed above the AT produces a metabolic acidosis, shortening exercise duration, and producing dyspnea and rapid fatigue. These are all common clinical symptoms in CHF. Although the concept of the AT remains controversial from both semantic and theoretical viewpoints, it represents a reproducible means of quantifying exercise performance, and has the advantage over $\dot{V}O_2$max of not requiring a maximal effort if expressed on an absolute basis (e.g., $\dot{V}O_2$ in L/min at ml/[kg · min] at the AT). In this population, it is advisable to quantify the threshold on an absolute basis rather than as a percentage of $\dot{V}O_2$max, since patients do not always attain maximal effort. Many clinical centers now measure these parameters as a routine follow-up in CHF. Some have demonstrated that the oral administration of an inotropic agent and a peripheral vasodilator delays the increase in blood lactate, thus increasing the $\dot{V}O_2$ achieved at the AT.

Response to Graded Exercise

Upon exertion, patients with CHF demonstrate a supra-normal end-diastolic pressure. A reduced stroke volume is largely due to a diminished systolic reserve; consequently, the EF is low both at rest and during exercise when compared to normal subjects. Some investigators report an increase in EDV during exercise in CHF. However, this is not always seen; differences in underlying pathology, and body position (supine vs. upright) may account for the varying responses.

Although some patients with CHF can increase their EF during exercise, the common observation in patients with primary or secondary cardiomyopathy is that the EF either remains unchanged or decreases during exercise. When gas-exchange is monitored, patients typically demonstrate an early AT, a low $\dot{V}O_2$ peak and a low O_2 pulse. They also ventilate less than 50% of their maximum voluntary ventilation (V_E/MVV), suggesting that they fail to exhaust their ventilatory reserve. Figure 1 depicts actual data from cardiopulmonary exercise testing, using time-averaged (15 seconds), breath-by-breath sampling; the anaerobic (also called the "ventilatory") threshold and $\dot{V}O_2$max are compared between a well-trained subject and a patient with CHF. The well-trained subject attains a well-defined centrally-limited O_2 consumption plateau, observed, with a ventilatory threshold of at least 20 ml/(kg · min). In the case of CHF, both the $\dot{V}O_2$max and the AT is low, and the total exercise time and peak workrate (watts) are correspondingly reduced. In many cases the heart rate response during submaximal exercise is more pronounced in CHF, likely a consequence of a reduced stroke volume.

IMPACT OF PHARMACOLOGIC INTERVENTION

Potential improvements in exercise performance could be accomplished by augmenting systolic performance (via inotropic agents), and unloading the ventricle and enhancing peripheral blood flow (via diuretics and/or vasodilators). However, recent data suggest that exercise performance ($\dot{V}O_2$max, lactate production) is not improved immediately after such treatment, despite improvements in central hemodynamics; such changes are only observed after long-term ACE inhibitor

Table 2 Common Gas-Exchange Measurements: Definitions, Normal Ranges, and Response in Congestive Heart Failure

Variable	Definition	Normal Range	Typical CHF Response
$\dot{V}O_2$ max	Upper limit for O_2 consumption obtained despite increase in work rate. Functional limit of cardiovascular system.	Male: 4.2–0.0032 (age) L/min (SD ± 0.4); 60–0.55 (age) ml/(kg · min) (SD ± 7.5) Female: 2.6–0.014 (age) L/min (SD ± 0.4); 48–0.37 (age) ml/(kg · min) (SD ± 7.0)	Most laboratories report $\dot{V}O_2$max values of 14–20; ml/(kg · min); $\dot{V}O_2$max values are poorly related to resting EF; See Table 3 for classifications
$\dot{V}O_2$ slope ($\dot{V}O_2$/WR)	Aerobic contribution to exercise; low slope implies greater anaerobic contribution to work.	8.6–12 (ml/min per watt)	Slope reduced
O_2 pulse ($\dot{V}O_2$/HR)	Proportional to avO_2 when SV is constant. Varies with age, sex, height, hemoglobin; higher in endurance trained. Can reflect changes in SV at maximum exercise if avO_2 is constant.	10–14 (males) 7–10 (female)	Decreased at maximal exercise
Anaerobic threshold (AT)	Noninvasive index of the nonlinear increase in blood lactate. Disproportionate increase in $\dot{V}E$ vs. $\dot{V}O_2$, or other criteria (see text)	Percentage (% $\dot{V}O_2$max): 45–65% Absolute (ml/(kg · min): >25 ml/(kg · min).	Percentage values: similar to normals Absolute values: usually <15
$\dot{V}E$/MVV (dyspnea index)	Index providing analysis of the balance between demand and capacity of ventilatory system	65–80%	Often <50%
HR_{max}	Maximal heart rate obtained during maximal-effort exercise test. Age dependent.	$HR_{max} = 210 - 0.65$ age $= 220 -$ age	Can be reduced despite evidence of maximal effort
RER_{max} ($\dot{V}CO_2$/$\dot{V}O_2$)	Indicates substrate utilization (1.0 = complete carbohydrate metabolism). Rest = 0.75–0.85.	Values >1.10–1.15 indicate similar or higher maximal effort reached (when used in conjunction with other criteria—see text)	
VD/VT	Physiologic dead space/tidal volume ratio. Indicates matching of ventilation to perfusion. Falls with exercise, high in obstructive lung disease.	25–40% at rest 5–20 during exercise	High: due to increased dead space in CHF and evidence of poor matching

CHF = Congestive heart failure
RER = respiratory gas exchange ratio
$\dot{V}CO_2$ = carbon dioxide production
$\dot{V}O_2\dot{V}E$ = ventilation
SV = stroke volume

HR = heart rate
MVV = maximum voluntary ventilation
VD = dead space
VT = tidal volume

therapy. These findings suggest that a short-term *functional* change in the periphery (increased vasodilatory reserve and ventricular unloading) may be sufficient to improve hemodynamics, but that long-term *structural* changes (intrinsic skeletal muscle function) are necessary to augment exercise performance. The mechanism behind these observations remains to be elucidated.

EXERCISE TRAINING IN CHF

Aerobic exercise training offers intriguing possibilities for patients with stable CHF. The rationale for training is simple: many of the adaptations induced by aerobic conditioning should ameliorate the peripheral abnormalities (e.g., chronic deconditioning) that limit exercise performance in these patients (see Table 2). However, a high degree of supervision and follow-up is required because of a high incidence of arrhythmias and a risk of rapid cardiac decompensation.

There are few well controlled studies involving stable CHF patients and training. However, in patients with poor LV function (EF < 25%), improvements in both submaximal and maximal exercise performance have been observed. As in the normal population, most improvements reflect local adaptations of peripheral

Table 3 Classification of Functional Impairment

Class	Severity	Maximal Aerobic Power ($\dot{V}o_2$max) ml/(kg · min)	$\dot{V}o_2$ at Anaerobic Threshold (ml/ [kg · min])
A	Mild to none	>20	>14
B	Mild to moderate	16–20	11–14
C	Moderate to severe	10–16	8–11
D	Severe	6–10	5–8
E	Very severe	<6	<4

From Weber KT, Janicki JS. Cardiopulmonary exercise testing: Physiologic principles and clinical applications. Philadelphia: WB Saunders, 1986:153; with permission.

function that directly alter exercise tolerance and clinical status. During submaximal exercise, trained patients demonstrate a lower heart rate and venous lactate at any given work rate. This is also reflected by a reduction in ratings of perceived exertion, and in some cases, increased oxygen consumption. Studies have also reported an increased vagal tone and lower norepinephrine spillover following training in CHF. These are significant clinical findings, because of the close relationship between catecholamine levels and mortality. In addition, they suggest training may reverse the sympathetic imbalance and modulate baroreceptor activity in CHF. Local changes in the skeletal muscle following training in CHF include a reduced peripheral vascular resistance and augmented peak limb blood flow, in addition to an increased skeletal muscle oxidative capacity.

These physiologic changes are accompanied by improved quality of life scores; gains in quality of life may occur before physiologic benefits are realized. Since quality of life is profoundly affected in CHF, exercise training offers a rapid and successful intervention.

RECOMMENDATIONS

For the clinician, exercise testing adds considerable precision to patient classification, and it is an excellent tool for examining the efficacy of therapeutic intervention, and the underlying pathophysiology of chronic heart failure. The reversal of peripheral impairments that limit exercise performance have led many to suggest that in most cases, activity should not be restricted for CHF patients. Exercise training is now regarded as a useful potential intervention, and it should certainly be considered in carefully chosen patients.

SUGGESTED READING

Braunwald E, Ross J, Sonnenblick EH. Mechanisms of contraction of the normal and failing heart. Boston: Little, Brown, 1976.
Coats AJS, Adamopoulos S, Radaelli A, et al. Controlled trial of physical training in chronic heart failure: Exercise performance, hemodynamics ventilation and autonomic function. Circulation 1992; 85:2119–2131.
Myers J, Froelicher VR. Hemodynamic determinants of exercise capacity in chronic heart failure. Ann Intern Med 1991; 115:377–386.
Parmely WW. Pathophysiology and current therapy of congestive heart failure. J Am Coll Cardiol 1989; 13:771–785.
Weber KT, Janicki JS. Cardiopulmonary exercise testing: Physiologic principles and clinical applications. Philadelphia: WB Saunders, 1986.

EXERCISE AND CARDIAC TRANSPLANTATION

TERENCE KAVANAGH, M.D., F.R.C.P.(C), F.A.C.C., F.C.C.P.

The introduction of the immunosuppressant agent cyclosporine (Sandimmune), coupled with improved surgical techniques, has led to a tripling of heart transplantation procedures worldwide during the 1980s, the number increasing from 700 in 1984 to approximately 3,000 in 1988. Thereafter this figure has plateaued at about 3,000 annually, due almost entirely to the shortage of donor hearts. Nevertheless, the success rate continues to improve, with current 1, 5 and 10 year survival rates of 80%, 68%, and 56%, respectively.

THE HEART TRANSPLANT PATIENT

The typical heart transplant recipient is a 44-year-old male who is suffering from "end-stage" heart disease, either from a cardiomyopathy or severe ischemia, and has endured a prolonged period of invalidism, with all its attendant adverse effects on mood, morale, and the musculoskeletal system. Individuals in this age group can be assumed to have high personal expectations, usually coupled with significant career and family responsibilities. The first major step in the recovery process is the surgical procedure itself. Yet mere survival, no matter how devoutly desired and enthusiastically acclaimed in the first few postoperative months, is not enough. Complete operative success can be claimed only if the patient regains the physical and mental capacity to pursue a full, active, and enjoyable life. There is now ample evidence that a formal, medically prescribed, and supervised exercise rehabilitation program can go a long way towards achieving this goal.

Physiology of Heart Transplantation

The prescription of an exercise program for the heart transplant patient requires an understanding of the physiologic changes brought about by the implantation of a healthy, but nevertheless denervated, heart into a failing circulatory system. Immediately after the transplantation procedure, cardiac function is slightly impaired, both as a result of myocardial anoxia following the brain death of the donor and the subsequent period of organ preservation. Right- and left-sided chamber filling pressures are elevated. However, within days the myocardium recovers, pulmonary hypertension regresses, and the intravascular pressures normalize. Thereafter, any significant return of these abnormalities is seen only after the onset of an episode of transplant rejection. The following description, therefore, pertains to the patient who has recovered from surgery and has no signs of rejection.

The resting heart rate (HR) is rapid, usually between 90 and 110 beats per minute, due to absence of the normal vagal influence on the sinoatrial node. The HR does not alter in response to the Valsalva maneuver, carotid sinus massage, or a change in body position from lying to standing. Any minor fluctuations in HR that may occur over a 24 hour period are the result of variations in the levels of circulating catecholamines. Apart from this relative tachycardia, resting ventricular performance is within normal limits, as measured by ventricular ejection fraction, myocardial contractility, and contractile reserve. There is, however, some mild impairment of diastolic function, as demonstrated by a slower relaxation time, possibly the result of increased myocardial stiffness.

An elevation of resting systolic and diastolic blood pressure (BP) is a common finding as early as 2 to 3 weeks after cardiac transplantation, and ultimately it may require medical treatment. The precise mechanism remains unclear, although now it appears likely that it is a side effect of cyclosporine therapy rather than an intrinsic feature of cardiac transplantation.

The denervated heart is supersensitive to endogenous catecholamines, partly due to the loss of presynaptic uptake following sympathetic denervation and partly the result of an "up-regulation" of myocardial beta-adrenoreceptors. Levels of atrial natriuretic peptide (ANP) are persistently one-and-a-half to two times higher than normal. This substance plays a role in maintaining sodium and water balance, as well as

regulating aldosterone secretion and arterial vasomotor tone. The trigger for its release is stretching of the atrial walls. Since atrial pressures are not necessarily elevated in the transplanted heart, a high atrial pressure is unlikely to explain the increase in ANP. It may be due to the increased surface area of the atria, which now includes the donor atria and the remnant of the recipient atria. Alternatively, it may be a response to water retention as a result of steroid immunosuppressant therapy. The clinical significance of elevated ANP levels is unknown.

Response to Exercise

Heart transplant patients compete regularly in the World Transplant Games; some have taken part in long-distance runs, including the Boston Marathon, and there is even a report of an individual playing professional soccer. Thus there is no doubt that such individuals can perform heavy bouts of exercise. However, the mechanism by which the denervated heart responds to physical effort is atypical. In the normal subject, an increase in cardiac output demanded by a bout of physical exercise is met initially by a rapid increase in HR and then, as the intensity of work escalates, by an augmentation in stroke volume (SV). The denervated heart, beating at the high intrinsic rate of the sino-atrial node and lacking any direct neural influence, cannot respond by immediate acceleration. It thus relies entirely on the Frank-Starling mechanism to increase SV in the early stages of exercise. Thereafter, and with increasing effort, the HR, contractility, and ejection fraction increase in response to climbing levels of catecholamines. The tendency for HR to continue to rise after the cessation of exercise, and its tardy return to resting levels in the recovery period, mirror the gradual fall in catecholamine concentrations (Fig. 1). These chrono-

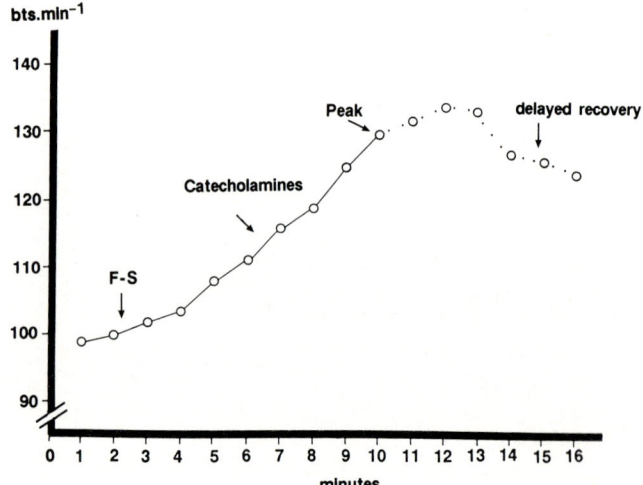

Figure 1 Typical transplanted denervated heart rate response to increasing effort. Note the high resting rate, the delayed rate of acceleration during effort, the delayed deceleration during recovery, and the tendency for the rate to continue to rise after the termination of effort (peak exercise).

tropic and inotropic responses are enhanced by the increased myocardial catecholamine sensitivity; by the same token, they are severely attenuated by beta-blockade.

Peak work rate and oxygen intake, measured either on the treadmill or cycle ergometer, are generally reported as being lower in heart transplant patients than in age-matched controls. There is some debate as to whether this is due to impaired cardiopulmonary performance, or to the loss of lean tissue mass with its attendant muscle weakness. It seems likely that both central and peripheral mechanisms are involved. Maximal HR is lower than in normals, as is SV, with the result that maximal cardiac output is reduced by approximately 25%. There is also a suggestion, at least in some patients, that impairment of pulmonary diffusing capacity may be partially responsible for the diminished peak oxygen intake. Minute ventilation, although greater than normal at low work rates, is significantly less than in normal subjects at peak effort. Finally, as stated previously, there is significant (10% to 15%) reduction in lean body mass, due to the prolonged period of preoperative physical inactivity and the side effect of immunosuppressant steroid therapy.

The reduction in maximal physical performance may be a manifestation of subclinical episodes of graft rejection, rather than an indication of suboptimal cardiac function. Animal studies lend some credence to this argument. For instance, the peak heart rates and performance times of denervated, autotransplanted racing greyhounds (in which the heart is removed and then reimplanted in the same animal) are only slightly less than in sham-operated controls.

With regard to isometric exercise, the normal response is an increase in peripheral resistance, a rise in systolic and diastolic BP, and an increase in HR. In the heart transplant patient, BP reacts in an identical fashion; peripheral resistance increases, but there is no acceleration in HR.

Other Considerations

The development of hypertension has already been mentioned as a potential problem in the long-term management of the heart transplant patient. Acute episodes of graft rejection are also an ever-present threat, and although they may be heralded by clinical, electrocardiographic, radiologic, and echocardiographic changes, they are most accurately detected by endomyocardial biopsy. Intercurrent infections due to immunosuppression, particularly of the cytomegalovirus variety, are another possibility.

Accelerated coronary atherosclerosis is a serious late complication, and by the fifth postoperative year some 50% of patients will show angiographic evidence of this condition. Although there is recent evidence that partial autonomic reinnervation can occur in some patients, and occasional anginal-type symptoms have been observed in individuals who have developed post-transplant coronary disease, it is generally accepted that reinnervation does not occur in the human heart.

Consequently, one cannot rely on angina as a symptom of myocardial ischemia. Furthermore, reports suggest that exercise-induced ST segment depression is frequently absent despite ischemia. Whether this is due to the typical low peak HR attained by transplant patients, or to a difference in pathophysiology between transplant vasculopathy and native coronary atherosclerosis, remains unclear.

The denervated heart is not immune from arrhythmias. Indeed, a number of studies have indicated that both atrial and ventricular ectopic beats are common. These may increase in frequency during bouts of acute rejection, or with the advent of accelerated coronary atherosclerosis. In long-term survivors, the development of a sinus tachycardia of 130 beats per minute or higher, or the incidence of repeated bouts of supraventricular tachycardia, have been identified as adverse prognostic signs, sometimes preceding sudden death.

EXERCISE TRAINING PROGRAM

The Hospital Inpatient Phase

Six days after surgery, and as soon as their condition is stable, patients commence physical therapy. Passive range of motion exercises, as well as breathing and postural exercises, are followed by active upper and lower limb mobilization, initially in the supine position and then seated in a chair. Patients progress from sitting to standing exercises, and by the fifth day are walking in the room. At this time they may also begin to use a cycle ergometer, pedaling at zero resistance for 3 to 5 minutes. Direct monitoring is by BP and electrocardiogram (ECG), and the intensity of effort is held in the 11 to 13 range on the Borg categoric scale ("fairly light" to "somewhat hard" exercise). As performance improves, the duration of exercise and the power outputs on the ergometer are increased, corridor walking is permitted, and by the time of discharge, usually 3 weeks after surgery, a low-level incremental exercise test may be carried out either on the cycle ergometer or on the treadmill, with power output increments of one MET every 1 to 2 minutes. Such a test allows the prescription of a walking or stationary cycling program that can be followed during the early (4 to 8 week) outpatient phase. During this period, the medical staff is occupied primarily with detecting and treating complications, adjusting drug regimens, and performing routine investigations, but the enthusiastic therapist will take every opportunity in this phase to motivate and attune the patient to the restorative value of long-term outpatient exercise rehabilitation.

The Exercise Test

The exercise test can be carried out either on a treadmill or on a cycle ergometer. The protocol varies with the laboratory, but in general calls for continuous progressive increments in work rate of one to two METs to maximal effort, usually attained within 10 to 14 minutes. The exercise ECG is monitored continuously, and the Borg Categoric Rating of Perceived Exertion (RPE) is noted at the end of each test stage. The BP is measured just prior to exercise, every 2 minutes, at peak effort, and in recovery. It is preferable to analyze expired air for ventilation ($\dot{V}_E$), oxygen intake ($\dot{V}O_2$), carbon dioxide output ($\dot{V}CO_2$), and gas exchange ratio (RER) using a metabolic chart. This permits determination of true maximal effort, as demonstrated by the achievement of an oxygen intake plateau. It also enables measurement of the ventilatory threshold ($\dot{V}_T$), a level of effort that correlates well with the intensity required for endurance training, and that is usually attainable even in those patients who have been unable or unwilling to exert a maximal effort. The $\dot{V}_T$ is estimated from a number of variables that include, in respect to a progressive increase of oxygen intake, a disproportionate increase in the minute ventilation, the ventilatory equivalent for oxygen, and $\dot{V}CO_2$ (Fig. 2).

Because of their severely deconditioned state, only about 50% of cardiac transplant patients are likely to meet the oxygen plateau criteria of a maximal exercise test. Corroborative evidence of maximal effort is therefore sought in a respiratory gas exchange ratio greater than 1.10. The indications for stopping a test before the demonstration of a plateau are as recommended by the American College of Sports Medicine. Since an ischemic state cannot manifest itself as anginal pain, particular attention must be paid to such symptoms as excessive dyspnea, lightheadedness, faintness or "feeling odd," and increasing atrial or ventricular ectopic beats on the exercise ECG.

Outpatient Phase

The training mode depends on the experience and preference of the rehabilitation team, but should adhere to the accepted principle that cardiovascular fitness is achieved most consistently by dynamic activity, which involves large muscle groups and can be accurately quantified and monitored, e.g., walking/jogging, cycling, swimming, circuit training. I usually prescribe walking, progressing to jogging, with stationary cycling or swimming either on a temporary or permanent basis for those who have problems ambulating.

In view of the heart transplant patient's poor chronotropic response to effort, the use of a predetermined HR to define exercise training intensity is inappropriate. In the Toronto Rehabilitation Centre's program we use 60% to 70% of the peak $\dot{V}O_2$ as measured on the exercise test, confirmed by the $\dot{V}O_2$ at which the $\dot{V}_T$ occurred, as well as a perceived exertion rating of 14 on the original Borg RPE scale. In a typical case, this calls for an initial walking pace of 11 to 14 min/km. The initial exercise prescription is for 1.6 km at this pace, carried out five times weekly. The distance is then increased by 1.6 km every 2 weeks, maintaining the same pace until, by 6 weeks, the patient is walking 4.8 km, five times weekly. The pace is then quickened by 1 minute per 1.6 km until 4.8 km is accomplished in 45 minutes (typically within 4 months of starting the

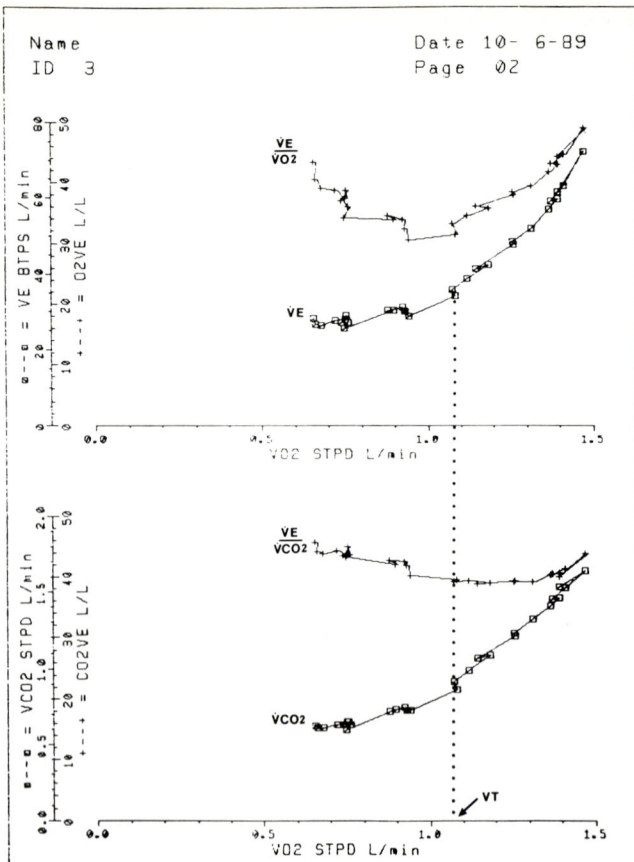

Figure 2 The ventilatory threshold (VT) is identified, relative to oxygen intake, ($\dot{V}O_2$) at the upward inflection of the curves for the ventilatory equivalent for oxygen ($\dot{V}E/\dot{V}O_2$); the minute ventilation ($\dot{V}E$), and the carbon dioxide output ($\dot{V}CO_2$); note that the ventilatory equivalent for carbon dioxide ($\dot{V}E/\dot{V}CO_2$) curve is still flat at the VT.

program). Thereafter, 50 meter bouts of slow jogging paced at 7.5 min/km are introduced at the start of every 100 m, then every 400 m, 200 m, 100 m, and so on until ultimately the entire 4.8 km is completed in 36 minutes. The more highly motivated subjects are progressed to 6.4 km, or 32 km weekly, maintaining the same pace of 7.5 min/km. After the first 6 weeks, if the pace cannot be increased, the exercise prescription is adjusted so as to obtain a training session that lasts from 30 to 60 minutes.

The following points should be emphasized:

1. Exercise diaries should be filled out for each workout, recording distance walked, pace, and any unusual symptoms such as excessive breathlessness, fatigue, or lightheadedness; patients should be taught the significance and interpretation of the latter. Pulse rates before and after exercise should be recorded, and the presence of extrasystoles noted. Any medication changes should also be noted.
2. Accurate pacing and the use of the Borg RPE scale should be stressed.
3. Training should be reduced or stopped during episodes of rejection or infection.

Table 1 Effects of Exercise Training after Cardiac Transplantation: Published Reports

Author	No. of Patients	Exercise Protocol	Training Duration	Physiologic Benefits
Squires et al, 1983	2	Treadmill and stationary cycle, 3× weekly	8 wk	Systolic BP and Borg RPE ↓ at equal submax. workloads
Savin et al, 1983	5	Stationary cycling, 5× weekly	16 wk	Peak work rate ↑, peak O_2 intake ↑, submax. heart rates ↓
Niset et al, 1988	62	Stationary cycling and calisthenics, 3–5× weekly	12 mo	Peak work rate ↑, peak O_2 intake ↑, peak HR ↑, max RER ↓, submax. minute ventilation ↓, blood lactates ↓
Kavanagh et al, 1988	36	Walk/jog, 5× weekly	24 mo	*Resting:* Lean body mass ↑, HR ↓, systolic BP ↓, diastolic BP ↓ *Submax:* HR ↓*, diastolic BP ↓, minute ventilation ↓, RPE ↓ *Maximal:* HR ↑, work rate ↑, O_2 intake ↑, minute ventilation ↑, systolic BP ↑*, diastolic BP ↓
Keteyian et al, 1990	19	Treadmill, stationary cycling, rowing, arm ergometry, stair-stepping, 3× weekly	10 wk	Peak HR ↑, peak work rate ↑, peak O_2 intake ↑, peak minute ventilation ↑, diastolic BP ↓
Keteyian et al, 1991	12 trained; 5 controls	Treadmill, stationary cycling, rowing, arm ergometry, stair-stepping, 3× weekly	10 wk	Peak HR ↑, peak O_2 intake ↑, peak minute ventilation ↑
Ehrman et al, 1992	11	Treadmill, stationary cycling, rowing, arm ergometry, stair-stepping, 3× weekly	8 wk	Peak O_2 intake ↑, peak HR ↑, ventilatory threshold ↑

*Highly compliant patients.

4. As with patients suffering from ischemic heart disease, and in view of the propensity for the donor heart to develop coronary atherosclerosis, advice and counseling should be given regarding smoking, a low-fat diet, and weight control. Close attention should be paid to BP and to lipid and glucose levels.

Initially some patients may need supervision or possibly telemetry during exercise sessions, but these are a minority. Most will be able to train at home without risk, attending a supervised class only once a week, and eventually only once a month. During the first 6 to 12 months there are frequent return visits to the transplant unit or the local hospital for routine follow-up testing, and this gives ample opportunity for the rehabilitation team to carry out exercise testing and to assess the patient's progress and adherence to the training regimen.

BENEFITS OF TRAINING

The benefits of training have been outlined in a number of reports (Table 1). To date, all of the exercise training regimens utilized have been aerobic in type. In view of the fact that peripheral factors may play a large part in the heart transplant patient's deconditioned state, it would seem appropriate to employ a resistance training program, in conjunction with the more usual dynamic exercise program.

RECOMMENDATIONS

Published studies have shown that an exercise rehabilitation program can induce a good training effect, although complete restoration of physiologic function may not be possible. The prescription of exercise must take into account the denervated heart's peculiar response to effort, and must rely on perceived exertion and metabolic measurements rather than on target HRs for defining intensity of training.

The routine use of a comprehensive exercise rehabilitation program following cardiac transplantation is fully justified on physiologic, psychological, and vocational grounds. It is a safe and effective way to maximize the benefits of surgery. It is also tempting to speculate on the favorable effects of a rehabilitation program that includes not only exercise training, but also dietary advice and weight control on: (1) the incidence and severity of post-transplant coronary atherosclerosis, (2) the extent and degree of post-transplantation hypertension, and (3) the incidence of bouts of intercurrent infection and rejection in the immunosuppressed patient.

SUGGESTED READING

Ehrman J, Keteyian S, Fedel F, et al. Ventilatory threshold after exercise training in orthotopic heart transplant patients. J Cardiopul Rehabil 1992; 12:126–130.

Kavanagh T. Exercise and therapy of the cardiac transplant patient. In: Miller HS, ed. Exercise and the heart in health and cardiac disease. New York: Marcel Dekker, 1991.

Kavanagh T, Yacoub M, Campbell R, Mertens D. Marathon running after cardiac transplantation: a case report. J Cardiopul Rehabil 1986; 6:16–20.

Kavanagh T, Yacoub MH, Mertens DJ, et al. Cardiorespiratory responses to exercise training after orthotopic cardiac transplantation. Circulation 1988; 77:162–171.

Kavanagh T, Yacoub MH, Mertens DJ, et al. Exercise rehabilitation after heterotopic cardiac transplantation. J Cardiopul Rehabil 1989; 9:303–310.

Kaye MP. The registry of the International Society for Heart and Lung Transplantation: Tenth official report – 1993. J Heart Lung Transplant 1993; 12:541–548.

Keteyian S, Ehrman J, Fedel F, Rhoads K. Heart rate-perceived exertion relationship during exercise in orthotopic heart transplant patients. J Cardiopul Rehabil 1990; 10:287–293.

Keteyian S, Shepard R, Ehrman J, et al. Cardiovascular responses of heart transplant patients to exercise training. J Appl Physiol 1991; 70:2627–2631.

Niset G, Cousty-Degré C, Degré S. Psychosocial and physical rehabilitation after heart transplantation: 1-year follow-up. Cardiology 1988; 75:311–317.

Savin WM, Gordon E, Green S, et al. Comparison of exercise training effects in cardiac denervated and innervated humans. J Am Coll Cardiol 1983; 1:722.

Squires RW, Arthur PR, Gau GT, et al. Exercise after cardiac transplantation: a report of two cases. J Cardiac Rehabil 1983; 3:570–574.

EXERCISE AND OPTIMIZATION OF LIPID PROFILE

J. LARRY DURSTINE, Ph.D.

Recent advances in the understanding of lipid and lipoprotein metabolism have taken place. Much of this new knowledge comes from a better understanding of the interactions between the various lipoproteins and the many environmental and genetic factors that influence lipid and lipoprotein synthesis and catabolism. These factors alter the lipoprotein metabolic pathways and ultimately lipoprotein composition. Some of the factors to be considered include gender, age, body fat distribution, dietary composition, cigarette smoking, medication use, and routine participation in physical activity. Intervention programs, such as regular involvement in physical activity, can have an impact on blood lipid and lipoprotein composition and reduce the risk of developing premature cardiovascular disease. This chapter focuses on lipoprotein metabolism, physical activity, factors related to exercise, and the quantity of physical activity necessary to induce a favorable change in lipoprotein composition in normal and hyperlipoproteinemic persons.

LIPOPROTEIN METABOLISM

Since lipids are not soluble in an aqueous solution, they must combine with various apolipoproteins and form micelle lipid-protein complexes or lipoproteins for movement throughout the body. The resulting molecules are round in shape, have measurable dimensions, and contain triglyceride (TG), phospholipid, various apolipoproteins, and free and esterified cholesterol. Although several lipoprotein classification systems exist, separation into different gravitational density ranges by ultracentrifugation is the most common approach. The prominent lipoprotein classes include chylomicron, derived from intestinal absorption of exogenous TG; very-low-density lipoprotein (VLDL or pre-β-lipoprotein), derived from the liver for the transport of endogenous TG; low-density lipoprotein (LDL or β-lipoprotein), representing a final stage in the catabolism of VLDL; and high-density lipoprotein (HDL or α-lipoprotein), involved in the reverse transport of cholesterol. Several other lipoprotein subfractions exist and in recent years have received attention regarding a person's risk of developing premature coronary artery disease (CAD). These subfractions include intermediate-density lipoprotein (IDL), an intermediate step in VLDL catabolism, lipoprotein(a) [Lp(a)] situated within the upper density range of LDL, and two separate HDL subfractions: HDL_2 and the more dense HDL_3 (for a detailed description of these lipoprotein classes see Table 1).

Movement of lipids such as cholesterol and TG between the intestine, liver, and extrahepatic tissue is completed by a complex transport system with plasma lipoproteins as the prominent element. Accordingly, several lipoprotein metabolic pathways have been characterized. One sequence of steps is defined for the delivery of cholesterol to extrahepatic tissue. This is termed the *LDL receptor pathway*, whereas the sequence of steps for returning cholesterol from peripheral tissue is described as *reverse cholesterol transport*. Disturbance of these pathways can result in altered plasma lipoprotein profiles and modified CAD risk.

Dietary TG is absorbed by the small intestine, packaged into large chylomicron particles, and released into the vascular system by way of the lymphatic system. In the cardiovascular system, these chylomicron particles react with lipoprotein lipase (LPL): an enzyme that is bound to the capillary wall of most extrahepatic tissue, functions in the removal of TG from the core of chylomicrons and enhances TG uptake into surrounding tissues. The remainder of the molecule forms chylomicron remnants that are metabolized by the liver. TG synthesized in the liver is packaged into the center of VLDL molecules. These molecules are released into the cardiovascular system, where they react with LPL, forming VLDL remnants and IDL molecules. IDL is the

precursor of LDL particles. The breakdown of VLDL into LDL provides for the direct transport of cholesterol by the LDL receptor pathway. Transfer of LDL cholesterol (LDL-C) to cells is mediated by LDL receptors, located on the surface of most cell types. LDL molecules contain a specific protein (apolipoprotein B-100); this protein enables the cellular LDL receptor to recognize the LDL molecule and bind with it. The LDL receptor and molecule are then internalized into the cell, where the LDL molecule is exposed to lysosomal enzymes. Within the cell, cholesterol is freed from the LDL molecule and is used in metabolic processes such as hormone synthesis and/or the formation of cell membranes. The cholesterol freed within the cell also initiates a negative feedback system, causing a reduction in cellular cholesterol synthesis; it promotes the storage of excess cholesterol and suppresses cellular LDL receptor synthesis, thus preventing further uptake of LDL molecules.

Whereas chylomicrons, VLDL, IDL, and LDL are involved in movement of lipids from the intestine and/or liver to peripheral tissues, HDL is involved in the reverse transport of cholesterol by HDL (HDL-C) from peripheral tissues to the liver, where it is catabolized and excreted into the small intestine as bile salt. After release from the liver or the small intestine and/or formation from LPL catabolism of chylomicrons and VLDL, HDL generally reacts quickly with the enzyme lecithin:cholesterol acyltransferase (LCAT). This enzyme esterifies and internalizes free cholesterol into the core of an HDL_3 particle. The action of LCAT and the movement of cholesterol into the HDL_3 core enhances the development of a chemical gradient, leading to continual uptake of cholesterol by the HDL_3 molecule. As the center of the HDL_3 particle expands from lipid accumulation, the density range of the particle shifts to that of the less dense HDL_2 particle. The resulting HDL_2 molecule continues to expand, but as the core lipid content increases, other enzymatic reactions begin. One reaction is the transfer of cholesteryl ester to chylomicron and VLDL remnants, in exchange for TG. This process is facilitated by the enzyme cholesteryl ester transfer protein (CETP). This enzyme allows the cholesteryl ester that originated by the LCAT reaction to be transferred from HDL_2 to chylomicron and VLDL remnants where it can be moved to the liver for catabolism. At the same time that the cholesteryl ester is transferred to the chylomicron and VLDL remnants, TG is moved from these remnants to the HDL_2 particle. The increased TG content of the HDL_2 provides a good substrate for the liver enzyme hepatic lipase (HL). Thus, the small dense HDL_3 particle that originates in the liver, the intestine and/or by LPL action is altered by LCAT, forming HDL_2. This molecule continues additional processing, mediated by CEPT and HL; in the liver it is transformed back into HDL_3 and released into the circulatory system to commence the process again. At this point there exist several other possible pathways for the removal of HDL-C from the circulation. One pathway involves the direct action of HL, resulting in the uptake

Table 1 Characteristics of Plasma Lipoproteins and Lipids

Lipid/Lipoprotein	Source	Composition						Related to CAD Risk	Desired Fasting Plasma Concentration
		Protein (%)	Total Lipid (%)	Percentage of Total Lipid					
				TG	Phos	Chol Ester	Free Chol		
Chylomicron	Intestine	1–2	98–99	88	8	3	1	+ +	Trace of Chol
VLDL	Major: Liver Minor: Intestine	7–10	90–93	56	20	15	8	+	<30 mg · dl^{-1} of Chol
IDL	Major: VLDL Minor: Chylomicron	11	89	29	26	34	9	+	Trace of Chol
LDL	Major: VLDL Minor: Chylomicron	21	79	13	28	48	10	+ + +	<130 mg · dl^{-1} of Chol*
HDL$_2$	HDL$_2$	33	67	16	43	31	10	– –	(HDL$_2$ plus HDL$_3$)
HDL$_3$	Major: Liver and Intestine Minor: VLDL and Chylomicron Remnants	57	43	13	46	29	6	– –	>45 mg · dl^{-1} of Chol*
Chol	Liver and Diet		100			70–75	25–30	+ + +	<200 mg · dl^{-1} of Chol
TG	Liver and Diet		100	100				+ +	<150 mg · dl^{-1} of TG

*Values are for cholesterol associated each lipoprotein.
CAD = Coronary Artery Disease; Phos = Phospholipid; TG = Triglyceride; Chol = Cholesterol; + = Positively Related to CAD; – = Negatively Related to CAD.

of blood HDL-C and transfer to the liver cholesterol pool. Another pathway is hepatic apolipoprotein E receptor mediated removal of HDL. Essentially, large HDL_2 particles rich with cholesteryl ester and containing apolipoprotein E are withdrawn from the circulation by liver LDL receptor mediated endocytosis. Presently, additional research is necessary to delineate the precise conditions necessary for each of these processes to take place.

Although environmental factors affect lipoprotein metabolism and composition, genetic factors also play a role in determining blood lipid and lipoprotein composition. Generally, when genetic factors are implicated, an elevation of blood lipid and lipoprotein concentrations can result. Terms such as dyslipidemia, hyperlipidemia, hypertriglyceridemia, hypercholesterolemia, and hyperlipoproteinemia are often used to describe these conditions. A clear distinction should be drawn between these several terms. Dyslipidemia is a broad term used to describe any of the following conditions. Hyperlipidemia indicates pathologically elevated blood lipids, including TG and cholesterol. Hypertriglyceridemia denotes only a pathologically elevated TG level, whereas hypercholesterolemia implies only a pathologically elevated blood cholesterol. Hyperlipoproteinemia or dyslipoproteinemia denotes pathologically elevated lipoproteins. Hyperlipoproteinemia is either associated with genetic abnormalities or is secondary to an underlying disease such as diabetes mellitus, renal insufficiency, hypothyroidism, biliary obstruction, dysproteinemia, or nephrotic liver disease. The present system of classification for hyperlipoproteinemias was initially proposed by Fredrickson et al in 1967. This system is based on laboratory measurements of blood lipid and lipoprotein concentrations and does not necessarily define genetic abnormalities or the underlying pathophysiology. Although this original classification of disorders did not consider HDL, subsequent epidemiologic, clinical, and biochemical findings leave little reservation concerning the diagnostic importance of HDL-C. Essentially, six hyperlipoproteinemic phenotypes exist (Type I, IIa, IIb, III, IV, and V). Since hyperlipoproteinemic Types I, III, and V collectively constitute only a small portion of all hyperlipidemic conditions, the principle focus is upon the diagnosis of hypertriglyceridemia (Type IV, defined as elevated VLDL and TG), hypercholesterolemia (Type IIa, defined as increased LDL and cholesterol) and mixed hyperlipidemia (Type IIb, defined as increased LDL, VLDL, cholesterol, and TG). Phenotype, laboratory definitions, and characteristics of these various forms of hyperlipoproteinemia are summarized in Table 2.

LIPIDS, LIPOPROTEINS, AND ENDURANCE EXERCISE

Both cross-sectional and longitudinal research designs have been used to evaluate the effects of physical activity on plasma lipids and lipoproteins. Although cross-sectional designs afford a quick means of studying the effects of regular participation in physical activity, this approach allows little control over such parameters as diet and the volume of exercise training and is often susceptible to large within-subject variations. Consequently, cause-effect relationships are difficult to establish and quantify. Longitudinal designs allow for the control of many factors that affect lipid and lipoprotein metabolism such as diet and the volume of exercise training that has been completed. This type of study is better able to establish and quantify cause-effect relationships. Unfortunately, longitudinal studies are costly and the exercise training volume that can be completed by sedentary subjects after several months is usually lower in longitudinal studies than that reported in cross-sectional or observational studies. In addition, some differences of lipid and lipoprotein metabolism exist between aerobic and resistive physical activity programs. Regardless of these problems, most exercise studies show some modification in plasma lipid and lipoprotein concentrations.

Lipids

Cholesterol

Although some early observational studies reported either lower or higher cholesterol concentrations in physically active individuals when compared to their inactive counterparts, most recent observational and longitudinal studies indicate that physical activity does not effect any change in total plasma cholesterol. This lack of effect seems true, regardless of age or gender. Some studies have reported an inverse relationship between maximal aerobic power and cholesterol concentration, but these relationships cease to exist when the data are adjusted for age and body mass. Consequently, factors such as body mass, the distribution and percentage of body fat, gender, dietary intake, and plasma volume must all be considered when evaluating the effects of physical activity on total plasma cholesterol.

Triglyceride

Regular participation in physical activity is generally associated with lower TG concentrations. This relationship persists even after adjustment of data for age, body mass, gender, and body composition. In some cases endurance athletes have not had significantly lower TG concentrations than inactive controls (especially in women). In these instances, the lack of difference was likely due to lower than average TG values for the inactive comparison group. Following endurance training, TG concentrations are generally reduced. This reduction is related to the pretraining TG concentration and the volume of physical activity completed during the training program. The response is thought to reflect both the immediate effects of a single session of activity as well as the impact of regular participation in physical activity.

Table 2 Hyperlipoproteinemic Characteristics

Phenotype	Definition	Associated with Genetic Conditions	Circumstances Associated with Secondary Hyperlipoproteinemia	Premature CAD Risk	Frequency in Population
Type I	Hyperchylomicronemia and absolute deficiency of LPL Plasma cholesterol normal TG greatly increased	Familial LPL deficiency Apolipoprotein C-II deficiency	Dysglobulinemia, pancreatitis, inadequately controlled diabetes mellitus	Normal?	Very rare
Type IIa	LDL increased Cholesterol greatly increased TG normal	Familial hypercholesterolemia LDL receptor abnormal Familial combined hyperlipidemia	Hypothyroidism, nephrosis, anorexia nervosa, dysglobulinemia	Very elevated	0.1–0.5%
Type IIb	LDL increased VLDL increased Cholesterol increased TG increased	Polygenic hypercholesterolemia Familial hypercholesterolemia Familial combined hyperlipidemia		Elevated	5%
Type III	Floating Beta lipoproteins VLDL increased VLDL-cholesterol to VLDL–TG ratio >0.35 Apo E-II homozygote on isoelectric focusing Cholesterol increased TG increased	Familial dysbetalipoproteinemia	Diabetes mellitus, hypothyroidism, dysglobulinemia	Very elevated	Rare
Type IV	VLDL increased Cholesterol normal or increased TG increased	Familial hypertriglyceridemia Familial combined hyperlipidemia	Glycogen storage disease, hypothyroidism, disseminated lupus, erythematosus, diabetes mellitus, nephrotic syndrome, renal failure, ethanol abuse	Elevated	1.5%
Type V	Chyomicrons and VLDL increased LDL present reduced Cholesterol increased TG greatly increased	Familial hypertriglyceridemia Familial multiple lipoprotein type hyperlipidemia	Poorly controlled diabetes mellitus, glycogen storage disease, hypothyroidism, dysglobulinemia, nephrotic syndrome, pregnancy, estrogen administration (either contraceptive or therapeutic) in women with familial hypertriglyceridemia	Elevated	1%

Lipoproteins

Chylomicrons

Since the postprandial half-life of the chylomicron is less than 5 minutes, chylomicrons are found only in the fasting plasma of persons with an absolute deficiency of LPL. Few studies have evaluated the effect of physical activity on chylomicron metabolism. Observational results indicate that chylomicron clearance after a high-fat meal is faster in highly trained endurance athletes than in inactive controls. LPL activity is increased in conjunction with this enhanced removal of blood chylomicrons.

VLDL

Both the cholesterol and the TG associated with the VLDL molecule are reduced after exercise training. The mechanism responsible could be catabolism of TG, a reduced hepatic synthesis and release into the circulation, or some mix of both. Although evidence favors increased catabolism of the VLDL molecule, some indications suggest a reduced hepatic synthesis of VLDL. When catabolism of the VLDL molecule is evident, it is most likely a result of increased LPL action. The mechanisms for reduced TG synthesis remains unclear.

LDL and Subfractions

Results from observational and longitudinal endurance training studies have reported that LDL-C concentrations are either lower than or similar to inactive controls. When LDL-C concentrations are lower, the change usually ranges between 3% and 8%, being inversely related to the volume of exercise that has been completed. As was true with total cholesterol, exercise training could result in weight loss, plasma volume expansion, or an altered dietary intake, and all of these variables must be considered when reductions in LDL-C occur after exercise training.

There are at least three LDL subspecies within the LDL classification: the small LDL molecule, the large LDL molecule, and the IDL molecule. The smaller apolipoprotein B rich LDL and IDL particles have particular atherogenic characteristics. Few exercise studies have been completed in this area. Unfortunately, the results of observational and longitudinal studies do not agree. Observational results indicate that the mass of small LDL particles is significantly lower in runners, with no differences in the mass of the larger LDL and IDL particles. Since endurance runners have smaller LDL particle mass, their risk of premature CAD would be reduced. Unfortunately, longitudinal endurance training studies do not indicate any changes in these subfractions. The explanation may be in the volume of training completed. After 1 year of participating in a longitudinal study subjects completed a training volume of approximately 13 to 16 km/week. This volume of work is less than the work completed (approximately 64 km/week) by runners from the observational study.

HDL and Subfractions

HDL-C is inversely associated with a risk of developing CAD prematurely. In addition, this lipoprotein displays a strong relationship with regular exercise. Nearly all cross-sectional studies have observed a positive correlation between the performance of endurance exercise and a higher HDL-C concentration (usually a 20% to 30% increase over controls) is rather consistent. Furthermore, a dose-response relationship between the volume of exercise completed and the change in HDL-C concentration has been implied. When the HDL-C subfractions (HDL_2-C and HDL_3-C) have been reported, the increase in HDL-C has been attributed to an increased HDL_2-C, without significant change in HDL_3-C. The findings from longitudinal endurance training studies have not been as consistent. Approximately one-half of the exercise training studies have reported no change in HDL-C concentrations. Presently, there are no clear explanations for this inconsistency. Likely explanations include the length of the training period, the volume of training completed, changes in body composition, dietary intake, weight loss, and the pretraining HDL-C concentration.

HDL subfractions can be measured in several ways: the specific lipid component of each subfraction (i.e., HDL_2-C and HDL_3-C), the specific mass of each HDL_2 and HDL_3 particle, or by (use of nondenaturing polyacrylamide gradient gel electrophoresis) the fractionation of HDL_2 into two specific particles (HDL_{2a} and HDL_{2b}) and of HDL_3 into three particles (HDL_{3a}, HDL_{3b}, HDL_{3c}). Various associations between these HDL subclasses have been described including an inverse relation between HDL_{2a} and HDL_{2b}. In addition, HDL_{3b} is positively related to a risk of premature CAD. Presently, only one longitudinal exercise training study has evaluated these subfractions. The effects of weight-loss, induced by diet or exercise, were evaluated during a 1 year period in moderately overweight men. After adjustment of the data for weight-loss, HDL_{2b} was significantly decreased only in the exercisers. Further investigations are necessary in this area, but these results support the beneficial effects of routine physical activity on plasma lipoproteins and the reverse transport of cholesterol.

Lipoprotein(a)

While Lp(a) and LDL have similarities in structure and composition, Lp(a) is more dense than LDL and has apolipoprotein(a) bound by covalent disulphide bonds to apolipoprotein B-100. Human plasminogen and the amino acid sequence of this apolipoprotein are strikingly similar, and this likeness has led many to speculate that Lp(a) may mimic plasminogen and interfere with the fibrinolytic functions of plasminogen and/or plasmin, thus fostering thrombotic events. Consequently, Lp(a) has been associated with an increased CAD risk. Since present knowledge suggests that Lp(a) is a heritable trait and not metabolically linked with LDL, intervention programs that modify plasma LDL concentrations usually have no effect on Lp(a) values.

Few studies have been completed, but the available results from observational and longitudinal exercise studies support the premise that physical activity has little or no effect on Lp(a).

Enzymes

Enzymes are involved in the breakdown of lipid-rich lipoproteins (LPL action), in the conversion of HDL_2 to HDL_3 (HL and LCAT action) and in the transfer of lipids from one lipoprotein class to another lipoprotein class (CETP action). Most observational and longitudinal exercise studies have reported higher LPL activity among individuals routinely involved in physical activity. Cross-sectional studies of active and inactive subjects have observed lower HL activity in active subjects. However, these differences did not persist after adjustment of the data for adiposity. The results from longitudinal exercise studies are contradictory with either reductions or no change in HL activity being reported. Nevertheless, when HL activity failed to change significantly during a trial, HL was still correlated negatively with the change in HDL_2-C concentration. LCAT activity has consistently been higher in active than in inactive groups, whereas longitudinal exercise studies have reported either no change or only slight increases in LCAT activity in physically active groups. Evaluation of the effects of exercise on CETP activity has only recently begun. One cross-sectional study observed higher CETP activity in runners and cyclists than in inactive controls. Nonetheless, another recent longitudinal study found lower CETP concentrations in men and women completing a 9 or 12 month endurance training program despite an increase in HDL-C. CETP concentrations were decreased, whether or not weight loss occurred, and the results showed no significant correlation with lean body mass or body fat.

Findings from these various studies generally support the beneficial effects of physical activity in reducing blood lipids and/or the redistribution of blood lipids among the lipoproteins. Many of these enzyme adaptations support an increased reverse cholesterol transport in persons who are regularly involved in physical activity. Furthermore, these results provide insight into likely explanations regarding previous observations of lipoprotein profiles after exercise training. Chylomicron and TG removal was enhanced as a result of increased LPL activity, and in some cases reverse cholesterol transport was enhanced as a result of increased CETP activity when decreased or no change in HDL-C concentration was reported.

LIPIDS, LIPOPROTEINS, AND RESISTANCE EXERCISE

The use of resistance exercise training has become more prevalent in recent years. However, observational and longitudinal studies relative to lipid and lipoprotein changes have been inconsistent. There are many reasons for these contradictions including small sample sizes,

lack of distinction between various resistance training programs (powerlifting, Olympic weight lifting and body building), failure to account for anabolic steroid use, and changes in plasma volume, body composition, or dietary composition. Because of these confounding influences, it is difficult to draw conclusions from much of this early work. Nevertheless, recent published studies have taken greater care to develop appropriate experimental designs, and as a result have established the benefits of regular participation in resistance exercise programs and its effect on lipoprotein metabolism. Recent studies employed programs of low resistance and a high number of repetition (8 to 16) per set with short rest periods (50 to 80 seconds) between exercises. This type of protocol mimics endurance exercise training more closely than does powerlifting and is thus more likely to improve the lipid and lipoprotein profile. Since the energy requirements during resistance training are lower than those imposed by endurance exercise, adaptations to lipid and lipoprotein metabolism in response to resistance training tend to be less than those found after endurance training. Some early resistance training studies found changes in TG, cholesterol, LDL-C, and HDL-C concentrations, but they failed to correct for such factors as plasma volume expansion and alterations in body composition. Recent published longitudinal studies have found no changes in plasma lipids and lipoprotein concentrations after resistance training.

OTHER FACTORS RELATED TO EXERCISE AND OPTIMIZATION OF THE LIPID AND LIPOPROTEIN PROFILE

Dietary Intake and Weight Loss

Reductions in the dietary intake of lipids and restricted energy intake resulting in weight loss does aid in the lowering of blood lipids and lipoproteins. Lipid and lipoprotein concentrations can be changed by a reduction in total dietary intake of energy, cholesterol, the percentage of fat ingested relative to other nutrients, and the type of fat ingested. Reductions in dietary fat indirectly affect plasma cholesterol by decreasing hepatic cholesterol levels. The outcome is an increase in the number of and/or activity of hepatic LDL receptors, and an augmented hepatic uptake of LDL-C that would elicit a lower total plasma cholesterol concentration. Reductions in dietary fat and increases in dietary carbohydrate can reduce HDL-C and increase TG concentrations. These dietary responses for HDL-C and TG are diminished when accompanied by physical activity. Weight loss as a result of a restricted intake of food energy is negatively associated with total cholesterol and LDL-C concentrations and HL activity, and is positively associated with HDL-C and HDL_2-C concentrations. A restriction of energy intake has been associated with reduced HDL-C concentrations in obese women, whereas in distance runners HDL-C concentrations are augmented by dietary restriction. Consequently, reductions in dietary fat and a reduced energy intake resulting in weight loss should optimize changes in lipid and lipoprotein profiles when combined with increased physical activity.

Medications

A number of medications affect lipid and lipoprotein concentrations. Beta blockers with the exception of those with intrinsic sympathomimetic activity (ISA) increase TG concentrations and reduce HDL-C concentrations. Oral contraceptives tend to increase levels of serum cholesterol, but this effect is a function of the relative amounts of estrogen and progesterone in the various preparations. Progesterone decreases TG as well as HDL-C concentrations. Although their effect on CAD risk is currently under investigation, the use of estrogens, especially in postmenopausal women, tends to raise HDL-C and VLDL TG concentrations, whereas in some cases the use of estrogen by men will reduce HDL-C concentration. Diuretics adversely affect plasma lipid and lipoprotein concentrations primarily by increasing total plasma cholesterol, VLDL-C, LDL-C, and TG concentrations without an effect on HDL-C concentration. Studies of diabetic subjects indicate that plasma TG is reduced and HDL-C concentrations is increased by oral hypoglycemic agents or insulin therapy. Presently, few studies have examined the interaction of these medications with longitudinal exercise training. Some preliminary results suggest that exercise training may attenuate the increased TG concentration and reduced HDL-C concentrations associated with the use of beta-blocking medication. Thus, it is possible that exercise may counteract the effect of some medications.

Hyperlipoproteinemia

Clinical management of dyslipidemic patients reduces CAD morbidity and mortality. Although secondary causes of dyslipidemia should be identified and treated, diet and drug therapy are the mainstay of treatment for lipid and lipoprotein disorders; most professionals would use exercise training as a secondary or a supportive therapy. Drugs have various actions on lipoprotein metabolism: nicotinic acid suppresses VLDL synthesis by the liver; the fibric acid derivatives (gemfibrozil [Lopid] and clofibrate [Atromid]) increase LPL activity and result in an increased catabolism of VLDL and IDL; the bile acid sequestrants (cholestyramine [Questran] and colestipol [Colestid]), the HMG CoA reductase inhibitors, and dextrothyroxine (Choloxin) reduce plasma cholesterol by increasing hepatic LDL receptor activity; and probucol (Lorelco) may increase lipid clearance by the macrophage pathway. Since there are many possible metabolic deficiencies that result in abnormal lipid and lipoprotein profiles, the effect of exercise on such patients may differ substantially from the effect found in patients free of these afflictions. For example, exercise training is unlikely to benefit patients with LPL deficiency, nor will it increase HDL concentration in patients with hypoalphalipoprotein syndrome (an ail-

ment due to an inability to produce normal amounts of alpha lipoprotein). Other than hypertriglyceridemic men (where reductions in TG have been reported) few randomized exercise studies have been completed in patients with dyslipoproteinemia. Thus, the effect of exercise training on other dyslipoproteinemic conditions is unclear. However, if intervention programs that stress a restriction of energy intake, a decreased dietary fat intake, and a reduced body fat and body mass are accompanied by a physical activity program, total plasma cholesterol and LDL-C concentrations should fall, while the HDL-C concentration would either stay the same or increase. If exercise is not included, HDL-C concentration is likely to decrease, and the reduction of TG concentration is less consistently found.

Volume of Physical Activity Necessary for Change

Concern is often expressed regarding the volume of exercise training necessary to produce a change in lipid and lipoprotein concentrations. Since many factors affect lipid and lipoprotein metabolism and many of these factors are interrelated, the issue is complex. Longitudinal exercise training studies suggest there may be an energy expenditure threshold that differs for different lipids and lipoproteins. For example, TG concentrations are lower in hypertriglyceridemic men after just 2 weeks of exercise on consecutive days, whereas the total plasma cholesterol concentration usually remains unchanged even after 1 year of exercise training when the data have been corrected for changes in body mass, body composition, and plasma volume. On the other hand HDL-C concentrations are frequently increased by exercise regimens requiring 4 to 5 megajoules (1,000 to 1,200 kcal) of energy expenditure per week and training is sustained for at least 12 weeks. In addition, a dose–response relationship between exercise and change in HDL-C concentration has been reported. Inactive subjects may also have a lower threshold than physically active persons for change in HDL-C concentration. Although information is limited, inactive individuals who begin moderate physical activity programs (i.e., walking or stationary bicycling) may in time expect a change in blood lipid and lipoprotein metabolism as well as composition.

SUGGESTED READING

Durstine JL, Haskell WL. Effects of exercise-training on plasma lipids and lipoproteins. In: Hollozy JO, ed. Exercise and sport science review. Vol. 22. Baltimore: Williams & Wilkins, 1994:477.

Haskell WL, Durstine JL. Impact of exercise training on lipoprotein metabolism. In: Devlin J, Horton ES, Vranic M, eds. Diabetes mellitus and exercise. Great Britain: Smith-Gordon, 1992:205.

Kokkinos PF, Hurley BF. Strength training and lipoprotein-lipid profiles: a critical analysis and recommendations for further study. Sports Med 1990; 9:266–272.

Shepherd J. Lipoprotein metabolism: An overview. Ann Acad Med 1992; 21:106–113.

Superko HR. Exercise training, serum lipids, and lipoprotein particles: is there a change threshold. Med Sci Sports Exerc 1991; 23:677–685.

Superko HR. Advances in lipoprotein metabolism: applications in the cardiac rehabilitation setting. In: Pashkow FJ, Dafoe WA, eds. Clinical cardiac rehabilitation: a cardiologist's guide. Baltimore: Williams & Wilkins, 1993:196.

Superko HR, Haskell WL. The role of exercise training in the therapy of hyperlipoproteinemia. Cardiol Clin 1987; 5:285–310.

Tall AR. Plasma high density lipoproteins: metabolism and relationship to atherogenesis. J Clin Invest 1990; 86:379–384.

Tikkanen MJ. Plasma lipoproteins and atherosclerosis. J Diabetes Complications 1990; 4:35–38.

EXERCISE-INDUCED BRONCHIAL OBSTRUCTION

KIERAN J. KILLIAN, M.D., F.R.C.P.(C)

Understanding asthma is a prerequisite to the optimal management of exercise-induced bronchial obstruction. Approximately 4% to 12% of the general population experience constriction of airway smooth muscle, hypersecretion from nasal and airway glands, and conjunctival irritation within 5 to 15 minutes of exposure to common allergens such as house dust, animal dander, tree, grass, or ragweed pollen. Bronchoconstriction improves within 1 hour, to be followed in 4 to 6 hours by a bronchoconstriction that is now accompanied by an influx of inflammatory cells with mucosal congestion. The late response is commonly absent in those with a small early response. Individuals afflicted with these responses are known as extrinsic asthmatics. There are other individuals where no allergic responses can be demonstrated who nevertheless react to nonspecific irritants such as dusts, cigarette smoke, and fumes. These individuals are known as intrinsic asthmatics. At one time or other in the course of life, up to 10% of the population suffer from this disability, and persistent life-long affliction is found in up to 5% of people.

PATHOLOGY AND PATHOPHYSIOLOGY

Characteristic pathologic features include a thickening of basement membranes, smooth muscle hypertrophy, and the presence of metachromatic cells and eosinophils in the airways. Characteristic physiologic features include airway hyperresponsiveness with variable airway obstruction. Characteristic clinical features include variable dyspnea with wheezing, itching, sneezing, hypersecretion of mucus, nasal obstruction, and conjunctivitis.

AIRWAY RESPONSIVENESS

Airway responsiveness varies across the population, from relatively unresponsive normal subjects to the highly responsive asthmatic population. The degree of responsiveness is a continuum and any distinction between asthmatics and normals is arbitrary. A cutoff criterion such as a 20% reduction of (forced expired volume over/second) FEV_1 with 8 mg/ml of methacholine for the asthmatic population is helpful, but in evaluating the individual, attention should be focused on the intensity of the stimulus in conjunction with the level of responsiveness. A small stimulus and a high degree of responsiveness is equivalent to a large stimulus and a low level of responsiveness. The propensity to bronchoconstrict in response to all nonspecific stimuli is determined by the magnitude of airway responsiveness. Reducing responsiveness has become the central focus of management, and has primacy over treatment of the bronchoconstrictor response.

The aim of treatment is to reduce the airway responsiveness of the asthmatic, preferably until it lies within the normal range. This is generally achieved by the use of inhaled steroids at a dosage titrated to achieve an acceptable reduction in airway responsiveness, characterized by infrequent bronchoconstriction; this state is recognized by an absence of the characteristic symptoms such as breathing discomfort, accompanied by wheezing and tightness, in association response to specific or nonspecific stimuli. The dosage of inhaled steroid is adjusted to maintain this quasi normalized clinical state. Stopping the inhaled steroid is subsequently possible in some asthmatics.

The exposure to specific allergens with the generation of a late response results in increasing airway responsiveness, sometimes for long periods of time. This requires an increase in the dose of inhaled steroid to reduce responsiveness back to an appropriate level. Similar increases in responsiveness follow certain viral infections of the upper and lower airway. Effective management includes avoidance of allergen, protection of the airway where exposure cannot be avoided using Sodium Chromoglycate, and readjustment of the dose of inhaled steroid to bring airway responsiveness within the normal range. During severe exacerbations, systemic steroids are required at a dosage titrated to reverse the bronchoconstrictor response quickly; the usual requirement is 30 to 40 mg prednisone per day. However, the dose of systemic steroid therapy should be high and adequate rather than low and ineffective. There are few side effects to short-term systemic steroid therapy and a very high dose may be needed in some asthmatics.

MEASUREMENT OF AIRWAY RESPONSIVENESS

Airway responsiveness may be estimated clinically from the magnitude of exposure required to induce symptoms. However, it is difficult to assess the amount of dust, smoke, fumes, or exercise required to induce asthma. The precise measurement requires the inhalation of incrementally increasing doses of methacholine, until the forced expired volume measured over 1 sec (FEV_1) declines by 20% from its baseline value. The methacholine may be delivered as a single breath or more commonly by a nebulizer during 2 minutes of quiet breathing. The dose is doubled every 5 minutes, until the measured FEV_1 has declined by 20% relative to the response seen with a control inhalation of phosphate buffered saline. The doses used range from 0.03 to 256 mg/ml. In most of the general population, a 20% reduction in the FEV_1 cannot be achieved by 256 mg/ml. Such subjects are clearly unresponsive. Most subjects recognized as asthmatic have a 20% reduction in FEV_1 at a dosage of less than 8 mg/ml methacholine, they are clearly responsive. Between 8 and 256 mg/ml, the subjects require a high intensity challenge to cause the airways to react. Subjects with a methacholine PC20 of < 2 mg/ml commonly experience exercise-induced asthma. With a methacholine PC20 > 2 mg/ml, exercise-induced asthma is less common and is usually seen only with more extreme bouts of exercise or unfavorable conditions such as cold and dry air.

NATURE OF EXERCISE-INDUCED ASTHMA

The inspired air must be conditioned, so that when it reaches the alveoli the air contains 6% water and is warmed to 37°C. These conditions, mandatory to protecting the alveolar surfaces against desiccation and cooling, are achieved by transfer of heat and water from the conducting airways to the inspired air. The magnitude of the required conditioning is proportional to the magnitude of ventilation, and to the temperature and water content of inspired air. Cooling and drying of the airway is a nonspecific stimulant, causing the airways to bronchoconstrict. The extent of any exercise-induced asthma depends on the magnitude of ventilation, the condition of the inspired air, temperature and dryness, and the magnitude of airway responsiveness. Failure to demonstrate exercise-induced asthma formally in a laboratory setting is common, because the protocols for the demonstration of exercise-induced asthma vary from laboratory to laboratory with a corresponding variation in the stimulus to bronchoconstriction. The intensity of ventilation may not be sufficiently high to provoke a response; the inspired air is also commonly warm; and the humidity is commonly high. Failure to demonstrate exercise-induced asthma in the laboratory does not exclude exercise-induced asthma. The measurement of nonspecific airway responsiveness to methacholine is an alternative, because this technique is carefully standardized, reproducible, and reliable in most laboratories. However, measurement of the response to both methacholine and exercise is the ideal.

CLINICAL PRESENTATION OF EXERCISE-INDUCED ASTHMA

Classically, exercise is accompanied by a bronchodilator response, mediated by poorly defined neural responses and local mediators. Bronchodilation persists into the immediate postexercise period. There is then a bronchoconstrictor response, beginning approximately 5 minutes after the completion of exercise. The bronchoconstrictor response is maximal at 10 minutes postexercise and regresses over the subsequent hour. Repeat bouts of exercise lead to an attenuation of the response. With sustained exercise, the bronchodilator responses that are seen early in exercise recede and bronchoconstriction may be seen during the period of exercise itself. Many asthmatics note subtle difficulties with breathing during exercise. Experimentally, asthmatics detect very small changes in airway caliber before the usual decline in spirometric measurements (peak flow rates or the FEV_1).

MANAGEMENT OF EXERCISE-INDUCED ASTHMA

The patient is encouraged to exercise in a manner conducive to her or his selected lifestyle. The central focus of management is an educated patient, with a thorough understanding of the mechanism of asthma in general and of exercise-induced asthma in particular. The patient should be in control of management and have access to all appropriate medication, including systemic steroids. Pharmacologic interventions are taken to normalize function and to reduce any expected responses. The first goal is to decrease the level of nonspecific airway responsiveness. This reduces the propensity to and frequency of exercise-induced asthma. Formal skin testing against known allergens is essential if relevant allergens are to be avoided. Continuous exposure to allergens, particularly household pets, is heavily discouraged in the event of positive skin test responses. A reduction in allergen exposure reduces airway responsiveness. If transient and occasional contact with an allergen cannot be avoided, the airway should be protected during such exposure, using Sodium Chromoglycate repeated in adequate dosage every 4 hours throughout exposure. Protection with beta-adrenergic agents such as salbutamol should be avoided, because of the danger of intense exposure and the risk of severe late responses, which are less amenable to correction. Following viral infections, the dose of inhaled steroid is increased, because increases in airway responsiveness are to be anticipated. Early and adequate treatment of any exacerbations of asthma are advised; systemic steroids may be required if the condition appears severe.

The specific treatment of exercise-induced asthma requires that treatment be initiated prior to exercising. No medication is superior to the prophylactic use of a beta-adrenergic agent such as salbutamol, fenoterol, or terbutaline. The patient should be aware that the duration of the bronchodilator response does not necessarily coincide with airway protection from exercise-induced asthma. The period of protection may be as little as half the duration of the bronchodilator response. Increasing the dose of the beta-agonist will increase the period of protection, but repeated dosage may be required if the period of exercise is particularly prolonged. Where beta-adrenergic agents cannot be used, Sodium Chromoglycate may be substituted. It is effective, but the dose required varies from asthmatic to asthmatic (20 mg is the recommended dose for exercise-induced asthma). For patients with severe exercise-induced asthma a combination of beta-adrenergic agents with Sodium Chromoglycate may be an effective treatment. Anecdotal reports suggest that the addition of anticholinergic agents may also be useful, but these cannot as yet be firmly recommended. Sedating antihistamines, delivered by the unusual route of inhalation, have some limited benefit. All medication should be given by inhalation in preference to oral administration. By following this approach, most patients with exercise-induced asthma can be effectively managed.

SUGGESTED READING

Anderson SD. Drugs and the control of exercise-induced asthma. Eur Respir J 1993; 6:1090–1092.

Anderson SD, Schoeffel RE, Black JL, Daviskas E. Airway cooling as the stimulus to exercise-induced asthma: A re-evaluation. Eur J Respir Dis 1985; 67:20–30.

Bar-Yishay E, Godfrey S. Exercise-induced asthma. In Weiss EB, Stein M, eds. Bronchial asthma: Mechanisms and therapeutics. 3rd Ed. Boston: Little Brown, 1993:612.

EXERCISE RECONDITIONING IN PATIENTS WITH CHRONIC AIRFLOW LIMITATION

DENIS E. O'DONNELL, M.D., F.R.C.P.(I), F.R.C.P.(C), F.C.C.P.
KATHERINE A. WEBB, M.Sc.

Despite welcome trends in reduced tobacco consumption, chronic airflow limitation (CAL) due to chronic bronchitis and emphysema remains a major cause of disability and death and is one of the most important causes of work incapacity and restricted activity in the industrialized world. Since CAL is essentially irreversible in its advanced stages, prevention is of paramount importance. For those patients with established disease, management strategies at present focus largely on halting functional decline. Pharmacotherapy, although useful for relieving breathlessness, does not halt the rate of decline of dynamic expiratory flow rates with time in CAL. Regular exercise conditioning has been advocated as a counter measure to increasing functional disability in CAL for many years. The simple rationale behind this recommendation is that such a measure would effectively break the vicious cycle of reduced habitual activity, global skeletal muscle deconditioning, and progressive exertional breathlessness with curtailed exercise capacity. In this chapter, we outline our experience with exercise reconditioning in CAL with particular reference to the efficacy of this modality as an adjunct to patient management.

BRIEF OVERVIEW OF THE LITERATURE

Research into the effect of exercise training in CAL has focused primarily on the physiologic rationale for the intervention. Interpretation of the literature is confounded by: (1) a paucity of prospective randomized controlled studies, (2) small study sample sizes, (3) variability in the mode, frequency, duration, and intensity of training regimens, (4) uncertainty with respect to the clinical stability of patients at the onset of training, (5) variability in disease severity and the existence of comorbid conditions among study patients, and (6) failure to consider subjective outcome parameters.

On surveying the literature, it is clear that patients with CAL can attain physiologic training effects similar to those seen in sedentary healthy normal individuals, although training responses are less consistently observed in patients with more advanced disease. Reported cardiovascular training effects in CAL include decreases in resting heart rates (HR) and HRs at standardized submaximal work rates, with concomitant increases in stroke volume (SV). However, evidence for associated cytochemical alterations in the peripheral muscles is sparse in CAL. Reductions in mean resting pulmonary arterial and systemic blood pressures have also been reported. Improvements in maximal oxygen consumption ($\dot{V}O_2$max) and aerobic capacity have been found in some studies but not in others. Finally, reductions in ventilatory requirements at a standardized submaximal work rate have been variously reported. In one study, such a reduction was shown to be associated with a diminished lactate load after training.

Regardless of the controversy over the physiologic rationale for training, there is general agreement that most patients with CAL who undergo supervised exercise training will benefit in terms of improved symptomatology and exercise performance. The safety of exercise training, even in elderly patients with chronic ventilatory insufficiency, is firmly established.

FACTORS LIMITING EXERCISE IN CAL

Recently, we systematically examined the factors contributing to exercise limitation in 125 consecutive patients entering our exercise training program (Table 1). The majority of patients (66%) stopped exercise because of breathlessness well before they had reached the physiologic boundaries of their maximal ventilatory or circulatory capacities. Patients who stopped primarily because of breathlessness had significantly greater airflow obstruction (a reduced forced expired volume in one second [FEV_1]). It is noteworthy that 30% of the sample stopped exercise, either entirely or partially, because of a high intensity of perceived leg effort. In patients with less severe disease, perception of heightened leg effort or fatigue has been recognized as the most frequently encountered symptom limiting exercise. Given this information, it follows that any intervention that reduces the intensity of perceived leg effort or breathlessness should improve exercise capacity in CAL. Since improvement in exercise capacity is an important goal in deconditioned patients, some understanding of the source and mechanisms of the symptoms that limit exercise is required if this goal is to be achieved.

Mechanisms of Breathlessness in CAL

The precise neurophysiologic origins of breathlessness in CAL remain unknown. However, the circumstances under which breathlessness is encountered in CAL are well identified. Breathlessness occurs when: (1) ventilation is increased, (2) the impedances against which the ventilatory muscles must contract are increased, or (3) the ventilatory muscles are functionally weakened. During exercise, all three conditions occur. First, ventilation increases in response to the increased metabolic load. Second, the ventilatory muscles are intrinsically loaded by increased resistance and particularly by elastic loads resulting from dynamic increases in air-trapping. Third, this "dynamic hyperinflation" greatly compromises the ability of the ventilatory muscles to generate pressure and results in functional weakness. The net result is that the ventilatory muscles are forced to operate at a large fraction of their maximal force generating capacity at any given work rate when compared to normals. The major consequence of these adverse mechanical factors (increased loading and weakness) is that the amplitude of central motor command output from the respiratory center must increase greatly in order to maintain ventilation in pace with metabolic demands. It is currently postulated that motor command output can be perceived directly at the cortical level as "sense of effort." There is ample evidence that the sense of inspiratory muscle contractile effort contributes importantly to breathlessness in CAL. There is also evidence that regular exercise training in CAL can reduce ventilatory demands at a given external power output, either by improving aerobic power or increasing mechanical efficiency. This physiologic training effect translates directly into a reduced intensity of breathlessness for a given activity, which in turn leads to an improved exercise capacity.

Mechanisms of Increased Perceived Leg Effort

With the prolonged inactivity that results from exertional breathlessness, demonstrable reductions in static peripheral muscle strength and endurance are common in patients with CAL. Deprived of the conditioning stimulus of regular exercise, skeletal muscles undergo extensive structural and biochemical changes (i.e., reduced protein synthesis and a decreased capacity for oxidative metabolism). In patients with advanced CAL, peripheral muscle function may be further compromised by other problems such as poor nutrition, electrolyte disturbance, steroid myopathy, and chronic hypoxemia. Moreover, during acute exercise, gas-exchange abnormalities and circulatory compromise often lead to a greater reliance on anaerobic metabolism. This results in an acidic environment at the

Table 1 Exercise Limitation in 125 Patients with CAL Entering an Endurance Exercise Training Program

Reason for Stopping Exercise	No. (%)	FEV_1 (%pred)	$\dot{V}_E$ max (%MBC)	HRmax (%pred max)
Breathlessness	83 (66%)	37 ± 1*	72 ± 3	70 ± 1
Leg fatigue	19 (19%)	44 ± 4	68 ± 4	67 ± 2
Both breathlessness and leg fatigue	14 (11%)	50 ± 4	76 ± 5	69 ± 3
Other	9 (4%)	47 ± 4	70 ± 4	76 ± 4
Age-matched normals	10	104 ± 5	75 ± 11	80 ± 4

Values are means ± SEM.
*$p < 0.001$ Significant difference between CAL groups.
See text for abbreviations; pred = predicted; MBC = maximal breathing capacity.

peripheral muscle level at lower work rates than in normal subjects.

Both peripheral muscle deconditioning and abnormal muscle metabolism may ultimately result in a relative lack of responsiveness to neural activation, such that greater motor command output is necessary for a given external power output. As previously discussed, it is currently believed that an increased amplitude of motor output to the skeletal muscles (peripheral and ventilatory) can be appreciated directly as sense of effort. Exercise reconditioning should enhance responsiveness of the peripheral muscle unit by strengthening muscles and, in some instances, by improving aerobic power and hence the metabolic milieu. The resultant reduction in motor command output translates into a decrease in perceived leg effort and an improved exercise tolerance in those limited primarily by this symptom.

EXERCISE RECONDITIONING PROGRAM

The principal objective of exercise training (EXT), in our view, is to ameliorate breathlessness and perceived leg effort and thereby to improve exercise capacity. Our secondary objective is to achieve cardiovascular training effects where possible. The sequence of events within the training program includes: (1) patient selection, (2) patient assessment, (3) the setting of realistic goals for the patient, (3) implementation of an individualized training program, (4) post-program reassessment, (5) development of a home-based exercise regimen, and (6) appropriate follow-up of patients.

Patient Assessment

Patients meeting the selection criteria (Table 2) are assessed by a team consisting of an exercise physiologist, a physiotherapist, and a respirologist. A careful history and physical examination are obtained, with particular emphasis on the evaluation of handicap. The intensity of chronic activity-related breathlessness is assessed by using validated questionnaires. Chronic symptom intensity is scored by an objective observer using the Baseline Dyspnea Index (BDI) and by self-

Table 2 Selection Criteria for the Pulmonary Rehabilitation Candidate

---

Exertional breathlessness
Diminished exercise capacity
Stable pulmonary disease
Optimal bronchodilator medication
Current nonsmoker
No evidence of active:
   Ischemic heart disease
   Musculoskeletal problems
   Neurologic disorders
   Psychiatric illness
Sufficient motivation
Sufficient rehabilitation potential
Practical considerations (time, travel)

---

rated questionnaires such as an oxygen cost diagram. Specific factors that provoke breathlessness are identified so that specific interventions or advice can be offered (Table 3). Each patient's current pharmacotherapy and inhaler technique are carefully evaluated. All prospective participants in our EXT program undertake full pulmonary function testing and, in patients with more severe CAL, resting steady-state gas-exchange is measured. Exercise performance is assessed by the 6 minute walking distance and by cycle ergometry. Ventilatory and peripheral muscle strength and endurance are tested using validated techniques.

Exercise testing is particularly useful in identifying symptom limitations and symptom intensity. In this regard, breathlessness and leg effort are rated using a validated semiquantitative category scale (Borg Scale). The exercise test also allows an assessment of the major physiologic constraints in a particular patient; whether these be ventilatory, circulatory, neuromuscular, or musculoskeletal. In addition, exercise testing permits screening for active ischemic heart disease and oxygen desaturation.

Individualized Exercise Training Program

Before embarking on supervised EXT, every effort is made to optimize bronchodilator therapy (Table 3). Relief of breathlessness can be achieved with various bronchodilators in the presence of only small improvements in forced expiratory volumes or flow rates ($< 15\%$ change in FEV_1). The mechanisms of improvement have not been fully elucidated. In our experience, they are closely linked to reductions in gas trapping and concomitant enhancement of inspiratory muscle function. Preliminary evidence further suggests that the improved exercise tolerance and reduced breathlessness following high-dose anticholinergic therapy and oral theophylline therapy is closely linked to the reduction in thoracic gas volumes in CAL.

The EXT program is a multimodality exercise endurance training program, the ultimate aim of which is to achieve aerobic training of as large a muscle mass as possible. This is achieved through a variety of exercises, including walking, stair climbing, treadmill exercise, cycle ergometry, and weight training of the upper and lower extremities. Details of the exercise prescription are provided in Table 4. Training intensity is individualized and is carefully guided by targeted Borg ratings, based on the results of preliminary exercise testing. Using a graduated, stepwise approach, the patient is encouraged eventually to train at the highest attainable work rate for the longest tolerable duration. Since there is a close linear relationship between Borg ratings and $\dot{V}O_2$, minute ventilation ($\dot{V}_E$) and heart rate (HR), high targeted Borg ratings ensure an adequate training stimulus and correspond to high ventilatory levels, HRs and metabolic loads. We have abandoned traditional training HR targets, as these are less reliable in elderly and CAL populations. The supervised 8 week training program consists of three sessions per week, each session lasting 2 to 3 hours.

Adjuncts to Training

Oxygen Therapy

For patients whose oxygen saturation (SaO_2) falls to less than 90% on exercise, supplemental oxygen is provided to ensure adequate oxygenation ($SaO_2 > 90\%$ or $PaO_2 > 60$ mm Hg). In controlled studies of oxygen versus compressed air, oxygen has been shown to reduce breathlessness and perceived leg effort significantly, thus improving exercise tolerance. The mechanisms of relief of breathlessness are likely multifactorial, but are thought to relate primarily to blunted peripheral chemoreceptor responsiveness during oxygen treatment, or to a reduction in metabolic load ($\dot{V}CO_2$). Both effects result in a reduced ventilatory demand at a given work rate, which in turn is associated with a reduced symptom intensity. In hypoxemic patients, supplemental oxygen also reduces pulmonary vascular resistance, thereby reducing the right ventricular afterload and enhancing cardiac output. The net effect of improving oxygen delivery and/or utilization at the level of the peripheral muscles is that ionic status is favorably altered at this site. Thus, the muscle unit is more responsive to neural activation, and a reduced motor output translates into a reduced perceived leg effort for a given external power output.

Inspiratory Muscle Training

Specific inspiratory muscle training (IMT) has recently been advocated as a means of reducing breathlessness by improving the strength and endurance of

Table 3 Potential Problems to Address while Individualizing the Treatment Plan

Problems	Possible Solutions
Suboptimal pharmacotherapy	• Review inhaler technique and delivery systems • Beta-2 agonists (suggest anticipatory use) • Anticholinergics (try higher dosages) • Oral theophyllines (useful in some) • Steroids (only 10% of patients respond)
Anxiety, respiratory panic	• Counseling • Relaxation techniques • Pursed lip breathing • Anxiolytic therapy
Mucus congestion, morning cough	• Iodinated glycerol
Oxygen desaturation*	• Oxygen treatment • Portable oxygen delivery systems
Reduced muscle strength and/or endurance	• Specific muscle group training
Breathlessness with arm exercise	• Upper limb weight training • Arm ergometry
Inspiratory muscle weakness†	• Specific inspiratory muscle training

*Resting $PaO_2 < 55$ mm Hg (breathing room air), $PaO_2 < 60$ mm Hg when associated with cor pulmonale or polycythemia, or $SaO_2 < 90\%$ during exercise.
†Maximal inspiratory pressure <50% predicted after correcting for lung volume.

Table 4 Guidelines for Exercise Prescription in Patients with CAL

Type of exercise:	Continuous aerobic-type activities involving large muscle groups. Examples include walking, cycling, rowing, stair climbing.
Exercise intensity:	At least 50% of peak exercise capacity. Exercising at, or just below, the point of **symptom-limitation** (i.e., breathlessness, leg fatigue) is preferred since other indices of exercise intensity (i.e., oxygen consumption, HR, ventilation) tend to become more unreliable with advancing age.
Exercise duration:	Start with the maximum tolerable amount of exercise and increase gradually as able. Short intervals of exercise may be performed to complete a total of 20–30 minutes per day. Aim for 20–30 minutes of continuous activity.
Frequency of exercise:	Aim for 3–5 days per week. Maximum benefit is gained with daily exercise.
Exercise progression:	Start with a 10–15 minute **warm-up** consisting of gentle stretching and flexibility exercises and low intensity total body exercises. A **cool-down** of gentle stretching and flexibility exercises should end each exercise session.

A. EXERTIONAL BREATHLESSNESS

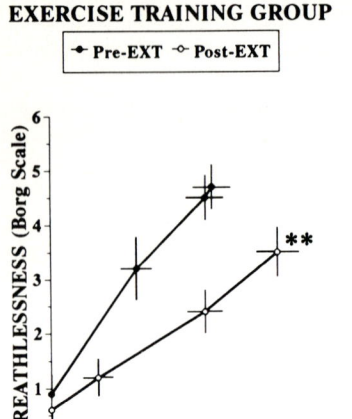

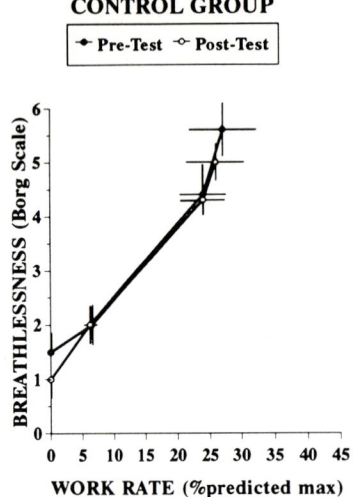

B. PERCEIVED LEG EFFORT

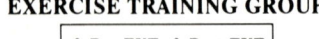
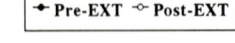

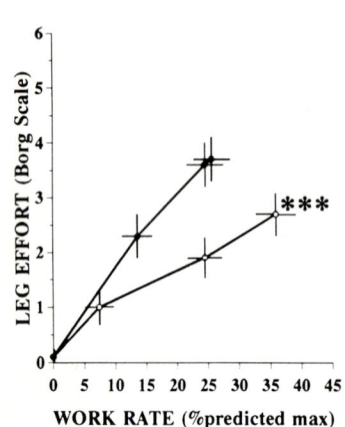

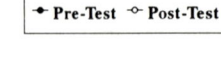
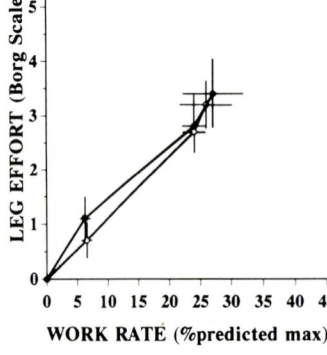

Figure 1 Following EXT, exertional breathlessness and perceived leg effort were significantly reduced while exercise capacity significantly improved in 23 patients with CAL. In a matched group of 13 CAL patients, no changes were noted after a control period without EXT. $**p < 0.01$, $***p < 0.001$ pre-EXT versus post-EXT.

these muscles. However, a recent meta-analysis of available controlled studies of IMT has failed to demonstrate significant objective or subjective improvement in the majority of patients with CAL. These negative results may be explained by the fact that in CAL, the respiratory muscles undergo adaptive structural and biochemical changes in response to long-standing intrinsic mechanical loading (resistive and elastic). This results in a relative preservation of muscle function, at least under resting conditions. Nevertheless, some patients derive benefit from IMT in terms of reduced breathlessness and functional disability. Our practice is to offer specific IMT using an inspiratory threshold loading device to selected patients with demonstrable reductions of static inspiratory muscle strength (maximal inspiratory pressure <50% of predicted normal after correcting for lung volume).

Breathing Retraining

Of all the various breathing retraining techniques, we have found that pursed lip breathing (PLB) has consistently provided the most effective results. PLB is a breathing technique that many patients with advanced CAL adopt spontaneously to relieve breathlessness. Since PLB is particularly useful in relieving breathlessness during the phase of recovery from exercise, we instruct patients in this technique. It is very useful in allaying anxiety and aborting respiratory panic attacks in those so predisposed. The mechanisms of relief of breathlessness during PLB are largely unknown. Reduced dynamic compression of central airways on expiration or improved alveolar ventilation have previously been proposed as relieving mechanisms. We believe that symptom relief is closely linked to reduced thoracic gas trapping (and consequent improved muscle

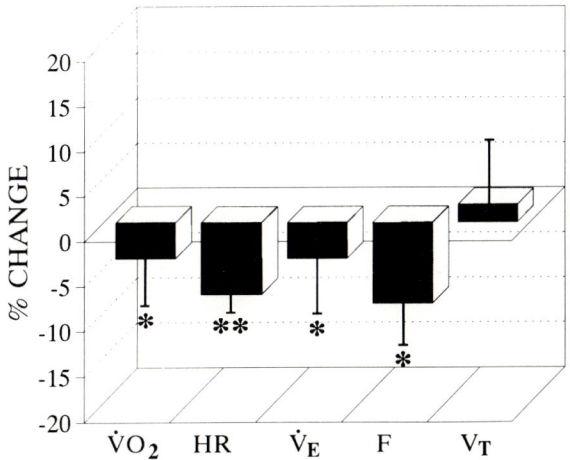

Figure 2 Physiologic training effects were noted at the highest equivalent work rate achieved during cycle exercise testing conducted before and after EXT. Post-EXT, significant ($*p < 0.05$, $**p < 0.01$) improvements were found in efficiency ($\dot{V}O_2$/work rate), heart rate (HR), ventilation ($\dot{V}_E$), and breathing frequency (F), with no change in tidal volume (V_T).

function); this is readily demonstrable in flow limited patients when the expiratory time is greatly prolonged (i.e., > 10 sec).

Educational Program

A structured educational program consisting of 12 2-hour sessions is provided in conjunction with EXT. These sessions consist of didactic, teaching, and group discussions conducted by physiotherapists experienced in every aspect of living with CAL. The course is designed to ensure that the patient is knowledgeable about the disease and its management. It is used to encourage patients to make important life-style modification decisions, such as beginning a regular schedule of home-based exercise.

Our Experience

Improved symptoms following EXT are amply demonstrated in a recent controlled study where we compared ratings of breathlessness using the BDI and a self-rated oxygen cost diagram in 23 patients with severe CAL ($FEV_1 = 38 \pm 2\%$ predicted; mean $\pm$ SEM) and in 13 age-matched control subjects ($FEV_1 = 36 \pm 3\%$ predicted) who did not undergo exercise training. Chronic activity-related breathlessness was significantly ($p < 0.001$) diminished in the training group after EXT. Similarly, Borg ratings of breathlessness and leg effort at a standardized work rate, together with exercise capacity, were significantly improved in trained patients, but not in controls (Fig. 1).

We have consistently observed a number of physiologic training effects following EXT (Fig. 2). Improved exercise capacity has been demonstrated by increased 6

minute walking distances (a 35% increase in 6 minute walking distance was shown in 102 consecutive patients entering our EXT program). Despite this increase, Borg ratings at walking cessation were significantly lower, by 18%. Exercise capacity as measured by endurance time or total cumulative work during cycle ergometry was also consistently increased. Increases in peripheral muscle strength and endurance were readily demonstrated (quadriceps strength increased 24% in 61 patients completing EXT). Improved cardiovascular function was evidenced by reductions in HR at given submaximal work rates (Fig. 2). Reductions in ventilatory demand as a result of improved mechanical efficiency or, less commonly, enhanced aerobic power were also shown (see Fig. 2). The physiologic consequence of EXT that contributed most significantly ($p < 0.05$) to the relief of breathlessness was the reduction in ventilatory requirement. However, improved breathlessness was also undoubtedly related to densensitization to dyspnea and habituation to the unpleasant sensations related to physical activity.

Patient Follow-Up

Supervised exercise training represents the first step in the rehabilitative process. It is imperative that a regular home-based exercise program be maintained so that the benefits of the program are not lost. Patients are provided with an individualized home-based exercise prescription, and follow-up appointments are arranged every 2 months to re-evaluate patient outcomes. The family physician plays a pivotal role in maintaining careful surveillance of the patients' status and in providing encouragement and much needed reinforcement with respect to the need for regular home exercise. Patients are encouraged to purchase treadmills or stationary bicycles for use in the home to assist them in their daily training. Where possible, graduates of the EXT program are advised to participate in self-help group meetings on a weekly basis, so that they can continue to derive psychosocial support in the group setting.

Acknowledgments. We thank Maureen McGuire, BSc, Reg PT, and Lorelei Samis, BSc, Reg PT, for their technical assistance in the Pulmonary Rehabilitation Program, St. Mary's of the Lake Hospital, Kingston, Ontario.

SUGGESTED READING

Carter R, Coast JR, Idell S. Exercise training in patients with chronic obstructive pulmonary disease. Med Sci Sports Exerc 1992; 24: 281–291.

Casaburi R, Patessio A, Ioli F, et al. Reductions in exercise lactic acidosis and ventilation as a result of exercise training in patients with obstructive lung disease. Am Rev Respir Dis 1991; 143:9–18.

Killian KJ, Leblanc P, Martin DH, et al. Exercise capacity and ventilatory, circulatory, and symptom limitation in patients with chronic airflow limitation. Am Rev Respir Dis 1992; 146:935–940.

Mahler DA, O'Donnell DE. Alternative modes of exercise training for pulmonary patients. J Cardiopulm Rehab 1991; 11:58–63.

Mahler DA, Weinberg DH, Wells CK, Feinstein AR. The measurement of dyspnea: contents, interobserver agreement, and physiologic correlates of two new clinical indexes. Chest 1984; 85:751–758.

O'Donnell DE, Webb KA. Exertional breathlessness in patients with chronic airflow limitation: the role of lung hyperinflation. Am Rev Respir Dis 1993; 148:1351–1357.

O'Donnell DE, Webb KA, McGuire MA. Benefits of exercise training in elderly patients with COPD. Geriatrics 1993; 48:59–66.

Paine R, Make BJ. Pulmonary rehabilitation for the elderly. Clin Geriatr Med 1986; 2:313–335.

EXERCISE AND DIABETES

WALTER VAN HELDER, M.D., Ph.D.

The role of exercise in patients with diabetes mellitus has been a topic of much interest for a long time. From the dawn of the art of medicine until the discovery of insulin, exercise and diet were the only possible therapeutic tools to alleviate diabetic symptoms. Exercise was recommended in this capacity by Aristotle as well as by other ancient thinkers. Shortly after the discovery of insulin, Lawrence reported that exercise could potentiate the hypoglycemic effect of insulin. For a long time it was not clear, however, whether exercise was beneficial for insulin-dependent as well as for non-insulin dependent patients. In addition, there was much confusion regarding appropriate types and duration of exercise, and various frequencies and intensities of exercise were prescribed for diabetic patients. A much clearer picture has emerged in the 1990s with respect to the value of exercise therapy in diabetic or prediabetic men and women, although many problems of exercising diabetics have yet to be resolved.

EXERCISE IN NON-INSULIN DEPENDENT DIABETES

It is now generally accepted that an appropriately prescribed exercise regimen benefits non-insulin dependent diabetes mellitus (NIDDM) patients. Numerous studies have reported that regular exercise benefits diabetic patients in several ways. One of the largest studies was conducted in Malmo, Sweden over a 6 year period; it involved approximately 7,000 males in their late forties. The sample included normal, NIDDM, and glucose tolerance impaired subjects. A combination of a controlled diet and regular exercise resulted in an improvement of glucose tolerance, a reduction in hyperinsulinemia, blood lipids, and blood pressure and an increased maximal oxygen uptake. One very important finding of this study was the safety of such carefully prescribed exercise therapy; the mortality was in fact 33% lower in exercising subjects than in the remainder of the cohort. Similar findings of improved glucose tolerance, decreased fasting plasma glucose, and improved aerobic fitness have been reported by a variety of other investigators, using various durations and modes of exercise.

Exercise has also been suggested as a safe and important therapeutic modality in gestational diabetes mellitus (GDM, a carbohydrate intolerance first manifested during pregnancy). The introduction of an exercise program can sometimes entirely eliminate the need for insulin in GDM. A less clear picture exists in the case of geriatric patients with NIDDM. Although exercise can induce weight loss, reduce stress and cholesterol levels, and improve cardiac functional status, it may or may not increase glucose tolerance and insulin sensitivity in elderly patients. Nonetheless, exercise has become an important therapeutic modality in general NIDDM population. It is believed that exercise confers additional beneficial effects on glycemic control beyond what might be anticipated from the improvement in physical fitness itself. Other important consequences of the prescribed exercise include weight loss, enhanced cardiovascular function, psychosocial benefits, and the prevention of a wide range of other diseases.

The physician must nevertheless also consider the potential risks of exercise, which are much more likely to occur in patients with severe or uncontrolled NIDDM: cardiac ischemia and arrhythmias, extensive increases of blood pressure during exercise, retinal haemorrhage, a worsening of hyperglycemia, and foot ulcers.

Patients with NIDDM should receive a careful clinical examination by their physician before beginning what should preferably be a custom-designed exercise program. Particular attention should be paid to the possibility of problems arising from coexisting cardiovascular or neurologic disease. The prescribed exercise should be continuous, aerobic activity carried out at 50% to 60% of the individual's maximal oxygen intake for 20 to 60 minutes on 3 to 5 days per week. The exercise should be as enjoyable as possible, in order to increase compliance with the regimen. Prolonged periods of boring and repetitive exercise should be avoided. Proper footwear should be used to avoid the Nemesis of diabetic athletes—ulceration of the foot—and the feet should be inspected daily for any signs of injury or infection.

EXERCISE IN INSULIN DEPENDENT DIABETICS

The evidence that exercise improves glycemic control in insulin dependent diabetes (IDDM) is not conclusive, despite some reports that it may improve insulin sensitivity and decrease insulin requirements.

This may be because many confounding factors play a role in glucose control when IDDM patients exercise. These include exaggerated glucogenic hormonal responses in IDDM. For instance, growth hormone opposes (counter-regulates) the action of insulin, and counter-regulatory hormones such as growth hormones, cortisol, and glucagon are released in differing amounts during various types of exercise (aerobic vs anaerobic and continuous vs intermittent activity), despite a matching of average power output and total duration. However, exercise is recommended for IDDM patients and even participation in competitive sports is possible if certain precautions are observed. Self-monitoring of blood glucose is very important and a proper adjustment (usually a decrease) of the injected insulin is required if hypoglycemia is not to result. The biggest benefits of exercise for IDDM patients are usually an improvement of cardiovascular fitness, psychosocial well-being, and the sense of personal achievement. The potential risks, in addition to those mentioned earlier in the section regarding NIDDM, are, among others: hypoglycemic episodes, higher than average risks of diabetic nephropathy and neuropathy, and proliferative retinopathy. Patients should always carry a quick-acting supply of carbohydrate (such as a candy bar) and consideration should be given to the use of multiple doses of a shorter-acting insulin preparation, since the variable absorption of intermediate or longer-acting insulin during exercise is much less predictable. The injection of insulin into the part of the body that will be involved in exercise is to be avoided. An extra intake of food energy may be needed to compensate for the additive and combined actions of injected insulin and exercise. Without such an increase, a further decrease of blood glucose levels is likely. Even people with diabetic complications may benefit from regular exercise, provided it is individualized, closely monitored by a specialist, and designed as a part of the whole therapeutic regimen with the interplay of medications, life-style, and diet.

RECOMMENDATIONS

Exercise is generally recommended for all classes of diabetic patients, provided that their individual condition does not preclude it. Exercise is indeed one of the most important therapeutic modalities in the treatment of diabetes. However, the type, duration, intensity, and regimen of exercise have a large influence on whether the prescribed exercise will be beneficial or detrimental to the diabetic individual. Going one step further, exercise that improves insulin-stimulated glucose uptake in normal human subjects can possibly prevent or postpone the onset of diabetes mellitus.

SUGGESTED READING

American Diabetes Association. Diabetes mellitus and exercise. Diabetes Care 1990; 13:804–805.
Cross MC, VanHelder WP, VanHelder T, Radomski MW. Growth hormone responses and sympathetic activity during heavy resistance exercise. Eur J Appl Physiol, in press.
Eriksson KF, Lindgarde F. Prevention of Type 2 (non-insulin-dependent) diabetes mellitus by diet and physical exercise. Diabetologia 1991; 34:891–898.
Graham C, Lasko-McCarthey P. Exercise options for persons with diabetic complications. Diabetes Educ 1992; 16:212–220.
Lawrence RD. The effects of exercise on insulin action in diabetes. Br Med J 1926; 1:648–650.
Reitman JS, Vasgner B, Klimes I, Nagulespuran M. Improvement of glucose homeostasis after exercise training in non-insulin dependent diabetes. Diabetes Care 1984; 7:434–441.
Rodnick KJ, Haskell WL, Swislocki AL, et al. Improved insulin action in muscle, liver and adispose tissue in physically trained human subjects. Am J Physiol 1987; 253:E489–E495.
Rogers MA, Yamamoto C, King DS, et al. Improvement in glucose tolerance after one week of exercise in patients with mild NIDDM. Diabetes Care 1988; 11:613–618.
Rosas T, Constantino N. Exercise as a treatment modality to maintain normoglycemia in gestational diabetes. J Perinat Neonatal Nurs 1992; 6:14–24.
Ruoff G. The management of non-insulin-dependent diabetes mellitus in the elderly. J Fam Pract 1993; 36:329–335.
Schneider SH, Khachadurian AK, Amorosa LF, et al. Ten-year experience with an exercise-based outpatient life-style modification program in the treatment of diabetes mellitus. Diabetes Care 1992; 15(suppl.4):1800–1810.
Shilo S, Shamoon H. Abnormal growth hormone response to hypoglycemia and exercise in adults with type I Diabetes. Isr J Med Sci 1990, 26:136–141.
Trovat M, Carta Q, Cavalot F. Influence of physical training on blood glucose tolerance, insulin secretion and insulin action in non-insulin-dependent diabetic patients. Diabetes Care 1984; 5:416–420.
VanHelder WP, Goode RC, Radomski W. Effects of anaerobic and aerobic exercise of equal duration and work expenditure on plasma growth hormone levels. Eur J Appl Physiol 1984; 52:255–257.
VanHelder WP, Radomski MW, Casey K. The role of oxygen availability: demand ratio in the regulation of growth hormone response to exercise. Eur J Appl Physiol 1987; 56:628–632.
VanHelder WP, Radomski MW, Goode RC. Growth hormone responses during intermittent weight lifting exercise in men. Eur J Appl Physiol 1984; 53:31–34.
Zinman B, Zuniga-Guajardo S, Kelly D. Comparison of the acute and long-term effects of exercise on glucose control in Type I Diabetes. Diabetes Care 1984; 7:515–519.

EXERCISE AND RENAL DISEASE

GEOFFREY E. MOORE, M.D.

Renal failure not only causes severe metabolic abnormality, but many patients also endure the burdens of concomitant disease, polypharmacy, and physical disability. Not surprisingly, a reduced quality of life, as well as increased morbidity and mortality are common in renal failure. Exercise intolerance is well documented; the average dialysis patient has a $\dot{V}o_2$max of about 20 ml/[kg · min] and an average transplant recipient has a $\dot{V}o_2$max of about 35 ml/[kg · min]. The very low aerobic powers seen in dialysis patients would seem to have an intimate link with disability, but are less well-correlated with a reduced quality of life. In normal individuals, a low aerobic power is a risk factor for cardiovascular and all-cause mortality. It is not known whether the same is true in patients with renal failure. Nevertheless, many dialysis patients are incapable of undertaking the common activities of daily living (ADL) and barely maintain their independence. Increasing functional capacity should thus be a major objective of exercise therapy for patients with renal failure.

Nearly all physiologic systems are impaired in end-stage renal disease (ESRD) patients who are being treated with dialysis. Common abnormalities include a reduced peak chronotropic response to exercise (the peak heart rate [HR] is usually about 70% of the age-predicted value), left-ventricular hypertrophy, severe anemia, autonomic dysfunction, secondary hyperparathyroidism, and uremic myopathy. In addition, about 30% of ESRD patients in the United States are diabetic. A sedentary existence and the resultant deconditioning is superimposed on these problems, all of which make exercise management extremely challenging.

Research has shown that aerobic training usually improves $\dot{V}o_2$max by about 20% to 25%, entirely by increasing oxygen extraction in muscle. Unlike normal individuals, dialysis patients do not increase their stroke volume (SV) or cardiac output after exercise training. The cause for this is unclear, but it may be related to left-ventricular concentric hypertrophy and decreased ventricular compliance, both secondary to hypertension. Low oxygen delivery to skeletal muscle can be improved by erythropoietin (EPO), which increases the hemoglobin level, $\dot{V}o_2$max and quality of life. In anemic patients, EPO should theoretically increase the hemoglobin and $\dot{V}o_2$max in equal proportions. However, hemoglobin commonly increases more than $\dot{V}o_2$, so it is likely that skeletal muscle fails to extract some of the available oxygen. Since $\dot{V}o_2$max correlates with muscle strength more closely than with hemoglobin in hemodialysis patients, it is thought that some skeletal muscular factor limits aerobic power. However, magnetic resonance spectroscopy data suggest that the intrinsic oxidative energy metabolism is normal. One plausible explanation for this paradox (normal intrinsic capacity, but subnormal performance) is a subnormal oxygen transfer from blood to muscle. A reduction in oxygen transfer is supported by biopsy findings of capillary/myofiber dissociation in skeletal muscle.

Additional benefits of exercise training include improved blood pressure control, improved lipid profiles, fewer muscle cramps during dialysis, and an improved psychological state (largely a reduction of depression and enhanced mood profiles). The mechanisms of these benefits are not known, but may be similar to those in the normal population (which are also poorly understood).

To increase functional capacity, one objective of exercise management in renal failure patients should be increasing $\dot{V}o_2$max. Since the subnormal capacity to extract oxygen may be related to muscle weakness and a loss of muscle capillaries, it is reasonable to try both resistance and aerobic training programs to improve functional capacity. This approach is based on the theory that resistance training will increase intrinsic strength, whereas aerobic training will increase the potential for oxygen extraction. Problems with executing such a plan include (1) a lack of data showing that this will work, (2) the interaction of exercise and EPO (increased hemoglobin) are unknown, (3) the lack of a method to distinguish deconditioning from debilitation, (4) a risk of fractures secondary to renal osteodystrophy when resistance training is undertaken, (5) the lack of a proven method to individualize goals of exercise training, and (6) the difficulty of integrating an exercise program into an already complex and intensive medical schedule. With so little surety of success, and despite what seem to be insurmountable obstacles, exercise provides the only possible chance to increase functional capacity in these patients, many of whom are on the verge of losing independence. So be gentle, go slowly, take reasonable precautions, but try something. The following suggestions are only a start.

APPROACH

In many ways, the plan of exercise training for renal failure patients is similar to exercise in other patient populations. Although there are no data documenting a dose/response relationship for renal failure patients, exercising less than 30 minutes three to four times a week may bring little benefit to any but the most deconditioned individuals. However, exercise in doses smaller than this may be of some benefit to very deconditioned patients. Most people prefer to exercise 3 to 6 days a week and enjoy their days off. Recent epidemiologic longevity data suggest this is an entirely reasonable approach, but I advocate daily exercise.

Exercise can play an integral role in patient care by reinforcing the perception of self-determination and participation in one's own health. Hemodialysis patients may struggle particularly hard with this concept, because dialysis is something doctors and nurses do *to* them. As medicine tends to encourage patients to accept greater responsibility for their own care, they need a tangible

686

reward for their efforts. Compliance with complex medical regimens is not tangible, and it is easy to make a mistake when you take several medicines several times each day. Exercise produces tangible results (albeit in a few weeks), it provides private time, and daily exercise becomes a routine part of living. We have very little contact with our patients, yet we must convey to them that regular exercise, smoking cessation, moderation in alcohol, a heart-healthy diet, and routine safety measures will bring more benefits than anything else they can do. No medication, no laboratory test, no procedure, no therapy has the potential to improve health and well-being as much as a patient's conscious decision to improve his or her life-style.

Exercise is not the key to good health in this class of patients. By itself, exercise improves their health only a little. However, if exercise is used as the keystone for several difficult life-style changes, it can improve health a great deal. Many ex-smokers attribute their success to their physician's continuous encouragement to stop. Many reformed alcoholics and substance abusers attribute their success to finding the will to stop. Switching from a sedentary to an active life-style is no less difficult than quitting smoking or substance abuse. Because successfully finding the will to change depends on *believing* in the importance of my advice, I advocate daily exercise.

Aerobic Training

In trying to combine aerobic and resistance training, a good target for aerobic exercise would be three to four times a week for a duration of 30 to 60 minutes per session. Intensity is most easily measured by perceived exertion, though HRs are a possible alternative. Use of target HRs is complicated in dialysis patients because of the large variation in plasma volume status (and thus cardiac preload and SV), which alter the HR response to exercise. This change in the HR-SV relationship, illustrated in Figure 1, is most problematic when exercise is performed during hemodialysis, but affects peritoneal dialysis patients to some degree as well. Standard exercise recommendations of 13 to 15 on the 20-point Borg scale of perceived exertion, or from 50% to 70% of peak HR are appropriate. Patients taking beta-adrenergic antagonists should use perceived exertion rather than HR. It is worth programming one "hard day" of interval-type training each week, both for variety and to introduce higher intensity training.

Resistance Training

Resistance training has been advocated for renal failure patients, since there is a correlation between muscle weakness and peak aerobic power. However, there are no data to guide management of strength training in any renal failure population. Presumably, strength training sessions should be performed two to three times per week, using resistances that yield 9 to 12 repetitions maximum. For isokinetic exercise, moderate speeds (90 to 120 degrees per second) are probably best

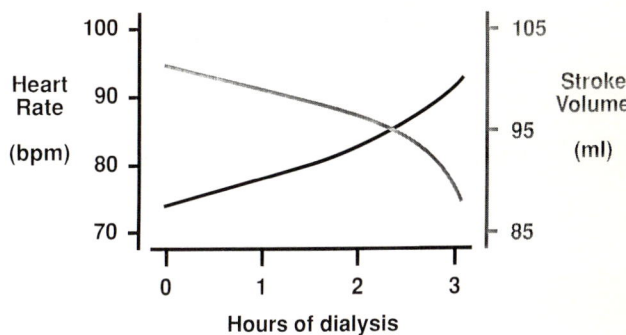

Figure 1 Effect of hemodialysis on stroke volume and heart rate. As fluid removal causes preload and stroke volume to decrease, a compensatory increase in heart rate occurs.

suited for dialysis patients. Slow speeds (<90 degrees per second) are potentially risky, and high speeds (>120 degrees per second) are probably too fast for most patients. As in aerobic exercise, it may be worth programming one "hard day" each week.

Extreme range of motion stretches and high resistance exercise are contraindicated in patients with severe renal osteodystrophy. Patients with poorly controlled renal osteodystrophy are at risk for fractures from osteitis fibrosa cystica—notably avulsion fractures of the quadriceps tendon. Patellar avulsion fractures may be due to the relatively high forces generated by the knee extensors in concert with reduced bone strength. Patients with secondary hyperparathyroidism for more than 4 years are at high risk for fractures, but any patient with a history of bone pain, tendon avulsions, alkaline phosphatase or a PTH concentration more than four times the upper limit of normality (or elevated for longer than 2 to 4 years) is probably at increased risk. In renal transplant patients, hyperparathyroidism is not usually corrected in the first year after transplantation. Corticosteroid therapy has not been reported to cause increased fractures after renal transplantation, but anecdotal experience suggests that it may contribute some risk. However, thousands of ESRD patients, including dialysis and transplant patients, have participated in clinical and experimental exercise testing and training. Fractures have occurred, but only in a few of these individuals.

Hemodialysis Patients

Hemodialysis is the mainstay of maintenance therapy for patients with chronic renal failure. Because of hemodynamic considerations, ESRD patients present a unique situation during exercise. Exercise testing is easier to perform when the patient is off dialysis, but exercise training is generally more effective while on dialysis (during the dialysis session) because monitoring is easier and participation rates are better. Fortunately, test results obtained off and on dialysis are similar, so exercise prescriptions may be based on tests performed at either time. Training during the first 2 hours of treatment allows exercise while patients are hemody-

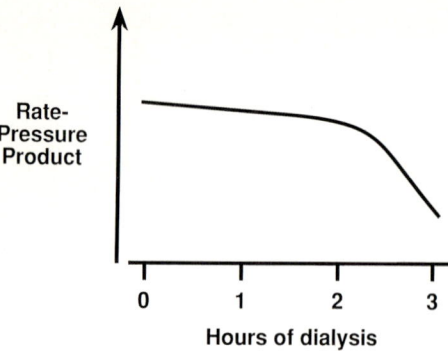

Figure 2 Effect of hemodialysis on rate-pressure product (at rest). After 2 hours of dialysis, many patients cannot maintain adequate heart rate compensation and become hypotensive.

Table 1 Recommended Program for Hemodialysis Patients

Stationary cycling on-dialysis
  5 min warm-up, 20–50 min cycling at RPE 13–15, 5 min
    cool-down
  3 sessions each week

Walk, cycle, roller blade, or swim off-dialysis
  5 min warm-up, 20–50 min activity at RPE 13–15, 5 min
    cool-down
  1–2 sessions each week

Calisthenics/strength training
  6–12 repetitions each lift
  1–3 sessions each week

namically stable (Fig. 2). Perceived exertion is preferred over HR monitoring as a means of judging exercise intensity, largely because of the hemodynamic changes that occur during dialysis and the resultant low peak HRs. Exercise program recommendations for hemodialysis patients are summarized in Table 1.

Peritoneal Dialysis Patients

Peritoneal dialysis is an attractive alternative to hemodialysis for patients who can administer their own treatments. It involves periodic infusion and drainage of dialysate into the patient's abdominal cavity, using the peritoneal pleura as the dialysis membrane. The volume of dialysate dwelling within the abdominal cavity is typically 0.5 to 1.5 L; the total volume, composition, and time that the dialysate remains within the abdomen is determined by individual requirements. Typically, a total volume of 6 to 10 L dwells within the abdominal cavity for a total duration of 6 to 12 hours. Bacterial peritonitis is the most common complication that prevents patients from using this modality. Also, the patients bear much more responsibility for their own management. The advantages are that dialysis is more "gentle" in fluid and solute exchange, the patient no longer has to attend a dialysis center three times a week, and some patients can dialyze while asleep at night, unencumbered with dialysis during the daytime.

Table 2 Recommended Program for Peritoneal Dialysis Patients

Walk, cycle, roller blade, or swim while peritoneum is empty
  5 min warm-up, 20–50 min activity at RPE 13–15, 5 min
    cool-down
  4–6 sessions each week

Calisthenics/strength training
  6–12 repetitions each lift
  1–3 sessions each week

Table 3 Recommended Program for Renal Transplant Recipients

Walk, jog, cycle, roller blade, or swim
  5 min warm-up, 20–50 min activity at RPE 13–15, 5 min
    cool-down
  4–6 sessions each week

Calisthenics/strength training
  6–12 repetitions each lift
  1–3 sessions each week

Exercise training for peritoneal dialysis patients is more flexible, because more modes of exercise are available. The only precaution is that the patient must avoid contaminating or traumatizing their dialysis catheter. Swimming would seem to be contraindicated, particularly since pool water contains *Pseudomonas aeruginosa*, but (depending upon the standard of pool hygiene) this may be more of a theoretical than a real problem. Care with the catheter cannot be overstressed. Patients are more comfortable when exercising with an empty peritoneum. Exercise program recommendations for peritoneal dialysis patients are summarized in Table 2.

Renal Transplant Patients

Renal transplantation is the best form of therapy, since this normalizes renal function; however, the secondary effects of life-long immunosuppression are the tradeoff. Graft rejection and infection are the largest causes of intercurrent illness and hospitalization in transplant recipients, and can interfere somewhat in an exercise program. One might wonder if the effects of exercise training on immunologic function alter the risk of infection or rejection, but experience suggests that they do not. As in dialysis patients, an exaggerated pressor response, arthritis flare-ups, and joint injuries are probably the greatest risks, and are almost surely to be encountered at some time during exercise therapy. Experience is that fractures are much less common. Myocardial infarction and sudden death are a rare risk of exercise in this population.

Renal transplantation resolves both the anemia and chronotropic insufficiency of ESRD. This increases aerobic power and may expose underlying cardiovascular problems such as angina. Cyclosporine worsens hypertension in heart transplant patients, but less so in renal transplant recipients. Nonetheless, an exaggerated hypertensive response is a consideration in transplant

Table 4 Risks and Benefits of Exercise Programs in End-Stage Renal Disease

Major risks
  Exaggerated hypertensive response to exercise
  Hypotension during exercise on hemodialysis
  Ischemia secondary to increased incidence of coronary artery disease
  Fractures secondary to renal osteodystrophy
  Hypoglycemia (30% of ESRD patients in the U.S. are diabetic)

Major benefits
  Increased strength and aerobic capacity
  Empowers patients with some control over health care
  Often improves management of hypertension and reduces medication requirements
  Reduced carpopedal spasm
  Improved coronary artery disease risk profile
  Improved scores on psychological tests—reduced depression, fatigue, anxiety
  Some patients like to sweat off fluid, and can liberalize fluid restrictions

Possible benefits
  Improved quality of life
  Increased bone density

recipients, particularly in patients with ESRD from hypertensive nephrosclerosis. Residual renal osteodystrophy and corticosteroid immunosuppression therapy may cause bone weakness. It has been suggested that exercise training may carry a short-term risk of fracture while enhancing bone remodeling, which may increase bone density over the long term. Transplant patients should avoid exercises with the potential of causing trauma to their graft. Exercise program recommendations for renal transplant recipients are summarized in Table 3.

RECOMMENDATIONS

Exercise therapy in ESRD patients should be directed towards increasing functional capacity and ADLs. To this end, both aerobic and strength training programs should be tried as a means of improving skeletal muscle performance (Table 4). The usual benefits of exercise training, such as improved blood pressure, improved lipid profile, and better psychological status can be expected in a majority of patients (Table 4). ESRD patients have many metabolic complications from their disease, and are at increased risk for injury because of these secondary illnesses. Nonetheless, given reasonable judgement and precautions, the traditional methods of exercise prescription are effective for patients with renal failure.

SUGGESTED READING

Converse RL Jr, Jacobsen TN, Toto RD, et al. Sympathetic overactivity in patients with chronic renal failure. New Engl J Med 1992; 327:1912–1918.

Diesel W, Noakes TD, Swanepoel C, Lambert M. Isokinetic muscle strength predicts maximum exercise tolerance in renal patients on chronic hemodialysis. Am J Kidney Dis 1990; 16:109–114.

Kempeneers GLG, Myburgh KH, Wiggins T, et al. Skeletal muscle limits the exercise tolerance of renal transplant recipients: effects of a graded exercise training programme. Am J Kidney Dis 1990; 14:57–65.

Moore GE, Bertocci LA, Painter PL. ^{31}P-Magnetic resonance spectroscopy assessment of subnormal oxidative metabolism of skeletal muscle in renal failure patients. J Clin Invest 1993; 91:420–424.

Moore GE, Brinker KR, Stray-Gundersen J, Mitchell JH. Determinants of $\dot{V}o_2$peak in patients with end-stage renal disease: on and off dialysis. Med Sci Sports Exerc 1993; 25:18–23.

Moore GE, Parsons DB, Stray-Gundersen J, et al. Uremic myopathy limits aerobic capacity of hemodialysis patients. Am J Kidney Dis 1993; 22:277–287.

Painter PL. Exercise in end-stage renal disease. Exerc Sports Sci Rev 1988; 16:305–339.

Robertson HT, Haley NR, Guthrie M, et al. Recombinant erythropoietin improves exercise capacity in anemic hemodialysis patients. Am J Kidney Dis 1990; 16:325–332.

Ryuzaki M, Konishi K, Kasuga A, et al. Spontaneous rupture of the quadriceps tendon in patients on maintenance hemodialysis—report of three cases with clinicopathological observations. Clin Nephrol 1989; 32:144–148.

EXERCISE AND ARTHRITIS

DOUGLAS B. McKEAG, M.D.

Osteoarthritis (also known as degenerative joint disease) is a pathological process of multifactorial etiology leading to cartilaginous degeneration with associated clinical symptoms. It is a process commonly regarded as the inevitable consequence of aging, a "wear and tear" manifestation and/or the result of abnormal joint mechanics. It is the most prevalent rheumatic disease, and the most common chronic disease in humans.

It is estimated that one in five American adults suffers from some type of disability ranging from difficulty in walking to problems in lifting things during the course of daily routine activities. This rate of functional disability increases with age, affecting over 50% of people aged 65 and over. A major factor of this disability seems related to the onset of osteoarthritis (OA). The pathological process is closely related to aging, but is different than the effects of aging itself. At present, 40.5 million adults are thought to have OA; 27 million have symptoms related to the disease. In populations of individuals in their eighth decade of life,

85% were diagnosed as having OA. The disease may begin as early as the second decade of life. It has been identified in 35% of people under the age of 30.

The economic impact of the disease is significant. Of all visits to the ambulatory care center, 10% are the result of symptoms related to OA. In-patient hospital care in the United States directly attributed to this disease has passed the $7 million mark.

What role does physical activity play in OA? As Eichner asks, "Are runners spoiling their joints to spare their hearts? Does running, with all of its pounding, cause osteoarthritis?"

Because we are just beginning to understand the disease process, we have had a rather poor and unorganized view of its causes. Are Eichner's questions merely hypothetical or do we now have evidence to suggest a relationship between exercise and OA? Are injuries incurred by athletes in the pursuit of sport predisposing these individuals to future OA? Our ability to answer this question is limited, because our ability to diagnose microscopic injury is limited. Sports medicine has done an excellent job of defining and standardizing the diagnosis of major sports-induced injury. Microscopic injury, however, remains difficult to diagnose, and it is probably through the study of microscopic injury that we will find answers to the above questions.

PATHOPHYSIOLOGY

Normal joints can sustain an impact loading force with no resulting detrimental effect. Energy from the impact is dissipated by the joint in two different ways: (1) throughout the articulation, by means of its movement and frictional surface, and (2) by absorption through its external muscle support.

Articulation characteristics that allow for relatively frictionless motion depend on synovial fluid lubrication. Low impact loads such as those seen with the activities of daily living are handled by the hyaluronic acid molecules normally present in human joints. Repetitive or high-impact loads augment this normal state of affairs with stimulation of a water-based transudate, generated by the synovial membrane. The normal human joint has a number of unique characteristics. It is hypothermic, with temperatures normally ranging from 32.4° to 34.6°C. This probably reflects a relative lack of blood supply to the joint. Hyaline cartilage that makes up the articular surface of major joints is basically avascular, aneural, and alymphatic. It is a hypocellular substance, made up of 5% cells by volume, and 75% to 80% water in an aggregated proteoglycan complex. It essentially acts as a water filled sponge during daily activity, especially in weight-bearing joints. The water is pushed out of this spongy parenchyma by external motion of the body and impact loading. This process is prevalent enough for many individuals to be 2 cm shorter at night than in the morning. Chondrocytes (cartilage cells) have the longest life cycle in the body. Matrix or parenchyma is made up of proteoglycan aggregates, each aggregate consisting of multiple proteoglycan mono-

mers. Each monomer comprises a long chain, random coil hyaluronic acid and glycosaminoglycans emerging as "brushes" from this coil. Numerous enzymes govern the biochemical systems, which regulate the degradation and generation of this matrix. The synovium serves as a rapid exchanger of water and solutes. It has a blood supply as well as innervation, and is a sensitive, highly reactive tissue.

Lubrication of the joint depends on the type of load involved. Bone distal to a joint absorbs most of the impact force presented to it. Bursae, or potential fluid-filled spaces, facilitate gliding of soft tissue structures across each other or bony prominences. Finally, tendons and ligaments offer elasticity and stabilization to the joint, maintaining normal biomechanics.

Consider how this normal physiologic joint must adapt to the difference between walking and running. A running human being generates two times the impact load at the ankle, six times at the knee, and two times at the hip as the same individual during walking. This assumes proper and correct biomechanics. Abnormal motion would produce even more impact load.

THE PROCESS OF OSTEOARTHRITIS

The sequence of events leading to OA remains controversial. Independent of the type of initiating event, the joint undergoes changes to a specific endpoint. The process may arrest at any point, continue to total joint destruction and disability, or reverse and repair itself. A part of the process of adaptation is architectural bony remodeling (Wolff's Law) secondary to repetitive stress (impact) load. Repetitive impact may stimulate increases in transudate within the joint in an attempt to decrease friction. Eventually, however, such an insult may lead to trabecular microfractures in the articular surface, traveling deep to subchondral bone. This bone then hypertrophies, giving the clinical symptom of stiffening and the clinical sign of a decreasing range of motion about the joint. These changes in turn lead to an increase in biomechanical stress about the joint, with further cartilaginous damage and a resultant degeneration of anatomy, physiology, and functionality of the joint. On a cellular basis, the pathophysiology can be summarized as follows: The increased stress and deterioration of biomechanics stimulate a decrease in the amount of mucopolysaccharide, reduce its aggregation, and cause an increase of water within the articular cartilaginous matrix. This whole process is mediated by lyzasomal enzymes. Chondrocytes increase their activity and attempt repair. If damage is minimal, with no continuing insult, the increase in chondrocyte activity may be enough to arrest the process and begin repair. Usually, however, cellular pathophysiology continues to develop and the articular surface becomes fibrillated; this decreases mechanical integrity and lubrication and increases friction (Fig. 1). The increased frictional forces predispose to further cartilaginous destruction of the matrix, with a thinning of that matrix. The subchondral bone proliferation mentioned above results in an increased area of load bearing (perhaps the body's attempt to take pressure off the area of insult). The hypertrophy of most structures about the joint in turn creates functional instability and further cystic changes in the trabecular bone.

SPORTS-RELATED OSTEOARTHRITIS: EXERCISE AS STRESSOR

Does exercise cause OA? Before one can answer additional research questions, especially questions in-

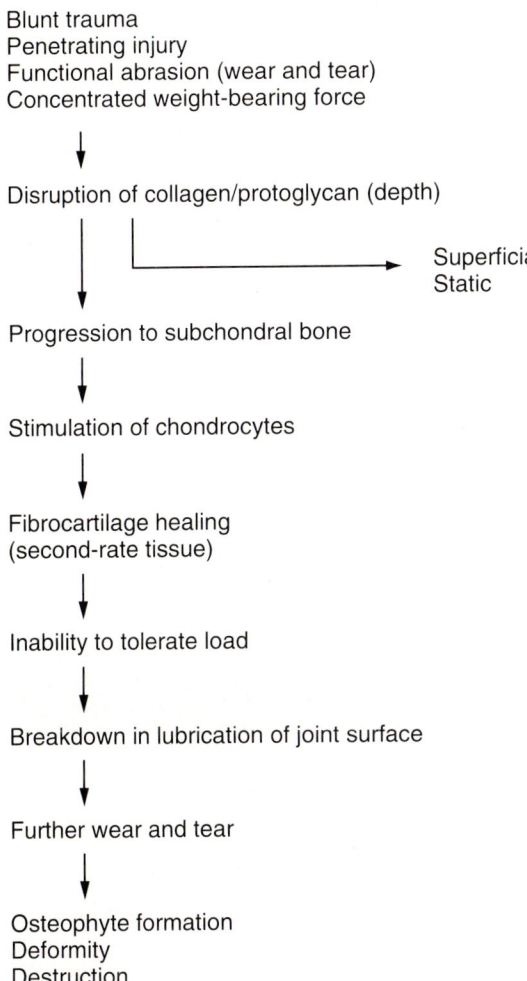

Figure 1 The progression of osteoarthritis.

volving the population characteristics of existing prospective studies, the following questions must be answered:

1. What is the state of the joint? Is it healthy or unhealthy? Is there some occult pathology affecting any of the structures about the joint/joints in question?

2. What is the "past medical history" of the joint? Has there been a previous injury that affects the joint now?

Dorr discusses several musculoskeletal injury processes that lead to OA in athletes:

(*a*) Repetitive, cyclic trauma coupled with acute injury.

(*b*) Torn meniscus, with resultant removal of the entire meniscus.

(*c*) A meniscectomy associated with an anterior cruciate ligament tear that results in a tricompartmental OA, involving the medial and lateral compartments of the knee as well as the patellofemoral joint. Arthritis is here considered as secondary to translation of the femur on the tibia.

(*d*) Juxta-articular and intra-articular fractures, which predispose a joint to arthritic changes. A somewhat weaker relationship exists with diaphyseal fractures.

Animal studies show that there is a risk of OA in different species depending on the type of activity performed. Table 1 summarizes these studies.

There remains a major problem in deciding whether exercise is a causative factor in human OA. There is as yet no prospective controlled study of the long-term effects of exercise on the musculoskeletal system.

Associated Factors

Table 2 lists a number of factors that may be associated with the development of sports-related osteoarthritis (SROA). Ten of these associations are discussed in detail because they have either a major influence, a major proven relationship (or lack of relationship), or a potential for a significant relationship in the future.

1. *Age*

As we look at general OA with clinical signs and proven radiographic findings (which tend to correspond with the diagnosis of "severe osteoarthritis"), the incidence increases exponentially with age. Age continues to be a major confounding variable in the unknown equation describing the etiology of osteoarthritis.

Table 1 Studies of the Risk of Development of Osteoarthritis (OA) in Animals

Species	Involved Joints	Type of Activity	Risk of OA
Dog (huskies)	Hip, shoulder	Sled pulling	Increased
Guinea-pigs	Knee	Running	Increased
Horses	Foreleg	Racing	Increased
Rabbits	Knee	Running	No change
		Impact joint loading	Increased
Sheep	Knee	Ambulation on cement	No change
Tigers and lions	Foreleg	Springing, running	Increased

Table 2 Factors Which May Be Associated with the Development of Sports-Related Osteoarthritis (SROA)

Possible Factors	Assertions
Biochemical factors	
Aging of articular cartilage	Loss of biophysical properties of articular cartilage (i.e., chondrocytes) may increase risk of OA
Subchondral microfracture	May evolve with repetitive strenuous exercise and later increase risk of OA
Bone growth/remodeling	May be decreased at site of previous fractures; remodeling may be affected by chronic exercise
Joint lubrication	May be decreased with excessive impact loading stress and later increase risk of OA
Local inflammation	May increase risk for development of early OA post-injury
Hormonal influences (i.e., steroids)	An imbalance may affect bone metabolism in such a way as to increase the risk of OA
Synovial fluid characteristics	Alterations in hyaluronic acid, sulfates, structural glycosaminoglycans and water content may increase risk of OA
Characteristics of the playing surfaces	
Asphalt	May increase OA
Clay	Unknown
Cement (concrete)	Increases stress-loading, which may increase risk of OA
Grass	May decrease injury and thereby decrease risk of early OA
Ice	Unknown
Tarton surface ("Astroturf")	May increase risk of injuries (i.e., turf toe) which may increase risk of premature OA
Water	May decrease the risk of OA by lessening stress and loading
Wood	May increase lower extremity injuries, which may increase risk of OA
Characteristics of Sport	
Contact vs. noncontact	May increase risk of OA with repetitive stress loading
Duration of participation	May increase injuries and development of premature OA
Onset and level of participation	
Childhood/adolescent	May increase long-term risk of OA
Adult	May increase risk of OA with overuse syndrome
Professional/competitive (amateur)/Recreational	An increased risk of OA may be associated with antecedent injuries or length of participation
Miscellaneous	
Nutrition	
Protein diets	May cause electrolyte loss and accelerate osteoporosis
Phosphate loading	Unknown effect, may deplete magnesium sources
Calcium deficient diets	May increase osteoporosis, which increase risk of OA
Medical therapy	Accurate diagnosis and management of injury may decrease OA
Pharmacologic therapy	Ceratin nonsteroidal anti-inflammatory drugs and steroids may have deleterious effects on cartilage. Ice, heat, and rest may decrease local inflammation and decreases risk of OA.
Surgical therapy	Surgically or biomechanically altered joints may be more susceptible to OA (i.e., meniscectomies) yet allow the individual to continue participation
Preventative Measures	
Coaching methods	Proper techniques may decrease stressload, prevent injury and therefore OA
Conditioning techniques	Well-conditioned athletes may have a decreased risk of OA
Training techniques	Overuse may increase risk of OA
Equipment design (i.e., headgear, shoes)	May decrease OA by decreasing stressloading or preventing injuries
Rehabilitation of injury (i.e., orthotics)	May decrease risk of OA and reinjury
Restricted participation post-injury	May decrease risk of premature OA in unstable, injured joints
Rule changes	Will hopefully decrease incidence of injuries and risk of OA

From Panush RS, Brown DG. Exercise and arthritis. Sports Med 1987; 4:54-64; with permission.

Changes in the articular cartilage associated with aging and OA are compared in Table 3. Too often, OA is considered a consequence of aging, but that is obviously not the case. Table 4 compares whole joint changes in the two processes. Although dramatic differences exist, most individuals with severe OA are elderly. Therefore, any attempt to understand SROA must consider advancing age as a major factor affecting OA. Conversely, early participation in sports at a very intense and frequent level, may increase the risk of OA in future life. Until there are prospective control studies of long-term effects, this can remain nothing more than an interesting observation.

2. *Gender*

Men and women appear to be affected equally. However, the age of initial involvement differs, females being affected earlier in life than males. Anatomic disease prevalence differs; male knees are most com-

Table 3 Comparison of Changes in Articular Cartilage in Aging and Osteoarthritis (OA)

Criterion	Aging	OA
Water content	Decreased	Increased
Glycosaminoglycans		
Chondroitin sulfate	Normal or slightly less	Decreased
Chondroitin sulfate 4/6 ratio†	Decreased	Increased
Keratan sulfate	Increased	Decreased
Hyaluronate	Increased	Decreased
Proteoglycans		
Aggregation	Normal	Diminished
Monomer size	Decreased	Decreased
Link protein	Fragmented	Normal
Proteases	"Normal"	Increased

Table 4 OA Versus Aging

OA	Aging
Highly anabolic and synthetic process	Normal metabolism
Enzymatic destruction of hard tissue	Normal enzymatic remodeling
Remodeling all tissues about joint, articular, and periarticular	Cartilage changes only
Chondrocyte mitosis	No mitosis
Intense increase synthesis collagen and proteoglycan	Normal rates synthesis, collagen and proteoglycan
Increased water content cartilage	No change
Fibrillation, focal, and progressive at weight-bearing sites	Fibrillation nonprogressive, non-weight-bearing sites
Eburnation, ivory-like	No eburnation
Osteophytes occur with other changes	Osteophytes only with excessive use
No increased collagen x link	Increased collagen x link
Inflammation	No inflammation
No pigment-cartilage	Pigment—cartilage

From Bland JH, Cooper SM. Osteoarthritis: A review of the cell biology involved and evidence for reversibility. Management nationally related to known genesis and pathophysiology. Arthritis Rheum 1984; 14:106-133; with permission.

monly affected, whereas females tend to be affected more in the first metatarsophalangeal (MTP) or distal interphalangeal joints. OA may be reduced by exercise therapy in osteoporotic postmenopausal females.

3. *Ethnicity*

A number of studies have compared the prevalence of OA in selected populations. For example, there appears to be an increased prevalence of OA among Native American Indians, but a decreased prevalence of OA of the hips in the Chinese population. Perhaps the extreme range of motion of squatting has a protective effect in the Chinese.

4. *Geography*

Geographic associations have been shown, with OA being less common in colder climates, such as Alaska and Finland. However, comparison of other data by latitude show no such difference.

5. *Body Habitus*

Obesity is a definite risk factor for OA of the knee, the great toe, and the hands. This does not seem true for OA of the hip.

6. *Bone Density*

Osteoporosis and osteopenia appear to slow the progress of arthritis. An increased density of bone leads to increased OA, perhaps through the mechanism of decreased shock absorption.

7. *Hyperuricemia*

Individuals with a high serum uric acid also show a slightly increased propensity towards OA.

8. *Hypertension*

An elevation in diastolic blood pressure appears to be associated with OA. Once again, a cause and effect relationship has not been proven.

9. *Hypercholesterolemia*

Curiously, there seems to be no association between hypercholesterolemia and OA.

10. *Trauma* is a major factor in the development of OA, because of its ability to change the biomechanics of activity and movement in an individual.

Subclinical trauma, often involving repetitive impact stress or an overuse syndrome, can lead to initial changes and pathology within a joint, which in turn predispose to OA. Prior injury affecting gait, joint alignment, or ligamentous stability is a definite risk factor for OA. Immobilization during treatment can lead to increased articular degeneration and fibrillation, which may progress to OA. Although trauma is a strong risk factor, findings remain conflicting and studies confounded. As an example, if we look at arthritis of the elbow, it appears that foundry workers using prongs to lift metal rods who undertake much movement about the elbow, develop OA of this region. However, pneumatic drillers also place a great impact load on their elbows, but show no increase in OA.

Ballet dancers, who place a great deal of stress on the lower extremity and specifically the ankle and foot, are susceptible to OA about the talar joint. However, dancing does not seem to affect the prevalence of OA at the first MTP joint, a common site for initial presentation of OA in women.

Single impact loading (e.g., parachutists) showed an increased prevalence of OA of the spine, a referred area of the body for impact loading, but no evidence of increased OA about the knee or ankle, considered as primary recipients of the initial impact.

Soccer involves quick changes of direction and a great deal of weight bearing in running and sprinting; Klunder showed the foot and hip of soccer players were affected, but not the knee. The patterns described above defy explanation based upon our present knowledge of the etiology of OA.

EXERCISE AS ETIOLOGIC AGENT

The alleged association between exercise and OA is not limited to one type of activity any more than arthritis is limited to one type of person. Many sport associations exist. Panush completed an exhaustive literature search on this subject. Table 5 summarizes his findings.

Running in its various forms (jogging and sprinting) is the quintessential activity to study the effects of exercise on the development of OA. It has been implicated as a direct cause of osteoarthritis, but has also been advocated as a treatment. Once again, it is important to emphasize the need for prolonged prospective studies of weight-bearing activity such as running in relation to the development of OA. Retrospective studies have shown definite effects in relating abnormal joints to arthritis. The effect of acute trauma on OA is summarized in Table 2. Bland asked the question, "Does running cause osteoarthritis in a normal joint?" The literature does not support a relationship between running and OA in normal individuals. McDermott studied 20 runners with chronic knee pain and found OA in six of them. Confounding variables including genu varus and a history of prior knee injuries were present in the general sample, but were more apparent in the six affected runners. Another study of adolescents tended to suggest that athletic activity during adolescence promoted OA of the hip in adulthood. Finnish champion elite runners were examined for radiographic evidence of OA and were compared with nonexercising controls. The incidence in the elite athletes was significantly less. The "controls" were hospital patients, perhaps not appropriate to compare with the experimental population.

Two cross-sectional studies compared runners versus sedentary, nonrunning controls. Panush concluded after looking at 17 middle-aged runners over a 12 year period, that there were no differences in arthritis between the two groups. Likewise Lane reported on 41 runners and an equal number of matched controls over 5 years, analyzing x-rays of the hands, lumbar spine, and

Table 5 Sport Participation and Associations with Osteoarthritis (SROA)

Sport	Site (Joint)
Ballet	Talus
	Ankle
	Cervical spine
	Hip
	Knee
	Metatarsophalangeal
Baseball	Elbow
	Shoulder
Boxing	Hand (Carpometacarpal)
Cricket	Finger
Football (American style)	Ankle
	Feet
	Knee
	Spine
Gymnastics	Elbow
	Shoulder
	Wrist
	Hip
Lacrosse	Ankle
	Knee
Martial arts	Spine
Parachuting	Ankle
	Knee
	Spine
Rugby	Knee
Running	Knee
	Hip
Skiing (downhill)	Thumb
Soccer	Ankle-foot
	Cervical spine
	Hip
	Knee
	Talus
	Talofibular
Weight-lifting	Spine
Wrestling	Cervical spine
	Elbow
	Knee

the knees, as well as obtaining a computed tomography (CT) scan of the first lumbar vertebrae. The results of this study indicated that runners had 40% more mineral content in the bone, but no increased prevalence of clinical OA.

Studies have also compared athletes in different disciplines. One study compared perceived OA symptoms in former runners and in former swimmers with an average age of 57 years. The former college runners were no more likely to have symptomatic OA than were former college swimmers. Finally, we have preliminary results from longitudinal data. The Stanford Arthritis Study is comparing runners and nonrunners. After 5 years, the runners appear to have less disability and visit the physician less often than their nonrunning counterparts. This may indicate that the runners have less disability, and that running may actually slow functional aspects of aging, as we have implied in the past. A 35 year Framingham follow-up study showed a strong relationship between obesity at a mean age of 37, and the development of OA of the knees as the mean age of 73. Once again, it is Eichner who poses the following thought provoking statement, "The question for the future is not 'Does running cause osteoarthritis?' but rather does sloth cause osteoarthritis?"

We may conclude that aerobic training involving major muscle groups helps decrease active inflammatory disease, including OA. This may occur as a result of decreasing obesity, increasing bone density, and/or increasing muscle strength and tone. Future investigations need to include: (1) prospective longitudinal studies; (2) noninvasive technology to monitor more closely early subclinical OA; (3) a better definition and quantifying of impact loading and physical stress, so that the actual intervention can be measured and replicated; (4) standardized definition of osteoarthritis and what it represents as a disease process; and (5) studies that control for other confounding variables and risk factors.

EXERCISE AS TREATMENT

Can exercise slow or even reverse the course of OA? Initially, a number of misconceptions need to be addressed:

1. OA is often thought to be a consequence of chronologic age. However, chronologic aging and OA are two separate processes.
2. OA is said to be secondary to "wear and tear." However, the literature indicates that normal wear and tear does not predispose to OA. The mammalian joint, spared grossly excessive impact loads, cannot be worn out. Lubrication is so efficient that there is little shear force. The joint has an extremely low coefficient of friction, approximating ice on ice.
3. Cartilage is believed not to heal or repair itself. However, this scientific dogma has been proven incorrect. An important milestone in this research was the finding by Mankin. As the severity of OA progresses, metabolic activity in the cartilage increases over the initial range of the Mankin-Dorfman histological/histochemical scale (Table 6). Although poorly responsive to trauma, articular cartilage can heal. Specifically, the "point of no return" appears to be a degree of pathophysiology reflected by a score of 10. The replacement cartilage may be a mix of fibro and hayline cartilage, however.
4. Chondrocytes are held to be effete cells that cannot replicate or change rates of synthesis and degradation of cartilage macromolecules. However, Mankin, reinforced by Bland, have shown that chondrocytes are indeed dynamic in their function. There is a definite cellular and tissue response to the onset of OA that is purposeful and is aimed at repair. Chondrocytes do not normally divide, but with appropriate stimuli, they do divide forming clones.
5. OA is regarded as an inexorable process. However, it appears that OA occasionally remits

Table 6 Histochemical/Histopathologic Scale for Grading the Severity of Osteoarthritis

I. Structure	
a. Normal	0
b. Surface irregularities	1
c. Surface and pannus irregularities	2
d. Clefts to the transitional zone	3
e. Clefts to the radial zone	4
f. Clefts to the calcified zone	5
g. Complete disorganization	6
II. Cells	
a. Normal	0
b. Diffuse hypercellularity	1
c. Cloning	2
d. Hypocellularity	3
III. Safranin-O Staining	
a. Normal	0
b. Slight reduction	1
c. Moderate reduction	2
d. Severe reduction	3
e. No dye noted	4
IV. Tidemark Integrity	
a. Intact	0
b. Crossed by blood vessels	1

From Mankin HJ, et al. Biochemical and metabolic abnormalities in articular cartilage from osteoarthritic human hips. J Bone Joint Surg 1971; 53A: 523-537; with permission.

spontaneously. Surgical intervention has demonstrated that with precise planning, OA of the hip and of the knee can be arrested and reversed by changing biomechanical factors.

The Standard treatment of arthritis is aimed primarily at reducing joint pain, with use of non-weight-bearing exercises to strengthen the supporting muscles. Often, patients are told not to exercise, for fear of increasing their symptoms. Adjunct to such treatment is the use of medications (nonsteroidal anti-inflammatory medications and/or ice), and, if necessary, surgery to correct biomechanical abnormalities. Recent studies have shown that patients with OA can tolerate weight-bearing exercises, especially walking.

Cartilage can repair itself, and the process of OA is subject to arrest and reversal. Chondrocytes are metabolically active, and will attempt repair, increasing the amount of proteoglycan, Type 2 collagen within the matrix of the cartilage. There is also a potential for hyaline fibrocartilaginous healing, dependent on motion and hydrostatic pressure changes induced by weight-bearing exercise. Secondary deficits such as decreased muscle strength in the periarticular muscles, decreased flexibility, weight gain, and decreased aerobic power impede any therapeutic regimen. One needs to consider exercise as a unique modality and as a means of diminishing certain arthritic signs and symptoms: (1) correction of disuse atrophy and weakness by programs to maintain and develop musculoskeletal fitness, (2) increase of periarticular muscle strength, to protect

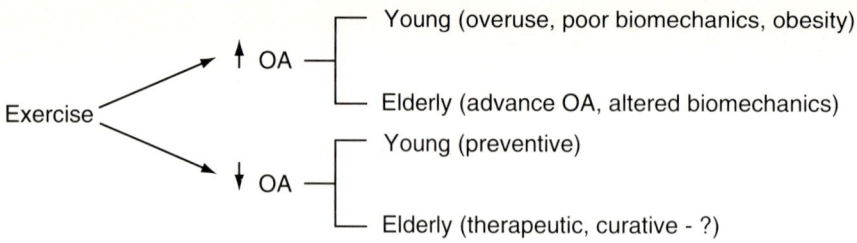

Figure 2 Summary of relation between exercise and osteoarthritis.

joints from injury and biomechanical insult, (3) increase of intra-articular nutrient diffusion by the pumping action of weight-bearing exercise, and (4) stimulation of cartilage via the compressive action of weight bearing.

PRINCIPLES OF TREATMENT

The major goal of a therapeutic regimen is to shift the osteoarthritic process from degradation and catabolic activity to synthesis and anabolic activity. Major risk factors need to be identified and controlled. Early recognition of the disease process will increase the chances of a positive therapeutic result. Routine rest periods interspersed between short episodes of weight-bearing activity promote cartilage repair. The rest needs to be non-weight bearing and take place two to four times per day. Home physical therapy, specifically stretching prior to weight-bearing exercise, and the application of ice or cryotherapy after exercise, is important in controlling post-exercise induced inflammation. Exercise can take the form of postural as well as simple aerobic weight-bearing exercises. Alleviation of symptoms and signs with the use of medications (NSAID and corticosteroids) is an important backup.

The physician should consider two precautions before allowing an osteoarthritic patient to begin such an aggressive exercise program. First, acute inflammation or joint swelling is an absolute contraindication to the initiation of such a program until the acute inflammation has subsided. Secondly, all individuals contemplating such an exercise program should undergo a complete physical examination, including a graded exercise stress test to identify occult cardiac disease and determine an appropriate target heart rate.

OSTEOARTHRITIS REVERSAL

We have recently reported the use of magnetic resonance imaging as a noninvasive means of monitoring intervention in mild to moderate OA. Computer en-

hancement of the knee joint, and specifically the articular surface on both the tibia and femur, will allow us to monitor in vivo the natural history and effects of weight-bearing exercise intervention on early subclinical OA.

Figure 2 summarizes our current knowledge of the relationship between exercise and the chronic disease process known as osteoarthritis.

SUGGESTED READING

Bland JH. The reversibility of osteoarthritis: A review. Am J Med 1983; 74:16–26.

Bland JH, Cooper SM. Osteoarthritis: A review of the cell biology involved and evidence for reversibility. Management nationally related to known genesis and pathophysiology. Arthritis Rheum 1984; 14(2):106–133.

Eichner ER. Does running cause osteoarthritis? Phys Sportsmed 1989; 17(3):147–154.

Felson DT, Anderson JJ, Naimark A, et al. Obesity and knee osteoarthritis. The Framingham study. Ann Intern Med 1988; 109:18–24.

Hammerman D. Aging and the musculoskeletal system. In: Hazzard WR, Andres R, Bierman EL, Blass JP, eds. Principles of geriatric medicine and gerontology. 2nd Ed. New York: McGraw-Hill (in press).

Lane NE, Bloch DA, Wood PD, et al. Aging, long-distance running, and the development of musculoskeletal disability. A controlled study. Am J Med 1987; 82:772–780.

Mankin HJ. The reaction of articular cartilage to injury and osteoarthritis. Part I. N Engl J Med 1974; 291:1285–1292.

Mankin HJ. The reaction of articular cartilage to injury and osteoarthritis. Part II. N Engl J Med 1974; 291:1335–1340.

Maskowitz RW. Primary osteoarthritis: Epidemiology, clinical aspects, and general management. Am J Med 1987; 83:5–10.

McKeag, DB. The relationship of osteoarthritis and exercise. Clin Sports Med 1992; 11:471–487.

McKeag, DB, Smith BWH, Edminster R, et al. Estimating the severity of osteoarthritis with magnetic resonance spectroscopy. Arthritis Rheum 1992; 21:227–238.

Panush RS, Brown DG. Exercise and arthritis. Sports Med 1987; 4:54–64.

Panush RS, Schmidt C, Caldwell JR, et al. Is running associated with degenerative joint disease? JAMA 1986; 255:1152–1154.

Sartorius DJ. Magnetic resonance imaging of the musculoskeletal system. J Musculoskeletal Med 1990; 29–45.

Semble EL, Loeser RF, Wise CM. Therapeutic exercise for rheumatoid arthritis and osteoarthritis. Arthritis Rheum 1990; 20:32–40.

EXERCISE AND OSTEOPOROSIS

JILL A. KANALEY, Ph.D.
MARK L. HARTMAN, M.D.
ARTHUR WELTMAN, Ph.D

Osteoporosis is a major public health problem in the United States that is responsible for at least 1.5 million fractures each year. The most frequent cause of bone fractures is low bone mass. Aging typically results in an approximate 3% bone loss per decade in both males and females. Osteoporosis is an age-related condition with a higher incidence in women compared to men. Among some of the many reasons for the higher incidence of osteoporosis in women are: (1) lower dietary intake of calcium, (2) participation in weight reducing diets, (3) pregnancy and lactation draining calcium reserves, (4) bone mineral loss associated with cessation of ovarian function at menopause, and (5) a lower peak bone density in young women than found in young men.

Peak bone mass is attained during the third decade of life and bone loss begins shortly thereafter. The pattern of bone mineral loss over time in women can be modeled as biphasic with a protracted slow phase and a transient accelerated phase. At approximately 40 years of age, the slow phase of cortical bone loss begins with accelerated bone loss at the onset of menopause (Fig. 1). The slow phase of trabecular bone loss may begin even earlier due to either a constant loss with increasing age or an accelerated loss after menopause (Fig. 2). In both sexes, the onset of trabecular bone loss occurs at least a decade earlier than the onset of cortical bone loss. During the course of their lifetime, women lose about 50% of their cancellous bone and 30% of their cortical bone; men lose about 30% and 20%, respectively. Therefore, maximizing the peak bone mass at a young age is essential since once bone mass falls below a critical level, the structural integrity of the bone diminishes and the risk of fracture increases. Further, confounding the study of age-related bone loss, cross-sectional studies have shown differences in the pattern of bone mineral decrease in the lumbar spine, femoral neck, and femoral shaft.

The age-related loss of bone mass is attributed to an imbalance in remodeling. Bone loss occurs when osteo-clasts create an excessively deep cavity, when osteoblasts fail to refill a normal resorption cavity, or when both occur. There is a proportional loss of both trabecular and cortical bone. The peripheral skeleton, approximately 80% of skeletal mass, is made primarily of cortical bone. The axial skeleton is about 20% of the skeletal mass and is composed of approximately 70% trabecular bone. Trabecular bone is more susceptible to incomplete remodelling and consequently more prone to fractures. Factors determining bone mass include age, race, sex, cigarette use, nutritional status, alcohol intake, muscular strength, body composition, and several hormones (e.g., parathyroid hormone, growth hormone, vitamin D_3, thyroid, gonadal, and adrenal hormones). Regular physi-

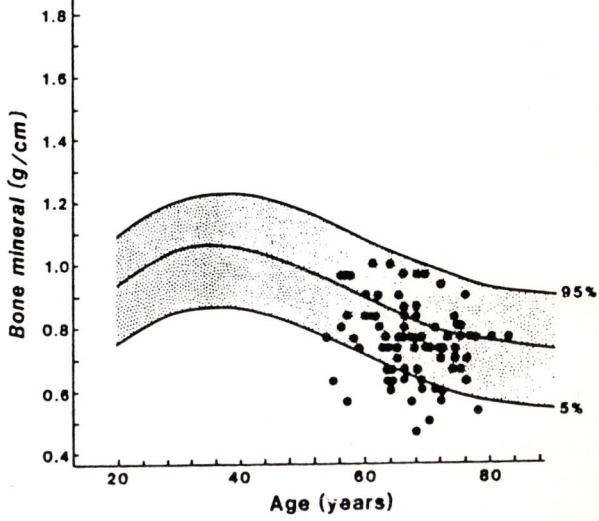

Figure 1 Individual values for bone mineral density (BMD) of midradius in 76 women with osteoporosis and one or more vertebral-compression fractures (●). Center line denotes age regression for normal women, and upper and lower lines represent 90% confidence limits. (From Riggs BL, Wahner HW, Dunn WL, et al. Differential changes in bone mineral density of the appendicular and axial skeleton with aging. J Clin Invest 1981; 67:328-335; with permission.)

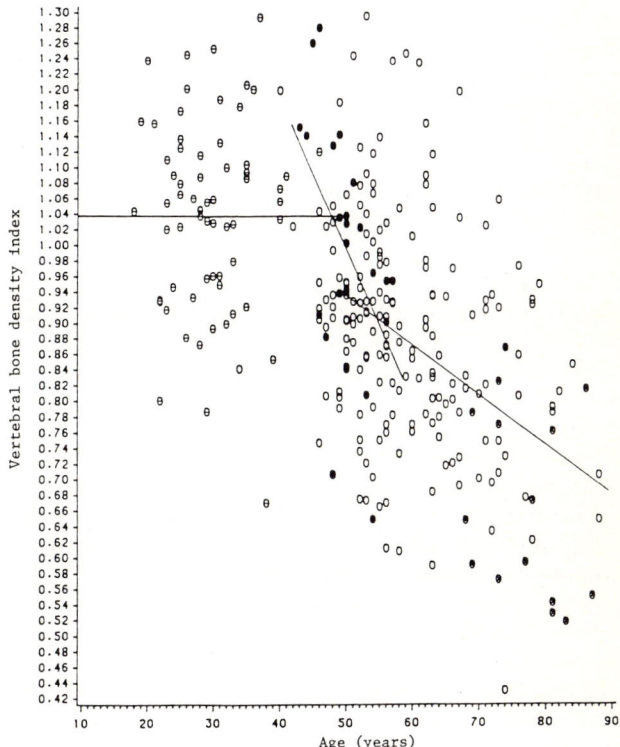

Figure 2 Plot of vertebral bone density versus age. Separate regression lines drawn for three menopausal groups: ⊖ premenopausal; ● perimenopausal; ○ postmenopausal; ⊗ vertebral fractures. (From Hui SL, Slemenda CW, Johnston CC, Apledorn CR. Effects of age and menopause on vertebral bone density. Bone and Mineral 1987; 2:141-146; with permission.)

cal activity is also believed to effect bone mineral density (BMD). Cross-sectional studies report higher BMD in athletic individuals compared to age-matched sedentary controls, and prospective studies find that exercise training either increases BMD or retards bone loss.

SKELETAL LOADING, EXERCISE, AND BONE MASS

Skeletal loading is a determinant of bone mineral density. Bone accommodates to the forces applied within physiologic and structural limits, by altering its amount and distribution of mass (Wolff's law). The architecture of bone is determined primarily by genetic predisposition; however, it can be altered by mechanical stress, which is a strong stimulus for bone remodeling. A minimal level of strain is necessary to maintain bone mass. All forces imposed on bone produce strain and will determine the strength and shape of that bone. The magnitude of the bone tissue response is influenced by the hormonal milieu and the nutritional status. Cross-sectional data show relationships between physical activity and bone density, and between muscular strength and bone density. Bone mass is also higher in athletic women, and bone density is increased (or bone loss retarded) with exercise training. However, effects may be limited to the specific bones that were mechanically loaded. Physical activity that applies stress beyond that encountered in daily living may stimulate bone formation. Whether this stimulus is only effective in the years of bone deposition is unclear.

TRAINING RESULTS IN AN INCREASE IN BONE MINERAL DENSITY

Exercise training and physical activity may result in an increase in BMD. One cross-sectional study reported a relationship between spine and hip BMD and routine daily activities in 151 women (age 35-65 years); hours of walking per day were positively correlated with lumbar BMD ($r = 0.23$, $p < 0.01$) and femoral neck BMD ($r = 0.25$, $p < 0.003$). For each hour of daily walking, there was an 0.8% increase in lumbar spine BMD and a 1.9% increase in femoral neck BMD. Unfortunately, this study did not take oral contraceptive use, hormone replacement therapy, or menopausal status into account. When sedentary women were compared with women who exercised aerobically in excess of 2.5 hours per week, and women who supplemented their 2.5 hours of aerobic exercise with muscle-building activities (Fig. 3), lumbar spine BMD was found to be significantly greater in the muscle-building group. Similarly, when body builders, runners, and swimmers are compared with physically inactive eumenorrheic women, the average bone mineral content (BMC) was consistently greatest in the body builders. Unfortunately, these studies were cross-sectional in design and the possibility exists that a greater percentage of women with high initial BMD may "self select" muscle building exercise.

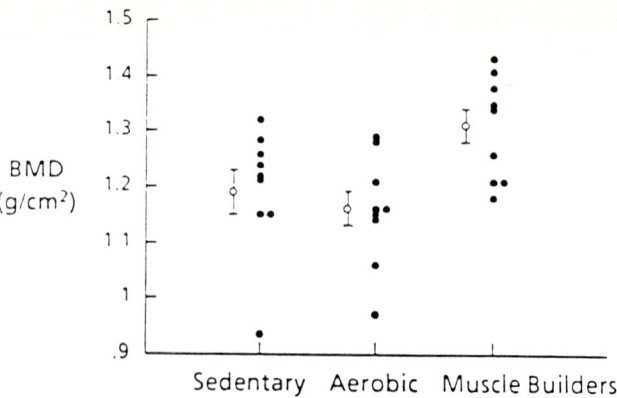

Figure 3 Bone mineral content (g/cm^2) of the lumbar spine was determined by dual-photon absorptiometry in healthy young women. Individual measurements are depicted by small closed circles for sedentary women, aerobic exercisers, and muscle builders. Group means are shown by open circles with SEM bars. (From Davee AM, Rosen CJ, Robert A, Adler RA. Exercise patterns and trabecular bone density in college women. J Bone Min Res 1990; 5:245-250; with permission.)

Strength training is effective in increasing regional BMD and bone remodeling in middle-aged and older men. A 16 week strength training program in 11 men increased muscle strength by 45%, femoral neck BMD by a significant $3.8 \pm 1.0\%$ and lumbar spine BMD by $2.0 \pm 0.9\%$ (not statistically significant). In addition, there were significant increases in osteocalcin and in skeletal alkaline phosphatase isoenzyme levels (which mark bone formation), but not in the enzyme markers of bone resorption.

Several recent prospective studies have examined the effects of strength training on BMD in premenopausal eumenorrheic women. Twelve months of Nautilus training was shown to result in a nonsignificant increase in lumbar spine BMD (0.81%) compared with a nonsignificant decrease of 0.5% in a matched control group. Although a small change in BMD was observed, these authors concluded that moderate weight lifting may not be a practical treatment for osteoporosis, even in a highly motivated population.

Snow-Harter et al compared the effects of 8 months of jogging or weight lifting on BMD. In the 31 women who completed the study, weight training increased strength in all muscle groups, whereas, no strength gains were found in the runners. Both training protocols increased lumbar BMD (running—1.3% and weight training—1.2%, respectively, P = NS), but no change in BMD at the proximal femur was found (Fig. 4). Both training groups had greater post-training lumbar BMD than control (no exercise) subjects. Thus, bone mass can be increased by diverse modes of weight-bearing activity, although longer training periods may be needed to see differentiation between these modes of exercise.

It has been hypothesized that BMD is related to the strength of muscles whose body insertions are located close to the sites where BMD is measured. BMD at the hip was found to correlate independently with muscle strength and body mass but not with age. Biceps strength

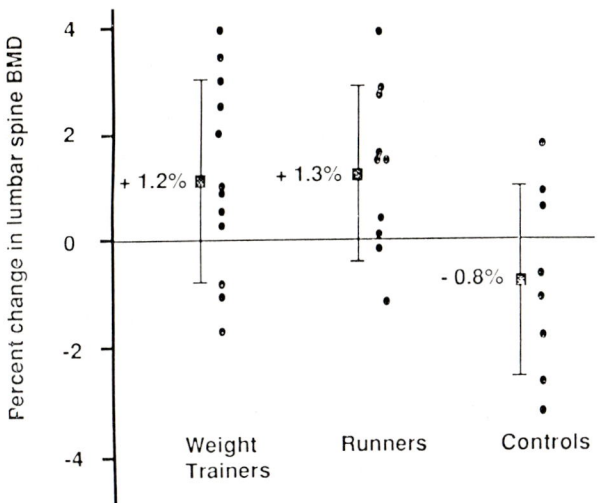

Figure 4 The filled circles represent the percentage change in lumbar spine bone mineral density (BMD) compared to baseline for individual subjects following 8 months of exercise training. The square notes the mean percentage change for each group, and the error bars represent 1 SD. The percentage change in the weight training and running groups was significantly different from zero ($p < 0.05$). (From Snow-Harter C, Bouxsein ML, Lewis BL, et al. Effects of resistance and endurance exercise on bone mineral status of young women: a randomized exercise intervention trial. J Bone Min Res 1992; 7:761-769; with permission.)

was an independent predictor of BMD at the hip, and grip strength best predicted lumbar spine density. The femoral neck BMD was significantly correlated with back strength and body mass, whereas trochanter and overall hip BMD were significantly related to biceps, and back and hip adductor strength. Hip BMD was not related to the strength of the quadriceps groups or to the hip flexors, extensor, or abductors. Muscle strength accounted for only 15% to 20% of the total variance in bone density of young women. Therefore, it seems that the relationship of muscle strength to bone density is more than a simple matter of direct muscle attachments to bone.

In contrast, some reports have suggested that exercise training does not alter BMD. Rockwell et al reported that 9 months of strength training in a small sample of eumenorrheic women significantly increased muscular strength (by 57%) but there was a 4% decrease in lumbar spine BMD and a significant increase in parathyroid hormone (PTH) levels relative to control subjects. Possibly, strength training initially alters bone turnover and a longer study is required to demonstrate a gain of bone mass. Peterson et al also observed that 1 year of weight training in middle-aged women significantly increased strength, but did not increase bone mass. The stress of daily ambulation in itself may be sufficient for maintenance of BMD at the femoral neck, Ward's triangle, and trochanter. The BMD at these sites is no greater in trained eumenorrheic runners than in sedentary eumenorrheic control subjects. These data imply that once an appropriate level of ambulation is

established, increasing exercise may not provide additional benefit unless the level of mechanical stress is also increased.

The type of exercise that stimulates bone formation remains unclear. Traditionally, weight-bearing activity, such as walking, running, and dancing have been promoted to minimize menopause-related bone loss. These recommendations were based on the theory that mechanical loading stress stimulated bone formation. For example, jogging produces a force 1 to 1.75 times the body weight, whereas weight-lifting activity specifically loads the lumbar spine five to six times the body weight. Sports that involve frequent jumping create large forces on impact and this may also be important. BMD has been reported to be significantly greater in the total body, femoral neck, Ward's triangle, and lumbar spine in college varsity volleyball players and gymnasts compared with swimmers and inactive controls. More than three-quarters of the gymnasts tested were either oligomenorrheic or amenorrheic, and yet they had significantly greater BMD than eumenorrheic swimmers and control subjects. Thus, athletes who participate in weight-bearing or high impact sports may have a higher BMD despite the negative influence of amenorrhea. The duration of involvement in high-impact activity may also be important. Grove and Londeree observed no differences in BMD in sedentary, early postmenopausal women whether they engaged in low- or high-impact exercise over a 1 year period. However, both forms of exercise reduced age-related bone loss relative to controls. These data support the notion that high-impact activity may have a greater impact on premenopausal than on postmenopausal women (in whom rates of bone resorption are increased). Unfortunately, this study did not control for estrogen supplementation, which may have confounded their results.

TRAINING SLOWS THE RATE OF AGE-RELATED BONE LOSS

Physical activity slows the rate of age-related bone loss and preserves lean body mass in women. The BMC of the mid-shaft of the radius is higher in women with a high level of physical activity than in those who are less active. BMC does not differ between women who are moderately active and those with low levels of activity. The relationship between activity level and BMC is significant in the premenopausal but not in the postmenopausal women. The rapid losses in BMC after menopause most likely overwhelm any beneficial effects of increased physical activity.

Other investigators have also found associations between physical activity and lumbar spine BMD ($r = 0.41$) or peak skeletal mass ($r = 0.51$). A reduced rate of bone loss in the arms of both pre- and postmenopausal women has also been shown. The greatest effects of exercise were on the radius and ulna, although the rates of bone loss from the left humerus were also reduced in the exercise group. Earlier studies suggested that age-related bone loss may be slowed by exercise programs that combine increased mechanical loading with increased physical fitness.

Increased aerobic power ($\dot{V}o_2$ max) has been associated with greater bone mass. Muscle strength, physical fitness, and body mass exert independent effects on bone mass, with age mediating its effect indirectly through associated changes in these factors. For example, age is not an independent predictor of femoral neck bone mass, suggesting that the reduction in proximal femoral bone mass with increasing age is due to decreased physical loading of the skeleton rather than a direct effect of aging.

In summary, the literature is equivocal with respect to the effects of exercise and skeletal loading on BMD. Any effects of exercise are confounded by both gender and age. Most studies support the concept that exercise protects bone mass, but the optimal exercise program to accomplish this goal has yet to be elucidated.

EXERCISE, GONADAL STEROIDS AND BONE MASS

Reproductive Hormone Abnormalities in Premenopausal Women Athletes

High levels of exercise training induce hormonal changes that possibly have adverse effects on bone density. In women, estrogens have profound effects on bone mineralization, whereas progesterone may impact trabecular bone density. Decreased estrogen production in premenopausal women is associated with vertebral bone loss and increased bone remodeling. Chronic exercise training reduces serum concentrations of estro-gen and progesterone in some premenopausal women, and athletes with reduced circulating levels of gonadal steroids show diminished lumbar spine BMD. It is speculated that hypoestrogenemia and/or hypoprogesteronemia associated with oligomenorrhea and amenorrhea is largely responsible for the lower BMD. Anovulatory menstrual cycles and low progesterone levels have been related to trabecular bone loss in normally menstruating women.

Drugs that inhibit ovulation also increase bone turnover. Administration of a superactive GnRH agonist (nafarelin) daily for 6 months to 47 healthy eumenorrheic women, as a means of contraception, inhibited ovulation, decreased the mean serum estradiol concentrations to levels observed during the early follicular phase of the menstrual cycle (162 pmol/L), and resulted in biochemical changes consistent with increased bone turnover (increased serum calcium, phosphate, and osteocalcin concentrations, and decreased serum PTH levels).

We examined the relationship between reproductive hormones and BMD of the lumbar spine and proximal femur among 43 female runners (age 18 to 40 years) classified as either eumenorrheic ($n = 24$), oligomenorrheic ($n = 8$), or amenorrheic ($n = 11$) (Fig. 5). Lumbar spine BMD and concentrations of progesterone and 17β-estradiol were higher in the control and eumenorrheic runner groups than in the oligomenorrheic and amenorrheic runner groups. None of the steroid hormones were significantly related to BMD in the oligo/amenorrheic groups, but progesterone was significantly correlated with lumbar BMD in the eumenorrheic runners (Fig. 6). We concluded that circulating levels of gonadal steroid hormones influence axial BMD in

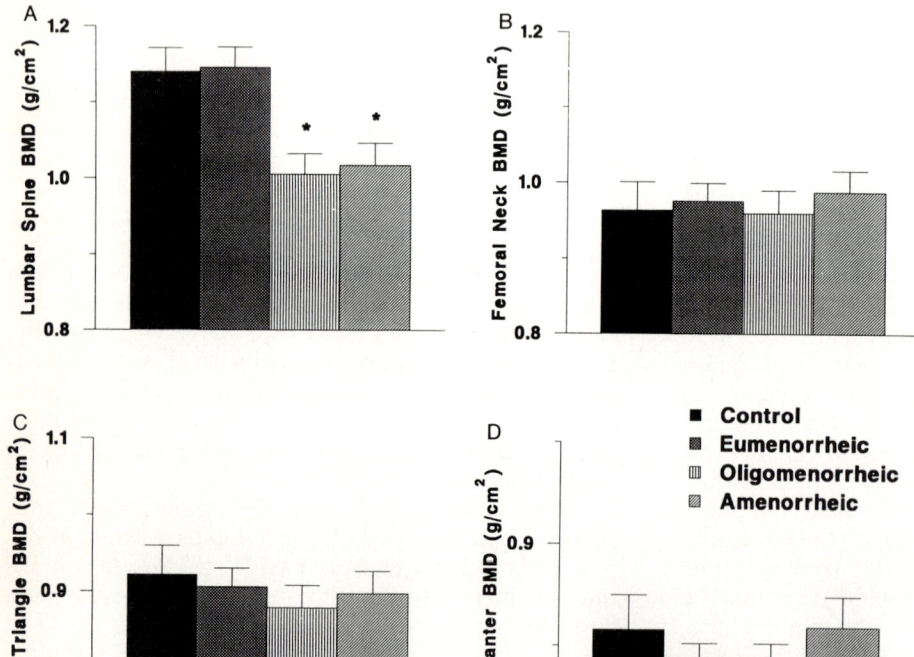

Figure 5 Comparison of bone mineral density (BMD) values at lumbar spine *(A)*, femoral neck *(B)*, Ward's triangle *(C)*, and trochanter *(D)* in nonrunner control group and eumenorrheic, oligomenorrheic, and amenorrheic runner groups. Means ± SE. *oligomenorrheic and amenorrheic < controls, eumenorrheics ($p < 0.05$). (From Snead DB, Weltman A, Weltman JY, et al. Reproductive hormones and bone mineral density in women runners. J Appl Physiol 1992; 72:2149-2156; with permission.)

eumenorrheic runners. A subsample of 32 women runners, classified as eumenorrheic ($n = 19$) or oligo/amenorrheic ($n = 13$) were compared with a group of eumenorrheic control subjects ($n = 9$). Dietary intake and the eating disorders inventory subscale scores were similar among groups; however, in the oligomenorrheic and amenorrheic runners, there was an inverse trend between eating disorders subscale scores (for bulimia and an attitude of ineffectiveness) and femoral BMD ($r = -0.62$ to -0.71, $p < 0.05$). Therefore, although self-reported dietary intake and/or eating behaviors do not predict reproductive dysfunction in women runners, eating behaviors may be associated with lower BMD in oligo/amenorrheic runners.

The reversibility of decreased bone mass associated with amenorrhea is still unclear. When amenorrheic runners resume regular menses (due to reduced training intensity or injury preventing training), there is a partial restoration of BMD. Athletes who remained amenor-

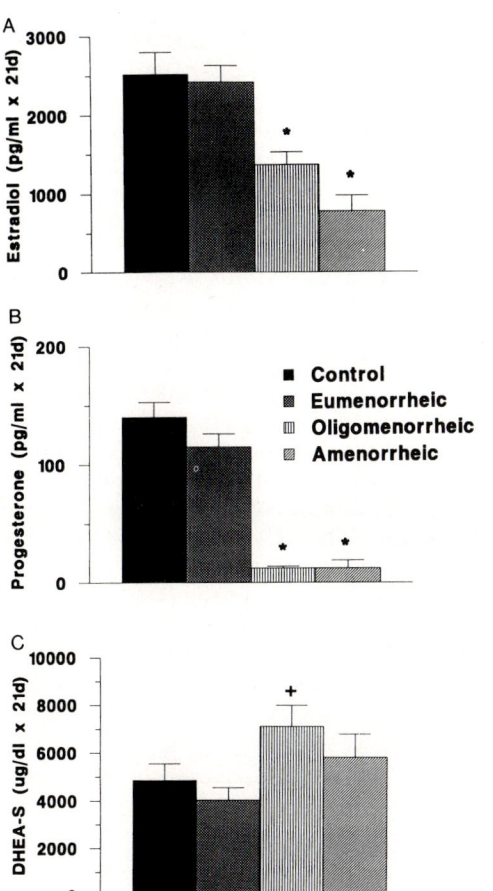

Figure 6 Integrated area under the curve (21 days) for 17β-estradiol *(A)*, progesterone *(B),* and dehydroepiandrosterone sulfate (DHEA-S) *(C)*, concentrations of runner control group and eumenorrheic, oligomenorrheic and amenorrheic runner group. Means ± SE. *oligomenorrheic, amenorrheic < control, eumenorrheic; + oligomenorrheic > eumenorrheic ($p < 0.05$). (From Snead DB, Weltman A, Weltman JY, et al. Reproductive hormones and bone mineral density in women runners. J Appl Physiol 1992; 72:2149-2156; with permission.)

rheic during the study period had a 3.4% loss of vertebral BMD while vertebral BMD was significantly increased (6.3%) in those who regained menses, although BMD was still less than in controls. Residual defects in bone density from previous oligomenorrhea or amenorrhea seem to be limited to the vertebrae. This is in contrast with postmenopausal osteoporosis, where decreased bone mass is seen at both the radius and vertebrae. Prior menstrual history is nevertheless the best predictor of trabecular bone density and some amenorrheic athletes may not be able to restore bone density mass.

Although estrogen/progesterone replacement therapy can maintain bone mass and decrease the fracture rate in postmenopausal women, few data exist regarding the effect of estrogen/progesterone replacement therapy in premenopausal women with oligomenorrhea or amenorrhea. Oral contraceptive use in eumenorrheic premenopausal women either slightly elevates or has no effect on BMD. In seven amenorrheic athletes, De Cree et al demonstrated a 9.5% increase in lumbar spine BMD after 8 months of treatment with a contraceptive dose of cyproterone acetate (2 mg) (which has potent progestational activity) plus 50 μg of ethinyl estradiol. In contrast, control subjects showed only a 1.6% increase in lumbar spine BMD. It remains unclear whether there is an interaction between the amount and type of exercise, menstrual function, and benefit from estrogen/progesterone replacement therapy in premenopausal women.

Male Runners

Although the study of bone loss has focussed on women, there is concern that male runners may also be susceptible to bone loss. Male runners (148 km/week) had significantly lower vertebral BMD (1.12 ± 0.03 g cm^{-2}) than non-runners (1.24 ± 0.04 g cm^{-2}) ($p < 0.05$); however, the BMD at sites of predominantly cortical bone did not differ significantly between the two groups. The low vertebral BMD values obtained in this study are similar to those reported by others for amenorrheic female runners and may reflect the hormonal changes that accompany endurance training. Spinal BMD did not differ between male runners and sedentary control subjects, but in the lower legs, BMD was significantly ($p < 0.05$) greater for the 24 to 32 km/week group than in the control and 8 to 16 km/week groups. Tibial BMD showed no further increase when running more than 32 km/week and even tended to decrease, such that the tibial BMD was similar for the 96 to 129 km/week and control group. The cross-sectional area of the tibia and fibula, normalized for body mass, tended to be greater as weekly distance increased and it was significantly greater in the 64 to 88 km/week runners than in the control group. Trunk BMD tended to be lower in runners who ran more than 64 km/week. The average BMD of the trunk in the 96 to 120 km/week runners was ~6% and ~9% lower than the 24 to 32 km/week and control groups, respectively. These findings suggest that running volume affects both BMD and cross-sectional area of certain load bearing bones in male runners. Serum testosterone concentrations were unrelated to running distance, suggesting that other factors may mediate these effects.

Lumbar BMC has also been negatively correlated with the distance run ($r = -0.37$, $p < 0.0001$) (Fig. 7). The weekly distance run remained significantly and negatively related to the BMC of the lumbar spine and the proximal femur when body mass index (BMI) and age were added to the multiple regression model. Male long distance runners had significantly lower BMC of the lumbar spine, proximal femur, distal forearm, and total body than the nonrunners. For those individuals who ran more than 100 km/week, the lumbar BMC averaged 19% less than that of nonrunning controls. After adjustment for differences in body mass index (BMI) and body height, the BMC in the elite runners remained significantly lower in those weight-bearing bones with a high proportion of trabecular bone. Serum concentrations of gonadal steroids and gonadotropin were nevertheless within the normal range. The low BMC was correlated with biochemical markers of bone turnover, which were 20% to 30% higher in the elite runners than in the nonrunners. However, an increased bone turnover does not necessarily indicate whether the net balance of remodeling is positive or negative.

Postmenopausal Women

It is difficult to separate the effects of age and menopause on bone loss. The loss of trabecular bone is accelerated around the onset of menopause and slows somewhat thereafter, although rates of bone loss remain above premenopausal levels (Fig. 2). At menopause, bone loss increases to 9% per decade. Ballard et al reported that in postmenopausal women a high physical activity group (activities with an intensity of 8.5 METs or greater) had a significantly higher BMC at the distal third of the radius compared to a low physical activity group. In addition, an estrogen replacement therapy group had a higher bone mass than a group that did not receive estrogen therapy. They speculated that the combination of physical activity and estrogen replacement therapy would produce a more positive effect on forearm bone than either treatment alone.

In postmenopausal women, bone loss is slowed or prevented by exercise. Intensive bone-loading exercise prevents radial bone loss, but brisk walking does not. However, normal daily walking is associated with a greater lumbar spine and femoral neck BMD. Aerobic exercise and/or strength training for 1 year increases the bone calcium index compared to a control group, but the type of exercise seems unimportant. In women with a low initial bone density, an exercise program alone is ineffective in preventing further bone loss.

A 5 year longitudinal study of men and women examined the association of long-term physical training with changes in lumbar bone mineralization; decreases in BMD over time were statistically significant in both runners and control subjects. Fourteen members of a running club (aged 55 to 77 years) and 14 matched sedentary control subjects underwent computerized tomography scans of the first lumbar vertebra at baseline and after 5 years. Despite significant decreases in lumbar spine BMD in both runners and control subjects, the runners maintained a greater BMD over the study period. The decrease in BMD was most pronounced in individuals who decreased their running habits. In both men and women, highly significant correlations ($r = 0.78$ and 0.91, respectively, $p < 0.002$) were found between changes in lumbar BMD and the average time spent running (min/week). Although regular running appeared to reduce age-related bone loss both in women and men, substantial decreases in physical weight-bearing activity were associated with important bone loss in the lumbar spine.

A well-controlled study reported that short-term weight-bearing exercise training increased BMC in postmenopausal women (aged 55 to 70 years). Bone mineral content increased 5.2% over 9 months of training, whereas there was no change (-1.4%) in the control group. After 22 months of exercise, BMC was increased 6.1%. After 13 months of decreased activity, however, bone mass was only 1.1% above baseline. Thus, long-term training can maintain the increase in bone mass, but detraining quickly causes the BMC to revert to baseline. These findings support the Lanyon hypothesis that bone mass will increase to meet the demand from mechanical loading, but only for as long as the stimulus is

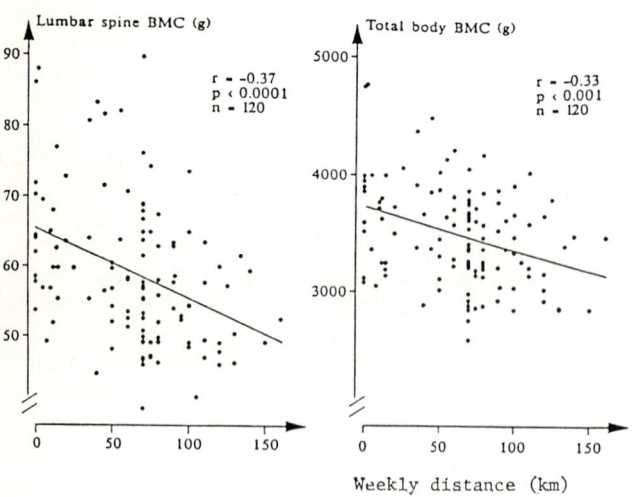
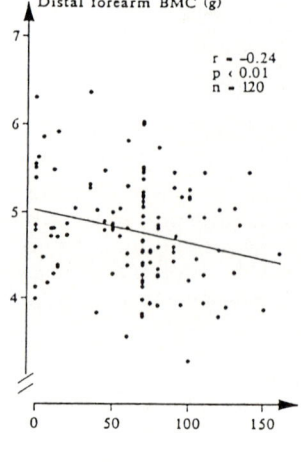

Figure 7 Bone mineral content in the lumbar spine, total body and distal forearm as a function of the weekly running distance in 120 men. (From Hetland ML, Haarbo J, Christiansen C. Low bone mass and high bone turnover in male long distance runners. J Clin Endocrinol Metab 1993; 77: 770-775; with permission.)

continued. Adequate activity must be maintained if the bone adaptations to training are to persist.

In early postmenopausal women who are not receiving estrogen replacement therapy, weight training is effective in maintaining or increasing BMD at the lumbar spine, and femoral neck and BMC at the distal wrist. Following 9 months of weight training, lumbar spine BMD was significantly greater in the weight-trained group than the control group. Values in the control group decreased by 3.6%, whereas those in the weight-training group increased by 1.6%; no effect was detected at the femoral neck or distal wrist site. These positive findings are similar to those of Dalsky and colleagues, who found a 5.2% increase in vertebral BMD over a 9 month period of walking, jogging, and stair climbing.

Nonloading exercises seem to be ineffective in preventing vertebral bone loss in postmenopausal women. Using a backpack with weights equivalent to 30% of maximal strength, back raises were carried out 3 times/5 days a week for 2 years. Lumbar spine density did not change significantly in either the control or the exercise group, although back extensor strength increased significantly more in the exercise group than in the control group.

Estrogen Replacement Therapy

Estrogen alone or in combination with progesterone retards postmenopausal bone loss. It is most beneficial if prescribed in the early postmenopausal years before irreversible bone loss has occurred. Long-term (3 years) estrogen replacement therapy initiated soon after menopause resulted in a 3.7% increase in forearm BMC; a 5.7% decrease was seen in the placebo group. Subsequent discontinuation of estrogen replacement therapy resulted in bone loss identical to that seen in a group that was not receiving estrogen replacement therapy. Long-term estrogen replacement therapy users (19 years) had a greater spinal BMD (1.219 g/cm^2) than nonusers (1.092 g/cm^2; $p < 0.01$). All types of estrogen replacement therapy increased lumbar and femoral BMD compared with control subjects. Transdermal estrogen replacement therapy is effective in increasing both forearm and lumbar spine BMD compared to placebo groups. An 18 month comparison of oral estrogen (0.625 mg daily) and transdermal estrogen (0.05 mg) replacement therapy revealed significant vertebral BMD increases at 6, 12, and 18 months with transdermal estrogen replacement therapy and at 12 and 18 months with oral estrogen replacement therapy (Fig. 8). The minimum effective dose for bone sparing is 0.625 mg of conjugated equine estrogen and doubling the dose does not provide any additional benefit. Bone resorption is diminished when circulating levels of estradiol reach a value of 60 pg/ml, similar to that seen the last days of the early follicular phase. Transdermal estrogen replacement therapy may protect against bone loss with serum estradiol concentrations of 45 to 50 pg/ml.

Heikkinen et al found that physical exercise with estrogen treatment did not result in further increases in BMD. One cross-sectional study reported that control subjects had a 3.3% lower total body BMC, whereas the

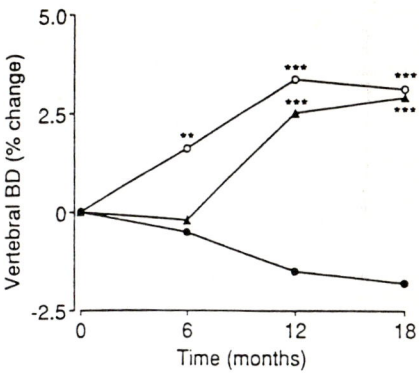

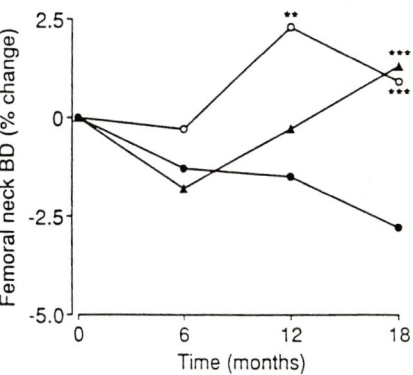

Figure 8 Bone density changes (median % initial value) in lumbar spine *(A)* and femoral neck *(B)*. ● Untreated; ○ transdermal estrogen replacement therapy; △ oral hormone replacement therapy. **$p < 0.01$, ***$p < 0.001$ versus untreated. (From Stevenson JC, Cust MP, Gangar KF, et al. Effects of transdermal versus oral hormone replacement therapy on bone density in spine and proximal femur in postmenopausal women. Lancet 1990; 335:265-269; with permission.)

physical activity group and drug group had a 2.3% and 1.6% greater BMC, respectively. In addition, exercise and high dietary calcium may preferentially alter bone density at different skeletal sites. The women who exercised maintained the trabecular BMD of the spine, whereas, the women who remained sedentary lost bone at this site, with dietary calcium having no effect. Calcium intake affected the BMD of the femur. Women who consumed high amounts of dietary calcium maintained femoral BMD, whereas those on moderate amounts showed a decrease. There was no effect of either intervention on the BMD of the distal radius or on total body calcium. This implies that women should be encouraged to adopt a combination of a calcium-rich diet and weight-bearing exercise to maintain the health of their skeleton. In women under the age of 75 who had taken estrogen for 7 years or longer, the bone density (average of all sites) was 11.2% greater than in women who had never received estrogen. This was associated with a reduction in hip fractures of approximately 44% at the femoral neck and 52% at the trochanter. In women over the age of 75 who received 7 or more years of estrogen therapy, bone density was only 3.2% higher than in women who had never taken estrogen. The authors concluded that at least 7 years of estrogen replacement therapy after menopause are necessary for a long-term protective effect on BMD and that even therapy of this duration may be insufficient to protect women 75 years old and older from fracture.

REFERENCES

Aloia JF, Vaswani AN, Yeh JK, Cohn SH. Premenopausal bone mass is related to physical activity. Arch Intern Med 1988; 148:121–123.

Ballard JE, McKeown BC, Graham HM, Zinkgraf SA. The effect of high level physical activity (8.5 METs or greater) and estrogen replacement therapy upon bone mass in postmenopausal females, aged 50-68 years. Int J Sports Med 1990; 3:208–214.

Bilanin JE, Blanchard MS, Russek-Cohen E. Lower vertebral bone density in male long distance runners. Med Sci Sport Exerc 1989; 21:66–70.

Chow R, Harrison JE, Notarius C. Effect of two randomised exercise programmes on bone mass of healthy postmenopausal women. Br Med J 1987; 295:1441–1444.

Christiansen C, Rii BJ. Hormonal replacement therapy and the skeletal system. Maturitas 1990; 12:247–257.

Dalsky GP, Stocke KS, Ehsani AA, et al. Weight-bearing exercise training and lumbar bone mineral content in postmenopausal women. Ann Intern Med 1988; 108:824–828.

Dalsky GP. The role of exercise in the prevention of osteoporosis. Compr Ther 1989; 15:30–37.

Davee AM, Rosen CJ, Robert A, Adler RA. Exercise patterns and trabecular bone density in college women. J Bone Min Res 1990; 5:245–250.

De Cree C, Lewin R, Ostyn M. Suitability of cyproterone acetate in the treatment of osteoporosis associated with athletic amenorrhea. Int J Sports Med 1988; 9:187–192.

Drinkwater BL, Nilson K, Chestnut CH III, et al. Bone mineral content of amenorrheic and eumenorrheic athletes. N Engl J Med 1984; 311:277–281.

Drinkwater BL, Nilson K, Otts, Chestnut CH III. Bone mineral density after resumption of menses in amenorrheic women. JAMA 1986; 256:380–382.

Fehling PC, Rector A, Alekel L, et al. A comparison of bone mineral densities at axial and appendicular sites among collegiate athletes. Med Sci Sport Exerc 1993; 25(Suppl):S199.

Felson DT, Zhang Y, Hannan MT, et al. The effect of postmenopausal estrogen therapy on bone density in elderly women. N Engl J Med 1993; 329:1141–1146.

Gleeson PB, Protas EJ, LeBlanc AD, et al. Effects of weight lifting on bone mineral density in premenopausal women. J Bone Min Res 1990; 5:153–158.

Grove KA, Londeree BR. Bone density in postmenopausal women: High impact vs low impact exercise. Med Sci Sport Exerc 1992; 24:1190–1193.

Gudmundsson JA, Ljunghall S, Bergquist C, et al. Increased bone turnover during gonadotropin-releasing hormone superagonist-induced ovulation inhibition. J Clin Endocrinol Metab 1987; 65:159–163.

Heikkinen J, Kurttila-Matero E, Kyllonen E, et al. Moderate exercise does not enhance the positive effect of estrogen on bone mineral density in postmenopausal women. Calcif Tissue Int 1991; 49(Suppl):83–84.

Heinrich CH, Going SB, Pamenter RW, et al. Bone mineral content of cyclically menstruating female resistance and endurance trained athletes. Med Sci Sport Exerc 1989; 22:558–563.

Hetland ML, Haarbo J, Christiansen C. Low bone mass and high bone turnover in male long distance runners. J Clin Endocrinol Metab 1993; 77:770-775.

Hui SL, Slemenda CW, Johnston CC, Apledorn CR. Effects of age and menopause on vertebral bone density. Bone Miner 1987; 2:141-146.

Johnston CC Jr, Hui Sl, Witt RM, et al. Early menopausal changes in bone mass and sex steroids. J Endocrinol Metab 1985; 61:905–911.

MacDougall JD, Webber JE, Martin J, et al. Relationship among running mileage, bone density, and serum testosterone in male runners. Am J Physiol 1992; 73:1165–1170.

Mazess RB, Barden HS. Bone density in premenopausal women: Effects of age, dietary intake, physical activity, smoking, and birth-control pills. Am J Clin Nutr 1991; 53:132–142.

Menkes A, Mazel S, Redmond RA, et al. Strength training increases regional bone mineral density and bone remodeling in middle-aged and older men. J Appl Physiol 1993; 74:2478–2484.

Michel BA, Bloch DA, Fries JF. Weight-bearing exercise, overexercise, and lumbar bone density over age 50 years. Arch Intern Med 1989; 149:2325–2329.

Moore M, Bracker M, Sartoris D, et al. Long-term estrogen replacement therapy in postmenopausal women sustains vertebral bone mineral density. J Bone Min Res 1990; 5:659–663.

Nelson ME, Fisher EC, Dilmanian FA, et al. A l-y walking program and increased dietary calcium in postmenopausal women: Effects on bone. Am J Clin Nutrit 1991; 53:1304–1311.

Peterson SE, Peterson MD, Raymond G, et al. Muscular strength and bone density with weight training in middle-aged women. Med Sci Sports Exerc 1991; 23:499–504.

Pocock N, Eisman J, Gwinn T, et al. Muscle strength, physical fitness, and weight but not age predict femoral neck bone mass. J Bone Min Res 1989; 4:441–448.

Prior JC, Vigna YM, Schechter MT, Burgess AE. Spinal bone loss and ovulatory disturbances. N Eng J Med 1990; 323:1221–1227.

Pruitt LA, Jackson RD, Bartels RL, Lehnhard HJ. Weight-training effects on bone mineral density in early postmenopausal women. J Bone Min Res 1992; 7:179–185.

Reginster JY, Sarlet N, Deroisy R, et al. Minimal levels of serum estradiol prevent postmenopausal bone loss. Calcif Tissue Int 1992; 51:340–343.

Riggs BL, Wahner HW, Dunn WL, et al. Differential changes in bone mineral density of the appendicular and axial skeleton with aging: Relationship to spinal osteoporosis. J Clin Invest 1981; 67:328–335.

Riggs BL, Melton LJ III. The prevention and treatment of osteoporosis. N Engl J Med 1992; 327:620–627.

Rockwell JC, Sorensen AM, Baker S, et al. Weight training decreases vertebral bone density in premenopausal women: A prospective study. J Clin Endocrinol Metab 1990; 71:988–993.

Sinaki M, Wahner HW, Offord KP, Hodgson SF. Efficacy of nonloading exercises in prevention of vertebral bone loss in postmenopausal women: a controlled trial. Mayo Clin Proc 1989; 64:762–769.

Smith EL, Gilligan C, McAdam M, et al. Deterring bone loss by exercise intervention in premenopausal and postmenopausal women. Calcif Tissue Int 1989; 44:312–321.

Snead DB, Weltman A, Weltman JY, et al. Reproductive hormones and bone mineral density in women runners. J Appl Physiol 1992; 72:2149–2156.

Snow-Harter C, Marcus R. Exercise, bone mineral density, and osteoporosis. In: Holloszy JO, ed. Exercise and sports sciences review. Philadelphia: Williams & Wilkins, 1991, p 351.

Snow-Harter C, Bouxsein ML, Lewis BL, et al. Effects of resistance and endurance exercise on bone mineral status of young women: a randomized exercise intervention trial. J Bone Min Res 1992; 7:761-769.

Stevenson JC, Cust MP, Gangar KF, et al. Effects of transdermal versus oral hormone replacement therapy on bone density in spine and proximal femur in postmenopausal women. Lancent 1990; 335:265-269.

Stillman RJ, Lohman TG, Slaughter MH, Massey BH. Physical activity and bone mineral content in women aged 30 to 85 years. Med Sci Sport Exerc 1986; 18:576-580.

Zylstra S, Hopkins A, Erk M, et al. Effect of physical activity on lumbar spine and femoral neck bone densities. Int J Sports Med 1989; 10:181-186.

PHYSIOTHERAPY IN SPORTS MEDICINE

SCOTT M. HASSON, Ed.D., P.T., F.A.C.S.M.

This chapter describes the role of the sports physiotherapist in the prevention, evaluation, and treatment of musculoskeletal dysfunction. The etiology, prevention, and treatment of specific injuries are discussed in other chapters.

ETIOLOGY AND PREVENTION OF MUSCULOSKELETAL DYSFUNCTION

The physiotherapist acts as an advisor to athletes, coaches, athletic trainers, and physicians in regards to the prevention of acute traumatic and chronic overuse musculoskeletal dysfunction. The certified sports physiotherapist is trained in conditioning techniques and is familiar with equipment modifications that will minimize acute trauma. In addition, and in my opinion most importantly, the physiotherapist is able to recognize normal and abnormal patterns of motion that have a high probability of causing an overuse injury.

Acute Traumatic Injuries

Acute traumatic injuries occur when an external or internal force is applied that is too great for the target tissue to withstand. Injuries are very specific to individual sports, and protective wear has been developed to minimize injuries, such as the helmets worn in American football. The joints are the most commonly injured structures. Sports physiotherapists work with team physicians, coaches, and athletic trainers to devise braces and joint taping to prevent an acute injury or reduce the likelihood of a recurrent injury. Even though taping and bracing of joints have become common, there are little data to support the view that these interventions make a difference on first time or repeat injuries. Another method of preventing acute traumatic injury is through muscle and joint conditioning. Sports physiotherapists again work closely with trainers and coaches in developing specific muscle strengthening exercise regimens to help protect hyper- or hypomobile joints. In addition, the sports physiotherapist may help to develop specific training programs to improve muscle flexibility. This type of conditioning is usually incorporated into warm-ups, cool-downs, or during drills. Very little research has been performed to determine the effectiveness of specific muscle and joint conditioning programs in preventing injuries. I personally believe that such conditioning may be helpful in reducing injuries. However, with high velocity impact sports, the magnitude of the internal and external forces generated often exceed the tensile breaking limits of the musculoskeletal system.

In my opinion, external bracing and taping do very little to prevent a first time or recurrent injury. Protective pads and helmets, however, do prevent serious injuries and should be worn throughout a contest. Specific muscle strengthening and joint conditioning may also play a role in decreasing initial or recurrent injuries, although a valid human model of research does not presently exist.

Overuse Injuries

The normal mechanics of motion can and do cause overuse injuries. Most overuse injuries occur because the motion incorporates an eccentric muscle action. As an individual repeats the motion, "mechanical fatigue" may develop. Mechanical fatigue is very different from the metabolic fatigue that is observed with higher intensity muscle action of either concentric or isometric type. It occurs when the muscle is challenged repeatedly by significant intensities of eccentric muscle action. The intensity of eccentric action that causes mechanical fatigue depends on the individual's physical condition and the mechanics of the motion. Individuals who train with eccentric loads are less likely to develop a musculotendinous overuse injury or delayed onset muscle soreness. Proper biomechanics of motion usually place the muscle and joint in a position where the transmission and absorption of force are optimal. When the mechanics of motion deviate from this optimal relationship, overuse injuries become more prevalent. Intensity is not the only factor determining when mechanical fatigue may occur. Frequency and duration of muscle action are also critical components. In fact, I view the major determinant of mechanical fatigue and thus injury to be the total amount of work performed, which incorporates intensity, frequency, and duration. However, trained individuals are less likely to develop difficulties than are untrained individuals when presented with an equal physical challenge.

Trained athletes develop overuse injuries when the intensity, frequency, and/or mechanics of eccentric muscle action go beyond the limit of tensile strength of the musculotendinous junction. Regardless of the cause of injury, the muscle and musculotendinous regions undergo an inflammatory response, with tissue swelling. If uncontrolled and untreated, the result is delayed onset discomfort. If the primary area of injury is muscle, the discomfort abates after 72 to 96 hours. If the injury is primarily to the tendon, the discomfort is of much longer duration and healing of the tissue is much slower. The differences in the two tissues are the extent of supportive vascularity and the speed of actual healing and repair processes. Muscle is much more vascular than tendon. The inflammatory and repair response is also much more vigorous. Muscle tissue heals without scarring, unless a tear has occurred. When a muscle tear occurs, this is classed as macrotrauma. In microtrauma induced by mechanical fatigue, the sarcomeres of the muscle cell are disrupted and the myofilaments are damaged. Nevertheless, the myotube is spared and repair of the muscle is a very "natural" process. However, tendon tissue that has undergone either macrotrauma or microtrauma, is less likely to be restored to a fully normal tissue. The healing response is much slower in tendon, because of the limited vascularity and the tissue generated does not have the same constituents as previously. Elastic fibers are not laid down with as much prevalence and the fibrous repair tissue lacks the original architecture of the tendon. The repair is a scar with more cross-linking and fewer parallel fibers than are normally observed in tendinous tissue. The most prevalent overuse injuries that are of a chronic nature incorporate tendinous structures (e.g., lateral epicondylitis).

Overuse injuries may be preventable by proper training techniques and evaluation of the mechanics of the sports motion. Training of the athlete or a nonathletic individual must incorporate sound principles of exercise prescription, with an appropriate regulation of intensity, frequency, duration, and mode of activity. As described above, the total amount of eccentric muscle work performed is the major factor determining the risk of overuse injuries. Elimination of all eccentric activity is not possible in training and athletic endeavors. Therefore, the total work and mode of exercise must be modified when initiating new or changing existing training activities. The amount of work that is performed in a given time can be modified by altering the intensity, frequency and/or duration of the activity. The duration and frequency are probably easier to modify than intensity for most activities. Studies from our laboratory indicate that during a bout of eccentric muscle action, the individual can perceive the onset of "mechanical fatigue." If activity continues beyond this perception point, the result is typically muscle injury, weakness, and eventually delayed onset muscle soreness. One of our experimental overuse research models involving extensor carpi radialis brevis results in a "lateral epicondylitis-like condition," with muscle and tendon involvement. Yet, exercising to the point of fatigue is commonly used in endurance and power training in order to achieve physiologic adaptations. It seems reasonable to believe that in order to get positive adaptations of musculotendinous tensile strength, the tissues must be stressed near to fatigue.

Is it necessary for damage to occur in order to gain the adaptation? This is an important, unanswered question. The answer may be different for muscle as compared to tendon. If a training bout causes muscle damage, subsequent exercise bouts to a similar total workload cause neither muscle damage nor delayed onset muscle soreness. Therefore, training appears to be a possible way to gain a physiologic adaptation that will prevent repeated injury of muscle. However, it is not known what effect proper training would have on preventing overuse musculotendinous injuries.

In my opinion, training is the best way to prevent overuse injuries. However, training incorporating too much duration and frequency at too high an intensity is the most common cause of overuse injuries. The athlete balances upon a fine line in many sports. Unfortunately, there is really no research on the human model to determine what intensity, frequency, and duration is too much or too little. Athletes are dependent on their own experiences and those of their coaches, trainers, and therapists.

EVALUATION AND TREATMENT OF MUSCULOSKELETAL DYSFUNCTION

The physiotherapist in conjunction with the physician is responsible for evaluating musculoskeletal dysfunction of acute, traumatic, and chronic overuse etiology. The certified sports physiotherapist is usually trained to undertake both emergency diagnosis and care on the field and differential diagnosis of acute and chronic musculoskeletal dysfunction and derangements. The physiotherapist is also trained in the use of modalities to control pain, inflammation, and promote tissue healing. In addition, and in my opinion most importantly, the physiotherapist is able to develop therapeutic exercise programs to improve general strength and endurance, and to treat specific problems of muscle weakness, contractures, and joint hypo- and hypermobility. Finally, the physiotherapist uses techniques of massage and manual therapy in the treatment of pain, soft tissue and joint dysfunction, and derangement.

Acute Traumatic Injuries

Acute traumatic injuries arise primarily when an external or internal force is applied that is too great for the target tissue to handle. The results are broken bones, torn ligaments, joint disruption, and soft tissue injury. Evaluation seeks to differentiate the level of injury. In professional and major university settings roentgenographic technology is available on the field to differentiate ligament, joint, and soft tissue injury from fractures. However, in grade school, high school, most college, and other recreational settings roentgenographic equipment is not available. Here, on-site medical and professional personnel must assess quickly and accurately the type and severity of injury, determining whether continued play is recommended. This involves inspection and palpation of the damaged area. Key features in differential evaluation are the location of the injury, and how the damaged tissue responds. For example, if the location of the injury is mid-leg, a deformity points to a probable fracture. However, if the location of the injury is at the knee joint and immediate swelling occurs, the tissue damaged is probable ligamentous in type, with associated joint disruption. In both instances, return to immediate play is not recommended! One other quick point is the recognition of life-threatening injuries, such as those affecting the head and spine. In these cases, immediate attention should be rendered and immobilization might be recommended, even before a thorough evaluation. When head and spine injuries occur, play for the athlete should be suspended, even if the injuries are deemed minor following evaluation.

Treatment for acute traumatic injuries depends on the type of injury. In most cases of ligamentous injury and joint disruption, the area is initially immobilized—rested (R), iced (I), compressed (C), and elevated (E). With muscle tears and deep contusions, a similar regimen is followed to reduce swelling and limit motion. The usual course of these "macrotraumas" is immediate bleeding in the affected tissue region, with resultant tissue and/or joint swelling. The athlete may have a sharp acute pain with the injury, followed by a continuous throbbing pain associated with the tissue swelling. The immediate treatment described above (RICE) is continued for 12 to 24 hours, with the possible exception of initiating active motion (depending on the pain response). In my own practice, I push for early motion of joints and areas of soft tissue injury. The range of motion (ROM) may be severely restricted, and the pain pattern guides patients and therapists as to the amount of movement that should be performed. With most acute traumatic joint and soft tissue injuries, I continue to promote ice and manual compression (ice massage) and continued progressive ROM over the next few days. Nonsteroidal antiinflammatory drugs (NSAIDs) may be appropriate, beginning 24 hours after the injury (bleeding has abated in the first few hours), and continuing along with ice, massage, and therapeutic exercise. The result is decreased tissue swelling and pain, and in my opinion an earlier return to activity. I do not recommend the use of moist heat or deeper tissue heating modalities for these injuries; the risk of increased swelling and tissue damage from self application of moist heat far outweighs the benefit of minor pain relief and increased blood flow. Blood flow increases (arterial and venous) are much greater during active movement as compared to passive tissue heating. In addition, I do not advocate electrical stimulation either to induce muscle contractions or to relieve pain. Active motion is controlled by the patient, and the subjective established ROM remains intact. Also, this type of pain (acute, arising from damaged tissue) is not well controlled by electrical stimulation. Finally, I do advocate ultrasound (US) treatment, but in a pulsed, nonthermal mode. Pulsed US applied 24 hours after muscle injury decreases discomfort and augments muscle strength. Animal studies have shown that pulsed mode US causes a fluid streaming effect within musculotendinous tissue, resulting in decreased inflammation and interstitial swelling.

Overuse Injuries

Overuse injuries arise primarily when mechanical fatigue occurs, as the muscle and tendon are challenged repeatedly by eccentric muscle action of significant intensity. Microtrauma develop in the muscle and musculotendinous regions. These tissues undergo an inflammatory response, with interstitial swelling. Differential diagnosis is needed to determine the structure at fault. In most cases, this involves (1) medical history; (2) evaluation of active and passive ROM, strength, and sensation; and (3) specialized tests, including palpation and evaluation of specific motions focusing on pain production and functional limitations. Thermography, computed tomography (CT) and magnetic resonance imaging (MRI) scans are possible laboratory tools to evaluate these soft tissue injuries. However, the ability of these instruments to detect and assess the severity of a musculotendinous overuse lesion is controversial. Regardless of accuracy, such equipment is not available to most physiotherapists and many physicians. The physiotherapists and physicians who work with athletes must thus be highly skilled in the clinical differential diagnosis of musculoskeletal overuse injuries. Key features in differential diagnosis are the location of the injury, determined from history and palpation; the presence of pain during specific passive and active motions; and the presence of pain during complex functional tasks that are now limited because of pain. Many patients begin to develop dysfunction in other joints and body segments because of the primary injury. Therefore, when evaluating an overuse injury, the physiotherapist also assesses distal and proximal joints about the injury site.

The treatment of chronic overuse injuries depends on the type of injury. In most cases, the area is initially immobilized and rested by use of a splint. Exercise during this initial "rest" period must be questioned, since the cause of the injury was activity. A current study in our laboratory is evaluating the effect of "controlled regimented" exercise on lateral epicondylitis. The rationale for combining immobilized rest with controlled bouts of exercise is to allow the tissue to heal, but to minimize disuse and muscle and connective tissue atrophy. The exercise incorporated into the program is designed to affect the target muscle-tendon structure (i.e., extensor carpi radialis brevis); it incorporates both concentric and eccentric muscle action at very low loads. This type of exercise allows the muscle to become innervated, and promotes gliding between the fascial planes of neighboring muscles. This is similar to the idea of dynamically controlled mobilization after flexor tendon repair in zone 2 of the hand. In addition to rest and controlled mobilization, specific modalities are used to reduce inflammation in the tendinous structure. Since tendon undergoes a very different inflammatory and healing process than muscle, therapy for tendinitis must be independent of the vascular system. Ice, pulsed US with and without corticosteroid medication, and iontophoresis of corticosteroid medication have all been used with some success. The usual course of these overuse injuries is damage of the musculotendinous region without local bleeding. Delayed onset muscle soreness may begin 18 to 24 hours after the offending activity. Pain about the tendon, and tendon to bone junction may occur during this period, or it may manifest itself 24 to 48 hours later. Controlled mobilization, ice, and the delivery of corticosteroid by US or iontophoresis is begun immediately and may continue for 2 to 3 weeks. The range of mobilization may be somewhat restricted; the pain pattern guides the patient and therapist as to the amount of movement that should be performed during therapeutic exercise. NSAIDs may be appropriate during the initial 2 to 3 weeks of treatment, but the effect on the inflammation is not as dramatic as with muscle injuries. These initial weeks allow tendon healing, decrease tissue swelling and pain, and minimize tissue atrophy. As with acute traumatic injuries, I do not recommend the use of moist heat or deeper tissue heating modalities for chronic overuse injuries, for the reasons described earlier.

After the initial 2 to 3 weeks of rehabilitation, a more aggressive therapeutic exercise program can be initiated, with the goal of strengthening the muscle, tendon, and supportive connective tissue. In addition, I continue to use ice and occasionally US or iontophoresis as required. The exercise program I use is resistive in type, incorporating low-load concentric and eccentric muscle action. The selection of an appropriate intensity, frequency, and duration is critical, since reinjury is a real possibility. Initially, I tend to be on the conservative side, but progress the exercise in a fairly rapid fashion once I feel comfortable with the patient's ability and the injury itself. This "second phase" may take several months before the patient no longer experiences pain and is ready to return to full-time work and/or recreation.

The patient must accept that the process of healing of overuse injuries takes time and excellent compliance. Too quick a return to the offending activity may exacerbate the original problem. However, it is not necessary for the patient to stop all exercise and play. With assistance from the physiotherapist, the patient should look for alternative exercise and recreational activities. The treatment of an overuse injury should be oriented toward the etiology, with an initial emphasis on healing of the damaged tissue, followed by a conditioning of the target tissue. Patience must be practiced in order to insure a good result.

EXERCISE AND MUSCLE SORENESS

ALLAN H. GOLDFARB, Ph.D.
BRIAN T. BOYER, M.S.

Two types of soreness can occur as a result of exercise. The soreness that occurs during and immediately after exercise is thought to be of metabolic origin. The build-up of metabolic factors such as lactic acid, ammonia, and hydrogen ions that alters pH is believed to stimulate pain afferents. Soreness that typically develops 24 hours after exercise and peaks 48 to 72 hours after cessation of the exercise is called delayed onset muscle soreness (DOMS). DOMS usually diminishes gradually after peaking, although pain may persist for 4 to 7 days. Activities that are novel or unaccustomed often result in DOMS.

The pain associated with DOMS is frequently experienced with palpation or muscular contraction. The severity of DOMS is a function of the intensity and duration of the exercise and can be accompanied by a decrease in force production and/or a decreased range of motion (ROM). Elevated levels of blood proteins, creatine kinase (CK), or lactate dehydrogenase have been used as indicators of muscle damage and are related to DOMS.

Eccentric exercise (lengthening contractions) is more likely to cause DOMS than are concentric contractions. Activities such as downhill running, controlled lowering of a weight, skiing, and jumping all have extensive eccentric components. Eccentric contractions use fewer motor units than concentric contractions at a given work load. Since fewer muscle fibers are being recruited during eccentric contractions, a greater work load or force is sustained by each muscle fiber. This greater force is thought to result in disruption of both myofibrillar elements and connective tissue within the muscle.

The theory that DOMS results from muscle tissue and/or connective tissue damage has now gained considerable acceptance. Support has been documented by leakage of muscle enzymes into the blood, and by morphologic evidence such as Z band streaming and alterations in the structural integrity of the sarcomere.

The most common method for evaluating DOMS is by self report questionnaires. Individuals are asked to rate their perceptions of muscle soreness, using an ordinal scale ranging from one to 10. Verbal descriptors are usually associated with a particular numerical value on the rating scale. Individuals are asked to indicate their soreness after palpation or movement of the affected body part.

In an attempt to reduce the subjectivity associated with the use of soreness questionnaires, researchers have also attempted to quantify soreness using a strain gauge that measures force applied by a wooden probe. Force is applied over a superficial muscle site and the subject is asked to indicate when the feeling changes from pressure to discomfort. However, activation of pressure and pain afferents may elicit similar sensations of pain, which can lead to erroneous interpretations. Furthermore, force scores do not correlate significantly with subjective assessments of pain.

Researchers have also attempted to relate DOMS to biochemical measures within muscle and blood. Since tissue damage is associated with DOMS, markers of muscle damage and connective tissue damage have been utilized as indicators of DOMS. The leakage of certain muscle proteins such as CK, lactate dehydrogenase, or myoglobin out of the muscle and into the blood can occur when the integrity of the muscle membrane is compromised. Following exercise that commonly results in DOMS, there is a delayed increase in the blood concentration of these enzymes. However, it is not known whether the increase in the concentration of these enzymes is directly related to the processes that induce DOMS; certainly, blood CK levels can increase independent of DOMS.

One theory that has purported to explain the mechanism of DOMS resulting from eccentric loading is that of acute inflammation. Since an acute inflammatory response results in a series of events similar to what has been observed following eccentrically-induced muscle damage and connective tissue damage, inflammation has been implicated as a mechanism of DOMS. The classic signs of inflammation include redness, swelling, heat, pain, and decreases in ROM. Many of these symptoms are also associated with DOMS, supporting a linkage between the two phenomena. In further support of this theory, studies using both animals and humans have reported infiltration of neutrophils, mononuclear cells (lymphocytes, monocytes), and mast cells into damaged tissue following eccentric muscle activity. The data imply an activation of the acute inflammatory response following eccentric muscle contraction. In contrast, an acute inflammatory response is not always evident following eccentric muscle contraction, which induces tissue damage. The relationship between DOMS and acute inflammation therefore remains equivocal.

TREATMENT

The inflammatory response and DOMS are both associated with pain. Muscle pain is thought to be mediated by activation of type III and IV afferent fibers. Mechanical as well as chemical stimuli can activate these pain receptors, which are located in the sheaths surrounding muscle fibers, in tendons, and within muscle fibers. It has been hypothesized that activation of type III and IV afferent fibers generates DOMS.

Type III and IV afferent nerve fibers can be activated by chemicals such as bradykinin, serotonin, histamine, and potassium. Other substances can also modulate the activity of pain receptor nerve endings. Products from arachidonic acid metabolism, particularly prostaglandins and leukotrienes can sensitize these receptors to noxious stimuli. Several of these substances are also mediators of the inflammatory process and are therefore candidates for generating the pain associated with DOMS.

Since several of these substances are believed to contribute to DOMS, treatment has often centered on preventing these chemicals from activating the afferent nerve endings. Corticosteroids such as cortisone (Cortone) and prednisolone are effective anti-inflammatory agents because they inhibit the activity of phospholipase A_2. Phospholipase A_2 is the enzyme that converts phospholipids to arachidonic acid. The inhibitory action of corticosteroids on phospholipase A_2 prevents the production of the precursor for both prostaglandins and leukotrienes. In addition, corticosteroids can inhibit the release of histamine, a chemical associated with the generation of pain.

The effectiveness of corticosteroids as a means of inhibiting the production of histamine, prostaglandins, and leukotrienes *in vivo* has not been studied extensively.

The supposed effectiveness of corticosteroids in relieving DOMS is thus based primarily on conjecture. Furthermore, the analgesia produced by corticosteroids may be accompanied by undesirable side effects with attendant risks that outweigh the analgesic benefits.

Nonsteroidal anti-inflammatory agents (NSAIDs) are another possible drug treatment for DOMS. NSAIDs block the inflammatory response at the site of acute inflammation by blocking the enzyme cyclooxygenase and inhibiting the formation of prostaglandins. Theoretically, the inhibition of prostaglandin formation could diminish DOMS. Although the ability of NSAIDs to reduce DOMS has been researched, the results of these studies have been equivocal. Several investigators have reported decreases in DOMS with use of NSAIDs. However, other investigators have been unable to demonstrate a reduction in DOMS with the use of NSAIDs.

Several factors may contribute to the conflicting results. The type, intensity, and duration of the exercise that has been performed influence the amount of tissue damage, the inflammatory response, and the extent of DOMS. Studies that have investigated NSAIDs have utilized different modes of exercise, making comparisons difficult. The effectiveness of NSAIDs in alleviating DOMS may also depend on the extent of muscle damage as well as the type and intensity of the exercise.

It is possible that by inhibiting prostaglandin synthesis, NSAIDs may shift the metabolism of arachidonic acid to the lipoxygenase pathway, with a resultant increase in the production of leukotrienes. Increased leukotriene production could in turn contribute to the sensation of DOMS. It is not known whether leukotriene production is increased with exercise that results in DOMS. Studies are needed to determine if leukotrienes are involved in DOMS, and whether the administration of NSAIDs alters leukotriene concentrations at times when exercise induces DOMS. There is a need for research using anti-inflammatory agents that block both the cyclooxygenase and lipoxygenase pathways in order to determine whether these chemicals are responsible for DOMS.

The time at which a therapeutic dosage of NSAIDs is given may also affect its ability to diminish or prevent DOMS. The sensitization of pain associated with DOMS may last over an extended period of time. Blocking the synthesis of prostaglandins and their metabolites after hyperalgesia has been established may be ineffective in reducing DOMS. Several studies have examined the effect of administering NSAIDs on DOMS after exercising. This may explain why most investigations have found that the administration of NSAIDs after exercise was not efficacious in reducing DOMS. This contention is supported by a study that demonstrated that the administration of indomethacin (Indocin) before and during exercise gave mice some protection against muscle injury, whereas administration of indomethacin after exercise did not elicit a protective response.

Currently, few studies have examined whether the administration of NSAIDs before exercise is effective in relieving DOMS. Administration of 1,200 mg of ibuprofen (Advil, Motrin, Nuprin, three doses over a 24 hour period, with the initial dose given 4 hours before exercise) significantly reduced soreness for up to 48 hours after exercise. However, if the same amount of ibuprofen was given 24 hours after exercise, it was only effective in reducing DOMS 24 hours later.

In contrast, administration of 50 mg of flurbiprofen (three times per day before and after exercise did not result in decreases in DOMS. This study found that muscle soreness ratings were decreased in the second testing session independent of the flurbiprofen treatment. The time between the two treatments was 3 weeks. This study confirmed previous investigations in showing that prior exercise protected against DOMS. It is important to note that even a single bout of eccentric exercise can help to reduce the amount of DOMS.

The varied responses to NSAIDs treatment exhibited in these studies may have been further confounded by such factors as the type and intensity of exercise utilized; subject selection; the efficacy of the administered drug as an inhibitor of prostaglandin synthesis; and the timing of NSAID dosage.

A number of nonpharmacologic treatments have been used to alleviate DOMS. Static stretching before and after exercise has been recommended as a means of diminishing DOMS, but the basis for this recommendation is not currently documented. Preliminary investigations using ultrasound treatment and topical analgesics have shown some promise in temporarily reducing soreness. Other types of treatment, such as massage and electrical stimulation, have many proponents within the athletic community, although their claims have not been substantiated through definitive research.

Although pharmacologic agents and other treatment modalities may be effective in attenuating DOMS, the treatment of DOMS is not always advisable. The sensation of DOMS serves as a protective mechanism, helping to minimize use of the affected muscles. During this time, synthesis and repair of damaged muscle and connective tissue can occur. If DOMS is alleviated, the muscles and connective tissues that have been damaged may be used once again, with further damage or delay to the repair processes. Rest of the affected muscles and connective tissue is often recommended as the most appropriate treatment for DOMS. The healing process can be inhibited by NSAIDs, since the presence of products of arachidonic acid metabolism may play an integral role in the repair of exercise-induced tissue damage. Research has indicated that the treatment of muscle injuries by anti-inflammatory agents may inhibit the healing process.

PREVENTION

DOMS is associated with a decreased ability to generate force, reductions in the ROM of affected joints, and changes in movement patterns. It would be desirable to minimize DOMS in order to maintain proper performance. Recently, investigators have found that pretreatment with ibuprofen helped to reduce the decrements in isometric, concentric, and eccentric force that are usually associated with DOMS after exercise. Additionally, the presence of DOMS often leads the affected individual to adopt an abnormal movement pattern in an attempt to avoid the sensation of intense pain. Such changes in biomechanics may result in an alteration of certain movement patterns, and may contribute to injury.

Although DOMS can be reduced after a single bout of unaccustomed exercise, it is more advisable to prevent DOMS by the adoption of proper training procedures. The development of muscle soreness is significantly diminished after repeating a bout of the same exercise. The reduction in DOMS occurs particularly when the second exercise bout is preceded by an initial exercise bout of shorter duration and intensity. Furthermore, the effects of a single bout of exercise in preventing DOMS during subsequent exercise persist for up to 6 weeks after the initial exercise bout. It has been hypothesized that muscle tissue rapidly adapts to exercise-induced tissue damage through changes in muscle fibers, connective tissue elements, and neural inputs, thereby protecting the muscle from further injury during subsequent exercise. Rapid adaptation of the muscle to overload resulting from exercise can diminish muscle damage; plasma levels of muscle enzymes; the decrement of force generation; and DOMS.

RECOMMENDATIONS

Research suggests that DOMS results from tissue damage produced by novel or unaccustomed exercise. Delayed muscle soreness may serve to prevent muscle contraction, in order to promote the healing process associated with adaptation to exercise. Therefore, when DOMS is experienced, it is advisable to engage in activities that do not utilize the affected muscle groups. If activity using sore muscles is unavoidable, the intensity of exercise should be reduced in order to minimize its impact on the adaptation process. If physical performance is essential and will be adversely affected by the presence of DOMS, prophylactic doses of NSAIDs should be given 24 to 48 hours before the initial exercise bout.

In order to minimize the extent of DOMS after exercise, individuals should engage in low-intensity, short duration activities when initiating a particular type of exercise. The intensity and duration of exercise can be increased, gradually, thereby allowing the muscles to adapt to the increasing demands of physical performance. In addition, repeated bouts of eccentric contractions involving the use of specific muscle groups over a period of time may afford some protection against DOMS when these muscle groups are used to perform unaccustomed or infrequent activities.

SUGGESTED READING

Armstrong RB. Mechanisms of exercise-induced delayed onset muscle soreness: a brief review. Med Sci Sports Exerc 1984; 16:529–538.

Byrnes WC, Clarkson PM. Delayed onset muscle soreness and training. Clin Sports Med 1986; 5:605–614.

Clarkson PM, Tremblay I. Exercise-induced muscle damage, repair, and adaptation in humans. J Appl Physiol 1988; 65:1–6.

Ebbeling CB, Clarkson PM. Exercise-induced muscle damage and adaptation. Sports Med 1989; 7:207–234.

Evans WJ, Cannon JG. The metabolic effects of exercise-induced muscle damage. Exerc Sport Sci Rev 1991; 19:99–125.

Hasson SM, Daniels JC, Divine JG, et al. Effect of ibuprofen use on muscle soreness, damage, and performance: a preliminary investigation. Med Sci Sports Exerc 1993; 25:9–17.

Smith LL. Acute inflammation: the underlying mechanism in delayed onset muscle soreness? Med Sci Sports Exerc 1991; 23:532–551.

Smith LL. Causes of delayed onset muscle soreness and the impact on athletic performance: a review. J Appl Sports Sci Res 1992; 6:135–141.

Stauber WT. Eccentric action of muscles: physiology, injury, and adaptation. Exerc Sport Sci Rev 1989; 17:157–185.

EXERCISE AND CANCER

LAUREL TRAEGER MacKINNON, Ph.D., F.A.C.S.M.

Cancer is the second leading cause of death, after heart disease, in many Western countries. Although genetic predisposition is an important factor in many forms of cancer, it is generally accepted that life-style and environment are also important determinants of cancer incidence. It has been estimated that perhaps as many as 50% to 60% of cancer deaths in developed countries could be prevented by changes in life-style and environmental factors such as avoidance of cigarette smoking, reduction of alcohol consumption, alteration of diet and reduced exposure to environmental and occupational carcinogens. This implies that, like heart disease, the incidence and risk of cancer could be appreciably reduced by modifying these risk factors.

Given the prevalence of cancer in Western societies, and the interest in exercise in the context of preventive medicine, it is surprising that more attention has not been focused on whether physical activity influences the incidence of cancer. Although limited, recent evidence suggests that regular moderate exercise, as often recommended for general health, is associated with a reduced incidence of certain forms of cancer. Epidemiologic data suggest that physical activity is associated with lower rates of colorectal cancer in men and women, and reproductive system cancers in women. In addition, animal models show a relationship between voluntary physical activity and reduced growth of experimentally-induced tumors.

Exercise has recently been considered as adjunct therapy in cancer patients. The initial motivation for using exercise in this context was to maintain functional capacity in patients. However, recent reports suggest that moderate exercise training may also have beneficial effects on psychological factors and may possibly counteract some of the negative side-effects of treatment.

EPIDEMIOLOGIC STUDIES

Epidemiologic studies over extended periods (i.e., 10 to 20 years) have reported a reduced risk of combined-sites cancer as well as some specific types of cancer in physically active groups. Occupational and recreational (leisure) physical activity have each been associated with a reduced risk of cancer, although at present, the relationship appears stronger for occupational activity. This may be due to the greater number of studies using large sample sizes that have focused on occupational compared with recreational activity levels.

Both retrospective and prospective approaches have examined the relationship between physical activity and incidence of cancer. Physical activity has been defined and quantified by several methods in these studies, including standardized job classifications that include estimates of average occupational physical activity; measures of subject fitness level such as cardiovascular endurance (aerobic power, $\dot{V}O_2max$) or resting heart rate; subject recall of past and present physical activity patterns; and recording of subject activity patterns over time in longitudinal studies. There is a great potential for misclassification of physical activity level in the first three methods; the last method provides a more valid measure of long-term activity patterns. Moreover, recall of past activity patterns or measures of current fitness level do not consistently reflect the total lifetime exposure to exercise, which is the relevant statistic for diseases such as cancer, which usually develop over decades.

The relative risk of cancer (RR) associated with a sedentary life-style is in the range 1.3 to 2.0 (i.e., approximately 25% to 50% reduction in cancer risk due to physical activity). These relative risk values are similar to those observed for physical activity as a means of protection against heart disease. There appears to be a dose-response relationship between the amount of physical activity undertaken and the combined-sites cancer risk; the relative risk decreases progressively with increasing weekly physical activity. The greatest reduction of risk has been noted between the lowest level (< 2 megaJoules, 500 kcal per week of combined occupational and leisure activity) and the moderately active level (2 to 4 megaJoules, 500 to 1,000 kcal per week) of activity. The statistical association between physical activity and cancer incidence is essentially unchanged after adjustment for potential confounding factors such as age, body mass, dietary factors, cigarette smoking, and sociodemographic variables.

Sedentary living has been associated with a higher relative risk of all-sites cancer in males compared with females (RR of 1.8 vs. 1.3, respectively). It is not clear whether this reflects a true gender-difference or is due to methodologic problems. For example, there are few studies that included subjects of both sexes; studies that included both sexes had relatively small female sample sizes, with fewer cancer-related deaths and thus lower statistical power. Alternatively, physical activity patterns may not be as diverse in women, since relatively few women are classified into the highest activity groups. In addition, assessment of physical activity often does not include activities such as housework, which may selectively underestimate the lifetime physical activity of women in traditional households.

Although physical activity may reduce the relative risk of combined-sites cancer, the effect is not uniform across sites, but appears to be site specific. The most consistent evidence to date is for colorectal cancer, with relative risk values of 1.2 to 2.0 attributable to physical inactivity. Physical activity is most clearly associated with a reduced incidence of cancer of the transverse and descending colon, whereas such activity does not appear to be protective against cancer of the ascending colon and rectum. The association between physical activity and a reduced incidence of colon cancer is consistent across total, occupational, or recreational measures of physical activity, and persists after adjustment for potential confounding variables.

There are proportionately fewer studies on the relationship between physical activity and other types of cancer. The risk of reproductive system cancer has been reported to be lower in physically active compared with inactive women. Both recreational and nonrecreational activity appear related to a reduced incidence of breast cancer. Adjustment for potential confounding variables such as family history and the number of pregnancies does not appear to alter the association, although long-term effects of physical activity on body mass, fat levels, and sex hormones have been implicated as causal factors. There are inconsistent data on physical activity and the incidence of prostate cancer in men. Some studies have reported a moderately increased relative risk (RR of 1.1 to 1.5) among males employed in sedentary compared with active occupations. However, other studies have failed to find a statistical association after adjustment for confounding variables such as body mass index, alcohol consumption, and cigarette smoking.

At present, there are too few studies to support any relationship between physical activity and cancer at other sites. Although the risk of combined-sites cancer appears to be lower in physically active groups, this trend is not apparent when delineating specific sites other than those discussed above.

POSSIBLE MECHANISMS

A variety of mechanisms have been proposed to explain the association between physical activity and a reduced incidence of cancer. The general term cancer represents several diseases with varied etiology, and more than one mechanism may be involved. Moreover, the role of a particular mechanism in influencing the incidence of cancer may be specific to the site and type of cancer.

Exercise may reduce the risk of colon cancer by enhancing peristalsis, presumably via parasympathetic (vagal) stimulation. The net effect would be to decrease intestinal transit time, limiting exposure of the bowel to potential carcinogens in feces. Regular physical activity may influence the level of circulating sex hormones that are causal factors in certain forms of cancer, such as breast and other reproductive system cancers in women and prostate cancer in men. Endurance exercise training has been associated with lower levels of estrogens (in women), testosterone (in men), and prolactin (in both sexes). Exercise may influence the risk of cancer by controlling body mass and fat levels; excess body fat is considered a contributing factor to several forms of cancer, including endometrial, breast, and colon cancers. Individuals who choose to exercise or to work in physically active occupations may be more likely to adopt healthy life-styles, reducing risk factors such as smoking and high-fat diets.

Soluble factors involved in regulation of the immune system and/or tumor growth (e.g., prostaglandins, cytokines interleukin-1 and tumor necrosis factor) appear to be released during exercise. Exercise also stimulates antitumor cytotoxic activity in immune cells (e.g., natural killer cells, monocytes) that are involved in the early natural defense against tumor growth.

Regular physical activity is considered an effective technique for the management of daily stress, which may have a positive effect on resistance to cancer. Regular exercise lowers circulating levels of, and downregulates cellular receptors to, stress hormones such as catecholamines. Some stress hormones have been implicated as mediators of stress-induced alterations in resistance to tumor growth in experimental animal models. It is possible that, by altering the response to stress, physical activity may augment the body's natural defenses against tumor growth. Finally, there may be some common genetic factors (e.g., somatotype) that predispose certain individuals to both physical activity and a lower risk of cancer.

EXPERIMENTAL ANIMAL STUDIES

Studies on humans are limited to retrospective and prospective epidemiologic approaches that may not clearly define or control confounding variables. Although the direct relevance of animal models to human cancer may be questioned, data from experimental animal studies provide important corroborative evidence of a link between exercise and cancer.

Studies over the past 50 years have consistently shown that exercise inhibits growth of experimentally-induced tumors. In nearly all studies showing reduced or delayed tumor growth, exercise training was begun several days or weeks before introduction of the tumor. Resistance to tumor growth appears to persist only with continued physical activity. Voluntary access to physical activity or moderate enforced exercise appear to be most effective in delaying or suppressing tumor growth; intense enforced exercise may act as a stressor, negating any positive effects of increased physical activity.

In animal models, the positive effects of exercise on resistance to tumor growth appear to be related only partially to diet and body composition. For example, growth rate and body mass are often lower in exercised compared with free-eating sedentary animals; a low growth rate by itself may inhibit tumor growth. However, studies that included pair-weighted sedentary control animals generally show lower rates of tumor growth beyond what can be explained by a suppression of growth alone. It has been suggested that physical activity may stimulate the immune response to tumor implantation; however, recent data do not support a correlation between excise-induced resistance to tumor growth and immune cell antitumor activity.

PRESCRIBING EXERCISE FOR THE CANCER PATIENT

Although the use of exercise in the treatment of cancer has not been widely studied, there is reason to expect beneficial effects of moderate exercise in cancer patients. Moderate exercise within the range that can be tolerated by cancer patients may counteract decrements in functional capacity and lean body mass resulting from the disease, consequent bed rest, and/or treatment. Moderate exercise is also generally associated with an enhanced psychological state, which may help the cancer patient cope with side effects of treatment such as nausea.

There is evidence that some cancer patients may be capable of improving functional capacity after exercise training. Moderate exercise training, such as stationary cycling at 60% to 85% of maximum exercise capacity ($\dot{V}o_2max$) for 20 to 30 minutes three times per week, has been shown to increase $\dot{V}o_2max$ in breast cancer patients; the degree of improvement is similar to that expected in a nonpatient group. Equally important, however, were an improvement in mood state, a reduction of nausea, and prevention of the gains in body mass and fat that usually accompany chemotherapy. It is not yet clear whether these results can be generalized to patients with other forms of cancer.

Exercise prescription for the cancer patient should be based on general recommendations for exercise in individuals with low functional capacity (i.e., low impact, low intensity exercise that progresses gradually). Exercise prescription must be individualized for the cancer patient, taking into consideration the generally low functional capacity (approximately 3 to 6 METS) resulting from disease and muscular atrophy, the type and

Table 1 Exercise for Cancer Patients

Intensity	Low intensity 40–60% $\dot{V}o_2max$ or HRR initially $<80\%$ $\dot{V}o_2max$ or HRR after initial stage RPE may be best indicator of intensity (RPE of 10–14)
Duration	15–60 min depending on functional capacity Adjust daily according to symptoms and treatment Interval rather than continuous training when appropriate
Frequency	Daily if possible, with at least three sessions per week Avoid exercise within 24 hr of chemotherapy

Mode of activity	Combination of: (1) low impact rhythmic aerobic activities using large muscle groups, (2) muscular strength exercises such as low intensity calisthenics or resistance exercise, and (3) exercises to maintain muscular flexibility and joint range of motion:
	
	Aerobic activities such as:
	  Walking
	  Stationary cycling
	  Water activities (aquaerobics, swimming)
	  Very low impact aerobic dance
	  Gardening
	  Ballroom dance
	
	Resistance exercise such as:
	  Calisthenics using body weight as resistance
	  Higher repetition (>10), low resistance (e.g., hydraulic and pin weight machines, small free weights)
	
	Muscular flexibility exercise such as:
	  Slow static stretching
	  Range of motion exercises

$\dot{V}o_2max$ = measure of maximum aerobic exercise capacity or cardiorespiratory endurance; % HRR = % of heart rate reserve, calculated as e.g., $[0.40 \times (220 - age - resting\ HR) + resting\ HR]$; RPE = rating of perceived exertion using Borg scale of 7 (very, very light) to 19 (very, very hard).

frequency of medical treatment, and the potential side effects of treatment (Table 1). Contraindications to exercise in cancer patients include: intravenous chemotherapy within the previous 24 hours; excessive fatigue and/or muscular weakness; chest pain, irregular pulse, or dysrhythmias; vomiting or severe diarrhea within the previous 24 to 36 hours; dizziness or faintness; nausea during exercise; and abnormal heart rate or blood pressure responses during exercise (e.g., a decrease of blood pressure with increasing work rate).

Some types of cancer or cancer treatment may interfere with the normal adaptations to exercise training. For example, tumors have a high metabolic rate, and coupled with poor patient appetite, they may limit the proportion of daily energy intake available for physical activity. Muscle wasting due to inactivity and decreased protein synthesis may limit muscular adaptations to exercise (e.g., muscular strength gains, mitochondrial adaptations). Low hemoglobin levels and dehydration resulting from therapy will influence the patient's cardiovascular endurance, and thus the ability to sustain prolonged exercise.

The site of the cancer, the symptoms of the disease, and/or side-effects of treatment (e.g., nausea, weakness) may limit the patient's ability to exercise frequently or for long duration, and may influence the choice of exercise mode. For example, in patients with actual or potential bone metastases, exercise should be non-weight bearing (e.g., stationary cycling or water-based activities). Patients may fatigue easily, and it may be advisable to base the exercise prescription on the patient's subjective rating of perceived exertion (RPE) by using the Borg scale rather than to adopt a preset exercise intensity (e.g., a fixed percentage of $\dot{V}O_2max$ or heart rate reserve). Use of interval (alternating exercise and rest periods) rather than continuous training may be more appropriate, especially during the early stages of an exercise program. Finally, the type and timing of medication must be considered, since exercise has been shown to exacerbate cardiac and pulmonary lesions resulting from some types of treatment. It is generally recommended that cancer patients not exercise within 24 hours of chemotherapy.

Further work is needed to determine the physiological and psychological responses to moderate exercise training in patients with different types of cancer and at different stages of the disease. The question of whether regular exercise alters the outcome of the disease has not yet been addressed. The present limited data suggest that, regardless of an effect on outcome, moderate regular exercise may be a relatively inexpensive adjunct therapy with potential benefits for patients during and after treatment.

RECOMMENDATIONS

Although the epidemiologic and experimental data are far from complete, evidence to date suggests that regular moderate physical activity affords some degree of protection against certain forms of cancer. Even if the reduction in cancer risk attributable to physical activity is relatively small, given the prevalence of inactive life-styles coupled with the high incidence of cancer in most developed countries, there is reason to expect a significant impact on public health from the encouragement of regular moderate physical activity among the general population.

SUGGESTED READING

Bartram HP, Wynder EL. Physical activity and colon cancer risk? Physiological considerations. Am J Gastroenterol 1989; 84:109–112.

Frisch RE, Wyshak G, Albright NL, et al. Lower prevalence of breast cancer and cancers of the reproductive system among former college athletes compared to non-athletes. Br J Cancer 1985; 52:885–891.

Kohl HW, LaPorte RE, Blair SN. Physical activity and cancer: An epidemiological perspective. Sports Med 1988; 6:222–237.

MacVicar MG, Winningham ML. Promoting the functional capacity of cancer patients. Cancer Bull 1986; 38:236–239.

Pollock ML, Wilmore JH. Exercise in health and disease: evaluation and prescription for prevention and rehabilitation. London: WB Saunders Company, 1990:89.

Shephard RJ. Exercise in the prevention and treatment of cancer: An update. Sports Med 1993; 15:258–280.

Sternfeld B. Cancer and the protective effect of physical activity: the epidemiological evidence. Med Sci Sports Exerc 1992: 24: 1195–1209.

Winningham ML, MacVicar MG, Burke CA. Exercise for cancer patients: Guidelines and precautions. Physician Sportsmed 1986; 14:125–134.

COSTS AND BENEFITS OF EXERCISE PRESCRIPTION

ROY J. SHEPHARD, M.D., Ph.D., D.P.E., F.A.C.S.M.

In the early postwar era, many governments and major corporations espoused free access to medical services as the unquestioned right of returning service personnel. Despite professed horror over the possibility of "socialized medicine," a combination of MEDICARE and company insurance plans now accounts for a major segment of medical practice, even in the United States.

However, there is increasing concern about ability to sustain such policies. An aging population, advances in medical technology, and occasionally unethical billing practices have led to a rapid escalation of medical expenditures. Costs in Canada increased to 9% of the gross national product, and overall government grants to hospitals and physicians were then capped. In the United States, costs have now reached 14% of an even larger gross national product, although there is little evidence of proportionate gains in either national health or industrial productivity. Indeed, some statistics suggest that the overall health of the U.S. population is poor relative to countries that spend much less on medical care.

Promotion of a healthy life-style is one possible way to contain medical costs. Fitness enthusiasts have argued that regular physical activity is beneficial to both health and performance, yielding economic benefits to the state, the employer, and the individual. However, such schemes, like their medical predecessors, have been introduced largely on trust. This chapter critically examines the postulated costs and benefits of fitness programs.

Economists equate costs with either benefits or effectiveness of a program. The cost-benefit approach ascribes a dollar value to all suggested benefits of exercise, direct and indirect. The program costs, direct and indirect, are treated in similar fashion, and the two sets of figures are compared. The hope of the exercise enthusiast is that the benefits will exceed costs, encouraging continued investments in physical education for children, fitness programming for adults, and life-style enhancement schemes for all ages.

A cost/effectiveness analysis, in contrast, estimates the program expense needed to achieve a given outcome. Initially, we might ask how much it has cost to achieve a 20% participation of 45-year-old employees in a work-site exercise class, but as a program matures the focus might shift to a response variable such as a 15% gain in maximal oxygen intake, or a 1-year extension of quality-adjusted lifespan.

There are sound reasons why we should pursue a cost/effectiveness rather than a cost/benefit analysis. Cost/benefit analyses are notoriously difficult to carry out. Many items on the benefit side of the ledger are difficult to quantitate or are of unknown magnitude. If a patient "feels better," how much is this worth to the individual or to an employer? Will the patient then be less likely to worry the physician with minor psychosomatic complaints? And how much of any dollar value that we may ascribe to "feeling better" has already been counted under such headings as increased industrial productivity, reduced absenteeism, or a lesser abuse of alcohol and other drugs? Many postulated benefits of physical activity occur far into the future. A change in mortality from ischemic heart disease or cancer may be 30 or 40 years distant. It then becomes unclear how far our estimate of ultimate economic benefit should be discounted in order to reflect society's reluctance to pay now for future good. Rigid costing may provoke squabbles as to who should reap any economic rewards that derive from fitness programs. Often, the largest single cost is the time the patient has invested; an opportunity to pursue other interests that has been forgone. If the anticipated outcome is greater industrial productivity, unionized workers may argue that the exercise classes should be organized in company time, and upper echelon workers, also, may push for such benefits as reduced health insurance premiums if they participate in exercise programs. However, if the main gain is an enhanced sense of personal well-being, or an increase of social contacts, management may argue that exercise participants should meet all costs of both time and facilities. Perhaps the most important argument against a rigid cost/benefit analysis is ethical. One major element in most calculations is a reduced loss of future production, due to avoidance of chronic illness and premature death. Unfortunately, such a calculation draws an inappropriate distinction between the health of a chief executive– whose services may be valued at $1 million per year– and a short-order cook, a person who is easily replaced and earns only a hundredth of the executive's salary. Even worse, zero worth is ascribed to the survival of senior citizens and full-time care-givers.

Cost/effectiveness analysis avoids such ethical difficulties and can be used to make a rational choice between competing options such as exercise counseling by a family physician and large-scale industrial or community fitness promotion programs. But a cost/effectiveness approach creates other dilemmas. Benefit is disaggregated into its many components– for example, rival programs may spend $50,000 and $100,000, respectively, to extend a patient's life by 1 calendar year, but if the yardstick of effectiveness is changed to 1 year of quality-adjusted life, the respective costs may change to $150,000 and $105,000. A given program (for example, a physician-monitored jogging prescription) may also be very effective in yielding one type of dividend– for instance, an extension of longevity– but it may have little impact upon an alternative problem– for example, the social isolation of the older patient. A first step in cost/effectiveness analysis is therefore to rank the various postulated benefits of a program, and to decide which will be used in evaluating its effectiveness. The order of such a listing inevitably varies with the person who is proposing the investment and with the age of the suggested beneficiaries.

BENEFITS OF EXERCISE

Reduction of Medical Costs

School Programs

Physicians may sometimes be asked to advise School Boards on the health benefits of required school programs of physical education. Physical educators often point to the poor performance of North American students on current fitness test batteries, and argue the need to optimize physical function in growing children. But even if current field tests measured fitness accurately (and this is by no means certain), health-related fitness in the adult could probably be developed more readily by rigorous physical exercise at the age of 18 years than by long periods of classroom instruction at the age of 8 years.

Recent attention has focused on the prevalence of cardiac risk factors in quite young children, and a search has begun for tests to measure and programs to enhance "health-related" rather than "performance-related" fitness. But even if we redirect attention from performance to health-related fitness, there is only a limited tracking of cardiac risk factors from childhood to adult life. The prospects for a cost-effective enhancement of health in the classroom are correspondingly low. The most important (but often the most overlooked) facet of a school program is the molding of attitudes. Experiences of activity as a child strongly influence exercise behavior in the later years of life. Required school programs too often fail to promote enthusiasm for exercise. Indeed, a high proportion of participants become totally inactive once they reach an age where physical education is no longer a required subject.

The types of school programs with the greatest long-term impact likely involve noncompetitive, cooperative, and family-linked physical activities. Growing children should be given a chance to explore various activity options in order to find out those that are personally enjoyable and suited to body build and aptitudes.

Working Adults

Containment of medical costs can be one of the main economic benefits of a fitness program for the working adult. The direct costs of illness (physician visits, hospital stays, and medication) are of the same order as the indirect costs (loss of production due to chronic illness and premature mortality). However, the direct costs are incurred largely by senior citizens, whereas a major part of the indirect costs necessarily arise during "working" life. In dollar terms, the largest potential benefit comes from a reduction of the indirect costs of ill-health, particularly the loss of production due to premature

cardiovascular illness and death. Given the long-term nature of these gains, evidence of program benefit is often sought in a reduction of cardiac risk factors.

Senior Citizens

Some economists have argued that as lifespan is extended, seniors will become an increasing burden on pension funds. The estimated costs of prolonged survival vary enormously, depending on discount rates and assumptions about compulsory retirement. If the discount rate is low and there is a fixed age of retirement, it may be economically undesirable to extend lifespan, although this is hardly an ethical argument for scrapping a fitness program. Plainly, if those who have adopted a healthy life-style are allowed to work for a longer period, any arguments about increased pension costs become invalid.

Much of the expense of caring for seniors arises from major hospital costs during the final few weeks of life. Benefit should therefore be sought through exercise programs that increase functional independence and reduce the demands for terminal medical and institutional care. Functional independence seems to be fostered by programs that sustain or develop aerobic power, muscle strength, flexibility, and balance, while developing the social contacts that will assure support during intercurrent periods of acute illness. The risk factors for chronic disease are unlikely to be modified greatly in old age, but regular exercise can still partially reverse many of the effects of senescence, bringing about a substantial reduction of functional age. Demands for medical care may also be reduced by programs that improve mood-state and therefore perceived health.

Benefits to Industry

Industrial benefits of a work-site exercise program include an improved corporate image, the selective recruitment of premium employees, an improved quality and quantity of production, a reduced absenteeism rate, lower medical insurance payments, and a reduced incidence of industrial injuries. In some recent analyses, the largest item has been a reduced turnover among physically active employees. The cost of such turnover ranges from perhaps a million dollars to replace a key executive to near zero when a new floor-sweeper is hired. Most analyses have been carried out on white-collar workers at times when turnover has been encouraged by low rates of unemployment, and the benefit may therefore have been overstated relative to the average value for a postindustrial society.

Any impact of fitness programming on turnover depends on the uniqueness of the corporate initiative. If identical facilities and program are available at a rival company, a work-site fitness class may have little influence on employee turnover. Moreover, there has been no critical analysis of the effectiveness of fitness programs relative to alternative tactics for reducing employee turnover (for example, escalating pension rights or stock-sharing options).

The impact of an exercise and health facility on corporate image is difficult to assess, as is the claim that high achievers are selectively recruited to the company concerned. Both factors likely depend on the uniqueness of the work-site program. The reported decrease of absenteeism among participants in work-site fitness programs is generally quite small (0.5 to 2.0% of payroll costs), and is limited to enthusiastic exercise participants. Likewise, in a white-collar, postindustrial corporation, a reduction of compensable accidents is unlikely to be a major dividend of an exercise program. Economic gains must be sought in the areas of quality and quantity of production; our controlled studies of two insurance companies suggested that the net impact amounted to a 2.7% gain of productivity, *averaged across the entire company.*

Personal Benefits

In addition to a search for health and extended social contacts, many class participants perceive esthetic and ascetic gains (the body beautiful/enhanced self-image; activity as a means to physical and mental toughness), a pleasurable sense of vertigo, the enjoyment of competition, and an opportunity for detente. The dollar value that the patient places on each of these benefits varies with the individual's age and social background. In adolescence, the exerciser generally focuses on excitement and competition, but in older age groups, fitness, health, and a sense of well-being are the main perceived benefits of physical activity.

EFFECTIVENESS

The impact of a fitness program on community health depends on the prevalence of need, the likelihood that this need will be met by the program, and the likelihood that those in need will participate. Marathon running might be a rather effective method of avoiding a future heart attack. But if likely participation is 1 in 10,000 of the population, and few of those involved have major cardiac risk factors, the effectiveness of the program in preventing heart disease is quite low. In contrast, a required school sports program may improve long-term health attitudes in only 25% of school pupils, yet if the participation rate is close to 100%, the impact on future health will be much greater than that of an optional community program, attended by a small minority of people who are already committed to a healthy life-style.

The prevalence of need becomes an important issue when looking at either medical or industrial benefits. A large fraction of total medical costs is generated by a small proportion of patients, and these seem unlikely candidates for a fitness program. Likewise, most of the absenteeism experience of large corporations is attributable to about 20 percent of employees, and unfortu-

nately this particular group are the least likely to enroll in an exercise program.

In addition to problems in recruiting susceptible individuals, many fitness programs have a disappointing overall adherence rate. General practitioners are often disillusioned by the time they must devote to keep patients active in physical fitness activities. Work-site fitness programs typically recruit some 20% of the labor force, and long-term attendance drops to around 10%. Campbell's Cross-Canada Fitness Survey showed that only 2-4% of the Canadian population exercise at the work-site, despite a decade of vigorous promotion of such initiatives by the Canadian Federal and the Provincial governments. Moreover, the long-term impact of such programs on cardiac risk factors is small. Cigarette and alcohol consumption are reduced, and age-related changes in aerobic power and percentage body fat are slowed, but there is little change in serum lipid profile, probably because the total additional weekly energy expenditure fails to reach the threshold for such an effect. It seems inherently improbable that the usual exercise-class (30 to 45 minutes 2-3 times per week) could have a major impact on health, although there may be a beneficial influence on the attitudes of both program participants and other employees. In particular, drop-outs from a work-site program are sometimes stimulated to begin exercising elsewhere.

Individual perceptions of program effectiveness can be gauged from participation rates. The time people are prepared to invest in specific activities (or the equivalent travel distance to a recreational site) also provides a simple measure of personally perceived benefits. A third method of evaluation is to ask how much the individual would be willing to pay over and above the current cost of participation. Unfortunately, such evaluations are not very stable. Participants are usually prepared to invest more for a first than for a second or a third experience of a given activity.

The Canada Fitness Survey of 1981 and Campbell's survey of 1988 both found that walking was by far the most popular form of exercise for Canadians, and U.S. surveys have had similar findings. In Canada, commonly perceived intentions have been to begin swimming, jogging or running, and tennis. However, there has been a distinct gap between these stated intentions and the expensive commercial and equipment-intensive pursuits that have developed in recent years—downhill, cross-country, and water skiing, sailboarding, and various types of racquet sports.

Information on the therapeutic effectiveness of alternative programs is mainly intuitive. We have already noted the types of exercise that seem likely to form positive health habits in schoolchildren. In working adults, substantial protection against premature death is obtained from sustained brisk walking and from stair-climbing, although more vigorous pursuits give somewhat larger gains (Table 1). However, sports offer no inherent advantage over other equally energetic leisure pursuits. In old age, the range of therapeutic options narrows and benefit may be anticipated

Table 1 Effectiveness of Various Types of Physical Activity in Preventing a First Clinical Attack of Myocardial Infarction

	Percentage of Subjects Showing this Type of Activity	
Type of Activity	Attacked Subjects	Matched Controls
Active recreation	2.10	3.99
Keeping fit	1.26	3.36
Vigorous getting about	0.42	4.41
Heavy work	7.98	16.39
Climbing > 450 stairs/day	0	1.68
Total reporting physical activity	10.50	25.21

Based on data of Morris et al. (1980) for 238 attacked subjects and 476 matched controls.

from any program that increases body movement and is fun.

Program Costs

Program costs include promotion, facilities, equipment, leadership, and lost opportunity. Outdoor pursuits may also create environmental costs.

Participation has increased in North America over the past decade, but it is unclear whether this trend has now plateaued or whether the attempts at exercise promotion by such agencies as ParticipACTION in Canada and the U.S. President's Council on Fitness have influenced the situation positively. Even if the effects of recent promotion and advertising have been positive, it is unlikely that further expenditures will yield a proportional increase of exercise participation, given a hard core of questionnaire respondents who indicate that "nothing" would make them more active. A further issue around motivation is whether it would be cheaper to promote some types of physical activity than others. Is it more economical to advertise a work-site program than to promote exercise through a physician's private office or formal community-based classes? The physician starts with the advantage of acceptance as a health counselor. Likewise, existing publicity channels can be used to advertise a work-site program, and in such a setting much of the necessary labor can be provided by volunteers.

Facilities vary enormously in cost, depending on their purpose and utilization rates (Table 2). When advising an individual patient, the choice of option will be guided by the questioner's preferences and disposible income. In the corporate context, some multimillion dollar work-site facilities have a low cost-effectiveness as a means of health promotion, but achieve their unofficially intended objective of providing a substantial tax-free fringe benefit to top executives. Flexible hours of work and imaginative scheduling of exercise classes are important to a full utilization of corporate facilities by lower echelon employees. The apparent cost also depends on the location of the facility (downtown, suburban, or rural) and methods of corporate accounting.

Table 2 Cost of Exercise Facilities

Expected Number of Participants	Recommended Facility	Cost per Participant (year)
< 400	Campus wide, with full-time supervisor	$300–500
5–50	Minimal facility, tests & ex. prescription only	$150–500
75–250	150-300m² facility, part-time or full-time supervisor	$365–500
400–850	600-1,200m² facility, full-time supervisor	$300–500

Based on data summarized by Shephard (1986).

Some company balance-sheets allow "free" occupancy of unused space, but others assess the full commercial cost of equivalent space.

Year-round use is important to the effectiveness of community operations—outdoor swimming or cross-country skiing facilities may be esthetically appealing, but they are costly because of a very short operating season. A full costing of a publicly operated community facility should include not only the immediate expense of construction, but also an appropriate allowance for serviced land, parking, and access roads, and a consideration of the economic impact of the facility (whether positive or negative) on the surrounding environment. If all such costs are included, the relative expense of work-site and community programs may change dramatically. Popular options of the type advocated by many physicians, such as walking and cycling, have the lowest facility cost. Often, the community expense associated with such activities amounts to no more than the maintenance, snow-ploughing, and sanding of sidewalks.

School Boards should incorporate a wide variety of experiences into their exercise programs, so that growing children can discover pursuits that they enjoy. But this approach inevitably increases the cost of equipment and facilities. Occupancy of school facilities can be increased, and the unit cost can be reduced if such facilities are open to the local community at off-peak hours.

Equipment may be owned by the program or by the participant. Unfortunately, the sale of sports clothing and exercise equipment has been exploited by entrepreneurs, who have created a demand for fashionable items. These are not required for effective exercise, but have often become a barrier to participation by less-wealthy patients. Even walking and jogging are thought to require an expensive cupboard filled with athletic shoes designed for various terrains, speeds of movement, and seasons, whereas very effective health-giving exercise could be obtained by buying and keeping in repair a solid $40 to $50 pair of leather Oxford shoes.

Likewise, it is suggested that the cyclist needs a stable of racing, mountain, touring, and town bicycles, purchased at a cost of $2000 to $3000 per unit, whereas very good health-giving exercise would be possible using a simple second-hand bicycle purchased for $30 or less at a police auction. Large amounts of money can be spent on such items as designer jeans and track pants, with little effect on the patient's health. In fact, walking or cycling is quite possible while wearing a minimum of normal clothing.

Trained leadership is important to program safety, but adds substantially to the cost of exercise. Adherence may be increased by a good class-leader. However, the most popular forms of physical activity (cycling and walking) need no formal leadership. Equally, the cost of work-site and community programs can be reduced (and sometimes the effectiveness can be enhanced) through the involvement of well-trained lay class-leaders.

Lost opportunity is commonly the largest cost on a personal exercise balance sheet. Membership at a commercial exercise facility may cost $300 to $600 per year, $2 to $4 per session if the patient attends 150 times over a year. However, if we assume an hour of participation and an hour of travel to and from the facility, the opportunity cost at a typical wage of $15/h is ten times as great ($30/session). Notice also that the opportunity cost rises disproportionately as exercise eats into the individual's remaining free time. It is hardly surprising that school boards argue "their" curricular time is too precious to be invested in required physical activity programs, and that most patients cite "lack of time" as the main barrier to their involvement in exercise classes. For both school-children and working adults there are plainly important cost advantages to an on-site program (where the element of travel time is eliminated). Nevertheless, walking and cycling are even cheaper forms of exercise, since they can be built into the normal structure of the day (such as the journey to and from school or work).

An interesting commentary on this analysis of opportunity costs is that many patients still prefer recreation at a lakeside resort to participation in an apparently convenient work-site program. There are two possible explanations for this paradox—the journey to and from the recreational site may have become an integral part of the pleasurable experience, or the quality of recreation (a significant component of its effectiveness) may be perceived as much higher in the rural setting.

COST-EFFECTIVENESS

We could carry out elaborate and speculative analyses correlating costs and effectiveness for each of many potential exercise options, finally comparing the "best" forms of exercise with alternative tactics. In the case of school programs, necessary evidence on the prime component of effectiveness, the development of adult attitudes, is currently lacking. The first step in advising school authorities should therefore be to demand statistics on the value of various required and voluntary school programs as a means of developing positive attitudes towards exercise among the adult population.

In adults, the cheapest forms of exercise by far are walking and cycling. Moreover, these activities rate highly in terms of both current and likely future participation rates, and they have a demonstrated therapeutic effectiveness against such concerns as premature death and disability from cardiac disease. Their low risk also enhances the perceived benefit, and relative to many alternative options, benefits are less likely to be attenuated as novelty wears off. It therefore seems unnecessary to undertake sophisticated analyses that would merely confirm the decision already reached by the sensible consumer—that walking and cycling are the most cost-effective exercise options. Rather, the challenge is to accept this wisdom, to advocate incorporation of the necessary trails and parkways into the design of our future towns and cities, and to encourage those of our patients who are still sedentary to use such facilities.

SUGGESTED READING

American College of Sports Medicine. Guidelines for graded exercise testing and exercise prescription. Philadelphia: Lea & Febiger, 1986.

Blair SN, Piserchia PV, Wilbur CS, Crowder JH. A public health intervention model for work-site health promotion: Impact on exercise and physical fitness in a health promotion plan after 24 months. JAMA 255:921–926; 1986.

Pate R, Shephard RJ. Characteristics of physical fitness in youth. In: Gisolfi CV, Lamb DR, eds. Youth, exercise and sports. Indianapolis: Benchmark Press, 1989:1.

Shephard RJ. The economic benefits of enhanced fitness. Champaign, Ill: Human Kinetics Publishers, 1986.

Shephard RJ. Fitness boom or bust? A Canadian perspective. Res Quart 59:265–269, 1986.

Shephard RJ. Current perspectives on the economics of fitness and sport with particular reference to worksite programmes. Sports Med 7:286–309, 1989.

Stephens T. Secular trends in adult physical activity—Exercise boom or bust? Res Quart 58:94–105, 1987.

Walsh RG. Recreation economic decisions: Comparing benefits and costs. State College, Pa: Venture Publishing, 1986.

INDEX